PORTH'S
Essentials of
Pathophysiology

FIFTH EDITION

TOMMIE L. NORRIS, DNS, RN

AACN Leadership for Academic Nursing Fellow
Dean, Benjamín León School of Nursing
Miami Dade College
Miami, Florida

Contributing Author:

RUPA LALCHANDANI TUAN, PhD

Assistant Professor
Department of Cellular and Molecular Pharmacology
University of California, San Francisco
San Francisco, California

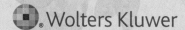

Philadelphia • Baltimore • New York • London
Buenos Aires • Hong Kong • Sydney • Tokyo

Not authorised for sale in United States, Canada, Australia, New Zealand, Puerto Rico, and U.S. Virgin Islands.

Vice President and Publisher: Julie K. Stegman
Director of Nursing Content Publishing: Renee Gagliardi
Senior Acquisitions Editor: Jonathan Joyce
Director of Product Development: Jennifer K. Forestieri
Senior Development Editor: Meredith L. Brittain
Editorial Coordinator: Tim Rinehart
Marketing Manager: Brittany Clements
Editorial Assistant: Molly Kennedy
Design Coordinator: Stephen Druding
Art Director, Illustration: Jennifer Clements
Production Project Manager: Joan Sinclair
Manufacturing Coordinator: Karin Duffield
Prepress Vendor: S4Carlisle Publishing Services

Fifth Edition

Library of Congress Cataloging-in-Publication Data

ISBN-13: 978-1-975107-19-2

ISBN-10: 1-975107-19-5

Library of Congress Control Number: 2019911909

shop.lww.com

To my husband, Stephen Sr., and children—Richie, Robby,
Stephen Jr., and Rachel—who always inspire me.
To those pursuing or continuing a love for healthcare,
with a special thanks for your dedication, compassion, and selflessness.

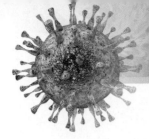

Contributors

Contributors to Essentials of Pathophysiology, Fourth Edition

Jacqueline M. Akert, RNC, MSN, WHNP-BC
Nurse Practitioner
Women's Health Aurora Health Care
Waukesha, Wisconsin
(Chapters 40, 41 with Patricia McCowen Mehring)

Diane Book, MD
Associate Professor, Neurology
Co-Director Stroke & Neurovascular
 Program
Froedtert Hospital & Medical College
 of Wisconsin
Milwaukee, Wisconsin
(Chapter 37)

Freddy W. Cao, MD, PhD
Clinical Associate Professor
College of Nursing
University of Wisconsin–Milwaukee
Milwaukee, Wisconsin
(Chapters 18, 34)

Paula Cox-North, PhD, ARNP
Clinical Assistant Professor
Hepatitis & Liver Clinic
Harborview Medical Center
University of Washington School of Nursing
Seattle, Washington
(Chapters 29, 30)

Herodotos Ellinas, MD, FAAP, FACP
Assistant Professor
Department of Anesthesiology
Med–Anesthesia and PGY-1 Program
 Director
Medical College of Wisconsin
Milwaukee, Wisconsin
(Chapters 11, 12, 13)

Jason R. Faulhaber, MD
Assistant Program Director, Fellowship
 in Infectious Diseases
Division of Infectious Diseases,
 Carilion Clinic
Assistant Professor, Virginia Tech,
 Carilion School of Medicine
Adjunct Professor, Department of
 Biomedical Sciences, Jefferson
 College of Health Sciences
Roanoke, Virginia
(Chapters 15, 16)

Anne M. Fink, RN, PhD
Postdoctoral Research Associate
College of Nursing
University of Illinois–Chicago
Chicago, Illinois
(Chapters 19, 20 with Karen M. Vuckovic)

Susan A. Fontana, PhD, APRN-BC
Associate Professor and Family Nurse
 Practitioner
College of Nursing
University of Wisconsin–Milwaukee
Milwaukee, Wisconsin
(Chapter 38)

Kathleen E. Gunta, MSN, RN, OCNS-C
Clinical Nurse Specialist
Aurora St. Luke's Medical Center
Milwaukee, Wisconsin
(Chapter 43)

Nathan A. Ledeboer, PhD, D(ABMM)
Associate Professor of Pathology
Medical College of Wisconsin
Milwaukee, Wisconsin
(Chapter 14)

Kim Litwack, PhD, RN, FAAN, APNP
Associate Dean for Academic Affairs
Family Nurse Practitioner
Advanced Pain Management
University of Wisconsin–Milwaukee
Milwaukee, Wisconsin
(Chapter 35)

Glenn Matfin, MSc (Oxon), MB, ChB, FACE, FACP, FRCP
Medical Director
International Diabetes Center
Clinical Professor of Medicine
University of Minnesota
Minneapolis, Minnesota
(Chapters 10, 31, 32, 33, 39)

Patricia McCowen Mehring, RNC, MSN, WHNP
Nurse Practitioner
Women's Health
Milwaukee, Wisconsin
(Chapters 40, 41 with Jacqueline M. Akert)

Carrie J. Merkle, PhD, RN, FAAN
Associate Professor
College of Nursing
The University of Arizona
Tucson, Arizona
(Chapters 1, 2, 3, 4, 7)

Kathleen Mussatto, PhD, RN
Nurse Scientist
Herma Heart Center
Children's Hospital of Wisconsin
Assistant Clinical Professor of
 Surgery
Medical College of Wisconsin
Milwaukee, Wisconsin
*(Chapter 19, Heart Disease in Infants
 and Children)*

Debra Bancroft Rizzo, RN, MSN, FNP-BC
Nurse Practitioner
Division of Rheumatology
University of Michigan
Ann Arbor, Michigan
(Chapter 44)

Jonathan Shoopman, MD
Assistant Professor of Anesthesiology
 and Critical Care
Medical College of Wisconsin
Milwaukee, Wisconsin
(Chapters 22, 23)

Gladys Simandl, RN, PhD
Professor
Columbia College of Nursing
Milwaukee, Wisconsin
(Chapters 45, 46)

Aoy Tomita-Mitchell, PhD
Associate Professor
Department of Surgery
Children's Research Institute
Medical College of Wisconsin
Milwaukee, Wisconsin
(Chapters 5, 6)

Karen M. Vuckovic, RN, PhD, ACNS-BC
Assistant Clinical Professor
College of Nursing
University of Illinois–Chicago
Chicago, Illinois
(Chapters 19, 20 with Anne M. Fink)

Jill M. Winters, RN, PhD, FAHA
President and Dean
Columbia College of Nursing
Milwaukee, Wisconsin
(Chapter 9)

Contributors to Porth's Pathophysiology, Tenth Edition

Sawsan Abuhammad, PhD
Assistant Professor, Maternal and Child Health
Jordan University of Science and Technology
Irbid, Jordan
Chapter 42: Structure and Function of the Male Genitourinary System

Maeghan Arnold, MNSc, APRN, AGACNP-BC
Clinical Instructor
Practice Department
College of Nursing
University of Arkansas for Medical Sciences
Little Rock, Arkansas
Chapter 20: Disorders of Hearing and Vestibular Function

Michele R. Arwood, DNP, MSN, BSN, CNS-BC, NE-BC, CJCP
System Director, Quality and Accreditation
Baptist Memorial Health Care Corporation
Memphis, Tennessee
Chapter 8: Disorders of Fluid and Electrolyte and Acid Base Balance
Chapter 29: Structure and Function of the Respiratory System

Trina Barrett, DNP, RN, CNE, CCRN
Assistant Professor
College of Nursing
University of Tennessee Health Science Center
Memphis, Tennessee
Chapter 3: Cellular Adaptation, Injury, and Death

Cynthia Bautista, PhD, CCRN, SCRN, CCNS, ACNS-BC, FNCS
Associate Professor
Marion Peckham Egan School of Nursing and Health Studies
Fairfield University
Fairfield, Connecticut
Chapter 13: Organization and Control of Neural Function

Chapter 14: Somatosensory Function, Pain, Headache, and Temperature
Chapter 15: Disorders of Motor Function
Chapter 16: Disorders of Brain Function

Hallie Bensinger, DNP, APN, FNP-BC
Kaplan Nurse Consultant
New York, New York
Chapter 44: Structure and Function of the Female Reproductive System
Chapter 45: Disorders of the Female Reproductive System

Jami S. Brown, DHEd, RN, CNN
Assistant Professor
College of Nursing
University of Tennessee Health Science Center
Memphis, Tennessee
Chapter 34: Acute Kidney Injury and Chronic Kidney Disease

Melissa Brown, MS, RN
Instructional Academic Staff
College of Nursing
University of Wisconsin–Milwaukee
Milwaukee, Wisconsin
Chapter 43: Disorders of the Male Reproductive System

Jacqueline Rosenjack Burchum, DNSc, FNP-BC, CNE
Associate Professor
College of Nursing
University of Tennessee Health Science Center
Memphis, Tennessee
Chapter 21: Blood Cells and Hematopoietic System
Chapter 23: Disorders of Red Blood Cells

Kathy Diane Butler, DNP, APRN, FNP/GNP-BC, NP-C
Clinical Associate Professor
College of Nursing
University of Memphis
Memphis, Tennessee
Chapter 49: Disorders of Musculoskeletal Function: Developmental and Metabolism Disorders, Activity Intolerance, and Fatigue

Freddy W. Cao, MD, PhD
Clinical Associate Professor
College of Nursing
University of Wisconsin–Milwaukee
Milwaukee, Wisconsin
Chapter 36: Structure and Function of the Gastrointestinal System
Chapter 37: Disorders of Gastrointestinal Function
Chapter 38: Disorders of Hepatobiliary and Exocrine Pancreas Function

Jaclyn Conelius, PhD, FNP-BC, FHRS
Associate Professor & FNP Track Coordinator
Marion Peckham Egan School of Nursing & Health Studies Fairfield University
Fairfield, Connecticut
Chapter 28: Disorders of Cardiac Conduction and Rhythm

Herodotos Ellinas, MD, FAAP/FACP
Associate Professor
Department of Anesthesiology
Residency Program Director
Medical College of Wisconsin
Milwaukee, Wisconsin
Chapter 27: Disorders of Cardiac Function, and Heart Failure and Circulatory Shock

Deena Garner, DNP, RN
Clinical Instructor
Practice Department
College of Nursing
University of Arkansas for Medical Sciences
Little Rock, Arkansas
Chapter 20: Disorders of Hearing and Vestibular Function

Sandeep Gopalakrishnan, PhD
Assistant Professor
College of Nursing
University of Wisconsin–Milwaukee
Milwaukee, Wisconsin
Chapter 7: Stress and Adaptation
Chapter 9: Inflammation, Tissue Repair, and Wound Healing
Chapter 12: Disorders of the Immune Response

Lisa Hight, EdD
Professor of Biology
General Education–Biomedical Sciences – Biology
Baptist College of Health Sciences
Memphis, Tennessee
Chapter 51: Structure and Function of the Skin
Chapter 52: Disorders of Skin Integrity and Function

Deborah L. Hopla, DNP, APRN-BC, FAANP
Associate Professor
Director MSN/FNP and DNP Programs
Amy V. Cockcroft Leadership Fellow
Department of Nursing
School of Health Sciences
Francis Marion University
Florence, South Carolina
Chapter 46: Sexually Transmitted Infections

Teresa Kessler, PhD, RN, ACNS-BC, CNE
Professor, Kreft Endowed Chair for the Advancement of Nursing Science
College of Nursing and Health Professions
Valparaiso University
Valparaiso, Indiana
Chapter 8: Disorders of Fluid, Electrolyte, and Acid–Base Balance

Christine Paquin Kurtz, DNP
Associate Professor
Nursing and Health Professions
College of Nursing
Valparaiso University
Valparaiso, Indiana
Chapter 17: Sleep and Sleep-Wake Disorders

Elizabeth M. Long, DNP, APRN-BC, CNS
Assistant Professor
School of Nursing
Lamar University
Beaumont, Texas
Chapter 18: Disorders of Thought, Emotion, and Memory

Tracy McClinton, DNP, AG-ACNP, BC
Assistant Professor
College of Nursing
University of Tennessee Health Science Center
Memphis, Tennessee
Chapter 30: Respiratory Tract Infections, and Neoplasms
Chapter 31: Disorders of Ventilation and Gas Exchange

Linda C. Mefford, PhD, MSN, APRN, NNP-BC, RNC-NIC
Associate Professor of Nursing
Lansing School of Nursing and Clinical Sciences
Bellarmine University
Louisville, Kentucky
Chapter 26: Disorders of Blood Flow and Blood Pressure Regulation
Chapter 32: Structure and Function of the Kidney
Chapter 33: Disorders of Renal Function
Chapter 40: Mechanisms of Endocrine Control
Chapter 41: Disorders of Endocrine Control

Sarah Morgan, PhD, RN
Clinical Associate Professor
College of Nursing
University of Wisconsin–Milwaukee
Milwaukee, Wisconsin
Chapter 47: Structure and Function of the Musculoskeletal System

Chapter 48: Disorders of Musculoskeletal Function: Trauma, Infection, Neoplasms
Chapter 50: Disorders of Musculoskeletal Function: Rheumatic Disorders

Nancy A. Moriber, PhD, MSN, BSN, CRNA, APRN
Assistant Professor
Nurse Anesthesia
School of Nursing
Fairfield University
Fairfield, Connecticut
Chapter 11: Innate and Adaptive Immunity

Emma Murray, DNP, APRN, ACNP-BC
Assistant Professor
College of Nursing
University of Tennessee Health Science Center
Memphis, Tennessee
Chapter 30: Respiratory Tract Infections, Neoplasms, and Childhood Disorders
Chapter 31: Disorders of Ventilation and Gas Exchange

Cheryl Neudauer, PhD, MEd
Faculty
Department of Biology
Minneapolis Community and Technical College
Minneapolis, Minnesota
Chapter 2: Cell and Tissue Characteristics

Stephanie Nikbakht, DNP, PPCNP-BC
Assistant Professor
College of Nursing
University of Tennessee Health Science Center
PNP, Division of Genetics
Le Bonheur Children's Hospital
Memphis, Tennessee
Chapter 30: Respiratory Tract Infections, Neoplasms, and Childhood Disorders

Alyssa Norris, MS, RD, LDN, CLC
Clinical Dietitian II
Nutrition Therapy
Le Bonheur Children's Hospital
Memphis, Tennessee
Chapter 39: Alterations in Nutritional Status

Keevia Porter, DNP, NP-C
Assistant Professor
College of Nursing
University of Tennessee Health Science Center
Memphis, Tennessee
Chapter 35: Disorders of the Bladder and Lower Urinary Tract

Michelle Rickard, DNP, CPNP-AC
Assistant Professor
College of Nursing
University of Tennessee Health Science Center
Memphis, Tennessee
Chapter 6: Neoplasia

Archie Sims, MSN
Nurse Practitioner
Hospitalist
Palmetto Health Tuomey
Sumter, South Carolina
Chapter 1: Concepts of Health and Disease

Diane Smith, DNP, FNP-BC
Clinical Professor
University of Wisconsin–Milwaukee
Milwaukee, Wisconsin
Chapter 19: Disorders of Visual Function

Ansley Grimes Stanfill, PhD, RN
Assistant Professor
College of Nursing
University of Tennessee Health Science Center
Memphis, Tennessee
Chapter 4: Genetic Control of Cell Function and Inheritance
Chapter 5: Genetic and Congenital Disorders

Sharon Stevenson, DNP, APRN, PPCNP-BC
Clinical Assistant Professor
Practice Department
College of Nursing
University of Arkansas for Medical Sciences
Little Rock, Arkansas
Chapter 20: Disorders of Hearing and Vestibular Function

James Mark Tanner, DNP, RN
Assistant Clinical Professor
BSN Program Director
UAMS College of Nursing
University of Arkansas for Medical Sciences
Little Rock, Arkansas
Chapter 25: Structure and Function of the Cardiovascular System

Janet Tucker, PhD, RNC-OB
Assistant Professor
Loewenberg College of Nursing
University of Memphis
Memphis, Tennessee
Chapter 39: Alterations in Nutritional Status

Reba A. Umberger, PhD, RN, CCRN-K
Assistant Professor
College of Nursing
University of Tennessee Health Science Center
Memphis, Tennessee
Chapter 10: Mechanisms of Infectious Disease
Chapter 32: Structure and Function of the Kidney
Chapter 33: Disorders of Renal Function

Melody Waller, PhD, RN
Assistant Professor
College of Nursing
University of Tennessee Health Science Center
Memphis, Tennessee
Chapter 44: Structure and Function of the Female Reproductive System
Chapter 45: Disorders of the Female Reproductive System

Paige Wimberley, PhD, APRN, CNS-BC, CNE
Associate Professor
College of Nursing and Health Professions
Arkansas State University
Jonesboro, Arkansas
Chapter 22: Disorders of Hemostasis
Chapter 24: Disorders of White Blood Cells and Lymphoid Tissues

Sachin Yende, MD, MS
Professor
Department of Critical Care Medicine and Clinical and Translational Sciences
University of Pittsburgh
Pittsburgh, Pennsylvania
Chapter 10: Mechanisms of Infectious Disease

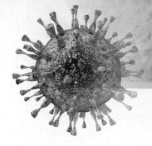

Reviewers

Jennifer Armfield, DNP, RN, ACNP-BC
Assistant Clinical Professor
School of Nursing
Northern Arizona University
Flagstaff, Arizona

Debbie Ciesielka, DEd, MSN, ANP-BC
Associate Professor, MSN Program Coordinator
Department of Nursing
Clarion University
Clarion, Pennsylvania

Karen Cooper, MSN
Assistant Professor
Research College of Nursing
Kansas City, Missouri

Catherine Hogan, PhD, MPH, RN
Assistant Professor
Catherine MacAuley School of Nursing
Maryville University
St. Louis, Missouri

Angela Jupiter-McCon, PhD
Associate Professor
Joseph and Nancy Fail School of Nursing
William Carey University
Hattiesburg, Mississippi

Katie R. Katz, DNP, FNP-BC, RN
Assistant Professor
School of Nursing
Radford University
Radford, Virginia

Keerat Kaur, PhD
Adjunct Professor
School of Nursing & Healthcare Professions
College of New Rochelle
New Rochelle, Texas

Christine Kessel, PhD, MSN, RN, CNE
Interim Dean, Professor
Department of Nursing
Trinity College of Nursing & Health Sciences
Rock Island, Illinois

Heather LaPoint, RN, MSN-Ed, CNE, CCRN-E
Assistant Professor
Department of Nursing
State University of New York at Plattsburgh
Plattsburgh, New York

Debra Marsala, DNS, ANP
Adjunct Instructor
Division of Nursing
Keuka College
Keuka Park, New York

Sandra Nash, PhD, RN
Assistant Professor
Western Illinois University
Macomb, Illinois

Catherine Pankonien, DNP, RNC-NIC
Assistant Professor
Wilson School of Nursing
Midwestern State University
Wichita Falls, Texas

Diane Ryan, PhD, AGPCNP
Associate Professor
Department of Nursing
Daemen College
Amherst, New York

Jennifer Sipe, MSN, CRNP
Assistant Professor
School of Nursing and Health Sciences
La Salle University
Philadelphia, Pennsylvania

Monica Sousa, EdD, ACNS-BC, APRN
Associate Professor
Department of Nursing
Western Connecticut State University
Danbury, Connecticut

Ann Tritak, EdD, RN
Associate Dean, DNP Program Director
School of Nursing
Felician University
Lodi, New Jersey

Renee Wenzlaff, DNP, RN
Associate Professor
School of Nursing
Milwaukee School of Engineering
Milwaukee, Wisconsin

Jean Yockey, PhD, FNP, RN, CNE
Assistant Professor
Department of Nursing
University of South Dakota
Vermillion, South Dakota

Preface

This book was written with the intent of presenting the subject matter of pathophysiology as the foundation for all future studies in the health sciences. The text provides necessary content for the beginning student to build upon while also serving those furthering their education by reinforcing the link between comprehending complex disease process and clinical decision-making. This text will serve as a reference long after the coursework is completed.

This edition considers the many technologic advances allowing health care providers to diagnose earlier and with more accuracy. A diverse array of contributors for *Porth's Pathophysiology*, 10th Edition (from which this *Essentials* book is derived)was selected based on subject expertise.

This text focuses on the scientific basis upon which the practice components of the health professions are based. The evidence-based information provides data for best practices, ultimately improving health care outcomes.

A holistic conceptual framework uses body systems as an organizing structure and demonstrates how the systems are interrelated. Selection of content was based on common causes of morbidity and mortality across the life span, and recent advances in the fields of genetics, epigenetics, immunology, microbiology, and molecular biology are included. Content is presented in a manner that is logical and understandable for students. One goal of the new edition is to provide critical information needed to understand complex health alterations while delivering the content in a reader-friendly format. The chapters are arranged so that fundamental concepts such as cellular adaptation, inflammation and repair, genetic control of cell function and inheritance, and immunologic processes appear in the early chapters before the specific discussions of particular disease states.

Strengths of the text include the expanded chapters on health and disease; nutrition; sleep and sleep disorders; and thought, emotion, and mood disorders. Advances in health care are presented through the inclusion of international studies, World Health Organization guidelines, updated standards, and the health variants of diverse populations.

Organization

Many of the units have an introductory chapter that contains essential information about the structure and function of the body systems that are being discussed in the unit. Each such chapter provides the foundation for understanding the pathophysiology content presented in the subsequent chapters. The chapter outline that appears at the beginning of each chapter provides an overall view of the chapter content and organization.

Features of This Book

This book includes the following special features to help you master the essential content.

Objectives

Objectives appear at the beginning of each chapter to provide a focus for your study. After you have finished each of these areas of content, you may want to go back and make sure that you have met each of the objectives.

Learning Objectives

After completing this chapter, the learner will be able to meet the following objectives:

1. Contrast disorders due to multifactorial inheritance with those caused by single-gene inheritance.
2. Cite the most susceptible period of intrauterine life for development of defects because of teratogenic agents.
3. State the cautions that should be observed when considering use of drugs during pregnancy, including the possible effects of alcohol abuse, vitamin A derivatives, and folic acid deficiency on fetal development.
4. Describe the process of genetic assessment.
5. Describe screening methods used for prenatal diagnosis including specificity and risks.

Key Terms and Glossary

To enable you to better use and understand the vocabulary of your profession, throughout the text you will encounter key terms in bold purple. This is a signal that a word and the ideas associated with it are important to learn. In addition, a glossary is provided to help you expand your vocabulary and improve your comprehension of what you are reading. The glossary contains concise definitions of the key terms. If you are unsure of the meaning of a term you encounter in your reading, check the glossary in the back of the book before proceeding.

Lysosomes play an important role in the normal metabolism of certain substances in the body. In some inherited diseases known as **lysosomal storage disorders**, a specific lysosomal enzyme is absent or inactive, preventing digestion of certain cellular substances and allowing them to build up in cells.[6] There are approximately 50 lysosomal storage disorders, each caused by a lack of activity of one or more lysosomal enzymes, and each disorder is rare.

Boxes

Boxes are used throughout the text to summarize and highlight key information.

"Key Points" Boxes

One of the ways to approach learning is to focus on the major ideas or concepts. Because health care is an applied science, it is imperative that rather than trying to memorize a list of related and unrelated bits of information, you understand the content and relate it to cases you encounter. Health care providers must apply these concepts in the clinical setting, which requires an understanding of the underlying etiology, histology, symptoms, risk factors, and hallmark features of a particular disease. As you have probably already discovered, it is impossible to memorize everything that is in a particular section or chapter of the book. It has been said that pathophysiology is a new language for many students. So not only does your brain have to figure out where to store all the information, it must also be able to retrieve the information when you need it. This is best accomplished by understanding rather than memorizing information. Most important of all, memorized lists of content can seldom, if ever, be applied directly to an actual clinical situation. The "Key Points" boxes guide you in identifying the major ideas or concepts that form the foundation for truly understanding the major areas of content. When you understand the concepts in the "Key Points" boxes, you will have a framework for remembering and using the facts given in the text.

KEY POINTS

Cellular Adaptations

- Cells are able to adapt to increased work demands or threats to survival by changing their size (atrophy and hypertrophy), number (hyperplasia), and form (metaplasia).
- Normal cellular adaptation occurs in response to an appropriate stimulus and ceases once the need for adaptation has ceased.

"Summary Concepts" Boxes

The "Summary Concepts" boxes at the end of each main section provide a review and a reinforcement of the important content that has been covered. Use the summaries to ensure that you have covered and understood what you have read.

 SUMMARY CONCEPTS

Neonates are protected against antigens in early life as a result of passive transfer of maternal IgG antibodies through the placenta and IgA antibodies in colostrum and breast milk. Many changes occur with aging, but the exact mechanisms are not completely understood. However, the elderly population is more prone to infection and autoimmune disorders secondary to altered response in both innate and adaptive immune function.

"Understanding" Boxes

"Understanding" boxes focus on the physiologic processes and phenomena that form the basis for understanding disorders presented in the text. This feature breaks a process or phenomenon down into its component parts and presents it in a sequential manner, providing an insight into the many opportunities for disease processes to disrupt the sequence.

UNDERSTANDING ➔ **The Complement System**

The complement system provides one of the major effector mechanisms of both humoral and innate immunity. The system consists of a group of proteins (complement proteins C1 through C9) that are normally present in the plasma in an inactive form. Activation of the complement system is a highly regulated process, involving the sequential breakdown of the complement proteins to generate a cascade of cleavage products capable of proteolytic enzyme activity. This allows for tremendous amplification because each enzyme molecule activated by one step can generate multiple activated enzyme molecules at the next step. Complement activation is inhibited by proteins that are present on normal host cells; thus, its actions are limited to microbes and other antigens that lack these inhibitory proteins.

The reactions of the complement system can be divided into three phases: **(1)** the initial activation phase, **(2)** the early-step inflammatory responses, and **(3)** the late-step membrane attack responses.

1 **Initial Activation Phase** There are three pathways for recognizing microbes and activating the complement system: (1) the alternative pathway, which is activated on microbial cell surfaces in the absence of antibody and is a component of innate immunity; (2) the classical pathway, which is activated by certain types of antibodies bound to antigen and is part of humoral immunity; and (3) the lectin pathway, which is activated by a plasma lectin that binds to mannose on microbes and activates the classical system pathway in the absence of antibody.

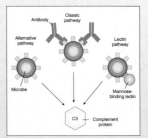

Tables and Charts

Tables and charts are designed to present complex information in a format that makes it more meaningful and facilitates recall of the information. Tables, which have two or more columns, are often used for the purpose of comparing or contrasting information. Charts, which have one column, are used to summarize information.

TABLE 20-1 Common Disorders Affecting the Vestibular System

Type of Disorder	Pathology
Acoustic neuroma	A noncancerous growth or tumor on the vestibulocochlear nerve
Benign paroxysmal positional vertigo	Disorder of otoliths
Ménière disease	Dislodgement of otoliths that participate in the receptor function of the vestibular system
Motion sickness	Repeated stimulation of the vestibular system such as during car, air, and boat travel
Labyrinthitis	Acute viral or bacterial infection of the vestibular pathways
Vestibular migraine	Dizziness or vertigo occurs with or without headache; related to the neurotransmitter serotonin

Illustrations and Photos

The detailed, full-color illustrations will help you to build your own mental image of the content that is being presented. Each drawing has been developed to fully support and build upon the ideas in the text. Some illustrations are used to help you picture the complex interactions of the multiple phenomena that are involved in the development of a particular disease; others can help you to visualize normal function or understand the mechanisms that enable the disease processes to exert their effects. In addition, photographs provide a realistic view of selected pathologic processes and lesions.

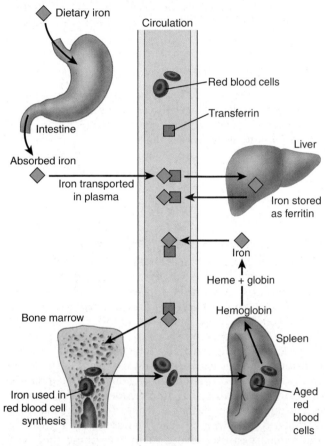

FIGURE 23-3. Diagrammatic representation of the iron cycle, including its absorption from the gastrointestinal tract, transport in the circulation, storage in the liver, recycling from aged red cells destroyed in the spleen, and use in the bone marrow synthesis of red blood cells.

Concept Mastery Alerts

Concept Mastery Alerts clarify fundamental nursing concepts to improve the reader's understanding of potentially confusing topics, as identified by Misconception Alerts in Lippincott's Adaptive Learning Powered by prepU.

Concept Mastery Alert

Smoking is an independent risk factor for the development of coronary artery disease and should be avoided, but it has not been identified as a direct cause of hypertension.

Interactive Learning Resources

Interactive learning tools available online enrich learning and are identified with icons in the text.
- **Concepts in Action Animations** bring physiologic and pathophysiologic concepts to life, explaining concepts that are difficult to understand.
- **Interactive Tutorials** include graphics and animations and provide interactive review exercises.

Review Exercises

The Review Exercises at the end of each chapter are designed to help you integrate and synthesize material and to help you verify your understanding of the material presented. If you are unable to answer a question, reread the relevant section in the chapter. (Answers are available for instructors at http://thepoint.lww.com/PorthEssentials5e.)

Review Exercises

1. A 32-year-old woman with diabetes is found to have a positive result on a urine dipstick test for microalbuminuria. A subsequent 24-hour urine specimen reveals an albumin excretion of 50 mg (an albumin excretion >30 mg/day is abnormal).
   A. Use the structures of the glomerulus in Figure 32-5 to provide a possible explanation for this finding. Why specifically test for the albumin rather than the globulins or other plasma proteins?
   B. Strict control of blood sugars and treatment of hypertension have been shown to decrease the progression of kidney disease in person with diabetes. Explain the physiologic rationale for these two types of treatments.

2. A 54-year-old man, seen by his physician for an elevated blood pressure, was found to have a serum creatinine of 2.5 and BUN of 30. He complains that he has been urinating more frequently than usual, and his first morning urine specimen reveals dilute urine with a specific gravity of 1.010.
   A. Explain the elevation of serum creatinine in terms of renal function.
   B. Explain the inability of people with early renal failure to produce concentrated urine as evidenced by the frequency of urination and the low specific gravity of his first morning urine specimen.

Appendix

The appendix "Lab Values" provides rapid access to normal values for many laboratory tests, as well as a description of the prefixes, symbols, and factors (*e.g.*, micro, μ, 10^{-6}) used for describing these values. Knowledge of normal values can help you to put abnormal values in context.

A Comprehensive Package for Teaching and Learning

To further facilitate teaching and learning, a carefully designed ancillary package has been developed to assist faculty and students.

Instructor Resources

Tools to assist you with teaching your course are available upon adoption of this text on thePoint at http://thepoint.lww.com/PorthEssentials5e.

- A **Test Generator** features NCLEX-style questions mapped to chapter learning objectives.
- An extensive collection of materials is provided for each book chapter:
  - **Pre-lecture Quizzes** (and answers) allow you to check students' reading.
  - **PowerPoint Presentations** provide an easy way to integrate the textbook with your students' classroom experience; multiple-choice and true/false questions are included to promote class participation.
  - **Guided Lecture Notes** walk you through the chapter, learning objective by learning objective, with integrated references to the PowerPoint presentations.
  - **Discussion Topics** (and suggested answers) can be used in the classroom or in online discussion boards to facilitate interaction with your students.
  - **Assignments** (and suggested answers) include group, written, clinical, and Web assignments to engage students in varied activities and assess their learning.
  - **Case Studies** with related questions (and suggested answers) give students an opportunity to apply their knowledge to a client case similar to one they might encounter in practice.
  - **Answers to the Review Exercises** in the book facilitate review of student responses to these exercises.
- Sample **Syllabi** are provided for 14-week and 28-week courses.
- An **Image Bank** lets you use the photographs and illustrations from this textbook in your course materials.
- An **ebook** serves as a handy resource.
- **Strategies for Effective Teaching** provide general tips for instructors related to preparing course materials and meeting student needs.
- **Dosage Calculation Quizzes** and **Drug Monographs** are convenient references.
- Access to all **Student Resources** is provided so that you can understand the student experience and use these resources in your course as well.

Student Resources

An exciting set of free learning resources is available on thePoint to help students review and apply vital concepts. Multimedia engines have been optimized so that students can access many of these resources on mobile devices. Students can access all these resources at http://thepoint.lww.com/PorthEssentials5e using the codes printed in the front of their textbooks.

- **NCLEX-Style Review Questions** for each chapter help students review important concepts and practice for NCLEX.
- **Interactive learning resources** appeal to a variety of learning styles. As mentioned previously in this preface, icons in the text direct readers to relevant resources:
  - **Concepts in Action Animations** bring physiologic and pathophysiologic concepts to life, explaining concepts that are difficult to understand.
  - **Interactive Tutorials** include graphics and animations and provide interactive review exercises.
- **Journal Articles** offer access to current articles relevant to each chapter and available in Wolters Kluwer journals to familiarize students with nursing literature.
- **Learning Objectives** from the book.
- A **Spanish–English Audio Glossary** provides helpful terms and phrases for communicating with patients who speak Spanish.

Adaptive Learning Powered by PrepU

Lippincott's Adaptive Learning Powered by prepU helps every student learn more, while giving instructors the data they need to monitor each student's progress, strengths, and weaknesses. The adaptive learning system allows instructors to assign quizzes or students to take quizzes on their own that adapt to each student's individual mastery level. Visit http://thePoint.lww.com/prepU to learn more.

A Comprehensive, Digital, Integrated Course Solution: *Lippincott CoursePoint*

The same trusted solution, innovation, and unmatched support that you have come to expect from *Lippincott CoursePoint* is now enhanced with more engaging learning tools and deeper analytics to help prepare students for practice. This powerfully integrated digital learning solution combines learning tools, case studies, real-time data, and the most trusted nursing education content on the market to make curriculum-wide learning more efficient and to meet students where they are at in their learning. And now, it is easier than ever for instructors and students to use, giving them everything they need for course and curriculum success!

Lippincott CoursePoint includes:

- Engaging course content provides a variety of learning tools to engage students of all learning styles.
- A more personalized learning approach gives students the content and tools they need at the moment they need it, giving them data for more focused remediation and helping to boost their confidence and competence.
- Powerful tools, including varying levels of case studies, interactive learning activities, and adaptive learning powered by PrepU, help students learn the critical thinking and clinical judgment skills to help them become practice-ready nurses.
- Unparalleled reporting provides in-depth dashboards with several data points to track student progress and help identify strengths and weaknesses.
- Unmatched support includes training coaches, product trainers, and nursing education consultants to help educators and students implement CoursePoint with ease.

Acknowledgments

The expertise of the contributors for *Porth's Pathophysiology*, 10th Edition (from which this *Essentials* book is derived) keeps the book at the forefront of advances in science and medicine. Their attention to detail and desire to share current, relevant, and essential information with learners are primary strengths of the text. For the fifth edition, several chapters were merged to improve flow of content, and chapters that include new discoveries were added. Thanks also to Dr. Rupa Lalchandani Tuan for her time and talent in helping to ensure the accuracy of the information and assisting in condensing it to reflect only essential content needed to understand disease processes.

I would like to thank Jonathan Joyce, senior acquisitions editor, for keeping us on task so the project remained on track. Many thanks go to Meredith Brittain, senior development editor, for her edits and comments that kept the focus of this book consistent. I also want to thank Jennifer Forestieri, director of product development, who stepped in to help, and especially for all her encouragement. Thanks also to Tim Rinehart, who provided the chapter tracking updates.

Lastly, I want to thank my family for their inspiration during this difficult time of transition in my life. I also want to thank all the professors who have kept in touch with me throughout this project, cheering me forward to produce a text that is understandable yet concise and that meets the learning needs of today's health care professional.

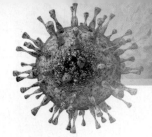

Contents

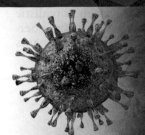
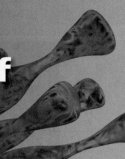
C H A P T E R 1

Concepts of Health and Disease

Learning Objectives

After completing this chapter, the learner will be able to meet the following objectives:

1. Compare the World Health Organization definition of health to the *Healthy People 2020* definition.
2. Define *pathophysiology*.
3. Describe the process of disease to include etiology, pathogenesis, morphologic changes, clinical manifestations, diagnosis, and clinical course.
4. Define the term *epidemiology*.
5. Compare the meaning of the terms *incidence* and *prevalence* as they relate to measures of disease frequency.
6. Differentiate primary, secondary, and tertiary levels of prevention.
7. Compare morbidity and mortality.

The term *pathophysiology*, which is the focus of this book, may be defined as the physiology of altered health. The term combines the words *pathology* and *physiology*. Pathology (from the Greek *pathos*, meaning "disease") deals with the study of the structural and functional changes in cells, tissues, and organs of the body that cause or are caused by disease. Physiology deals with the functions of the human body. Thus, pathophysiology deals not only with the cellular and organ changes that occur with disease but also with the effects that these changes have on total body function (Fig. 1-1). Examples of atrophy of the brain (Fig. 1-1A) and hypertrophy of the myocardium (Fig. 1-1B) illustrate pathophysiologic changes from a cerebrovascular accident to long-standing unmanaged hypertension and how this impacts the myocardium. Pathophysiology also focuses on the mechanisms of the underlying disease and provides information to assist with planning preventive as well as therapeutic health care measures and practices such as following a healthy diet, exercising, and being compliant with prescribed medications. This chapter is intended to orient the reader to the concepts of health and disease, various terms that are used throughout the book, the sources of data and what they mean, and the broader aspects of pathophysiology in terms of the health and well-being of populations.

In most organisms, the cell is the smallest functional unit that has the characteristics necessary for life. Cells combine to form tissues based on their embryonic origin. These tissues combine to form organs. Although cells of different tissues and organs vary in structure and function, certain characteristics are common to all cells. Because most disease processes start at the cellular level, we need to understand cell function to understand disease processes. This chapter discusses the structural parts of cells, cell functions and growth, movement of substances such as ions across the cell membrane, and tissue types.

Functional Components of the Cell

Most organisms, including humans, contain **eukaryotic** cells that are made up of internal membrane-bound compartments called **organelles** ("small organs" within cells); an example of an organelle is the nucleus. This is in contrast to prokaryotes, such as bacteria, that do not contain membrane-bound organelles. When seen under a microscope, three major components of a eukaryotic cell become evident—the nucleus, the **cytoplasm**, and the cell membrane (Fig. 2-1).

Protoplasm

Biologists call the intracellular fluid **protoplasm**. Protoplasm is composed of water, proteins, lipids, carbohydrates, and electrolytes.[1]

- Water makes up 70% to 85% of the cell's protoplasm.[1]
- Proteins make up 10% to 20% of the protoplasm. Proteins are polar and soluble in water. Examples of proteins include **enzymes** necessary for cellular reactions, structural proteins, ion channels, and receptors.[1]
- Lipids make up 2% to 3% of the protoplasm. Lipids are nonpolar and insoluble in water. They are the main parts of cell membranes surrounding the outside and inside of cells. Examples of lipids include phospholipids and cholesterol. Some cells also contain large quantities of triglycerides. In fat cells, triglycerides can make up as much as 95% of the total cell mass.[1] Carbohydrates make up approximately 1% of the protoplasm. These serve primarily as a rapid source of energy.[1]
- The major intracellular electrolytes include potassium, magnesium, phosphate, sulfate, and bicarbonate ions. Small quantities of the electrolytes sodium, chloride, and calcium ions are also present in cells. These electrolytes participate in reactions that are necessary for the cell's **metabolism**, and they help generate and send signals in neurons, muscle cells, and other cells.
  Two distinct regions of protoplasm exist in the cell:
- The **karyoplasm** or nucleoplasm is inside the nucleus.
- The cytoplasm is outside the nucleus. The cytosol is the fluid of the cytoplasm (cytoplasm = cytosol + organelles).

KEY POINTS

The Functional Organization of the Cell

- Organelles in the cytoplasm perform functions within cells similar to how organs in the body perform functions within the organism.
- The nucleus is the largest and most visible organelle in the cell. The nucleus is the control center for the cell. In eukaryotic cells, it contains genetic information that we inherit from our parents.[1]
- Other organelles include the mitochondria, which help to make energy molecules that cells can use, and the lysosomes and **proteasomes**, which function as the cell's digestive system. Ribosomes, which are not surrounded by membranes, are the cellular structures that make proteins; those proteins may help to make other molecules needed for cell function.

The Nucleus

The cell nucleus is a rounded or elongated structure near the center of the cell (see Fig. 2-1). All eukaryotic cells have at least one nucleus. Some cells contain more than one nucleus; osteoclasts (a type of bone cell) usually contain 12 or more nuclei.[1]

The nucleus can be thought of as the control center for the cell because it contains the instructions to make proteins, and proteins can then make other molecules needed for cellular function and survival.[1] The nucleus contains deoxyribonucleic acid (DNA), which contains genes. Genes contain the instructions for cellular function and survival. For example, the insulin gene contains instructions to make insulin protein. In addition, genes are units of inheritance that pass information from parents to their children.

The nucleus also is the site for the **synthesis** of the three main types of ribonucleic acid (RNA). These RNA molecules move from the nucleus to the cytoplasm and carry out the synthesis of proteins. These three types of RNA are as follows:

- Messenger RNA (mRNA), which is made from genetic information transcribed from the DNA in a process called transcription. mRNA travels to ribosomes in the cytoplasm so these instructions can be used to make proteins.
- Ribosomal RNA (rRNA) is the RNA component of ribosomes, the site of protein production.
- Transfer RNA (tRNA) transports amino acids to ribosomes so that mRNA can be turned into a sequence of amino acids. This process, known as translation, uses the mRNA template to link amino acids to synthesize proteins.[1]

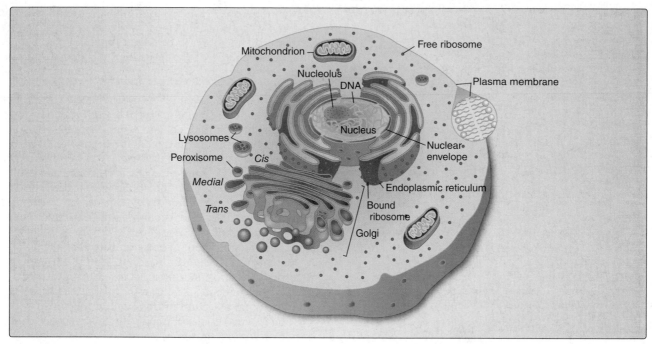

FIGURE 2-1. Cell organelles. DNA, deoxyribonucleic acid. (Reprinted from Leeper-Woodford. (2016). *Lippincott illustrated reviews: Integrated systems* (Fig. 2.1, p. 39). Philadelphia, PA: Wolters Kluwer, with permission.)

The Cytoplasm and Its Organelles

The cytoplasm includes the fluid and organelles outside the nucleus but within the cell membrane surrounding the cell. Cytoplasm is a solution that contains water, electrolytes, proteins, fats, and carbohydrates.[1] Pigments may also accumulate in the cytoplasm. Some pigments are normal parts of cells. One example is melanin, which gives skin its color. Some pigments are not normal parts of cells. For example, when the body breaks down old red blood cells, pigments in red blood cells are changed to the pigment bilirubin, which the body can excrete. Embedded in the cytoplasm are various organelles that function as the organs of the cell. In addition to the nucleus, which was discussed in the previous section, these organelles include the ribosomes, the endoplasmic reticulum (ER), the Golgi complex, lysosomes, **peroxisomes**, proteasomes, and mitochondria.[1]

Ribosomes

The ribosomes are the sites of protein synthesis in the cell. There are two subunits of ribosomes that are made up of rRNA and proteins. During protein synthesis, the two ribosomal subunits are held together by a strand of mRNA.[1] These active ribosomes either stay within the cytoplasm (Fig. 2-2) or are attached to the membrane of the ER, depending on where the protein will be used.[1]

Endoplasmic Reticulum

The ER is an extensive system of paired membranes and flat **vesicles** that connect various parts of the inner cell (see Fig. 2-2).[1] Two forms of ER exist in cells—rough and smooth.

Rough ER has ribosomes attached, and the ribosomes appear under a microscope as "rough" structures on the ER membrane. Proteins made by the rough ER usually become

parts of organelles or cell membranes, or are secreted from cells as a protein. For example, the rough ER makes (1) digestive enzymes found in lysosomes and (2) proteins that are secreted, such as the protein hormone insulin.

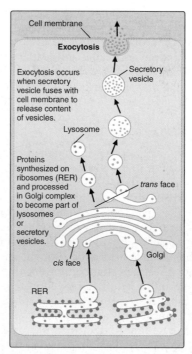

FIGURE 2-2. Endoplasmic reticulum (ER), ribosomes, and Golgi apparatus. The rough ER (RER) consists of intricately folded membranes studded with ribosomes. Ribosomes are made of protein and ribosomal ribonucleic acid organized together. Golgi apparatus processes proteins synthesized on ribosomes. (Reprinted from Leeper-Woodford. (2016). *Lippincott illustrated reviews: Integrated systems* (Fig. 2.3, p. 41). Philadelphia, PA: Wolters Kluwer, with permission.)

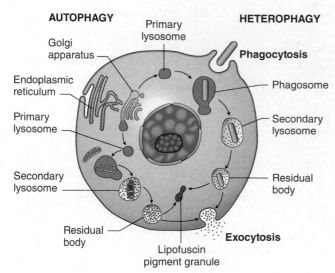

FIGURE 2-3. The processes of autophagy and heterophagy, showing the primary and secondary lysosomes, residual bodies, extrusion of residual body contents from the cell, and lipofuscin-containing residual bodies.

The smooth ER is free of ribosomes and has a smooth structure when viewed through a microscope. Because it does not have ribosomes attached, the smooth ER does not participate in protein synthesis. Instead, the smooth ER is involved in the synthesis of lipids including steroid hormones. The smooth ER of the liver is involved in storage of extra glucose as glycogen as well as metabolism of some hormone drugs.

If proteins build up in the ER faster than they can be removed, the cell is said to experience "ER stress." The cell responds by slowing down protein synthesis and restoring homeostasis. Abnormal responses to ER stress, which can cause inflammation and even cell death, have been implicated in inflammatory bowel disease,[2] a genetic form of diabetes mellitus,[3] and a disorder of **skeletal muscle** known as myositis,[4] as well as many other diseases.

Golgi Complex

The Golgi apparatus, sometimes called the Golgi complex, consists of four or more stacks of thin, flattened vesicles or sacs (see Fig. 2-3).[1] Substances produced in the ER are carried to the Golgi complex in small, membrane-covered transfer vesicles. The Golgi complex modifies these substances and packages them into **secretory granules** or vesicles. In addition to making secretory granules, the Golgi complex is thought to make large carbohydrate molecules that combine with proteins produced in the rough ER to form glycoproteins. The Golgi apparatus can receive proteins and other substances from the cell surface by a **retrograde** transport mechanism. Several bacterial toxins, such as Shiga and cholera toxins, and plant toxins, such as ricin, that have cytoplasmic targets have exploited this retrograde pathway.[1]

Lysosomes and Peroxisomes

Lysosomes can be thought of as the digestive system or the stomach of the cell. These small, membrane-enclosed sacs contain powerful enzymes that can break down excess and worn-out cell parts as well as foreign substances that are taken into the cell (*e.g.*, bacteria taken in by **phagocytosis**). All of the lysosomal enzymes require an acidic environment, and the lysosomes maintain a pH of approximately 5 in their interior compared to the pH of the cytoplasm, which is approximately 7.2, protecting other cellular structures from being broken down by these enzymes should leakage occur. **Primary lysosomes** are membrane-bound intracellular organelles that contain a variety of enzymes that have not yet entered the digestive process. They receive their enzymes as well as their membranes from the Golgi apparatus. Primary lysosomes become secondary lysosomes after they fuse with membrane-bound vacuoles that contain material to be digested. Lysosomes break down phagocytosed material by either **heterophagy** or **autophagy** (Fig. 2-3).

Heterophagy (*hetero*, different; *phagy*, eat) refers to digestion of a substance phagocytosed from the cell's external environment.[5] An infolding of the cell membrane takes external materials into the cell to form a surrounding phagocytic vesicle, or **phagosome**. Primary lysosomes then fuse with phagosomes to form secondary lysosomes. Heterophagocytosis is most common in phagocytic white blood cells such as neutrophils and macrophages.

Autophagy involves the digestion of damaged cellular organelles, such as mitochondria or ER, which the lysosomes must remove if the cell's normal function is to continue.[5] Autophagocytosis is most common in cells undergoing **atrophy** (cell **degeneration**).

Lysosomes play an important role in the normal metabolism of certain substances in the body. In some inherited diseases known as **lysosomal storage disorders**, a specific lysosomal enzyme is absent or inactive, preventing digestion of certain cellular substances and allowing them to build up in cells.[6] There are approximately 50 lysosomal storage disorders, each caused by a lack of activity of one or more lysosomal enzymes, and each disorder is rare.

In Tay–Sachs disease, an autosomal recessive disorder, cells do not make hexosaminidase A, a lysosomal enzyme needed for degrading the GM_2 ganglioside found in nerve cell membranes. Its accumulation in the nervous system and retina of the eye causes the most damage.[6]

Smaller than lysosomes, round membrane-bound organelles called peroxisomes contain a special enzyme that degrades peroxides (*e.g.*, hydrogen peroxide) in the control of free radicals.[6] In liver cells, peroxidases help make bile acids.[5]

Proteasomes

Three major cellular mechanisms are involved in the breakdown of proteins, or **proteolysis**.[5] One of these is by the previously described lysosomal **degradation**. The second mechanism is the **caspase pathway** that is involved in apoptotic cell death. The third method of proteolysis occurs within an organelle called the proteasome. Proteasomes are small organelles made up of protein complexes in the cytoplasm and nucleus. These organelles recognize misformed and misfolded proteins that have been targeted for degradation.

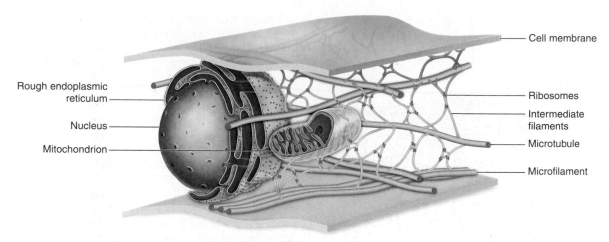

Cell membrane

Rough endoplasmic reticulum

Nucleus

Mitochondrion

Ribosomes

Intermediate filaments

Microtubule

Microfilament

FIGURE 2-4. Cytoskeleton. The cytoskeleton is made up of microfilaments, microtubules, and intermediate filaments. (Reprinted with permission from Wingerd B. (2014). *The human body* (3rd ed., Fig. 3.10, p. 55). Philadelphia, PA: Wolters Kluwer.)

Mitochondria

The mitochondria are the "power plants" of the cell because they contain enzymes that can change carbon-containing nutrients into energy that is easily used by cells. This multistep process is often referred to as **cellular respiration** because it requires oxygen.[1] Cells store most of this energy as high-energy phosphate bonds in substances such as adenosine triphosphate (ATP) and use the ATP as energy in various cellular activities. Mitochondria are found close to the site of energy use in the cell (*e.g.,* near the **myofibrils** in muscle cells). A large increase in mitochondria occurs in skeletal muscle repeatedly stimulated to contract.

Mitochondria contain their own DNA and ribosomes and are self-replicating. Mitochondrial DNA (mtDNA) is inherited from the mother and thought to be linked to certain diseases and aging. mtDNA is a double-stranded, circular molecule that contains the instructions to make 13 of the proteins needed for mitochondrial function. The DNA of the nucleus contains the instructions for the structural proteins of the mitochondria and other proteins needed for cellular respiration.[5,7]

Most cells in the body can be affected by mtDNA mutations.[5]

Mitochondria also function as key regulators of apoptosis, or programmed cell death. In cancer, there is too little apoptosis and in neurodegenerative diseases, there is too much apoptosis.

The Cytoskeleton

In addition to its organelles, the cytoplasm contains a *cytoskeleton*, or the skeleton of the cell. The cytoskeleton is a network of microtubules, microfilaments, intermediate filaments, and thick filaments (Fig. 2-4).[5] The cytoskeleton controls cell shape and movement.

Microtubules

Microtubules are formed from protein subunits called **tubulin.** Microtubules are long, stiff, hollow structures shaped like cylinders.[7] Microtubules can rapidly disassemble in one location and reassemble in another. This constant reassembling forms elements of the cytoskeleton by continuously shortening and lengthening the tubulin **dimers,** a process known as dynamic instability.[6]

Microtubules function in the development and maintenance of cell formation. Microtubules participate in transport mechanisms inside cells, including transport of materials in the long axons of neurons and melanin in skin cells. Microtubules are also part of other cell structures such as **cilia** and flagella[7] (Fig. 2-5).

Another important role of microtubules is participating in **mitosis** (cell division). Some cancer drugs (*e.g.,* vinblastine and vincristine) bind to microtubules and inhibit cell division.[8]

Cilia and Flagella

Flagella and cilia (*plural*) are microtubule-filled cellular extensions surrounded by a membrane that is continuous with the cell membrane. Eukaryotic flagellated cells are generally classified as having only one flagellum (*singular*), whereas ciliated cells typically have a large number of cilia.[7] In humans, sperm cells are the only cell type with flagella. Cilia are found on surfaces of many epithelial linings, including the nasal sinuses and bronchi in the upper respiratory system. Damage to cilia or ciliated cells causes a cough, which is then used to help remove these substances from the airways.

Genetic defects can result in incorrect assembly of cilia.[7] For example, primary ciliary dyskinesia, also called **immotile cilia syndrome,** causes problems in the cilia of the respiratory tract so that inhaled bacteria cannot be removed, leading to a chronic lung disease called **bronchiectasis.** Genetic defects can also cause fertility problems by affecting the cilia in the fallopian tubes or the flagella on sperm.[7,9] A condition called **polycystic kidney disease** is linked to a genetic defect in the cilia of the renal tubular cells.

Microfilaments

Microfilaments are thin, thread-like cytoplasmic structures. There are three classes of microfilaments:

1. Thin microfilaments, which are similar to thin actin filaments in muscle

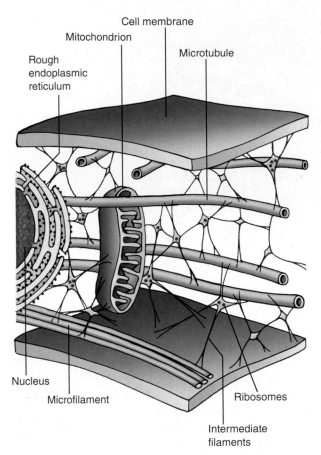

Cell membrane

Mitochondrion

Microtubule

Rough endoplasmic reticulum

Nucleus

Microfilament

Ribosomes

Intermediate filaments

FIGURE 2-5. Microtubules and microfilaments of the cell. The microfilaments are associated with the inner surface of the cell and aid in cell motility. The microtubules form the cytoskeleton and maintain the position of the organelles.

2. Intermediate filaments, which are a group of filaments with diameters between those of the thick and thin filaments

3. Thick myosin filaments, which are in muscle cells but may also exist temporarily in other cells[5]

Muscle contraction depends on the interaction between the thin actin filaments and thick myosin filaments. Microfilaments are also present in the microvilli of the intestine. The intermediate filaments help support and maintain the shape of cells.[5] The **neurofibrillary tangles** found in the brain in Alzheimer disease are formed by aggregated microtubule-associated proteins and result in abnormal cytoskeletons in neurons.

The Cell (Plasma) Membrane

The cell is surrounded by a thin membrane that separates the intracellular contents from the extracellular environment. (Note that this is different from a cell wall.) Cell walls add structure and strength. Human cells do not have cell walls because of the development of tissues, organs, and organ systems, which must have the ability to communicate.

The cell membrane is one of the most important parts of the cell acting as a **semipermeable** structure that helps determine what can and cannot enter and exit cells. The cell membrane contains receptors for hormones, neurotransmitters, and other chemical signals, as well as transporters that allow ions to cross the membrane during electrical signaling in cells (such as neurons and muscle cells). It also helps regulate cell growth and division.

The cell membrane is a dynamic and fluid structure made up of organized lipids, carbohydrates, and proteins (Fig. 2-6). The main part of the membrane is the lipid bilayer, made up mostly of phospholipids, with glycolipids and cholesterol.[7] This lipid bilayer is a mostly impermeable barrier to all but lipid-soluble substances.

Phospholipid molecules are arranged so their **hydrophilic**, water-loving heads face outward on each side of the membrane, where there is watery extracellular or intracellular fluid, and their **hydrophobic** tails project toward the middle of the membrane.

Although the lipid bilayer provides the basic structure of the cell membrane, proteins carry out most of the functions. The way proteins are associated with the cell

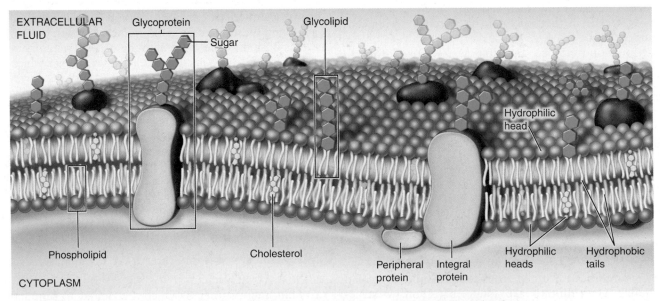

FIGURE 2-6. Structure of the cell membrane showing the hydrophilic (polar) heads and the hydrophobic (fatty acid) tails. (From McConnell T. H., Hull K. L. (2011). *Human form, human function: Essentials of anatomy & physiology* (p. 67). Philadelphia, PA: Lippincott Williams & Wilkins.)

membrane often determines their function. The **integral proteins**, called **transmembrane proteins**, cross the entire lipid bilayer and function on both sides of the membrane or transport molecules across it. Many transmembrane proteins form ion channels and are selective for which substances move through them. Mutations in channel proteins, often called **channelopathies**, can cause genetic disorders.[10] For example, cystic fibrosis involves an abnormal chloride channel, which causes the epithelial cell membrane to be impermeable to the chloride ion. The defective chloride secretion with excessive sodium and water causes abnormally thick and viscid respiratory secretions, blocking the airways. Water channels or pores called **aquaporins** are also transmembrane proteins in the cell membrane. Changes in water transport through aquaporin can cause diseases, including diabetes insipidus. Carriers are another type of transmembrane protein that allows substances to cross membranes. Glucose transporters are examples of carriers, and changes in the movement of glucose through these carriers are involved in diabetes mellitus.[8]

The **peripheral proteins** are temporarily bound to one side or the other of the membrane and do not pass into the lipid bilayer, and they have functions involving the inner or outer side of the membrane where they are found. Several peripheral proteins are receptors for chemical signals or are involved in intracellular signaling systems.

SUMMARY CONCEPTS

The cell is a self-sufficient structure that functions similarly to the total organism. In most cells, a single nucleus controls cell function. It contains DNA, which provides the information necessary to make the various proteins the cell needs to stay alive and to transmit genetic information from one generation to another. The nucleus also is where RNA is made. The three types of RNA (mRNA, rRNA, and tRNA) move to the cytoplasm to make proteins.

The cytoplasm contains the cell's organelles and cytoskeleton. Ribosomes are sites for protein synthesis in the cell. The ER transports substances from one part of the cell to another and makes proteins (rough ER), carbohydrates, and lipids (smooth ER). Golgi bodies modify substances made in the ER and package them into secretory granules for transport within the cell or for export from the cell. Lysosomes, which are viewed as the digestive system of the cell, contain enzymes that digest worn-out cell parts and foreign materials. The proteasome digests misformed and misfolded proteins. The mitochondria serve as power plants for the cell because they change nutrient energy into ATP to power cell activities. Mitochondria contain their own DNA, which is important for making mitochondrial RNAs and proteins used in oxidative metabolism. The cytoplasm also contains microtubules, microfilaments, intermediate filaments, and thick filaments.

Microtubules help determine cell shape, provide a means of moving organelles through the cytoplasm, and help move cilia and **chromosomes** during cell division. Actin microfilaments and myosin thin filaments interact so that muscle cells can contract.

The cell membrane is a lipid bilayer that surrounds the cell and separates it from its surrounding external environment. Although the lipid bilayer provides the basic structure of the cell membrane, proteins carry out most of the specific functions of the cell membrane. Peripheral proteins often function as receptor sites for signaling molecules, and transmembrane proteins frequently form transporters for ions and other substances.

Integration of Cell Function and Replication

Cell Communication

Cells in multicellular organisms need to communicate with each other to coordinate their function and control their growth. The human body has several ways of sending information between cells. These include direct communication between neighboring cells through gap junctions, autocrine and **paracrine** signaling, and endocrine or synaptic signaling.[7]

- **Autocrine** signaling (*auto*: self) occurs when a cell releases a chemical into the extracellular fluid that affects its own activity (Fig. 2-7).
- Paracrine signaling acts mainly on nearby cells.
- Endocrine signaling relies on hormones carried in the bloodstream to cells throughout the body.
- Synaptic signaling occurs in the nervous system, where neurotransmitters are released from neurons to act only on neighboring cells at **synapses.**

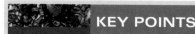

KEY POINTS

Cell Communication

- Cells communicate with each other and with the internal and external environments in a number of ways; for example, electrical and chemical signaling systems control electrical potentials, the overall function of a cell, and gene activity needed for cell division and cell replication.

- Chemical messengers bind to protein receptors on the cell surface or inside of cells in a process called **signal transduction**.

- Cells can regulate their responses to chemical messengers by increasing or decreasing the number of receptors.

UNDERSTANDING → Cell Metabolism

Cell metabolism is the process that changes the calorie-containing nutrients (carbohydrates, proteins, and fats) into ATP, which provides for the energy needs of the cell. ATP is formed through three major pathways: **(1)** the glycolytic pathway, **(2)** the citric acid cycle, and **(3)** the electron transport chain. Without oxygen, cells will use the glycolytic pathway in the cytosol and make two molecules of ATP from one glucose molecule. With oxygen and mitochondria, cells will make much more ATP per glucose molecule.

Cells start the energy metabolism process with the anaerobic glycolytic pathway in the cytoplasm, and if oxygen is present, the pathway moves into the mitochondria for the aerobic pathway. Both pathways involve oxidation–reduction reactions involving an electron donor, which is oxidized in the reaction, and an electron acceptor, which is reduced in the reaction. In energy metabolism, the breakdown products of carbohydrate, fat, and protein metabolism donate electrons and are oxidized, and the coenzymes nicotinamide adenine dinucleotide (NAD$^+$) and flavin adenine dinucleotide (FAD) accept electrons and are reduced.[7]

1

Anaerobic Metabolism. Glycolysis (*glycol*, sugar; **lysis,** breaking down) is the process by which energy is released from glucose. It is an important energy provider for cells that lack mitochondria, the cell organelles where aerobic metabolism occurs. Glycolysis also provides energy in situations when delivery of oxygen to the cell is delayed or impaired (*e.g.,* in skeletal muscle during the first few minutes of exercise).

Glycolysis, which occurs in the cytoplasm of the cell, involves the splitting of the six-carbon glucose molecule into 2 three-carbon molecules of pyruvic acid. Because the reaction that splits glucose requires two molecules of ATP, there is a net gain of only two molecules of ATP from each molecule of glucose that is metabolized. The process is anaerobic and does not require oxygen (O_2) or produce carbon dioxide (CO_2). When O_2 is present, pyruvic acid moves into the mitochondria, where it enters the aerobic citric acid cycle. Under anaerobic conditions, such as cardiac arrest or circulatory shock, pyruvate is converted to lactic acid, allowing glycolysis to continue as a means of supplying cells with ATP when O_2 is lacking.

Converting pyruvate to lactic acid is reversible, and after the oxygen supply has been restored, lactic acid is converted back to pyruvate and used for energy or to make glucose.

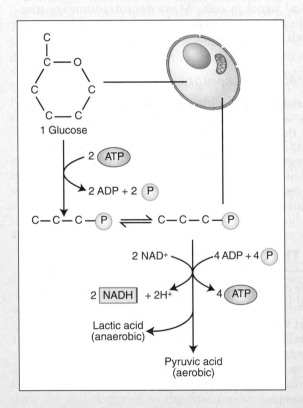

② Aerobic Metabolism

Aerobic metabolism occurs in the cell's mitochondria and involves the citric acid cycle and the electron transport chain. It is here that the carbon compounds from the fats, proteins, and carbohydrates in our diet are broken down and their electrons combined with oxygen to form carbon dioxide, water, and ATP. Unlike lactic acid, which is an end product of anaerobic metabolism, carbon dioxide and water are generally harmless and easily eliminated from the body.[7]

Under aerobic conditions, both of the pyruvate molecules formed by the glycolytic pathway enter the mitochondria, where pyruvate combines with acetyl coenzyme to form acetyl coenzyme A (acetyl-CoA). The formation of acetyl-CoA begins the reactions in the citric acid cycle, also called the **tricarboxylic acid** or **Krebs cycle**. Some reactions release CO_2, and some transfer electrons from the hydrogen atom to NADH or FADH. In addition to pyruvate from the glycolysis of glucose, fatty acid and amino acid breakdown products can also enter the citric acid cycle. Fatty acids, which are the major source of fuel in the body, are oxidized to acetyl-CoA for entry into the citric acid cycle.[1,6,7]

Oxidative metabolism takes place in the electron transport chain in the mitochondria.[1,6,7] At the end of the citric acid cycle, each glucose molecule has yielded four new molecules of ATP (two from glycolysis and two from the citric acid cycle). In fact, the main function of these earlier stages is to make the electrons (e^-) from glucose and other nutrients available for oxidation. Oxidation of the electrons carried by NADH and $FADH_2$ is accomplished through a series of enzyme reactions in the mitochondrial electron transport chain. During these reactions, protons (H^+) combine with O_2 to form water (H_2O), and large amounts of energy are released and used to add a high-energy phosphate bond to ADP, converting it to ATP. Because the formation of ATP involves the addition of a high-energy phosphate bond to ADP, the process is sometimes called **oxidative phosphorylation**. There is a net yield of 36 molecules of ATP from one molecule of glucose (2 from glycolysis, 2 from the citric acid cycle, and 32 from the electron transport chain). In general, the net amount of ATP formed from each gram of protein that is metabolized is less than for glucose, whereas ATP formed from fat is greater (*e.g.*, each 16-carbon fatty acid molecule makes about 129 molecules of ATP).

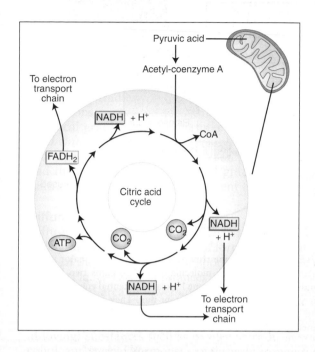

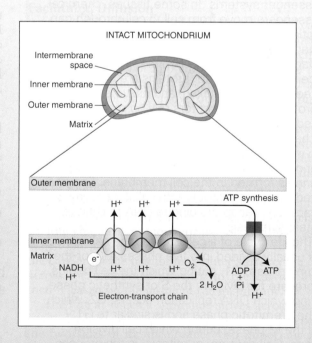

UNDERSTANDING → Membrane Potentials

Electrochemical potentials are present across the membranes of virtually all cells in the body. Some cells, such as nerve and muscle cells, are capable of generating rapidly changing electrical impulses, and these impulses are used to transmit signals along their membranes. In other cells, such as glandular cells, membrane potentials are used to signal the release of hormones or activate other functions of the cell. Generation of membrane potentials relies on **(1)** diffusion of current-carrying ions, **(2)** development of an electrochemical equilibrium, **(3)** establishment of an RMP, and **(4)** triggering of action potentials.

1

Diffusion Potentials A diffusion potential is a potential difference generated across a membrane when a current-carrying ion, such as the potassium (K^+) ion, diffuses down its concentration gradient. Two conditions are necessary for this to occur: (1) the membrane must be selectively permeable to a particular ion and (2) the concentration of the diffusible ion must be greater on one side of the membrane than on the other.

The magnitude of the diffusion potential, measured in mV, depends on the size of the concentration gradient. The sign (+ or –) or polarity of the potential depends on the diffusing ion. It is negative on the inside when a positively charged ion such as K^+ diffuses from the inside to the outside of the membrane, carrying its charge with it.

2

Equilibrium Potentials
An equilibrium potential is the membrane potential that exactly balances and opposes the net diffusion of an ion down its concentration gradient. As a cation diffuses down its concentration gradient, it carries its positive charge across the membrane, thereby generating an electrical force that will eventually retard and stop its diffusion. An electrochemical equilibrium is one in which the *chemical forces driving diffusion* and the *repelling electrical forces* are exactly balanced so that no further diffusion occurs. The equilibrium potential (EMF, electromotive force) can be calculated by inserting the inside and outside ion concentrations into the Nernst equation.

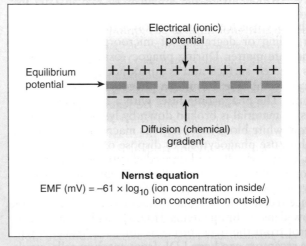

Nernst equation
EMF (mV) = $-61 \times \log_{10}$ (ion concentration inside/ion concentration outside)

The Nernst Equation for Calculating an Equilibrium Potential

The following equation, known as the *Nernst equation*, can be used to calculate the equilibrium potential (EMF in mV of a univalent ion at body temperature of 37°C).

$$\text{EMF (mV)} = -61 \times \log_{10} \text{(ion concentration inside / ion concentration outside)}$$

For example, if the concentration of an ion inside the membrane is 100 mmol/L and the concentration outside the membrane is 10 mmol/L, the EMF (mV) for that ion would be $-61 \times \log_{10}$ (100/10 [$\log_{10}$ of 10 is 1]). Therefore, it would take 61 mV of charge inside the membrane to balance the diffusion potential created by the concentration difference across the membrane for the ion.

The EMF for potassium ions using a normal estimated intracellular concentration of 140 mmol/L and a normal extracellular concentration of 4 mmol/L is –94 mV:

$$-94 = -61 \times \log_{10} \text{(mmol inside / mmol outside)}$$

This value assumes the membrane is permeable only to potassium. This value approximates the –70 to –90 mV *RMP* for nerve fibers measured in laboratory studies.

When a membrane is permeable to several different ions, the diffusion potential reflects the sum of the equilibrium potentials for each of the ions.

③ Resting Membrane Potential The RMP, which is necessary for electrical excitability, is present when the cell is not transmitting impulses. Because the resting membrane is permeable to K^+, it is essentially a K^+ equilibrium potential. This can be explained in terms of the large K^+ concentration gradient (*e.g.*, 140 mEq/L inside and 4 mEq/L outside), which causes the positively charged K^+ to diffuse outward, leaving the nondiffusible, negatively charged intracellular anions (A^-) behind. This causes the membrane to become polarized, with negative charges aligned along the inside and positive charges along the outside. The Na^+/K^+ membrane pump, which removes three Na^+ from inside while returning only two K^+ to the inside, contributes to the maintenance of the RMP.

④ Action Potentials Action potentials involve rapid changes in the membrane potential. Each action potential begins with a sudden change from the negative RMP to a positive threshold potential, causing an opening of the membrane channels for Na^+ (or other ions of the action potential). Opening of the Na^+ channels allows large amounts of the positively charged Na^+ ions to diffuse to the interior of the cell, causing the membrane potential to undergo depolarization or a rapid change to positive on the inside and negative on the outside. This is quickly followed by closing of Na^+ channels and opening of the K^+ channels, which leads to a rapid efflux of K^+ from the cell and reestablishment of the RMP.

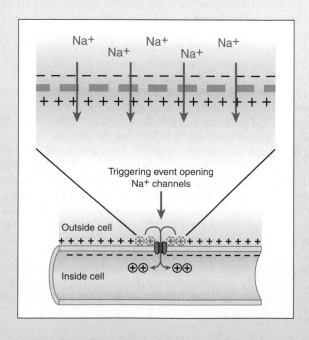

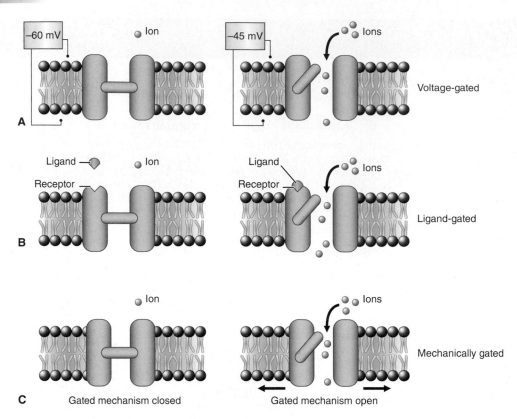

FIGURE 2-14. Gated ion channels that open in response to a specific stimulus. (**A**) Voltage-gated channels are controlled by a change in membrane potential. (**B**) Ligand-gated channels are controlled by binding of a ligand to a receptor. (**C**) Mechanically gated channels, which are controlled by mechanical stimuli such as stretching, often have links that connect to the cytoskeleton.

Electrical potentials are measured in volts (V) or millivolts (mV; see later). Electrical potentials describe the ability of separated electrical charges of opposite polarity (+ and –) to do work. The potential difference is the difference between the separated charges. The terms *potential difference* and *voltage* are synonymous.[5]

Voltage is always measured by comparing two points in a system. For example, the voltage in a car battery (6 or 12 V) is the potential difference between the two battery terminals. Because the total amount of charge that can be separated by a cell membrane is small, the potential differences in cells are small and are measured in mV, or 1/1000th of a volt (Fig. 2-15).

Potential differences across the cell membrane can be measured by inserting a very fine electrode into the cell and another into the extracellular fluid surrounding the cell and connecting the two electrodes to a voltmeter. If cells are not stimulated and are at rest, this difference is called the *resting membrane potential* (RMP). The cell is said to be polarized at rest because the two sides of the membrane have different voltages. In most resting cells, sodium, calcium, and chloride ions are higher outside the cell, and potassium is higher inside the cell.

If sodium or calcium channels are stimulated to open in resting cells, then these positively charged ions will diffuse down their concentration gradients from the outside of the cell, where they have a higher concentration, to the inside of the cell, where they have a lower concentration. This brings positive charge into the cell, causing the cell to be less negative (or more positive). Now, the difference between the inside and outside of the cell is less, so it is less polarized. This is called **depolarization**.

If chloride channels are stimulated to open in resting cells, then negatively charged chloride ions will also diffuse from the outside of the cell to the inside of the cell. However, this brings negative charge into the cell, causing the cell to be more negative (or less positive). Now, the difference between the inside and outside of the cell is more, so it is more polarized. This is called *hyperpolarization*.

If potassium channels are stimulated to open in resting cells, then positively charged potassium ions will diffuse down their concentration gradients from the inside of the cell, where they have a higher concentration, to the outside of the cell, where they have a lower concentration. This removes positive charge from the inside of the cell, causing the cell to be more negative (or less positive). Now the difference between the inside and outside of the cell is more, so it is more polarized. This is called hyperpolarization (note that like chloride diffusion, the inside of the cell is more negative, but chloride adds negative charge to the inside of the cell, and potassium diffusion removes positive charge from the inside of a cell). If cells are first depolarized (*e.g.*, by sodium or calcium diffusing into cells) and then potassium diffuses out of cells, removing the positive charge of potassium from the inside of the cell would be called *repolarization*.

To summarize, at rest, specific ions have higher concentrations on one side of the membrane, resulting in differences in charge and chemical gradients on either side of the membrane. This establishes the RMP, where the two sides of the membrane are polarized. Ion channels can then be stimulated to open or close, changing where the ions (and their charges) move. If the inside of the cell becomes less negative, cells are considered depolarized. If the inside of the cell becomes more negative, cells are considered hyperpolarized (or repolarized if it was first depolarized).

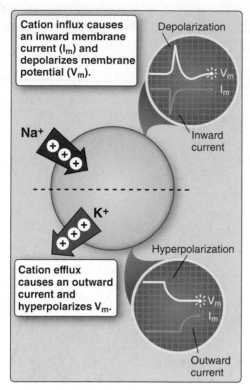

FIGURE 2-15. Membrane potential changes and ion currents. (Reprinted from Preston R. R., Wilson T. (2013). *Lippincott's illustrated reviews: Physiology* (Fig. 2.8, p. 20). Philadelphia, PA: Wolters Kluwer, with permission.)

Graded Potentials

In neurons, **dendrites** receive signals that change which ion channels are open. If sodium or calcium channels are opened, then the dendrites and cell body are depolarized, because this would result in positive charge traveling into the cell. This is called a graded potential because it is graded to the strength of the signal (stronger signals result in greater depolarization). If there is enough signal and depolarization, then an action potential is stimulated in the axon so that this signal can be passed to the next cell.

Action Potential

In neurons, if a graded potential is strong enough, then an action potential is generated in the axon of the neuron. The ion movement in graded potentials causes changes in voltage, and this stimulates voltage-gated sodium channels to open in the axon. Sodium ions rush into the cell, causing it to be less negative resulting in depolarization. This stimulates nearby voltage-gated potassium channels to open, and potassium ions cause a positive charge resulting in repolarization. This sequence continues until the signal reaches the axon terminal. Some neurons in the central nervous system (CNS) have gap junctions with target neurons, and ions diffuse into the target neuron to stimulate the neuron. At the axon terminal, the depolarization from the action potential causes calcium channels to open. Calcium diffuses in to stimulate a chain of reactions that stimulate exocytosis of neurotransmitter.

SUMMARY CONCEPTS

Movement of materials across the cell's membrane is needed for survival of the cell. Diffusion is a process by which substances such as ions move down a concentration gradient, from an area of greater concentration to an area of lower concentration. Osmosis is the diffusion of only water molecules through a membrane down the concentration gradient for water, from where water is more concentrated (where there are fewer solutes) to where water is less concentrated (where there are more solutes). Protein-assisted diffusion allows small, hydrophilic (water-loving) substances such as ions or glucose to cross the cell's membrane with the assistance of a transport protein that spans the membrane (a channel or a carrier protein). Another type of transport, called active transport, requires the cell to input energy to move substances against a concentration gradient, from an area of lower concentration to an area of higher concentration. Two types of active transport exist, primary and secondary, both of which require carrier proteins. The Na^+/K^+–ATPase pump is the best-known active transporter. Endocytosis is a process by which cells engulf materials from the surrounding medium. Small particles are ingested by a process called pinocytosis and larger particles by phagocytosis. Some particles require bonding with a ligand, and this process is called receptor-mediated endocytosis. Exocytosis involves the removal of large particles from the cell and is essentially the reverse of endocytosis.

Ion channels are integral transmembrane proteins that span the width of the cell membrane and are either open (leakage channels) or gated to open or close (ligand-, voltage-, and mechanically gated channels).

Electrochemical potentials exist across the membranes of many cells in the body because there are higher concentrations of specific ions on either side of the cell membrane. For example, in most cells, sodium, calcium, and chloride ions are higher outside the cell, and potassium ions are higher inside the cell. When most cells are at rest, there is more negative charge inside the cell than the outside, and the cell is said to be polarized. This is RMP, established by the difference in electrical charge and chemical gradients. When cells are stimulated, ion channels can open or close, changing the ability for specific ions to diffuse. Ion diffusion that causes the inside of the cell to become more positive causes depolarization. Ion diffusion that causes the inside of the cell to become more negative causes hyperpolarization or repolarization if the cell was first depolarized.

Body Tissues

Although all cells share certain characteristics, their structures and functions are specialized depending on where they are found in the body. For example, muscle, skin, and nervous cells are structurally distinct from one another and perform vastly different functions. Groups of cells that work together are called tissues. Four categories of tissue exist:

1. Epithelial tissue
2. Connective (supportive) tissue
3. Muscle tissue
4. Nervous tissue

These tissues do not exist in isolated units but combine with other tissues to form the organs of the body. This section provides a brief overview of the cells in each of these four tissue types, the structures that hold these cells together, and the extracellular matrix in which they live.

Cell Differentiation

After conception, the fertilized egg undergoes a series of cell divisions, leading to approximately 200 different cell types. The formation of different types of cells and the placement of these cells into tissue types is called **cell differentiation**, a process controlled by a system that switches genes on (to increase transcription) and off (to decrease transcription).

Embryonic cells must differentiate (become different) to develop into all of the various cell types and organ systems. Cells must then remain different after the signal that initiated cell **differentiation** is gone. The process of cell differentiation is controlled by cell memory, which is maintained by proteins in the individual cells of a particular cell type. This means that after differentiation has occurred, the tissue type does not change back to an earlier stage of differentiation.

Although most cells differentiate into specialized cell types, many tissues contain a few partially differentiated **stem cells.**[1] These stem cells, which are still capable of cell division, serve as a reserve source for specialized cells throughout the life of the organism and make regeneration possible in some tissues.

KEY POINTS

Organization of Cells into Tissues
- Cells are organized into larger functional units called *tissues*. Tissues associate with other tissues to form the various organs of the body.

Embryonic Origin of Tissue Types

All of the approximately 200 different types of body cells can be classified into four basic or primary tissue types: (1) epithelial, (2) connective, (3) muscle, and (4) nervous (Table 2-1). These basic tissue types

TABLE 2-1 Classification of Tissue Types

Tissue Type	Location
Epithelial Tissue	
Covering and lining of body surfaces	
Simple epithelium	
Squamous	Lining of blood vessels, body cavities, alveoli of the lungs
Cuboidal	Collecting tubules of the kidney; covering of the ovaries
Columnar	Lining of the intestine and gallbladder
Stratified epithelium	
Squamous keratinized	Skin
Squamous nonkeratinized	Mucous membranes of the mouth, esophagus, and vagina
Cuboidal	Ducts of the sweat glands
Columnar	Large ducts of the salivary and mammary glands; also found in the conjunctiva
Transitional	Bladder, ureters, renal pelvis
Pseudostratified	Tracheal and respiratory passages
Glandular	
Endocrine	Pituitary gland, thyroid gland, adrenal and other glands
Exocrine	Sweat glands and glands in the gastrointestinal tract
Neuroepithelium	Olfactory mucosa, retina, tongue
Reproductive epithelium	Seminiferous tubules of the testis; cortical portion of the ovary
Connective Tissue	
Embryonic connective tissue	
Mesenchymal	Embryonic mesoderm
Mucous	Umbilical cord (Wharton jelly)
Adult connective tissue	
Loose or areolar	Subcutaneous areas
Dense regular	Tendons and ligaments
Dense irregular	Dermis of the skin
Adipose	Fat pads, subcutaneous layers
Reticular	Framework of lymphoid organs, bone marrow, liver
Specialized connective tissue	
Bone	Long bones, flat bones
Cartilage	Tracheal rings, external ear, articular surfaces
Hematopoietic	Blood cells, myeloid tissue (bone marrow)
Muscle Tissue	
Skeletal	Skeletal muscles
Cardiac	Heart muscles
Smooth	Gastrointestinal tract, blood vessels, bronchi, bladder, and others
Nervous Tissue	
Neurons	Central and peripheral neurons and nerve fibers
Supporting cells	Glial and ependymal cells in the CNS; Schwann and satellite cells in the PNS

CNS, central nervous system; PNS, peripheral nervous system.

are often described by their embryonic origin. The embryo is essentially a three-layered tubular structure (Fig. 2-16):

1. The outer layer of the tube is called the **ectoderm**.
2. The middle layer of the tube is called the **mesoderm**.
3. The inner layer of the tube is called the **endoderm**.

All of the adult body tissues develop from these three cellular layers. Epithelial tissues develop from all three embryonic layers, connective tissue and muscle tissue develop mainly from the mesoderm, and nervous tissue develops from the ectoderm.

Epithelial Tissue

Epithelial tissue covers the body's outer surface and lines the internal closed cavities (including blood vessels) and body tubes that connect with the exterior of the body (gastrointestinal, respiratory, and genitourinary tracts). Epithelial tissue also forms the secretory portion of glands and their ducts.

Epithelial tissue develops from all three embryonic layers.[5]

Most epithelia of the skin, mouth, nose, and anus develop from the outer ectoderm.

1. The endothelial lining of blood vessels develops from the middle mesoderm.
2. Linings of the respiratory tract, gastrointestinal tract, and glands of the digestive system develop from the inner endoderm.
3. Many types of epithelial tissue retain the ability to differentiate and undergo rapid **proliferation** for replacing injured cells.

The cells that make up epithelial tissue have three general characteristics:

- They have three distinct surfaces: (1) a free surface or apical surface, (2) a **lateral** surface (on the sides of cells), and (3) a **basal** surface (at the base of the tissue).
- The basal surface of epithelial cells is attached to a basement membrane (below the epithelial cells, like a basement is below a house).
- Cells in epithelial tissues are close to neighboring cells and are joined to neighboring cells by cell-to-cell adhesion molecules (Fig. 2-17).[5]

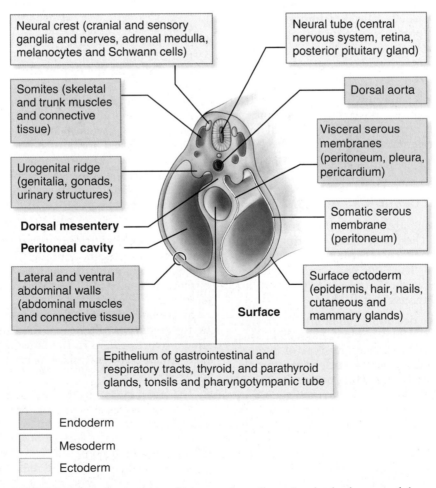

Neural crest (cranial and sensory ganglia and nerves, adrenal medulla, melanocytes and Schwann cells)

Neural tube (central nervous system, retina, posterior pituitary gland)

Somites (skeletal and trunk muscles and connective tissue)

Dorsal aorta

Urogenital ridge (genitalia, gonads, urinary structures)

Visceral serous membranes (peritoneum, pleura, pericardium)

Dorsal mesentery

Somatic serous membrane (peritoneum)

Peritoneal cavity

Lateral and ventral abdominal walls (abdominal muscles and connective tissue)

Surface

Surface ectoderm (epidermis, hair, nails, cutaneous and mammary glands)

Epithelium of gastrointestinal and respiratory tracts, thyroid, and parathyroid glands, tonsils and pharyngotympanic tube

Endoderm

Mesoderm

Ectoderm

FIGURE 2-16. Cross section of human embryo illustrating the development of the somatic and visceral structures.

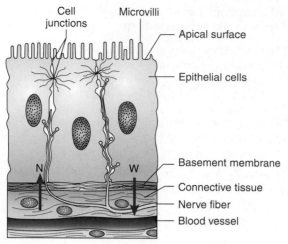

Cell junctions · Microvilli
Apical surface
Epithelial cells
Basement membrane
Connective tissue
Nerve fiber
Blood vessel
N · W

FIGURE 2-17. Typical arrangement of epithelial cells in relation to underlying tissues and blood supply. Epithelial tissue has no blood supply of its own but relies on the blood vessels in the underlying connective tissue for nutrition (N) and elimination of wastes (W).

Epithelial tissue is **avascular** (*a*, without; *vascular*, refers to blood vessels). Therefore, epithelial tissues receive oxygen and nutrients from the capillaries of the connective tissue on which the epithelial tissue rests (see Fig. 2-17).

To survive, epithelial tissue must be kept moist. Even the skin **epithelium**, which seems dry, is kept moist by a waterproof layer of skin cells called **keratinocytes**, which make **keratin**; keratin prevents evaporation of moisture from deeper skin cells.

Basement Membrane

Underneath all types of epithelial tissue is an extracellular matrix, called the **basement membrane**. A basement membrane consists of (1) the basal lamina and (2) an underlying reticular layer. The terms **basal lamina** and *basement membrane* are often used interchangeably.[6]

Cell Junctions and Cell-to-Cell Adhesions

Cells of epithelial tissue are tightly joined together by specialized junctions. These specialized junctions enable the cells to form barriers to prevent the movement of water, solutes, and cells from one body compartment to the next. Three basic types of intercellular junctions are observed in epithelial tissues (Fig. 2-18):

1. **Continuous tight** or **occluding junctions** (*i.e.*, zonula occludens), which are found only in epithelial tissue, bind neighboring cells together. This type of intercellular junction prevents materials such as macromolecules in the intestines from passing between cells and entering the bloodstream or body cavities.[5]
2. **Adhering junctions** are sites of strong adhesion between neighboring cells. The main role of adhering junctions is to prevent cells separating from each other. Adhering junctions are found in epithelial tissue and between cardiac muscle cells.

3. **Gap junctions** are sites of strong adhesion between neighboring cells with channels that link the cytoplasm of the two neighboring cells (like a tunnel between cells). Gap junctions are found in epithelial tissue and in many other types of cell-to-cell communication. For example, gap junctions allow ions to move between cells as part of electrical signals (*e.g.*, in **smooth muscle** or cardiac muscle).[5,7]

Types of Epithelial Tissues

Epithelial tissues are classified according to the:

1. Shape of the cells: squamous (thin and flat), cuboidal (cube shaped), and columnar (resembling a column)
2. Number of layers that are present: simple, stratified, and **pseudostratified** (Fig. 2-19)[6]

Simple Epithelium

Simple epithelium contains a single layer of cells, all of which rest on the basement membrane. Simple squamous epithelium is adapted for **filtration**. In filtration, some substances are able to pass, whereas others cannot.

- Simple epithelium lines the blood vessels, lymph nodes, and alveoli of the lungs.
- A single layer of squamous (thin and flat) epithelium lines the heart and blood vessels and is called the **endothelium**.
- A similar type of layer forms the **serous** membranes that line the pleural, pericardial, and peritoneal cavities and cover the organs of these cavities. This type of layer is called the **mesothelium**.
- **Simple cuboidal epithelium** is found on the surface of the ovary and in the thyroid.
- **Simple columnar epithelium** lines the intestine.
- One specialized form of a simple columnar epithelium has hair-like projections called cilia, often with mucus-secreting cells called **goblet cells**. This form of simple columnar epithelium lines the airways of the respiratory tract.[5]

Stratified and Pseudostratified Epithelia

Stratified epithelium contains more than one layer of cells, with only the deepest layer resting on the basement membrane. It is designed to protect body surfaces.

Stratified squamous keratinized epithelium makes up the epidermis of the skin. Keratin is a tough, fibrous (like a fiber) protein in the outer cells of skin. A stratified squamous keratinized epithelium is made up of many layers.

- The layers closest to the basement membrane and underlying tissues are cuboidal or columnar.
- Cells become more irregular and thinner as they move closer to the surface of the skin.
- Surface cells become filled with keratin and die, are sloughed off, and then are replaced by deeper cells.

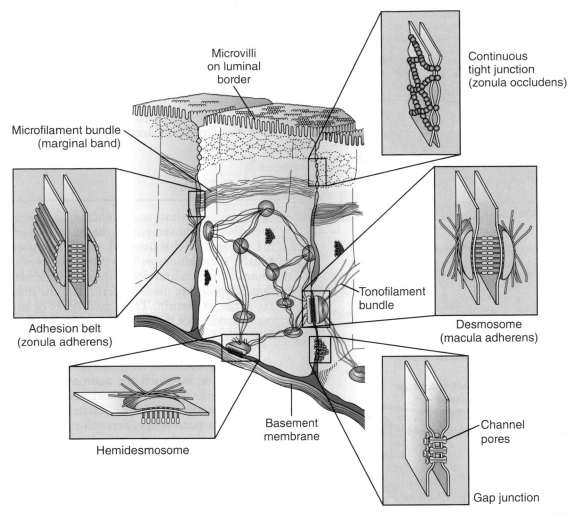

FIGURE 2-18. Three types of intercellular junctions found in epithelial tissue: the continuous tight junction (zonula occludens); the adhering junction, which includes the adhesion belt (zonula adherens), desmosomes (macula adherens), and hemidesmosomes; and the gap junction.

A stratified squamous nonkeratinized epithelium is found on moist surfaces such as the mouth and tongue. Stratified cuboidal and columnar epithelia are found in the ducts of salivary glands and the larger ducts of the mammary glands.[5] In smokers, the normal columnar ciliated epithelial cells of the trachea and bronchi are often replaced with stratified squamous epithelium cells that are better able to withstand the irritating effects of cigarette smoke.

Pseudostratified epithelium is a type of epithelium in which all of the cells are in contact with the underlying intercellular matrix, but some do not extend to the surface. A pseudostratified ciliated columnar epithelium with goblet cells forms the lining of most of the upper respiratory tract. **Transitional epithelium** is a stratified epithelium characterized by cells that can change shape and become thinner when the tissue is stretched. Such tissue can be stretched without pulling the superficial cells apart. Transitional epithelium is well adapted for the lining of organs that are constantly changing their volume, such as the urinary bladder.

Glandular Epithelium

Glandular epithelial tissue is formed by cells specialized to produce a fluid secretion.[5] This process usually occurs with the intracellular synthesis of macromolecules. The macromolecules are usually stored in the cells in small, membrane-bound vesicles called secretory granules. For example, glandular epithelial cells can make, store, and secrete proteins (*e.g.*, insulin), lipids (*e.g.*, adrenocortical hormones, secretions of the sebaceous glands), and complexes of carbohydrates and proteins (*e.g.*, saliva).

Exocrine glands use ducts to secrete substances outside of the body or into body cavities, such as the sweat glands and lactating mammary glands. **Endocrine glands** are ductless and secrete hormones directly into the bloodstream.

4. Injury from biologic agents
5. Injury from nutritional imbalances

Injury from Physical Agents

Physical agents responsible for cell and tissue injury include mechanical forces, extremes of temperature, and electrical forces. They are common causes of injuries because of environmental exposure, occupational and transportation accidents, and physical violence and assault.

Mechanical Forces

Injury or trauma because of mechanical forces occurs as a result of body impact with another object. The body or the mass can be in motion or, as sometimes happens, both can be in motion at the time of impact. These types of injuries split and tear tissue, fracture bones, injure blood vessels, and disrupt blood flow.

Extremes of Temperature

Extremes of heat and cold cause damage to the cell, its organelles, and its enzyme systems. Exposure to low-intensity heat (43°C to 46°C), such as occurs with partial-thickness burns and severe heat stroke, causes cell injury by causing vascular injury, accelerating cell metabolism, inactivating temperature-sensitive enzymes, and disrupting the cell membrane. With more intense heat, **coagulation** of blood vessels and tissue proteins occurs. Exposure to cold increases blood **viscosity** and induces vasoconstriction by direct action on blood vessels and through reflex activity of the sympathetic nervous system. The resultant decrease in blood flow may lead to hypoxic tissue injury, depending on the degree and duration of cold exposure. Injury from freezing probably results from a combination of ice crystal formation and vasoconstriction. The decreased blood flow leads to capillary stasis and arteriolar and capillary thrombosis. **Edema** results from increased capillary permeability.

Electrical Injuries

Electrical injuries can affect the body through extensive tissue injury and disruption of neural and cardiac impulses. Voltage, type of current, amperage, pathway of the current, resistance of the tissue, and interval of exposure determine the effect of electricity on the body.[12]

Alternating current is usually more dangerous than direct current because it causes violent muscle contractions, preventing the person from releasing the electrical source and sometimes resulting in fractures and dislocations. In electrical injuries, the body acts as a conductor of the electrical current.[12] The current enters the body from an electrical source, such as an exposed wire, and passes through the body and exits to another conductor, such as the moisture on the ground or a piece of metal the person is holding. The pathway that a current takes is critical because the electrical energy disrupts impulses in excitable tissues. Current flow through the brain may interrupt impulses from respiratory centers in the brainstem, and current flow through the chest may cause fatal cardiac arrhythmias.

The resistance to the flow of current in electrical circuits transforms electrical energy into heat. This is why

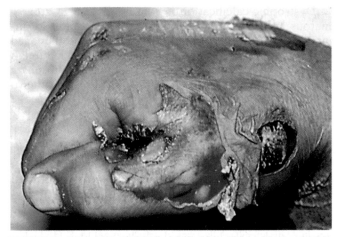

FIGURE 3-5. Electrical burn of the skin. The person was electrocuted after attempting to stop a fall from a ladder by grasping a high-voltage electrical line. (From Strayer D. S., Rubin E. (2015). *Cell injury*. In Rubin R., Strayer D. S. (Eds.), *Rubin's pathology: Clinicopathologic foundations of medicine* (7th ed., Fig. 8-21, p. 352). Philadelphia, PA: Lippincott Williams & Wilkins.)

the elements in electrical heating devices are made of highly resistive metals. Much of the tissue damage produced by electrical injuries is caused by heat production in tissues that have the highest electrical resistance. Resistance to electrical current varies from the greatest to the least in bone, fat, tendons, skin, muscles, blood, and nerves. The most severe tissue injury usually occurs at the skin sites where the current enters and leaves the body (Fig. 3-5). After electricity has penetrated the skin, it passes rapidly through the body along the lines of least resistance—through body fluids and nerves. Degeneration of vessel walls may occur, and thrombi may form as current flows along the blood vessels. This can cause extensive muscle and deep tissue injury. Thick, dry skin is more resistant to the flow of electricity than thin, wet skin. It is generally believed that the greater the skin resistance, the greater is the amount of local skin burn, and the less the resistance, the greater are the deep and systemic effects.

Radiation Injury

Electromagnetic radiation comprises a wide spectrum of wave-propagated energy, ranging from ionizing gamma rays to radiofrequency waves (Fig. 3-6). A photon is a particle of radiation energy. Radiation energy above the ultraviolet (UV) range is called *ionizing radiation* because the photons have enough energy to knock electrons off atoms and molecules. *Nonionizing radiation* refers to radiation energy at frequencies below those of visible light. *UV radiation* represents the portion of the spectrum of electromagnetic radiation just above the visible range.[12] It contains increasingly energetic rays that are powerful enough to disrupt intracellular bonds and cause sunburn.

Ionizing Radiation

Ionizing radiation impacts cells by causing ionization of molecules and atoms in the cell. This is accomplished

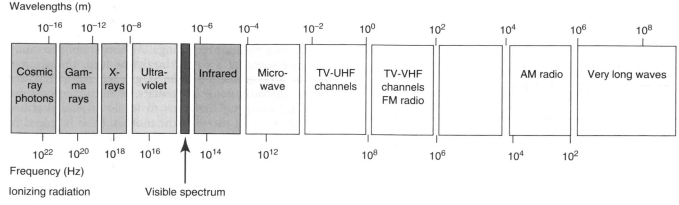

FIGURE 3-6. Spectrum of electromagnetic radiation.

by releasing free radicals that destroy cells and by directly hitting the target molecules in the cell.[13] It can immediately kill cells, interrupt cell replication, or cause a variety of genetic mutations, which may or may not be lethal. Most radiation injury is caused by localized irradiation that is used in the treatment of cancer. Except for unusual circumstances such as the use of high-dose irradiation that precedes bone marrow transplantation, exposure to whole-body irradiation is rare.

The injurious effects of ionizing radiation vary with the dose, dose rate (a single dose can cause greater injury than divided or fractionated doses), and the differential sensitivity of the exposed tissue to radiation injury. Because of the effect on deoxyribonucleic acid (DNA) synthesis and interference with mitosis, rapidly dividing cells of the bone marrow and intestine are much more vulnerable to radiation injury than tissues such as bone and skeletal muscle. Over time, occupational and accidental exposure to ionizing radiation can result in increased risk for the development of various types of cancers, including skin cancers, leukemia, osteogenic sarcomas, and lung cancer. This is especially true when the person is exposed to radiation during childhood.[13]

Many of the clinical manifestations of radiation injury result from acute cell injury, dose-dependent changes in the blood vessels that supply the irradiated tissues, and fibrotic tissue replacement. The cell's initial response to radiation injury involves swelling, disruption of the mitochondria and other organelles, alterations in the cell membrane, and marked changes in the nucleus. The endothelial cells in blood vessels are particularly sensitive to irradiation. During the immediate postirradiation period, only vessel dilation is apparent (*e.g.*, the initial **erythema** of the skin after radiation therapy). Later or with higher levels of radiation, destructive changes occur in small blood vessels such as the capillaries and venules. Acute reversible **necrosis** is represented by such disorders as radiation cystitis, dermatitis, and diarrhea from enteritis. More persistent damage can be attributed to acute necrosis of tissue cells that are not capable of regeneration and chronic ischemia. Chronic effects of radiation damage are characterized by **fibrosis** and scarring of tissues and organs in the irradiated area (*e.g.*, interstitial fibrosis of the heart and lungs after irradiation of the chest). Because the radiation delivered

in radiation therapy inevitably travels through the skin, radiation dermatitis is common. There may be necrosis of the skin, impaired wound healing, and chronic radiation dermatitis.

Ultraviolet Radiation

UV radiation causes sunburn and increases the risk of skin cancers. The degree of risk depends on the type of UV rays, the intensity of exposure, and the amount of protective melanin pigment in the skin. Skin damage produced by UV radiation is thought to be caused by reactive oxygen species (ROS) and by damage to melanin-producing processes in the skin.[14] UV radiation also damages DNA, resulting in the formation of pyrimidine dimers (*i.e.*, the insertion of two identical pyrimidine bases into replicating DNA instead of one). Other forms of DNA damage include the production of single-stranded breaks and formation of DNA–protein cross-links. Normally, errors that occur during DNA replication are repaired by enzymes that remove the faulty section of DNA and repair the damage. The importance of DNA repair in protecting against UV radiation injury is evidenced by the vulnerability of people who lack the enzymes needed to repair UV-induced DNA damage. In a genetic disorder called *xeroderma pigmentosum*, an enzyme needed to repair sunlight-induced DNA damage is lacking. This autosomal recessive disorder is characterized by extreme photosensitivity and an increased risk of skin cancer in sun-exposed skin.[14]

Nonionizing Radiation

Nonionizing radiation includes infrared light, ultrasound, microwaves, and laser energy. Unlike ionizing radiation, which can directly break chemical bonds, nonionizing radiation exerts its effects by causing vibration and rotation of atoms and molecules.[12] All of this vibrational and rotational energy is eventually converted to thermal energy. Low-frequency nonionizing radiation is used widely in radar, television, industrial operations (*e.g.*, heating, welding, melting of metals, processing of wood and plastic), household appliances (*e.g.*, microwave ovens), and medical applications (*e.g.*, diathermy). Isolated cases of skin burns and thermal injury to deeper tissues have occurred in industrial settings and from improperly used household microwave ovens. Injury from

Translation

After the mRNA is processed (adding nucleic acids to the ends and splicing out the exons), it is a mature molecule and is passed into the cytoplasm of the cell, where translation occurs. Translation is the synthesis of a protein using the mRNA template. All proteins are made from amino acids, which are joined end to end to form the long polypeptide chains of protein molecules. Each polypeptide chain may have more than 300 amino acids in it. Translation requires the coordinated actions of mRNA, rRNA, and tRNA to make such a complex molecule (Fig. 4-5). The mRNA provides the information needed for placing the amino acids in their proper order for each specific type of protein. During protein synthesis, mRNA contacts and passes through the ribosome (binding to rRNA), during which it "reads" the directions for protein synthesis. As mRNA passes through the ribosome, tRNA delivers the appropriate amino acids for attachment to the growing polypeptide chain. Each of the 20 different tRNA molecules transports its specific amino acid to the ribosome for incorporation into the developing protein molecule.

Next, this new polypeptide chain must fold up into its unique three-dimensional conformation. The folding of many proteins is made more efficient by special classes of proteins called *molecular chaperones*.[5] These proteins also assist in the transport to the site in the cell where the protein will carry out its function and help to prevent misfolding of existing proteins. Disruption of these chaperoning mechanisms causes intracellular molecules to become denatured and insoluble. These denatured proteins tend to stick to one another, precipitate, and form **inclusion** bodies, which is a pathologic process that occurs in Parkinson, Alzheimer, and Huntington diseases.

During folding, other modifications can occur. A newly synthesized polypeptide chain may also need to combine with one or more polypeptide chains from the same or an adjacent chromosome, bind small **cofactors** for its activity, or undergo appropriate enzyme modification. Other modifications may involve cleavage of the protein, which can happen to remove a specific amino acid sequence or to split the molecule into smaller chains.

Regulation of Gene Expression

Only about 2% of the genome encodes instructions for the synthesis of proteins; the remainder consists of noncoding regions that are structural or serve to determine where, when, and in what quantity proteins are made. The degree to which a gene or particular group of genes are actively being transcribed is called *gene expression*. A phenomenon termed *induction* is an important process by which gene expression is increased.

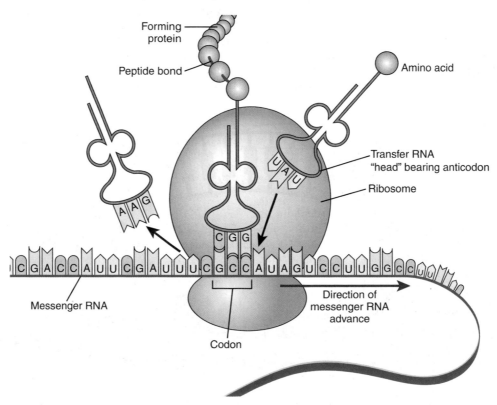

FIGURE 4-5. Protein synthesis. A messenger RNA (mRNA) strand is shown moving along a small ribosomal subunit in the cytoplasm. As the mRNA codon passes along the ribosome, a new amino acid is added to the growing peptide chain by the transfer RNA (tRNA). As each amino acid is bound to the next by a peptide bond, its tRNA is released.

Gene repression is a process by which a regulatory gene acts to reduce or prevent gene expression. Activator and repressor sites commonly monitor levels of the synthesized product and regulate gene transcription through a negative feedback mechanism. Whenever product levels decrease, gene transcription is induced, and when levels increase, it is repressed.

Although control of gene expression occurs in many ways, many of the regulatory events occur at the transcription level. The initiation and regulation of transcription require the collaboration of a battery of proteins, collectively termed *transcription factors*.[6] Transcription factors are a class of proteins that bind to their own specific DNA region and function to increase or decrease transcriptional activity of the genes. Transcription factors are one component that allows neurons and liver cells to use the same DNA yet still have completely different structures and functions. Some of these, referred to as *general transcription factors*, are required for transcription of all genes. Others, termed *specific transcription factors*, have more specialized roles, activating genes only at specific stages of development. For example, the PAX family of transcription factors is involved in the development of such embryonic tissues as the eye and portions of the nervous system.[7]

SUMMARY CONCEPTS

Genes determine the types of proteins and enzymes made by the cell and therefore control both inheritance and day-to-day cell function. Genetic information is stored in a stable macromolecule called DNA. The genetic code is determined by the arrangement of the nitrogenous bases of the four nucleotides (i.e., adenine, guanine, thymine [or uracil in RNA], and cytosine). Gene mutations represent accidental errors in duplication, rearrangement, or deletion of parts of the genetic code. Fortunately, most mutations are corrected by DNA repair mechanisms in the cell. The vast majority of DNA is identical across human populations, with only 0.01% creating the individual differences in physical traits and behavior.

A second type of nucleic acid called RNA is used to create a protein from the DNA code. There are three major types of RNA: messenger RNA (mRNA), ribosomal RNA (rRNA), and transfer RNA (tRNA). Transcription of mRNA is initiated by RNA polymerase and other associated factors that bind to the DNA at a specific site called the promoter region. Once transcribed, mRNA undergoes processing before moving to the cytoplasm of the cell. Translation occurs in the cytoplasm when the mRNA binds to the ribosome (rRNA) to create a polypeptide. tRNA acts as a carrier system for delivering the appropriate amino acids to the ribosomes.

The degree to which a gene or a particular group of genes is active is called gene expression. Gene expression involves a set of complex interrelationships, including RNA transcription and posttranslational processing. The initiation and regulation of RNA transcription are controlled by transcription factors that bind to specific DNA regions and function to regulate gene expression of the many different types of cells in the body. Posttranslational processing involves the proper folding of the newly synthesized polypeptide chain into its unique three-dimensional conformation. Special classes of proteins called molecular chaperones make the folding of many proteins more efficient. Posttranslational processing may also involve the combination of polypeptide chains from the same or an adjacent chromosome, the binding of small cofactors, or enzyme modification.

Chromosomes

Most of the genetic information in a cell is organized, stored, and retrieved in structures called *chromosomes*. Although the chromosomes are visible only in dividing cells, they retain their integrity between cell divisions. The chromosomes are arranged in pairs where one member of the pair is inherited from the father and the other member is inherited from the mother. Each species has a characteristic number of chromosomes. In the human, 46 chromosomes are present, and these are arranged into 23 pairs. Of the 23 pairs of human chromosomes, 22 are called *autosomes*, and each has been given a numeric designation for classification purposes (Fig. 4-6). The pairs of autosomal chromosomes each contain similar genes and have similar sequences and are therefore called *homologous chromosomes*. They are not identical, however, because one comes from the father and one comes from the mother.

The sex chromosomes, which make up the 23rd pair of chromosomes, determine the sex of a person. Human males have an X and Y chromosome (*i.e.*, an X chromosome from the mother and a Y chromosome from the father); human females have two X chromosomes (*i.e.*, one from each parent). The much smaller Y chromosome contains the *male-specific region* that determines male sex.[8] But only one X chromosome in the female is active in controlling the expression of genetic traits. Whether the active X chromosome is derived from the mother or father is determined within a few days after conception. The selection of either X is random for each possible cell line. Thus, the tissues of normal women have on average 50% maternally derived and 50% paternally derived active X chromosomes. This is known as the *Lyon principle*.[9]

UNDERSTANDING → DNA-Directed Protein Synthesis

Deoxyribonucleic acid (DNA) contains the information to direct the synthesis of the many thousands of proteins that are contained in the different cells of the body. A second type of nucleic acid—ribonucleic acid (RNA)—participates in the actual assembly of the proteins.

There are three types of RNA: messenger RNA (mRNA), ribosomal RNA (rRNA), and transfer RNA (tRNA) that participate in **(1)** the transcription of the DNA instructions for protein synthesis and **(2)** the translation of those instructions into the assembly of the polypeptides that make up the various proteins.

The genetic code is a triplet of four bases (adenine [A], thymine [T], guanine [G], and cytosine [C], with thymine in DNA being replaced with uracil [U] in RNA) that control the sequence of amino acids in a protein molecule that is being synthesized. The triplet RNA code is called a codon.

1

Transcription Transcription occurs when the DNA is copied into a complementary strand of mRNA. Transcription is initiated by an enzyme called *RNA polymerase*, which binds to a promoter site on DNA. Many other proteins, including transcription factors, function to increase or decrease transcriptional activity of the genes. After mRNA has been transcribed, it detaches from DNA and is processed by adding nucleotide sequences to the beginning and end of the molecule, and introns are spliced out. Changes to the splicing allow the production of a variety of mRNA molecules from a single gene. Once mRNA has been processed, it diffuses through the nuclear pores into the cytoplasm, where it is translated into protein.

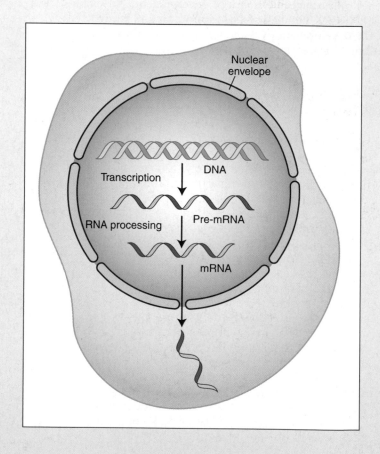

2 **Translation** Translation begins when the mRNA carrying the instructions for a particular protein comes in contact with a ribosome and binds to a small subunit of the rRNA. It then travels through the ribosome while the tRNA delivers and transfers the correct amino acid to its proper position on the growing peptide chain. There are 20 types of tRNA, one for each of the 20 different types of amino acid. In order to be functional, the newly synthesized protein must be folded into its functional form, modified further, and then routed to its final position in the cell.

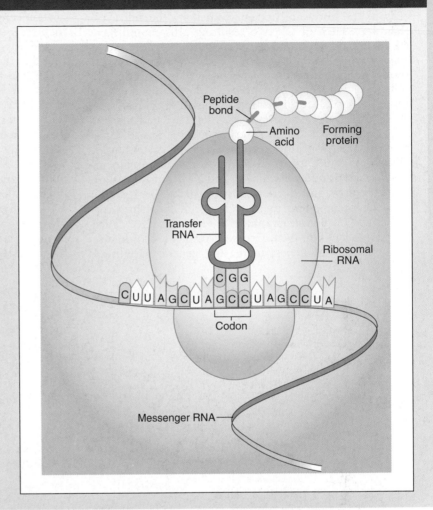

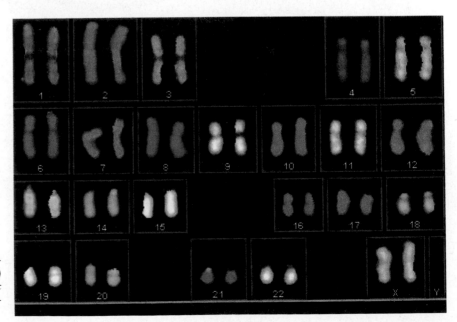

FIGURE 4-6. Karyotype of human chromosomes. (From Rubin R., Strayer D. (Eds.) (2012). *Rubin's pathology: Clinicopathologic foundations of medicine* (6th ed., p. 221). Philadelphia, PA: Lippincott Williams & Wilkins.)

Cell Division

Two types of cell division occur in humans and many other animals: mitosis and meiosis. Mitosis involves the replication of DNA to duplicate somatic cells in the body and is represented by the cell cycle (Fig. 4-7). Each of the two resulting cells should have an identical set of 23 pairs of chromosomes. Meiosis is limited to replicating germ cells (Fig. 4-8). It results in the formation of gametes or reproductive cells (*i.e.*, ovum and sperm), each of which has only a single set of 23 chromosomes. Meiosis is typically divided into two distinct phases, meiosis I and meiosis II. As in mitosis, the first step of meiosis I is to replicate the DNA during interphase. During metaphase I, all homologous autosomal chromosomes pair up, forming a tetrad of *bivalents*. The X and Y chromosomes are not **homologs** and do not form bivalents. Because the bivalents are lined up, an interchange of chromatid segments can occur in metaphase I. This process is called *crossing-over* (Fig. 4-9). Crossing-over allows for new combinations of genes, increasing genetic variability.

After telophase I, each of the two daughter cells contains one member of each homologous pair of chromosomes and a sex chromosome (23 double-stranded chromosomes). During anaphase of **meiosis II**, the 23 double-stranded chromosomes (two **chromatids**) divide at their centromeres. Each subsequent daughter cell will then receive 23 single-stranded chromatids.

Meiosis, occurring only in the gamete-producing cells found in the testes or ovaries, has a different outcome in males and females. In males, meiosis (spermatogenesis) results in four viable daughter cells called *spermatids* that differentiate into sperm cells. In females, gamete formation or **oogenesis** is quite different. After the first meiotic division of a primary **oocyte**, a secondary oocyte and another structure called a *polar body* are formed. This small polar body contains little cytoplasm, but it may undergo a second meiotic division, resulting in two polar bodies. The secondary oocyte undergoes its second meiotic division, producing one mature oocyte and another polar body. Four viable sperm cells are produced during spermatogenesis, but only one ovum is produced by oogenesis.

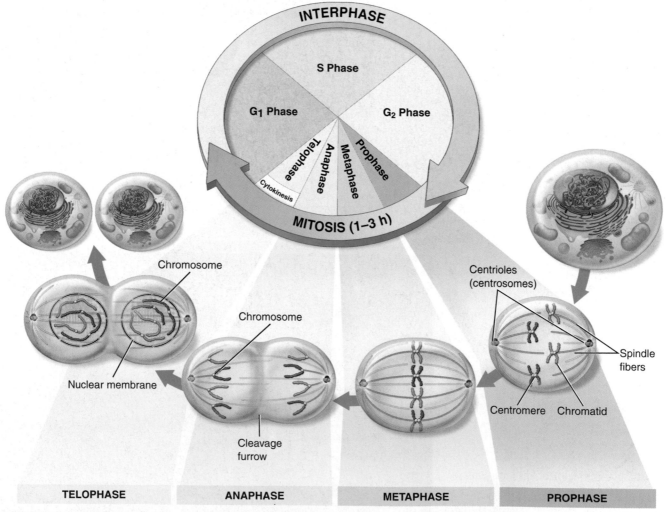

FIGURE 4-7. Mitosis. Mitosis consists of division of the nucleus and is made up of four steps: telophase, anaphase, metaphase, and prophase. (From McConnell T. H., Hull K. L. (2011). *Human form human function: Essentials of anatomy & physiology* (p. 79, Fig. 3.12). Philadelphia, PA: Lippincott Williams & Wilkins.)

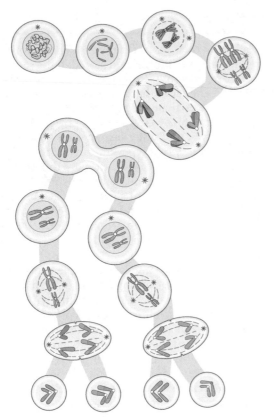

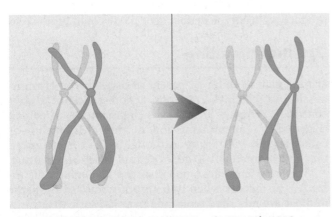

FIGURE 4-8. Meiosis. Meiosis is the cell division that produces gametes or reproductive cells. (From *Stedman's Medical Dictionary* (2015). Philadelphia, PA: Lippincott Williams & Wilkins.)

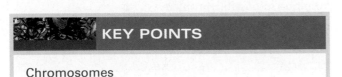

FIGURE 4-9. Crossing-over of DNA at the time of meiosis.

KEY POINTS

Chromosomes

- DNA is organized into 23 pairs of chromosomes. There are 22 pairs of autosomes, which are alike for males and females, and one pair of sex chromosomes, with XX pairing in females and XY pairing in males.

- Cell division requires the duplication of chromosomes. Duplication of chromosomes in a somatic cell line is completed by the process of mitosis, in which each daughter cell receives 23 pairs of chromosomes. Meiosis is limited to replicating germ cells and results in daughter cells that each have a single set of 23 chromosomes.

Chromosome Structure

Cytogenetics is the study of the structure and numeric characteristics of the cell's chromosomes. Chromosome studies can be done on any tissue or cell that grows and divides in culture, but white blood cells or buccal (cheek) samples are frequently used for this purpose. After the cells have been cultured, a drug called *colchicine* is used to arrest mitosis in metaphase so that the chromosomes can be easily seen. A chromosome spread is prepared by fixing and spreading the chromosomes on a slide, and they are stained to show banding patterns specific to each chromosome. The chromosomes are photographed, and the photomicrographs of each of the chromosomes are cut out and arranged in pairs according to a standard classification system (see Fig. 4-7). The completed picture is called a **karyotype**, and the procedure for preparing the picture is called *karyotyping*.

In the metaphase spread, each chromosome takes the form of an "X" or "wishbone" pattern. The two chromatids are connected by a *centromere*. Human chromosomes are divided into three types according to the position of the centromere. If the centromere is in the center and the arms are of approximately the same length, the chromosome is said to be *metacentric*; if it is not centered and the arms are of clearly different lengths, it is *submetacentric*; and if it is near one end, it is *acrocentric*. The short arm of the chromosome is designated as "p" for "petite," and the long arm is designated as "q" for no other reason than it is the next letter of the alphabet.[10] The arms of the chromosome are indicated by the chromosome number followed by the p or q designation (*e.g.*, 15p). Chromosomes 13, 14, 15, 21, and 22 have small masses of chromatin called *satellites* attached to their short arms by narrow stalks. At the ends of each chromosome are special DNA sequences called *telomeres*. Telomeres allow the end of the DNA molecule to be replicated completely.

The banding patterns of a chromosome are used in describing the position of a gene on a chromosome. Each arm of a chromosome is divided into regions, which are numbered from the centromere outward (*e.g.*, 1, 2). The regions are further divided into bands, which are also numbered (Fig. 4-10). These numbers are used in designating the position of a gene on a chromosome. For example, Xp22 refers to band 2, region 2 of the short arm (p) of the X chromosome.

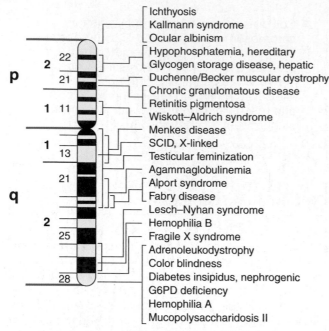

FIGURE 4-10. Localization of representative inherited diseases on the X chromosome. G6PD, glucose-6-phosphate dehydrogenase; SCID, severe combined immunodeficiency (syndrome). (From Rubin R., Strayer D. (Eds.) (2015). *Rubin's pathology: Clinicopathologic foundations of medicine* (7th ed., Fig. 6.32, p. 282). Philadelphia, PA: Lippincott Williams & Wilkins.)

SUMMARY CONCEPTS

The genetic information in a cell is organized in structures called chromosomes. In humans, the 46 chromosomes are arranged into 23 pairs. Twenty-two of these pairs are autosomes. Sex chromosomes make up the 23rd pair. Two types of cell division occur, meiosis and mitosis. Mitotic division occurs in somatic cells and results in two daughter cells, each with 23 pairs of chromosomes. Meiosis is limited to replicating germ cells and results in the formation of gametes or reproductive cells (ovum and sperm), each of which has only a single set of 23 chromosomes. A karyotype is a photographic arrangement of a person's chromosomes. It is prepared by special laboratory techniques in which cells are cultured, fixed, and stained to display identifiable banding patterns.

Patterns of Inheritance

The characteristics inherited from a person's parents are carried within genes found along the length of the chromosomes. Alternate forms of the same gene are possible, and each may produce a different aspect of a trait.

Definitions

Genetics has its own set of definitions. The **genotype** of a person is the genetic information stored in the sequence of base pairs. The **phenotype** refers to the recognizable traits, physical or biochemical, that are associated with a specific genotype. But more than one genotype may have the same phenotype. Some brown-eyed people are carriers of the code for blue eyes, and other brown-eyed people are not. Phenotypically, these two types of brown-eyed people appear the same, but genotypically they are different.

The position of a gene on a chromosome is called its *locus*, and alternate forms of a gene at the same locus are called alleles. When only one pair of genes is involved in the transmission of information, the term *single-gene trait* is used. Single-gene traits follow the mendelian laws of inheritance.

Polygenic inheritance involves multiple genes at different loci, with each gene exerting a small effect in determining a trait. Multiple pairs of genes, many with alternate codes, determine most human traits. Polygenic traits are predictable, but with less reliability than single-gene traits. *Multifactorial* inheritance is similar to polygenic inheritance in that multiple alleles at different loci affect the outcome; the difference is that multifactorial inheritance also includes environmental effects on the genes.

Many other gene–gene interactions are known. These include *epistasis*, in which one gene masks the phenotypic effects of another gene; *multiple alleles*, in which more than one allele affects the same trait (*e.g.*, ABO blood types); *complementary genes*, in which each gene is mutually dependent on the other; and *collaborative genes*, in which two different genes influencing the same trait interact to produce a phenotype neither gene alone could produce.

Genetic Imprinting

Certain genes exhibit a "parent of origin" type of transmission in which the parental genomes do not always contribute equally in the development of a person (Fig. 4-11). The transmission of this phenomenon is called *genetic imprinting*. Although rare, it is estimated that approximately 100 genes exhibit genetic imprinting.

A related chromosomal disorder is *uniparental disomy*. This occurs when two chromosomes of the same number are inherited from one parent. Normally, this is not a problem except in cases where a chromosome has been imprinted by a parent. In this case, the offspring will have only one working copy of the chromosome, resulting in possible problems.

KEY POINTS

Transmission of Genetic Information

■ The transmission of information from one generation to the next is vested in genetic material transferred from each parent at the time of conception.

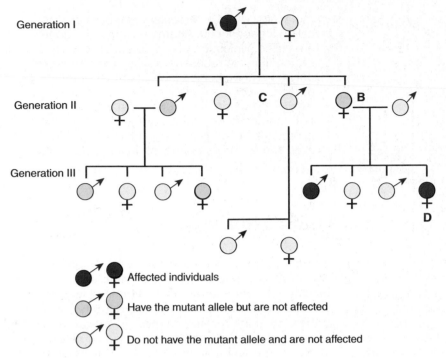

FIGURE 4-11. A three-generation pedigree of genetic imprinting. In generation I, male *A* has inherited a mutant allele from his affected mother (not shown); the gene is "turned off" during spermatogenesis, and therefore, none of his offspring (generation II) will express the mutant allele, regardless of whether they are carriers. However, the gene will be "turned on" again during oogenesis in any of his daughters (*B*) who inherit the allele. All offspring (generation III) who inherit the mutant allele will be affected. All offspring of normal children (*C*) will produce normal offspring. Children of female *D* will all express the mutation if they inherit the allele.

■ Mendelian, or single-gene, patterns of inheritance are transmitted from parents to their offspring in a predictable manner. Polygenic inheritance, which involves multiple genes, and multifactorial inheritance, which involves multiple genes as well as environmental factors, are less predictable.

Mendel Laws

A main feature of inheritance is predictability: given certain conditions, the likelihood of the occurrence or recurrence of a specific trait in the offspring is remarkably predictable. The units of inheritance are the genes, and the pattern of single-gene transmission can often be predicted using Mendel laws of genetic transmission. Since Gregor Mendel's original work was published in 1865, new discoveries have led to some modification of the original laws, but many of the basic principles still hold true.

Mendel discovered the basic pattern of inheritance by conducting carefully planned experiments with simple garden peas. Experimenting with several phenotypic traits in peas, Mendel proposed that inherited traits are transmitted from parents to offspring by means of independently inherited factors—now known as genes—and that these factors are transmitted as recessive and dominant traits. Mendel labeled dominant factors (his round peas) "A" and recessive factors (his wrinkled peas) "a." Geneticists continue to use capital letters to designate dominant traits and lowercase letters to identify recessive traits. The possible combinations that can occur with transmission of single-gene dominant and recessive traits can be described by constructing a figure called a *Punnett square* using capital and lowercase letters (Fig. 4-12).

The observable traits of single-gene inheritance are inherited by the offspring from the parents. The germ cells (*i.e.*, sperm and ovum) of both parents undergo meiosis, in which the number of chromosomes is divided into half (from 46 to 23) and each germ cell receives only one allele from each pair (*i.e.*, Mendel first law). According to Mendel second law, the alleles from the different gene loci segregate independently and recombine randomly in the offspring. People in whom the two alleles of a given pair are the same (AA or aa) are called *homozygotes*. *Heterozygotes* have different alleles (Aa) at a gene locus. A *recessive trait* is one expressed only in a **homozygous** (aa) pairing; a *dominant trait* is one expressed in either a homozygous (AA) or a **heterozygous** (Aa) pairing. If the trait follows simple mendelian inheritance, then all people with a dominant allele in either one or two copies will show the phenotype for that trait. For example, the genes for blond hair are recessive and those for brown hair are dominant. Therefore, only people with a genotype having two alleles for blond hair would be blond; people with either one or two brown alleles would have brown hair.

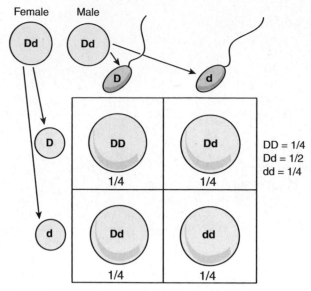

Female   Male

DD = 1/4
Dd = 1/2
dd = 1/4

FIGURE 4-12. The Punnett square showing all possible combinations for transmission of a single-gene trait (dimpled cheeks). The example shown is when both parents are heterozygous (Dd) for the trait. The alleles carried by the mother are on the left, and those carried by the father are on the top. The D allele is dominant, and the d allele is recessive. The DD and Dd offspring have dimples, and the dd offspring does not.

Sometimes, the person who is heterozygous for a recessive trait (Aa) is called a *carrier*. That individual will not exhibit the phenotype for the recessive trait, but they "carry" the allele for the recessive trait. If they have offspring with someone who exhibits and is homozygous for the recessive trait, or with someone who is also a carrier, then that offspring could also exhibit the recessive trait. Such a situation might occur when two people who have a phenotype of brown eyes have a child with blue eyes. Brown (B) eyes are dominant to blue eyes (b), so both parents had to be genotypically heterozygous (Bb).

Pedigree

A pedigree is a graphic method (see Figs. 4-11 and 4-12) for portraying a family history for an inherited trait. It is constructed from a carefully obtained family history and is useful for tracing the pattern of inheritance for a particular trait.

SUMMARY CONCEPTS

Inheritance patterns can calculate the likelihood of the occurrence or recurrence of a specific genetic trait. The genotype refers to information stored in the genetic code of a person, whereas the phenotype represents the recognizable traits, physical and biochemical, associated with the genotype. The specific region of the DNA

molecule where a particular gene is located is called a gene locus. Alternate forms of a gene are called alleles. Traits can be either recessive or dominant. A recessive trait is one expressed only when two copies (homozygous) of the recessive allele are present. Dominant traits are expressed when either one (heterozygous) or two (homozygous) copies of the dominant allele is present. A pedigree is a graphic method for portraying a family history of an inherited trait.

Gene Technology

The past several decades have seen phenomenal advances in the field of genetics. These advances have included the completion of the Human Genome Project, the establishment of the International HapMap Project to map the haplotypes of variations in the human genome, and the development of methods for applying the technology of these projects to the diagnosis and treatment of disease. Many health care professions also have established clinical competencies for their specific professions regarding genetics, because the application of genetic technology is becoming more evident in all areas of disease screening and management. Multiple new genetic diagnostics in use are able to assess people for various genetic alterations. Information obtained from these technologies greatly assists in planning the care and pharmacologic management of many types of diseases. Health care professionals need to be able to answer questions and explain to people and families the results of testing and how this knowledge may or may not influence the course of one's health.

Genetic Mapping

Genetic mapping is the assignment of genes to a specific locus or to specific parts of the chromosome. Another type of mapping strategy, the *haplotype* map, focuses on identifying the slight variations in the human genome that affect a person's susceptibility to disease and responses to environmental factors such as microbes, toxins, and drugs.

The Human Genome Project

The Human Genome Project, initiated in 1990 and completed in 2003, sought to identify all the genes in the human genome. The international project was charged with both determining the precise locations of genes and also exploring technologies that would enable the sequencing of large amounts of DNA with high accuracy and low cost. Some of what was discovered was quite unexpected, including the revelation that humans have a mere 30,000 genes, rather than the 100,000 that were initially predicted from the number of different proteins in our body. Another surprising finding was mentioned earlier in this chapter. On average, any two unrelated people will still share 99.9% of their DNA sequence, indicating that the remarkable diversity among people is carried in about 0.1% of our DNA.

Genetic Mapping Methods

Many methods have been used for developing genetic maps. The most important ones are family linkage studies, gene dosage methods, and hybridization studies. Often, the specific assignment of a gene locus is made using information from several mapping techniques.

Linkage Studies

Linkage studies assume that genes occur in a linear array along the chromosomes. During meiosis, the paired chromosomes of the germ cells sometimes exchange genetic material because of crossing-over (see Fig. 4-8). This exchange usually involves more than one gene; large blocks of genes (representing large portions of the chromosome) are usually exchanged. Although the point at which one block separates from another occurs randomly, the closer together two genes are on the same chromosome, the greater the chance is that they will be passed on together to the offspring. When two inherited traits occur together at a rate greater than would occur by chance alone, they are said to be *linked*. Linkage analysis can be used clinically to identify affected people in a family with a known genetic defect.

Hybridization Studies

A recent biologic discovery revealed that two somatic cells from different species, when grown together in the same culture, occasionally fuse to form a new hybrid cell. Two types of hybridization methods are used in genomic studies: somatic cell hybridization and in situ hybridization.

Somatic cell hybridization involves the fusion of human somatic cells with those of a different species (typically, the mouse) to yield a cell containing the chromosomes of both species. Because these hybrid cells are unstable, they begin to lose chromosomes of both species during subsequent cell divisions. This makes it possible to obtain cells with different partial combinations of human chromosomes. The proteins of these cells are then studied with the understanding that for a protein to be produced, a certain chromosome must be present and, therefore, the coding for that protein must be located on that chromosome.

In situ hybridization involves the use of specific sequences of DNA or RNA to locate genes that do not express themselves in cell culture. DNA and RNA can be chemically tagged with radioactive or fluorescent markers. These chemically tagged DNA or RNA sequences are used as probes to detect gene location. If the probe matches the complementary DNA of a chromosome segment, it hybridizes and remains at the precise location (therefore the term in situ) on a chromosome. Radioactive or fluorescent markers are used to find the location of the probe.

Haplotype Mapping

As work on the Human Genome Project progressed, many researchers reasoned that identifying the common patterns of DNA sequence variations in the human genome would be possible. An international project, known as the *International HapMap Project*, was organized with the intent of developing a haplotype map of these variations.[4] Sites in the DNA sequence where people differ at a single DNA base are called *single nucleotide polymorphisms* (SNPs, pronounced "snips"). A haplotype consists of the many closely linked SNPs on a single chromosome that generally are passed as a block from one generation to another in a particular population. One of the motivating factors behind the HapMap Project was the realization that the identification of a few SNPs was enough to uniquely identify the haplotypes in a block. The specific SNPs that identify the haplotypes are called *tagging SNPs*. This approach reduces the number of SNPs required to examine an entire genome and makes genome scanning methods much more efficient in finding regions with genes that contribute to disease development. Much attention has focused on the use of SNPs indicating disease susceptibility in one population versus another, as well as determining appropriate medications and therapies based on genotype.

Recombinant DNA Technology

The term *recombinant DNA* refers to a combination of DNA molecules that are not found together in nature. Recombinant DNA technology makes it possible to identify the DNA sequence in a gene and produce the protein product encoded by a gene. The specific nucleotide sequence of a DNA fragment can often be identified by analyzing the amino acid sequence and mRNA codon of its protein product. Short sequences of base pairs can be synthesized, radioactively labeled, and subsequently used to identify their complementary sequence. In this way, identifying both normal and abnormal gene structures is possible.

Gene Isolation and Cloning

The gene isolation and cloning methods used in recombinant DNA technology rely on the fact that the genes of all organisms, from bacteria through mammals, are based on a similar molecular organization. *Gene cloning* requires cutting a DNA molecule apart, modifying and reassembling its fragments, and producing copies of the modified DNA, its mRNA, and its gene product. The DNA molecule is cut apart by using a bacterial enzyme, called a *restriction enzyme*, that binds to DNA wherever a particular short sequence of base pairs is found and cleaves the molecule at a specific nucleotide site. In this way, a long DNA molecule can be broken down into smaller, discrete fragments, one of which contains the gene of interest. Many restriction enzymes are commercially available that cut DNA at different recognition sites.

The fragments of DNA can then often be replicated through insertion into a unicellular organism, such as a bacterium. To do this, a cloning **vector** such as a bacterial virus or a small DNA circle that is found in most bacteria, called a *plasmid*, is used. Viral and plasmid vectors replicate autonomously in the host bacterial cell. During gene cloning, a bacterial vector and the DNA fragment are mixed and joined by a special enzyme called a *DNA ligase*. The recombinant vectors formed are then introduced into a suitable culture of bacteria, and the bacteria are allowed to replicate and express the recombinant vector gene.

Pharmaceutical Applications

The methods of recombinant DNA technology can also be used in the treatment of disease. For example, recombinant DNA technology is used in the manufacture of human insulin that is used to treat diabetes mellitus. Recombinant DNA corresponding to the A chain of human insulin was isolated and inserted into plasmids that were in turn used to transform *Escherichia coli*. The bacteria then synthesized the insulin chain. A similar method was used to obtain the B chains. The A and B chains were then mixed and allowed to fold and form disulfide bonds, producing active insulin molecules. Human growth hormone has also been produced in *E. coli*. More complex proteins are produced in mammalian cell culture using recombinant DNA techniques. These include erythropoietin, which is used to stimulate red blood cell production; factor VIII, which is used to treat hemophilia; and tissue plasminogen activator, which is frequently administered after a heart attack to dissolve thrombi.

DNA Fingerprinting

The technique of DNA fingerprinting also uses recombinant DNA technology, as well as basic principles of medical genetics.[11] Using restriction enzymes, DNA is first cleaved at specific regions (Fig. 4-13). The DNA fragments are separated according to size by electrophoresis and denatured (by heating or treating chemically) so that all the DNA is single stranded. The single-stranded DNA is then transferred to nitrocellulose paper, baked to attach the DNA to the paper, and treated with a series of radioactive probes. After the radioactive probes have been allowed to bond with the denatured DNA, radiography is used to reveal the labeled DNA fragments.

When used in forensic pathology, this procedure is applied to specimens from the suspect and the forensic specimen. This can be done with even very small samples of DNA (a single hair or a drop of blood or saliva) using amplification by *polymerase chain reaction*. The DNA banding patterns between samples are analyzed to see if they match. With conventional methods of analysis of blood and serum enzymes, a 1 in 100 to 1000 chance exists that the two specimens match because of chance. With DNA fingerprinting, these odds are 1 in 100,000 to 1 million.

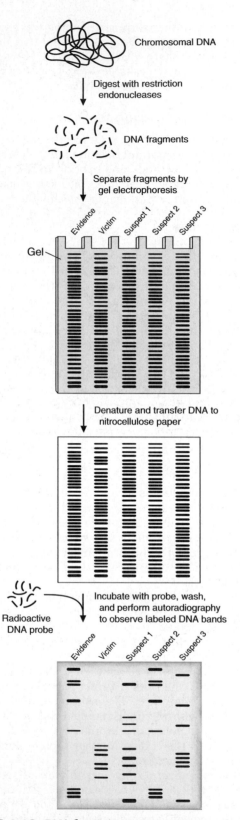

FIGURE 4-13. DNA fingerprinting. Restriction enzymes are used to break chromosomal DNA into fragments, which are then separated by gel electrophoresis, denatured, and transferred to nitrocellulose paper; the DNA bands are labeled with a radioactive probe and observed using autoradiography. (Modified from Smith C., Marks A. D., Lieberman M. (2005). *Marks' basic medical biochemistry* (2nd ed., p. 309). Philadelphia, PA: Lippincott Williams & Wilkins.)

Gene Therapy

Although quite different from inserting genetic material into a unicellular organism such as bacteria, techniques are available for inserting genes into the genome of intact multicellular plants and animals. Promising delivery vehicles for these genes are the adenoviruses. These viruses are ideal vehicles because their DNA does not become integrated into the host genome. However, repeated inoculations are often needed because the body's immune system usually targets cells expressing adenovirus proteins. This type of therapy remains one of the more promising methods for the treatment of genetic disorders such as cystic fibrosis, certain cancers, and many infectious diseases.

Two main approaches are used in gene therapy: transferred genes can replace defective genes, or they can selectively inhibit the expression of deleterious genes. **Cloned** DNA sequences are usually the compounds used in gene therapy. However, the introduction of the cloned gene into the multicellular organism can influence only the few cells that get the gene. An answer to this problem would be the insertion of the gene into a sperm or ovum; after fertilization, the gene would be replicated in all of the differentiating cell types. Even so, techniques for cell insertion are limited. Not only are moral and ethical issues involved, but these techniques cannot direct the inserted DNA to attach to a particular chromosome or supplant an existing gene by knocking it out of its place.

RNA Interference Technology

One approach of gene therapy focuses on the previously described replacement of missing genes. However, several genetic disorders are due not to missing genes but to faulty gene activity. With this in mind, some scientists are approaching the problem by using *RNA interference* (RNAi) to stop genes from making unwanted disease proteins.[12] RNAi is a naturally occurring process in which small pieces of double-stranded RNA (small interfering RNA) suppress gene expression. Scientists believe that RNAi may have originated as a defense against viral infections and potentially harmful genomic invaders. In viral infections, RNAi would serve to control the infection by preventing the synthesis of viral proteins.

With the continued refinement of techniques to silence genes, RNAi has already had a major impact on molecular biology. For example, it has given scientists the ability to practice reverse genomics, in which a gene's function can be inferred through silencing its expression. Increasingly, pharmaceutical companies are using RNAi to identify disease-related drug targets. There also is considerable interest in harnessing RNAi for therapeutic purposes, including the treatment of human immunodeficiency virus infection and hepatitis C. Before this can occur, however, the therapeutic methods must be shown to be safe and effective, and obstacles to delivering the RNAi into targeted cells must be overcome. It is difficult for RNA to cross the cell membrane, and enzymes in the blood quickly break it down.

SUMMARY CONCEPTS

Genomic mapping is a method used to assign genes to particular chromosomes or parts of a chromosome. Linkage studies assign a chromosome location to genes based on their close association with other genes of known location or their tendency to be inherited together. A haplotype consists of the many closely linked SNPs on a single chromosome that generally are passed as a block from one generation to another in a particular population. The International HapMap Project has been developed to map the SNPs on the human genome with the anticipation that it may be useful in the prediction and management of disease.

Genetic engineering has provided the methods for manipulating nucleic acids and recombining genes (recombinant DNA) into hybrid molecules that can be inserted into unicellular organisms and reproduced many times over. As a result, proteins that formerly were available only in small amounts can now be made in large quantities once their respective genes have been isolated. DNA fingerprinting, which relies on recombinant DNA technologies and those of genetic mapping, is often used in forensic investigations. A newer strategy for management of genetic disorders focuses on gene silencing by using RNAi to stop genes from making unwanted disease proteins.

Review Exercises

1. The Human Genome Project has revealed that humans have only 30,000 to 35,000 genes. Only about 2% of the genome encodes instructions for protein synthesis, whereas 50% consists of repeat sequences that do not code proteins.

   A. Use this information to explain how this small number of protein-encoding genes is able to produce the vast array of proteins needed for organ and structural development in the embryo, as well as those needed for normal function of the body in postnatal life.

2. A child about to undergo surgery is typed for possible blood transfusions. His parents are told that he is type O positive. Both his mother and father are type A positive.

   A. How would you explain this variation in blood type to the parents?

3. **More than 100,000 people die of adverse drug reactions each year; another 2.2 million experience serious reactions, whereas others fail to respond at all to the therapeutic actions of drugs.**

   A. Explain how the use of information about single nucleotide polymorphisms might be used to map individual variations in drug responses.

4. **Human insulin, prepared by recombinant DNA technology, is used for the treatment of diabetes mellitus.**

   A. Explain the techniques used for the production of a human hormone with this technology.

REFERENCES

1. Meselson M., Stahl F. W. (1958). The replication of DNA in Escherichia coli. *Proceedings of the National Academy of Sciences of the United States of America* 44(7), 671–682.
2. Biterge B., Schneider R. (2014). Histone variants: Key players of chromatin. *Cell and Tissue Research* 356(3), 457–466. doi:10.1007/s00441-014-1862-4.
3. Clapier C. R., Iwasa J., Cairns B. R., et al. (2017). Mechanisms of action and regulation of ATP-dependent chromatin-remodelling complexes. *Nature Reviews Molecular Cell Biology* 18(7), 407–422. doi:10.1038/nrm.2017.26.
4. The International HapMap Consortium. (2003). The International HapMap Project. *Nature* 426(6968), 789–796. doi:10.1038/nature02168.
5. Brandvold K. R., Morimoto R. I. (2015). The chemical biology of molecular chaperones—Implications for modulation of proteostasis. *Journal of Molecular Biology* 427(18), 2931–2947. doi:10.1016/j.jmb.2015.05.010.
6. Spitz F., Furlong E. E. (2012). Transcription factors: From enhancer binding to developmental control. *Nature Reviews Genetics* 13(9), 613–626. doi:10.1038/nrg3207.
7. Blake J. A., Ziman M. R. (2014). Pax genes: Regulators of lineage specification and progenitor cell maintenance. *Development* 141(4), 737–751. doi:10.1242/dev.091785.
8. Hughes J. F., Rozen S. (2012). Genomics and genetics of human and primate y chromosomes. *Annual Review of Genomics and Human Genetics* 13, 83–108. doi:10.1146/annurev-genom-090711-163855.
9. Rubin R., Strayer D. (Eds.) (2012). *Rubin's pathology: Clinicopathologic foundations of medicine*. Philadelphia, PA: Lippincott Williams & Wilkins.
10. Strayer D. S., Rubin E. (2015). *Rubin's pathology clinicopathologic foundations of medicine* (7th ed.). Philadelphia, PA: Wolters Kluwer.
11. Thompson R., Zoppis S., McCord B. (2012). An overview of DNA typing methods for human identification: Past, present, and future. *Methods in Molecular Biology* 830, 3–16. doi:10.1007/978-1-61779-461-2_1.
12. Fischer S. E. (2015). RNA interference and microRNA-mediated silencing. *Current Protocols in Molecular Biology* 112(26), 1–5. doi:10.1002/0471142727.mb2601s112.

Genetic and Congenital Disorders

Learning Objectives

After completing this chapter, the learner will be able to meet the following objectives:

1. Contrast disorders due to multifactorial inheritance with those caused by single-gene inheritance.
2. Cite the most susceptible period of intrauterine life for development of defects because of teratogenic agents.
3. State the cautions that should be observed when considering use of drugs during pregnancy, including the possible effects of alcohol abuse, vitamin A derivatives, and folic acid deficiency on fetal development.
4. Describe the process of genetic assessment.
5. Describe screening methods used for prenatal diagnosis including specificity and risks.

Congenital defects, sometimes called birth defects, are abnormalities of a body structure, function, or metabolism that are present at birth. They affect more than 185,000 infants discharged from the hospital in the United States each year and are the leading cause of infant death.[1] Congenital defects may be caused by genetic factors or environmental factors that are active during embryonic or fetal development. Although congenital defects caused by genetic factors are present at birth, they may not make their appearance until later in life. This chapter provides an overview of genetic and congenital disorders and is divided into three parts:

1. Genetic and chromosomal disorders
2. Disorders due to environmental agents
3. Diagnosis and counseling

Genetic and Chromosomal Disorders

Most genetic disorders are caused by changes in the deoxyribonucleic acid (DNA) sequence that alters the synthesis of a single gene product. Other genetic disorders are a result of chromosomal aberrations such as deletion or duplication errors, or are due to an abnormal number of chromosomes.

The genes on each chromosome are arranged in strict order, with each gene occupying a specific location or *locus*. The two members of a gene pair, one inherited from the mother and the other from the father, are called *alleles*. If the members of a gene pair are identical (*i.e.*, code the exact same gene product), the person is homozygous, and if the two members are different, the person is heterozygous. The genetic composition of a person is called a genotype, whereas the phenotype is the observable expression of a genotype in terms of physical or biochemical traits. If the trait is phenotypically seen in the heterozygote, the allele is said to be *dominant*. If it is phenotypically seen only in the homozygote, the allele is *recessive*. Many genes have more than one normal allele (alternate forms) at the same locus. This is called a *polymorphism*. Although most traits follow a dominant or recessive pattern, it is possible for both alleles of a gene pair to be phenotypically seen in the heterozygote, a condition called *codominance*. Blood group inheritance (*e.g.*, AO, BO, AB) is an example of both codominance and polymorphism.

A gene *mutation* is a biochemical event such as nucleotide change, deletion, or insertion that produces a new allele for a particular gene. A single mutant gene may be expressed in many different parts of the body. Marfan syndrome, for example, is a single gene defect in a connective tissue protein that has widespread effects involving skeletal, eye, and cardiovascular structures. The disorder may be inherited as a family trait or arise as a sporadic case because of a new mutation.

Single-Gene Disorders

Single-gene disorders are caused by a defective or mutant allele at a single gene locus and follow mendelian patterns of inheritance. Single-gene disorders are characterized by their patterns of transmission, which usually are obtained through a family genetic history. The patterns of inheritance depend on whether the phenotype is dominant or recessive and whether the gene of concern is located on an autosomal or sex chromosome. In addition to disorders caused by mutations of genes located on the chromosomes within the nucleus, another (but more rare) class of disorders involves the mitochondrial genome and shows a maternal pattern of inheritance.

Virtually all single-gene disorders lead to the formation of an abnormal protein or the decreased production of a gene product. These changes can result in many different types of systemic alterations. Table 5-1 lists some of the common single-gene disorders and their manifestations.

Autosomal Dominant Disorders

In autosomal dominant disorders, a single mutant allele from an affected parent is transmitted to an offspring regardless of sex. The affected parent has a 50% chance of transmitting the disorder to each offspring (Fig. 5-1). The unaffected relatives of the parent or unaffected siblings of the offspring do not transmit the disorder. In many conditions, the age of onset is delayed, and the signs and symptoms of the disorder do not appear until later in life.

Autosomal dominant disorders also may manifest as a new mutation. Many autosomal dominant mutations are accompanied by reduced reproductive capacity; therefore, the defect is not repeated in future generations. If an autosomal defect is accompanied by a total inability to reproduce, essentially all new cases of the

TABLE 5-1 Some Disorders of Mendelian or Single-Gene Inheritance and Their Significance

Disorder	Significance
Autosomal Dominant	
Achondroplasia	Short-limb dwarfism
Adult polycystic kidney disease	Chronic kidney disease
Huntington chorea	Neurodegenerative disorder
Familial hypercholesterolemia	Premature atherosclerosis
Marfan syndrome	Connective tissue disorder with abnormalities in the skeletal, ocular, cardiovascular systems
Neurofibromatosis (NF)	Neurogenic tumors: fibromatous skin tumors, pigmented skin lesions, and ocular nodules in NF-1; bilateral acoustic neuromas in NF-2
Osteogenesis imperfecta	Brittle bone disease due to defects in collagen synthesis
Spherocytosis	Disorder of red blood cells
von Willebrand disease	Bleeding disorder
Autosomal Recessive	
Cystic fibrosis	Disorder of membrane transport of chloride ions in exocrine glands causing lung and pancreatic disease
Glycogen storage diseases	Excess accumulation of glycogen in the liver and hypoglycemia (von Gierke disease); glycogen accumulation in striated muscle in myopathic forms
Oculocutaneous albinism	Hypopigmentation of skin, hair, eyes as a result of inability to synthesize melanin
Phenylketonuria	Lack of phenylalanine hydroxylase with hyperphenylalaninemia and impaired brain development
Sickle cell disease	Red blood cell defect
Tay–Sachs disease	Deficiency of hexosaminidase A; severe mental and physical deterioration beginning in infancy
X-Linked Recessive	
Bruton-type hypogammaglobulinemia	Immunodeficiency
Hemophilia A	Bleeding disorder
Duchenne dystrophy	Muscular dystrophy
Fragile X syndrome	Intellectual disability

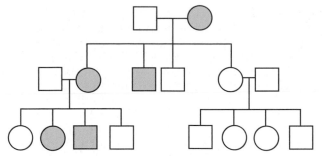

FIGURE 5-1. Simple pedigree for inheritance of an autosomal dominant trait. *Squares* represent males, *circles* represent females. The *shaded symbols* represent an affected parent with a mutant gene. An affected parent with an autosomal dominant trait has a 50% chance of passing the mutant gene on to each child regardless of sex.

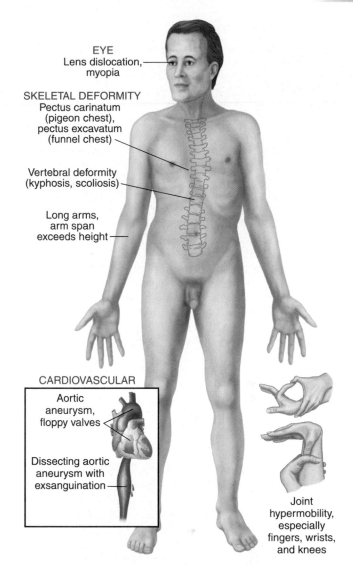

FIGURE 5-2. Clinical features of Marfan syndrome.

disorder will be due to new mutations. If the defect does not affect reproductive capacity, it is more likely to be inherited from a parent.

Although there is a 50% chance of inheriting a dominant genetic disorder from an affected parent, there can be wide variation in **gene penetrance** and expression. When a person inherits a dominant mutant gene but fails to exhibit the associated phenotype, the trait is described as having *reduced penetrance*. The person who has a mutant gene but does not express it is an important exception to the rule that unaffected persons do not transmit an autosomal dominant trait. These people can transmit the gene to their descendants and so produce a "skipped generation" in their family history. Autosomal dominant disorders also can display *variable expressivity*, meaning that they can be expressed differently in people who carry the mutant gene. Polydactyly or supernumerary digits, for example, may be expressed in either the fingers or the toes.[2] Other disorders of autosomal inheritance, Marfan syndrome and neurofibromatosis (NF), are described here.

Marfan Syndrome

Marfan syndrome is an autosomal dominant disorder of the connective tissue. The basic biochemical abnormality in Marfan syndrome affects *fibrillin I*, a major component of microfibrils found in the extracellular matrix.[3] Fibrillin I is coded by the *FBNI* gene, which maps to chromosome 15q21. The prevalence of Marfan syndrome is estimated to be 1 per 5000. Approximately 70% to 80% of cases are familial and the remainder are sporadic, arising from new mutations in the germ cells of the parents.[3]

Marfan syndrome affects several organ systems, including the eyes; the cardiovascular system; and the skeletal system (bones and joints).[3] There is a wide range of variation in the phenotype for the disorder. The skeletal deformities include a long, thin body with exceptionally long extremities and long, tapering fingers, sometimes called *arachnodactyly* or *spider fingers*; hyperextensible joints; and a variety of spinal deformities, including **kyphosis** and scoliosis (Fig. 5-2). Chest deformities, pectus excavatum (*i.e.*, deeply depressed sternum) or pigeon chest deformity, often are present and may require surgery. The most common eye disorder is

bilateral dislocation of the lens because of weakness of the suspensory ligaments. Myopia and predisposition to retinal detachment also are common. However, the most life-threatening aspects of the disorder are the cardiovascular defects, which include mitral valve **prolapse**, progressive dilation of the aortic valve ring, and weakness of the aorta and other arteries. Dissection and rupture of the aorta may lead to premature death.

The diagnosis of Marfan syndrome is based on major and minor diagnostic criteria that include skeletal, cardiovascular, and ocular deformities. There is currently no cure for Marfan syndrome. Treatment plans include regular assessment of the at-risk systems.

Neurofibromatosis

NF is a condition that causes tumors to develop from the Schwann cells of the neurologic system.[4] There are at least two genetically and clinically distinct forms of the disorder:

1. Type 1 NF (NF-1), also known as *von Recklinghausen disease*.

2. Type 2 bilateral acoustic NF (NF-2).[4,5]

Both of these disorders result from a genetic defect in a tumor suppressor gene that regulates cell differentiation and growth. The gene for NF-1 has been mapped to the long arm of chromosome 17 and the gene for NF-2 to chromosome 22.[4,6]

Type 1 NF is a common disorder, characterized by **cutaneous** and subcutaneous neurofibromas that develop in late childhood or adolescence.[4] The cutaneous neurofibromas, which vary in number from a few to many hundreds, manifest as soft, **pedunculated** lesions that project from the skin. They are the most common type of lesion, often are not apparent until puberty, and are present in greatest density over the trunk (Fig. 5-3). The subcutaneous lesions grow just below the skin. They are firm and round and may be painful. Plexiform neurofibromas involve the larger peripheral nerves. They tend to form large tumors that cause severe disfigurement of the face, overgrowth of an extremity, or skeletal deformities such as scoliosis. Pigmented nodules of the iris (Lisch nodules), which are specific for NF-1, usually are present after 6 years of age.[7] They do not present any clinical problem but are useful in establishing a diagnosis.

A second major component of NF-1 is the presence of large (usually ≥15 mm in diameter), flat cutaneous pigmentations, known as *café au lait spots*. They are usually a uniform light brown in whites and darker brown in people of color, with sharply demarcated edges. Although small single lesions may be found in normal children, larger lesions or six or more spots greater than 1.5 cm in diameter suggest NF-1.[8] The skin pigmentations become more evident with age as the melanosomes in the epidermal cells accumulate melanin.

Children with NF-1 are also susceptible to neurologic complications including an increased incidence of learning disabilities, attention deficit disorders, abnormalities of speech, and complex partial and generalized tonic–clonic seizures. Malignant neoplasms are also a significant problem in people with NF-1. One of the major complications of NF-1, occurring in 3% to 5% of people, is the appearance of a neurofibrosarcoma.[4] NF-1 is also associated with increased incidence of other neurogenic tumors, including meningiomas, optic gliomas, and pheochromocytomas.

Type 2 NF is characterized by tumors of the acoustic nerve. Most often, the disorder is asymptomatic through the first 15 years of life. This type of NF occurs less frequently, at a rate of 1 in 50,000 people. The most frequent symptoms are headaches, hearing loss, and **tinnitus**. There may be associated intracranial and spinal meningiomas.

Autosomal Recessive Disorders

Autosomal recessive disorders are manifested only when both members of the gene pair are affected (homozygous). In this case, both parents may be unaffected but are carriers of the defective gene. Autosomal recessive disorders affect both sexes. The occurrence risks in each pregnancy are one in four for an affected child, two in four for a carrier child, and one in four for a normal (noncarrier, unaffected), homozygous child (Fig. 5-4). *Consanguineous mating* (mating of two related people), or inbreeding, increases the chance that two people who mate will be carriers of an autosomal recessive disorder.

With autosomal recessive disorders, the age of onset is frequently early in life. In addition, the symptomatology tends to be more uniform than with autosomal dominant disorders. Autosomal disorders are characteristically caused by loss-of-function mutations, many of which impair or eliminate the function of an enzyme. In the case of a heterozygous carrier, the presence of a mutant gene usually does not produce symptoms because equal amounts of normal and defective enzymes are synthesized. This "margin of safety" ensures that cells with half their usual amount of enzyme function normally. By contrast, the inactivation of both alleles in a homozygote results in complete loss of enzyme activity. Autosomal recessive disorders include almost all inborn errors of metabolism. Enzyme disorders that impair catabolic pathways result in an accumulation of dietary substances (*e.g.*, phenylketonuria [PKU]) or cellular constituents (*e.g.*, lysosomal storage diseases). Other disorders result from a defect in the enzyme-mediated synthesis of an essential protein (*e.g.*, the cystic fibrosis transmembrane conductance regulator in cystic fibrosis). Two examples of autosomal recessive disorders that are not covered elsewhere in this book are PKU and Tay–Sachs disease.

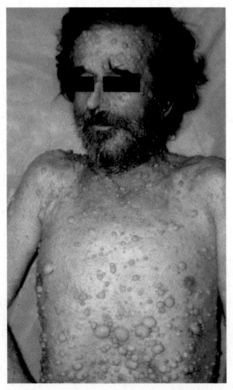

FIGURE 5-3. Neurofibromatosis type 1. Multiple cutaneous neurofibromas are noted on the face and trunk. (From Strayer D. S., Rubin E. (Eds.) (2015). *Rubin's pathology: Clinicopathologic foundations of medicine* (7th ed., Fig. 6-20C, p. 269). Philadelphia, PA: Lippincott Williams & Wilkins.)

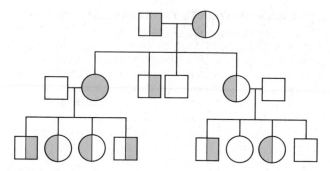

FIGURE 5-4. Sample pedigree for inheritance of an autosomal recessive trait. *Squares* represent males, *circles* represent females. When the symbols are *half shaded*, then that parent is a carrier of an autosomal recessive trait. When both parents are carriers, on each conception, there is a 25% chance of having an affected child (*full-shaded circle* or *square*), a 50% chance of a carrier child, and a 25% chance of a nonaffected or noncarrier child, regardless of sex.

Phenylketonuria

PKU is a rare autosomal recessive metabolic disorder that affects approximately 1 in every 10,000 to 15,000 infants in the United States. The disorder is caused by a deficiency of the liver enzyme phenylalanine hydroxylase, which allows toxic levels of the amino acid, phenylalanine, to accumulate in tissues and the blood.[9] If untreated, the disorder results in mental retardation, microcephaly, delayed speech, and other signs of impaired neurologic development.

Because the symptoms of PKU develop gradually and are difficult to assess, all infants are screened for abnormal levels of serum phenylalanine.[5] Infants with the disorder are treated with a special diet that restricts phenylalanine intake to prevent mental retardation as well as other neurodegenerative effects. Infants with elevated phenylalanine levels should begin treatment by 7 to 10 days of age, indicating the need for early diagnosis.[9]

Tay–Sachs Disease

Tay–Sachs disease is a variant of a class of lysosomal storage diseases, known as the *gangliosidoses*, in which there is failure to break down the GM2 gangliosides of cell membranes.[10] Tay–Sachs disease is inherited as an autosomal recessive trait and occurs 10 times more frequently in offspring of Eastern European (Ashkenazi) Jews as compared to the general population, although targeted carrier screening efforts have shown success in reducing rates for this population.[11]

The GM2 ganglioside accumulates in the lysosomes of all organs in Tay–Sachs disease, but is most prominent in the brain neurons and retina.[10] Microscopic examination reveals neurons ballooned with cytoplasmic vacuoles, each of which constitutes a markedly distended lysosome filled with gangliosides.[10] In time, there is progressive destruction of neurons, including in the cerebellum, basal ganglia, brainstem, spinal cord, and autonomic nervous system. Involvement of the retina is detected by ophthalmoscopy as a cherry-red spot on the **macula**.[10]

Infants with Tay–Sachs disease appear normal at birth but begin to manifest progressive weakness, muscle flaccidity, and decreased responsiveness at approximately 6 to 10 months of age.[10] This is followed by rapid deterioration of motor and mental function, often with development of generalized seizures. Retinal involvement leads to visual impairment and eventual blindness. Death usually occurs before 4 to 5 years of age.[10] Analysis of the blood serum for the lysosomal enzyme, hexosaminidase A, which is deficient in Tay–Sachs disease, allows for accurate identification of genetic carriers for the disease.[11]

X-Linked Recessive Disorders

Sex-linked disorders are almost always associated with the X chromosome, and the inheritance pattern is predominantly recessive. Remember that the sex chromosomes for human females are XX and human males are XY. Because of the presence of a normal X, female heterozygotes (carriers) rarely experience the effects of a recessive defective gene, whereas all males who receive the gene are typically affected as they only have the mutant copy.

The common pattern of inheritance in a family is one in which an unaffected mother is a carrier of the mutant allele. She is not affected herself because she has one normal X that is dominant over the mutant recessive X. Because she will contribute one of these two X chromosomes to each of her offspring, she has a 50% chance of transmitting the mutant gene to her sons (who only have one X and will be affected), and her daughters have a 50% chance of being carriers of the mutant gene (who have two X chromosomes and so will not be affected because of the presence of a normal X) (Fig. 5-5).

When the affected son procreates, he only has his mutant X or a normal Y to pass on to the next generation. In order to have a daughter, the father donates his only X chromosome, which combines with one of the mother's two X chromosomes, resulting in a XX child. Because his X is mutated, he transmits the mutant gene to 100% of his daughters, who then become carriers. Because the genes of the Y chromosome are unaffected, the affected male does not transmit the defect to any of his sons, and they will not be carriers or transmit the disorder to their children.

Although rare, females can be affected with an X-linked recessive disorder. In order for this to happen, an affected male would need to have a child with a carrier female. In this case, 50% of the sons would be affected, and 50% of the daughters would be affected. The remaining daughters would be carriers like their mother. X-linked recessive disorders include color blindness, glucose-6-phosphate dehydrogenase deficiency, hemophilia A, and X-linked **agammaglobulinemia**.

X-Linked Dominant Disorders

X-linked dominant disorders are not as common as X-linked recessive disorders affecting both males and females that inherit a copy of the mutated X chromosome.

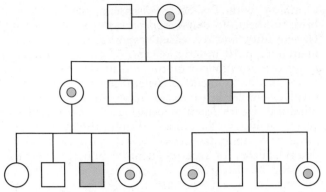

FIGURE 5-5. Sample pedigree for inheritance of an X-linked recessive trait. X-linked recessive traits are expressed phenotypically in the male offspring, whereas females are typically carriers for the trait. A *small shaded circle* represents a carrier female and the *larger shaded square*, the affected male. A carrier female will transmit her carrier status to 50% of her daughters and 50% of her sons will be affected. The affected male passes the mutant gene to all of his daughters, who become carriers of the trait. The affected male will have no affected sons.

For the females, the mutant X chromosome is dominant to the normal X chromosome. Although both sexes are affected, many times the mutation will be embryonic lethal for males (who only have the mutated X and a normal Y) or for homozygous mutant females. Affected females who are heterozygous with one mutant X chromosome and one normal X chromosome will transmit the disorder to 50% of their offspring regardless of sex. Affected males will have 100% affected daughters or 100% normal sons. This is explained because all sons inherited their father's Y chromosome, but the daughters inherited the mutated X chromosome from their father. Examples of X-linked dominant disorders include fragile X syndrome and Rett syndrome.

Fragile X Syndrome

Fragile X syndrome is a single-gene disorder that causes intellectual disability.[12] The mutation occurs at Xq27 on the fragile site and is characterized by amplification of a cytosine, guanine, guanine (CGG) repeat.[13] The disorder, which affects approximately 1 in 1250 males and 1 in 2500 females, is the most common form of inherited intellectual disability.[12]

Pathogenesis

The fragile X gene has been mapped to the long arm of the X chromosome, designated the *FMR1* (fragile X mental retardation 1) site.[13] The gene product, the fragile X mental retardation protein (FMRP), is a widely expressed cytoplasmic protein. It is most abundant in the brain and testis, the organs most affected by the disorder. Each gene contains a promoter region and an instruction region that carries the directions for protein synthesis. The promoter region of the *FMR1* gene contains repeats of a specific CGG triplet code that, when normal, controls gene activity. Once the repeat exceeds a threshold length for the disease, no FMRP is produced, resulting in the fragile X phenotype.[13]

Clinical Manifestations and Diagnosis

Affected boys are intellectually disabled and share a common physical phenotype that includes a long face with large mandible and large, everted ears. Hyperextensible joints, a high-arched palate, and mitral valve prolapse, which are observed in some cases, mimic a connective tissue disorder.[12] Some physical abnormalities may be subtle or absent. Because girls have two X chromosomes, they are more likely to have relatively normal cognitive development, or they may show a learning disability in a particular area.

Diagnosis of fragile X syndrome is based on mental and physical characteristics. DNA tests can be done to confirm the presence of an abnormal *FMR1* gene. Fragile X screening is now often offered along with routine prenatal screening to determine if the woman is a carrier.

KEY POINTS

Single-Gene Disorders

■ Genetic disorders can be inherited as autosomal dominant disorders, in which the phenotype is seen in both the homozygous dominant or heterozygous genotype, or as autosomal recessive disorders, in which the phenotype is only seen in the homozygous recessive genotype.

■ Sex-linked disorders almost always are associated with the X chromosome and are predominantly recessive.

Inherited Multifactorial Disorders

Multifactorial disorders are caused by the influence of multiple genes along with environmental factors. These traits do not follow the same clear-cut pattern of inheritance as do single-gene disorders because the appearance of the disorder phenotype will be dependent on environmental changes in addition to genetic mutations. Disorders of multifactorial inheritance can be present at birth, or they may be expressed later in life. Congenital disorders that are thought to arise through multifactorial inheritance include cleft lip or palate, clubfoot, congenital dislocation of the hip, congenital heart disease, pyloric **stenosis**, and urinary tract malformation. Environmental factors are thought to play an even greater role in disorders of multifactorial inheritance that develop in adult life, such as coronary artery disease, diabetes mellitus, hypertension, and cancer.

Although multifactorial traits cannot be predicted with the same degree of accuracy as mendelian single-gene mutations, characteristic patterns do exist for congenital disorders. First, multifactorial congenital malformations tend to involve a single organ or tissue derived from the same embryonic developmental field. Second, the risk of recurrence in future pregnancies is high for the same or a similar defect. For instance, this means that parents of a child with a cleft palate defect have an increased risk of having another child with a cleft palate defect. Third, first-degree relatives of an affected person have an increased risk (as compared with the general population) of having a child with the disease. The risk increases with increasing numbers of the incidence of the defect among relatives.

Cleft Lip and Cleft Palate

Cleft lip with or without cleft palate is one of the most common birth defects, occurring in about 0.1% of all pregnancies.[14] It is also one of the more conspicuous birth defects, resulting in an abnormal facial appearance and defective speech.

Developmentally, the defect has its origin at about the 35th day of gestation when the frontal prominences of the craniofacial structures fuse with the **maxillary** process to form the upper lip.[14] This process is under the control of many genes, and disturbances in these (whether hereditary or environmental) at this time may result in cleft lip with or without cleft palate (Fig. 5-6). The defect may also be caused by **teratogens** (*e.g.*, rubella, anticonvulsant drugs) and is often encountered in children with chromosomal abnormalities.

Cleft lip and palate defects may vary from a small notch in the vermilion border of the upper lip to complete separation involving the palate and extending into the floor of the nose. The clefts may be unilateral or bilateral and may involve the alveolar ridge. The condition may be accompanied by deformed, supernumerary, or absent teeth. Isolated cleft palate occurs in the midline and may involve only the uvula or may extend into or through the soft and hard palates.

A child with cleft lip or palate may require years of special treatment by medical and dental specialists. The immediate problem in an infant with cleft palate is feeding.

Nursing at the breast or nipple depends on suction developed by pressing the nipple against the hard palate with the tongue. Although infants with cleft lip usually have no problems with feeding, those with cleft palate usually require specially constructed, soft artificial nipples with large openings and a squeezable bottle. As the child ages, speech may be impaired because of these issues.

Major advances in the care of children born with cleft lip and palate have occurred within the last quarter of the 20th century.[15] Surgical closure of the lip is usually performed by 3 months of age, with closure of the palate usually done before 1 year of age. Depending on the extent of the defect, additional surgery may be required as the child grows.

Chromosomal Disorders

Chromosomal disorders form a major category of genetic disease, accounting for a large proportion of early miscarriages, congenital malformations, and intellectual disability. The study of chromosomal disorders is called *cytogenetics*.

During mitosis in human somatic cells, the chromosomes replicate so that each cell receives a total of 23 pairs of chromosomes. But in germ cells undergoing meiosis, these pairs are reduced so that each daughter cell only receives 23 individual chromosomes. At the time of conception, the set of 23 individual chromosomes in the ovum and the set of 23 individual chromosomes in the sperm join to produce an offspring with 23 pairs, or 46 total chromosomes.

Chromosomal abnormalities are commonly described according to the shorthand description of the karyotype. In this system, the total number of chromosomes is given first, followed by the sex chromosome complement, and then the description of any abnormality. For example, a male with trisomy 21 is designated 47,XY,+21.

Structural Chromosomal Abnormalities

The aberrations underlying chromosomal disorders can be an abnormal number of chromosomes, but there can also be alterations to the structure of one or more chromosomes. Structural changes in chromosomes usually result from breakage in one or more of the chromosomes during meiosis followed by rearrangement or deletion of chromosome parts. Among the factors believed to cause chromosome breakage are exposure to radiation sources such as x-rays, influence of certain chemicals, extreme changes in the cellular environment, and viral infections.

Several patterns of chromosome breakage and rearrangement can occur (Fig. 5-7). There can be a *deletion* of the broken portion of the chromosome. When one chromosome is involved, the broken parts may be *inverted*. *Isochromosome formation* occurs when the centromere of the chromosome separates horizontally instead of vertically. *Ring formation* results when deletion is followed by uniting of the chromatids to form a ring. *Translocation* occurs when there are simultaneous breaks in two chromosomes from different pairs, with

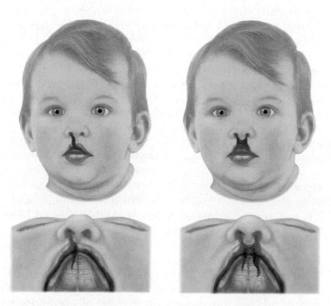

Unilateral Bilateral

FIGURE 5-6. Cleft lip and cleft palate.

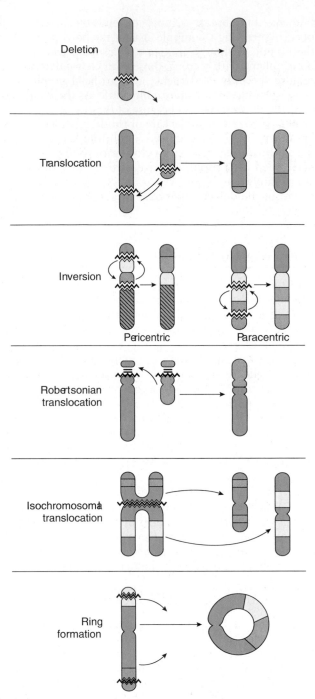

Deletion

Translocation

Inversion

Pericentric   Paracentric

Robertsonian
translocation

Isochromosomal
translocation

Ring
formation

FIGURE 5-7. Structural abnormalities in the human chromosome. The deletion of a portion of a chromosome leads to loss of genetic material and shortened chromosome. A **reciprocal translocation** involves breaks on two nonhomologous chromosomes, with exchange of the acentric segment. An **inversion** requires two breaks in a single chromosome. If the breaks are on opposite sides of the centromere, the inversion is **pericentric**; it is **paracentric** if the breaks are on the same arm. A **robertsonian translocation** occurs when two nonhomologous acrocentric chromosomes break near their centromeres, after which the long arms fuse to form one large metacentric chromosome. **Isochromosomes** arise from faulty centromere division, which leads to duplication of the long arm (iso q) and deletion of the short arm, or the reverse (iso p). Ring chromosomes form involve breaks in both telomeric portions of a chromosome, deletion of the acentric fragments, and fusion of the remaining centric portion. (From Rubin R, Strayer D. S. (Eds.) (2015). *Rubin's pathology: Clinicopathologic foundations of medicine* (7th ed., Fig. 6-8, p. 253). Philadelphia, PA: Lippincott Williams & Wilkins.)

exchange of chromosome parts. With a balanced reciprocal translocation, no genetic information is lost; therefore, persons with translocations usually are normal.

Centric fusion or *robertsonian translocation* involves two acrocentric chromosomes in which the centromere is near the end, most commonly chromosomes 13 and 14, or 14 and 21. Typically, the break occurs near the centromere affecting the short arm in one chromosome and the long arm in the other. Transfer of the chromosome fragments leads to one long and one extremely short fragment. The short fragment is usually lost during subsequent divisions. In this case, the person has only 45 chromosomes, but the amount of genetic material that is lost is so small that it often goes unnoticed. Difficulty, however, arises during meiosis; the result is gametes with an unbalanced number of chromosomes. The chief clinical importance of this type of translocation is that carriers of a robertsonian translocation involving chromosome 21 are at high risk for producing a child with Down syndrome.

The manifestations of aberrations in chromosome structure depend to a great extent on the amount of genetic material that is lost or displaced. Many cells sustaining major unrestored breaks are eliminated within the next few replication cycles because of deficiencies that may in themselves be fatal. This is beneficial because it prevents the damaged cells from becoming a permanent part of the organism or, if it occurs in the gametes, from giving rise to grossly defective zygotes.

Numeric Disorders Involving Autosomes

Having an abnormal number of chromosomes is referred to as **aneuploidy**. Many times, this happens when there is a failure of the chromosomes to separate during oogenesis or spermatogenesis. This can occur in either the autosomes or the sex chromosomes and is called *nondisjunction* (Fig. 5-8). Nondisjunction gives rise to germ cells that have an even number of chromosomes.[16,17] The products of conception formed from this even number of chromosomes have an uneven number of chromosomes, 45 or 47. *Monosomy* refers to the presence of only one member of a chromosome pair. The defects associated with monosomy of the autosomes are severe and often cause miscarriage in utero.

Polysomy, or the presence of more than two chromosomes to a set, occurs when a germ cell (either egg or sperm) containing more than 23 chromosomes is involved in conception. In contrast to Down syndrome, most other trisomies are much more severe, and these infants rarely survive beyond the first years of life.[6]

Down Syndrome

First described in 1866 by John Langdon Down, trisomy 21, or Down syndrome, causes a combination of birth defects including some degree of intellectual disability, characteristic facial features, and other health problems. It is the most common chromosomal disorder.

Approximately 95% of cases of Down syndrome are caused by nondisjunction or an error in cell division during meiosis, resulting in a trisomy of chromosome 21. A rare form of Down syndrome can occur in the offspring of people in whom there has been a robertsonian

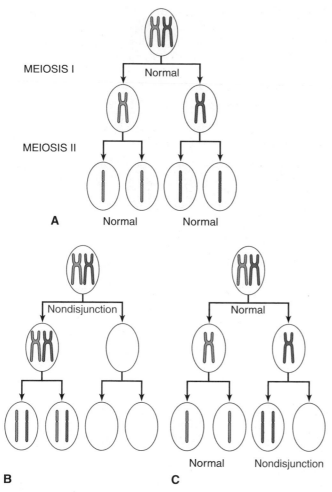

MEIOSIS I

Normal

MEIOSIS II

A   Normal   Normal   Normal

Nondisjunction   Normal

B   **C**   Normal   Nondisjunction

FIGURE 5-8. Nondisjunction as a cause of disorders of chromosomal numbers. (**A**) Normal distribution of chromosomes during meiosis I and II. (**B**) If nondisjunction occurs at meiosis I, the gametes contain either a pair of chromosomes or a lack of chromosomes. (**C**) If nondisjunction occurs at meiosis II, the affected gametes contain two of copies of one parenteral chromosome or a lack of chromosomes.

nasal bridge; small folds on the inner corners of the eyes (epicanthal folds) and upward slanting of the eyes; small, low-set, and malformed ears; a fat pad at the back of the neck; an open mouth; and a large, protruding tongue (Fig. 5-9). The child's hands usually are short and stubby, with fingers that curl inward, and there usually is only a single palmar (*i.e.*, simian) crease. There is excessive space between the large and second toes. There often are accompanying congenital heart defects and an increased risk of gastrointestinal malformations. In addition, there is an increased risk of Alzheimer disease among older people with Down syndrome.

There are several prenatal screening tests that can be done to determine the risk of having a child with Down syndrome.[19] The most commonly used are blood tests that measure maternal serum levels of α-fetoprotein (AFP), human chorionic gonadotropin (hCG), **unconjugated** estriol, inhibin A, and pregnancy-associated plasma protein A (PAPP-A) (see section on Diagnosis and Counseling). The results of three or four of these tests, together with the woman's age, often are used to determine the probability of a pregnant woman having a child with Down syndrome. Between 10 and 13 weeks, women can have an ultrasound that assesses for nuchal translucency (sonolucent space on the back of the fetal

translocation (see Fig. 5-7) involving the long arm of chromosome 21q and the long arm of one of the acrocentric chromosomes (most often 14 or 22). The translocation adds to the normal long arm of chromosome 21. Therefore, the person with this type of Down syndrome has 46 chromosomes, but a trisomy of the long arm of chromosome 21 (21q).[18]

The risk of having a child with Down syndrome increases with maternal age. The reason for the correlation between maternal age and nondisjunction is unknown, but is thought to reflect some aspect of aging of the oocyte. Although men continue to produce sperm throughout their reproductive life, women are born with all the oocytes they ever will have. These oocytes may change as a result of the aging process and are likely to have chromosomal abnormalities.

A child with Down syndrome has specific physical characteristics that are evident at birth. These features include a small and rather square head. There is a flat facial profile, with a small nose and somewhat depressed

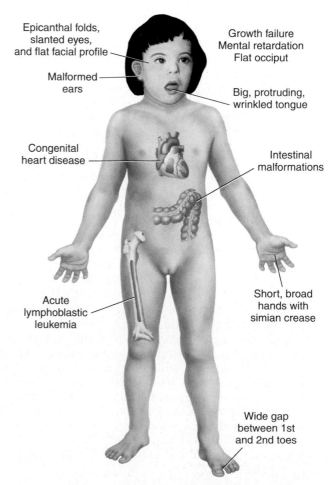

Epicanthal folds, slanted eyes, and flat facial profile

Malformed ears

Congenital heart disease

Acute lymphoblastic leukemia

Growth failure
Mental retardation
Flat occiput

Big, protruding, wrinkled tongue

Intestinal malformations

Short, broad hands with simian crease

Wide gap between 1st and 2nd toes

FIGURE 5-9. Clinical features of a child with Down syndrome.

neck). The fetus with Down syndrome tends to have a greater area of translucency as compared to a chromosomally normal infant. But the definitive diagnosis of Down syndrome in the fetus is through chromosome analysis using chorionic villus sampling, amniocentesis, or percutaneous umbilical blood sampling, which is discussed later in this chapter.

Numeric Disorders Involving Sex Chromosomes

Chromosomal disorders associated with the sex chromosomes are much more common than those related to the autosomes, except for trisomy 21. Furthermore, imbalances in the number (either excesses or deletions) are much better tolerated than those chromosomal abnormalities involving the autosomes. This is related in a large part to two factors that are peculiar to the sex chromosomes:

1. All but one X chromosome is inactivated.
2. There are very few genes that are carried on the Y chromosome.

Although females normally receive both a paternal and a maternal X chromosome, the clinical manifestations of X chromosome abnormalities can be quite variable because of the process of X inactivation.[20] In somatic cells of females, only one X chromosome is transcriptionally active and creates protein from the DNA template. The other chromosome is inactive. The process of X inactivation, which is random, occurs early in embryonic life and is usually complete at about the end of the first week of development. After one X chromosome has become inactivated in a cell, all cells descended from that cell will have the same active and inactive X chromosome. Although much of one X chromosome is inactivated in females, several regions do contain genes that escape inactivation and can continue to be expressed by both X chromosomes. These genes may explain some of the variations in clinical symptoms seen in cases of numeric abnormalities of the X chromosome.

Turner Syndrome

Turner syndrome describes an absence of all (45,X/0) or part of the X chromosome. Some women with Turner syndrome may have part of the X chromosome, and some may display a **mosaicism** where one or more additional cell lines are active. This disorder affects approximately 1 of every 2500 live births and is the most frequently occurring genetic disorder in women.[20]

Characteristically, a female with Turner syndrome is short in stature, but her body proportions are normal (Fig. 5-10). Females with Tuner syndrome lose the majority of their oocytes by the age of 2 years. Therefore, they do not menstruate and show no signs of secondary sex characteristics. There are variations in the syndrome, with abnormalities ranging from essentially a normal phenotype to cardiac abnormalities such as bicuspid aortic valve and **coarctation** of the aorta, and a small webbed neck.[20]

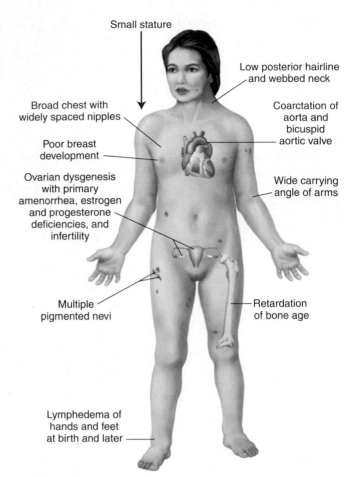

FIGURE 5-10. Clinical features of Turner syndrome.

Labels: Small stature; Low posterior hairline and webbed neck; Broad chest with widely spaced nipples; Coarctation of aorta and bicuspid aortic valve; Poor breast development; Ovarian dysgenesis with primary amenorrhea, estrogen and progesterone deficiencies, and infertility; Wide carrying angle of arms; Multiple pigmented nevi; Retardation of bone age; Lymphedema of hands and feet at birth and later

Because the phenotype can be somewhat variable, the diagnosis of Turner syndrome often is delayed until late childhood or early adolescence in girls who do not present with all of the classic features of the syndrome. It is important to diagnose girls with Turner syndrome as early as possible, so treatment plans can be implemented and managed throughout their lives. Growth hormone therapy generally can result in a gain of 6 to 10 cm in final height. Estrogen therapy, which is instituted around the normal age of puberty, is used to promote development and maintenance of secondary sexual characteristics.[20]

Klinefelter Syndrome

Klinefelter syndrome is a condition of testicular **dysgenesis** accompanied by the presence of one or more extra X chromosomes in excess of the normal male XY complement.[19] Most males with Klinefelter syndrome have one extra X chromosome (47,XXY). In rare cases, there may be more than one extra X chromosome (48,XXXY). The presence of the extra X chromosome in the 47,XXY male results from nondisjunction during meiotic division in one of the parents, but the cause of the nondisjunction is unknown. Advanced maternal age increases the risk, but only slightly. Klinefelter syndrome occurs in approximately 1 per 700 newborn male infants.[19]

Although the presence of the extra chromosome is fairly common, it is still a rare diagnosis as the phenotype is again variable. Many men live their lives without being aware that they have an additional chromosome. For this reason, it has been suggested that the term *Klinefelter syndrome* be replaced with *47,XXY male.*[19]

Phenotypic changes common to Klinefelter syndrome include enlarged breasts, sparse facial and body hair, small testes, and the inability to produce sperm (Fig. 5-11). Regardless of the number of X chromosomes present, the male phenotype is retained. The condition often goes undetected at birth. The infant usually has normal male genitalia, but at puberty, the testes do not respond to stimulation from the gonadotropins and undergo degeneration. This leads to a tall stature with abnormal body proportions in which the lower part of the body is longer than the upper part. Later in life, the body build may become heavy, with a female distribution of subcutaneous fat and variable degrees of breast enlargement. There may be deficient secondary male sex characteristics, such as a voice that remains feminine in pitch and sparse beard and pubic hair. Although the intellect usually is normal, most 47,XXY males have some degree of language impairment.[19]

Adequate management of Klinefelter syndrome requires a comprehensive neurodevelopmental evaluation. Males with Klinefelter syndrome have congenital hypogonadism and decreased sperm count. **Androgen** therapy is usually initiated when there is evidence of a testosterone deficit. If sperm are present, cryopreservation may be useful for future family planning.[19] However, genetic counseling is advised because of the increased risk of autosomal and sex chromosomal abnormalities.

Mitochondrial Gene Disorders

The mitochondria contain their own DNA, which is distinct from the DNA contained in the cell nucleus. Although the majority of inherited disorders come from nuclear DNA abnormalities, there are multiple disease causing rearrangements and mutations that can occur in mitochondrial DNA (mtDNA). This DNA is packaged in a double-stranded circular chromosome and contains 37 genes: 2 ribosomal RNA genes, 22 transfer RNA genes, and 13 structural genes encoding subunits of the mitochondrial respiratory chain enzymes, which participate in oxidative phosphorylation and generation of adenosine triphosphate.

Because mtDNA is inherited only from the mother, all disorders of mtDNA are also inherited on the maternal line. Ova contain numerous mitochondria in their abundant cytoplasm, whereas spermatozoa contain few, if any, mitochondria. Thus, the mtDNA in the zygote is derived solely from the mother. The zygote and its daughter cells have many mitochondria, allowing for a mixture of normal and mutant DNA. The clinical expression of a disease produced by a given mutation of mtDNA depends on the total content of mitochondrial genes and the proportion that is mutant.

mtDNA mutations generally affect tissues that are dependent on oxidative phosphorylation to meet their high needs for metabolic energy. Thus, mtDNA mutations frequently affect the neuromuscular system and produce disorders such as encephalopathies, myopathies, retinal degeneration, loss of extraocular muscle function, and deafness. The range of mitochondrial diseases is broad, however, and may include liver dysfunction, bone marrow failure, and pancreatic islet cell dysfunction and diabetes, among other disorders. Table 5-2 describes representative examples of disorders due to mutations in mtDNA.

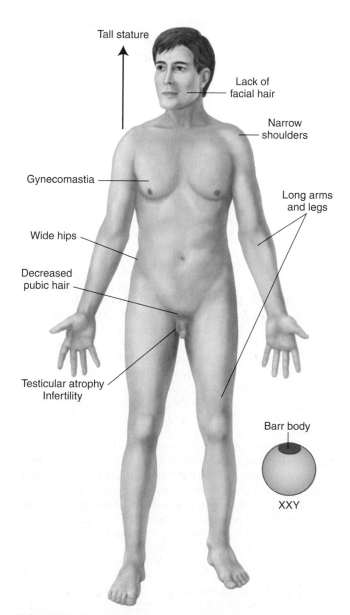

Tall stature

Lack of facial hair

Narrow shoulders

Gynecomastia

Long arms and legs

Wide hips

Decreased pubic hair

Testicular atrophy Infertility

Barr body

XXY

FIGURE 5-11. Clinical features of Klinefelter syndrome.

TABLE 5-2 Some Disorders of Organ Systems Associated with Mitochondrial DNA Mutations

Disorder	Manifestations
Chronic progressive external ophthalmoplegia	Progressive weakness of the extraocular muscles
Deafness	Progressive sensorineural deafness, often associated with aminoglycoside antibiotics
Kearns–Sayre syndrome	Progressive weakness of the extraocular muscles of early onset with heart block, retinal pigmentation
Leber hereditary optic neuropathy	Painless, subacute, bilateral visual loss, with central blind spots (scotomas) and abnormal color vision
Leigh disease	Proximal muscle weakness, sensory neuropathy, developmental delay, ataxia, seizures, dementia, and visual impairment due to retinal pigment degeneration
MELAS	Mitochondrial *e*ncephalomyopathy (cerebral structural changes), *l*actic *a*cidosis, and *s*trokelike syndrome, seizures, and other clinical and laboratory abnormalities; may manifest only as diabetes mellitus
MERRF	*M*yoclonic *e*pilepsy, *r*agged *r*ed *f*ibers in muscle, ataxia, sensorineural deafness
Myoclonic epilepsy with ragged red fibers	Myoclonic seizures, cerebellar ataxia, mitochondrial **myopathy** (muscle weakness, fatigue)

 SUMMARY CONCEPTS

Genetic disorders can affect a single gene (mendelian inheritance) or several genes (polygenic inheritance). Single-gene mutations may be present on an autosome or on the X chromosome, and they may be expressed as a dominant or recessive trait. In autosomal dominant disorders, the affected parent has a 50% chance of transmitting the disorder to each offspring. Autosomal recessive disorders are manifested only when both members of the gene pair are affected. Usually, both parents are unaffected but are carriers of the defective gene. Their chances of having an affected child are one in four; of having a carrier child, two in four; and of having a noncarrier, unaffected child, one in four. X-linked recessive disorders, which are associated with the X chromosome, are typically transmitted by an unaffected carrier mother, who carries one normal X chromosome and one mutant X chromosome. She has a 50% chance of transmitting the defective gene to her sons, who are affected, and her daughters have a 50% chance of being carriers of the mutant gene. Because of a normal paired gene, female heterozygotes rarely experience the effects of a defective gene. X-linked dominant disorders are less common than X-linked recessive, but do exist. Multifactorial inheritance disorders are caused by multiple genes and, in many cases, environmental factors.

Chromosomal disorders result from a change in chromosome number or structure. A change in chromosome number is called *aneuploidy.* *Monosomy* involves the presence of only one member of a chromosome pair. *Polysomy* refers to the presence of more than two chromosomes in a set. Alterations in chromosome structure involve deletion or addition of genetic material, or a translocation of genetic material from one chromosome pair to another.

The mitochondria contain their own DNA, which is distinct from nuclear DNA. This mtDNA is only inherited maternally. Disorders of mitochondrial genes interfere with oxidative phosphorylation and the production of cellular energy. The range of mitochondrial gene disorders is diverse, with neuromuscular disorders predominating.

Disorders due to Environmental Influences

The developing embryo is subject to many nongenetic influences. After conception, development is influenced by the environmental factors that the embryo shares with the mother. The physiologic status of the mother—her hormone balance, her general state of health, her nutritional status, and the drugs she takes undoubtedly influences the development of the unborn child. For example, maternal smoking is associated with lower than normal neonatal weight. Maternal use of alcohol is known to cause fetal abnormalities. Various drugs can cause early miscarriage. Measles and other infectious agents cause congenital malformations. Other agents, such as radiation, can cause chromosomal and genetic defects and produce developmental disorders.

Period of Vulnerability

The embryo's development is most easily disturbed during the period when differentiation and development of the organs are taking place. This time interval, which is often referred to as the period of *organogenesis*, extends from day 15 to day 60 after conception. Environmental influences during the first 2 weeks after fertilization may interfere with implantation and result in abortion or early **resorption** of the products of conception. Each organ has a critical period during which it is highly susceptible to environmental derangements (Fig. 5-12).

Teratogenic Agents

A teratogenic agent is a chemical, physical, or biologic agent that produces abnormalities during embryonic or fetal development. Maternal disease or altered metabolic state also can affect the development of the embryo or fetus. Theoretically, teratogenic agents can cause birth defects in three ways:

1. By direct exposure of the pregnant female and the embryo or fetus to the agent.
2. Through exposure of the soon to be pregnant female to an agent that has a slow clearance rate, such that a teratogenic dose is retained during early pregnancy.

3. As a result of **mutagenic** effects of an environmental agent that occur before pregnancy, causing permanent damage to a female's or a male's reproductive cells.

For the purposes of discussion, teratogenic agents have been divided into three groups: radiation, drugs and chemical substances, and infectious agents. Chart 5-1 lists commonly identified agents in each of these groups.

Radiation

Heavy doses of ionizing radiation are teratogenic and mutagenic and have the capacity to effect inheritable changes in genetic materials. Specifically, excessive levels of radiation have been shown to cause microcephaly, skeletal malformations, and mental retardation. There is no evidence that *diagnostic* levels of radiation (*e.g.*, from a chest x-ray) cause congenital abnormalities, but all efforts to shield the fetus are taken when possible. In situations where a study is necessary for the woman's health, the benefits to her of having proper diagnostic imaging must outweigh potential theoretical risks to the fetus.

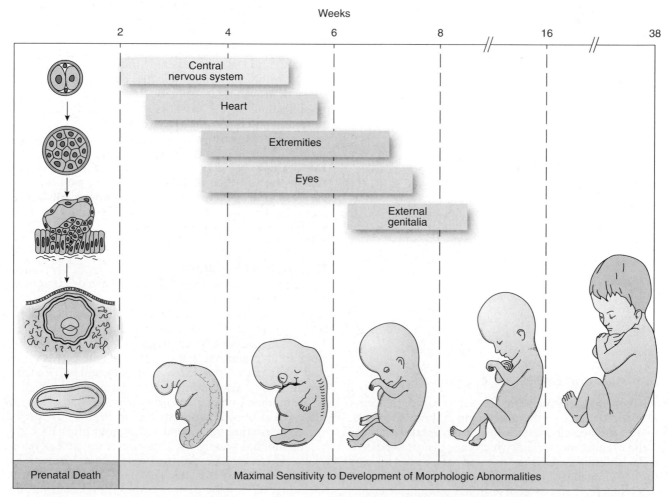

FIGURE 5-12. Sensitivity of specific organs to teratogenic agents at critical periods in embryogenesis. Exposure to adverse influences in the preimplantation and early postimplantation stages of development (*far left*) leads to prenatal death. Periods of maximal sensitivity to teratogens (*horizontal bars*) vary for different organ systems, but overall are limited to the first 8 weeks of pregnancy. (From Strayer D. S., Rubin E. (Eds.) (2015). *Rubin's pathology: Clinicopathologic foundations of medicine* (7th ed., Fig. 6-2, p. 246). Philadelphia, PA: Lippincott Williams & Wilkins.)

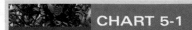

CHART 5-1

TERATOGENIC AGENTS*

Radiation

Drugs and Chemical Substances

Alcohol

Anticoagulants

  Warfarin

Antibiotics

  Quinolones

  Tetracycline

Antiepileptics

Anti-hypertension

  Angiotensin-converting enzyme inhibitors,
  angiotensin II receptor blockers

Antipsychotics

  Lithium

Cancer drugs

  Aminopterin

  Methotrexate

  6-Mercaptopurine

Isotretinoin (Accutane)

Thalidomide

Infectious Agents

Viruses

  Cytomegalovirus

  Herpes simplex virus

  Measles (rubella)

  Mumps

  Varicella-zoster virus (chickenpox)

Nonviral factors

  Syphilis

  Toxoplasmosis

*Not inclusive.

Chemicals and Drugs

Environmental chemicals and drugs can cross the placenta and cause damage to the developing embryo and fetus. Some of the best-documented environmental teratogens are the organic mercurials, which cause neurologic deficits and blindness. Certain fish and water sources may be contaminated by mercury. The precise mechanisms by which chemicals and drugs exert their teratogenic effects are largely unknown. They may produce cytotoxic (cell killing), antimetabolic, or growth-inhibiting effects to the embryonic and fetal development.

Drugs top the list of chemical teratogens. Many drugs can cross the placenta and expose the fetus to both the pharmacologic and teratogenic effects. Factors that affect placental drug transfer and drug effects on the fetus include the rate at which the drug crosses the placenta, the duration of exposure, and the stage of placental and fetal development at the time of exposure. Lipid-soluble drugs tend to cross the placenta more readily and enter the fetal circulation. The molecular weight of a drug also influences the rate and amount of drug transferred across the placenta.

Several medications have been considered teratogenic. However, perhaps the best known of these drugs is thalidomide, which has been shown to give rise to a full range of malformations, including phocomelia (*i.e.*, short, flipper-like appendages) of all four extremities. Other drugs known to cause fetal abnormalities are those used in the treatment of cancer, the anticoagulant drug warfarin, several of the anticonvulsant drugs, ethyl alcohol, and cocaine. More recently, vitamin A and its derivatives (the retinoids) have been targeted for concern because of their teratogenic potential. Concern over the teratogenic effects of vitamin A derivatives arose with the introduction of the acne drug isotretinoin (Accutane).

In 1983, the U.S. Food and Drug Administration (FDA) established a system for classifying drugs according to probable risks to the fetus. According to this system, drugs are put into five categories: A, B, C, D, and X. Drugs in category A are the least dangerous, and categories B, C, and D are increasingly more dangerous. Those in category X are contraindicated during pregnancy because of proven teratogenicity. Recently, the FDA added modifications to the categories with narrative descriptions and potential reproductive risks.[21]

Because many drugs are suspected of causing fetal abnormalities, and even those that were once thought to be safe are now being viewed critically, it is recommended that women in their childbearing years avoid unnecessary use of drugs. This pertains to nonpregnant women as well as pregnant women because many developmental defects occur early in pregnancy.

Fetal Alcohol Syndrome

A drug that is often abused and can have deleterious effects on the fetus is alcohol. The term *fetal alcohol syndrome* (FAS) refers to a group of physical, behavioral, and cognitive fetal abnormalities that occur secondary to drinking alcohol while pregnant.[21] Alcohol, which is lipid soluble and has a molecular weight between 600 and 1000, passes freely across the placental barrier. Concentrations of alcohol in the fetus are at least as high as in the mother. Unlike many other teratogens, the harmful effects of alcohol are not restricted to the sensitive period of early gestation but extend throughout pregnancy.

Alcohol has widely variable effects on fetal development. There may be prenatal or postnatal growth retardation; central nervous system (CNS) involvement, including neurologic abnormalities, developmental delays, behavioral dysfunction, intellectual impairment, and skull and brain malformation; and a characteristic set of facial features that include small palpebral **fissures** (*i.e.*, eye openings), a thin vermilion border (upper lip), and an elongated, flattened midface and

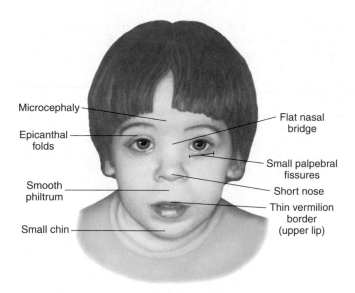

Microcephaly

Epicanthal folds

Smooth philtrum

Small chin

Flat nasal bridge

Small palpebral fissures

Short nose

Thin vermilion border (upper lip)

FIGURE 5-13. Clinical features of fetal alcohol syndrome.

philtrum (*i.e.*, the groove in the middle of the upper lip) (Fig. 5-13).[22] The facial features of FAS may not be as apparent in the newborn but become more prominent as the infant develops. As the children grow into adulthood, the facial features become more subtle, making diagnosis of FAS in older people more difficult. Each of these defects can vary in severity, probably reflecting the timing of alcohol consumption in terms of the period of fetal development, amount of alcohol consumed, and hereditary and other environmental influences.

The amount of alcohol that can be safely consumed during pregnancy is unknown. Even small amounts of alcohol consumed during critical periods of fetal development may be teratogenic. For example, if alcohol is consumed during the period of organogenesis, a variety of skeletal and organ defects may result. If alcohol is consumed later in gestation, when the brain is undergoing rapid development, there may be behavioral and cognitive disorders in the absence of physical abnormalities. Chronic alcohol consumption throughout pregnancy may result in a variety of effects, ranging from physical abnormalities to growth retardation and compromised CNS functioning. Evidence suggests that short-lived high concentrations of alcohol, such as those that occur with binge drinking, may be particularly significant, with abnormalities being unique to the period of exposure.[22] Because of the possible effect on the fetus, it is recommended that women abstain completely from alcohol during pregnancy.

Infectious Agents

Many microorganisms cross the placenta and enter the fetal circulation, often producing multiple malformations. The acronym TORCH stands for *t*oxoplasmosis, *o*ther, *r*ubella (*i.e.*, German measles), *c*ytomegalovirus, and *h*erpes, which are the agents most frequently implicated in fetal anomalies.[16] Other infections that can cause fetal anomalies include varicella-zoster virus infection, listeriosis, leptospirosis, Epstein–Barr virus infection, tuberculosis, and syphilis.[16] Human immunodeficiency virus and human parvovirus (B19) have been suggested as

KEY POINTS

Teratogenic Agents

■ Teratogenic agents such as radiation, chemicals and drugs, and infectious organisms are agents that produce abnormalities in the developing embryo.

■ The stage of development of the embryo determines the susceptibility to teratogens. The period during which the embryo is most susceptible to teratogenic agents is the time during which rapid differentiation and development of body organs and tissues are taking place, usually from days 15 to 60 postconception.

other potential additions to the list. Common clinical and pathologic manifestations include growth retardation and abnormalities of the brain (microcephaly, hydrocephalus), eye, ear, liver, hematopoietic system (anemia, thrombocytopenia), lungs (pneumonitis), and heart (myocarditis, congenital heart disorders).[16] These manifestations will vary among symptomatic newborns, however, and only a few present with multisystem abnormalities.

Folic Acid Deficiency

Although most birth defects are related to exposure to a teratogenic agent, deficiencies of nutrients and vitamins also may be a factor. Folic acid deficiency has been implicated in the development of neural tube defects (NTDs) (*e.g.*, anencephaly, spina bifida, encephalocele). Studies have shown a significant decrease in NTDs when folic acid was taken long term by women of reproductive age. Therefore, it is recommended that all women of childbearing age receive 400 µg (0.4 mg) of folic acid daily and then continue upon becoming pregnant.

SUMMARY CONCEPTS

A teratogenic agent is one that produces abnormalities during embryonic or fetal life. It is during the early part of pregnancy (15 to 60 days after conception) that environmental agents are most apt to produce their deleterious effects on the developing embryo. A number of environmental agents can be damaging to the unborn child, including radiation, drugs and chemicals, and infectious agents. Because many drugs have the potential for causing fetal abnormalities, often at an early stage of pregnancy, it is recommended that women of childbearing age avoid unnecessary use of drugs.

Diagnosis and Counseling

Genetic Assessment

Assessment of genetic risk and prognosis usually is directed by a clinical geneticist, often with the aid of laboratory and clinical specialists. A detailed family history (*i.e.*, pedigree), a pregnancy history, and detailed accounts of the birth process and postnatal health and development are included. A careful physical examination of the affected child and often of the parents and siblings usually is needed. Laboratory tests, including chromosomal analysis and biochemical studies, often precede a definitive diagnosis.

Prenatal Screening and Diagnosis

The purpose of prenatal screening and diagnosis is not only to detect fetal abnormalities but also to allay anxiety and provide assistance to prepare for a child with a specific disability. Prenatal screening cannot be used to rule out all possible fetal abnormalities. It is limited to determining whether the fetus has (or probably has) predesignated conditions as indicated by late maternal age, family history, or well-defined risk factors.

There are multiple methods that can assist in diagnosing a fetus regarding genetic disorders, including ultrasonography, maternal serum (blood) screening tests, amniocentesis, chorionic villus sampling, and percutaneous umbilical fetal blood sampling (Fig. 5-14). Prenatal diagnosis can also provide the information needed for prescribing prenatal treatment for the fetus or making appropriate plans for the birth of a child with a known disease.

Ultrasonography

Ultrasonography is a noninvasive diagnostic method that uses reflections of high-frequency sound waves to visualize soft tissue structures. Since its introduction in 1958, it has been used during pregnancy to determine the number of fetuses, fetal size and position, amount of amniotic fluid, and placental location. But improved resolution and real-time units have enhanced the ability of ultrasound scanners to detect congenital anomalies. Ultrasonography makes possible the in utero diagnosis of cardiac defects, hydrocephalus, spina bifida, facial

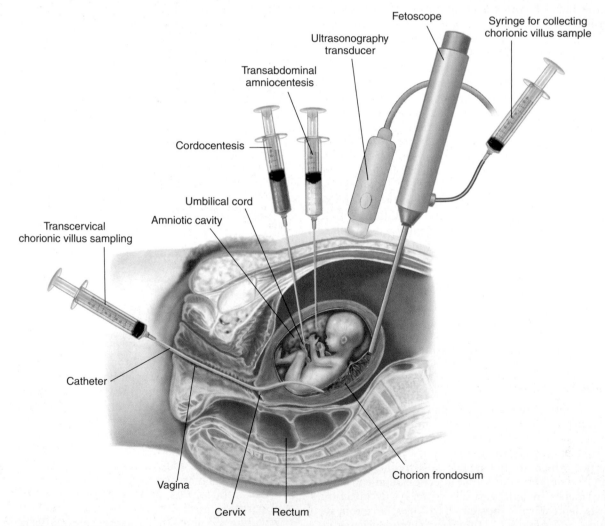

FIGURE 5-14. Methods of prenatal screening.

defects, congenital heart defects, congenital diaphragmatic hernias, disorders of the gastrointestinal tract, skeletal anomalies, and various other defects. Three-dimensional sonography has become useful in better assessing facial profiles and abdominal wall defects. A fetal echocardiogram can be done as follow-up for possible cardiac anomalies. Fetal magnetic resonance imaging can be done to better assess skeletal, neurologic, and other anomalies. Intrauterine diagnosis of congenital abnormalities permits better monitoring, further workup and planning with appropriate specialties, preterm delivery for early correction, selection of cesarean section to reduce fetal injury, and, in some cases, intrauterine therapy.

Maternal Serum Markers

Maternal blood testing began in the early 1980s. Current maternal testing favors first trimester screening for all women between 11 and 13 weeks combining nuchal translucency seen on sonogram with PAPP-A level, hCG level, and maternal age to determine a risk for trisomy 21, 13, and 18. PAPP-A, which is secreted by the placenta, has been shown to play an important role in promoting cell differentiation and proliferation in various body systems. When used along with maternal age, free β-hCG, and ultrasonographic measurement of nuchal translucency, serum PAPP-A levels can reportedly detect 85% to 95% of affected pregnancies with a false-positive rate of approximately 5%.

The quad screen checks for markers of four substances—AFP, hCG, estriol, and inhibin A—providing a formula for the probability of carrying a child with a chromosomal abnormality.

AFP is a major fetal plasma protein made initially by the yolk sac, gastrointestinal tract, and liver. Fetal plasma levels of AFP peak at approximately 10 to 13 weeks' gestation and decrease until the third trimester when the level peaks again. Maternal and amniotic fluid levels of AFP are elevated in pregnancies where the fetus has an NTD or certain other malformations such as an **anterior** abdominal wall defect. Although NTDs have been associated with elevated levels of AFP, decreased levels have been associated with Down syndrome.

A complex glycoprotein, hCG, is produced exclusively by the outer layer of the trophoblast shortly after implantation in the uterine wall. It increases rapidly in the first 8 weeks of gestation, declines steadily until 20 weeks, and then plateaus. The single maternal serum marker that yields the highest detection rate for Down syndrome is an elevated level of hCG. Inhibin A, which is secreted by the corpus luteum and fetoplacental unit, is also a maternal serum marker for fetal Down syndrome.

Unconjugated estriol is produced by the placenta from precursors provided by the fetal adrenal glands and liver. It increases steadily throughout pregnancy to a higher level than that normally produced by the liver. Unconjugated estriol levels are decreased in Down syndrome and trisomy 18.

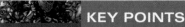

KEY POINTS

Diagnosis and Counseling

■ Sonography, first trimester screening, quad screening, amniocentesis, chorionic villi sampling, and percutaneous umbilical cord blood sampling are important procedures that allow prenatal diagnosis and management.

Amniocentesis

Amniocentesis is an invasive diagnostic procedure that involves the withdrawal of a sample of amniotic fluid from the pregnant uterus usually using a transabdominal approach (see Fig. 5-14). The procedure is useful in women with elevated risk on first trimester screen or quad screen, abnormal fetal findings on sonogram, or in parents who are carriers or with a strong family history of an inherited disease. Ultrasonography is used to gain additional information and to guide the placement of the amniocentesis needle. The amniotic fluid and cells that have been shed by the fetus are studied. Amniocentesis can be performed on an outpatient basis starting at 15 weeks. For chromosomal analysis, the fetal cells are grown in culture and the result is available in 10 to 14 days.

Chorionic Villus Sampling

Chorionic villus sampling is an invasive diagnostic procedure that obtains tissue that can be used for fetal chromosome studies, DNA analysis, and biochemical studies. Sampling of the chorionic villi usually is done after 10 weeks' gestation. Performing the test before 10 weeks is not recommended because of the danger of limb reduction defects in the fetus. The chorionic villi are the site of exchange of nutrients between the maternal blood and the embryo—the chorionic sac encloses the early amniotic sac and fetus, and the villi are the primitive blood vessels that develop into the placenta. The sampling procedure can be performed using either a transabdominal or transcervical approach (see Fig. 5-14).

Percutaneous Umbilical Cord Blood Sampling

Percutaneous umbilical cord blood sampling is an invasive diagnostic procedure that involves the transcutaneous insertion of a needle through the uterine wall and into the umbilical artery. It is performed under ultrasonographic guidance and can be done any time after 16 weeks' gestation. It is used for prenatal diagnosis of hemoglobinopathies, coagulation disorders, metabolic and cytogenetic disorders, and immunodeficiencies. Fetal infections such as rubella and toxoplasmosis can be detected through measurement of immunoglobulin M antibodies or direct blood cultures. Because the procedure carries a greater risk of pregnancy loss compared to amniocentesis, it is usually reserved for situations in which rapid cytogenetic analysis is needed or in which diagnostic information cannot be obtained by other methods.

Cytogenetic and DNA Analyses

Amniocentesis and chorionic villus sampling yield cells that can be used for cytogenetic and DNA analyses. Cytogenetic studies are used for fetal karyotyping to detect abnormalities of chromosome number and structure in the fetus. Karyotyping also reveals the sex of the fetus. This may be useful when an inherited defect is known to affect only one sex.

Analysis of DNA can be done on cells extracted from the amniotic fluid, chorionic villi, or fetal blood from percutaneous umbilical sampling. These analyses are used to detect genetic defects that cause inborn errors of metabolism, such as Tay–Sachs disease, glycogen storage diseases, and familial hypercholesterolemia. Prenatal diagnoses are possible for more than 70 inborn errors of metabolism.

The newest realm of fetal diagnosis involves looking at fetal DNA in the maternal blood. Some private companies and many research institutions are exploring the efficacy of looking at fetal DNA for sex determination and other genetic testing. More research is needed before this will be offered to all women.

 SUMMARY CONCEPTS

Genetic and prenatal diagnosis and counseling are done in an effort to determine the risk of having a child with a genetic or chromosomal disorder. They often involve a detailed family history (*i.e.*, pedigree), examination of any affected and other family members, and laboratory studies including chromosomal analysis and biochemical studies. These examinations are usually done by a genetic counselor and a specially prepared team of health care professionals. Prenatal screening and diagnosis are used to detect fetal abnormalities. Ultrasonography is used for fetal anatomic imaging. It is used for determination of fetal size and position and for the presence of structural anomalies. Maternal serum screening is used to identify pregnancies that are at increased risk for some disorders. Amniocentesis and chorionic villus sampling may be used to obtain specimens for cytogenetic and biochemical studies.

Review Exercises

1. A 23-year-old woman with sickle cell disease and her husband want to have a child but worry that the child will be born with the disease.

   A. What is the mother's genotype in terms of the sickle cell gene? Is she heterozygous or homozygous?
   B. If the husband is found not to have the sickle cell gene, what is the probability of their child having the disease or being a carrier of the sickle cell trait?

2. A couple has a child who was born with a congenital heart disease.

   A. Would you consider the defect to be the result of a single gene or a polygenic trait?
   B. Would these parents be at greater risk of having another child with a heart defect or would they be at equal risk of having a child with a defect in another organ system, such as cleft palate?

3. A couple has been informed that their newborn child has the features of Down syndrome, and it is suggested that genetic studies be performed.

   A. The child is found to have trisomy 21. Use Figure 5-8, which describes the events that occur during meiosis, to explain the origin of the third chromosome 21.
   B. If the child had been found to have the robertsonian chromosome, how would you explain the origin of the abnormal chromosome?

4. An 8-year-old boy has been diagnosed with mitochondrial myopathy. His major complaints are those of muscle weakness and exercise intolerance. His mother gives a report of similar symptoms, but to a much lesser degree.

   A. Explain the cause of this boy's symptoms.
   B. Mitochondrial disorders follow a non-mendelian pattern of inheritance. Explain.

5. A 26-year-old woman is planning to become pregnant.

   A. What information would you give her regarding the effects of medications and drugs on the fetus? What stage of fetal development is associated with the greatest risk?
   B. What is the rationale for ensuring that she has an adequate intake of folic acid before conception?

REFERENCES

1. Centers for Disease Control and Prevention. (2007). Birth defects and congenital abnormalities. [Online]. Available: https://www.cdc.gov/nchs/fastats/birth-defects.htm. Accessed November 15, 2017.
2. Malik S. (2014). Polydactyly: Phenotypes, genetics and classification. *Clinical Genetics* 85(3), 203–212. doi:10.1111/cge.12276.

3. Verstraeten A., Alaerts M., Van Laer L., et al. (2016). Marfan syndrome and related disorders: 25 years of gene discovery. *Human Mutation* 37(6), 524–531. doi:10.1002/humu.22977.

4. Hirbe A. C., Gutmann D. H. (2014). Neurofibromatosis type 1: A multidisciplinary approach to care. *Lancet Neurology* 13(8), 834–843. doi:10.1016/S1474-4422(14)70063-8.

5. Berry S. A., Brown C., Grant M., et al. (2013). Newborn screening 50 years later: Access issues faced by adults with PKU. *Genetics in Medicine* 5(8), 591–599. doi:10.1038/gim.2013.10.

6. Kresak J. L., Walsh M. (2016). Neurofibromatosis: A review of NF1, NF2, and schwannomatosis. *Journal of Pediatric Genetics* 5(2), 98–104. doi:10.1055/s-0036-1579766.

7. Abdolrahimzadeh B., Piraino D. C., Albanese G., et al. (2016). Neurofibromatosis: An update of ophthalmic characteristics and applications of optical coherence tomography. *Clinical Ophthalmology* 10, 851–860. doi:10.2147/OPTH.S102830.

8. Bernier A., Larbrisseau A., Perreault S. (2016). Cafe-au-lait macules and neurofibromatosis type 1: A review of the literature. *Pediatric Neurology* 60, 24.e1–29.e1. doi:10.1016/j.pediatrneurol.2016.03.003.

9. Al Hafid N., Christodoulou J. (2015). Phenylketonuria: A review of current and future treatments. *Translational Pediatrics* 4(4), 304–317. doi:10.3978/j.issn.2224-4336.2015.10.07.

10. Patterson M. C. (2013). Gangliosidoses. *Handbook of Clinical Neurology* 113, 1707–1708. doi:10.1016/B978-0-444-59565-2.00039-3.

11. Lew R. M., Burnett L., Proos A. L., et al. (2015). Ashkenazi Jewish population screening for Tay-Sachs disease: The international and Australian experience. *Journal of Paediatrics and Child Health* 51(3), 271–279. doi:10.1111/jpc.12632.

12. Kidd S. A., Lachiewicz A., Barbouth D., et al. (2014). Fragile X syndrome: A review of associated medical problems. *Pediatrics* 134(5), 995–1005. doi:10.1542/peds.2013-4301.

13. Bagni C., Oostra B. A. (2013). Fragile X syndrome: From protein function to therapy. *American Journal of Medical Genetics*. Part A 161A(11), 2809–2821. doi:10.1002/ajmg.a.36241.

14. Seto-Salvia N., Stanier P. (2014). Genetics of cleft lip and/or cleft palate: Association with other common anomalies. *European Journal of Medical Genetics* 57(8), 381–393. doi:10.1016/j.ejmg.2014.04.003.

15. Smith D. M., Losee J. E. (2014). Cleft palate repair. *Clinics in Plastic Surgery* 41(2), 189–210. doi:10.1016/j.cps.2013.12.005.

16. Strayer D. S., Rubin E. (Eds.) (2015). *Rubin's pathology: Clinicopathologic foundations of medicine* (7th ed.). Philadelphia, PA: Wolters Kluwer.

17. Asim A., Kumar A., Muthuswamy S., et al. (2015). Down syndrome: An insight of the disease. *Journal of Biomedical Science* 22, 41. doi:10.1186/s12929-015-0138-y.

18. Groth K. A., Skakkebaek A., Host C., et al. (2013). Clinical review: Klinefelter syndrome—A clinical update. *Journal of Clinical Endocrinology and Metabolism* 98(1), 20–30. doi:10.1210/jc.2012-2382.

19. Milbrandt T., Thomas E. (2013). Turner syndrome. *Pediatrics in Review* 34(9), 420–421. doi:10.1542/pir.34-9-420.

20. Burkey B. W., Holmes A. P. (2013). Evaluating medication use in pregnancy and lactation: What every pharmacist should know. *Journal of Pediatric Pharmacology and Therapeutics* 18(3), 247–258. doi:10.5863/1551-6776-18.3.247.

21. Memo L., Gnoato E., Caminiti S. (2013). Fetal alcohol spectrum disorders and fetal alcohol syndrome: The state of the art and new diagnostic tools. *Early Human Development* 89(Suppl 1), S40–S43. doi:10.1016/S0378-3782(13)70013-6.

22. Burdge G. C., Lillycrop K. A. (2012). Folic acid supplementation in pregnancy: Are there devils in the detail? *British Journal of Nutrition* 108(11), 1924–1930. doi:10.1017/S0007114512003765.

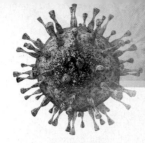

Neoplasia

Characteristics of Benign and Malignant Neoplasms

Terminology
Benign Neoplasms
Malignant Neoplasms
  Cancer Cell Characteristics
  Invasion and Metastasis
  Tumor Growth

Etiology of Cancer

Genetic and Molecular Basis of Cancer
  Cancer-Associated Genes
  Epigenetic Mechanisms
  Molecular and Cellular
    Pathways
  Role of the Microenvironment
  Carcinogenesis
Host and Environmental Factors
  Heredity
  Hormones
  Immunologic Mechanisms
  Chemical Carcinogens
  Radiation
  Oncogenic Viruses

Clinical Manifestations

Tissue Integrity
Systemic Manifestations
  Anorexia and Cachexia
  Fatigue and Sleep Disorders
  Anemia

Screening, Diagnosis, and Treatment

Screening
Diagnostic Methods
  Tumor Markers
  Cytologic and Histologic Methods
  Staging and Grading of Tumors
Cancer Treatment
  Surgery
  Radiation Therapy
  Chemotherapy
  Hormonal Therapy
  Biotherapy

Childhood Cancers

Incidence and Types
  Embryonal Tumors
Biology of Childhood Cancers
Diagnosis and Treatment
  Radiation Therapy
  Chemotherapy

Learning Objectives

After completing this chapter, the learner will be able to meet the following objectives:

1. Relate the properties of cell differentiation to the development of a cancer cell clone and the behavior of the tumor.
2. Trace the pathway for hematologic spread of a metastatic cancer cell.
3. Use the concepts of growth fraction and doubling time to explain the growth of cancerous tissue.
4. Describe various types of cancer-associated genes and cancer-associated cellular and molecular pathways.
5. Describe genetic events and epigenetic factors that are important in tumorigenesis.
6. State the importance of cancer stem cells, angiogenesis, and the cell microenvironment in cancer growth and metastasis.
7. Characterize the mechanisms involved in anorexia and cachexia, fatigue, sleep disorders, anemia, and venous thrombosis experienced by people with cancer.
8. Define the term *paraneoplastic syndrome* and explain its pathogenesis and manifestations.
9. Compare the different screening mechanisms for cancer.
10. Differentiate among the three types of cancer treatment (curative, control, and palliative), considering the risks and benefits of each approach.
11. Cite the most common types of cancer affecting infants, children, and adolescents.
12. Describe how cancers that affect children differ from those that affect adults.

Cancer is a leading cause of death in adults worldwide, second only to cardiovascular disease.[1] It is the second leading cause of death in school-aged children in the United States.[2] Exposure to external factors such as tobacco, ultraviolet radiation, unhealthy diet, infectious agents, and carcinogens as well as internal factors such as gender, ethnicity, and genetics affect the incidence of cancer.[3] Research has led to an enhanced understanding of the causes of cancer and improved screening tools and prevention modalities.[3] Survival rates are affected by the type of cancer, stage at diagnosis, and what or if treatment is available.[4] Review of previous chapters on cell differentiation, growth, and division will provide a foundation for understanding this chapter.

This chapter is divided into five sections:

- Characteristics of benign and malignant neoplasms
- Etiology of cancer
- Clinical manifestations
- Diagnosis and treatment
- Childhood cancers

Characteristics of Benign and Malignant Neoplasms

Terminology

Traditionally, by definition, a *tumor* is a swelling that can be caused by a number of conditions, including inflammation and trauma. In addition, the term has been used to define a mass of cells that arises because of overgrowth. Although not synonymous, the terms *tumor* and *neoplasm* often are used interchangeably. The term *neoplasm* refers to an abnormal mass of tissue in which the growth exceeds and is uncoordinated with that of the normal tissues. Unlike normal cellular adaptive processes such as hypertrophy and hyperplasia, neoplasms do not obey the laws of normal cell growth. They serve no useful purpose, they do not occur in response to an appropriate stimulus, and they continue to grow at the expense of the host. Neoplasms usually are classified as benign or malignant. Neoplasms that contain well-differentiated cells (cell differentiation is the process whereby proliferating cells become progressively more specialized cell types) that are clustered together in a single mass are considered to be **benign**. These tumors usually do not cause death unless their location or size interferes with vital functions. In contrast, *malignant neoplasms* are less well differentiated and have the ability to break loose, enter the circulatory or lymphatic system, and form secondary malignant tumors at other sites.

Tumors usually are named by adding the suffix *-oma* to the **parenchymal** tissue type from which the growth originated.[5] Thus, a benign tumor of glandular epithelial tissue is called an *adenoma*, and a benign tumor of bone tissue is called an *osteoma*. The term *carcinoma* is used to designate a malignant tumor of epithelial tissue origin. In the case of a malignant tumor of glandular epithelial tissue, the term *adenocarcinoma* is used.

Oncology is the study of tumors and their treatment. Table 6-1 lists the names of selected benign and malignant tumors according to tissue types.

TABLE 6-1 Names of Selected Benign and Malignant Tumors According to Tissue Types

Tissue Type	Benign Tumors	Malignant Tumors
Epithelial		
Surface	Papilloma	Squamous cell carcinoma
Glandular	Adenoma	Adenocarcinoma
Connective		
Fibrous	Fibroma	Fibrosarcoma
Adipose	Lipoma	Liposarcoma
Cartilage	Chondroma	Chondrosarcoma
Bone	Osteoma	Osteosarcoma
Blood vessels	Hemangioma	Hemangiosarcoma
Lymph vessels	Lymphangioma	Lymphangiosarcoma
Lymph tissue		Lymphosarcoma
Muscle		
Smooth	Leiomyoma	Leiomyosarcoma
Striated	Rhabdomyoma	Rhabdomyosarcoma
Neural Tissue		
Nerve cell	Neuroma	Neuroblastoma
Glial tissue	Glioma	Glioblastoma, astrocytoma, medulloblastoma, oligodendroglioma
Nerve sheaths	Neurilemmoma	Neurilemmal sarcoma
Meninges	Meningioma	Meningeal sarcoma
Hematologic		
Granulocytic		Myelocytic leukemia
Erythrocytic		Erythrocytic leukemia
Plasma cells		Multiple myeloma
Lymphocytic		Lymphocytic leukemia or lymphoma
Monocytic		Monocytic leukemia
Endothelial Tissue		
Blood vessels	Hemangioma	Hemangiosarcoma
Lymph vessels	Lymphangioma	Lymphangiosarcoma

TABLE 6-2 Characteristics of Benign and Malignant Neoplasms

Characteristics	Benign	Malignant
Cell characteristics	Well-differentiated cells that resemble cells in the tissue of origin	Cells are undifferentiated, with anaplasia and atypical structure that often bears little resemblance to cells in the tissue of origin
Rate of growth	Usually progressive and slow; may come to a standstill or regress	Variable and depends on level of differentiation; the more undifferentiated the cells, the more rapid the rate of growth
Mode of growth	Grows by expansion without invading the surrounding tissues; usually encapsulated	Grows by invasion, sending out processes that infiltrate the surrounding tissues
Metastasis	Does not spread by metastasis	Gains access to blood and lymph channels to metastasize to other areas of the body

Benign and malignant neoplasms usually are distinguished by the following:

- Cell characteristics
- Rate of growth
- Manner of growth
- Capacity to invade and metastasize to other parts of the body
- Potential for causing death

The characteristics of benign and malignant neoplasms are summarized in Table 6-2.

Benign Neoplasms

Benign tumors are composed of well-differentiated cells that resemble the cells of the tissues of origin and are characterized by a slow, progressive rate of growth that may come to a standstill or regress.[6] For unknown reasons, benign tumors have lost the ability to suppress the genetic program for cell proliferation but have retained the program for normal cell differentiation. They grow by expansion and remain localized to their site of origin, lacking the capacity to infiltrate, invade, or metastasize to distant sites. Because they expand slowly, they develop a surrounding rim of compressed connective tissue called a *fibrous capsule*.[5] The capsule is responsible for a sharp line of demarcation between the benign tumor and the adjacent tissues, a factor that facilitates surgical removal.

Benign tumors are usually much less of a threat to health and well-being than malignant tumors, and they usually do not cause death unless they interfere with vital functions because of their anatomic location. For instance, a benign tumor growing in the cranial cavity can eventually cause death by compressing brain structures. Benign tumors also can cause disturbances in the function of adjacent or distant structures by producing pressure on tissues, blood vessels, or nerves. Some benign tumors are also known for their ability to cause alterations in body function by abnormally producing hormones.

KEY POINTS

Benign and Malignant Neoplasms

- A neoplasm, benign or malignant, represents a new growth.
- Benign neoplasms are well-differentiated tumors that resemble the tissues of origin but have lost the ability to control cell proliferation. They grow by expansion, are enclosed in a fibrous capsule, and do not cause death unless their location is such that it interrupts vital body functions.
- Malignant neoplasms are less well-differentiated tumors that have lost the ability to control both cell proliferation and differentiation. They grow in a disorganized and uncontrolled manner to invade surrounding tissues, have cells that break loose and travel to distant sites to form metastases, and inevitably cause suffering and death unless their growth can be controlled through treatment.

Malignant Neoplasms

Cancer is a disorder of altered cell differentiation and growth. The resulting process is called *neoplasia*, which means "new growth." Unlike changes in tissue growth that occur with hypertrophy and hyperplasia, the growth of a neoplasm tends to be uncoordinated and relatively autonomous in that it lacks normal regulatory controls over cell growth and division.

Malignant neoplasms, which invade and destroy nearby tissue and spread to other parts of the body, tend to grow rapidly and spread widely and have the potential to cause death. Because of their rapid rate of growth, malignant tumors may compress blood vessels and outgrow their blood supply, causing ischemia and tissue injury. Some malignancies secrete hormones or cytokines, release enzymes and toxins, or induce an inflammatory response that injures normal tissue as well as the tumor itself.

There are two categories of malignant neoplasms—solid tumors and hematologic cancers. Solid tumors initially are confined to a specific tissue or organ.

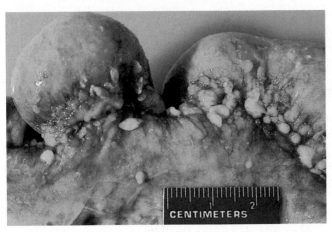

FIGURE 6-1. Peritoneal carcinomatosis. The mesentery attached to a loop of small bowel is studded with small nodules of metastatic ovarian carcinoma. (From Strayer D. S., Rubin R. (Eds.) (2015). *Rubin's pathology: Clinicopathologic foundations of medicine* (7th ed., Figure 5-8, p. 175). Philadelphia, PA: Lippincott Williams & Wilkins.)

As the growth of the primary solid tumor progresses, cells detach from the original tumor mass, invade the surrounding tissue, and enter the blood and lymph systems to spread to distant sites, a process termed **metastasis** (Fig. 6-1). Hematologic cancers involve cells normally found in the blood and lymph, thereby making them **disseminated** diseases from the beginning (Fig. 6-2).

Carcinoma in situ is a localized preinvasive lesion. As an example, in breast ductal carcinoma in situ, the cells have not crossed the basement membrane. Depending on its location, in situ lesions usually can be removed surgically or treated so that the chances of recurrence are small. For example, carcinoma in situ of the cervix is essentially 100% curable.

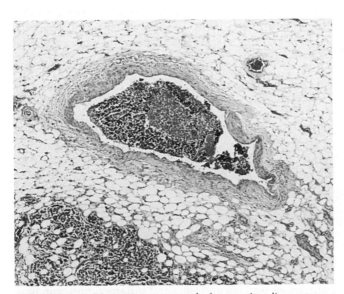

FIGURE 6-2. Hematogenous spread of cancer. A malignant tumor (**bottom**) has attached to adipose tissue and penetrated into a vein. (From Strayer D. S., Rubin R. (Eds.) (2015). *Rubin's pathology: Clinicopathologic foundations of medicine* (7th ed., Figure 5-9, p. 175). Philadelphia, PA: Lippincott Williams & Wilkins.)

Cancer Cell Characteristics

Cancer cells are characterized by two main features—abnormal and rapid proliferation and loss of differentiation. Loss of differentiation means that they do not exhibit normal features and properties of differentiated cells and hence are more similar to embryonic cells.

The term **anaplasia** describes the loss of cell differentiation in cancerous tissue.[5] Undifferentiated cancer cells are marked by a number of morphologic changes. The cells of undifferentiated tumors usually display greater numbers of cells in mitosis because of their high rate of proliferation. They also display atypical, bizarre mitotic figures, sometimes producing spindles (Fig. 6-3B). Advanced anaplastic cancer cells begin to resemble undifferentiated or embryonic cells more than they do their tissue of origin. The cytologic/histologic grading of tumors is based on the degree of differentiation and the number of proliferating cells. The closer the tumor cells resemble comparable normal tissue cells, both morphologically and functionally, the lower the grade. Accordingly, on a scale ranging from grades

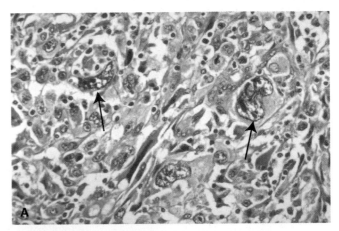

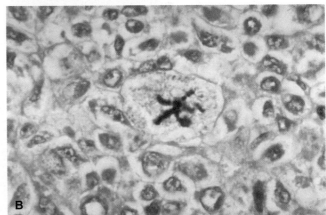

FIGURE 6-3. Anaplastic features of malignant tumors. (**A**) The cells of this anaplastic carcinoma are highly pleomorphic (*i.e.*, they vary in size and shape). The nuclei are hyperchromatic and are large relative to the cytoplasm. Multinucleated tumor giant cells are present (*arrows*). (**B**) A malignant cell in metaphase exhibits an abnormal mitotic figure. (From Strayer D. S., Rubin R. (Eds.) (2015). *Rubin's pathology: Clinicopathologic foundations of medicine* (7th ed., Figure 5-2, p. 171). Philadelphia, PA: Lippincott Williams & Wilkins.)

I to IV, grade I neoplasms are well differentiated, and grade IV are poorly differentiated and display marked anaplasia.[5]

The characteristics of altered proliferation and differentiation are associated with a number of other changes in cell characteristics and function that distinguish cancer cells from their normally differentiated counterparts. These changes are listed in Table 6-3.

Genetic Instability

Most cancer cells exhibit a characteristic called *genetic instability* that is often considered to be a hallmark of cancer. The concept arose after the realization that uncorrected mutations in normal cells are rare because of the numerous cellular mechanisms to prevent them. To account for the high frequency of mutations in cancer cells, it is thought that cancer cells have a "mutation phenotype" with genetic instability that contributes to the development and progression of cancer.[5] Characteristics of genetic instability include aneuploidy, in which chromosomes are lost or gained; intrachromosomal instability, which includes insertions, deletions, and amplifications; microsatellite instability, which involves short, repetitive sequences of deoxyribonucleic acid (DNA); and point mutations.

Growth Factor Independence

Another characteristic of cancer cells is their ability to proliferate even in the absence of growth factors. Breast cancer cells that do not express estrogen receptors are an example. Some cancer cells may produce their own growth factors, whereas others have abnormal receptors or signaling proteins that may inappropriately activate growth signaling pathways in the cells.

Cell Density–Dependent Inhibition

Cancer cells often lose *cell density–dependent inhibition*, which is the cessation of growth after cells reach a certain density. This is sometimes referred to as *contact inhibition* because cells often stop growing when they come into contact with each other. In wound healing, contact inhibition causes tissue growth to cease at the point where the edges of the wound come together. Cancer cells, however, tend to grow rampantly without regard for adjacent tissue.

Anchorage Dependence

Cancer cells also differ from their normal counterparts in attaining anchorage independence. Normal epithelial cells must be anchored to either neighboring cells or the underlying extracellular matrix to live and grow. Cancer cells, however, frequently remain viable and multiply without normal attachments to other cells and the extracellular matrix. Although the process of anchorage independence is complex and incompletely understood, recent studies have made progress in understanding the genes and mechanistic pathways involved.[7]

Cell-to-Cell Communication

Another characteristic of cancer cells is faulty cell-to-cell communication, a feature that may in turn contribute to other characteristics of cancer cells. Impaired cell-to-cell communication may interfere with formation of intercellular connections and responsiveness to membrane-derived signals. For example, changes in gap junction proteins, which enable cytoplasmic continuity and communication between cells, have been described in some types of cancer.[8]

Life Span

Cancer cells differ from normal cells by having an unlimited life span. If normal, noncancerous cells are harvested from the body and grown under culture conditions, most cells divide a limited number of times and fail to divide further. In contrast, cancer cells may divide an infinite number of times. Telomeres shorten with each cell division. When length is diminished sufficiently, chromosomes can no longer replicate, and cell division will not occur. Most cancer cells maintain high levels of telomerase, an enzyme that prevents telomere shortening. This keeps telomeres from aging and attaining the critically short length that is associated with cellular replicative senescence.

Antigen Expression

Cancer cells also express a number of cell surface molecules or **antigens** that are immunologically identified as foreign. The genes of a cell code these *tissue antigens*. Many transformed cancer cells revert to embryonic patterns of gene expression and produce antigens that are immunologically distinct from the antigens that are expressed by cells of the well-differentiated tissue from which the cancer originated. Some cancers express fetal

TABLE 6-3 Comparison of Normal Cell Characteristics with Those of Cancer Cells		
Characteristics	**Normal Cells**	**Cancer Cells**
Growth	Regulated	Unregulated
Differentiation	High	Low
Genetic stability	Stable	Unstable
Growth factor dependence	Dependent	Independent
Density dependent	High	Low inhibition
Cell-to-cell adhesion	High	Low
Anchorage dependence	High	Low
Cell-to-cell communication	High	Low
Cell life span	Limited	Unlimited
Antigen expression	Absent	May be present
Substance production (*e.g.*, proteases, hormones)	Normal	Abnormal
Cytoskeletal composition and arrangement	Normal	Abnormal

antigens that are not produced by comparable cells in the adult. Tumor antigens may be clinically useful as markers to indicate the presence, recurrence, or progressive growth of a cancer.

Production of Enzymes, Hormones, and Other Substances

Cancer cells may produce substances that normal cells of the tissue of origin either do not produce or secrete in lesser amounts. They may also secrete degradative enzymes that enable invasion and metastatic spread. Cancer cells may also assume hormone synthesis or production and secretion of procoagulant substances that affect clotting mechanisms.

Cytoskeletal Changes

Finally, cancer cells may show cytoskeletal changes and abnormalities. These may involve the appearance of abnormal intermediate filament types or changes in actin filaments and microtubules that facilitate invasion and metastasis. Actin, microtubules, and their regulatory proteins remain the focus of many cancer-related investigations.

Invasion and Metastasis

Unlike benign tumors, which grow by expansion and usually are surrounded by a capsule, cancer spreads by direct invasion and extension, seeding of cancer cells in body cavities, and metastatic spread through the blood or lymph pathways. The word *cancer* is derived from the Latin word meaning "crablike" because cancers grow and spread by sending crablike projections into the surrounding tissues. Most cancers synthesize and secrete enzymes that break down proteins and contribute to the infiltration, invasion, and penetration of the surrounding tissues. The lack of a sharp line of demarcation separating them from the surrounding tissue makes the complete surgical removal of malignant tumors more difficult than removal of benign tumors. Often, it is necessary for the surgeon to excise portions of seemingly normal tissue bordering the tumor for the pathologist to establish that cancer-free margins are present around the excised tumor and to ensure that the remaining tissue is cancer-free.

The *seeding* of cancer cells into body cavities occurs when a tumor sheds cells into these spaces. Most often, the peritoneal cavity is involved, but other spaces such as the pleural cavity, pericardial cavity, and joint spaces may also be involved. Seeding into the peritoneal cavity is particularly common with ovarian cancers. Similar to tissue culture, tumors in these sites grow in masses and are often associated with fluid accumulation (*e.g.*, ascites, pleural effusion).[5] Seeding of cancers into other areas of the body is often a postoperative complication after removal of a cancer. The term *metastasis* is used to describe the development of a secondary tumor in a location distant from the primary tumor.[5] Metastatic tumors frequently retain many of the characteristics of the primary tumor from which they were derived. This enables determination of the primary site of the tumor based on cellular characteristics of the metastatic tumor. Some tumors tend to metastasize early in their developmental course, whereas others do not metastasize until later.

Metastasis occurs through the lymph channels and the blood vessels.[5] In many types of cancer, the first evidence of disseminated disease is the presence of tumor cells in the lymph nodes that drain the tumor area. If they survive and grow, the cancer cells may spread from more distant lymph nodes to the thoracic duct and then gain access to the vasculature.

The term *sentinel node* is used to describe the initial lymph node to which the primary tumor drains.[5] Because the initial metastasis in breast cancer is almost always lymphatic, lymphatic spread and therefore extent of disease may be determined through lymphatic mapping and sentinel lymph node biopsy. This is done by injecting a radioactive tracer and/or blue dye into the tumor to determine the first lymph node in the route of lymph drainage from the cancer. Once the sentinel lymph node has been identified, it is examined to determine the presence or absence of cancer cells. The procedure is also used to map the spread of melanoma and other cancers that have their initial metastatic spread through the lymphatic system.

With hematologic spread, the blood-borne cancer cells may enter the venous flow that drains the site of the primary neoplasm. Cancer cells may also enter tumor-associated blood vessels that either infiltrate the tumor or are found at the periphery of the tumor. Before entering the general circulation, venous blood from the gastrointestinal tract, pancreas, and spleen is routed through the portal vein to the liver. The liver is therefore a common site for metastatic spread of cancers that originate in these organs. Although the site of hematologic spread usually is related to vascular drainage of the primary tumor, some tumors metastasize to distant and unrelated sites. One explanation is that cells of different tumors tend to metastasize to specific target organs that provide suitable microenvironments containing substances such as cytokines or growth factors that are needed for their survival.[5] For example, transferrin, a growth-promoting substance isolated from lung tissue, has been found to stimulate the growth of malignant cells that typically metastasize to the lungs. Other organs that are preferential sites for metastasis contain particular cytokines, growth factors, and other microenvironmental characteristics that facilitate metastatic tumor survival and growth.

To metastasize, a cancer cell must be able to break loose from the primary tumor, invade the surrounding extracellular matrix, gain access to a blood vessel, survive its passage in the bloodstream, emerge from the bloodstream at a favorable location, invade the surrounding tissue, begin to grow, and establish a blood supply (Fig. 6-4). However, there is also growing evidence for the significant role of the cancer cell ecosystem—which includes, but is not limited to, the extracellular matrix, neural cells, leukocytes, endothelial cells, adipocytes, fibroblasts, and macrophages—in enabling cancer cells to establish metastatic sites[5] (Fig. 6-5).

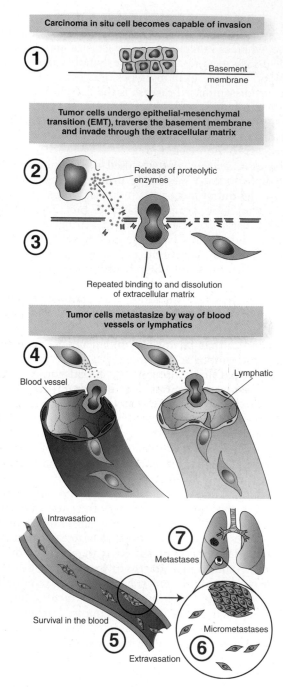

Carcinoma in situ cell becomes capable of invasion

① Basement membrane

Tumor cells undergo epithelial-mesenchymal transition (EMT), traverse the basement membrane and invade through the extracellular matrix

② Release of proteolytic enzymes

③ Repeated binding to and dissolution of extracellular matrix

Tumor cells metastasize by way of blood vessels or lymphatics

④ Blood vessel   Lymphatic

Intravasation

⑦ Metastases

Survival in the blood

Micrometastases

⑤ Extravasation   ⑥

FIGURE 6-4. Mechanisms of tumor invasion and metastasis. The mechanism by which a malignant tumor initially penetrates a confining basement membrane and then invades the surrounding extracellular environment involves several steps. (*1*) The tumor first acquires the ability to bind components of the extracellular matrix. These interactions are mediated by the expression of a number of adhesion molecules. (*2*) The tumor undergoes epithelial–mesenchymal transition (EMT) and traverses the basement membrane. (*3*) Proteolytic enzymes are then released from the tumor cells, and the extracellular matrix is degraded. (*4*) After moving through the extracellular environment, the invading cancer penetrates blood vessels and lymphatics by the same mechanisms. (*5*) After survival in blood vessels or lymphatics, the tumor exits the vascular system. (*6*) It establishes micrometastases at the site where it leaves the vasculature. (*7*) These micrometastases grow into gross masses of metastatic tumor. (From Strayer D. S., Rubin R. (Eds.) (2015). *Rubin's pathology: Clinicopathologic foundations of medicine* (7th ed., Figure 5-31, p. 196). Philadelphia, PA: Lippincott Williams & Wilkins.)

Tumor Growth

Once cells have an adequate blood supply, the rate of tissue growth in normal and cancerous tissue depends on three factors:

1. The number of cells that are actively dividing or moving through the cell cycle
2. The duration of the cell cycle
3. The number of cells that are being lost relative to the number of new cells being produced

One of the reasons cancerous tumors often seem to grow so rapidly relates to the size of the cell pool that is actively engaged in cycling. It has been shown that the cell cycle time of cancerous tissue cells is not necessarily shorter than that of normal cells. Rather, cancer cells do not die on schedule and growth factors prevent cells from exiting the cell cycle and entering the G_0 phase. Thus, a greater percentage of cells are actively engaged in cycling than occurs in normal tissue.

The ratio of dividing cells to resting cells in a tissue mass is called the *growth fraction*. The *doubling time* is the length of time it takes for the total mass of cells in a tumor to double. As the growth fraction increases, the doubling time decreases. When normal tissues reach their adult size, equilibrium between cell birth and cell death is reached. Cancer cells, however, continue to divide until limitations in blood supply and nutrients inhibit their growth.

SUMMARY CONCEPTS

Neoplasms may be either benign or malignant. Benign and malignant tumors differ in terms of cell characteristics, manner of growth, rate of growth, potential for metastasis, ability to produce generalized effects, tendency to cause tissue destruction, and capacity to cause death. The growth of a benign tumor is restricted to the site of origin, and the tumor usually does not cause death unless it interferes with vital functions. Malignant neoplasms grow in a poorly controlled fashion that lacks normal organization, spreads to distant parts of the body, and causes death unless tumor growth and metastasis are inhibited or stopped by treatment. There are two basic types of cancer: solid tumors and hematologic tumors. In solid tumors, the primary tumor is initially confined to a specific organ or tissue, whereas hematologic cancers are disseminated from the onset.

Cancer is a disorder of cell proliferation and differentiation. The term *anaplasia* is used to describe the loss of cell differentiation in cancerous tissue. Undifferentiated cancer cells are marked by a number of morphologic changes, including variations in size and shape, a condition referred to a *pleomorphism*. The characteristics of altered proliferation and differentiation are associated with a number of other changes in cell characteristics and cell function, including genetic instability; growth factor independence; loss of cell density–dependent inhibition, cohesiveness and adhesion, and anchorage dependence; faulty cell-to-cell communication; indefinite cell life span; expression of altered tissue antigens; abnormal secretion of degradative enzymes that enable invasion and metastatic spread or **ectopic** production of hormones; and abnormal cytoskeletal characteristics.

The spread of cancer occurs through three pathways: direct invasion and extension, seeding of cancer cells in body cavities, and metastatic spread through vascular or lymphatic pathways. Only a proportionately small clone of cancer cells is capable of metastasis. To metastasize, a cancer cell must be able to break loose from the primary tumor, invade the surrounding extracellular matrix, gain access to a blood vessel, survive its passage in the bloodstream, emerge from the bloodstream at a favorable location, invade the surrounding tissue, and begin to grow. The rate of growth of cancerous tissue depends on the ratio of dividing to resting cells (growth fraction) and the time it takes for the total cells in the tumor to double (doubling time).

Etiology of Cancer

The causes of cancers are very diverse and complex. It is useful to discuss causation in terms of:

1. The genetic and molecular mechanisms that are involved and that characterize the transformation of normal cells to cancer cells
2. The external and more contextual factors such as age, heredity, and environmental agents that contribute to the development and progression of cancer

Together, both mechanisms contribute to a multidimensional web of causation by which cancers develop and progress over time.

Genetic and Molecular Basis of Cancer

The molecular pathogenesis of most cancers is thought to originate with genetic damage or mutation with resultant changes in cell physiology that transform a normally functioning cell into a cancer cell. Epigenetic factors that involve silencing of a gene or genes may also be involved in the molecular pathogenesis of cancer. In recent years, an important role of cancer stem cells in the pathogenesis of cancer has been identified. Finally, the cellular microenvironment, which involves multiple cell types, the complex milieu of cytokines and growth factors, and the extracellular matrix, is now recognized as an important contributor to cancer development, growth, and progression.

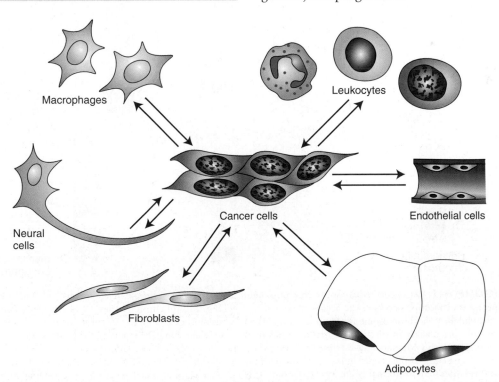

FIGURE 6-5. The cancer cell ecosystem. The developing tumor cells interact with the nonmalignant cells in their environment, via production of soluble and other mediators. (From Strayer D. S., Rubin R. (Eds.) (2015). *Rubin's pathology: Clinicopathologic foundations of medicine* (7th ed., Figure 5-32, p. 197). Philadelphia, PA: Lippincott Williams & Wilkins.)

Cancer-Associated Genes

Most cancer-associated genes can be classified into two broad categories based on whether gene overactivity or underactivity increases the risk of cancer. The category associated with gene overactivity involves *proto-oncogenes*, which are normal genes that become cancer-causing **oncogenes** if mutated. Proto-oncogenes encode for normal cell proteins such as growth factors, growth factor receptors, growth factor signaling molecules, and transcription factors that promote cell growth or increase growth factor–dependent signaling.

The category associated with gene underactivity comprises the *tumor suppressor genes*, which, by being less active, create an environment in which cancer is promoted. Tumor suppressor genes include the retinoblastoma (*RB*) gene, which normally prevents cell division, and the *TP53* gene, which normally becomes activated in DNA-damaged cells to initiate apoptosis.[5,9] Loss of *RB* activity may accelerate the cell cycle and lead to increased cell proliferation,[9] whereas inactivity of *TP53* may increase the survival of DNA-damaged cells. The *TP53* gene has become a reliable prognostic indicator.[10] There are a number of genetic events that can lead to oncogene formation or loss of tumor suppressor gene function.

Genetic Events Leading to Oncogene Formation or Activation

Chromosomal translocations have traditionally been associated with cancers such as Burkitt lymphoma and chronic myelogenous leukemia (CML). In Burkitt lymphoma, the *myc* **proto-oncogene**, which encodes a growth signal protein, is translocated from its normal position on chromosome 8 to chromosome 14 (Fig. 6-6C).[5] The outcome of the translocation in CML is the appearance of the so-called *Philadelphia chromosome* involving chromosomes 9 and 22 and the formation of an abnormal fusion protein, a hybrid oncogenic protein (bcr–abl) that promotes cell proliferation (Fig. 6-6A and B). Biotechnology and genomics are enabling the identification of gene translocations and an increased understanding of how these translocations, even within the same chromosome, contribute to tumorigenesis by the creation of abnormal fusion proteins that promote cell proliferation.

Another genetic event common in cancer is gene amplification. Multiple copies of certain genes may lead to overexpression, with higher-than-normal levels of proteins that increase cell proliferation. For example, the human epidermal growth factor receptor-2 (*HER-2/neu*) gene is amplified in many breast cancers; its presence indicates an aggressive tumor with a poor prognosis.[11]

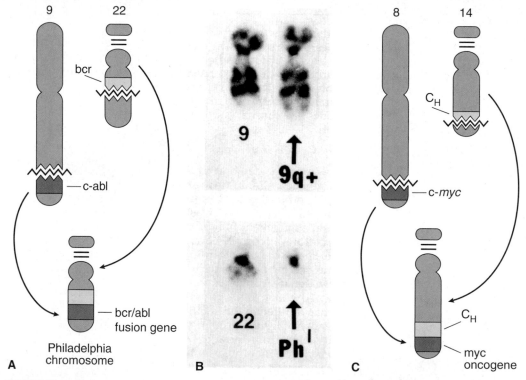

FIGURE 6-6. Oncogene activation by chromosomal translocation. (**A**) Chronic myelogenous leukemia. Reciprocal translocation occurs at the breaks at the ends of the long arms of chromosomes 9 and 22. This results in the Philadelphia chromosome (Ph[1]), which contains a new fusion gene coding for a hybrid oncogenic protein (bcr–abl), presumably involved in the pathogenesis of chronic myelogenous leukemia (CML). (**B**) Karyotypes of a person with CML showing the results of reciprocal translocations between chromosomes 9 and 22. The Philadelphia chromosome is recognized by a smaller-than-normal chromosome 22 (22q−). One chromosome 9 (9q+) is larger than its normal counterpart. (**C**) Burkitt lymphoma. Chromosomal breaks involve the long arms of chromosomes 8 and 14. The c-*myc* gene on chromosome 8 is translocated to a region on chromosome 14 adjacent to the gene coding for the constant region of an immunoglobulin heavy chain (C$_H$). (From Rubin R., Strayer D. S. (Eds.) (2012). *Rubin's pathology: Clinicopathologic foundations of medicine* (6th ed., p. 174). Philadelphia, PA: Lippincott Williams & Wilkins.)

Genetic Events Leading to Loss of Tumor Suppressor Gene Function

Tumor suppressor genes inhibit the proliferation of cells in a tumor. When this type of gene is inactivated, a genetic signal that normally inhibits cell proliferation is removed, thereby causing unregulated growth to begin. Multiple tumor suppressor genes have been found that connect with various types of cancer.[5] Of particular interest in this group is the *TP53* gene, which is on the short arm of chromosome 17 and codes for the p53 protein. Mutations in the *TP53* gene have been associated with lung, breast, and colon cancer.[10] The *TP53* gene also appears to initiate apoptosis in radiation- and chemotherapy-damaged tumor cells.

Although a single mutation generally plays an important role in oncogene activation, the malfunction of tumor suppressor genes may require "two hits" to contribute to total loss of function, as suggested by the *two-hit hypothesis* of carcinogenesis (Fig. 6-7).[5] The first "hit" may be a point mutation in an allele of a particular chromosome; later, a second "hit" occurs that involves the companion allele of the gene.

Epigenetic Mechanisms

In addition to mechanisms that involve DNA and chromosomal structural changes, there are molecular and cellular mechanisms, termed *epigenetic mechanisms*, that involve changes in the patterns of gene expression without a change in the DNA. Epigenetic mechanisms may "silence" genes, such as tumor suppressor genes, so that even though the gene is present, it is not expressed and a cancer-suppressing protein is not made. The epigenetic mechanisms that alter expression of genes associated with cancer are still under investigation.

Molecular and Cellular Pathways

There are numerous molecular and cellular mechanisms with a myriad of associated pathways and genes that are known or suspected to facilitate the development of cancer. Genes that increase susceptibility to cancer or facilitate cancer include defects in DNA repair mechanisms, defects in growth factor signaling pathways, evasion of apoptosis, avoidance of cellular senescence, development of sustained angiogenesis, and metastasis and invasion. In addition, associated genetic mutations are involved that enable invasion of and survival in neighboring tissue, as well as evasion of immune detection and attack.

DNA Repair Defects

Genetic mechanisms that regulate repair of damaged DNA have been implicated in the process of oncogenesis (Fig. 6-8). The DNA repair genes affect cell proliferation

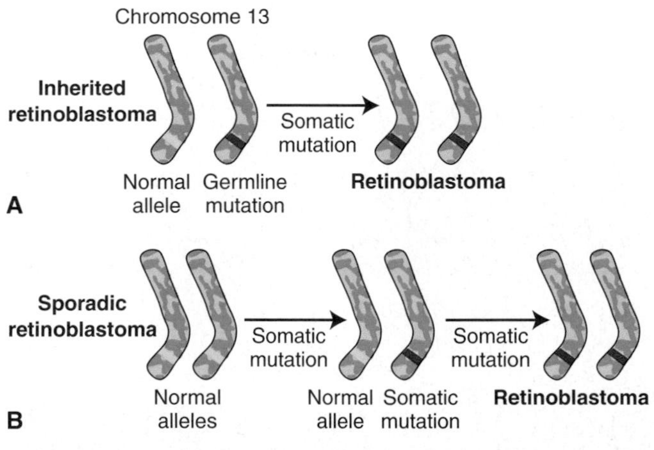

FIGURE 6-7. The "two-hit" origin of retinoblastoma. **(A)** A child with the inherited form of retinoblastoma is born with a germline mutation in one allele of the retinoblastoma gene located on the long arm of chromosome 13. This mutation is not sufficient for tumorigenesis, but the absence of two wild-type alleles weakens protection from tumor development in the event that the remaining allele becomes altered. Then, a second somatic mutation in the retina leads to the inactivation of the y functioning *RB* allele and the subsequent development of a retinoblastoma. **(B)** In sporadic cases of retinoblastoma, the child is born with two normal *RB* alleles. It requires two independent somatic mutations to inactivate *RB* gene function and allow for the appearance of a neoplastic clone. (From Strayer D., Rubin R. (Eds.) (2015). *Rubin's pathology: Clinicopathologic foundations of medicine* (7th ed., Figure 5-40, p. 208). Philadelphia, PA: Lippincott Williams & Wilkins.)

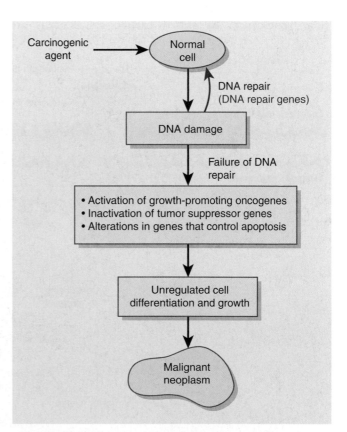

FIGURE 6-8. Flowchart depicting the stages in the development of a malignant neoplasm resulting from exposure to an oncogenic agent that produces deoxyribonucleic acid (DNA) damage. When DNA repair genes are present (*red arrow*), the DNA is repaired and gene mutation does not occur.

and survival indirectly through their ability to repair damage in proto-oncogenes, genes impacting apoptosis, and tumor suppressor genes.[5]

Defects in Growth Factor Signaling Pathways
A relatively common way in which cancer cells gain autonomous growth is through mutations in genes that control growth factor signaling pathways. These signaling pathways connect the growth factor receptors to their nuclear targets.[5] The pathway that regulates gene growth and division is explained in Figure 6-9.

Evasion of Apoptosis
Faulty apoptotic mechanisms have an important role in cancer. The failure of cancer cells to undergo apoptosis in a normal manner may be due to a number of problems. There may be altered cell survival signaling, overly active Ras proteins, *TP53* mutations, downregulation of death receptors (*e.g.*, tumor necrosis factor [TNF]–related apoptosis-inducing ligand), stabilization of the mitochondria, inactivation of proapoptotic proteins (*e.g.*, methylation of caspase-8), overactivity of nuclear factor kappa B, heat shock protein production, or failure of immune cells to induce cell death.[12] Alterations in apoptotic and antiapoptotic pathways, genes, and proteins have been found in many cancers.

Evasion of Cellular Senescence
Another normal cell response to DNA damage is cellular senescence. As stated earlier, cancer cells are characterized by longer life because of high levels of telomerase that prevent cell aging and senescence. High levels of telomerase and prevention of telomere shortening may also contribute to cancer and its progression because senescence is considered to be a normal response to DNA damage in cells as well as a tumor suppressor mechanism, and in model systems, short telomeres limit cancer growth.[13]

Development of Sustained Angiogenesis
Even with all the aforementioned genetic abnormalities, tumors cannot enlarge unless angiogenesis occurs and supplies them with the blood vessels necessary for survival. Angiogenesis is required not only for continued tumor growth but also for metastasis. The molecular basis for the angiogenic switch is unknown, but it appears to involve increased production of angiogenic factors or loss of angiogenic inhibitors. The mutation of the *TP53* gene seems to encourage angiogenesis. Angiogenesis is also influenced by hypoxia and release of proteases that are involved in regulating the balance between angiogenic and antiangiogenic factors.[5]

Invasion and Metastasis
Finally, multiple genes and molecular and cellular pathways are known to be involved in invasion and metastasis. There is evidence that cancer cells with invasive properties are actually members of the cancer stem cell population. This evidence suggests that genetic programs that are normally operative in stem

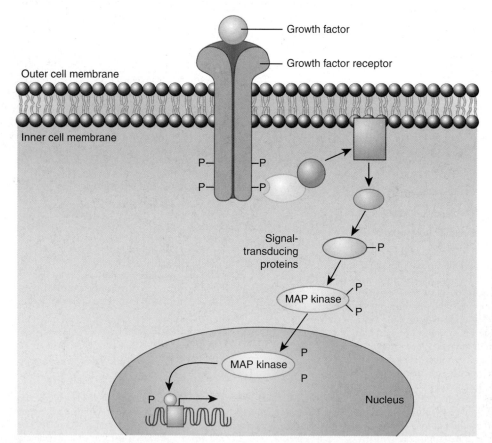

FIGURE 6-9. Pathway for genes regulating cell growth and replication. Stimulation of a normal cell by a growth factor results in activation of the growth factor receptor and signaling proteins that transmit the growth-promoting signal to the nucleus, where it modulates gene transcription and progression through the cell cycle. Many of these signaling proteins exert their effects through enzymes called *kinases* that phosphorylate proteins. MAP, mitogen-activated protein.

cells during embryonic development may become operative in cancer stem cells, enabling them to detach, cross tissue boundaries, escape death by detaching from tissue from which they belong (**anoikis**), and colonize new tissues. The *MET* proto-oncogene, which is expressed in both stem cells and cancer cells, is a key regulator of invasive growth. Findings suggest that adverse conditions such as tissue hypoxia, which are commonly present in cancerous tumors, trigger this invasive behavior by activating the MET tyrosine kinase receptor.

Role of the Microenvironment

Traditionally, the molecular and cellular biology of cancer has focused on the cancer itself. More recently, the important role of the microenvironment in the development of cancer and metastasis has been described. The microenvironment of the cancer cell consists of multiple cell types, including macrophages, fibroblasts, endothelial cells, and a variety of immune and inflammatory cells; the extracellular matrix; and the primary signaling substances such as cytokines, chemokines, and hormones. For example, signaling of the cytokine transforming growth factor-beta (TGF-β) is known to be important in the cellular pathway, leading to cancer cell formation or suppression.[14] The ability of TGF-β to cause the cancer to progress and metastasize, however, depends on the microenvironment of various cell types and cross talk of signals among the cell types. In some cases, the phenotype of a cancer cell can actually normalize when it is removed from the tumor microenvironment and placed in a normal environment and vice versa. Finally, essential steps needed for tumor growth and metastasis, such as angiogenesis and metastatic tumor survival, depend on the microenvironment.

Carcinogenesis

The process by which carcinogenic (cancer-causing) agents cause normal cells to become cancer cells is hypothesized to be a multistep mechanism that can be divided into three stages: initiation, promotion, and progression (Fig. 6-10). *Initiation* is the first step and describes the exposure of cells to a carcinogenic agent that causes them to be vulnerable to cancer transformation.[5] The carcinogenic agents can be chemical, physical, or biologic and produce irreversible changes in the genome of a previously normal cell. Because the effects of initiating agents are irreversible, multiple divided doses may achieve the same effects as a single exposure to the same total dose or to small amounts of highly carcinogenic substances. The cells most susceptible to mutagenic alterations are those that are actively synthesizing DNA.

Promotion is the second step that allows for prolific growth of cells triggered by multiple growth factors and chemicals.[5] Promotion is reversible if the promoter substance is removed. Cells that have been irreversibly initiated may be promoted even after long latency periods.

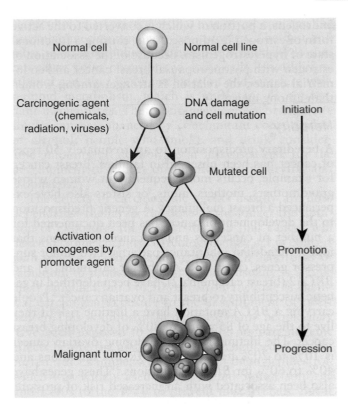

FIGURE 6-10. The processes of initiation, promotion, and progression in the clonal evolution of malignant tumors. Initiation involves the exposure of cells to appropriate doses of a carcinogenic agent; promotion, the unregulated and accelerated growth of the mutated cells; and progression, the acquisition of malignant characteristics by the tumor cells. DNA, deoxyribonucleic acid.

The latency period varies with the type of agent, the dosage, and the characteristics of the target cells. Many chemical carcinogens are called *complete carcinogens* because they can initiate and promote neoplastic transformation. *Progression* is the last step of the process that manifests when tumor cells acquire malignant phenotypic changes that promote invasiveness, metastatic competence, autonomous growth tendencies, and increased karyotypic instability.

Host and Environmental Factors

Because cancer is not a single disease, it is reasonable to assume that it does not have a single cause. More likely, cancer occurs because of interactions among multiple risk factors or repeated exposure to a single carcinogenic agent. Among the traditional risk factors that have been linked to cancer are heredity, hormonal factors, immunologic mechanisms, and environmental agents such as chemicals, radiation, and cancer-causing viruses. More recently, there has been interest in obesity as a risk factor for cancer. A strong and consistent relationship has been reported between obesity and mortality from all cancers among men and women.[15] Obese people tend to produce increased amounts of

TABLE 6-4 Common Paraneoplastic Syndromes

Type of Syndrome	Associated Tumor Type	Proposed Mechanism
Endocrinologic		
Syndrome of inappropriate antidiuretic hormone (ADH)	Small cell lung cancer, others	Production and release of ADH by tumor
Adrenocorticotropic hormone (ACTH)–Cushing syndrome	Small cell lung cancer, bronchial carcinoid cancers	Production and release of ACTH by tumor
Humoral hypercalcemia	Squamous cell cancers of the lung, head, neck, ovary	Production and release of polypeptide factor with close relationship to parathyroid hormone
Hematologic		
Venous thrombosis	Pancreatic, lung, most solid tumor metastatic cancers	Production of procoagulation factors
Nonbacterial thrombolytic endocarditis and anemia of malignancy	Advanced cancers	
Neurologic		
Eaton–Lambert syndrome	Small cell lung cancer	Autoimmune production of antibodies to motor end-plate structures
Myasthenia gravis	Thymoma	Autoimmune-generating abnormal neuron transmission
Dermatologic		
Cutaneous syndromes	Gastric carcinoma and other	Possibly caused by production of growth factors (epidermal) by tumor cells
Acanthosis nigricans	Cancers	Sometimes occur prior to cancer
Pemphigus		
Ichthyosis		
Extramammary Paget		Damage to renal glomerulus
Renal		
Nephrotic syndrome	Renal cancers	

than any other malignant neoplasms, ovarian cancers are associated with the accumulation of fluid in the peritoneal cavity. Abdominal discomfort, swelling and a feeling of heaviness, increase in abdominal girth, which reflect the presence of peritoneal effusions or ascites, shortness of breath, and increased urinary urgency or frequency are common presenting symptoms in ovarian cancer.[29]

Systemic Manifestations

Many of the clinical manifestations of cancer, including anorexia and cachexia, fatigue and sleep disorders, and anemia, are not directly related to the presence of a tumor mass but to altered metabolic pathways and the presence of circulating cytokines and other mediators. Although research has produced amazing insights into the causes and cures for cancer, much still is needed regarding management of the associated side effects of the disease.[5]

Anorexia and Cachexia

Many cancers are associated with weight loss and wasting of body fat and muscle tissue, accompanied by profound weakness, anorexia, and anemia. This wasting syndrome is often referred to as the *cancer anorexia–cachexia syndrome*.[30] It is a common manifestation of most solid tumors, with the exception of breast cancer. It has been estimated that it is a significant cause of morbidity and mortality in 50% to 80% of people with advanced cancer and is responsible for death in up to 20% of cases.[31] The condition is more common in children and older adults and becomes more pronounced as the disease progresses. People with cancer cachexia also respond less well to chemotherapy and are more prone to toxic side effects.

Although anorexia, reduced food intake, and abnormalities of taste are common in people with cancer and often are accentuated by treatment methods, the extent of weight loss and protein wasting cannot be explained in terms of diminished food intake alone. In contrast to starvation because of lack of food intake, where weight is preferentially lost from the fat compartment, in cachexia, it is lost from both the fat and skeletal muscle compartments.[30] Furthermore, the protein loss that occurs with starvation is divided equally between skeletal muscle and **visceral** proteins, whereas in cachexia, visceral proteins are relatively well preserved. Finally, and more important, weight loss that occurs with starvation is usually reversed by refeeding, whereas oral or parenteral nutritional supplementation does not reverse cachexia.

The mechanisms of cancer cachexia appear to reside in a hypermetabolic state and altered nutrient metabolism that are specific to the tumor-bearing state. The production of glucose (**gluconeogenesis**) from lactate contributes to the hypermetabolic state of cachectic people. The increased expression of mitochondrial uncoupling proteins that uncouple the oxidative phosphorylation process results in energy being lost as heat.

Abnormalities in fat and protein metabolism have also been reported. In people with cancer cachexia, amino acids are not spared and there is depletion of lean body mass, a condition thought to contribute to decreased survival time.

The acute-phase response is known to be activated by cytokines such as TNF-α and IL-1 and IL-6, suggesting that they may also play a role in cancer cachexia.[25] High serum levels of these cytokines have been observed in people with cancer, and their levels appear to correlate with progression of the tumor. TNF-α, secreted primarily by macrophages in response to tumor cell growth or gram-negative bacterial infections, was the first cytokine associated with cachexia and wasting to be identified. It causes anorexia by suppressing satiety centers in the hypothalamus and increasing the synthesis of lipoprotein lipase, an enzyme that facilitates the release of fatty acids from lipoproteins so that they can be used by tissues. IL-1 and IL-6 share many of the features of TNF-α in terms of the ability to initiate cachexia.

Fatigue and Sleep Disorders

Fatigue and sleep disturbances are two of the most frequent side effects experienced by people with cancer.[27] Cancer-related fatigue is characterized by feelings of tiredness, weakness, and lack of energy and is distinct from the normal tiredness experienced by healthy people in that it is not relieved by rest or sleep. It occurs both as a consequence of the cancer itself and as a side effect of cancer treatment. Cancer-related fatigue may be an early symptom of malignant disease and has been reported by more than a third of people at the time of diagnosis.[27] Furthermore, the symptom often remains for months or even years after treatment.

Although cancer-related fatigue and sleep disorders are distinct conditions, they are closely linked in terms of prevalence and symptoms.[27] People with cancer report poor sleep quality, disturbed initiation and maintenance of sleep, insufficient sleep, nighttime awakening, and restless sleep. As with fatigue, precipitating factors include the diagnosis of cancer, type and stage of cancer, pain, and side effects of treatment (e.g., nausea, vomiting).

Anemia

Anemia is common in people with various types of cancers. It may be related to blood loss, hemolysis, impaired red blood cell production, or treatment effects.[5] For example, drugs used in the treatment of cancer are cytotoxic and can decrease red blood cell production. Also, there are many mechanisms through which erythrocyte production can be impaired in people with malignancies, including nutritional deficiencies, bone marrow failure, and a blunted erythropoietin response to hypoxia. Inflammatory cytokines generated in response to tumors decrease erythropoietin production, resulting in a decrease in erythrocyte production.

SUMMARY CONCEPTS

There probably is no single body function left unaffected by the presence of cancer. Because tumor cells replace normally functioning parenchymal tissue, the initial manifestations of cancer usually reflect the primary site of involvement. Cancer compresses blood vessels, obstructs lymph flow, disrupts tissue integrity, invades serous cavities, and compresses visceral organs. It may result in the development of effusion (i.e., fluid) in the pleural, pericardial, or peritoneal spaces and generalized manifestations such as anorexia and cachexia, fatigue and sleep disorders, and anemia. Many of these manifestations are compounded by the side effects of methods used to treat the disease.

Screening, Diagnosis, and Treatment

Screening

Screening represents a secondary prevention measure for the early recognition of cancer in an otherwise asymptomatic population.[2] Screening can be achieved through observation (e.g., skin, mouth, external genitalia), palpation (e.g., breast, thyroid, rectum and anus, prostate, lymph nodes), and laboratory tests and procedures (e.g., Papanicolaou [Pap] smear, colonoscopy, mammography). It requires a test that will specifically detect early cancers or premalignancies, is cost-effective, and results in improved therapeutic outcomes.[5] For most cancers, stage at presentation is related to curability, with the highest rates reported when the tumor is small and there is no evidence of metastasis. For some tumors, however, metastasis tends to occur early, even from a small primary tumor. More sensitive screening methods such as tumor markers are being developed for forms of cancer. Lung cancer guidelines were developed by the American Cancer Society and recommend the initiation of discussions with healthy people aged 55 to 74 years who have a minimum of 30 pack-year smoking history and who have stopped smoking in the last 15 years or continue to smoke.[32]

Cancers for which current screening or early detection has led to improvement in outcomes include cancers of the breast (mammography), cervix (Pap smear), colon and rectum (rectal examination, fecal occult blood test, and colonoscopy), prostate (prostate-specific antigen [PSA] testing and transrectal ultrasonography), and malignant melanoma (self-examination). Although not as clearly defined, it is recommended that screening for other types of cancers such as cancers of the thyroid, testicles, ovaries, lymph nodes, and oral cavity be done at the time of periodic health examinations.

Diagnostic Methods

The methods used in the diagnosis and staging of cancer are determined largely by the location and type of cancer suspected. A number of procedures are used in the diagnosis of cancer, including blood tests for tumor markers, cytologic studies and tissue biopsy, endoscopic examinations, ultrasonography, x-ray studies, magnetic resonance imaging, computed tomography, and positron-emission tomography.

Tumor Markers

Tumor markers are antigens expressed on the surface of tumor cells or substances released from normal cells in response to the presence of tumor.[5,33] Some substances, such as hormones and enzymes, that are produced normally by the involved tissue become overexpressed as a result of cancer. Other tumor markers, such as oncofetal proteins, are produced during fetal development and are induced to reappear later in life as a result of benign and malignant neoplasms. Tumor markers are used for screening, establishing prognosis, monitoring treatment, and detecting recurrent disease.[33] Table 6-5 identifies some of the more commonly used tumor markers and summarizes their source and the cancers associated with them.

The serum markers that have proved most useful in clinical practice are human chorionic gonadotropin (hCG), cancer antigen (CA) 125, PSA, α-fetoprotein (AFP), carcinoembryonic antigen (CEA), and *cluster of differentiation* (CD) blood cell antigens.[5] A hormone normally produced by the placenta, hCG, is used as a marker for diagnosing, prescribing treatment, and following the disease course in people with high-risk gestational trophoblastic tumors. PSA is used as a marker in prostate cancer, and CA 125 is used as a marker in ovarian cancer. Markers for leukemia and lymphomas are grouped by so-called CD antigens. The CD antigens help to distinguish among T and B lymphocytes, monocytes, granulocytes, and NK cells and immature variants of these cells.[5]

Some cancers express fetal antigens that are normally present only during embryonal development.[5] The two that have proved most useful as tumor markers are AFP and CEA. AFP is synthesized by the fetal liver, yolk sac, and gastrointestinal tract and is the major serum protein in the fetus. Elevated levels are encountered in people with primary liver cancers and have also been observed in some testicular, ovarian, pancreatic, and stomach cancers. CEA normally is produced by embryonic tissue in the gut, pancreas, and liver and is elaborated by a number of different cancers. Depending on the serum level adopted for significant elevation, CEA is elevated in approximately 60% to 90% of colorectal carcinomas, 50% to 80% of pancreatic cancers, and 25% to 50% of gastric and breast tumors.[5] As with most other tumor markers, elevated levels of CEA and AFP are found in

TABLE 6-5 Tumor Markers

Marker	Source	Associated Cancers
Antigens		
AFP	Fetal yolk sac and gastrointestinal structures early in fetal life	Primary liver cancers; germ cell cancer of the testis
CA 15-3	Breast tissue protein	Tumor marker for tracking breast cancer; liver, lung
CA 27-29	Breast tissue protein	Breast cancer recurrence and metastasis
CEA	Embryonic tissues in gut, pancreas, liver, and breast	Colorectal cancer and cancers of the pancreas, lung, and stomach
Hormones		
hCG	Hormone normally produced by placenta	Gestational trophoblastic tumors; germ cell cancer of testis
Calcitonin	Hormone produced by thyroid parafollicular cells	Thyroid cancer
Catecholamines (epinephrine, norepinephrine) and metabolites	Hormones produced by chromaffin cells of the adrenal gland	Pheochromocytoma and related tumors
Specific Proteins		
Monoclonal immunoglobulin	Abnormal immunoglobulin produced by neoplastic cells	Multiple myeloma
PSA	Produced by the epithelial cells lining the acini and ducts of the prostate	Prostate cancer
Mucins and Other Glycoproteins		
CA 125	Produced by Müllerian cells of ovary	Ovarian cancer
CA 19-9	Produced by alimentary tract epithelium	Cancer of the pancreas, colon
Cluster of Differentiation		
CD antigens	Present on leukocytes	Used to determine the type and level of differentiation of leukocytes involved in different types of leukemia and lymphoma

AFP, α-fetoprotein; CA, cancer antigen; CD, cluster of differentiation; CEA, carcinoembryonic antigen; hCG, human chorionic gonadotropin; PSA, prostate-specific antigen.

other, noncancerous conditions, and elevated levels of both depend on tumor size, so that neither is useful as an early screening test for cancer.

As diagnostic tools, tumor markers have limitations. Nearly all markers can be elevated in benign conditions, and most are not elevated in the early stages of malignancy. Hence, tumor markers have limited value as screening tests. Furthermore, they are not in themselves specific enough to permit a diagnosis of a malignancy, but once a malignancy has been diagnosed and shown to be associated with elevated levels of a tumor marker, the marker can be used to assess response to therapy. Examples of tumor markers that assist in evaluating peoples' response to therapy, and if a recurrence of breast cancer may be occurring, are CA 15-3 and CA 27-29, both antigens that are found in breast tissue.[3] Extremely elevated levels of a tumor marker can indicate a poor prognosis or the need for more aggressive treatment. Perhaps the greatest value of tumor markers is in monitoring therapy in people with widespread cancer. The level of most cancer markers tends to decrease with successful treatment and increase with recurrence or spread of the tumor.

Cytologic and Histologic Methods

Histologic and cytologic studies are laboratory methods used to examine tissues and cells. Several sampling approaches are available, including cytologic smears, tissue biopsies, and needle aspiration.[5]

Papanicolaou Test

The Pap test is a cytologic method used for detecting cancer cells. It consists of a microscopic examination of a properly prepared slide by a cytotechnologist or pathologist for the purpose of detecting the presence of abnormal cells. The usefulness of the Pap test relies on the fact that cancer cells lack the cohesive properties and intercellular junctions that are characteristic of normal tissue. Without these characteristics, cancer cells tend to exfoliate and become mixed with secretions surrounding the tumor growth. Although the Pap test is widely used as a screening test for cervical cancer, it can be performed on other body secretions, including nipple drainage, anal washings, pleural or peritoneal fluid, and gastric washings.

Tissue Biopsy

Tissue biopsy, which is of critical importance in diagnosing the correct cancer and histology, involves the removal of a tissue specimen for microscopic study. Biopsies are obtained in a number of ways, including needle biopsy; endoscopic methods, such as bronchoscopy or cystoscopy, which involve the passage of an endoscope through an orifice and into the involved structure; or laparoscopic methods. In some instances, a surgical incision is made from which biopsy specimens are obtained. Excisional biopsies are those in which the entire tumor is removed. The tumors usually are small, solid, palpable masses. If the tumor is too large to be completely removed, a wedge of tissue from the mass can be excised for examination. Appropriate preservation of the specimen includes prompt immersion in a fixative solution such as formalin, with preservation of a portion of the specimen in a special fixative for electron microscopy, or prompt refrigeration to permit optimal hormone, receptor, and other types of molecular analysis. A quick frozen section may be done to determine the nature of a mass lesion or evaluate the margins of an excised tumor to ascertain that the entire neoplasm has been removed.[5]

Fine needle aspiration is another approach that is widely used. The procedure involves aspirating cells and attendant fluid with a small-bore needle. The method is most commonly used for the assessment of readily **palpable** lesions in sites such as the thyroid, breast, and lymph nodes. Modern imaging techniques have also enabled the method to be extended to deeper structures such as the pelvic lymph nodes and pancreas.

Immunohistochemistry

Immunohistochemistry involves the use of antibodies to facilitate the identification of cell products or surface markers.[5] For example, certain anaplastic carcinomas, malignant lymphomas, melanomas, and sarcomas look very similar under the microscope, but must be accurately identified because their treatment and prognosis are quite different. Antibodies against intermediate filaments have proved useful in such cases because tumor cells often contain intermediate filaments characteristic of their tissue of origin.[5] Immunohistochemistry can also be used to determine the site of origin of metastatic tumors. Many people with cancer present with metastasis. In cases in which the origin of the metastasis is obscure, immunochemical detection of tissue-specific or organ-specific antigens can often help to identify the tumor source. Immunohistochemistry can also be used to detect molecules that have prognostic or therapeutic significance. For example, detection of estrogen receptors on breast cancer cells is of prognostic and therapeutic significance because these tumors respond to antiestrogen therapy.

Microarray Technology

Microarray technology uses "gene chips" that can simultaneously perform miniature assays to detect and quantify the expression of large numbers of genes.[5] The advantage of microarray technology is the ability to analyze a large number of changes in cancer cells to determine overall patterns of behavior that could not be assessed by conventional means. DNA arrays are now commercially available to assist in making clinical decisions regarding breast cancer treatment. In addition to identifying tumor types, microarrays have been used for predicting prognosis and response to therapy, examining tumor changes after therapy, and classifying hereditary tumors.[5]

Staging and Grading of Tumors

The two basic methods for classifying cancers are *grading* according to the histologic or cellular characteristics of the tumor and *staging* according to the clinical spread of the disease. Both methods are used to determine the course of the disease and aid in selecting an

Hormonal Therapy

Hormonal therapy consists of administration of drugs designed to disrupt the hormonal environment of cancer cells. The actions of hormones and antihormones depend on the presence of specific receptors in the tumor. Among the tumors that are known to be responsive to hormonal manipulation are those of the breast, prostate, and endometrium. Additionally, other cancers, such as Kaposi sarcoma and renal, liver, ovarian, and pancreatic cancer, can be treated with hormonal therapy. The theory behind the majority of hormone-based cancer treatments is to deprive the cancer cells of the hormonal signals that otherwise would stimulate them to divide.

Biotherapy

Biotherapy involves the use of immunotherapy and biologic response modifiers as a means of changing the person's own immune response to cancer.[38] The major mechanisms by which biotherapy exerts its effects are modifications of host responses or tumor cell biology.

Immunotherapy

The use of immunotherapy has proven to be an effective treatment strategy of malignancy and has less toxicity than chemotherapy regimens.[39] Immunotherapy is a treatment that uses one's own immune system to treat cancer by either stimulating the immune system to attack cancer cells or improving the individual's immune system.[40] Immunotherapy may be used as a single-agent treatment or used in conjunction with other treatment modalities.[40]

Types of cancer immunotherapy include monoclonal antibodies, immune inhibitors, cancer vaccines, and nonspecific immunotherapies.[40] *Monoclonal antibodies* are made in the laboratory and target specific proteins or antigens often found on cancer cells allowing for an attack on specific cells.[40] *Immune inhibitors* allow the body to recognize molecules on specific immune cells in order to create an immune response.[40] *Cancer vaccines* are one of the latest biologic response modifiers that act by stimulating the immune system to fight a specific infection or disease, most often cancer-causing viruses such as hepatitis B and HPV.[41,42]

Biologic Response Modifiers

Biologic response modifiers can be grouped into three types: cytokines, which include the interferons and ILs; monoclonal antibodies; and hematopoietic growth factors. The interferons appear to inhibit viral replication and also may be involved in inhibiting tumor protein synthesis and in prolonging the cell cycle, increasing the percentage of cells in the G_0 phase. Interferons stimulate NK cells and T-lymphocyte killer cells. Interferon-γ has been approved for the treatment of hairy cell leukemia, AIDS-related Kaposi sarcoma, and CML and as adjuvant therapy for people at high risk for recurrent melanoma.[5,43]

The ILs are cytokines that affect communication between cells by binding to receptor sites on the cell surface membranes of the target cells. Of the 18 known ILs, IL-2 has been the most widely studied. A recombinant human IL-2 (aldesleukin) has been approved by the Food and Drug Administration and is being used for the treatment of metastatic renal cell and melanoma.[43]

SUMMARY CONCEPTS

The methods used in the diagnosis of cancer vary with the type of cancer and its location. Because many cancers are curable if diagnosed early, health care practices designed to promote early detection are important. Histologic studies are done in the laboratory using cells or tissue specimens. There are two basic methods of classifying tumors: grading according to the histologic or tissue characteristics and clinical staging according to spread of the disease. The TNM system for clinical staging of cancer takes into account tumor size, lymph node involvement, and presence of metastasis.

Treatment plans that use more than one type of therapy, often in combination, are providing cures for a number of cancers that a few decades ago had a poor prognosis and are increasing the life expectancy in other types of cancer. Surgical procedures are more precise and less invasive, preserving organ function and resulting in better quality-of-life outcomes. Newer radiation equipment and novel radiation techniques permit greater and more controlled destruction of cancer cells while sparing normal tissues. Cancer chemotherapy has evolved as one of the major systemic treatment modalities for cancer. Unlike surgery and radiation, chemotherapy is a systemic treatment that enables drugs to reach the site of the tumor as well as other distant sites. The major classifications of chemotherapy drugs are the direct DNA-interacting (alkylating agents, antitumor antibiotics, and topoisomerase inhibitors) and indirect DNA-interacting (antimetabolites and mitotic spindle inhibitors) agents. Cancer chemotherapeutic drugs may also be classified as either cell cycle specific or cell cycle nonspecific depending on whether they exert their action during a specific phase of the cell cycle. Other systemic agents include hormonal and molecularly targeted agents that block specific enzymes and growth factors involved in cancer cell growth.

Childhood Cancers

Cancer in children is relatively rare, accounting for about 1% of all malignancies in the United States.[1] Although rare, cancer remains the second leading cause of death among school-age children in the United States.[1] Common cancers that occur in children include leukemia, non-Hodgkin and Hodgkin lymphomas, and bone cancers (osteosarcoma and Ewing sarcoma). The overall survival rate for children is 85%.[2]

Incidence and Types

The spectrum of cancers that affect children differs markedly from those that affect adults. Although most adult cancers are of epithelial cell origin (*e.g.*, lung cancer, breast cancer, colorectal cancers), childhood cancers differ in that they generally involve the hematopoietic system, nervous system, soft tissues, bone, and kidneys.[44]

During the first year of life, embryonal tumors such as Wilms tumor, RB, and neuroblastoma are among the most common types of tumors. Embryonal tumors along with acute leukemia, non-Hodgkin lymphoma, and gliomas have a peak incidence in children 2 to 5 years of age. As children age, especially after they pass puberty, bone malignancies, Hodgkin lymphoma, **gonadal** germ cell tumors (testicular and ovarian carcinomas), and various carcinomas such as thyroid cancer and malignant melanoma increase in incidence.

Embryonal Tumors

A number of the tumors of infancy and early childhood are embryonal in origin, meaning that they exhibit features of organogenesis similar to that of embryonic development. Because of this characteristic, these tumors are frequently designated with the suffix "blastoma" (*e.g.*, nephroblastoma [Wilms tumor], RB, and neuroblastoma).[2] Wilms tumor and neuroblastoma are particularly illustrative of this type of childhood tumor.

Neuroblastoma

Neuroblastomas arise from the primordial neural crest tissue in the sympathetic nervous system and adrenal medulla.[45] It is the second most common solid malignancy in childhood after brain tumors. Neuroblastoma is also an extremely malignant neoplasm, particularly in children with advanced disease. In children younger than 2 years, neuroblastoma generally presents with large abdominal masses, fever, and possibly weight loss. Bone pain suggests metastatic disease. About 90% of the tumors, regardless of location, secrete **catecholamines**, which is an important diagnostic feature (*i.e.*, elevated blood levels of catecholamines and elevated urine levels of catecholamine metabolites).[45]

Biology of Childhood Cancers

As with adult cancers, there probably is no single cause of childhood cancer. Although a number of genetic conditions are associated with childhood cancer, such conditions are relatively rare, suggesting an interaction between genetic susceptibility and environmental exposures. There are some inheritable conditions that increase susceptibility to childhood and even adult cancer. An example is Down syndrome, which actually increases the risk of acute lymphoblastic leukemia (ALL) and acute myelogenous leukemia (AML).[2,46]

Although constituting only a small percentage of childhood cancers, the biology of a number of these tumors illustrates several important biologic aspects of neoplasms, such as the two-hit theory of recessive tumor suppressor genes (*e.g.*, *RB* gene mutation in RB); defects in DNA repair; and the histologic similarities between organogenesis and oncogenesis. Syndromes associated with defects in DNA repair include xeroderma pigmentosum, in which there is increased risk of skin cancers owing to defects in repair of DNA damaged by ultraviolet light. The development of childhood cancers has also been linked to genomic imprinting. The inactivation is determined by whether the gene is inherited from the mother or father. For example, the maternal allele for the insulin-like growth factor-2 (IGF-2) gene normally is inactivated (imprinted). In some Wilms tumors, loss of imprinting (reexpression of the maternal allele) can be demonstrated by overexpression of the IGF-2 protein, which is an embryonal growth factor.[47]

Diagnosis and Treatment

Early detection often leads to less therapy and improved outcomes. Because of generalized symptoms experienced by children such as prolonged fever, fatigue, and bone pain, diagnosis is often delayed. When these symptoms are experienced in the setting of persistent lymphadenopathy, unexplained weight loss, growing masses (especially in association with weight loss), and abnormalities of the central nervous system (CNS) function, they should be viewed as warning signs of cancer in children. Because these signs and symptoms of cancer are often similar to those of common childhood diseases, it is easy to miss a cancer diagnosis in the early stages.

Diagnosis of childhood cancers involves many of the same methods used in adults. Histologic examination is usually an essential part of the diagnostic procedure. Accurate disease staging is especially beneficial in childhood cancers, in which the potential benefits of treatment must be carefully weighed against potential long-term effects.

The treatment of childhood cancers is complex, intensive, prolonged, and continuously evolving. It usually involves appropriate multidisciplinary and multimodal therapies, as well as the evaluation for recurrent disease and late effects of the disease and therapies used in its treatment.

Two modalities are frequently used in the treatment of childhood cancer, with chemotherapy being the most widely used, followed, in order of use, by surgery, radiation therapy, and biologic agent therapy. Chemotherapy is more widely used in the treatment of children with cancer than in adults because children better tolerate the acute adverse effects and, in general, pediatric tumors are more responsive to chemotherapy than adult cancers.[48]

With improvement in treatment methods, the number of children who survive childhood cancer continues to increase. However, therapy may produce late sequelae, such as impaired growth, neurologic dysfunction, hormonal dysfunction, cardiomyopathy, pulmonary fibrosis, and the risk of second malignancies. Thus, one of the growing challenges is providing appropriate health care to survivors of childhood and adolescent cancers.[49]

Radiation Therapy

Radiation therapy poses the risk of long-term effects for survivors of childhood cancer. The late effects of radiation therapy are influenced by the organs and tissues included in the treatment field, type of radiation administered, daily fractional and cumulative radiation dose, and age at treatment. There is increased risk of melanoma, squamous cell carcinoma, and basal cell carcinoma. Musculoskeletal changes are also common after radiation. Even with current methods, survivors may have changes leading to pain and altered musculoskeletal function.

Chemotherapy

Chemotherapy also poses the risk of long-term effects for survivors of childhood cancer. Potential late effects of alkylating agents include dose-related gonadal injury (hypogonadism, infertility, and early menopause).[49] Alkylating agent therapy has also been linked to dose-related secondary AML, pulmonary fibrosis, kidney disease, and bladder disorders. Anthracyclines, including doxorubicin and daunomycin, which are widely used in the treatment of childhood cancers, can result in cardiomyopathy and eventual congestive heart failure.[49] The late effects of cisplatin and carboplatin, the most frequently used nonclassic alkylators, are nephrotoxicity, ototoxicity, and neurotoxicity. Although combination chemotherapy increases the effectiveness of treatment, it may also be associated with increased risk of side effects if the agents have a similar spectrum of toxicity. Intrathecal combination chemotherapy to prevent relapse of ALL in the CNS, which is a sanctuary for ALL cells, is known to cause significant and persistent cognitive impairment in many children.

SUMMARY CONCEPTS

Although most adult cancers are of epithelial cell origin, most childhood cancers usually involve the hematopoietic system, nervous system, or connective tissue. Heritable forms of cancer tend to have an earlier age of onset, a higher frequency of multifocal lesions in a single organ, and bilateral involvement of paired organs or multiple primary tumors. The early diagnosis of childhood cancers often is missed because the signs and symptoms mimic those of other childhood diseases. With improvement in treatment methods, the number of children who survive childhood cancer is continuing to increase. As these children approach adulthood, there is continued concern that the lifesaving therapy they received during childhood may produce late effects, such as impaired growth, cognitive dysfunction, hormonal dysfunction, cardiomyopathy, pulmonary fibrosis, and risk of secondary malignancies.

Review Exercises

1. A 30-year-old woman has experienced heavy menstrual bleeding and is told she has a uterine tumor called a *leiomyoma*. She is worried she has cancer.

   A. What is the difference between a leiomyoma and leiomyosarcoma?
   B. How would you explain the difference to her?

2. Among the characteristics of cancer cells are lack of cell differentiation, impaired cell-to-cell adhesion, and loss of anchorage dependence.

   A. Explain how each of these characteristics contributes to the usefulness of the Pap smear as a screening test for cervical cancer.

3. A 12-year-old boy is seen at the pediatric cancer clinic with osteosarcoma. His medical history reveals that his father had been successfully treated for RB as an infant.

   A. Relate the genetics of the RB gene and the "two-hit" hypothesis to the development of osteosarcoma in the son of the man who had RB.

4. A 48-year-old man presents at his health care clinic with complaints of leg weakness. He is a heavy smoker and has had a productive cough for years. Subsequent diagnostic tests reveal he has a small cell lung cancer with brain metastasis. His proposed plan of treatment includes chemotherapy and radiation therapy.

   A. What is the probable cause of the leg weakness, and is it related to the lung cancer?
   B. Relate this man's smoking history to the development of lung cancer.
   C. Explain the mechanism of cancer metastasis.
   D. Explain the mechanisms whereby chemotherapy and irradiation are able to destroy cancer cells while having a lesser or no effect on normal cells.

5. A 17-year-old-girl is seen by a guidance counselor at her high school because of problems in keeping up with assignments in her math and science courses. She tells the counselor that she had leukemia when she was 2 years old and was given radiation treatment to the brain. She confides that she

has always had more trouble with learning than her classmates and thinks it might be due to the radiation. She also relates that she is shorter than her classmates, and this has been bothering her.

A. Explain the relationship between cranial radiation therapy and decreased cognitive function and short stature.
B. What other neuroendocrine problems might this girl have as a result of the radiation treatment?

REFERENCES

1. Centers for Disease Control and Prevention. (2016). Deaths and mortality. [Online]. Available: https://www.cdc.gov/nchs/fastats/deaths.htm. Accessed October 26, 2017.
2. Center for Disease Control and Prevention. (2014). Child health. [Online]. Available: https://www.cdc.gov/nchs/fastats/child-health.htm. Accessed October 20, 2017.
3. American Cancer Society. (2017). Cancer facts & figures: 2017. [Online]. Available: https://www.cancer.org/content/dam/cancer-org/research/cancer-facts-and-statistics/annual-cancer-facts-and-figures/2017/cancer-facts-and-figures-2017.pdf. Accessed November 8, 2017.
4. American Cancer Society. (2015). Global cancer facts & figures (3rd ed.). [Online]. Available: https://www.cancer.org/content/dam/cancer-org/research/cancer-facts-and-statistics/global-cancer-facts-and-figures/global-cancer-facts-and-figures-3rd-edition.pdf. Accessed November 14, 2017.
5. Rubin R., Strayer D. S. (Eds.) (2014). *Rubin's pathology: Clinicopathologic foundations of medicine* (7th ed.). Philadelphia, PA: Lippincott Williams & Wilkins.
6. Cermeno E. A., Garcia A. J. (2016). Tumor-initiating cells: Emerging biophysical methods of isolation. *Current Stem Cell Reports* 2(1), 21–32.
7. Paoli P., Giannoni E., Chiarugi P. (2013). Anoikis molecular pathways and its role in cancer progression. *Biochemica et Biophysica Acta* 1833, 3481–3498.
8. Herve J. C., Derangeon M. (2013). Gap-junction-mediated cell-to-cell communication. *Cell and Tissue Research* 352(1), 21–31.
9. Manning A. L., Dyson N. J. (2012). RB: Mitotic implications of a tumor suppressor. *Nature Reviews Cancer* 12(3), 220–226.
10. Aloni-Grinstein R., Shetzer Y., Kaufman T., et al. (2014). P53: The barrier to cancer stem cell formation. *FEBS Letters* 588(16), 2580–2589.
11. Zhou H., Wang H., Yu G., et al. (2017). Synergistic inhibitory effects of an engineered antibody-like molecule ATF-Fc and trastuzumab on tumor growth and invasion in a human breast cancer xenograft mouse model. *Oncology Letters* 14, 5189–5196.
12. Rahman N. (2014). Realizing the promise of cancer predisposition genes. *Nature* 505, 302–308.
13. Maclejowski J., deLange T. (2017). Telomeres in cancer: Tumour suppression and genome stability. *Nature Reviews. Molecular Cell Biology* 18(3), 175–186.
14. Ribatti D. (2017). The concept of immune surveillance against tumors: The first theories. *Oncotarget* 8(4), 7175–7180.
15. Flegal K. M., Kit B. K., Orpana H., et al. (2013). Association of all-cause mortality with overweight and obesity using standard body mass index categories: A systematic review and meta-analysis. *Journal of the American Medical Association* 309(1), 71–82.
16. Brown S. B., Hankinson S. E. (2015). Endogenous estrogens and the risk of breast, endometrial and ovarian cancers. *Steroids* 99, 8–10.
17. Campbell C. D., Eichler E. E. (2013). Properties and rates of germline mutation in humans. *Trends in Genetics* 29(10), 575–584.
18. Kleinerman R. A., Schonfeld S. J., Tucker M. A. (2012). Sarcomas in hereditary retinoblastoma. *Clinical Sarcoma Research* 2(15), 1–7.
19. Plawski A., Banasiewicz T., Borun P., et al. (2013). Familial adenomatous polyposis of the colon. *Hereditary Cancer in Clinical Practice* 11(1), 15.
20. Center for Disease Control. (2016). Cancers linked to tobacco use make up 40% of all cancers diagnosed in the United States. Available: https://www.cdc.gov/media/releases/2016/p1110-vital-signs-cancer-tobacco.html. Accessed April 10, 2019.
21. Hemeryck L. Y., Vanhaecke L. (2016). Diet-related DNA adduct formation in relation to carcinogenesis. *Nutrition Reviews* 74(8), 475–489.
22. Moore S. C., Lee M., Weiderpass E. L., et al. (2016). Association of leisure-time physical activity with risk of 26 types of cancer in 1.44 million adults. *Journal of the American Medical Association* 176(6), 816–825.
23. Poskanzer D. C., Herbst A. (1977). Epidemiology of vaginal adenosis and adenocarcinoma associated with exposure to stilbestrol in utero. *Cancer* 39, 1892–1895.
24. Jablon S., Kato H. (1972). Studies of the mortality of A-bomb survivors: Radiation dose and mortality, 1950–1970. *Radiation Research* 50, 649–698.
25. Aoyagi T., Terracina K. P., Matsubara H., et al. (2015). Cancer cachexia, mechanism and treatment. *World Journal of Gastrointestinal Oncology* 7(4), 17–29.
26. Ruddon R. W. (Ed.) (1995). *Cancer biology.* New York, NY: Oxford University Press.
27. Bower J. E. (2014). Cancer-related fatigue-mechanisms, risk factors, and treatments. *National Review of Clinical Oncology* 11, 597–609.
28. Morgensztern D., Waqar S., Subramanian J., et al. (2012). Prognostic impact of malignant pleural effusion at presentation in patients with metastatic non-small-cell lung cancer. *Journal of Thoracic Oncology* 7, 1485–1489.
29. Gilbert L., Sampalis J., Karp I., et al. (2012). Assessment of symptomatic women for early diagnosis of ovarian cancer: Results from the prospective DOvE pilot project. *Lancet* 13, 285–291.
30. Muliawati Y., Haroen H., Rotty L. (2012). Cancer anorexia—cachexia syndrome. *The Indonesian Journal of Internal Medicine* 44(2), 154–162.
31. Mirsadraee S., Oswal D., Alizadeh Y., et al. (2012). The 7th lung cancer TNM classification and staging system: Review of the changes and implications. *World Journal of Radiology* 4(4), 128–134.
32. Wender R., Fontham E. T., Barrera E., et al. (2013). American Cancer Society lung cancer screening guidelines. *A Cancer Journal for Clinicians* 63, 106–117.
33. Duffy M. J. (2013). Tumor markers in clinical practice: A review focusing on common solid cancers. *Medial Principles and Practice* 22, 4–11.
34. Liang J., Gao P., Wang Z., et al. (2012). The integration of macroscopic tumor invasion of adjacent organs into TNM staging system for colorectal cancer. *PLoS One* 7(12), e52269.

35. Fu D., Calvo J. A., Samson L. D. (2012). Balancing repair and tolerance of DNA damage caused by alkylating agents. *Nature* 12, 104–120.

36. Yang F., Teves S. S., Kemp C. J., et al. (2014). Doxorubicin, DNA torsion, and chromatin dynamics. *Biochimica et Biophysica Acta* 1845, 84–89.

37. Mukhtar E., Adhami V. M., Kukhtar H. (2016). Targeting microtubules by natural agents for cancer therapy. *Molecular Cancer Therapeutics* 13(2), 275–284.

38. Kuroki M., Miyamoto S., Morisaki T., et al. (2012). Biological response modifiers used in cancer biotherapy. *Anticancer Research* 32, 2229–2234.

39. Myint Z. W., Goil G. (2017). Role of modern immunotherapy in gastrointestinal malignancies: A review of current clinical progress. *Journal of Hematology and Oncology* 10, 86–98.

40. American Cancer Society. (2017). Treatment and support. [Online]. Available: https://www.cancer.org/treatment.html. Accessed November 18, 2017.

41. Ott P. A., Fritsch E. F., Wu C. J., et al. (2014). Vaccines and melanoma. *Hematology Oncology Clinics of North America* 28, 559–569.

42. Joura E. A., Giuliano A. R., Iversen E. E., et al. (2015). A 9-valent HPV vaccine against infection and intraepithelial neoplasia in women. *The New England Journal of Medicine* 372(8), 711–723.

43. Lin F., Young H. (2014). Interferons: Success in anti-viral immunotherapy. *Cytokine and Growth Factor Reviews* 25, 369–376.

44. Siegel R. L., Miller K. D., Jemal A. (2018). Cancer statistics, 2018. *CA: A Cancer Journal for Clinicians* 68, 7–30.

45. Cheung N. V., Dyer M. A. (2013). Neuroblastoma: Developmental biology, cancer genomics and immunotherapy. *Nature Reviews. Cancer* 13, 397–411.

46. Bruwier A., Chantrain C. F. (2012). Hematological disorders and leukemia in children with Down syndrome. *European Journal of Pediatrics* 171, 1301–1307.

47. Harris L. K., Westwood M. (2012). Biology and significance of signaling pathways activated by IGF-II. *Growth Factors* 30(1), 1–12.

48. American Cancer Society. (2016). What are the differences between cancers in adults and children? [Online]. Available: https://www.cancer.org/cancer/childhood-non-hodgkin-lymphoma/about/differences-children-adults.html. Accessed March 2, 2018.

49. Robinson L. L., Hudson M. M. (2014). Survivors of childhood and adolescent cancer: Life-long risks and responsibilities. *Nature Reviews Cancer* 14, 61–70.

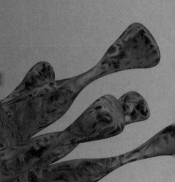

UNIT 3 — Disorders of Integrative Function

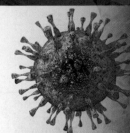

CHAPTER 7

Stress and Adaptation

Learning Objectives

After completing this chapter, the learner will be able to meet the following objectives:

1. Describe the concept of homeostasis.
2. Describe the components of a control system, including the function of a negative feedback system.
3. Explain the interactions among components of the nervous system in mediating the stress response.
4. Describe the stress responses of the autonomic nervous system, the endocrine system, the immune system, and the musculoskeletal system.
5. Explain adaptation and its physiologic purpose.
6. Discuss Selye's *general adaptation syndrome.*
7. Describe the physiologic and psychological effects of a chronic stress response.
8. Describe the characteristic of posttraumatic stress disorder.
9. List five nonpharmacologic methods of treating stress.

Stress has become an increasingly discussed topic in today's world. The concept is discussed extensively in the health care fields and is found in economics, political science, business, and education. In the popular press, the physiologic response to stress is often implicated as a contributor to a variety of individual physical and mental challenges and societal problems. The 2017 American Psychological Association's (APA) Stress in America survey identified various sources of stress and its effect on the overall health and well-being of Americans living in the Unites States. Interestingly, it identified that 57% of Americans reported that the current political climate is a significant source of stress. Other significant stressors included stress related to personal safety and future, police violence toward minorities, work and economy, terrorism, mass shootings, and gun violence. Technology and social media have changed the way people around the world access information. According to the APA, 8 in 10 Americans are attached to their devices on any typical day and are considered as constant checkers of information on their personal electronic devices, and this activity with technology is considered as a source of stress. The above-mentioned stressors affect the health of our society, and the percentage of Americans reported to have at least one symptom of stress (headache, anxiety, depression, etc.) increased from 71% in August 2016 to 80% in January 2017.[1]

In 1910, when Sir William Osler delivered his Lumleian Lectures on "angina pectoris," he described the relationship of stress and strain to angina pectoris.[2] Approximately 15 years later, Walter Cannon, well known for his work in physiology, began to use the word *stress* in relation to his laboratory experiments on the "fight-or-flight" response. It seems possible that the term emerged from his work on the homeostatic features of living organisms and their tendency to "bound back" and "resist disruption" when acted on by an "external force."[3] Cannon referred to the concept of a stable internal environment as *homeostasis*, which is achieved through a system of carefully coordinated physiologic processes that oppose change.[4] Cannon pointed out that these processes were largely automatic and emphasized that homeostasis involves resistance to both internal and external disturbances.

At about the same time, Hans Selye, who became known for his research and publications on stress, began using the term *stress* in a very special way to mean an orchestrated set of bodily responses to any form of noxious stimulus.[5]

The content in this chapter has been organized into three sections: homeostasis, the stress response and adaptation to stress, and disorders of the stress response.

Homeostasis

The concepts of stress and adaptation have their origin in the complexity of the human body and the interactions between its cells and its many organ systems. These interactions require that a level of homeostasis or constancy be maintained during the many changes that occur in the internal and external environments. In effecting a state of constancy, homeostasis requires feedback control systems that regulate cellular function and integrate the function of the different body systems.

Constancy of the Internal Environment

Claude Bernard, a 19th-century physiologist, was the first to describe clearly the central importance of a stable internal environment, which he termed the *milieu intérieur*.[6] Bernard recognized that body fluids surrounding the cells (extracellular fluids) and the various organ systems provide the means for exchange between the external and the internal environments. It is from this internal environment that body cells receive their nourishment, and it is into this fluid that they secrete their wastes. Even the contents of the gastrointestinal tract and lungs do not become part of the internal environment until they have been absorbed into the extracellular fluid. A multicellular organism is able to survive only as long as the composition of the internal environment is compatible with the survival needs of the individual cells. For example, even a small change in the pH of the body fluids can disrupt the metabolic processes of the individual cells.

Control Systems

The ability of the body to function and maintain homeostasis under conditions of change in the internal and external environment depends on the thousands of physiologic *control systems* that regulate body function. A homeostatic control system consists of a collection of interconnected components that function to keep a physical or chemical parameter of the body relatively constant. The body's control systems regulate cellular function, control life processes, and integrate functions of the different organ systems.

Of recent interest have been the neuroendocrine control systems that influence behavior. Biochemical messengers that exist in our brain serve to control nerve activity, regulate information flow, and, ultimately, influence behavior.[7] These control systems mediate the physical, emotional, and behavioral reactions to stressors that, taken together, are called the *stress response*.

Just like any control system, each stress response involves a *sensor* to detect the change, an *integrator* to sum all incoming data and compare them with "normal," and *effector(s)* to try to reverse the change. For instance, a hiker's eyes (sensor) see a snake (stressor), and the cerebral cortex (integrator) of the individual determines that the snake is a threat and activates the heart, respiratory muscles, and many other organs (effectors) to assist in escape.

More complex stressors invoke more complex control systems, and sometimes, the stress response cannot restore balance and homeostasis. For instance, adverse physical and psychological experiences early in life (prenatal and childhood periods) can impact one's adult health.[8] The impact may appear decades later, in the form of mental health issues, immune dysregulations, cardiovascular diseases, cancer, and so on.[8] Therefore, it is important to identify early negative experiences and treat them, not only for the current health of the child but also for the future health of the adult.[9]

KEY POINTS

Homeostasis

■ Homeostasis is the purposeful maintenance of a stable internal environment by coordinated physiologic processes that oppose change.

■ The physiologic control systems that oppose change operate by negative feedback mechanisms consisting of a sensor that detects a change, an integrator/comparator that sums and compares incoming data with a set point, and an effector system that returns the sensed function to within the range of the set point.

Feedback Systems

Most control systems in the body operate by *negative feedback mechanisms*, which function in a manner similar to the thermostat on a heating system. When the monitored function or value decreases below the set point of the system, the feedback mechanism causes the function or value to increase. When the function or value is increased above the set point, the feedback mechanism causes it to decrease (Fig. 7-1). For example, in the negative feedback mechanism that controls blood glucose levels, an increase in blood glucose stimulates an increase in insulin, which enhances the removal of glucose from the blood. When glucose has been taken up by cells and blood glucose levels fall, insulin secretion is inhibited and glucagon and other counterregulatory mechanisms stimulate the release of glucose from the glycogen stores of liver, which causes the blood glucose to return to normal. The same is true for all endocrine hormones that are connected to the pituitary for their stimulating hormone and the hypothalamus for their releasing hormone. For example, when thyroxine (T_4) in the thyroid is low, it triggers the pituitary to increase thyroid-stimulating hormone (TSH), which then increases T_4 secretion from the thyroid.

The reason most physiologic control systems function under negative rather than *positive feedback mechanisms* is that a positive feedback mechanism interjects instability rather than stability into a system. It produces a cycle in which the initiating stimulus produces more of the same. For example, in a hypothetical positive feedback system, exposure to an increase in environmental temperature would invoke compensatory mechanisms designed to increase rather than decrease body temperature.

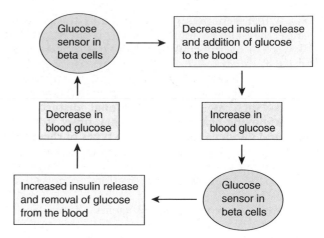

FIGURE 7-1. Illustration of negative feedback control mechanisms using blood glucose as an example.

contribute directly to the production or exacerbation of a disease, or it may contribute to the development of behaviors such as smoking, overeating, and drug abuse that increase the risk of disease.[10]

The Stress Response

In the early 1930s, the world-renowned endocrinologist Hans Selye was the first to describe a group of specific anatomic changes that occurred in rats that were exposed to a variety of different experimental stimuli. He came to an understanding that these changes were manifestations of the body's attempt to adapt to stimuli. Selye described *stress* as "a state manifested by a specific syndrome of the body developed in response to any stimuli that made an intense systemic demand on it."[11] In his early career as an experimental scientist, Selye noted that a triad of adrenal enlargement, thymic atrophy, and gastric ulcers appeared in rats he was using for his studies. These same three changes developed in response to many different or nonspecific experimental challenges. He assumed that the hypothalamic–pituitary–adrenal (HPA) axis played a pivotal role in the development of this response. To Selye, the response to stressors was a process that enabled the rats to resist the experimental challenge by using the function of the system best able to respond to it. He labeled the response the *general adaptation syndrome* (GAS): *general* because the effect was a general systemic reaction, *adaptive* because the response was in reaction to a stressor, and *syndrome* because the physical manifestations were coordinated and dependent on each other.[11]

According to Selye, the GAS involves three stages: the alarm stage, the resistance stage, and the exhaustion stage. The *alarm stage* is characterized by a generalized stimulation of the sympathetic nervous system and the HPA axis, resulting in the release of catecholamines and cortisol. During the *resistance stage*, the body selects the most effective and economic channels of defense. During this stage, the increased cortisol

SUMMARY CONCEPTS

Physiologic and psychological adaptation involves the ability to maintain the constancy of the internal environment (homeostasis) and behavior in the face of a wide range of changes in the internal and external environments. It involves control and negative feedback systems that regulate cellular function, control life's processes, regulate behavior, and integrate the function of the different body systems.

Stress and Adaptation

The increased focus on health promotion has heightened interest in the roles of stress and biobehavioral stress responses in the development of disease. Stress may levels, which were present during the first stage, drop because they are no longer needed. If the stressor is prolonged or overwhelms the ability of the body to defend itself, the *exhaustion stage* ensues, during which resources are depleted and signs of "wear and tear" or systemic damage appear.[12] Selye contended that many ailments, such as various emotional disturbances, mildly annoying headaches, insomnia, upset stomach, gastric and duodenal ulcers, certain types of rheumatic disorders, and cardiovascular and kidney diseases, appear to be initiated or encouraged by the "body itself because of its faulty adaptive reactions to potentially injurious agents."[13]

The events or environmental agents responsible for initiating the stress response were called *stressors*. According to Selye, stressors could be endogenous, arising from within the body, or exogenous, arising from outside the body.[13] In explaining the stress response, Selye proposed that two factors determine the nature of the stress response—the properties of the stressor and the conditioning of the person being stressed. Selye indicated that not all stress was detrimental; hence, he coined the terms *eustress* and *distress*.[12] He suggested that mild, brief, and controllable periods of stress could be perceived as positive stimuli to emotional and intellectual growth and development. It is the severe, protracted, and uncontrolled situations of psychological and physical distress that are disruptive of health.[13] For example, the joy of becoming a new parent and the sorrow of losing a parent are completely different experiences, yet their stressor effect—the nonspecific demand for adjustment to a new situation—can be similar.

It is increasingly clear that the physiologic stress response is far more complicated than can be explained fully by a classic stimulus–response mechanism. Stressors tend to produce different responses in different people or in the same person at different times, indicating the influence of the adaptive capacity of the person, or what Selye called *conditioning factors*. These conditioning factors may be internal (*e.g.*, genetic predisposition, age, sex) or external (*e.g.*, exposure to environmental agents, life experiences, dietary factors, level of social support).[13] The relative risk for development of a stress-related pathologic process seems, at least in part, to depend on these factors.

Neuroendocrine Responses

The manifestations of the stress response are strongly influenced by both the nervous and endocrine systems. The neuroendocrine systems integrate signals received along the neurosensory pathways and from circulating mediators that are carried in the bloodstream. In addition, the immune system both affects and is affected by the stress response. Table 7-1 summarizes the action of hormones involved in the neuroendocrine responses to stress. The results of the coordinated release of these neurohormones include the mobilization of energy, a sharpened focus and awareness, increased cerebral blood flow and glucose utilization, enhanced cardiovascular and respiratory functioning, redistribution of blood flow to the brain and muscles, modulation of the immune response, inhibition of reproductive function, and a decrease in appetite.[14]

The stress response is a normal, coordinated physiologic system not only meant to increase the probability of survival but also designed to be an acute response—turned on when necessary to bring the body back to a stable state and turned off when the challenge to homeostasis abates. Therefore, under normal circumstances, the neural responses and the hormones that are released during the response do not persist long enough to cause damage to vital tissues. Since the early 1980s, the term *allostasis* has been used by some investigators to

TABLE 7-1 Hormones Involved in the Neuroendocrine Responses to Stress

Hormones Associated with the Stress Response	Source of the Hormone	Physiologic Effects
Catecholamines (*e.g.*, NE, epinephrine)	LC, adrenal medulla	Produce a decrease in insulin release and an increase in glucagon release resulting in increased glycogenolysis, gluconeogenesis, lipolysis, proteolysis, and decreased glucose uptake by the peripheral tissues; an increase in heart rate, cardiac contractility, and vascular smooth muscle contraction; and relaxation of bronchial smooth muscle
Corticotropin-releasing factor	Hypothalamus	Stimulates ACTH release from the anterior pituitary and increased activity of the LC neurons
Adrenocorticotropic hormone (ACTH)	Anterior pituitary	Stimulates the synthesis and release of cortisol
Glucocorticoid hormones (*e.g.*, cortisol)	Adrenal cortex	Potentiate the actions of epinephrine and glucagon; inhibit the release and/or actions of the reproductive hormones and thyroid-stimulating hormone; and produce a decrease in immune cells and inflammatory mediators
Mineralocorticoid hormones (*e.g.*, aldosterone)	Adrenal cortex	Increase sodium absorption by the kidney
Antidiuretic hormone (*e.g.*, vasopressin)	Hypothalamus, posterior pituitary	Increases water absorption by the kidney; produces vasoconstriction of blood vessels; and stimulates the release of ACTH

LC, locus coeruleus; NE, norepinephrine.

describe the physiologic changes in the neuroendocrine, autonomic, and immune systems that occur in response to either real or perceived challenges to homeostasis.

 Concept Mastery Alert

The persistence or accumulation of the allostatic changes (*e.g.*, immunosuppression, activation of the sympathetic nervous and renin–angiotensin–aldosterone systems) has been called an *allostatic load* or *overload*, and this concept has been used to measure the cumulative effects of stress on humans.[15]

The integration of the components of the stress response, which occurs at the level of the central nervous system (CNS), is complex and not completely understood. It relies on communication along neuronal pathways of the cerebral cortex, the limbic system, the thalamus, the hypothalamus, the pituitary gland, and the reticular activating system (RAS; Fig. 7-2). The cerebral cortex is involved with vigilance, cognition, and focused attention and the limbic system with the emotional components (*e.g.*, fear, excitement, rage, anger) of the stress response. The thalamus functions as the relay center and is important in receiving, sorting out, and distributing sensory input. The hypothalamus coordinates the responses of the endocrine and autonomic nervous systems (ANSs). The RAS modulates mental alertness, ANS activity, and skeletal muscle tone, using input from other neural structures. The musculoskeletal tension that occurs during the stress response reflects increased activity of the RAS and its influence on the reflex circuits that control muscle tone. Adding to the complexity of this system is the fact that the individual brain circuits that participate in the mediation of the stress response interact and regulate the activity of each other. For example, reciprocal connections exist between neurons in the hypothalamus that initiate release of corticotropin-releasing factor (CRF) and neurons in the locus coeruleus (LC) associated with release of norepinephrine (NE). Thus, NE stimulates the secretion of CRF, and CRF stimulates the release of NE.[15]

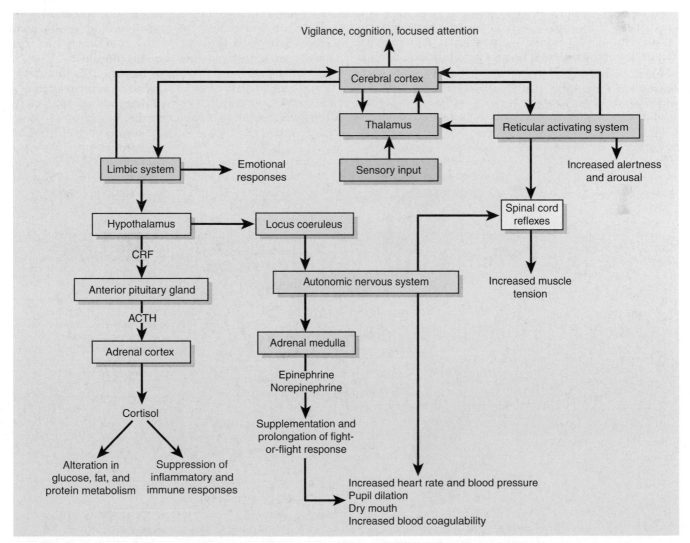

FIGURE 7-2. Neuroendocrine pathways and physiologic responses to stress. ACTH, adrenocorticotropic hormone; CRF, corticotropin-releasing factor.

Locus Coeruleus

Central to the neural component of the neuroendocrine response to stress is an area of the brain stem called the LC.[15] The LC is densely populated with neurons that produce NE and is thought to be the central integrating site for the ANS response to stressful stimuli (Fig. 7-3). The LC–NE system has afferent pathways to the hypothalamus, the limbic system, the hippocampus, and the cerebral cortex.

The LC–NE system confers an adaptive advantage during a stressful situation. The sympathetic nervous system manifestation of the stress reaction has been called the *fight-or-flight response*. This is the most rapid of the stress responses and represents the basic survival response of our primitive ancestors when confronted with the perils of the wilderness and its inhabitants. The increase in sympathetic activity in the brain increases attention and arousal and thus may intensify memory. The heart and respiratory rates increase, the hands and feet become moist, the pupils dilate, the mouth becomes dry, and the activity of the gastrointestinal tract decreases.

Corticotropin-Releasing Factor

CRF is central to the endocrine component of the neuroendocrine response to stress (see Fig. 7-3). CRF is a small peptide hormone secreted by the paraventricular nucleus (PVN) of the hypothalamus. It is both an important endocrine regulator of pituitary and adrenal activity and a neurotransmitter involved in ANS activity, metabolism, and behavior.[15] Receptors for CRF are distributed throughout the brain as well as in many peripheral sites. CRF secreted from the hypothalamus in response to stress stimulus induces secretion of adrenocorticotropic hormone (ACTH) from the anterior pituitary gland. ACTH, in turn, stimulates the adrenal gland to synthesize and secrete the glucocorticoid hormones (*e.g.*, cortisol).

The glucocorticoid hormones have a number of direct or indirect physiologic effects that mediate the stress response, enhance the action of other stress hormones, or suppress other components of the stress system. In this regard, cortisol acts not only as a mediator of the stress response but also as an inhibitor, such that overactivation of the stress response does not occur.[15] Cortisol maintains blood glucose levels by antagonizing the effects of insulin and enhances the effect of catecholamines on the cardiovascular system. It also suppresses osteoblast activity, **hematopoiesis**, collagen synthesis, and immune responses. All of these functions are meant to protect the organism against the effects of a stressor and to focus energy on regaining balance in the face of an acute challenge to homeostasis.

Angiotensin II

Stimulation of the sympathetic nervous system also activates the peripheral renin–angiotensin–aldosterone system, which mediates a peripheral increase in vascular tone and renal retention of sodium and water. These changes contribute to the physiologic changes that occur with the stress response and, if prolonged, may contribute to pathologic changes. Angiotensin II, peripherally delivered or locally produced, also has CNS effects; angiotensin II type 1 (AT$_1$) receptors are widely distributed in the hypothalamus and LC. Through these

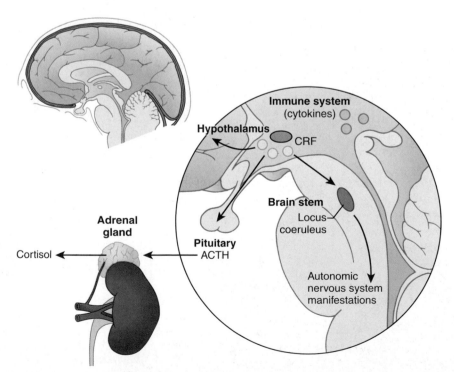

FIGURE 7-3. Neuroendocrine–immune system regulation of the stress response. ACTH, adrenocorticotropic hormone; CRF, corticotropin-releasing factor.

receptors, angiotensin II enhances CRF formation and release, contributes to the release of ACTH from the pituitary, enhances stress-induced release of vasopressin from the posterior pituitary, and stimulates the release of NE from the LC.[15]

Other Hormones

A wide variety of other hormones, including growth hormone, thyroid hormone, and the reproductive hormones, also are responsive to stressful stimuli. Systems responsible for reproduction, growth, and immunity are directly linked to the stress system, and the hormonal effects of the stress response profoundly influence these systems. Studies have shown that in females, stress and severe trauma can cause menstrual irregularities, anovulation, and amenorrhea.[14] In males, stress can induce decreased spermatogenesis, ejaculatory disorders, decreased levels of testosterone, and infertility.[16]

Although growth hormone is initially elevated at the onset of stress, the prolonged presence of cortisol leads to suppression of growth hormone, insulin-like growth factor 1, and other growth factors, exerting a chronically inhibitory effect on growth. In addition, CRF directly increases somatostatin, which in turn inhibits growth hormone secretion. Although the connection is speculative, the effects of stress on growth hormone may provide one of the vital links to understanding failure to thrive in children.

Stress-induced cortisol secretion also is associated with decreased levels of TSH and inhibition of conversion of thyroxine (T_4) to the more biologically active triiodothyronine (T_3) in peripheral tissues. Both changes may serve as a means to conserve energy at times of stress.

Antidiuretic hormone (ADH) released from the posterior pituitary is also involved in the stress response, particularly in hypotensive stress or stress due to fluid volume loss. ADH, also known as *vasopressin*, increases water retention by the kidneys and produces vasoconstriction of blood vessels. In addition, vasopressin synthesized in parvocellular neurons of the hypothalamus and transported to the anterior pituitary appears to synergize the capacity of CRF to stimulate the release of ACTH.

The neurotransmitter serotonin or 5-hydroxytryptamine (5-HT) also plays a role in the stress response through neurons that innervate the hypothalamus, amygdala, and other limbic structures. Administration of 5-HT receptor **agonists** to laboratory animals was shown to increase the secretion of several stress hormones. Other hormones that have a possible role in the stress response include vasoactive intestinal peptide, neuropeptide Y, cholecystokinin, and substance P. These hormones have well characterized physiologic roles in periphery, but they are also found in the CNS, and literature supports that they are involved in the stress response.[17]

Oxytocin is a neuropeptide/neurohormone produced in the PVN and supraoptic nucleus of the hypothalamus. A large body of literature suggests that oxytocin plays a significant role in reducing stress-related physiologic consequences. Exogenous delivery of oxytocin via intranasal route has shown reduction in psychosocial stress reactivity, fear and anxiety, and increases reward processing.[18]

Immune Responses

The hallmark of the stress response, as first described by Selye, are the endocrine–immune interactions (*i.e.*, increased corticosteroid production and atrophy of the thymus) that are known to suppress the immune response. In concert, these two components of the stress system, through endocrine and neurotransmitter pathways, produce the physical and behavioral changes designed to adapt to acute stress. Much of the literature regarding stress and the immune response focuses on the causal role of stress in immune-related diseases. It has also been suggested that the reverse may occur. That is, emotional and psychological manifestations of the stress response may be a reflection of alterations in the CNS resulting from the immune response (see Fig. 7-3). Immune cells such as monocytes and lymphocytes can penetrate the blood–brain barrier and take up residence in the brain, where they secrete chemical messengers called *cytokines* that influence the stress response.

The exact mechanism by which stress produces its effect on the immune response is unknown and probably varies from person to person, depending on genetic and environmental factors. The most significant arguments for interaction between the neuroendocrine and immune systems derive from evidence that the immune and neuroendocrine systems share common signal pathways (*i.e.*, messenger molecules and receptors), that hormones and neuropeptides can alter the function of immune cells, and that the immune system and its mediators can modulate neuroendocrine function.[15] Receptors for a number of CNS-controlled hormones and neuromediators reportedly have been found on lymphocytes. Among these are receptors for glucocorticoids, insulin, testosterone, prolactin, catecholamines, estrogens, acetylcholine, and growth hormone, suggesting that these hormones and neuromediators influence lymphocyte function. For example, cortisol is known to suppress immune function, and pharmacologic doses of cortisol are used clinically to suppress the immune response. It has been observed that the HPA axis is activated by cytokines such as interleukin-1, interleukin-6, and tumor necrosis factor-α that are released from immune cells.

A second possible route for neuroendocrine regulation of immune function is through the sympathetic nervous system and the release of catecholamines. The lymph nodes, thymus, and spleen are supplied with ANS nerve fibers. Centrally acting CRF activates the ANS through multisynaptic descending pathways, and circulating epinephrine acts synergistically with CRF and cortisol to inhibit the function of the immune system.

Not only is the quantity of immune expression changed because of stress, but the quality of the response is changed as well. Stress hormones differentially stimulate the proliferation of subtypes of T lymphocyte helper cells. Because these T helper cell subtypes secrete different cytokines, they stimulate different aspects of the immune response. One subtype tends to stimulate T lymphocytes and the cellular-mediated immune response, whereas a second type tends to activate B lymphocytes and humoral-mediated immune responses.[15]

KEY POINTS

Stress and Adaptation

- Stress is a state manifested by symptoms that arise from the coordinated activation of the neuroendocrine and immune systems, which Selye called the general adaptation syndrome.

- The hormones and neurotransmitters (catecholamines and cortisol) are released during the stress response function to alert the individual to a threat or challenge to homeostasis, to enhance cardiovascular and metabolic activity in order to manage the stressor, and to focus the energy of the body by suppressing the activity of other systems that are not immediately needed.

- Adaptation is the ability to respond to challenges of physical or psychological homeostasis and to return to a balanced state.

- The ability to adapt is influenced by previous learning, physiologic reserve, time, genetic endowment, age, health status and nutrition, sleep–wake cycles, and psychosocial factors.

Coping and Adaptation to Stress

The ability to adapt to a wide range of environments and stressors is not peculiar to humans. According to René Dubos (a microbiologist noted for his study of human responses to the total environment), "adaptability is found throughout life and is perhaps the one attribute that distinguishes most clearly the world of life from the world of inanimate matter."[19] Living organisms, no matter how primitive, do not submit passively to the impact of environmental forces.

Adaptation

Human beings, because of their highly developed nervous system and intellect, usually have alternative mechanisms for adapting and have the ability to control many aspects of their environment. The availability of antiseptic agents, immunizations, and antibiotics eliminates the need to respond to common infectious agents. At the same time, modern technology creates new challenges for adaptation and provides new sources of stress, such as noise and air pollution. Of particular interest

are the differences in the body's response to events that threaten the integrity of the body's physiologic environment and those that threaten the integrity of the person's psychosocial environment. Many of the body's responses to physiologic disturbances are controlled on a moment-by-moment basis by feedback mechanisms that limit their application and duration of action. For example, the baroreflex-mediated rise in heart rate that occurs when a person moves from the recumbent to the standing position is almost instantaneous and subsides within seconds. Furthermore, the response to physiologic disturbances that threaten the integrity of the internal environment is specific to the threat; the body usually does not raise the body temperature when an increase in heart rate is needed. In contrast, the response to psychological disturbances is not regulated with the same degree of specificity and feedback control. Instead, the effect may be inappropriate and sustained.

Factors Affecting the Ability to Adapt

Adaptation implies that an individual has successfully created a new balance between the stressor and the ability to deal with it. The means used to attain this balance are called *coping strategies* or *coping mechanisms*. Coping mechanisms are the emotional and behavioral responses used to manage threats to our physiologic and psychological homeostasis. According to Lazarus, how we cope with stressful events depends on how we perceive and interpret the event.[20] Is the event perceived as a threat of harm or loss? Is the event perceived as a challenge rather than a threat? Physiologic reserve, time, genetics, age, health status, nutrition, sleep–wake cycles, hardiness, and psychosocial factors influence a person's appraisal of a stressor and the coping mechanisms used to adapt to the new situation (Fig. 7-4).

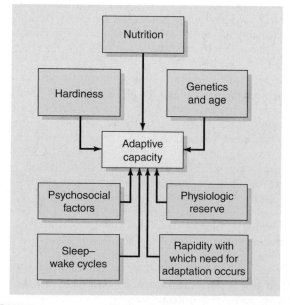

FIGURE 7-4. Factors affecting adaptation.

Physiologic and Anatomic Reserve

The safety margin for adaptation of most body systems is considerably greater than that needed for normal activities. The red blood cells carry more oxygen than the tissues can use, the liver and fat cells store excess nutrients, and bone tissue stores calcium in excess of that needed for normal neuromuscular function. The ability of body systems to increase their function given the need to adapt is known as the *physiologic reserve*. Many of the body organs, such as the lungs, kidneys, and adrenals, are paired to provide anatomic reserve as well. Both organs are not needed to ensure the continued existence and maintenance of the internal environment. Many people function normally with only one lung or one kidney. In kidney disease, for example, signs of renal failure do not occur until approximately 80% of the functioning nephrons have been destroyed.

Time

Adaptation is most efficient when changes occur gradually, rather than suddenly. It is possible, for instance, to lose a liter or more of blood through chronic gastrointestinal bleeding over a week without manifesting signs of shock. However, a sudden hemorrhage that causes rapid loss of an equal amount of blood is likely to cause hypotension and shock.

Genetics

Adaptation is further affected by the availability of adaptive responses and flexibility in selecting the most appropriate and economical response. The greater the number of available responses, the more effective is the capacity to adapt. Genetics can ensure that the systems that are essential to adaptation function adequately. Even a gene that has deleterious effects may prove adaptive in some environments. In Africa, the gene for sickle cell anemia persists in some populations because it provides some resistance to infection with the parasite that causes malaria.

Age

The capacity to adapt is decreased at the extremes of age. The ability to adapt is impaired by the immaturity of an infant, much as it is by the decline in functional reserve that occurs with age. For example, the infant has difficulty concentrating urine because of immature renal structures and therefore is less able than an adult to cope with decreased water intake or exaggerated water losses. A similar situation exists in the elderly owing to age-related changes in renal function.

Gender

Within the last decade, primarily because females have been included in basic science and clinical investigations, differences between the sexes in cardiovascular, respiratory, endocrine, renal, and neurophysiologic function have been found, and it has been hypothesized that sex hormones are the basis of these biologic differences. Technologic advances in cellular and molecular biology have made it clear, however, that there are fundamental differences in the locale and regulation of individual genes in the male and female genome. These differences have general implications for the prevention, diagnosis, and treatment of disease and specific implications for our understanding of the sex-based differences in response to life's stressors.

Given the nature of sex-based differences, it is not surprising that there are differences in the physiologic stress response in both the HPA axis and in the ANS. Premenopausal women tend to have a lower activation of the sympathetic nervous system than men in response to stressors. Gender-based differences in activation of the stress response may partially explain differences in susceptibility to diseases in which the stress response may play a causal role. These research results are not definitive but are intriguing and can serve as a springboard for further research.

Health Status

Physical and mental health status determines physiologic and psychological reserves and is a strong determinant of the ability to adapt. For example, people with heart disease are less able to adjust to stresses that require the recruitment of cardiovascular responses. Severe emotional stress often produces disruption of physiologic function and limits the ability to make appropriate choices related to long-term adaptive needs. Those who have worked with acutely ill people know that the will to live often has a profound influence on survival during life-threatening illnesses.

Nutrition

There are 50 to 60 essential nutrients, including minerals, lipids, certain fatty acids, vitamins, and specific amino acids. Deficiencies or excesses of any of these nutrients can alter a person's health status and impair the ability to adapt. The importance of nutrition to enzyme function, immune response, and wound healing is well known. On a worldwide basis, malnutrition may be one of the most common causes of immunodeficiency.

Among the problems associated with dietary excess are obesity and alcohol abuse. Obesity is a common problem. It predisposes a person to a number of health problems, including atherosclerosis and hypertension. Alcohol is commonly used in excess. It acutely affects brain function and, with long-term use, can seriously impair the function of the liver, brain, and other vital structures.

Circadian Rhythm

Sleep is considered to be a restorative function in which energy is restored and tissues are regenerated.[21] Sleep occurs in a cyclic manner, alternating with periods of wakefulness and increased energy use. Biologic rhythms play an important role in adaptation to stress, development of illness, and response to medical treatment. Many rhythms such as rest and activity, work and leisure, and eating and drinking oscillate with a frequency similar to that of the 24-hour light–dark solar day. The term **circadian**, from the Latin *circa* ("about") and *dies* ("day"), is used to describe these 24-hour **diurnal** rhythms.

Sleep disorders and alterations in the sleep–wake cycle have been shown to alter immune function, the normal circadian pattern of hormone secretion, and physical and psychological functioning.[21,22] The two most common manifestations of an alteration in the sleep–wake cycle are insomnia and sleep deprivation or increased somnolence. In some people, stress may produce sleep disorders, and in others, sleep disorders may lead to stress. Acute stress and environmental disturbances, loss of a loved one, recovery from surgery, and pain are common causes of transient and short-term insomnia. Air travel and jet lag constitute additional causes of altered sleep–wake cycles, as does shift work.

Hardiness

Studies by social psychologists have focused on individuals' emotional reactions to stressful situations and their coping mechanisms to determine those characteristics that help some people remain healthy despite being challenged by high levels of stressors. For example, the concept of *hardiness* describes a personality characteristic that includes a sense of having control over the environment, a sense of having a purpose in life, and an ability to conceptualize stressors as a challenge rather than a threat.[23] Many studies by nurses and social psychologists suggest that hardiness is correlated with positive health outcomes.[24]

Psychosocial Factors

Scientific interest in the social environment as a cause of stress has gradually broadened to include the social environment as a resource that modulates the relation between stress and health. Studies suggest that social support has direct and indirect positive effects on the health and well-being and serves as a **buffer** or modifier of the physical and psychosocial effects of stress.[25] Social support has been viewed in terms of the number of relationships a person has and the person's perception of these relationships. Close relationships with others can involve positive effects as well as the potential for conflict and may, in some situations, leave the person less able to cope with life stressors.

SUMMARY CONCEPTS

The stress response involves the activation of several physiologic systems (sympathetic nervous system, the HPA axis, and the immune system) that work in a coordinated fashion to protect the body against damage from the intense demands made on it. Selye called this response the *general adaptation syndrome*. The stress response is divided into three stages: the *alarm stage*, with activation of the sympathetic nervous system and the HPA axis; the *resistance stage*, during which the body selects the most effective defenses; and the *exhaustion stage*, during which physiologic resources are depleted and signs of systemic damage appear.

The activation and control of the stress response are mediated by the combined efforts of the nervous and endocrine systems. The neuroendocrine systems integrate signals received along neurosensory pathways and from circulating mediators that are carried in the bloodstream. In addition, the immune system both affects and is affected by the stress response.

Adaptation is affected by a number of factors, including experience and previous learning, the rapidity with which the need to adapt occurs, genetic endowment and age, health status, nutrition, sleep–wake cycles, hardiness, and psychosocial factors.

Disorders of the Stress Response

For the most part, the stress response is meant to be acute and time limited. The time-limited nature of the process renders the accompanying catabolic and immunosuppressive effects advantageous. It is the chronicity of the response that is thought to be disruptive to physical and mental health.

Stressors can assume a number of patterns in relation to time. They may be classified as acute time limited, chronic intermittent, or chronic sustained. An acute time-limited stressor is one that occurs over a short time and does not recur. A chronic intermittent stressor is one to which a person is chronically exposed. The frequency or chronicity of circumstances to which the body is asked to respond often determines the availability and efficiency of the stress responses. The response of the immune system, for example, is more rapid and efficient on second exposure to a pathogen than it is on first exposure. However, chronic exposure to a stressor can fatigue the system and impair its effectiveness.

Effects of Acute Stress

The reactions to acute stress are those associated with the ANS, the fight-or-flight response. The manifestations of the stress response—a pounding headache; a cold, moist skin; and a stiff neck—are all part of the acute stress response. Centrally, there is facilitation of neural pathways mediating arousal, alertness, vigilance, cognition, and focused attention, as well as appropriate aggression. The acute stress response can result from either psychologically or physiologically threatening events. In situations of life-threatening trauma, these acute responses may be lifesaving in that they divert blood from less essential to more essential body functions. Increased alertness and cognitive functioning enable rapid processing of information and arrival at the most appropriate solution to the threatening situation.

However, for people with limited coping abilities, either because of physical or mental health, the acute stress response may be detrimental (Chart 7-1). This is true of people with preexisting heart disease in whom the overwhelming sympathetic behaviors associated with the stress response can lead to arrhythmias. For people with other chronic health problems, such as headache disorder, acute stress may precipitate a recurrence. In healthy people, the acute stress response can redirect attention from behaviors that promote health, such as attention to proper meals and getting adequate sleep. For those with health problems, it can interrupt compliance with medication regimens and exercise programs. In some situations, the acute arousal state actually can be life-threatening, physically immobilizing the person when movement would avert catastrophe (*e.g.*, moving out of the way of a speeding car).

CHART 7-1

Possible Stress-Induced Health Problems
- Mood disorders
- Anxiety
- Depression
- PTSD
- Eating disorders
- Sleep disorders
- Diabetes type 2
- Hypertension
- Infection
- Exacerbation of autoimmune disorders
- Gastrointestinal problems
- Pain
- Obesity
- Eczema
- Cancer
- Atherosclerosis
- Migraine

Effects of Chronic Stress

The stress response is designed to be an acute self-limited response in which activation of the ANS and the HPA axis is controlled in a negative feedback manner.

As with all negative feedback systems, pathophysiologic changes can occur in the stress response system. Function can be altered in several ways, including when a component of the system fails, when the neural and hormonal connections among the components of the system are dysfunctional, and when the original stimulus for the activation of the system is prolonged or of such magnitude that it overwhelms the ability of the system to respond appropriately. In these cases, the system may become overactive or underactive.

Chronicity and excessive activation of the stress response can result from chronic illnesses as well as contribute to the development of long-term health problems. Chronic activation of the stress response is an important public health issue from both a health and a cost perspective. Stress is linked to a myriad of health disorders, such as diseases of the cardiovascular, gastrointestinal, immune, and neurologic systems, as well as depression, chronic alcoholism and drug abuse, eating disorders, accidents, and suicide.

Posttraumatic Stress Disorder

Posttraumatic stress disorder (PTSD) is a disabling syndrome caused by the chronic activation of the stress response as a result of experiencing a significant traumatic event. The person may remember the traumatic event, or PTSD may occur with no recollection of an earlier stressful experience. PTSD that is manifested 6 months after the traumatic event is called PTSD with delayed onset.[26] PTSD was formerly called *battle fatigue* or *shell shock* because it was first characterized in soldiers returning from combat. Although war is still a significant cause of PTSD, other major catastrophic events, such as weather-related disasters (hurricanes, earthquakes, and floods), airplane crashes, terrorist bombings, and rape or child abuse, also may result in the development of the disorder. In the United States, the most frequently reported traumatic events include physical and sexual assaults (with 52% prevalence) and accidents (with 50% prevalence).[26] People who are exposed to traumatic events are also at risk for development of major depression, panic disorder, generalized anxiety disorder, and substance abuse.[26] They may also have physical symptoms and illnesses (*e.g.*, hypertension, asthma, and chronic pain syndromes).

PTSD is characterized by a constellation of symptoms that are experienced as states of intrusion, avoidance, and hyperarousal. *Intrusion* refers to the occurrence of "flashbacks" during waking hours or nightmares in which the past traumatic event is relived, often in vivid and frightening detail. *Avoidance* refers to the emotional numbing that accompanies this disorder and disrupts important personal relationships. Because a person with PTSD has not been able to resolve the painful feelings associated with the trauma, depression is commonly a part of the clinical picture. Survivor guilt also may be a product of traumatic situations in which the person survived the disaster but loved ones did not. *Hyperarousal* refers to the presence of increased irritability, difficulty concentrating, an exaggerated startle reflex, and increased vigilance and concern over safety. In addition, memory problems, sleep disturbances, and excessive anxiety are commonly experienced by people with PTSD.

For a diagnosis of PTSD to be made, the person must have experienced, witnessed, or confronted a traumatic event, which caused a response in the person involving horror and fear. The triad of symptoms of intrusion, avoidance, and hyperarousal that characterize PTSD must be present together for at least 1 month, and the disorder must have caused clinically significant distress.[26] Although the pathophysiology of PTSD is not completely understood, the revelation of physiologic changes related to the disorder has shed light on why some people recover from the disorder, whereas others do not. Recent neuroanatomic studies have identified alterations in neural systems that are part of the amygdala and hippocampus that play a significant role in fear learning, threat detection, executive function and emotion regulation, and contextual processing.[26] Differences in hippocampal function and memory processes suggest a neuroanatomic basis for the intense problems suffered by people diagnosed with PTSD. People with PTSD demonstrate decreased cortisol levels, increased sensitivity of cortisol receptors, and an enhanced negative feedback inhibition of cortisol release with the dexamethasone suppression test, which mimics the effects of cortisol and directly inhibits the action of CRF and ACTH.

Little is known about the risk factors that predispose people to the development of PTSD. Health care professionals need to be aware that people who present with symptoms of depression, anxiety, and alcohol or drug abuse may in fact be suffering from PTSD. The patient history should include questions concerning the occurrence of violence, major loss, or traumatic events in the person's life.

Debriefing, or talking about the traumatic event at the time it happens, often is an effective therapeutic tool. Often concurrent pharmacotherapy with antidepressant and antianxiety agents is useful and helps the person participate more fully in therapy.

Treatment and Research of Stress Disorders

The change that occurs in the biochemical stress response system of people who have experienced some type of mistreatment as a child so that they are not able to respond effectively to stressors in the future is called the traumatic stress response.[27] Evidence supports that early intervention can assist the person in adapting new and effective coping mechanisms to better manage stress in the future.[27] Additionally, a study conducted with caregivers of a spouse or family member demonstrates that those who reported higher levels of caregiver stress also had poorer self-perceived health. When early

interventions for stress management were given to these caregivers, there were less negative self-identified behaviors.[28] Several studies have supported the use of early interventions to assist in managing stress. In fact, one study describes how resilience development was conducted with oncology nurses to decrease their burnout. Findings of the study indicated the program was successful and recommended to be implemented for all nurses.[28]

Treatment

The treatment of stress should be directed toward helping people avoid coping behaviors that impose a risk to their health and providing them with alternative stress-reducing strategies. People who are overwhelmed by the number of life stressors to which they have been exposed can use purposeful priority setting and problem solving. Other nonpharmacologic methods used for stress reduction are relaxation techniques, guided imagery, music therapy, massage, and biofeedback.

Relaxation

Practices for evoking the relaxation response are numerous. They are found in virtually every culture and are credited with producing a generalized decrease in sympathetic system activity and musculoskeletal tension. Herbert Benson, a physician who worked in developing the technique, described four elements integral to the various relaxation techniques: a repetitive mental device, a passive attitude, decreased mental tonus, and a quiet environment. He developed a noncultural method that is commonly used for achieving relaxation.[29]

Progressive muscle relaxation is one method of relieving tension. Tension can be defined physiologically as the inappropriate contraction of muscle fibers. Progressive muscle relaxation, which has been modified by a number of therapists, consists of systematic contraction and relaxation of major muscle groups. As the person learns to relax, the various muscle groups are combined. Eventually, the person learns to relax individual muscle groups without first contracting them.

Imagery

Guided imagery is another technique that can be used to achieve relaxation. One method is scene visualization, in which the person is asked to sit back, close the eyes, and concentrate on a scene narrated by the therapist. Whenever possible, all five senses are involved. The person attempts to see, feel, hear, smell, and taste aspects of the visual experience. Other types of imagery involve imagining the appearance of each of the major muscle groups and how they feel during tension and relaxation.

Music Therapy

Music therapy is used for both its physiologic and psychological effects. It involves listening to selected pieces of music as a means of ameliorating anxiety or stress, reducing pain, decreasing feelings of loneliness and isolation, buffering noise, and facilitating expression of emotion. Music usually is selected based on a person's musical preference and past experiences with music.

Biofeedback

Biofeedback is a technique in which a person learns to control physiologic functioning. It involves electronic monitoring of one or more physiologic responses to stress with immediate feedback of the specific response to the person undergoing treatment. Several types of responses are used: electromyography (EMG), electrothermal, and electrodermal.[30] The EMG response involves the measurement of electrical potentials from muscles to gain control over the contraction of skeletal muscles that occurs with anxiety and tension. The electrodermal sensors monitor skin temperature in the fingers or toes. The sympathetic nervous system exerts significant control over blood flow in the **distal** parts of the body such as the digits of the hands and feet. Consequently, anxiety often is manifested by a decrease in skin temperature in the fingers and toes. Electrodermal sensors measure conductivity of skin in response to anxiety.

Massage Therapy

Massage is the manipulation of the soft tissues of the body to promote relaxation and relief of muscle tension. The technique that is used may involve a soft stroking along the length of the muscle (effleurage), application of pressure across the width of a muscle (petrissage), deep massage movement applied by a circular motion of the thumbs or fingertips (friction), squeezing across the width of a muscle (kneading), or use of light slaps or chopping actions (hacking).[31]

Research

Research in stress has focused on personal reports of the stress situation and the physiologic responses to stress. A number of interview guides and written instruments are available for measuring the personal responses to stress and coping in adults.

Measurements of vital signs, ACTHs, glucocorticoids (cortisol) and glucose levels, and immunologic counts are all part of current research studies involving stress.

Research that attempts to establish a link between the stress response and disease needs to be interpreted with caution owing to the influence that individual differences have in the way people respond to stress. Not everyone who experiences stressful life events develops a disease. The evidence for a link between the stress response system and the development of disease in susceptible people is compelling but not conclusive.

 SUMMARY CONCEPTS

Stress in itself is neither negative nor deleterious to health. The stress response is designed to be time limited and protective, but in situations of prolonged activation of the response because of overwhelming or chronic stressors, it could be damaging to health. PTSD is an example of chronic activation of the stress response as a result of experiencing a severe trauma. In this disorder, memory of the traumatic event seems to be enhanced. Flashbacks of the event are accompanied by intense activation of the neuroendocrine system.

Treatment of stress should be aimed at helping people avoid coping behaviors that can adversely affect their health and providing them with other ways to reduce stress. Nonpharmacologic methods used in the treatment of stress include relaxation techniques, guided imagery, music therapy, massage techniques, and biofeedback.

Research in stress has focused on personal reports of the stress situation and the physiologic responses to stress. A number of interview guides and written instruments are available for measuring the personal responses to acute and chronic stressors. Methods used for studying the physiologic manifestations of the stress response include electrocardiographic recording of heart rate, blood pressure measurement, electrodermal measurement of skin resistance associated with sweating, and biochemical analyses of hormone levels.

Review Exercises

1. A 21-year-old college student notices that she frequently develops "cold sores" during the stressful final exam week.

   A. What is the association between stress and the immune system?

   B. One of her classmates suggests that she listen to music or try relaxation exercises as a means of relieving stress. Explain how these interventions might work in relieving stress.

2. A 75-year-old woman with congestive heart failure complains that her condition gets worse when she worries and is under stress.

   A. Relate the effects stress has on the neuroendocrine control of cardiovascular function and its possible relationship to a worsening of the woman's congestive heart failure.

   B. She tells you that she dealt with much worse stresses when she was younger and never had any problems. How would you explain this?

3. A 30-year-old woman who was rescued from a collapsed building has been having nightmares recalling the event, excessive anxiety, and loss of appetite and is afraid to leave her home for fear something will happen.

A. Given her history and symptoms, what is the likely diagnosis?

B. How might she be treated?

REFERENCES

1. American Psychological Association. (2017). *Stress in America: Coping with change.* Washington, DC: American Psychological Association.
2. Osler W. (1910). The Lumleian lectures in angina pectoris. *Lancet* 1, 696–700, 839–844, 974–977.
3. Cannon W. B. (1935). Stresses and strains of homeostasis. *American Journal of Medical Science* 189, 1–5.
4. Cannon W. B. (1939). *The wisdom of the body* (pp. 299–300). New York, NY: WW Norton.
5. Selye H. (1946). The general adaptation syndrome and diseases of adaptation. *Journal of Clinical Endocrinology* 6, 117–124.
6. Bernard C. (1878). *Leçons sur les phénomènes de la vie communs aux animaux et aux vegetaux.* Paris, France: Baillière JB.
7. Understanding the stress response. Chronic activation of this survival mechanism impairs health. (2016). Harvard Medical School. Harvard Health Publishing. Available: https://www.health.harvard.edu/staying-healthy/understanding-the-stress-response. Accessed February 24, 2018.
8. Momen N. C., Olsen J., Gissler M., et al. (2013). Early life bereavement and childhood cancer: A nationwide follow-up study in two countries. *BMJ Open* 3(5).
9. Finkelhor D., Shattuck A., Turner H., et al. (2013). Improving the adverse childhood experiences study scale. *Journal of the American Medical Association Pediatrics* 167(1), 70–75.
10. Schacter D. L., Gaesser B., Addis D. R. (2013). Remembering the past and imagining the future in the elderly. *Gerontology* 59(2), 143–151.
11. Selye H. (1976). *The stress of life* (rev. ed.). New York, NY: McGraw-Hill.
12. Selye H. (1974). *Stress without distress* (p. 6). New York, NY: New American Library.
13. Selye H. (1973). The evolution of the stress concept. *American Scientist* 61, 692–699.
14. Herman J. P., McKlveen J. M., Ghosal S., et al. (2016). Regulation of the hypothalamic-pituitary-adrenocortical stress response. *Comprehensive Physiology* 6(2), 603–621.
15. Hall J. E. (2015). *Guyten and Hall textbook of medical physiology* (13th ed.). Philadelphia, PA: Saunders.
16. Sengupta P., Dutta S., Krajewska-Kulak E. (2017). The disappearing sperms: Analysis of reports published between 1980 and 2015. *American Journal of Men's Health* 11(4), 1279–1304.
17. Yam K. Y., Naninck E. F., Schmidt M. V., et al. (2015). Early-life adversity programs emotional functions and the neuroendocrine stress system: The contribution of nutrition, metabolic hormones and epigenetic mechanisms. *Stress* 18(3), 328–342.
18. Sippel L. M., Allington C. E., Pietrzak R. H., et al. (2017). Oxytocin and stress-related disorders: Neurobiological mechanisms and treatment opportunities. *Chronic Stress (Thousand Oaks)* 1. doi:10.1177/2470547016687996.
19. Dubos R. (1965). *Man adapting* (pp. 256, 258, 261, 264). New Haven, CT: Yale University.
20. Lazarus R. (2011). Evolution of a model of stress, coping, and discrete emotions. In Rice V. H. (Ed.), *Handbook of stress, coping, and health* (2nd ed., pp. 195–222). Thousand Oaks, CA: Sage.
21. Buysse D. J. (2014). Sleep health: Can we define it? Does it matter? *Sleep* 37(1), 9–17.
22. Sollars P. J., Pickard G. E. (2015). The neurobiology of circadian rhythms. *Psychiatric Clinics of North America* 38(4), 645–665.
23. Hague A., Leggat S. G. (2010). Enhancing hardiness among health care workers: The perceptions of senior managers. *Health Services Management Research* 23(2), 54–59.
24. Jordan T. R., Khubchandani J., Wiblishauser M. (2016). The impact of perceived stress and coping adequacy on the health of nurses: A pilot investigation. *Nursing Research and Practice* 2016, 5843256.
25. Ozbay F., Johnson D. C., Dimoulas E., et al. (2007). Social support and resilience to stress: From neurobiology to clinical practice. *Psychiatry (Edgmont)* 4(5), 35–40.
26. Shalev A., Liberzon I., Marmar C. (2017). Post-traumatic stress disorder. *The New England Journal of Medicine* 376(25), 2459–2469.
27. De Bellis M. D., Woolley D. P., Hooper S. R. (2013). Neuropsychological findings in pediatric maltreatment: Relationship of PTSD, dissociative symptoms, and abuse/neglect indices to neurocognitive outcomes. *Child Maltreatment* 18(3), 171–183.
28. Kelley D. E., Lewis M. A., Southwell B. G. (2017). Perceived support from a caregiver's social ties predicts subsequent care-recipient health. *Preventive Medicine Reports* 8, 108–111.
29. Benson H. (1977). Systemic hypertension and the relaxation response. *The New England Journal of Medicine* 296, 1152–1154.
30. Strada E. A., Portenoy R. K. Psychological rehabilitative, and integrative therapies for cancer pain. In Savarese D. M. F. (Ed.), *UpToDate.* Available: https://www.uptodate.com/contents/psychological-rehabilitative-and-integrative-therapies-for-cancer-pain. Accessed February 24, 2018.
31. Salvo S. G. (2015). *Massage therapy: Principles and practice* (5th ed.). St. Louis, MO: Saunders.

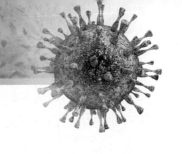

Disorders of Fluid, Electrolyte, and Acid–Base Balance

Learning Objectives

After completing this chapter, the learner will be able to meet the following objectives:

1. Differentiate the intracellular from the extracellular fluid compartments in terms of distribution and composition of water, electrolytes, and other osmotically active solutes.
2. Relate the concept of a concentration gradient to the processes of diffusion and osmosis.
3. Describe the control of cell volume and the effect of isotonic, hypotonic, and hypertonic solutions on cell size.
4. State the functions and physiologic mechanisms controlling body water levels and sodium concentration, including the effective circulating volume, sympathetic nervous system, renin–angiotensin–aldosterone system, and antidiuretic hormone.
5. Describe the relationship between antidiuretic hormone and aquaporin-2 channels in reabsorption of water by the kidney.
6. Compare the etiology, pathology, and clinical manifestations of diabetes insipidus and the syndrome of inappropriate antidiuretic hormone.
7. Characterize the distribution of potassium in the body and explain how extracellular potassium levels are regulated in relation to body gains and losses.
8. Relate the functions of potassium to the manifestations of hypokalemia and hyperkalemia.
9. Describe the associations among intestinal absorption, renal elimination, bone stores, and the functions of vitamin D and parathyroid hormone in regulating calcium, phosphorus, and magnesium levels.
10. Describe the intracellular and extracellular mechanisms for buffering changes in body pH.
11. Compare the roles of the kidneys and respiratory system in regulation of acid–base balance.
12. Describe the common causes of metabolic and respiratory acidosis and metabolic and respiratory alkalosis.
13. Contrast and compare the etiology and clinical manifestations of metabolic and respiratory acidosis and of metabolic and respiratory alkalosis.

Electrolytes significantly affect all cell functions and are maintained within a narrow range primarily by the kidneys. Hydrogen (H^+) concentration is controlled by buffers, and an imbalance results in either acidosis or alkalosis. Fluids and electrolytes are present in body cells, in the tissue spaces between the cells, and in the blood that fills the vascular compartment. Body fluids transport gases, nutrients, and wastes; help generate the electrical activity needed to power body functions; take part in the transformation of food into energy; and otherwise maintain the overall function of the body. Although fluid volume and composition remain relatively constant in the presence of a wide range of changes in intake and output, conditions such as environmental stresses and disease can interfere with mechanisms that regulate fluid volume, composition, and distribution. This chapter discusses the composition and compartmental distribution of body fluids; sodium and water balance, potassium balance, and calcium, phosphorus, and magnesium balance; and disorders of fluid and electrolyte balance.

The content related to H^+ balance has been organized into two sections: mechanisms of acid–base balance and disorders of acid–base balance.

Composition and Compartmental Distribution of Body Fluids

Body fluids are distributed between the intracellular fluid (ICF) and extracellular fluid (ECF) compartments. The *ICF compartment* consists of fluid contained within all cells in the body and constitutes approximately two thirds of the body water in healthy adults. The remaining one third of body water is in the *ECF compartment*, which contains all the fluids outside the cells, including those in the interstitial or tissue spaces and blood vessels (Fig. 8-1).

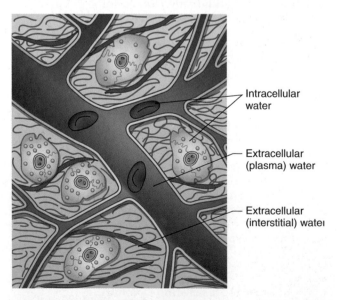

Intracellular water

Extracellular (plasma) water

Extracellular (interstitial) water

FIGURE 8-1. Distribution of body water. The extracellular space includes the vascular compartment and the interstitial spaces.

TABLE 8-1 Concentrations of Extracellular and Intracellular Electrolytes in Adults

Electrolyte	Extracellular Concentration*		Intracellular Concentration*	
	Conventional Units	SI Units (mmol/L)	Conventional Units	SI Units (mmol/L)
Sodium	135–145 mEq/L	135–145	10–14 mEq/L	10–14
Potassium	3.5–5.0 mEq/L	3.5–5.0	140–150 mEq/L	140–150
Chloride	98–106 mEq/L	98–106	3–4 mEq/L	3–4
Bicarbonate	24–31 mEq/L	24–31	7–10 mEq/L	7–10
Calcium	8.5–10.5 mg/dL	2.1–2.6	<1 mEq/L	<0.25
Phosphorus	2.5–4.5 mg/dL	0.8–1.45	Variable	Variable
Magnesium	1.8–3.0 mg/dL	0.75–1.25	40 mEq/kg[†]	20

*Values may vary among laboratories, depending on the method of analysis used.
†Values vary among various tissues and with nutritional status.

The ECF, including blood plasma and interstitial fluids, contains large amounts of sodium and chloride; moderate amounts of bicarbonate; and small amounts of potassium, magnesium, calcium, and phosphorus. The ICF contains almost no calcium; small amounts of sodium, chloride, bicarbonate, and phosphorus; moderate amounts of magnesium; and large amounts of potassium (Table 8-1).[1] Potassium is the most abundant intracellular electrolyte.

The cell membrane serves as the primary barrier to the movement of substances between the ECF and ICF compartments. Lipid-soluble substances (*e.g.*, oxygen [O_2] and carbon dioxide [CO_2]), which dissolve in the lipid bilayer of the cell membrane, pass directly through the membrane, whereas many ions (*e.g.*, sodium [Na^+] and potassium [K^+]) rely on transport mechanisms such as the Na^+/K^+ pump located in the cell membrane for movement across the membrane.[2] Because the Na^+/K^+ pump relies on adenosine triphosphate (ATP) and the enzyme adenosine triphosphatase (ATPase) for energy, it is often referred to as the Na^+/K^+-ATPase membrane pump. Water crosses the cell membrane by osmosis using transmembrane protein channels called *aquaporins*.[3]

Dissociation of Electrolytes

Body fluids contain water and electrolytes. Electrolytes are substances that dissociate in solution to form charged particles, or *ions*. For example, sodium chloride (NaCl) dissociates to form a positively charged Na^+ and a negatively charged Cl^- ion. Particles that do not dissociate into ions, such as glucose and urea, are called *nonelectrolytes*. Positively charged ions are called *cations* because they are attracted to the cathode of a wet electric cell, and negatively charged ions are called *anions* because they are attracted to the anode. The ions found in body fluids carry one charge (*i.e.*, monovalent ion) or two charges (*i.e.*, divalent ion). Positively charged cations are always accompanied by negatively charged anions. Thus, all body fluids contain equal amounts of anions and cations. However, cations and anions may be exchanged for one another, provided they carry the same charge. For example, H^+ may be exchanged for K^+, and HCO_3^- may be exchanged for Cl^-.

Diffusion and Osmosis

Diffusion

Diffusion is the movement of charged or uncharged particles along a concentration gradient. All molecules and ions are in constant random motion. It is the motion of these particles, each colliding with one another, that supplies the energy for diffusion. Because there are more molecules in constant motion in a concentrated solution, particles move from an area of higher concentration to one of lower concentration. Measurement units used to describe the amount of electrolytes and solutes in body fluids are discussed in Chart 8-1.

CHART 8-1

MEASUREMENT UNITS

The amount of electrolytes and solutes in body fluids is expressed as a concentration or amount of solute in a given volume of fluid, such as milligrams per deciliter (mg/dL), milliequivalents per liter (mEq/L), or millimoles per liter (mmol/L). The *milligrams per deciliter* measurement unit expresses the weight of the solute in one tenth of a liter (dL) or 100 mL of solution. The concentration of electrolytes, such as calcium, phosphate, and magnesium, is often expressed in mg/dL.

The *milliequivalent* is used to express the charge equivalency for a given weight of an electrolyte. Electroneutrality requires that the total number of cations in the body equals the total number of anions. When cations and anions combine, they do so according to their ionic charge, not according to their atomic

Another cause of lymphedema is infection and trauma involving the lymphatic channels and lymph nodes.

Clinical Manifestations

The effects of edema are determined largely by its location. Edema of the brain, larynx, or lungs is an acute, life-threatening condition. Although not life threatening, edema may interfere with movement, limiting joint motion. At the tissue level, edema increases the distance for diffusion of O_2, nutrients, and wastes. Edematous tissues usually are more susceptible to injury and development of ischemic tissue damage, including pressure ulcers. Edema can also compress blood vessels. *Pitting edema* occurs when the accumulation of interstitial fluid exceeds the absorptive capacity of the tissue gel. In this form of edema, tissue water becomes mobile and can be translocated with pressure exerted by a finger. *Nonpitting edema* usually reflects a condition in which plasma proteins have accumulated in the tissue spaces and coagulated. It is seen most commonly in areas of localized infection or trauma. The area often is firm and discolored.

Assessment and Treatment

Methods for assessing edema include daily weight, visual assessment, measurement of the affected part, and application of finger pressure to assess for pitting edema. Daily weight measured at the same time each day provides a useful index of water gain (1 L of water weighs 1 kg [2.2 lb]) because of edema. Visual inspection and measurement of the circumference of an extremity can also be used to assess the degree of swelling. Finger pressure can be used to assess the degree of pitting edema. If an indentation remains after the finger has been removed, pitting edema is identified. It is evaluated on a scale of +1 (minimal) to +4 (severe) (Fig. 8-5).

Treatment of edema usually is directed toward maintaining life when the swelling involves vital structures, correcting or controlling the cause, and preventing tissue injury. Edema of the lower extremities may respond to simple measures such as elevating the feet. Diuretic therapy commonly is used to treat edema associated with an increase in ECF volume. Serum albumin levels can be measured, and albumin may be administered intravenously to raise the plasma colloidal osmotic pressure when edema is caused by hypoalbuminemia.

Third-Space Accumulation

Third spacing represents the loss or trapping of ECF into the transcellular space. The serous cavities are part of the transcellular compartment (*i.e.*, third space) located in strategic body areas where there is continual movement of body structures—the pericardial sac, the peritoneal cavity, and the pleural cavity. The exchange of ECF among the capillaries, the interstitial spaces, and the transcellular space of the serous cavity uses the same mechanisms as capillaries elsewhere in the body. The serous cavities are closely linked with lymphatic drainage systems. The milking action of the moving structures, such as the lungs, continually forces fluid and plasma proteins back into the circulation, keeping these cavities empty. Obstruction to lymph flow causes fluid accumulation in the serous cavities. Third-space fluids represent an accumulation or trapping of body fluids that contribute to body weight but not to fluid reserve or function. Some causes of third spacing include systemic inflammatory response syndrome or leaky capillary syndrome in pancreatitis; hypoalbuminemia, which occurs with severe liver failure; and third-degree burns.[7]

The prefix *hydro-* may be used to indicate the presence of excessive fluid, as in *hydrothorax*, which means excessive fluid in the pleural cavity. The accumulation of fluid in the peritoneal cavity is called ascites. The transudation of fluid into the serous cavities is also referred to as effusion. Effusion can contain blood, plasma proteins, inflammatory cells (*i.e.*, pus), and ECF.

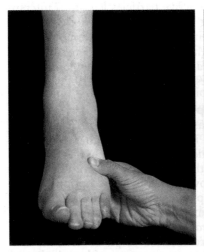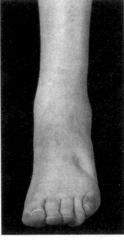

FIGURE 8-5. 3+ Pitting edema. (Adapted from Bickley L. S. (2017). *Bates' guide to physical examination and history taking* (12th ed., Figs. 12-24 and 12-25, p. 529). Philadelphia, PA: Wolters Kluwer.)

SUMMARY CONCEPTS

Body fluids, which contain water and electrolytes, are distributed between the ICF and ECF compartments. Two thirds of body fluids are contained in the body cells of the ICF compartment, and one third is contained in the vascular compartment, interstitial spaces, and third-space areas of the ECF compartment. The ICF has high concentrations of potassium, calcium, phosphorus, and magnesium, and the ECF high concentrations of sodium, chloride, and bicarbonate.

Electrolytes and nonelectrolytes move by diffusion across cell membranes that separate the ICF and ECF compartments. Water crosses the cell membrane by osmosis, using special protein channels called *aquaporins*. It moves from the side of the membrane that has the lesser number of particles and greater concentration of water to the side that has the greater number of particles and lesser concentration of water. The osmotic tension or effect that a solution exerts on cell volume in terms of causing the cell to swell or shrink is called *tonicity*.

Edema represents an increase in interstitial fluid volume. The physiologic mechanisms that contribute to the development of edema include factors that (1) increase capillary filtration pressure, (2) decrease capillary colloidal osmotic pressure, (3) increase capillary permeability, and (4) obstruct lymphatic flow. The effect that edema exerts on body function is determined by its location. Edema of the brain, larynx, or lungs is an acute, life-threatening situation, whereas swelling of the ankles and feet can be a normal discomfort that accompanies hot weather. Fluid can also accumulate in the transcellular compartment—the joint spaces, the pericardial sac, the peritoneal cavity, and the pleural cavity. Because this fluid is not easily exchanged with the rest of the ECF, it is often referred to as third-space fluid.

TABLE 8-2 Sources of Body Water Gains and Losses in the Adult

Gains		Losses	
Oral intake		Urine	1500 mL
As water	1000 mL	Insensible losses	
In food	1300 mL	Lungs	300 mL
Water of oxidation	200 mL	Skin	500 mL
		Feces	200 mL
Total	2500 mL	Total	2500 mL

Sodium and Water Balance

The movement of fluids between the ICF and ECF compartments occurs at the cell membrane and depends on ECF levels of water and sodium. Almost 93% of body fluids are made up of water, and sodium salts account for approximately 90% to 95% of ECF solutes.[2] Equivalent changes in sodium and water are such that the volume and osmolality of ECF are maintained within a normal range. Because the concentration of sodium controls ECF osmolality, changes in sodium are usually accompanied by proportionate changes in water volume.

Body Water Balance

Total body water (TBW) varies with sex and weight. These differences can be explained by differences in body fat, which is essentially water free (*i.e.*, fat is ~10% water by composition, compared with 75% for skeletal muscle). In young adult males, TBW approximates 60% of body weight, whereas TBW is approximately 50% for young adult females.[1] The TBW tends to decrease with old age because of more adipose tissue and less muscle.[1] Obesity produces further decreases in TBW because adipose tissue only contains about 10% water.[1]

Infants normally have more TBW than older children or adults. TBW constitutes approximately 75% of body weight in full-term infants and an even greater proportion in premature infants.[1] Infants have more than half of their TBW in the ECF compartment. The greater ECF water content of an infant can be explained in terms of its higher metabolic rate, larger surface area in relation to body mass, and inability to concentrate urine because of immature kidney structures. Because ECFs are more readily lost from the body, infants are more vulnerable to fluid deficit than older children and adults. As an infant grows older, TBW decreases, and by the second year of life, the percentages and distribution of body water approach those of an adult.[8]

Gains and Losses

Regardless of age, all healthy people require approximately 100 mL of water per 100 calories metabolized for dissolving and eliminating metabolic wastes. The metabolic rate increases approximately 12% for every 1°C (7% for every 1°F) increase in body temperature.[2] Fever also increases the respiratory rate, resulting in additional loss of water vapor through the lungs.

The main source of water gain is through oral intake and metabolism of nutrients. Water, including that obtained from liquids and solid foods, is absorbed from the gastrointestinal tract. Tube feedings and parenterally administered fluids are also sources of water gain. Metabolic processes also generate a small amount of water.

Normally, the largest loss of water occurs through the kidneys, with lesser amounts being lost through the skin, lungs, and gastrointestinal tract. Even when oral or parenteral fluids are withheld, the kidneys continue to produce urine as a means of ridding the body of metabolic wastes (*obligatory urine output*). The obligatory urine loss is approximately 300 to 500 mL/day. Water losses that occur through the skin and lungs are referred to as *insensible water losses*. The gains and losses of body water are summarized in Table 8-2.

Sodium Balance

Sodium is the most abundant cation in the body, averaging approximately 60 mEq/kg of body weight.[1] Most of the body's sodium is in the ECF compartment (135 to 145 mEq/L [135 to 145 mmol/L]), and only 10 to 14 mEq/L (10 to 14 mmol/L) is in the ICF compartment. The resting cell membrane is relatively impermeable to sodium; sodium that enters the cell is transported out of the cell against an electrochemical gradient by the Na^+/K^+-ATPase membrane pump.

KEY POINTS

Sodium and Water Balance

■ It is the amount of water and its effect on sodium concentration in the ECF that serves to regulate the distribution of fluid between the ICF and ECF compartments.

■ Hyponatremia or hypernatremia that is brought about by disproportionate losses or gains in sodium or water exerts its effects on the ICF compartment, causing water to move in or out of body cells. Many of the manifestations of changes in sodium concentration reflect changes in the intracellular volume of cells, particularly those in the nervous system.

Sodium functions mainly in regulating the ECF volume. As the major cation in the ECF compartment, Na^+ and its attendant anions (Cl^- and HCO_3^-) account for approximately 90% to 95% of the osmotic activity in the ECF. Because sodium is part of the sodium bicarbonate molecule, it is important in regulating acid–base balance. As a current-carrying ion, Na^+ contributes to the function of the nervous system and other excitable tissue.

Gains and Losses

Sodium normally enters the body through the gastrointestinal tract and is eliminated by the kidneys or lost from the gastrointestinal tract or skin. Sodium intake normally is derived from dietary sources. Body needs for sodium can be met by as little as 500 mg/day. The average salt intake is approximately 6 to 15 g/day, or 12 to 30 times the daily requirement. Sources of sodium are dietary intake, intravenous saline infusions, and medications that contain sodium.

Most sodium losses occur through the kidneys. The kidneys are extremely efficient in regulating sodium output, and when sodium is needed, the kidneys are able to reabsorb almost all the sodium that has been filtered by the glomerulus. This results in essentially sodium-free urine. Conversely, urinary losses of sodium increase as intake increases.

Usually less than 10% of sodium intake is lost through the gastrointestinal tract and skin. Although the sodium concentration of fluids in the upper part of the gastrointestinal tract approaches that of the ECF, sodium is reabsorbed as the fluids move through the lower part of the bowel, so that the concentration of sodium in the stool is only approximately 40 mEq/L (40 mmol/L). Sodium losses increase with conditions such as vomiting, diarrhea, **fistula** drainage, and gastrointestinal suction that remove sodium from the gastrointestinal tract. Sodium leaves the skin through the sweat glands. Sweat is a hypotonic solution containing both sodium and chloride. Although sodium losses because of sweating are usually negligible, they can increase greatly during exercise and periods of exposure to a hot environment.[2]

Mechanisms of Regulation

The major regulator of sodium and water balance is the maintenance of the *effective circulating volume*, also called the *effective arterial blood volume*. This is the vascular bed that perfuses the body. A low effective circulating volume activates feedback mechanisms that produce an increase in renal sodium and water retention, and a high effective circulating volume triggers feedback mechanisms that decrease sodium and water retention.

The effective circulating volume is monitored by a number of sensors that are located in both the vascular system and the kidney. These sensors are the **baroreceptors** because they respond to pressure-induced stretch of the vessel walls.[1] Baroreceptors are located in the low-pressure side of the circulation (walls of the cardiac atria and large pulmonary vessels) that respond primarily to fullness of the circulation. They are also present in the high-pressure arterial side of the circulation (aortic arch and carotid sinus) that respond primarily to changes in the arterial pressure. The activity of both types of receptors regulates water elimination by modulating sympathetic nervous system outflow and antidiuretic hormone (ADH) secretion.[1] The sympathetic nervous system responds to changes in arterial pressure and blood volume by adjusting the glomerular filtration rate and thus the rate at which sodium is filtered from the blood. Sympathetic activity also regulates tubular reabsorption of sodium and renin release. An additional mechanism related to renal sodium excretion is atrial natriuretic peptide (ANP), which is released from cells in the atria of the heart. ANP, which is released in response to atrial stretch and overfilling, increases sodium excretion by the kidney, which in turn pulls out more water.[1]

Pressure-sensitive receptors in the kidney, particularly in the afferent arterioles, respond directly to changes in arterial pressure through stimulation of the sympathetic nervous system and release of renin with activation of the renin–angiotensin–aldosterone system (RAAS).[1] The RAAS exerts its action through angiotensin II and aldosterone. Renin is a small protein enzyme that is released by the kidney in response to changes in arterial pressure, the glomerular filtration rate, and the amount of sodium in the tubular fluid. Most of the renin that is released leaves the kidney and enters the bloodstream, where it interacts enzymatically to convert a circulating plasma protein called *angiotensinogen* to angiotensin I.

Angiotensin I is rapidly converted to angiotensin II by the angiotensin-converting enzyme (ACE) in the small blood vessels of the lung. Angiotensin II acts directly on the renal tubules to increase sodium reabsorption. It also acts to constrict renal blood vessels, decreasing the glomerular filtration rate and slowing renal blood flow so that less sodium is filtered and more is reabsorbed.

Angiotensin II is also a powerful regulator of *aldosterone*, a hormone secreted by the adrenal cortex. Aldosterone acts at the level of the cortical collecting tubules of the kidneys to increase sodium reabsorption while increasing potassium elimination.[1]

Thirst and Antidiuretic Hormone

Two other mechanisms that contribute directly to the regulation of body water and indirectly to the regulation of sodium are thirst and ADH. Thirst is primarily a regulator of water intake and ADH a regulator of water

UNDERSTANDING ➡ Capillary Fluid Exchange

Movement of fluid between the vascular compartment and the interstitial fluid compartment occurs at the capillary level. The direction and amount of fluid that flows across the capillary wall are determined by **(1)** the hydrostatic pressure of the two compartments, **(2)** the colloidal osmotic pressures of the two compartments, and **(3)** the removal of excess fluid and osmotically active particles from the interstitial spaces by the lymphatic system.

1

Hydrostatic Pressure Hydrostatic pressure is the force exerted by a fluid. Inside the capillaries, the hydrostatic pressure is the same as the capillary filtration pressure, about 30 mm Hg at the arterial end and 10 mm Hg at the venous end. Interstitial fluid pressure is the force of fluid in the interstitial spaces pushing against the outside of the capillary wall. Evidence suggests that the interstitial pressure is slightly negative (−3 mm Hg), contributing to the outward movement of fluid from the capillary.

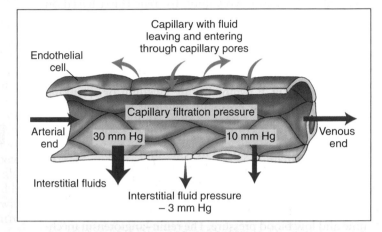

2

Colloidal Osmotic Pressure The colloidal osmotic pressure is the pulling force created by the presence of evenly dispersed particles, such as the plasma proteins, that cannot pass through the pores of the capillary membrane. Capillary colloidal osmotic pressure is about 28 mm Hg throughout the length of the capillary bed. Interstitial colloidal osmotic pressure (about 8 mm Hg) represents the pulling pressure exerted by the plasma proteins that leak through the pores of the capillary wall into the interstitial spaces. The capillary colloidal osmotic pressure, which is greater than both the hydrostatic pressure at the venous end of the capillary and the interstitial colloidal osmotic pressure, is largely responsible for the movement of fluid back into the capillary.

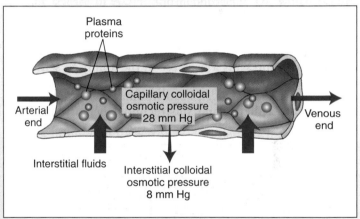

3

Lymph Drainage The lymphatic system represents an accessory system by which fluid can be returned to the circulatory system. Normally the forces moving fluid out of the capillary into the interstitium are greater than those returning fluid to the capillary. Any excess fluids and osmotically active plasma proteins that may have leaked into the interstitium are picked up by vessels of the lymphatic system and returned to the circulation. Without the function of the lymphatic system, excessive amounts of fluid would accumulate in the interstitial spaces.

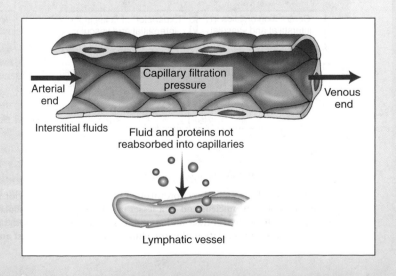

TABLE 8-6 Causes and Manifestations of Hyponatremia

Causes	Manifestations
Hypotonic Hyponatremia	**Laboratory Values**
Hypovolemic (Decreased Serum Sodium with Decreased ECF Volume)	Serum sodium levels below 135 mEq/L (135 mmol/L)
Use of excessively diluted infant formula	Hypotonic hyponatremia
Administration of sodium-free parenteral solutions	Serum osmolality 280 mOsm/kg
Gastrointestinal losses	Dilution of blood components, including hematocrit, BUN
Vomiting, diarrhea	Hypertonic hyponatremia
Sweating, with sodium-free fluid replacement	Serum osmolality >280 mOsm/kg
Repeated irrigation of body cavities with sodium-free solutions	**Signs Related to Hypoosmolality of ECFs and Movement of Water into Brain Cells and Neuromuscular Tissue**
Irrigation of gastrointestinal tubes with distilled water	Muscle cramps
Tap water enemas	Weakness
Use of nonelectrolyte irrigating solutions during prostate surgery	Headache
Third spacing (paralytic ileus, pancreatitis)	Depression
Diuretic use	Apprehension, feeling of impending doom
Mineralocorticoid deficiency (Addison disease)	Personality changes
Salt-wasting nephritis	Lethargy
Euvolemic (Decreased Serum Sodium with Normal ECF Volume)	Stupor, coma
Increased ADH levels	**Gastrointestinal Manifestations**
Trauma, stress, pain	Anorexia, nausea, vomiting
SIADH	Abdominal cramps, diarrhea
Use of medications that increase ADH	**Increased ICF**
Diuretic use	Fingerprint edema
Glucocorticoid deficiency	
Hypothyroidism	
Psychogenic polydipsia	
Endurance exercise	
MDMA ("ecstasy") abuse	
Hypervolemic (Decreased Serum Sodium with Increased ECF Volume)	
Decompensated heart failure	
Advanced liver disease	
Kidney failure without nephrosis	
Hypertonic Hyponatremia (Osmotic Shift of Water from the ICF to the ECF Compartment)	Manifestations largely related to hyperosmolality of ECFs
Hyperglycemia	

ADH, antidiuretic hormone; BUN, blood urea nitrogen; ECF, extracellular fluid; ICF, intracellular fluid; MDMA, 3,4-methylenedioxymethamphetamine; SIADH, syndrome of inappropriate antidiuretic hormone.

 Concept Mastery Alert

The cells of the brain and nervous system are the most seriously affected by increases in intracellular water. Symptoms include apathy, lethargy, and headache, which can progress to disorientation, confusion, gross motor weakness, and depression of deep tendon reflexes.

Seizures and coma occur when plasma sodium levels reach extremely low levels. These severe effects, which are caused by brain swelling, may be irreversible. If the condition develops slowly, signs and symptoms do not develop until plasma sodium levels approach 120 mEq/L (120 mmol/L) (*i.e.*, severe hyponatremia).[2] The term *water intoxication* is often used to describe the neurologic effects of acute hypotonic hyponatremia.

Diagnosis and Treatment

Diagnosis of hyponatremia is based on laboratory reports of a decreased plasma sodium concentration, plasma and urine osmolality, and urine sodium concentration; assessment of the person's volume status; presence of conditions that predispose to sodium loss or water retention; and signs and symptoms indicative of the disorder.

The treatment of hyponatremia with water excess focuses on the underlying cause. When hyponatremia is caused by water intoxication, limiting water intake or discontinuing medications that contribute to SIADH may be sufficient. Saline solution administration is used when hyponatremia is caused by sodium deficiency. Symptomatic hyponatremia (*i.e.*, neurologic manifestations) is often treated with hypertonic saline solution and a loop diuretic, such as furosemide, to increase water elimination. ADH V_2 receptor antagonists to the antidiuretic action of ADH (aquaretics) offer treatment for euvolemic hyponatremia.[15]

Hypernatremia

Hypernatremia implies a plasma sodium level above 145 mEq/L (145 mmol/L) and a serum osmolality greater than 295 mOsm/kg. Because sodium is functionally an impermeable solute, it contributes to tonicity and induces movement of water across cell membranes.

Hypernatremia is characterized by hypertonicity of ECF and almost always causes cellular dehydration.[2]

Etiology

Hypernatremia represents a deficit of water in relation to the body's sodium stores due to a net loss of water or sodium gain. Net water loss can occur through the urine, gastrointestinal tract, lungs, or skin. A defect in thirst or inability to obtain or drink water can interfere with water replacement. Rapid ingestion or infusion of sodium with insufficient time or opportunity for water ingestion can produce a disproportionate gain in sodium (Table 8-7). This can occur with critically ill people who present with multiple needs for fluid resuscitation and electrolyte balance. Hypernatremia is an independent risk factor linked highly with increased mortality.[17]

Hypernatremia almost always follows a loss of body fluids that have a lower-than-normal concentration of sodium, so that water is lost in excess of sodium. This can result from increased losses from the respiratory tract during fever or strenuous exercise, from watery diarrhea, or when osmotically active tube feedings are given with inadequate amounts of water. With pure water loss, each body fluid compartment loses an equal percentage of its volume. Because approximately one third of the water is in the ECF compartment and two thirds in the ICF compartment, more actual water volume is lost from the ICF than from the ECF compartment.[2]

Normally, water deficit stimulates thirst and increases water intake. Therefore, hypernatremia is more likely to occur in infants and in people who cannot express their thirst or obtain water to drink. With hypodipsia, or impaired thirst, the need for fluid intake does not activate the thirst response. Hypodipsia is particularly prevalent among older adults. In people with DI, hypernatremia can develop when thirst is impaired or access to water is impeded.

Clinical Manifestations

The clinical manifestations of hypernatremia caused by water loss are largely those of ECF loss and cellular dehydration (see Table 8-7). The severity of signs and symptoms is greatest when the increase in plasma sodium is large and occurs rapidly. Body weight decreases in proportion to the amount of water lost. Because blood plasma is roughly 90% to 93% water, the concentrations of blood cells and other blood components increase as ECF water decreases.

Thirst is an early symptom of water deficit, occurring when water losses are 0.5% of body water. Urine output is decreased and urine osmolality increased because of renal water-conserving mechanisms. Body temperature frequently is elevated, and the skin becomes warm and flushed. The vascular volume decreases, the pulse becomes rapid and thready, and blood pressure drops. Hypernatremia produces an increase in serum osmolality and pulls water out of body cells. As a result, the skin and mucous membranes become dry, and salivation and lacrimation are decreased. The mouth becomes dry and sticky, and the tongue becomes rough and fissured. Swallowing is difficult and subcutaneous tissues assume a firm, rubbery texture. Most significantly, water is pulled out of the cells in the CNS, causing decreased reflexes, agitation, headache, and restlessness. Coma and seizures may develop as hypernatremia progresses.

TABLE 8-7 Causes and Manifestations of Hypernatremia

Causes	Manifestations
Excessive Water Losses	**Laboratory Values**
Watery diarrhea	Serum sodium level above 145 mEq/L (145 mmol/L)
Excessive sweating	Increased serum osmolality
Increased respirations because of conditions such as tracheobronchitis	Increased hematocrit and BUN
Hypertonic tube feedings	**Thirst and Signs of Increased ADH Levels**
Diabetes insipidus	Polydipsia
Decreased Water Intake	Oliguria or anuria
Unavailability of water	High urine specific gravity
Oral trauma or inability to swallow	**Intracellular Dehydration**
Impaired thirst sensation	Dry skin and mucous membranes
Withholding water for therapeutic reasons	Decreased tissue turgor
Unconsciousness or inability to express thirst	Tongue rough and fissured
	Decreased salivation and lacrimation
Excessive Sodium Intake	**Signs Related to Hyperosmolality of ECFs and Movement of Water Out of Brain Cells**
Rapid or excessive administration of sodium-containing parenteral solutions	Headache
Near-drowning in salt water	Agitation and restlessness
	Decreased reflexes
	Seizures and coma
	Extracellular Dehydration and Decreased Vascular Volume
	Tachycardia
	Weak and thready pulse
	Decreased blood pressure
	Vascular collapse

ADH, antidiuretic hormone; BUN, blood urea nitrogen; ECF, extracellular fluid.

and failure to respond to drugs that act through calcium-mediated mechanisms.

The Chvostek and Trousseau tests can be used to assess for an increase in neuromuscular excitability and tetany.[28] The Chvostek sign is elicited by tapping the face just below the temple at the point where the facial nerve emerges. This causes spasm of the lip, nose, or face when the test result is positive. An inflated blood pressure cuff is used to test for the Trousseau sign. The cuff is inflated 10 mm Hg above systolic blood pressure for 3 minutes. Contraction of the fingers and hands (*i.e.*, carpopedal spasm) indicates the presence of tetany.

Chronic hypocalcemia is often accompanied by skeletal manifestations and skin changes. There may be bone pain, fragility, deformities, and fractures. The skin may be dry and scaling, the nails brittle, and hair dry. Development of cataracts is common.

Treatment

Acute hypocalcemia is an emergency, requiring prompt treatment. An intravenous infusion containing calcium is used when tetany or acute symptoms are present or anticipated because of a decrease in the plasma calcium level.[29]

Chronic hypocalcemia is treated with oral intake of calcium. Long-term treatment may require the use of vitamin D preparations, especially in persons with hypoparathyroidism and CKD. The active form of vitamin D is administered when the liver or kidney mechanisms needed for hormone activation are impaired. Synthetic PTH (1-34) can be administered by subcutaneous injection as replacement therapy in hypoparathyroidism.

Hypercalcemia

Hypercalcemia represents a total plasma calcium concentration greater than 10.5 mg/dL (2.6 mmol/L). Falsely elevated levels of calcium can result from prolonged drawing of blood with an excessively tight tourniquet. Increased plasma proteins may elevate the total plasma calcium but not affect the ionized calcium concentration.

Etiology

Hypercalcemia results when calcium movement into the circulation overwhelms the calcium regulatory hormones or the ability of the kidney to remove excess calcium ions (Table 8-11). The two most common causes of hypercalcemia are increased bone resorption because of neoplasms and hyperparathyroidism.[2] Hypercalcemia is a common complication of malignancy, occurring in approximately 10% to 20% of people with advanced disease and is called HCM.[30] A number of malignant tumors, including carcinoma of the lungs, have been associated with hypercalcemia. Some tumors destroy the

TABLE 8-11 Causes and Manifestations of Hypercalcemia

Causes	Manifestations
Increased Intestinal Absorption Excessive vitamin D Excessive calcium in the diet Milk-alkali syndrome	**Laboratory Values** Serum calcium level above 10.5 mg/dL (2.6 mmol/L)
Increased Bone Resorption Increased levels of parathyroid hormone Malignant neoplasms Prolonged immobilization	**Impaired Ability to Concentrate Urine and Exposure of Kidney to Increased Concentration of Calcium** Polyuria Polydipsia Flank pain Signs of acute and chronic renal insufficiency Signs of kidney stones
Decreased Elimination Thiazide diuretics Lithium therapy	**Gastrointestinal Manifestations** Anorexia Nausea, vomiting Constipation
	Neuromuscular Manifestations (Decreased Neuromuscular Excitability) Muscle weakness and atrophy Ataxia, loss of muscle tone
	Skeletal Manifestations Osteopenia Osteoporosis
	Central Nervous System Manifestations Lethargy Personality and behavioral changes Stupor and coma
	Cardiovascular Manifestations Hypertension Shortening of the QT interval Atrioventricular block on electrocardiogram

bone, whereas others produce **humoral** agents that stimulate osteoclastic activity, increase bone resorption, or inhibit bone formation.[30]

Less frequent causes of hypercalcemia are prolonged immobilization, increased intestinal absorption of calcium, excessive doses of vitamin D, or the effects of drugs such as lithium and thiazide diuretics. Children with hypercalcemia will need to expedite urinary excretion of calcium, which is the main treatment goal.[31] Prolonged immobilization and lack of weight bearing cause demineralization of bone and release of calcium into the bloodstream. Intestinal absorption of calcium can be increased by excessive doses of vitamin D or as a result of a condition called the *milk-alkali syndrome*. The milk-alkali syndrome is caused by excessive ingestion of calcium (often in the form of milk) and absorbable antacids and occurs in women who are overzealous in taking calcium preparations for osteoporosis prevention. Discontinuance of the antacid repairs the alkalosis and increases calcium elimination.

Drugs may elevate calcium levels. Lithium has caused hypercalcemia and hyperparathyroidism. Thiazide diuretics increase calcium reabsorption in the distal convoluted tubule of the kidney, and although they seldom cause hypercalcemia, they can unmask hypercalcemia from other causes such as underlying bone disorders and conditions that increase bone resorption.

Clinical Manifestations

The signs and symptoms associated with calcium excess reflect (1) changes in neural excitability, (2) alterations in smooth and cardiac muscle function, and (3) exposure of the kidneys to high concentrations of calcium (see Table 8-11). Neural excitability is decreased in people with hypercalcemia. There may be a dulling of consciousness, **stupor**, weakness, and muscle flaccidity. Behavioral changes range from subtle alterations in personality to acute psychoses. The heart responds to elevated levels of calcium with increased contractility and ventricular arrhythmias. Gastrointestinal symptoms reflect a decrease in smooth muscle activity and include constipation, anorexia, nausea, and vomiting. High calcium concentrations in the urine impair the ability of the kidneys to concentrate urine by interfering with the action of ADH. This causes salt and water diuresis and an increased sensation of thirst. Hypercalciuria also predisposes to the development of renal calculi. Pancreatitis is another potential complication of hypercalcemia and is probably related to stones in the pancreatic ducts.

Hypercalcemic crisis describes an acute increase in plasma calcium levels usually due to malignant disease and hyperparathyroidism.[8] In hypercalcemic crisis, cardiac dysrhythmias, oliguria, excessive thirst, volume depletion, fever, altered levels of consciousness, and a disturbed mental state accompany other signs of calcium excess.[8] Symptomatic hypercalcemia is associated with a high mortality rate; death often is caused by cardiac arrest.

Treatment

Treatment of calcemia is directed toward rehydration and increasing urinary excretion of calcium.[2,8] Fluid replacement is needed in situations of volume depletion.

Sodium excretion is accompanied by calcium excretion. Diuretics and NaCl can be administered to increase urinary elimination of calcium after the ECF volume has been restored. Loop diuretics are used rather than thiazide diuretics, which increase calcium reabsorption. Lowering of calcium is followed by measures to inhibit bone reabsorption. Dialysis can be used in people with hypercalcemia with renal failure and in people with heart failure in whom fluid overload is a concern.

Disorders of Phosphorus Balance

Phosphorus is mainly an intracellular anion. Approximately 85% of phosphorus is contained in bone, and 14% is located in cells. Approximately 1% is in the ECF compartment, and of that, only a minute proportion is in the plasma. In the adult, normal plasma phosphorus levels range from 2.5 to 4.5 mg/dL (0.8 to 1.45 mmol/L). These values are slightly higher in infants (3.7 to 8.5 mg/dL [01.2 to 02.7 mmol/L]) and children (4 to 5.4 mg/dL [1.3 to 1.7 mmol/L]), probably because of increased growth hormone and decreased gonadal hormones.

Phosphorus exists in two forms within the body—inorganic and organic. The inorganic form (phosphate [$H_2PO_4^-$ or HPO_4^{2-}]) is the principal circulating form of phosphorus and is routinely measured (and reported as phosphorus) for laboratory purposes.[2] Most of the intracellular phosphorus (~90%) is in the organic form (*e.g.*, nucleic acids, phospholipids, and ATP). Entry of phosphorus into cells is enhanced after glucose uptake because phosphorus is incorporated into the phosphorylated intermediates of glucose metabolism. Cell injury or atrophy leads to a loss of cell components that contain organic phosphate; regeneration of these cellular components results in withdrawal of inorganic phosphate from the ECF compartment.

Phosphorus plays a major role in bone formation; is essential to certain metabolic processes, including the formation of ATP and the enzymes needed for metabolism of glucose, fat, and protein; is a necessary component of several vital parts of the cell, being incorporated into the nucleic acids of deoxyribonucleic acid (DNA) and ribonucleic acid (RNA) and the phospholipids of the cell membrane; and serves as an acid–base buffer in the ECF and in the renal excretion of hydrogen ions. Delivery of O_2 by RBCs depends on organic phosphorus in ATP and 2,3-diphosphoglycerate (2,3-DPG). Phosphorus is also needed for normal function of other blood cells including the white blood cells and platelets.

Gains and Losses

Phosphorus is ingested in the diet and eliminated in the urine. Phosphorus is derived from many dietary sources, including milk and meats. Approximately 80% of ingested phosphorus is absorbed in the intestine, primarily in the jejunum. Absorption is diminished by concurrent ingestion of substances that bind phosphorus, including calcium, magnesium, and aluminum.

Phosphate is not bound to plasma proteins, and essentially all of the phosphate that is present in the

Carbon Dioxide and Bicarbonate Production

Body metabolism results in the production of approximately 15,000 mmol of CO_2 each day.[42] Carbon dioxide is transported in the circulation in three forms:

1. As a dissolved gas
2. As bicarbonate
3. As carbaminohemoglobin (see "Understanding: Carbon Dioxide Transport")

Collectively, dissolved CO_2 and HCO_3^- account for approximately 77% of the CO_2 that is transported in the ECF; the remaining CO_2 travels as carbaminohemoglobin.[37] Although CO_2 is a gas and not an acid, a small percentage combines with water to form H_2CO_3. This reaction that generates H_2CO_3 is catalyzed by *CA*, which is present in large quantities in RBCs, renal tubular cells, and other tissues. The rate of the reaction between CO_2 and water is increased approximately 5000 times by the presence of CA. Were it not for this enzyme, the reaction would occur too slowly to be of any significance in maintaining acid–base balance.

Because it is almost impossible to measure H_2CO_3, CO_2 measurements are commonly used when calculating pH. H_2CO_3 content of the blood can be calculated by multiplying the partial pressure of CO_2 (PCO_2) by its solubility coefficient (0.03). The concentration of H_2CO_3 in arterial blood, which normally has a PCO_2 of approximately 40 mm Hg, is 1.20 mEq/L (40 × 0.03 = 1.20), and that for venous blood, which normally has a PCO_2 of approximately 45 mm Hg, is 1.35 mEq/L.

Production of Fixed or Nonvolatile Acids and Bases

The metabolism of dietary proteins and other nutrients results in the generation of fixed or nonvolatile acids and bases.[39,43] Oxidation of the sulfur-containing amino acids results in the production of sulfuric acid. Oxidation of arginine and lysine produces HCl, and oxidation of phosphorus-containing nucleic acids yields phosphoric acid. Incomplete oxidation of glucose results in the formation of lactic acid, and incomplete oxidation of fats results in the production of ketoacids. The major source of base is the metabolism of amino acids such as aspartate and glutamate and of certain organic anions. Acid production normally exceeds base production during the breakdown of consumed foods in a person eating a diet of meat and vegetables.[3] A normal diet results in 50 to 100 mEq of H^+ each day as nonvolatile sulfuric acid.[6] A vegetarian diet, which contains large amounts of organic anions, results in the net production of base.[39]

Calculation of pH

Plasma pH can be calculated with the *Henderson–Hasselbalch equation*, which uses the pK_a of the bicarbonate buffer system (6.1) and $\log_{10}$ of the ratio of HCO_3^- to H_2CO_3[37-39]:

$$pH = 6.1 + \log_{10}(HCO_3^-/PCO_2 \times 0.03)$$

The pH designation was created to express the low value of H^+ more easily.[2] Plasma pH decreases when the ratio is less than 20:1 and increases when the ratio is greater than 20:1 (Fig. 8-13). Because it is the ratio of HCO_3^- or CO_2 that determines pH, pH can remain within a normal range as long as changes in HCO_3^- are accompanied by similar changes in CO_2, or vice versa. Plasma pH only indicates the balance or ratio, not where problems originate.[9]

Regulation of pH

The pH of body fluids (or change in H^+ concentration) is regulated by three major mechanisms:

1. Chemical buffer systems of the body fluids, which immediately combine with excess acids or bases to prevent large changes in pH
2. The lungs, which control the elimination of CO_2
3. The kidneys, which eliminate H^+ and both reabsorb and generate new HCO_3^-

Chemical Buffer Systems

The moment-by-moment regulation of pH depends on chemical buffer systems of the ICF and ECF. As previously discussed, a *buffer system* consists of a weak base and its conjugate acid pair or a weak acid and its conjugate base pair. In the process of preventing large changes in pH, the system trades a strong acid for a weak acid or a strong base for a weak base.

The three major buffer systems that protect the pH of body fluids are

1. The bicarbonate buffer system
2. Proteins
3. The transcellular H^+/K^+ exchange system[37,39]

These buffer systems act immediately to combine with excess acids or bases and prevent large changes in pH from occurring during the time it takes for the respiratory and renal mechanisms to become effective. Even though these buffer systems act immediately, they have a limited effect on pH and cannot correct large or long-term changes.

Bone represents an additional source of acid–base buffering.[10] Excess H^+ can be exchanged for Na^+ and K^+ on the bone surface, and dissolution of bone minerals with release of compounds such as sodium bicarbonate ($NaHCO_3$) and calcium carbonate ($CaCO_3$) into the ECF can buffer excess acids. As much as 40% of buffering of an acute acid load takes place in bone. The role of bone buffers is even greater in the presence of chronic acidosis. The consequences of bone buffering include demineralization of bone and predisposition to development of kidney stones because of increased urinary excretion of calcium. People with CKD are at particular risk for reduction in bone calcium because of acid retention.

Bicarbonate Buffer System

The HCO_3^- buffer system, which is the most powerful ECF buffer, uses H_2CO_3 as its weak acid and a bicarbonate salt such as $NaHCO_3$ as its weak base.[37,38]

UNDERSTANDING ➔ Carbon Dioxide Transport

Metabolism results in a continuous production of carbon dioxide (CO_2). As CO_2 is formed, it diffuses out of cells into tissue spaces and into the circulation. It is transported in the circulation in three forms: **(1)** dissolved in the plasma, **(2)** as bicarbonate, and **(3)** attached to hemoglobin.

1

Plasma About 10% of CO_2 produced is transported in the dissolved state to the lungs and exhaled. The amount of dissolved CO_2 that can be carried in plasma is determined by the partial pressure of the gas (PCO_2) and its solubility coefficient (0.03 mL/100 mL plasma for each 1 mm Hg PCO_2). Each 100 mL of arterial blood with a PCO_2 of 40 mm Hg contains 1.2 mL of dissolved CO_2. Carbonic acid (H_2CO_3) is formed from hydration of dissolved CO_2, which contributes to blood pH.

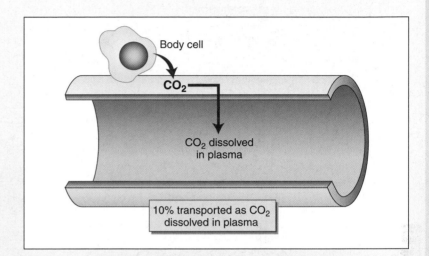

2

Bicarbonate Carbon dioxide in excess of that which can be carried in the plasma moves into RBCs where carbonic anhydrase (CA) catalyzes its conversion to carbonic acid (H_2CO_3). H_2CO_3 dissociates into H^+ and HCO_3^-. H^+ combines with hemoglobin and HCO_3^- diffuses into plasma, where it participates in acid–base regulation. The movement of HCO_3^- into plasma is via a transport system on the RBC membrane in which HCO_3^- ions are exchanged for chloride ions (Cl^-). Ventilation and kidney handling of HCO_3^- determine plasma HCO_3^- concentration.[7]

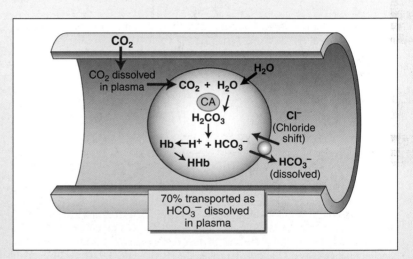

3

Hemoglobin Remaining CO_2 in RBCs combines with hemoglobin to form carbaminohemoglobin ($HbCO_2$).[2] This reversible reaction creates a loose bond so CO_2 can be released in capillaries and exhaled.

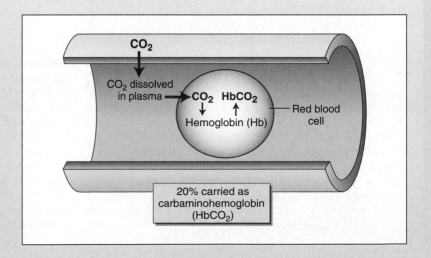

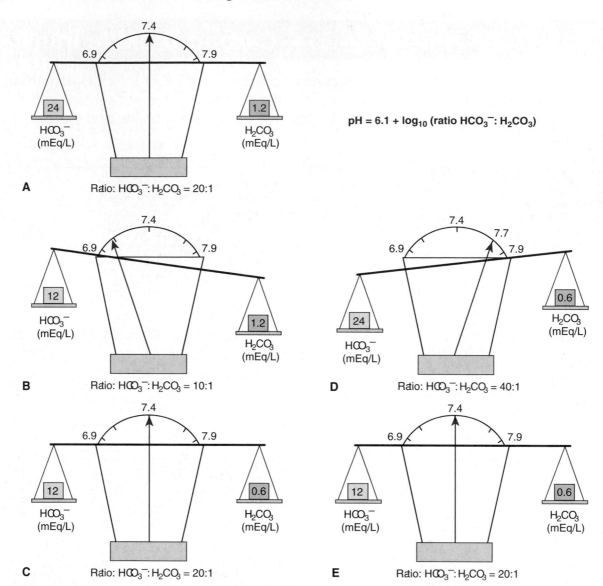

$$pH = 6.1 + \log_{10} (\text{ratio } HCO_3^- : H_2CO_3)$$

FIGURE 8-13. Normal and compensated states of pH and acid–base balance represented as a balance scale. **(A)** When the ratio of bicarbonate (HCO_3^-) to carbonic acid (H_2CO_3, arterial $CO_2 \times 0.03$) = 20:1, the pH = 7.4. **(B)** Metabolic acidosis with a HCO_3^-:H_3CO_3 ratio of 10:1 and a pH of 7.1. **(C)** Respiratory compensation lowers the H_3CO_3 to $0.^6$ mEq/L and returns the HCO_3^-:H_3CO_3 ratio to 20:1 and the pH to 7.4. **(D)** Respiratory alkalosis with a HCO_3^-:H_3CO_3 ratio of 40:1 and a pH of 7.7. **(E)** Renal compensation eliminates HCO_3^-, reducing serum levels to 12 mEq/L, returning the HCO_3^-:H_3CO_3 ratio to 20:1 and the pH to 7.4. Normally, these compensatory mechanisms are capable of buffering large changes in pH but do not return the pH completely to normal as illustrated here.

It substitutes the weak H_2CO_3 for a strong acid such as HCl ($NaHCO_3 + HCl \rightarrow H_2CO_3 + NaCl$) or the weak bicarbonate base for a strong base such as sodium hydroxide ($H_2CO_3 + NaOH \rightarrow HCO_3^- + H_2O$). The bicarbonate buffer system is a particularly efficient system because its components can be readily added or removed from the body.[37-39] Metabolism provides an ample supply of CO_2, which can replace any H_2CO_3 that is lost when excess base is added, and CO_2 can be readily eliminated when excess acid is added. Likewise, the kidney can conserve or form new HCO_3^- when excess acid is added, and it can excrete HCO_3^- when excess base is added.

Protein Buffer Systems

Proteins are the largest buffer system in the body.[37,38] They are **amphoteric** (can function either as acids or as bases) and contain many ionizable groups that can release or bind H^+. The protein buffers are largely located in cells, and H^+ ions and CO_2 diffuse across cell membranes for buffering by intracellular proteins. Due to slow movement of H^+ and HCO_3^- across cell membranes, buffering extracellular acid–base imbalances is delayed for several hours.[37] Albumin and plasma globulins are the major protein buffers in the vascular compartment.

Hydrogen–Potassium Exchange

The transcompartmental exchange of H^+ and K^+ is another important system for regulation of acid–base balance. H^+ and K^+ are positively charged and move freely between the ICF and ECF compartments. Excess H^+ in the ECF moves into the ICF in exchange for K^+, and excess K^+ in the ECF moves into the ICF in exchange for H^+. Thus, alterations in K^+ levels can affect acid–base balance, and changes in acid–base balance can influence K^+ levels. K^+ shifts tend to be more pronounced in metabolic acidosis than in respiratory acidosis.[3] Metabolic acidosis caused by an accumulation of nonorganic acids (*e.g.*, HCl that occurs in diarrhea and phosphoric acid that occurs in CKD) produces a greater increase in extracellular K^+ levels than does acidosis caused by an accumulation of organic acids (*e.g.*, lactic acid and ketoacids).

Respiratory Control Mechanisms

The second line of defense against acid–base disturbances when chemical buffers do not minimize H^+ changes is control of extracellular CO_2 by the lungs.[38,42] Increased ventilation decreases PCO_2 and decreased ventilation increases PCO_2. Blood PCO_2 and pH are important regulators of ventilation. **Chemoreceptors** in the brainstem and peripheral chemoreceptors in the carotid and aortic bodies sense changes in PCO_2 and pH and alter the ventilation rate.

When the H^+ concentration is above normal, the respiratory system is stimulated and ventilation is increased. This control of pH occurs within minutes and is maximal within 12 to 24 hours. Although the respiratory response is rapid, it does not completely return pH to normal. It is only about 50% to 75% effective as a buffer system.[37,38] But in acting rapidly it prevents large changes in pH from occurring while waiting for the more slowly reacting kidneys to respond.

Renal Control Mechanisms

The kidneys are the third line of defense in acid–base disturbances and play three major roles in regulating acid–base balance.[38,39] The first is through the excretion of H^+ from fixed acids that result from protein and lipid metabolism. The second is accomplished through the reabsorption of the HCO_3^- that is filtered in the glomerulus, so this important buffer is not lost in the urine. The third is the production of new HCO_3^- that is released back into the blood.[37–39] The kidneys also play a role in controlling pH: in conditions of acid load, ammonium ($NH4^+$) production and excretion allow for acid secretion and pH normalization.[38] The renal mechanisms for regulating acid–base balance begin to adjust the pH in hours and continue to function for days until the pH has returned to normal or near-normal range.

Hydrogen Ion Elimination and Bicarbonate Conservation

The kidneys regulate pH by excreting excess H^+, reabsorbing HCO_3^-, and producing new HCO_3^-. HCO_3^- is freely filtered in the glomerulus and reabsorbed in the tubules.[37,39] Loss of small amounts of HCO_3^- impairs the body's ability to buffer its daily load of metabolic acids. Because the amount of H^+ that can be filtered in the glomeruli is relatively small compared with HCO_3^-, its elimination relies on secretion of H^+ from the blood into the urine filtrate in the tubules.

Most H^+ secretion and HCO_3^- reabsorption take place in the proximal tubule.[42] It begins with a coupled Na^+/H^+ transport system in which H^+ is secreted into the tubular fluid and Na^+ is reabsorbed into the tubular cell (Fig. 8-14). The secreted H^+ combines with filtered HCO_3^- to form H_2CO_3. H_2CO_3 then decomposes into CO_2 and H_2O. The CO_2 and H_2O that are formed readily cross the luminal membrane and enter the tubular cell. Inside the cell, the reactions occur in reverse: CO_2 and H_2O combine to form a new H_2CO_3 molecule in a CA-mediated reaction. The H_2CO_3, in turn, is dissociated into HCO_3^- and H^+. HCO_3^- is then reabsorbed into the blood along with Na^+, and the newly generated H^+ is secreted into the tubular fluid to begin another cycle. Normally, only a few of the secreted H^+ ions remain in the tubular fluid because the secretion of H^+ is roughly equivalent to the number of HCO_3^- ions filtered in the glomerulus.

Tubular Buffer Systems

Because an extremely acidic urine filtrate would be damaging to the urinary tract, the minimum urine pH is about 4.5.[37,38] Once the urine reaches this level of acidity, H^+ secretion ceases. This limits the amount of unbuffered H^+ eliminated by the kidney and is accomplished by combining H^+ ions with intratubular buffers before they are excreted in the urine. There are two important intratubular buffer systems: the phosphate

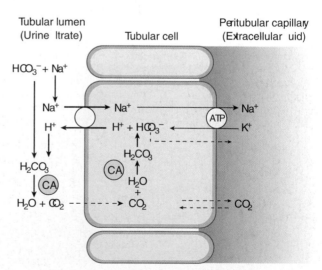

FIGURE 8-14. Hydrogen ion (H^+) secretion and bicarbonate ion (HCO_3^-) reabsorption in a renal tubular cell. Carbon dioxide (CO_2) diffuses from the blood or urine filtrate into the tubular cell, where it combines with water in a carbonic anhydrase (CA)–catalyzed reaction that yields carbonic acid (H_2CO_3). The H_2CO_3 dissociates to form H^+ and HCO_3^-. The H+ is secreted into the tubular fluid in exchange for Na^+. The Na^+ and HCO_3^- enter the extracellular fluid. ATP, adenosine triphosphate.

and ammonia buffer systems.[37,43] The HCO_3^- that is generated by these two buffer systems is new HCO_3^-, demonstrating one of the ways that the kidney is able to replenish the ECF stores of HCO_3^-.

The *phosphate buffer system* uses HPO_4^{2-} and $H_2PO_4^-$ that are present in the tubular filtrate. Both forms of phosphate are concentrated in the tubular fluid due to their relatively poor absorption and because of reabsorption of water from the tubular fluid. Another factor that makes phosphate effective as a urinary buffer is that urine pH is close to the pK of the phosphate buffer system. The process of H^+ secretion in the tubules is the same as that used for reabsorption of HCO_3^-. As long as there is excess HCO_3^- in the tubular fluid, most of the secreted H^+ combines with HCO_3^-. However, once all the HCO_3^- has been reabsorbed and is no longer available to combine with H^+, any excess H^+ combines with HPO_4^{2-} to form $H_2PO_4^-$ (Fig. 8-15). After H^+ combines with HPO_4^{2-}, it can be excreted as NaH_2PO_4, carrying the excess H^+ with it.

Another important but more complex buffer system is the *ammonia buffer system*. The excretion of H^+ and generation of HCO_3^- by the ammonia buffer system occur in three major steps:

1. The synthesis of ammonium (NH_4^+) from the amino acid glutamine in the proximal tubule
2. The reabsorption and recycling of NH_4^+ within the medullary portion of the kidney
3. The buffering of H^+ ions by NH_3 in the collecting tubules[37,39]

The metabolism of glutamate in the proximal tubule results in the formation of two NH_4^+ and two HCO_3^- ions[1,3] (Fig. 8-16). The two NH_4^+ ions are secreted into the tubular fluid by a countertransport mechanism in

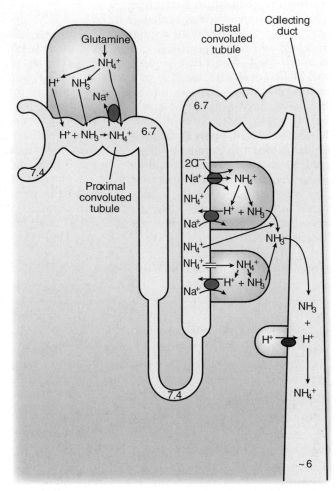

FIGURE 8-16. Acidification along the nephron. The pH of tubular urine decreases along the proximal convoluted tubule, rises along the descending limb of the loop of Henle, falls along the ascending limb, and reaches its lowest values in the collecting ducts. Ammonia (NH_3 + NH_4) is chiefly produced in proximal tubule cells and is secreted into the tubular urine. NH_4 is reabsorbed in the thick ascending limb and accumulates in the kidney medulla. NH_3 diffuses into acidic collecting duct urine, where it is trapped as NH_4. (From Rhodes R. A., Bell D. R. (2017). *Medical physiology: Principles for clinical medicine* (5th ed., Fig. 24.5, p. 492). Philadelphia, PA: Wolters Kluwer.)

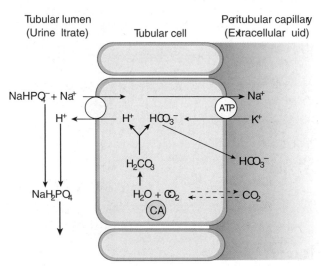

FIGURE 8-15. The renal phosphate buffer system. The monohydrogen phosphate ion (HPO_4^{2-}) enters the renal tubular fluid in the glomerulus. An H^+ combines with HPO_4^{2-} to form $H_2PO_4^-$ and is then excreted into the urine in combination with Na^+. The HCO_3^- moves into the extracellular fluid (ECF) along with the Na^+ that was exchanged during secretion of the H^+. ATP, adenosine triphosphate; CA, carbonic anhydrase.

exchange for Na^+. The two HCO_3^- ions move out of the tubular cell along with the reabsorbed Na^+ to enter the peritubular capillary system. So, for each molecule of glutamine metabolized in the proximal tubule, two NH_4^+ are secreted into the tubular filtrate, and two HCO_3^- are reabsorbed into the blood. HCO_3^- generated in this way constitutes a new HCO_3^-.

A significant portion of the NH_4^+ secreted by the proximal tubular cells is reabsorbed in the thick ascending loop of Henle where NH_4^+ substitutes K^+ on the $Na^+/K^+/2Cl^-$ cotransporter.[43] NH_4^+ is not lipid soluble and thus is trapped in the tubular fluid and excreted in urine. Note that the source of H^+ secreted by the cells of the collecting tubules is CO_2 and H_2O. Thus, for each H^+ produced in the cells and secreted, an additional new HCO_3^- is generated and added to the blood.

Under normal conditions, the amount of H^+ eliminated by the ammonia buffer system is about 50% of the acid excreted and 50% of new HCO_3^- regenerated.[37] However, with chronic acidosis, it can become the dominant mechanism for H^+ excretion and new HCO_3^- generation. The urine anion gap (AG), which is an indirect method for assessing urine NH_4^+ levels, can be used to assess kidney function in terms of H^+ elimination.

Potassium–Hydrogen Exchange

Hypokalemia is a potent stimulus for H^+ secretion and HCO_3^- reabsorption. When plasma K^+ levels fall, K^+ moves from ICF into ECF, whereas H^+ moves from ECF into ICF. A similar process occurs in the distal tubules of the kidney, where the H^+/K^+-ATPase exchange pump actively reabsorbs K^+ and secretes H^+.[37,39] Elevation in plasma K^+ levels has the opposite effect. Thus, acidosis tends to increase H^+ elimination and decrease K^+ elimination, with an increase in plasma potassium levels, whereas alkalosis tends to decrease H^+ elimination and increase K^+ elimination, with a decrease in plasma K^+ levels.[45]

Aldosterone also influences H^+ elimination by the kidney. It acts in the collecting duct to stimulate H^+ secretion indirectly, while increasing Na^+ reabsorption and K^+ secretion.

Chloride–Bicarbonate Exchange

Another mechanism that the kidneys use in regulating HCO_3^- is the chloride–bicarbonate anion exchange that occurs with Na^+ reabsorption. Cl^- is absorbed with Na^+ throughout the tubules. In situations of volume depletion, the kidneys substitute HCO_3^- for Cl^-, thereby increasing absorption of HCO_3^-. *Hypochloremic alkalosis* refers to an increase in pH induced by excess HCO_3^- reabsorption because of a decrease in Cl^- levels, and *hyperchloremic acidosis* refers to a decrease in pH because of decreased HCO_3^- reabsorption because of an increase in Cl^- levels.

Laboratory Tests

Laboratory tests that are used in assessing acid–base balance include arterial blood gases and pH, CO_2 content and HCO_3^- levels, base excess or deficit, and blood and urine AGs. Although useful in determining whether acidosis or alkalosis is present, measurements of the blood pH provide little information about the cause of an acid–base disorder.

Carbon Dioxide and Bicarbonate Levels

The PCO_2 of the arterial blood gas measurement assesses the respiratory component of acid–base balance. Arterial blood gases are used because venous blood gases are highly variable depending on metabolic demands of the tissues that empty into the sampled vein. H_2CO_3 levels can be determined from arterial blood gas measurements using PCO_2 and the solubility coefficient for CO_2 (normal arterial PCO_2 is 35 to 45 mm Hg). Arterial blood gases provide a measure of blood oxygen

(PO_2) levels, which can be important in assessing respiratory function.

CO_2 content refers to the total CO_2 in the blood, including dissolved CO_2, that is contained in HCO_3^- and that attached to hemoglobin (carbaminohemoglobin [CO_2HHb]). The normal range of venous HCO_3^- is 24 to 31 mEq/L (24 to 31 mmol/L) and of arterial HCO_3^- is 22 to 26 mEq/L (22 to 26 mmol/L).

Base Excess or Deficit

The total base excess or deficit, also referred to as the *whole blood buffer base*, measures the level of all the buffer systems of the blood—hemoglobin, protein, phosphate, and HCO_3^-. Base excess or deficit describes the amount of a fixed acid or base that must be added to a blood sample to achieve a pH of 7.4 (normal $\pm$ 2 mEq/L). Base excess or deficit can be viewed as a measurement of HCO_3^- excess or deficit and indicates a nonrespiratory change in acid–base balance. Base excess indicates metabolic alkalosis, and base deficit indicates metabolic acidosis.

Anion Gap

The AG describes the difference between the plasma concentration of the major measured cation (Na^+ and K^+) and the sum of the measured anions (Cl^- and HCO_3^-).[37,44] This difference represents the concentration of unmeasured anions, such as phosphates, sulfates, organic acids, and proteins (Fig. 8-17). Normally, AG ranges between 8 and 16 mEq/L1 (a value range of 12 to 20 mEq/L is normal when potassium is included in the calculation).[45] Because albumin is an anion, it is often measured and used in determining the AG in people with decreased albumin levels. For every 1 g/dL decline in plasma albumin concentration, a correction factor should be added to the gap that is calculated from the following formula: $AG = Na^+ - (Cl^- + HCO_3^-)$.[46] The AG is used in diagnosing causes of metabolic

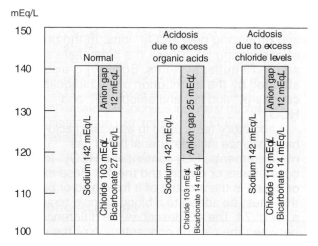

FIGURE 8-17. The anion gap in acidosis because of excess metabolic acids and excess plasma chloride levels. Unmeasured anions such as phosphates, sulfates, and organic acids increase the anion gap because they replace bicarbonate. This assumes there is no change in sodium content.

49. Rastegar M., Nagami G. T. (2017). Non-anion gap metabolic acidosis: A clinical approach to evaluation. *American Journal of Kidney Disease* 69(2), 296–301. Available: http://dx.doi.org/10.1053/j.ajkd.2016.09.013.

50. Ferreruela M., Raurich J. M., Ayerstaran L., et al. (2017). Hyperlactatemia in ICU patients: Incidence, causes, and associated mortality. *Journal of Critical Care* 42, 200–205. https://dx.doi.org/10.1016/jere.2017.07.039.

51. Bakker J., Nijsten M., Jansen T. C. (2013). Clinical use of lactate monitoring in critically ill patients. *Annals of Intensive Care* 3(12), 1–8. Available: http://www.annalsofintensivecare.com/content/3/1/12.

52. Garcia-Alvarez M., Marik P., Bellomo R. (2014). Sepsis-associated hyperlactatemia. *Critical Care* 18(503), 1–11. Available: http://ccforum.co/content/18/4/503.

53. Palmer B. F., Clegg D. J. (2015). Electrolyte and acid–base disturbances in patients with diabetes mellitus. *New England Journal of Medicine* 373, 548–559. doi:10.1056/NEJMra1503102.

54. Noor N. M., Basavaraju K., Sharpstone D. (2016). Alcoholic ketoacidosis: A case report and review of the literature. *Oxford Medical Case Reports* 3, 31–33. doi:10.1093/omcr/omw006.

55. Shivley R. M., Hoffman R. S., Manini A. F. (2017). Acute salicylate poisoning: Risk factors for severe outcome. *Clinical Toxicology* 55(3), 175–180. doi:10.1080/15563650.2016.1271127.

56. Santos F., Ordonez F. A., Claramunt-Taberner D., et al. (2015). Clinical and laboratory approaches in the diagnosis of renal tubular acidosis. *Pediatric Nephrology* 30, 2099–2107. doi:10.1007/s00467-015-3083-9.

57. Van der A. F., Joniau S., Van Den Braden M., et al. (2011). Metabolic changes after urinary diversion. *Advances in Urology* 2011, 1–5. doi:10.1155/2011/764325.

58. Berend K., deVries A. P. J., Gans R. O. B. (2015). Correspondence physiological approach to assessment of acid-base disturbances. *New England Journal of Medicine* 372, 193–195. doi:10.1056/NELMc1413880.

59. Malcolm O. T. (2015). Identification, treatment, and prevention of calcium-alkali syndrome in elderly patients. *The Consultant Pharmacist* 30(8), 444–454. doi:10.4140/TCP.n.2015.444.

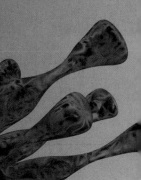

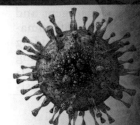

C H A P T E R 9

Inflammation, Tissue Repair, and Wound Healing

Learning Objectives

**After completing this chapter, the learner
will be able to meet the following objectives:**

1. State the physiologic reasons behind five cardinal signs of acute inflammation.
2. Describe the vascular changes in an acute inflammatory response.
3. Characterize the interaction of adhesion molecules, chemokines, and cytokines in leukocyte adhesion, migration, and phagocytosis in the cellular phase of inflammation.
4. List four types of inflammatory mediators and state their function.
5. Contrast acute and chronic inflammation.
6. Discuss the systemic manifestation of inflammation.
7. Compare labile, stable, and permanent cell types in terms of their capacity for regeneration.
8. Trace the wound-healing process through the inflammatory, proliferative, and remodeling phases.
9. Explain the effects of age; malnutrition; ischemia and oxygen deprivation; impaired immune and inflammatory responses; and infection, wound separation, and foreign bodies on wound healing.

Inflammation involves a wide variety of physiologic and pathologic responses intended to eliminate the initial cause of cell injury, remove the damaged tissue, and generate new tissue. It accomplishes this by destroying, enzymatically digesting, walling off, or otherwise neutralizing the harmful agents such as toxins, foreign agents, or infectious organisms.[1] These processes set the stage for the events that will eventually heal the damaged tissue. Thus, inflammation is intimately interwoven with the repair processes that replace damaged tissue or fill in the residual defects with fibrous scar tissue.

The pathogeneses of multiple diseases are now known to be linked to a dysregulated inflammatory response.[2-4] For example, the inflammatory response is attributed to the production of incapacitating bronchial asthma, the generation of atherosclerotic plaques that lead to

In contrast to acute inflammation, which is self-limiting, chronic inflammation is prolonged and usually is caused by persistent irritants, most of which are insoluble and resistant to phagocytosis and other inflammatory mechanisms. Chronic inflammation involves the presence of mononuclear cells (lymphocytes and macrophages) rather than granulocytes.

The systemic manifestations of inflammation include the systemic effects of the acute-phase response, such as fever and lethargy; increased ESR and levels of hsCRP and other acute-phase proteins; leukocytosis or, in some cases, leukopenia; and enlargement of the lymph nodes that drain the affected area.

 ## Tissue Repair and Wound Healing

Tissue Repair

Tissue repair, which overlaps the inflammatory process, is a response to tissue injury and represents an attempt to maintain normal body structure and function. It can take the form of regeneration in which the injured cells are replaced with cells of the same type, sometimes leaving no residual trace of previous injury, or it can take the form of replacement by connective tissue, which leaves a permanent scar. Both regeneration and repair by connective tissue replacement are determined by similar mechanisms involving cell migration, proliferation, and differentiation, as well as interaction with the ECM.[40]

Tissue Regeneration

Body organs and tissues are composed of two types of structures: parenchymal and **stromal**. The parenchymal tissues contain the functioning cells of an organ or body part (*e.g.*, hepatocytes, renal tubular cells). The stromal tissues consist of the supporting connective tissues, blood vessels, ECM, and nerve fibers.

Tissue regeneration involves replacement of the injured tissue with cells of the same type, leaving little or no evidence of the previous injury. The capacity for regeneration varies with the tissue and cell type. Body cells are divided into three types according to their ability to undergo regeneration: labile, stable, or permanent cells.[40] *Labile cells* are those that continue to divide and replicate throughout life, replacing cells that are continually being destroyed. They include the surface epithelial cells of the skin, oral cavity, vagina, and cervix; the columnar epithelium of the gastrointestinal tract, uterus, and fallopian tubes; the transitional epithelium of the urinary tract; and bone marrow cells. *Stable cells* are

those that normally stop dividing when growth ceases. However, these cells are capable of undergoing regeneration when confronted with an appropriate stimulus and are thus capable of reconstituting the tissue of origin. This category includes the parenchymal cells of the liver and kidney, smooth muscle cells, and vascular endothelial cells. *Permanent* or *fixed cells* cannot undergo mitotic division. The fixed cells include nerve cells, skeletal muscle cells, and cardiac muscle cells. These cells do not normally regenerate; once destroyed, they are replaced with fibrous scar tissue that lacks the functional characteristics of the destroyed tissue.

Fibrous Tissue Repair

Severe or persistent injury with damage to both the parenchymal cells and ECM leads to a situation in which the repair cannot be accomplished with regeneration alone. Under these conditions, repair occurs by replacement with connective tissue, a process that involves generation of granulation tissue and formation of scar tissue.

Granulation tissue is a glistening red, moist connective tissue that contains newly formed capillaries, proliferating fibroblasts, and residual inflammatory cells. The development of granulation tissue involves the growth of new capillaries (angiogenesis), fibrogenesis, and involution to the formation of scar tissue. Angiogenesis involves the generation and sprouting of new blood vessels from preexisting vessels. These sprouting capillaries tend to protrude from the surface of the wound as minute red granules, imparting the name *granulation tissue*. Eventually, portions of the new capillary bed differentiate into arterioles and venules.

Fibrogenesis involves the influx of activated fibroblasts. Activated fibroblasts secrete ECM components, including fibronectin, hyaluronic acid, proteoglycans, and collagen. Fibronectin and hyaluronic acid are the first to be deposited in the healing wound, and proteoglycans appear later. Because the proteoglycans are hydrophilic, their accumulation contributes to the edematous appearance of the wound. The initiation of collagen synthesis contributes to the subsequent formation of scar tissue.

Scar formation builds on the granulation tissue framework of new vessels and loose ECM. The process occurs in two phases: (1) emigration and proliferation of fibroblasts into the site of injury and (2) deposition of ECM by these cells. As healing progresses, the number of proliferating fibroblasts and new vessels decreases, and there is increased synthesis and deposition of collagen. Collagen synthesis is important to the development of strength in the healing wound site. Ultimately, the granulation tissue scaffolding evolves into a scar composed of largely inactive spindle-shaped fibroblasts, dense collagen fibers, fragments of elastic tissue, and other ECM components. As the scar matures, vascular degeneration eventually transforms the highly vascular granulation tissue into a pale, largely avascular scar.

Regulation of the Healing Process

Tissue healing is regulated by the actions of chemical mediators and growth factors that mediate the healing process as well as orchestrate the interactions between the extracellular and cell matrix.[40-43]

Chemical Mediators and Growth Factors

Chemical mediators and growth factors are released in an orderly manner from many of the cells that participate in tissue regeneration and the healing process. The chemical mediators include the ILs, interferons, TNF-α, and arachidonic acid derivatives (prostaglandins and LT) that participate in the inflammatory response.[19] The growth factors are hormone-like molecules that interact with specific cell surface receptors to control processes involved in tissue repair and wound healing.[44] They may act on adjacent cells or on the cell producing the growth factor. The growth factors are named for their tissue of origin, their biologic activity, or the cells on which they act.[44] The growth factors control the proliferation, differentiation, and metabolism of cells during wound healing. The growth factors assist in regulating the inflammatory process; serve as chemoattractants for neutrophils, monocytes (macrophages), fibroblasts, and epithelial cells; stimulate angiogenesis; and contribute to the generation of the ECM.

Extracellular Matrix

The ECM is secreted locally and assembles into a network of spaces surrounding tissue cells. There are three basic components of the ECM: fibrous structural proteins (*e.g.*, collagen and elastin fibers), water-hydrated gels (*e.g.*, proteoglycans and hyaluronic acid) that permit resilience and lubrication, and adhesive glycoproteins (*e.g.*, fibronectin and laminin) that connect the matrix elements to each other and to cells. The ECM occurs in two basic forms: (1) the *basement membrane* that surrounds epithelial, endothelial, and smooth muscle cells; and (2) the *interstitial matrix*, which is present in the spaces between cells in connective tissue and between the epithelium and supporting cells of blood vessels.

The ECM provides turgor to soft tissue and rigidity to bone; it supplies the substratum for cell adhesion; it is involved in the regulation of growth, movement, and differentiation of the cells surrounding it; and it provides for the storage and presentation of regulatory molecules that control the repair process. The ECM also provides the scaffolding for tissue renewal. Although the cells in many tissues are capable of regeneration, injury does not always result in restoration of normal structure unless the ECM is intact. The integrity of the underlying basement membrane, in particular, is critical to the regeneration of tissue. When the basement membrane is disrupted, cells proliferate in a haphazard way, resulting in disorganized and nonfunctional tissues.

Critical to the process of wound healing is the transition from granulation tissue to scar tissue, which involves shifts in the composition of the ECM. In the transitional process, the ECM components are degraded by proteases (enzymes) that are secreted locally by a variety of cells (fibroblasts, macrophages, neutrophils, synovial cells, and epithelial cells). Some of the proteases, such as the collagenases, are highly specific, cleaving particular proteins at a small number of sites.[45] This allows for the structural integrity of the ECM to be retained while cell migration occurs. Because of their potential to produce havoc in tissues, the actions of the proteases are tightly controlled. Research has focused on the unregulated action of the proteases in disorders such as cartilage matrix breakdown in arthritis and neuroinflammation in multiple sclerosis, and arterial stiffness causing increased peripheral resistance.[45]

Wound Healing

Injured tissues are repaired by regeneration of parenchymal cells or by connective tissue repair in which scar tissue is substituted for the parenchymal cells of the injured tissue. The primary objective of the healing process is to fill the gap created by tissue destruction and to restore the structural continuity of the injured part. When regeneration cannot occur, healing by replacement with a connective tissue scar provides the means for maintaining this continuity. Although scar tissue fills the gap created by tissue death, it does not repair the structure with functioning parenchymal cells. Because the regenerative capabilities of most tissues are limited, wound healing usually involves some connective tissue repair. The following discussion particularly addresses skin wounds.

Healing by Primary and Secondary Intention

Depending on the extent of tissue loss, wound closure and healing occur by *primary* or *secondary intention* (Fig. 9-8). A sutured surgical incision is an example

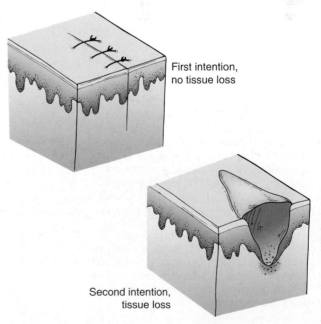

First intention, no tissue loss

Second intention, tissue loss

FIGURE 9-8. Healing of a skin wound by primary and secondary intention.

UNDERSTANDING ➤ Wound Healing

Wound healing involves the restoration of the integrity of injured tissue. The healing of skin wounds, which are commonly used to illustrate the general principles of wound healing, is generally divided into three phases: **(1)** the inflammatory phase, **(2)** the proliferative phase, and **(3)** the wound contraction and remodeling phase. Each of these phases is mediated through cytokines and growth factors.

1

Inflammatory Phase The inflammatory phase begins at the time of injury with the formation of a blood clot and the migration of phagocytic white blood cells into the wound site. The first cells to arrive, the neutrophils, ingest and remove bacteria and cellular debris. After 24 hours, the neutrophils are joined by macrophages, which continue to ingest cellular debris and play an essential role in the production of growth factors for the proliferative phase.

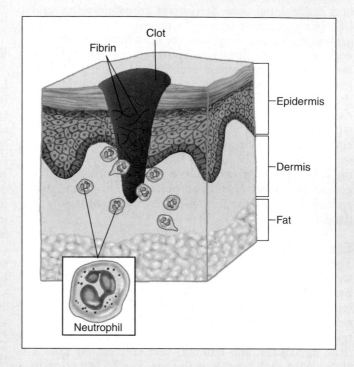

2

Proliferative Phase The primary processes during this phase focus on the building of new tissue to fill the wound space. The key cell during this phase is the *fibroblast*, a connective tissue cell that synthesizes and secretes the collagen, proteoglycans, and glycoproteins needed for wound healing. Fibroblasts also produce a family of growth factors that induce angiogenesis (growth of new blood vessels) and endothelial cell proliferation and migration. The final component of the proliferative phase is epithelialization, during which epithelial cells at the wound edges proliferate to form a new surface layer that is similar to that which was destroyed by the injury.

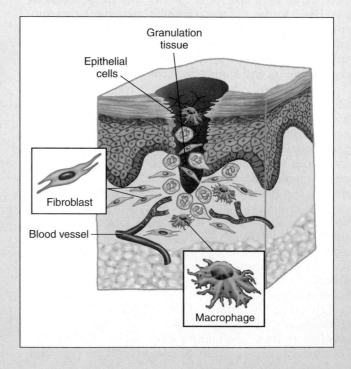

3 **Wound Contraction and Remodeling Phase** This phase begins approximately 3 weeks after injury with the development of the fibrous scar and can continue for 6 months or longer, depending on the extent of the wound. During this phase, there is a decrease in vascularity and continued remodeling of scar tissue by simultaneous synthesis of collagen by fibroblasts and lysis by collagenase enzymes. As a result of these two processes, the architecture of the scar is capable of increasing its tensile strength, and the scar shrinks so it is less visible.

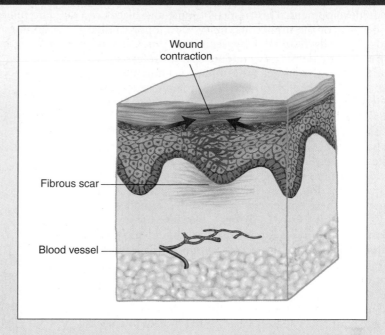

of healing by primary intention. Larger wounds (*e.g.*, burns and large surface wounds) that have a greater loss of tissue and contamination heal by secondary intention. Healing by secondary intention is slower than healing by primary intention and results in the formation of larger amounts of scar tissue. A wound that might otherwise have healed by primary intention may become infected and healed by secondary intention.

Phases of Wound Healing

Wound healing is commonly divided into three phases: (1) the inflammatory phase, (2) the proliferative phase, and (3) the maturational or remodeling phase.[1,28] The duration of the phases is fairly predictable in wound healing by primary intention. In wound healing by secondary intention, the process depends on the extent of injury and the healing environment.

Inflammatory Phase

The inflammatory phase of wound healing begins at the time of injury and is a critical period because it prepares the wound environment for healing. It includes hemostasis and the vascular and cellular phases of inflammation. Hemostatic processes are activated immediately at the time of injury. There is constriction of injured blood vessels and initiation of blood clotting through platelet activation and aggregation. After a brief period of constriction, the same vessels dilate and capillaries increase their permeability, allowing plasma and blood

components to leak into the injured area. In small surface wounds, the clot loses fluid and becomes a hard, desiccated scab that protects the area.

The cellular phase of inflammation follows and is evidenced by the migration of phagocytic white blood cells that digest and remove invading organisms, **fibrin**, extracellular debris, and other foreign matter. The neutrophils are the first cells to arrive and are usually gone by day 3 or 4. After approximately 24 hours, macrophages enter the wound area and remain for an extended period. Their functions include phagocytosis and release of growth factors that stimulate epithelial cell growth and angiogenesis and attract fibroblasts. When a large defect occurs in deeper tissues, neutrophils and macrophages are required to remove the debris and facilitate wound closure. Although a wound may heal in the absence of neutrophils, it cannot heal in the absence of macrophages.

Proliferative Phase

The proliferative phase of healing usually begins within 2 to 3 days of injury and may last as long as 3 weeks in wound healing by primary intention. The primary processes during this time focus on the building of new tissue to fill the wound space. The key cell during this phase is the *fibroblast*. The fibroblast is a connective tissue cell that synthesizes and secretes collagen and other intercellular elements needed for wound healing. Fibroblasts also produce a family of growth factors that induce angiogenesis and endothelial cell proliferation and migration.

As early as 24 to 48 hours after injury, fibroblasts and vascular endothelial cells begin proliferating to form the granulation tissue that serves as the foundation for scar tissue development. This tissue is fragile and bleeds easily because of the numerous, newly developed capillary buds. Wounds that heal by secondary intention have more necrotic debris and exudate that must be removed, and they involve larger amounts of granulation tissue. The newly formed blood vessels are semipermeable and allow plasma proteins and white blood cells to leak into the tissues.

The final component of the proliferative phase is epithelialization, which is the migration, proliferation, and differentiation of the epithelial cells at the wound edges to form a new surface layer that is similar to the one destroyed by the injury. In wounds that heal by primary intention, these epidermal cells proliferate and seal the wound within 24 to 48 hours.[41] Because epithelial cell migration requires a moist vascular wound surface and is impeded by a dry or necrotic wound surface, epithelialization is delayed in open wounds until a bed of granulation tissue has formed. When a scab has formed on the wound, the epithelial cells migrate between it and the underlying viable tissue; when a significant portion of the wound has been covered with epithelial tissue, the scab lifts off.

At times, excessive granulation tissue, sometimes referred to as *proud flesh*, may form and extend above the edges of the wound, preventing reepithelialization from taking place. Surgical removal or chemical cauterization of the defect allows healing to proceed.

As the proliferative phase progresses, there is continued accumulation of collagen and proliferation of fibroblasts. Collagen synthesis reaches a peak within 5 to 7 days and continues for several weeks, depending on wound size. By the second week, the white blood cells have largely left the area, the edema has diminished, and the wound begins to blanch as the small blood vessels become thrombosed and degenerate.

Remodeling Phase

The third phase of wound healing, the remodeling process, begins approximately 3 weeks after injury and can continue for 6 months or longer, depending on the extent of the wound. As the term implies, there is continued remodeling of scar tissue by simultaneous synthesis of collagen by fibroblasts and lysis by collagenase enzymes. As a result of these two processes, the architecture of the scar becomes reoriented to increase the tensile strength of the wound. Most wounds do not regain the full tensile strength of unwounded skin after healing is completed.

An injury that heals by secondary intention undergoes wound contraction during the proliferative and remodeling phases. As a result, the scar that forms is considerably smaller than the original wound. Cosmetically, this may be desirable because it reduces the size of the visible defect. However, contraction of scar tissue over joints and other body structures tends to limit movement and cause deformities. As a result of loss of elasticity, scar tissue that is stretched fails to return to its original length.

An abnormality in healing by scar tissue repair is *keloid* formation. Keloids are tumor-like masses caused by excess production of scar tissue (Fig. 9-9). The tendency toward development of keloids is more common in African Americans and seems to have a genetic basis.

KEY POINTS

Tissue Repair and Wound Healing

- Injured tissues can be repaired by regeneration of the injured tissue cells with cells of the same tissue or parenchymal type or by connective repair processes in which scar tissue is used to effect healing.

- Wound healing is impaired by conditions that diminish blood flow and oxygen delivery, restriction of nutrients essential for healing, and depression of inflammatory and immune responses by infection, wound separation, the presence of foreign bodies, and aging.

Factors That Affect Wound Healing

Many local and systemic factors influence wound healing. Among the causes of impaired wound healing are malnutrition; impaired blood flow and oxygen delivery; impaired inflammatory and immune responses; infection, wound separation, and foreign bodies; and age effects.[40,42] Specific disorders that slow wound healing include diabetes mellitus, peripheral artery disease, venous insufficiency, and nutritional disorders. Although many factors impair healing, science has found few ways to hasten the normal process of wound repair.

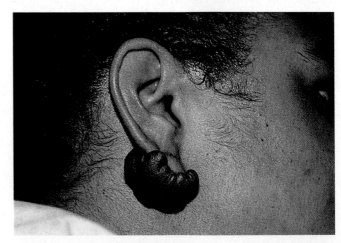

FIGURE 9-9. Keloid. A light-skinned black woman developed a keloid as a reaction to having her earlobe pierced. (From Strayer D. E., Rubin R. (Eds.) (2015). *Rubin's pathology: Clinicopathologic foundations of medicine* (7th ed., Fig. 3-18A, p. 129). Philadelphia, PA: Lippincott Williams & Wilkins.)

Malnutrition

Successful wound healing depends, in part, on adequate stores of proteins, carbohydrates, fats, vitamins, and minerals.[46] Protein deficiencies prolong the inflammatory phase of healing and impair fibroblast proliferation, collagen and protein matrix synthesis, angiogenesis, and wound remodeling. Carbohydrates are needed as an energy source for white blood cells. Carbohydrates also have a protein-sparing effect and help to prevent the use of amino acids for fuel when they are needed for the healing process. Fats are essential constituents of cell membranes and are needed for the synthesis of new cells.

Although most vitamins are essential cofactors for the daily functions of the body, vitamins A and C play an essential role in the healing process. Vitamin C is needed for collagen synthesis. In vitamin C deficiency, the by-products of collagen synthesis are not removed from the cell, new wounds do not heal properly, and old wounds may fall apart. Vitamin A functions in stimulating and supporting epithelialization, capillary formation, and collagen synthesis. The B vitamins are important cofactors in enzymatic reactions that contribute to the wound-healing process. Vitamin K plays an indirect role in wound healing by preventing bleeding disorders that contribute to **hematoma** formation and subsequent infection.

The macrominerals including sodium, potassium, calcium, and phosphorus, as well as the microminerals (trace minerals), such as copper and zinc, must be present for normal cell function. Zinc is a cofactor in a variety of enzyme systems responsible for cell proliferation. In animal studies, zinc has been found to aid in reepithelialization.

Blood Flow and Oxygen Delivery

For healing to occur, wounds must have adequate blood flow to supply the necessary nutrients and to remove the resulting waste, local toxins, bacteria, and other debris. Impaired wound healing caused by poor blood flow may occur as a result of wound conditions (*e.g.*, swelling) or preexisting health problems. Arterial disease and venous pathology are well-documented causes of impaired wound healing. In situations of trauma, a decrease in blood volume may cause a reduction in blood flow to injured tissues.

Molecular oxygen is required for collagen synthesis. Hypoxia is a serious factor in preventing wound healing because it has been shown to decrease fibroblast growth, collagen production, and angiogenesis.[47,48] Wounds in ischemic tissue become infected more frequently than wounds in well-vascularized tissue. PMNs and macrophages require oxygen for destruction of microorganisms that have invaded the area. Although these cells can accomplish phagocytosis in a relatively anoxic environment, they cannot digest bacteria.

Impaired Inflammatory and Immune Responses

Inflammation is essential to the first phase of wound healing, and immune mechanisms prevent infections that impair wound healing. Among the conditions that impair inflammation and immune function are disorders of phagocytic function, diabetes mellitus, and therapeutic administration of corticosteroid drugs.

Phagocytic disorders may be divided into extrinsic and intrinsic defects. Extrinsic disorders are those that reduce the total number of phagocytic cells (*e.g.*, immunosuppressive agents), impair the attraction of phagocytic cells to the wound site, interfere with the engulfment of bacteria and foreign agents by the phagocytic cells (*i.e.*, opsonization), or suppress the total number of phagocytic cells (*e.g.*, immunosuppressive agents). Intrinsic phagocytic disorders are the result of enzymatic deficiencies in the metabolic pathway for destroying the ingested bacteria by the phagocytic cell. The intrinsic phagocytic disorders include chronic granulomatous disease, an X-linked inherited disease in which there is a deficiency of the myeloperoxidase or NADPH oxidase enzymes. Deficiencies of these compounds prevent generation of superoxide and hydrogen peroxide needed for killing bacteria.

Many people with diabetes mellitus who have wounds do not respond well to traditional methods of wound treatment because of their high blood glucose levels.[48] Evidence shows delayed wound healing and complications such as prolonged infections in people with diabetes because of decreased chemotactic and phagocytic function.[48] Small blood vessel disease is also common among people with diabetes, impairing the delivery of inflammatory cells, oxygen, and nutrients to the wound site.

Infection, Wound Separation, and Foreign Bodies

Wound contamination, wound separation, and foreign bodies delay wound healing. Infection impairs all dimensions of wound healing.[49] It prolongs the inflammatory phase, impairs the formation of granulation tissue, and inhibits proliferation of fibroblasts and deposition of collagen fibers. All wounds are contaminated at the time of injury. Although body defenses can handle the invasion of microorganisms at the time of wounding, badly contaminated wounds can overwhelm host defenses. Trauma and existing impairment of host defenses also can contribute to the development of wound infections.

Approximation of the wound edges (*i.e.*, suturing of an incision type of wound) greatly enhances healing and prevents infection. Mechanical factors such as increased local pressure or **torsion** can cause wounds to pull apart, or *dehisce*. Foreign bodies tend to invite bacterial contamination and delay healing. Sutures are also foreign bodies, and although needed for the closure of surgical wounds, they are an impediment to healing. This is why sutures are removed as soon as possible after surgery.

Bite Wounds

Animal and human bites are particularly troublesome in terms of infection.[50] The animal inflicting the bite, the location of the bite, and the type of injury are all important determinants of whether the wound becomes infected. Cat bites (30% to 50%) are more apt to become infected with *Pasteurella multocida* compared with human bites.[50] Dog bites, for unclear reasons, become infected only approximately 5% of the time and generally either with *P. multocida* or *Capnocytophaga canimorsus*.[50] Bites inflicted by children are usually superficial and seldom become infected, whereas bites inflicted by adults have a much higher rate of infection. Puncture wounds are more likely to become infected than lacerations, probably because lacerations are easier to irrigate and debride.

The Effect of Age on Wound Healing

Wound Healing in Neonates and Children

Wound healing in children is similar to that in the adult population.[51] The child has a greater capacity for repair than the adult but may lack the reserves needed to ensure proper healing. A lack in reserves is evidenced by an easily upset electrolyte balance, a sudden change in temperature, and rapid spread of infection. The neonate and small child may have an immature immune system with no antigenic experience with organisms that contaminate wounds. The younger the child, the more likely the immune system is not fully developed.

Successful wound healing also depends on adequate nutrition. Children need sufficient calories to maintain growth and wound healing. The premature infant is often born with immature organ systems and minimal energy stores but high metabolic requirements—a condition that predisposes to impaired wound healing.

Children with certain comorbidities such as diabetes and malabsorption problems will be at higher risk for wound complication. Likewise, these children will be more apt to develop a skin breakdown or pressure sore. The Braden Q Scale is used to assess children's skin breakdown and is designed specifically for use with children.[52]

Wound Healing in Older Adults

A number of structural and functional changes occur in aging skin, including a decrease in dermal thickness, a decline in collagen content, and a loss of elasticity.[53] The observed changes in skin that occur with aging are complicated by the effects of sun exposure. Because the effects of sun exposure are cumulative, older adults show more changes in skin structure.

Wound healing is thought to be progressively impaired with aging. Older adults have reduced collagen and fibroblast synthesis, impaired wound contraction, and slower reepithelialization of open wounds.[54] Although wound healing may be delayed, most wounds heal, even in the debilitated older adult undergoing major surgical procedures.

Older adults are more vulnerable to chronic wounds, especially pressure, diabetic, and ischemic ulcers, compared to younger people, and these wounds heal more slowly. However, these wounds are more likely because of other disorders such as immobility, diabetes mellitus, or vascular disease, rather than aging.[54]

SUMMARY CONCEPTS

The ability of tissues to repair damage because of injury depends on the body's ability to replace the parenchymal cells and to organize them as

they were originally. Regeneration describes the process by which tissue is replaced with cells of a similar type and function. Healing by regeneration is limited to tissue with cells that are able to divide and replace the injured cells. Body cells are divided into types according to their ability to regenerate: labile cells, such as the epithelial cells of the skin and gastrointestinal tract, which continue to regenerate throughout life; stable cells, such as those in the liver, which normally do not divide but are capable of regeneration when confronted with an appropriate stimulus; and permanent or fixed cells, such as nerve cells, which are unable to regenerate. Scar tissue repair involves the substitution of fibrous connective tissue for injured tissue that cannot be repaired by regeneration.

Wound healing occurs by primary and secondary intention and is commonly divided into three phases: the inflammatory phase, the proliferative phase, and the maturational or remodeling phase. In wound healing by primary intention, the duration of the phases is fairly predictable. In wound healing by secondary intention, the process depends on the extent of injury and the healing environment. Wound healing can be impaired or complicated by factors such as malnutrition; restricted blood flow and oxygen delivery; diminished inflammatory and immune responses; and infection, wound separation, and the presence of foreign bodies. With infants and young children, wound healing is generally not impaired unless there is a hygiene issue and adolescents tend to have dry skin that can decrease the rate of wound healing.[55] Older adults experience dry skin and decreased subcutaneous fat that can lead to increased time with wound healing.[54]

Review Exercises

1. A 15-year-old boy presents with abdominal pain, a temperature of 38°C (100.5°F), and an elevated white blood cell count of 13,000/μL, with an increase in neutrophils. A tentative diagnosis of appendicitis is made.

   A. Explain the significance of pain as it relates to the inflammatory response.

   B. What is the cause of the fever and elevated white blood cell count?

   C. What would be the preferred treatment for this boy?

2. After a myocardial infarction, the area of heart muscle that has undergone necrosis

because of a lack of blood supply undergoes healing by replacement with scar tissue.

   A. Compare the functioning of the heart muscle that has been replaced by scar tissue with that of the normal surrounding heart muscle.

3. A 35-year-old man presents with a large abscess on his leg. He tells you he injured his leg while doing repair work on his house and he thinks there might be a wood sliver in the infected area.

   A. Explain the events that participate in formation of an abscess.

   B. He is told that incision and drainage of the lesion will be needed so healing can take place. Explain.

   C. He is reluctant to have the procedure done and asks whether an antibiotic would work as well. Explain why antibiotics alone are usually not effective in eliminating the microorganisms contained in an abscess.

REFERENCES

1. Rubin E., Strayer D. S. (2015). *Rubin's pathology: Clinicopathologic foundations of medicine* (7th ed.). Philadelphia, PA: Wolters Kluwer Health.
2. Kidane D., Chae W. J., Czochor J., et al. (2014). Interplay between DNA repair and inflammation, and the link to cancer. *Critical Reviews in Biochemistry and Molecular Biology* 49(2), 116–139.
3. Baune B. T. (2015). Inflammation and neurodegenerative disorders: Is there still hope for therapeutic intervention? *Current Opinion in Psychiatry* 28(2), 148–154.
4. Leonard B. E. (2015). Pain, depression and inflammation: Are interconnected causative factors involved? *Modern Trends in Pharmacopsychiatry* 30, 22–35.
5. Netea M. G., Balkwill F., Chonchol M., et al. (2017). A guiding map for inflammation. *Nature Immunology* 18(8), 826–831.
6. Sansbury B. E., Spite M. (2016). Resolution of acute inflammation and the role of resolvins in immunity, thrombosis, and vascular biology. *Circulation Research* 119(1), 113–130.
7. Lillico D. M., Zwozdesky M. A., Pemberton J. G., et al. (2015). Teleost leukocyte immune-type receptors activate distinct phagocytic modes for target acquisition and engulfment. *Journal of Leukocyte Biology* 98(2), 235–248.
8. Shoda T., Futamura K., Orihara K., et al. (2016). Recent advances in understanding the roles of vascular endothelial cells in allergic inflammation. *Allergology International* 65(1), 21–29.
9. Xiao L., Liu Y., Wang N. (2014). New paradigms in inflammatory signaling in vascular endothelial cells. *American Journal of Physiology: Heart and Circulatory Physiology* 306(3), H317–H325.
10. Henrot P., Foret J., Barnetche T., et al. (2018). Assessment of subclinical atherosclerosis in systemic lupus erythematosus: A systematic review and meta-analysis. *Joint, Bone, Spine* 85(2), 155–163.
11. Thomas M. R., Storey R. F. (2015). The role of platelets in inflammation. *Thrombosis and Haemostasis* 114(3), 449–458.
12. Hall J. E. (2011). *Guyton and Hall textbook of medical physiology* (12th ed.). Philadelphia, PA: Lippincott Williams & Wilkins.
13. Ross M. H., Pawlina W. (2011). *Histology: A text and atlas with correlated cell and molecular biology* (6th ed.). Philadelphia, PA: Lippincott Williams & Wilkins.
14. Theoharides T. C., Alysandratos K. D., Angelidou A., et al. (2012). Mast cells and inflammation. *Biochimica et Biophysica Acta* 1822(1), 21–33.
15. Pober J. S., Sessa W. C. (2014). Inflammation and the blood microvascular system. *Cold Spring Harbor Perspectives in Biology* 7(1), a016345.
16. Griffith J. W., Sokol C. L., Luster A. D. (2014). Chemokines and chemokine receptors: Positioning cells for host defense and immunity. *Annual Review of Immunology* 32, 659–702.
17. Rahmati M., Mobasheri A., Mozafari M. (2016). Inflammatory mediators in osteoarthritis: A critical review of the state-of-the-art, current prospects, and future challenges. *Bone* 85, 81–90.
18. Zanini M., Meyer E., Simon S. (2017). Pulp inflammation diagnosis from clinical to inflammatory mediators: A systematic review. *Journal of Endodontics* 43(7), 1033–1051.
19. Chen C., Wang D. W. (2015). Cytochrome P450-CYP2 family-epoxygenase role in inflammation and cancer. *Advances in Pharmacology* 74, 193–221.
20. Korotkova M., Lundberg I. E. (2014). The skeletal muscle arachidonic acid cascade in health and inflammatory disease. *Nature Reviews Rheumatology* 10(5), 295–303.
21. Stenson W. F. (2014). The universe of arachidonic acid metabolites in inflammatory bowel disease: Can we tell the good from the bad? *Current Opinion in Gastroenterology* 30(4), 347–351.
22. Gerber P. A., Gouni-Berthold I., Berneis K. (2013). Omega-3 fatty acids: Role in metabolism and cardiovascular disease. *Current Pharmaceutical Design* 19(17), 3074–3093.
23. Jain A. P., Aggarwal K. K., Zhang P. Y. (2015). Omega-3 fatty acids and cardiovascular disease. *European Review for Medical and Pharmacological Sciences* 19(3), 441–445.
24. Mori T. A. (2014). Omega-3 fatty acids and cardiovascular disease: Epidemiology and effects on cardiometabolic risk factors. *Food & Function* 5(9), 2004–2019.
25. Skarke C., Alamuddin N., Lawson J. A., et al. (2015). Bioactive products formed in humans from fish oils. *The Journal of Lipid Research* 56(9), 1808–1820.
26. van der Poll T., Herwald H. (2014). The coagulation system and its function in early immune defense. *Thrombosis and Haemostasis* 112(4), 640–648.
27. Morgan B. P., Harris C. L. (2015). Complement, a target for therapy in inflammatory and degenerative diseases. *Nature Reviews Drug Discovery* 14(12), 857–877.
28. Roos D. (2015). Complement and phagocytes—A complicated interaction. *Molecular Immunology* 68(1), 31–34.
29. Xu H., Chen M. (2016). Targeting the complement system for the management of retinal inflammatory and degenerative diseases. *The European Journal of Pharmacology* 787, 94–104.
30. Kalinska M., Meyer-Hoffert U., Kantyka T., et al. (2016). Kallikreins—The melting pot of activity and function. *Biochimie* 122, 270–282.
31. Turner M. D., Nedjai B., Hurst T., et al. (2014). Cytokines and chemokines: At the crossroads of cell signalling and inflammatory disease. *Biochimica et Biophysica Acta* 1843(11), 2563–2582.
32. Lee M. Y., Sun K. H., Chiang C. P., et al. (2015). Nitric oxide suppresses LPS-induced inflammation in a mouse asthma model by attenuating the interaction of IKK and Hsp90. *Experimental Biology and Medicine (Maywood, NJ)* 240(4), 498–507.
33. Sardon O., Corcuera P., Aldasoro A., et al. (2014). Alveolar nitric oxide and its role in pediatric asthma control assessment. *BMC Pulmonary Medicine* 14, 126.

34. Minihane A. M., Vinoy S., Russell W. R., et al. (2015). Low-grade inflammation, diet composition and health: Current research evidence and its translation. *The British Journal of Nutrition* 114(7), 999–1012.

35. Huang Y., Chen Z. (2016). Inflammatory bowel disease related innate immunity and adaptive immunity. *American Journal of Translational Research* 8(6), 2490–2497.

36. Rose C. D., Neven B., Wouters C. (2014). Granulomatous inflammation: The overlap of immune deficiency and inflammation. *Best Practice & Research: Clinical Rheumatology* 28(2), 191–212.

37. Sprung C. L., Dellinger R. P. (2015). Systemic inflammatory response syndrome criteria for severe sepsis. *The New England Journal of Medicine* 373(9), 880.

38. Kaur M. (2017). C-reactive protein: A prognostic indicator. *International Journal of Applied and Basic Medical Research* 7(2), 83–84.

39. Xu W., Chen B., Guo L., et al. (2015). High-sensitivity CRP: Possible link between job stress and atherosclerosis. *American Journal of Industrial Medicine* 58(7), 773–779.

40. Takeo M., Lee W., Ito M. (2015). Wound healing and skin regeneration. *Cold Spring Harbor Perspectives in Medicine* 5(1), a023267.

41. Janis J., Harrison B. (2014). Wound healing: Part II. Clinical applications. *Plastic and Reconstructive Surgery* 133(3), 383e–392e.

42. Kasuya A., Tokura Y. (2014). Attempts to accelerate wound healing. *Journal of Dermatological Science* 76(3), 169–172.

43. Martin P., Nunan R. (2015). Cellular and molecular mechanisms of repair in acute and chronic wound healing. *British Journal of Dermatology* 173(2), 370–378.

44. Barrientos S., Brem H., Stojadinovic O., et al. (2014). Clinical application of growth factors and cytokines in wound healing. *Wound Repair and Regeneration* 22(5), 569–578.

45. Tseng C. C., Chang S. J., Tsai W. C., et al. (2016). Increased incidence of rheumatoid arthritis in multiple sclerosis: A nationwide cohort study. *Medicine (Baltimore)* 95(26), e3999.

46. Quain A. M., Khardori N. M. (2015). Nutrition in wound care management: A comprehensive overview. *Wounds* 27(12), 327–335.

47. de Smet G. H. J., Kroese L. F., Menon A. G., et al. (2017). Oxygen therapies and their effects on wound healing. *Wound Repair and Regeneration* 25(4), 591–608.

48. Sidaway P. (2015). Diabetes: Epigenetic changes lead to impaired wound healing in patients with T2DM. *Nature Reviews Endocrinology* 11(2), 65.

49. Worster B., Zawora M. Q., Hsieh C. (2015). Common questions about wound care. *American Family Physician* 91(2), 86–92.

50. Rothe K., Tsokos M., Handrick W. (2015). Animal and human bite wounds. *Deutsches Ärzteblatt International* 112(25), 433–442; quiz 443.

51. Ball J., Bindler R., Cowen K. (2012). *Principles of pediatric nursing: Caring for children* (5th ed.). Boston, MA: Pearson.

52. Willock J., Habiballah L., Long D., et al. (2016). A comparison of the performance of the Braden Q and the Glamorgan paediatric pressure ulcer risk assessment scales in general and intensive care paediatric and neonatal units. *Journal of Tissue Viability* 25(2), 119–126.

53. Newton V. L., McConnell J. C., Hibbert S. A., et al. (2015). Skin aging: Molecular pathology, dermal remodelling and the imaging revolution. *Giornale Italiano di Dermatologia e Venereologia* 150(6), 665–674.

54. Gould L., Abadir P., Brem H., et al. (2015). Chronic wound repair and healing in older adults: Current status and future research. *Wound Repair and Regeneration* 23(1), 1–13.

55. Kyle T., Carman S. (2017). *Essentials of pediatric nursing* (3rd ed.). Philadelphia, PA: Wolters Kluwer.

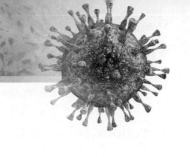

CHAPTER **10**

Mechanisms of Infectious Disease

Learning Objectives

After completing this chapter, the learner will be able to meet the following objectives:

1. Define the terms *host, agent, infectious disease, colonization, microflora, virulence, pathogen,* and *saprophyte.*
2. Describe the concept of host–microorganism interaction using the concepts of commensalism, mutualism, and parasitic relationships.
3. Describe the triad of infectious disease model.
4. Discuss modes of infectious disease transmission.
5. Describe the stages of an infectious disease.
6. Describe the factors that influence severity of an infectious disease.
7. Discuss clinical manifestations of a dysregulated host defense response to infection.
8. Explain the different methods for diagnosis of infectious disease.
9. List the infectious agents considered to pose the highest level of bioterrorism threat.
10. State an important concept in containment of infections because of bioterrorism and global travel.

All living organisms share two basic objectives in life: survival and reproduction. This principle applies equally to all members of the living world, including bacteria, viruses, fungi, and protozoa. To meet these objectives, organisms must extract essential nutrients for growth and proliferation from the environment.[1] The majority of the organisms found in the human body live in the gastrointestinal tract (over 300 different species) and are usually referred to as normal microflora. We now understand that microbial diversity plays a role in immune response and development of some immune-mediated diseases.[2] When pathogenic organisms surpass the barriers of our host defenses (*e.g.*, skin and mucous membranes), and the immune system is unable to eradicate them, they can produce harmful and potentially lethal consequences. The consequences of these invasions are collectively called *infectious diseases.*

Infectious Diseases

Infectious Disease Concepts

The study of infectious diseases is closely intertwined with the disciplines of microbiology, immunology, and epidemiology. Each of these disciplines (although there is an overlap) focuses on an aspect of the well-known triad of disease model (Fig. 10-1), which depicts the relationship between the agent, host, and environment. This model was first used in the study of infectious diseases. The host's immune response (covered in detail in the following chapter) and environmental factors involved in development of infectious disease will be described within the "Mechanisms of Infection" section later in this chapter.

Any organism capable of supporting the nutritional and physical growth requirements of another is called a *host*. Occasionally, *infection* and *colonization* are used interchangeably. However, the term *infection* describes the presence and multiplication within a host of another living organism, with subsequent injury to the host, whereas *colonization* describes the act of establishing a presence, a step required in the multifaceted process of infection.

One common misconception is that all interactions between microorganisms and humans are detrimental. The internal and external exposed surfaces of the human body are normally and harmlessly inhabited by a multitude of bacteria, collectively referred to as the normal *microflora*. Although the colonizing bacteria acquire nutrition, the host is not adversely affected by the relationship. This interaction is called *commensalism*, and the colonizing microorganisms are often referred to as *commensal flora*. The term *mutualism* is applied to an interaction in which both the microorganism and the host derive benefits from the interaction. For example, certain inhabitants of the human intestinal tract extract nutrients from the host and secrete essential vitamin by-products of metabolism (*e.g.*, vitamin K) that are absorbed and used by the host. A *parasitic relationship* is one in which only the infecting organism benefits from the relationship and the host either gains nothing or sustains injury from the interaction. If the host sustains injury or pathologic damage, the process is called an *infectious disease*.

The severity of an infectious disease can range from mild to life threatening. Severity depends on many variables, including the health of the host at the time of infection, the *virulence* (disease-producing potential) of the microorganism, and environmental conditions. Microorganisms capable of causing disease are called *pathogens*. Some microorganisms are highly virulent and frequently cause disease when a host is exposed to the microorganism. Table 10-1 includes a list of common pathogens that cause infectious disease in humans. Fortunately, there are few human pathogens in the microbial world. Most microorganisms are harmless *saprophytes*, free-living organisms obtaining their growth from dead or decaying organic material in the environment. All microorganisms, even saprophytes and members of the normal **flora**, can be *opportunistic pathogens*, capable of producing an infectious disease when the health and immunity of the host are weakened by illness, malnutrition, or medical therapy.

Agents of Infectious Disease

The agents of infectious disease include prions, viruses, bacteria, fungi, and parasites. A summary of the relevant characteristics of these human microbial pathogens is presented in Table 10-2.

Prions

In the past, *microbiologists* have assumed that all infectious agents possess a genome of either ribonucleic acid (RNA) or deoxyribonucleic acid (DNA) that codes to produce the essential proteins and enzymes necessary for survival and reproduction.[3] Prions, discovered in 1982, are protein particles that are able to transmit infection by self-propagation.[3,4] A number of prion-associated diseases have been identified, including Creutzfeldt–Jakob disease, multiple system atrophy, and kuru in humans. Animals are also affected, for example, bovine spongiform encephalopathy (or mad cow disease) in cattle.[5] The various prion-associated diseases produce very similar pathologic processes and symptoms in the hosts and are collectively called *transmissible neurodegenerative diseases* (see Fig. 10-2). All are characterized by a slowly progressive, noninflammatory neuronal degeneration, leading to loss of coordination (ataxia), dementia, and death over a period ranging from months to years. The conversion of a cellular precursor protein (PrP^C) into an abnormally folded protein (PrP^{SC}) causes the protein to behave differently. The PrP^{SC} is resistant to the action of proteases (enzymes that degrade excess or deformed proteins). Accumulation of these misfolded proteins becomes toxic to cells; however, as they aggregate, they become less toxic to the cell and can then be captured in plaques, tangles, or inclusion bodies.[4]

Prion diseases present significant challenges for management because of the pathogenic structure of PrP^{SC}. It is very stable and, therefore, is resistant to treatment. Studies investigating transmission of prion diseases in animals clearly demonstrate that prions replicate, leading researchers to investigate how proteins can reproduce in the absence of genetic material.[3] It is believed that PrP^{SC} aggregates into amyloid-like plaques in the

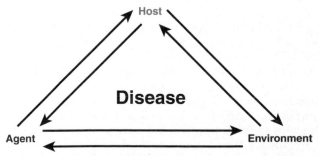

FIGURE 10-1. Triad of infectious disease model. Infectious diseases result from the interaction of an agent, a susceptible host, and environmental conditions that promote infection.

TABLE 10-1 Common Pathogens

Pathogen	Structural Characteristics	Functional Characteristics	Treatment	Common Diseases
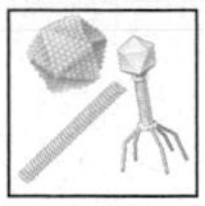 Viruses	DNA/RNA and protein coat	Cannot reproduce outside of cells	Antivirals, which slow viral replication	Influenza, the common cold, measles, HIV/AIDS
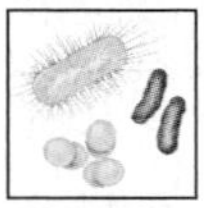 Bacteria	Microscopic cell without nucleus	Common on keyboards, water fountains, toilets, etc.	Antibiotics, which slow bacterial reproduction	Strep throat, some sinus and lung infections, some food poisoning
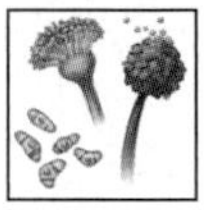 Fungi	Microscopic, unicellular (yeasts) or multicellular (molds)	Usually infect body surfaces and openings	Antifungals, which destroy the cell walls	Athlete's foot, yeast infections
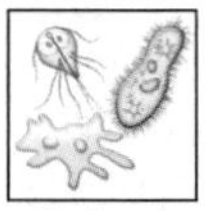 Protozoa	Microscopic, unicellular	Common in water supplies of developing countries	Antiprotozoal drugs, which interfere with protozoan metabolism	Malaria, sleeping sickness
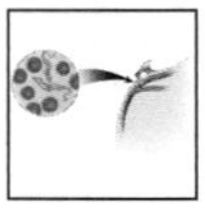 Worms	Multicellular	Prefer to live within body spaces and cells	Anthelmintics, which interfere with the worm's metabolism	Roundworms, tapeworms (helminths)
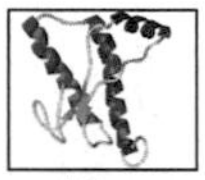 Prion	The protein (PrP) is found throughout the body; however, the PrP^{SC} in infectious materials is misfolded	Protein found in infected animals	Current research for effective treatment	Creutzfeldt–Jakob disease (associated with other neurodegenerative conditions)

Adapted with permission from McConnell T. H., Hull K. L. (2011). Human form, human function: Essentials of anatomy & physiology. Philadelphia, PA: Lippincott Williams & Wilkins. Prion image from Knipe D. M., Howley P. M. (2013). Fields virology (6th ed., Fig. 76.6, p. 2426). Philadelphia, PA: Lippincott Williams & Wilkins.

TABLE 10-2 Comparison of Characteristics of Human Microbial Pathogens

Organism	Defined Nucleus	Genomic Material	Size*	Intracellular or Extracellular	Motility
Prions	No	Unknown	55 kDa	E	–
Viruses	No	DNA or RNA	0.02–0.3	I	–
Bacteria	No	DNA	0.5–15	I/E	±
Mycoplasmas	No	DNA	0.2–0.3	E	–
Spirochetes	No	DNA	6–15	E	+
Rickettsiaceae	No	DNA	0.2–2	I	–
Chlamydiaceae	No	DNA	0.3–1	I	–
Yeasts	Yes	DNA	2–60	I/E	–
Molds	Yes	DNA	2–15 (hyphal width)	E	–
Protozoans	Yes	DNA	1–60	I/E	+
Helminths	Yes	DNA	2 mm to >1 m	E	+

*Micrometers unless indicated.

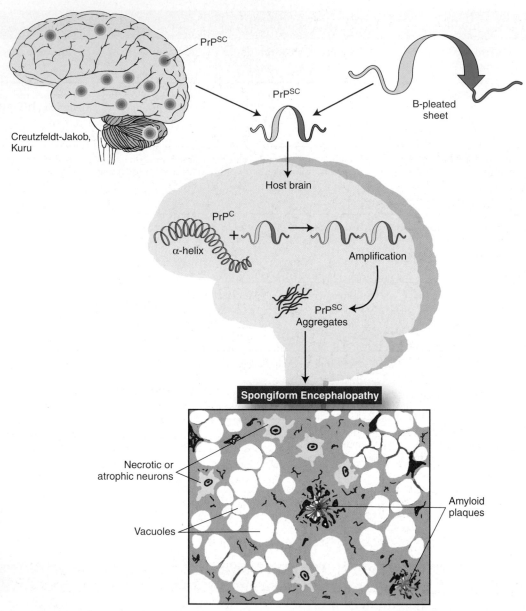

FIGURE 10-2. Molecular pathogenesis of prion disorders. (From Strayer D. S., Rubin R. (Eds.) (2015). *Rubin's pathology: Clinicopathologic foundations of medicine* (7th ed., Figure 32.71, p. 1452). Philadelphia, PA: Wolters Kluwer Health.)

brain and spreads within the axons of the nerve cells, causing progressively greater damage of host neurons and the eventual incapacitation of the host. Human transmission occurs primarily from eating infected meat or receiving an infected transplant organ or cornea.

Viruses

Viruses are the smallest obligate intracellular pathogens. They have no organized cellular structures but instead consist of a protein coat, or **capsid**, surrounding a nucleic acid core, or genome, of RNA *or* DNA—never both (Fig. 10-3). Some viruses are enclosed within a lipoprotein envelope derived from the cytoplasmic membrane of the parasitized host cell. Enveloped viruses include members of the herpesvirus group and paramyxoviruses (*e.g.*, influenza and poxviruses). Certain enveloped viruses are continuously shed from the infected cell surface enveloped in buds pinched from the cell membrane.

The viruses of humans and animals have been categorized according to various characteristics. These include the type of viral genome (single-stranded or double-stranded DNA or RNA), physical characteristics (*e.g.*, size, presence or absence of a membrane envelope), the mechanism of replication (*e.g.*, retroviruses), the mode of transmission (*e.g.*, arthropod-borne viruses, enteroviruses), target tissue, and the type of disease produced (*e.g.*, hepatitis A, B, C, D, and E viruses), to name a few.

Viruses are incapable of replication outside of a living cell. They must penetrate a susceptible living cell and use the biosynthetic structure of the cell to replicate.[3] The process of viral replication is shown in Figure 10-4. Not every viral agent causes lysis and death of the host cell during the course of replication. Some viruses enter the host cell where it remains in a latent, nonreplicating state for long periods without causing disease. The virus

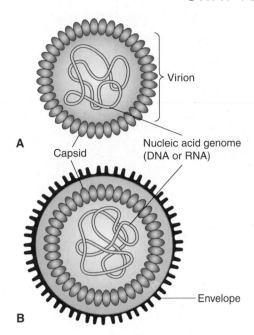

FIGURE 10-3. (A) The basic structure of a virus includes a protein coat surrounding an inner core of nucleic acid (DNA or RNA). (B) Some viruses may also be enclosed in a lipoprotein outer envelope.

may undergo active replication and produces symptoms of disease months to years later. Members of the herpesvirus group and adenovirus are examples of latent viruses. The resumption of the latent viral replication may produce symptoms of primary disease (*e.g.*, genital herpes) or cause an entirely different symptomatology (*e.g.*, shingles instead of chickenpox) (Fig. 10-5).

A family of viruses that has gained a great deal of attention is the *Orthomyxoviridae* or flu viruses. There has been attention focused on the hemagglutinin (H) subtype 5 and neuraminidase (N) subtype 1 or H5N1 variant, commonly known as the *avian influenza virus*, and the H1N1 variant, commonly known as *swine flu*.[6] The Centers for Disease Control and Prevention (CDC) recommends rapid influenza diagnostic tests using real-time polymerase chain reaction (PCR) by trained

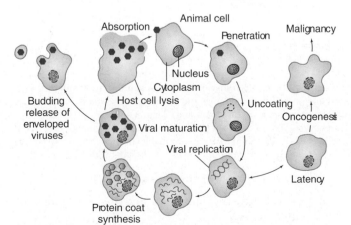

FIGURE 10-4. Schematic representation of the many possible consequences of viral infection of host cells, including cell lysis (poliovirus), continuous release of budding viral particles, or latency (herpesviruses) and oncogenesis (papovaviruses).

personnel.[6] Early infection control practices are important to prevent the spread of influenza.[6]

The retroviruses have a unique mechanism of replication. After entry into the host cell, the viral RNA genome is first translated into DNA by a viral enzyme called *reverse transcriptase*. The viral DNA copy is then integrated into the host chromosome where it exists in a latent state, similar to the herpesviruses. Reactivation and replication require a reversal of the entire process. In the case of HIV, when infected cells (CD4+ T cells) become activated, they release free virus by budding or cell–cell fusion. Lysis of CD4+ cells also releases HIV into the bloodstream, resulting in reduced CD4+ count and suppression of the immune response.[3]

In addition to causing infectious diseases, certain viruses also can transform normal host cells into malignant cells during the replication cycle. This group of viruses is referred to as *oncogenic* and includes certain retroviruses and DNA viruses, such as the herpesviruses, adenoviruses, and papovaviruses. Human papillomaviruses, members of the papovavirus family, cause cutaneous and genital warts, and several genotypes are associated with cervical cancer.

Bacteria

Bacteria are autonomously replicating unicellular organisms known as *prokaryotes* because they lack an organized nucleus. Compared with nucleated eukaryotic cells, the bacterial cells are small and structurally primitive.[3] They are the smallest of all living cells and contain no organized intracellular organelles, and the genome consists of only a single double-stranded circular chromosome of DNA, which is associated with RNA and proteins.[3] The **prokaryotic** cell is organized into an internal compartment called the *cytoplasm*, which contains the reproductive and metabolic machinery of the cell. The cytoplasm is surrounded by a flexible lipid membrane, called the *cytoplasmic membrane*.[3] This is in turn usually enclosed within a rigid cell wall. The structure and synthesis of the cell wall determine the microscopic shape of the bacterium (*e.g.*, spherical [cocci], helical [spirilla], or elongate [bacilli]). Further, bacteria can be divided into two types (gram-positive and gram-negative) based on their gram staining properties. Gram-positive bacteria produce a cell wall composed of a distinctive polymer known as *peptidoglycan*. This polymer is produced only by prokaryotes and is used as a target for some antibacterial therapies. Gram-negative bacteria produce an outer membrane composed of lipopolysaccharide, which can induce shock in the host.[3] Several bacteria synthesize an extracellular capsule composed of protein or polysaccharide. The capsule protects the organism from environmental hazards such as the immunologic defenses of the host.[3] Figure 10-6 shows a variety of bacterial morphologies.

Certain bacteria are motile as the result of external whiplike appendages called *flagella*. The flagella rotate like a propeller, transporting the organism through a liquid environment. Bacteria can also produce hairlike structures projecting from the cell surface called **pili** or **fimbriae**, which enable the organism to adhere to surfaces such as mucous membranes or other bacteria.

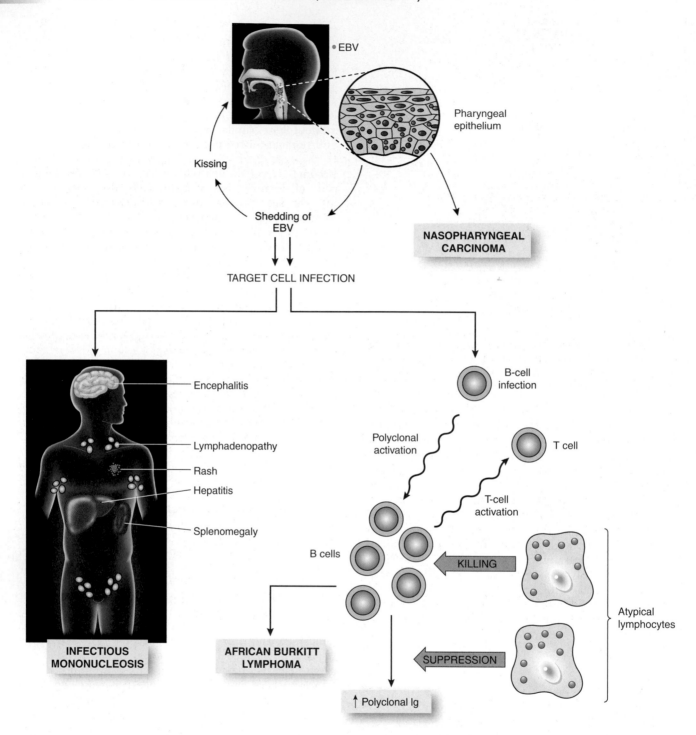

FIGURE 10-5. Role of Epstein–Barr virus (EBV) in infectious mononucleosis (IM), nasopharyngeal carcinoma, and Burkitt lymphoma. EBV invades and replicates within the salivary glands or pharyngeal epithelium and is shed into the saliva and respiratory secretions. Additionally, in some people, the virus transforms pharyngeal epithelial cells, which can cause nasopharyngeal carcinoma. Then in some people who are not immune from childhood exposure, EBV can cause IM. EBV can infect B lymphocytes and stimulate the production of atypical lymphocytes, which kill virally infected B cells and suppress immunoglobulin production. Some infected B cells can transform into malignant lymphocytes of Burkitt lymphoma. (From Strayer D. S., Rubin R. (Eds.) (2015). *Rubin's pathology: Clinicopathologic foundations of medicine* (7th ed., Figure 9.9, p. 383). Philadelphia, PA: Wolters Kluwer Health.)

Most prokaryotes reproduce asexually by **simple cellular** division. When the cocci divide in chains, they are called *streptococci*; in pairs, *diplococci*; and in clusters, *staphylococci*.[3] The growth rate of bacteria varies significantly among different species and depends greatly on physical growth conditions and the availability of nutrients.

In nature, bacteria rarely exist as single cells floating in an aqueous environment. Rather, bacteria prefer to stick to and colonize environmental surfaces, producing

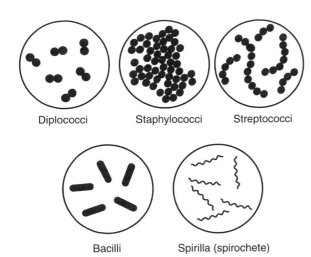

Diplococci   Staphylococci   Streptococci

Bacilli   Spirilla (spirochete)

FIGURE 10-6. The variety of bacterial morphology. Examples of bacteria-related disease: Streptococci are gram-positive aerobic organisms that cause skin infections such as impetigo, scarlet fever, pharyngitis, endocarditis, pneumonia, and potentially fatal toxic shock and sepsis. Salmonella and *Escherichia coli* are gram-negative, rod-shaped bacteria that cause food-borne illnesses. Spirilla bacteria are gram-negative bacteria that cause bacterial diarrhea and peptic ulcers. (From Houser H. J., Sesser J. R. (2016). *LWW's medical assisting exam review for CMA, RMA, and CMAS certification.* Philadelphia, PA: Wolters Kluwer.)

structured communities called *biofilms.*[7] The organization and structure of biofilms permit access to available nutrients and elimination of metabolic waste. Within the biofilm, individual organisms use chemical signaling as a form of primitive intercellular communication to represent the state of the environment. This is known as *quorum sensing.* These signals inform members of the community when sufficient nutrients are available for proliferation or when environmental conditions warrant dormancy or evacuation. Examples of biofilms abound in nature and are found on surfaces of aquatic environments and on humans.

Bacteria are extremely adaptable life forms and have a well-defined set of growth parameters, including nutrition, temperature, light, humidity, and atmosphere. Bacteria with extremely strict growth requirements are called *fastidious.* For example, *Neisseria gonorrhoeae,* the bacterium that causes gonorrhea, cannot live for extended periods outside the human body.[8] Some bacteria require oxygen for growth and metabolism and are called *aerobes.* Others cannot survive in an oxygen-containing environment and are called *anaerobes.* An organism capable of adapting its metabolism to aerobic or anaerobic conditions is called *facultatively anaerobic.*

Another means of classifying bacteria according to microscopic staining properties is the *acid-fast stain.* Because of their unique cell membrane fatty acid content and composition, certain bacteria are resistant to the decolorization of a primary stain when treated with a solution of acid alcohol. These organisms are termed *acid fast* and include a number of significant human pathogens, most notably *Mycobacterium tuberculosis.*[8]

For purposes of taxonomy (*i.e.,* identification and classification), each member of the bacterial kingdom is

categorized into a small group of biochemically and genetically related organisms called the *genus* and further subdivided into distinct individuals within the genus called *species.* The genus and species assignment of the organism is reflected in its name (*e.g., Staphylococcus* [genus] *aureus* [species]).

Spirochetes

The *spirochetes* are a category of bacteria that are mentioned separately because of their unusual cellular morphology and distinctive mechanism of motility. The spirochetes are gram-negative rods but are unique in that the cell's shape is helical and the length of the organism is many times its width. A series of filaments are wound about the cell wall and extend the entire length of the cell. These filaments propel the organism through an aqueous environment in a corkscrew motion.

Spirochetes are anaerobic organisms and comprise three genera: *Leptospira, Borrelia,* and *Treponema.* Each genus has saprophytic and pathogenic strains. The pathogenic leptospires infect a wide variety of wild and domestic animals. Infected animals shed the organisms into the environment through the urinary tract. Transmission to humans occurs by contact with infected animals or urine-contaminated surroundings. Leptospires gain access to the host directly through mucous membranes or breaks in the skin and can produce a severe and potentially fatal illness called *Weil syndrome.* In contrast, the borreliae are transmitted from infected animals to humans through the bite of an arthropod vector such as lice or ticks. Included in the genus *Borrelia* are the agents of relapsing fever (*Borrelia recurrentis*) and Lyme disease (*Borrelia burgdorferi*).

Pathogenic *Treponema* species require no intermediates and are spread from person to person by direct contact. The most important member of the genus is *Treponema pallidum,* the causative agent of syphilis.

Mycoplasmas

The mycoplasmas are unicellular prokaryotes capable of independent replication. These organisms are less than one third the size of bacteria. The cell is composed of cytoplasm surrounded by a membrane, but unlike bacteria, the mycoplasmas do not produce a rigid peptidoglycan cell wall. As a consequence, the microscopic appearance of the cell is highly variable, ranging from coccoid forms to filaments, and the mycoplasmas are resistant to cell wall–inhibiting antibiotics, such as penicillins and cephalosporins.

The mycoplasmas affecting humans are divided into three genera: *Mycoplasma, Ureaplasma,* and *Acholeplasma.* The first two require cholesterol from the environment to produce the cell membrane; the acholeplasmas do not. In the human host, mycoplasmas are commensals. However, a number of species are capable of producing serious diseases, including pneumonia (*Mycoplasma pneumoniae*), genital infections (*Mycoplasma hominis* and *Ureaplasma urealyticum*), maternally transmitted respiratory infections to infants with low birth weight (*U. urealyticum*), and potential complications during pregnancy.[8,9]

The human body is constantly exposed to potentially harmful microorganisms and foreign substances. A complete system composed of complementary and interrelated mechanisms defends against invasion by bacteria, viruses, and other foreign substances. Through recognition of specific patterns found on the surface of organisms and toxins, the body's immune system can distinguish itself from these foreign substances and tell the difference between potentially harmful and nonharmful agents. In addition, the immune system can defend against abnormal cells and molecules that periodically develop within the body. The skin and its epithelial layers in conjunction with the body's normal inflammatory processes make up the first line of the body's defense and confer *innate or natural immunity* to the host. Once these protective barriers have been crossed, the body relies upon a second line of defense known as the *adaptive immune response* to eradicate infection by invading organisms. The adaptive immune response develops slowly over time but results in the development of antibodies that can rapidly target specific microorganisms and foreign substances when a second exposure occurs.

This chapter covers immunity and the immune system, including a complete discussion of innate and adaptive immunity. Concepts related to key cellular processes, recognition systems, and effector responses integral to the immune system are also presented. In addition, developmental aspects of the immune system are discussed.

 ## The Immune Response

Immunity can be defined as the body's ability to defend against specific pathogens and/or foreign substances responsible for the development of disease. The immune response is initiated by the body's various defense systems. Some responses become active almost immediately, whereas others develop slowly over time. It is the coordinated interaction of these mechanisms that allows the body to maintain normal internal homeostasis. However, when these mechanisms are either depressed or become overactive, illness and disease can occur.

Innate immunity and adaptive immunity are complementary processes that work to protect the body. *Innate immunity*, the body's first line of defense, occurs early and more rapidly in response to foreign substances, whereas adaptive immunity is usually delayed unless the host has been previously exposed (Table 11-1).

Intact innate immune mechanisms are essential for the initiation of the adaptive immune response, requiring communication between the two systems. Dendritic cells (DCs) are an essential component of both innate and adaptive immunity and serve as the communication link between the two immune responses through the release of cytokines and chemokines.[1] As a result, innate immune cells are capable of communicating important information about the invading microorganism or foreign substance to the B and T lymphocytes, which are the key cells involved in adaptive immunity. These immune cells in turn recruit and activate additional phagocytes and molecules of the innate immune system to defend the host.

Cytokines and Their Role in Immunity

Cytokines, short-acting, biologically active, soluble substances, are an essential component of host defense mechanisms and the primary means with which cells of innate and adaptive immunity communicate. Chemokines are a subset of cytokines that consist of small protein molecules involved in both immune and inflammatory responses.[2] They are responsible for directing

Feature	Innate	Adaptive
Time of response	Immediate (minutes/hours)	Dependent upon exposure (first, delayed; second, immediate due to production antibodies)
Diversity	Limited to classes or groups of microbes	Very large; specific for each unique antigen
Microbe recognition	General patterns on microbes; nonspecific	Specific to individual microbes and antigens (antigen/antibody complexes)
Nonself recognition	Yes	Yes
Response to repeated infection	Similar with each exposure	Immunologic memory; more rapid and efficient with subsequent exposure
Defense	Epithelium (skin, mucous membranes), phagocytes, inflammation, fever	Cell killing; tagging of antigen by antibody for removal
Cellular components	Phagocytes (monocytes/macrophages, neutrophils), NK cells, DCs	T and B lymphocytes, macrophages, DCs, NK cells
Molecular components	Cytokines, complement proteins, acute-phase proteins, soluble mediators	Antibodies, cytokines, complement system

TABLE 11-1 Features of Innate and Adaptive Immunity

DC, dendritic cell; NK, natural killer.

the migration of leukocytes to both areas of injury and locations where immune responses have been activated such as lymph nodes, the spleen, Peyer patches, and the tonsils.[2] Chemokines can work together to antagonize or activate chemokine receptors. The source and function of the main cytokines that participate in innate and adaptive immunity are summarized in Table 11-2.

General Properties of Cytokines

Cytokines are low-molecular-weight, pro- or anti-inflammatory proteins secreted by cells of the innate and adaptive immune systems that regulate many of the actions of these cells. Most of the major cytokines are the interleukins (ILs), interferons (IFNs), and tumor necrosis factor alpha (TNF-α). Cytokines work by binding to specific receptors on the cells that they target and then activating intracellular processes.[3]

ILs are produced by both the macrophages and lymphocytes in the presence of an invading microorganism or when the process of inflammation is initiated. Their primary function is to enhance the acquired immune response or regulate through suppression or enhancement the inflammatory process. IFNs are cytokines that

TABLE 11-2 Cytokines and Chemokines of Innate and Adaptive Immunity

Cytokines	Source	Function
Interleukin-1 (IL-1)	Macrophages, endothelial cells, some epithelial cells	Wide variety of biologic effects; activates endothelium in inflammation; induces fever and acute-phase response; stimulates neutrophil production
Interleukin-2 (IL-2)	CD4$^+$, CD8$^+$ T cells	Growth factor for activated T cells; induces synthesis of other cytokines; activates cytotoxic T lymphocytes and NK cells
Interleukin-3 (IL-3)	CD4$^+$ T cells	Growth factor for progenitor hematopoietic cells
Interleukin-4 (IL-4)	CD4$^+$ T$_2$H cells, mast cells	Promotes growth and survival of T, B, and mast cells; causes T$_2$H cell differentiation; activates B cells and eosinophils; and induces IgE-type responses
Interleukin-5 (IL-5)	CD4$^+$ T$_2$H cells	Induces eosinophil growth and development
Interleukin-6 (IL-6)	Macrophages, endothelial cells, T lymphocytes	Stimulates the liver to produce mediators of acute-phase inflammatory response; also induces proliferation of antibody-producing cells by the adaptive immune system
Interleukin-7 (IL-7)	Bone marrow stromal cells	Primary function in adaptive immunity; stimulates pre-B cells and thymocyte development and proliferation
Interleukin-8 (IL-8)	Macrophages, endothelial cells	Primary function in adaptive immunity; chemoattracts neutrophils and T lymphocytes; regulates lymphocyte homing and neutrophil infiltration
Interleukin-10 (IL-10)	Macrophages, some T-helper cells	Inhibitor of activated macrophages and DCs; decreases inflammation by inhibiting T$_1$H cells and release of IL-12 from macrophages
Interleukin-12 (IL-12)	Macrophages, DCs	Enhances NK cell cytotoxicity in innate immunity; induces T$_1$H cell differentiation in adaptive immunity
Type I interferons (IFN-α, IFN-β)	Macrophages, fibroblasts	Inhibit viral replication; activate NK cells; and increase expression of MHC-I molecules on virus-infected cells
Interferon-γ (IFN-γ)	NK cells, CD4$^+$ and CD8$^+$ T lymphocytes	Activates macrophages in both innate immune responses and adaptive cell-mediated immune responses; increases expression of MHC-I and MHC-II and antigen processing and presentation
Tumor necrosis factor-α (TNF-α)	Macrophages, T cells	Induces inflammation, fever, and acute-phase response; activates neutrophils and endothelial cells; kills cells through apoptosis
Chemokines	Macrophages, endothelial cells, T lymphocytes	Large family of structurally similar cytokines that stimulate leukocyte movement and regulate the migration of leukocytes from the blood to the tissues
Granulocyte-monocyte CSF (GM-CSF)	T cells, macrophages, endothelial cells, fibroblasts	Promotes neutrophil, eosinophil, and monocyte maturation and growth; activates mature granulocytes
Granulocyte CSF (G-CSF)	Macrophages, fibroblasts, endothelial cells	Promotes growth and maturation of neutrophils consumed in inflammatory reactions
Monocyte CSF (M-CSF)	Macrophages, activated T cells, endothelial cells	Promotes growth and maturation of mononuclear phagocytes

CSF, colony-stimulating factor; DC, dendritic cell; Ig, immunoglobulin; MHC, major histocompatibility complex; NK, natural killer; T$_1$H, T-helper type 1; T$_2$H, T-helper type 2.

UNDERSTANDING ➔ Innate and Adaptive Immunity

The innate and adaptive immune systems mediate the body's defenses through an integrated system in which numerous cells and molecules function cooperatively to protect the host against foreign invaders. The innate immune system stimulates adaptive immunity. Although they use different mechanisms to recognize invading pathogens, both types of immunity use many of the same mechanisms, including destruction of the pathogen by phagocytosis and the complement system, to clear the organism from the body.

①

Innate Immunity Innate immunity (also called *natural immunity*) consists of the cellular and biochemical defenses that are normally in place before an encounter with an infectious agent and provide rapid protection against infection. The major effector components of innate immunity include epithelial cells, which block the entry of infectious agents and secrete antimicrobial enzymes, proteins, and peptides; phagocytic neutrophils and macrophages, which engulf and digest microbes; natural killer (NK) cells, which kill intracellular microbes and foreign agents; and the complement system, which amplifies the inflammatory response and uses the membrane attack response to lyse microbes. The cells of the innate immune system also produce chemical messengers that stimulate and influence the adaptive immune response.

The innate immune system uses pattern recognition receptors (PRRs), which recognize microbial structures that are shared by microbes and are often necessary for their survival, but are not present on human cells. Thus, the innate immune system is able to distinguish between self and nonself, but it does not distinguish between invading agents.

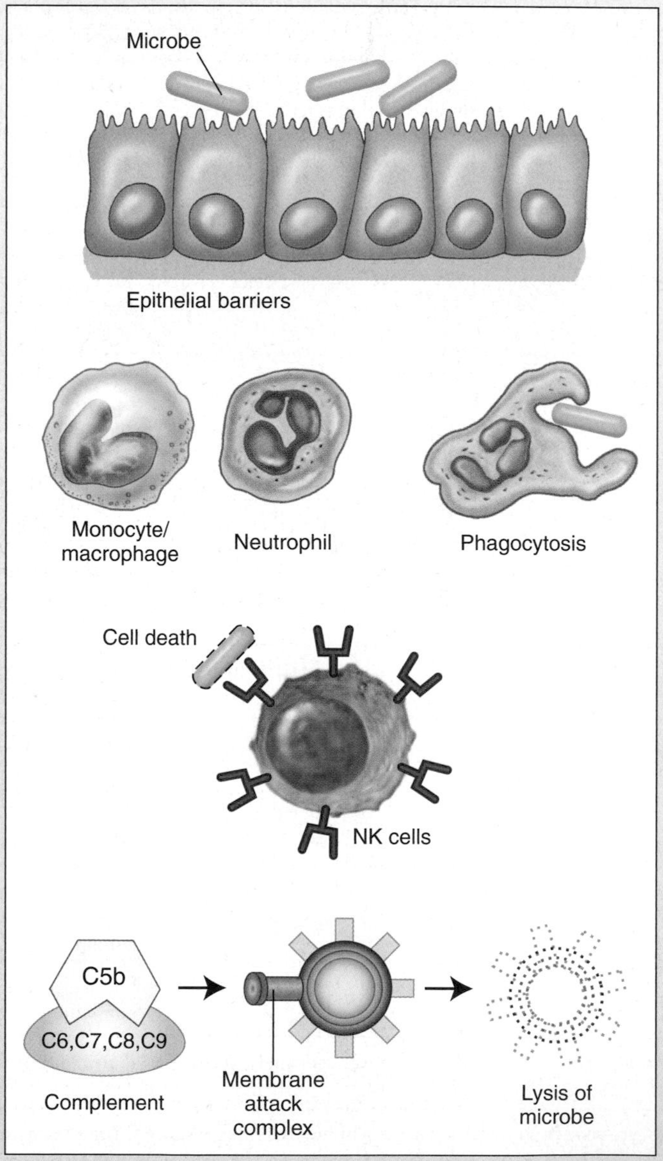

Microbe

Epithelial barriers

Monocyte/macrophage   Neutrophil   Phagocytosis

Cell death

NK cells

C5b

C6,C7,C8,C9

Complement   Membrane attack complex   Lysis of microbe

② **Adaptive Immunity** Adaptive immunity (also called *acquired immunity*) refers to immunity that is acquired through previous exposure to infectious and other foreign agents. A defining characteristic of adaptive immunity is the ability not only to distinguish self from nonself but also to recognize and destroy specific foreign agents based on their distinct antigenic properties. The components of the adaptive immune system are the T and B lymphocytes and their products. There are two types of adaptive immune responses, humoral and cell-mediated immunity.

Humoral immunity is mediated by the B lymphocytes (B cells) and is the principal defense against extracellular microbes and their toxins. The B cells differentiate into antibody-secreting plasma cells. The circulating antibodies then interact with and destroy the microbes that are present in the blood or mucosal surfaces.

Cell-mediated, or cellular, immunity is mediated by the cytotoxic T lymphocytes (T cells) and functions in the elimination of intracellular pathogens (*e.g.*, viruses). T cells develop receptors that recognize the viral peptides displayed on the surface of infected cells and then signal destruction of the infected cells.

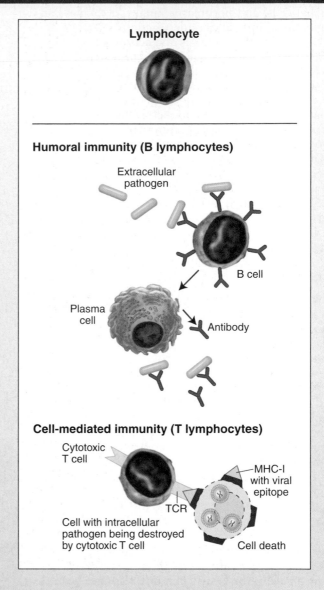

Lymphocyte

Humoral immunity (B lymphocytes)

Extracellular pathogen

B cell

Plasma cell

Antibody

Cell-mediated immunity (T lymphocytes)

Cytotoxic T cell

MHC-I with viral epitope

TCR

Cell with intracellular pathogen being destroyed by cytotoxic T cell

Cell death

---

primarily protect the host against viral infections and play a role in the modulation of the inflammatory response. Each type of IFN is produced by a specific cell of the immune response.[4]

All cytokines are secreted in a brief, self-limited manner. They are rarely stored as preformed molecules but instead are synthesized when the cells that produce them are activated. Some of the cytokines exhibit pleiotropism, which means they can act on many different cell types.[5] When these defenses malfunction, disease processes that originate in these tissues, such as asthma and psoriasis, can arise.

Concept Mastery Alert

Cytokines have the ability to act on different cell types so they are pleiotropic, not cell specific. They also have the ability to stimulate the same biologic factors as other cytokines or to overlap their effects. This is known as redundancy.

In addition to being pleiotropic and redundant, several different cell types are capable of producing the same cytokine. This allows cytokines to have a broader spectrum of activity. For example, IL-1 is a proinflammatory cytokine that is primarily produced by macrophages but can be produced by virtually all leukocytes, endothelial cells, and fibroblasts. Finally, cytokines can also function to initiate cascade reactions with one cytokine influencing the synthesis and actions of other cytokines. These effects may be localized or systemic, with the cytokines secreted into the bloodstream and transported to their site of action. Colony-stimulating factors (CSFs) are a unique subset of cytokines that participate in hematopoiesis and stimulate the production of large numbers of mature platelets, erythrocytes, lymphocytes, neutrophils, monocytes, eosinophils, basophils, and DCs. The CSFs were named according to the type of target cell on which they act (see Table 11-2). Although CSF is necessary for normal blood cell production, excess CSF is associated with several disease processes such as chronic obstructive pulmonary disease.[6] Recombinant CSF is being used to increase the success rates of bone marrow transplantations.

Chemokines

Chemokines are small protein molecules that are involved in immune and inflammatory cellular responses and function to control the migration of leukocytes to their primary site of action in the immune response.[2] The four distinct classes of chemokines are designated C, CC, CXC, and CX_3C.[7] The CC chemokines attract monocytes, lymphocytes, and eosinophils to sites of chronic inflammation. The CXC chemokines attract neutrophils to sites of acute inflammation.

Chemokines communicate with their target cells by activating G protein–coupled receptors in the cells. As a result, they are capable of activating different populations of leukocytes based upon the needs of the situation.[7] Chemokines are implicated in the development of a number of acute and chronic diseases, including atherosclerosis, rheumatoid arthritis, inflammatory bowel disease, allergic asthma and chronic bronchitis, multiple sclerosis, systemic lupus erythematosus, and human immunodeficiency virus (HIV) infection. They also play a role in the body's immune response against cancer cells through the enhancement of chemokines by activated T cells and other tumor-derived proteins.[8,9]

 SUMMARY CONCEPTS

Immunity is the body's defense against disease and invading microorganisms. Immune mechanisms can be divided into two types: innate and adaptive immunity. Innate immunity is the first line of defense and can distinguish between self and nonself through the recognition of cellular patterns on foreign substances and microbes. Adaptive immunity is part of the second line of defense and involves both humoral and cellular mechanisms that respond to cell-specific substances known

as antigens. The adaptive immune response is capable of amplifying and sustaining its responses, of distinguishing self from nonself, and finally of memory in that it can recognize the antigen on repeat exposure in order to quickly produce a heightened response on subsequent encounters with the same microorganism. The innate and adaptive immune responses work in concert with one another to ensure that the homeostasis is maintained.

Although cells of both the innate and adaptive immune systems communicate critical information about the invading microbe or pathogen by cell-to-cell contact, many interactions and cellular responses depend on the secretion of chemical mediators in the form of cytokines, chemokines, and CSFs. Cytokines are soluble proteins secreted by cells of both the innate and adaptive immune systems that mediate many of the functions of these cells. Chemokines are cytokines that stimulate the migration and activation of various immune and inflammatory cells. CSFs stimulate the growth and differentiation of bone marrow progenitors of immune cells and play a key role in hematopoiesis.

Innate Immunity

 **KEY POINTS**

Innate Immunity

■ Innate immunity consists of physical, chemical, cellular, and molecular defenses that are ready for activation and mediate rapid, initial protection against infection.

■ The innate immune response relies on the body's ability to distinguish structures present on the surface of pathogens known as pathogen-associated molecular patterns (PAMPs) from structures on human cells.

■ The phagocytic cells of the innate immune response express PRRs that bind with broad patterns shared by groups of microbes but that are not present on mammalian cells. Toll-like receptors (TLRs), a major type of PRR, are expressed on phagocytes and are potent activators of innate immune system cells and molecules.

■ Cytokines and chemokines that are released from activated leukocytes regulate the activities of innate immunity, stimulate the inflammatory process, and initiate the adaptive immune response.

Epithelial Barriers

Physical, mechanical, and biochemical barriers against microbial invasion are found in all common portals of entry into the body, including the skin and respiratory, gastrointestinal, and urogenital tracts. The intact skin is by far the most formidable physical barrier available to infection because of its design. It comprises closely packed cells that are organized in multiple layers that are continuously shed. In addition, a protective layer of protein, known as keratin, covers the skin. The skin has simple chemicals that create a nonspecific, salty, acidic environment and antibacterial proteins, such as the enzyme lysozyme, that inhibit the colonization of microorganisms and aid in their destruction.[10]

Epithelial cells destroy the invading organisms by secreting antimicrobial enzymes, proteins, and peptides. Specialized cells in these linings, such as the goblet cells in the gastrointestinal tract, secrete a viscous material comprising high-molecular-weight glycoproteins known as mucin, which when hydrated forms *mucus*. The mucins bind to pathogens, thereby trapping them and washing away potential invaders. In the lower respiratory tract, hair-like, mobile structures called cilia protrude through the epithelial cells and move microbes trapped in the mucus up the tracheobronchial tree and toward the throat. The physiologic responses of coughing and sneezing further aid in their removal from the body.

Microorganisms that are trapped by mucus are then subjected to various chemical defenses present throughout the body, including lysozymes and the complement system. Lysozyme is a hydrolytic enzyme found in tears, saliva, and human milk, which is capable of breaking down bacterial cell walls. The complement system is found in the blood and is essential for the activity of antibodies. It is composed of 20 different enzyme precursors, which when activated by antigen–antibody complexes cause bacteria to clump together so that they are more susceptible to phagocytic immune cells (Fig. 11-1). In addition, recent research has shown that complement plays a key role in bridging the innate–adaptive immune responses through the release of C3 complement protein.[11] In the stomach and intestines, death of microbes results from the action of digestive enzymes, acidic conditions, and the secretion of *defensins*, small positively charged peptides that quickly kill both gram-positive and gram-negative microorganisms by disrupting the microbial membrane.

When pathogens are able to breach the epithelial defenses, the innate immune response is initiated by the body's leukocytes, which recognize common surface receptors present on the invading microorganisms.

Cells of Innate Immunity

The cells of the innate immune response recognize microbes that share characteristics common to all of their surface receptors. Once recognized, the innate immune cells initiate a broad spectrum of responses that target the invading microorganisms. The key cells of innate immunity include neutrophils, macrophages, DCs, NK cells, and intraepithelial lymphocytes (IELs). They have both proinflammatory and anti-inflammatory effects on their targets and play an important role in priming adaptive immune responses.[12,13]

Neutrophils and Macrophages

The leukocytes involved in the innate immune response are derived from myeloid stem cells and are subdivided into two distinct groups based on the presence or absence of specific staining granules in their cytoplasm. Leukocytes that contain granules are classified as granulocytes and include neutrophils, eosinophils, and basophils. Cells that lack granules are classified as agranulocytes and include lymphocytes, monocytes,

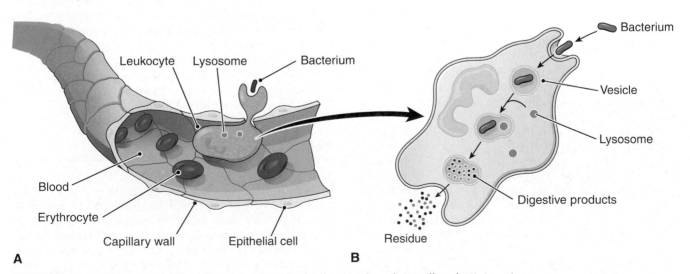

FIGURE 11-1. Phagocytosis. (**A**) A phagocytic white blood cell moves through a capillary that is in an infected area and engulfs the bacteria. (**B**) The lysosome digests the bacteria that were in a vesicle. (From Cohen B. J. (2013). *Memmler's the human body in health and disease* (12th ed.). Philadelphia, PA: Lippincott Williams & Wilkins.)

and macrophages. However, lymphocytes are derived from lymphoid precursors and are not part of the innate immune response.

Neutrophils, which are named for their neutral-staining granules, are the most abundant granulocytes found in the body and make up approximately 55% of all white blood cells. They are also known as polymorphonuclear neutrophils. They are phagocytic cells and are capable of amoeboid-like movement, which allows them to migrate throughout the body. They function as early responder cells in innate immunity. They are rare in the tissues and in body cavities and lie predominantly dormant in the blood and bone marrow until they are needed in the immune response.[14] Eosinophils have large coarse granules and normally comprise only 1% to 4% of the total white cell count. In contrast to neutrophils, these cells do not ingest cellular debris but rather antigen–antibody complexes and viruses. They frequently become active in parasitic infections and allergic responses. Basophils make up less than 1% of the total white cell count and contain granules that release a multitude of substances including histamine and proteolytic enzymes. Their function is not completely understood, but they are believed to play a role in allergy and parasitic infection as well.

The agranulocytes involved in innate immunity are part of the mononuclear phagocyte system and include the monocytes and macrophages. Monocytes are the largest in size of all the white blood cells but make up only 3% to 7% of the total leukocyte count. They are released from the bone marrow into the bloodstream where they migrate into tissues and mature into macrophages and DCs so that they can participate in the inflammatory response and phagocytize foreign substances and cellular debris. Macrophages have a long life span, reside in the tissues, and act as the first phagocyte that invading organisms encounter upon entering the host.[14]

Macrophages are essential for the clearance of bacteria that breach the epithelial barrier in the intestine and other organ systems. They have remarkable flexibility that allows them to efficiently respond to environmental signals. Once activated, these cells engulf and digest microbes that attach to their cell membrane. The ability of these phagocytic cells to initiate this response is dependent upon the repetitive structures known as pathogen-associated molecular patterns (PAMPs) and the receptors that can recognize them known as pattern recognition receptors (PRRs). Phagocytosis of invading microorganisms helps to limit the spread of infection until adaptive immune responses can become fully activated.

In addition to phagocytosis, macrophages and DCs process and present antigens in the initiation of the immune response acting as a major initiator of the adaptive immune response.[1] These cells secrete substances that initiate and coordinate the inflammatory response or activate lymphocytes. Macrophages can also remove antigen–antibody complexes and, under the influence of T cells, destroy malignant host or virus-infected cells.

Dendritic Cells

DCs are specialized, bone marrow–derived leukocytes found in lymphoid tissue and are the bridge between the innate and adaptive immune systems. DCs are relatively rare cells that are found mainly in tissues exposed to external environments such as the respiratory and gastrointestinal systems.[1] They are present primarily in an immature form that is available to directly sense pathogens, capture foreign agents, and transport them to secondary lymphoid tissues.[1] Once activated, DCs undergo a complex maturation process in order to function as key antigen-presenting cells (APCs) capable of initiating adaptive immunity.[1] They are responsible for the processing and presentation of antigens to the lymphocytes. DCs, like macrophages, also release several communication molecules that direct the nature of adaptive immune responses.

Natural Killer Cells and Intraepithelial Lymphocytes

NK cells and IELs are two other cell types involved in the innate immune response. NK cells have the innate ability to spontaneously kill target organisms. Both types of cells rely on the recognition of specific PAMPs on the cell surface of the microorganism.

NK cells are a **heterogeneous** population of lymphocytes that mediate spontaneous cytotoxicity against infected cells.[15] Because they have the unique ability to target microorganisms without previous exposure, they are considered to be part of the innate immune response despite being of lymphoid origin. They resemble large granular lymphocytes and are capable of killing some types of tumor and/or infected cells without previous exposure to surface antigens. However, they have been shown to play an equally important role in limiting the spread of infection and assisting in the development of adaptive immune responses through the production of cytokines.[15] NK cells can be excitatory or inhibitory, which ensures that only foreign cells are destroyed (see Fig. 11-2).[15] In addition to their role as phagocytes, NK cells assist in T-cell polarization, DC maturation, and innate immune control of viral infection through the secretion of immune modulators and antiviral cytokines. NK cells comprise approximately 10% to 15% of peripheral blood lymphocytes but do not bear T-cell receptors (TCR) or cell surface immunoglobulins (Igs).

Pathogen Recognition

The innate immune response plays a crucial role in the proinflammatory response to infection and relies upon the ability of host defenses to differentiate self from nonself so that only invading organisms are targeted. The leukocytes involved in this response recognize certain evolutionarily retained patterns present on the surface of pathogens and in response bind to its membrane and destroy the invading organism through the process of phagocytosis (Fig. 11-3).

Pattern Recognition

Invading pathogens contain structures in their cell membranes termed *PAMPs*, which are recognized by the cells of the innate immune system because these cells possess receptors known as *PRRs*. Upon PAMP recognition, PRRs come in contact with the cell surface and/or send intracellular signals to the host that trigger proinflammatory and antimicrobial responses including the synthesis and release of cytokines, chemokines, and cell adhesion molecules.[16] The PAMPs are made up of a combination of sugars, lipid molecules, proteins, or

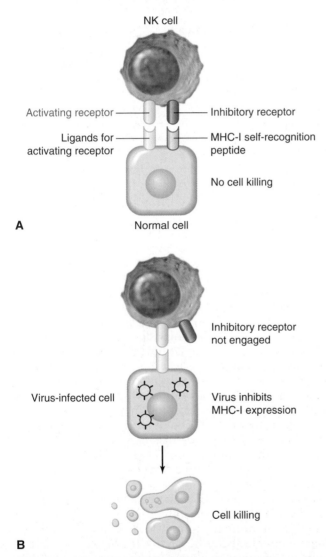

A

NK cell

Activating receptor

Inhibitory receptor

Ligands for activating receptor

MHC-I self-recognition peptide

No cell killing

Normal cell

Inhibitory receptor not engaged

Virus-infected cell

Virus inhibits MHC-I expression

Cell killing

B

FIGURE 11-2. Natural killer (NK) cell receptors. (**A**) NK cells express activating receptors that respond to ligands from virus-infected or injured cells and inhibiting receptors that bind to the class I major histocompatibility complex (MHC-I) self-recognition molecules expressed by normal cells. Normal cells are not killed because inhibitory signals from normal MHC-I molecules override activating signals. (**B**) In virus-infected or tumor cells, increased expression of ligands for activating receptors and reduced expression or alteration of MHC molecules interrupt the inhibitory signals, allowing activation of NK cells and lysis of target cells.

patterns of modified nucleic acids and are essential to the functioning and infectivity of the pathogen.

The ability of the innate immune response to limit microbes early in the infectious process results from the binding of pathogens to the PRRs on leukocytes, which in turn initiates the signaling events that lead to complement activation, phagocytosis, and autophagy. Once initiated, white blood cells, neutrophils, and monocytes migrate from the blood to the tissues, along with other body fluids causing peripheral edema. Blood monocytes mature into macrophages as they traverse the tissues and join the macrophages and DCs already present in the tissues. PRRs present on these cells become activated as well, amplifying the inflammatory response.

Toll-Like Receptors

TLRs derive their name from the study of the *Drosophila melanogaster* toll protein, which is responsible for the resistance of *Drosophila* to bacterial and fungal infections.[16] Structurally, TLRs are integral glycoproteins that possess an extracellular binding site and a cytoplasmic signaling toll/IL-1 domain that initiates the signaling cascade.[16] Binding of PAMP to a TLR induces a conformational change in the receptor activating intracellular processes. TLRs play essential roles in maintaining tissue homeostasis by regulating wound healing, tissue repair, and tissue regeneration. TLRs can be found in most of the bone marrow cells including the macrophages, DCs, neutrophils, T cells, B cells, and non–bone marrow cells including epithelial cells and fibrocytes. Ten different TLRs have been identified in humans, and they each recognize distinct PAMPs derived from various microorganisms including bacteria, viruses, fungi, and protozoa.[17]

Soluble Mediators of Innate Immunity

Although cells of the innate immune system communicate critical information about invading microorganisms and self–nonself recognition through cell-to-cell contact, soluble mediators are also essential for many other aspects of the innate immune response. Development of innate immune response is very much dependent upon the secretion of soluble molecules such as opsonins, cytokines, and acute-phase proteins.

Opsonins

Opsonins are molecules that coat negatively charged particles on cell membranes and as a result enhance the recognition and binding of phagocytic cells to microorganisms. The process by which the cellular particles on microbes are coated is called opsonization. Once the opsonin binds to the microbe, it is able to activate the phagocyte after attachment to a PRR on the phagocytic cell. There are several opsonins important in innate immunity and the acute inflammatory process including acute-phase proteins, lectins, and complement. Components of the adaptive immune response can also act as opsonins. For example, when the humoral response

Characteristics	Innate immunity	Adaptive immunity
Recognition	Molecular patterns common to microbes 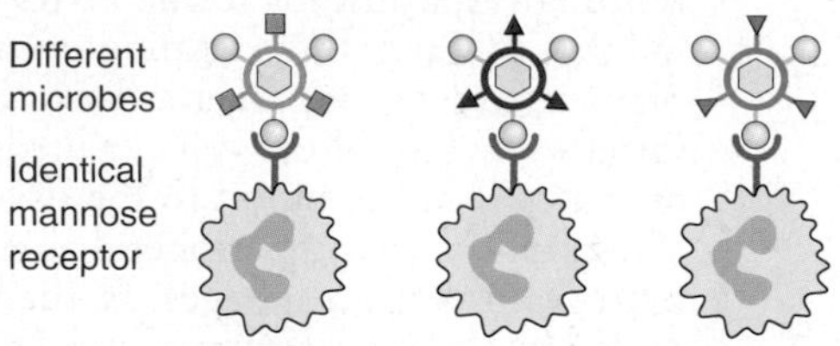 Different microbes Identical mannose receptor	Specific microbial molecules 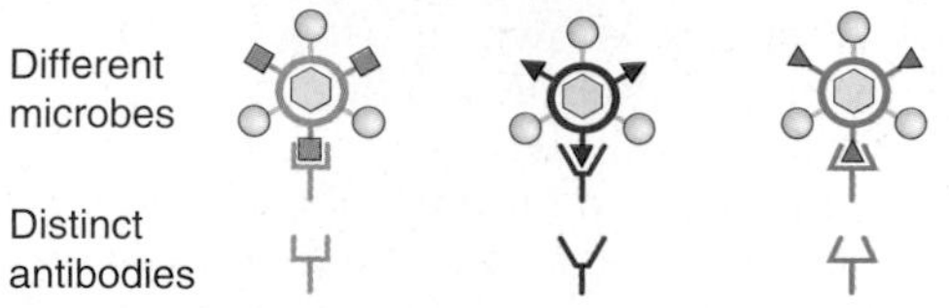 Different microbes Distinct antibodies
Receptors	Limited diversity expressed by germline genes 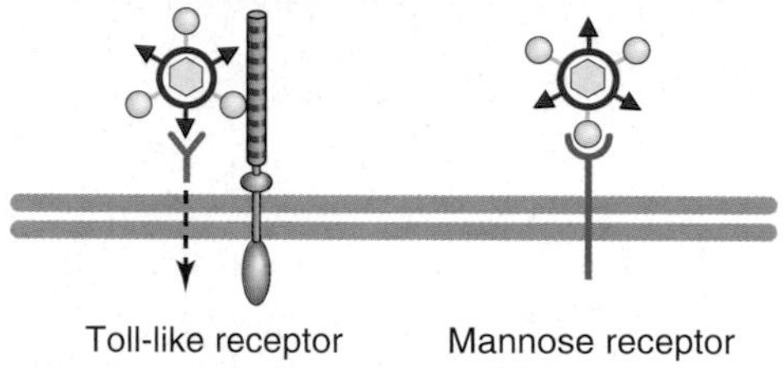 Toll-like receptor Mannose receptor	Great diversity expressed through recombination of somatic genes 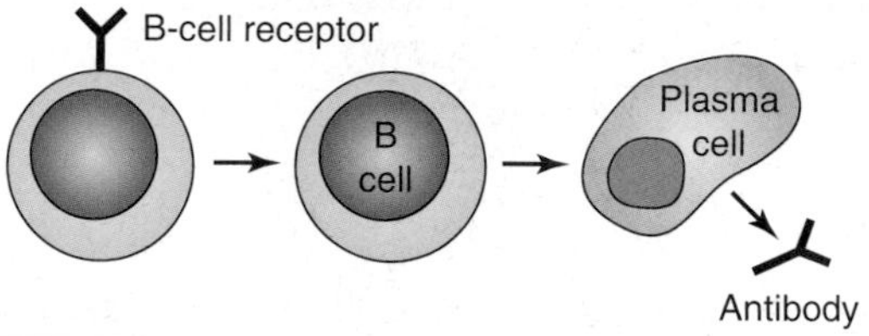 B-cell receptor B cell Plasma cell Antibody
Cellular expression	Effector cell types express identical receptors (*e.g.,* neutrophils express toll-like receptors).	Each clone of lymphocytes expresses unique receptors.
Self–nonself discrimination	Yes, by recognizing molecules unique to pathogen, NK cells recognize MHC-I self-recognizing molecules.	Yes, lymphocytes use MHC-I and -II and foreign peptides (*e.g.,* microbial peptides in recognition).

FIGURE 11-3. Recognition systems of innate and adaptive immunity. MHC, major histocompatibility complex; NK, natural killer.

is activated, IgG and IgM antibodies can coat cellular particles on pathogens and bind to Fc receptors on neutrophils and macrophages, enhancing the phagocytic function of innate cells.

Inflammatory Cytokines

Cytokines are low-molecular-weight proteins that serve as soluble chemical messengers and that mediate the interaction between immune and tissue cells. They are part of an integrated signaling network with extensive functions in both the innate (nonspecific) and adaptive immune defenses. The cytokines involved in innate immunity include TNF-α and lymphotoxin; IFN-γ, IFN-α, and IFN-β; IL-1, IL-6, and IL-12; and chemokines (see Table 11-2). These substances modify innate immunity by stimulating the development of cells involved in both innate and adaptive immunity, producing chemotaxis within leukocytes, and inhibiting viral replication. Once an innate immune phagocyte is activated by PRR–PAMP binding with a pathogen, cytokines are released into the surrounding tissues where they exert their effect. If large numbers of cells are activated, then cytokines may be able to stimulate inflammatory processes in tissues far from the initial site of infection. Under normal circumstances, the duration of activity of cytokines is relatively short so that a prolonged immune response does not occur.

TNF-α and lymphotoxins are cytokines that are structurally related and that have similar cytotoxic activities.[18] The two cytokines differ in that TNF-α can be secreted by a variety of immune cells, but the lymphotoxins are predominantly secreted by activated lymphocytes and NK cells. These cytokines regulate development of the lymphoid tissues and the inflammatory process by enhancing adhesion of immune cells to pathogens and stimulating the release of other cytokines/chemokines.[18] The IFNs are another family of cytokines that are critically involved in initiating and enhancing the cellular immune response to viral infection of host cells. In addition, they play a key role in amplifying the presentation of antigens to specific T cells forming the chemical bridge between the innate and adaptive immune response.[18] Type I IFN-α and IFN-β are secreted by virus-infected cells, whereas type II, immune or IFN-γ, are mainly secreted by T cells, NK cells, and macrophages.[18] IFNs activate macrophages, induce B cells to switch Ig type, alter T-helper response, inhibit cell growth, promote apoptosis, and induce an antiviral state in uninfected cells. Finally, ILs help to regulate the immune response by increasing the expression of adhesion molecules on endothelial cells, stimulating migration of leukocytes into infected tissues, and stimulating the production of antibodies by the cells of the adaptive immune response.

Acute-Phase Proteins

Two acute-phase proteins that are involved in the defense against infections are the mannose-binding lectin

(MBL) and C-reactive protein (CRP). MBL and CRP are produced in the liver and released in response to tissue injury and inflammation.[19,20] MBL binds specifically to mannose sugar residues, and CRP binds to both phospholipids and sugars that are found on the surface of microbes. These substances enhance the binding of phagocytic cells to suboptimally opsonized invading microorganisms. They also act as activators of the alternative complement pathway.

The Complement System

The complement system is a powerful effector mechanism of both innate and adaptive immunity that allows the body to localize infection and destroy invading microorganisms. The complement system is composed of groups of proteins found in the circulation and in various extracellular fluids. The proteins of the complement system normally circulate as inactive precursors. When activated by components of the immune response, a series of proteolytic and protein–protein interactions is initiated that ultimately culminates in opsonization of invading pathogens, migration of leukocytes to the site of invasion, initiation of a localized inflammatory reaction, and ultimately lysis of the pathogen.[21] For a complement reaction to occur, the complement components must be activated in the proper sequence. Inhibitor proteins and the instability of the activated complement proteins at each step of the process prevent uncontrolled activation of the complement system.

There are three parallel but independent activation pathways of the complement system during the innate immune response: the classical, the lectin, and the alternative pathways. The reactions of the complement systems can be divided into three phases:

1. Initiation or activation
2. Amplification of inflammation
3. Late-stage membrane attack response

The three pathways differ in the proteins used in the early stage of activation, but all ultimately converge on the key complement protein C3, which is essential for the amplification stage. Activated C3 then activates all subsequent complement molecules (C5 through C9), resulting in the ultimate lysis of cells.

The classic pathway is initiated by an antigen–antibody complex (either IgG or IgM mediated), which causes a specific reactive site on the antibody to be "uncovered" so that it can bind directly to the C1 molecule in the complement system.[22] Initially, a small amount of enzyme is produced, but with activation of successive complement proteins successively increasing, concentrations of proteolytic enzymes are produced. This process is known as *amplification*. In the lectin or alternative complement pathway, inactive circulating complement proteins are activated when they are exposed to microbial surface polysaccharides, MBL, CRP, and other soluble mediators that are integral to innate immunity.[23] Like the classic pathway, the lectin and alternative pathways

create a series of enzymatic reactions that cleave successive complement proteins in the pathway.

During the activation phase of the complement cascade, cleavage of C3 produces C3a and C3b. C3b is a key opsonin that coats bacteria and allows them to be phagocytized after binding to complement receptor on leukocytes. The presence of C3a triggers the migration of neutrophils into the tissues to enhance the inflammatory response. Production of C3a, C4a, and C5a also leads to activation of mast cells and basophils, causing them to release histamine, heparin, and other substances. These mediators of the inflammatory response increase tissue blood flow and increase localized capillary permeability, allowing leakage of fluids and protein into the area. In addition, they stimulate changes in the endothelial cells in order to stimulate chemotaxis of neutrophils and macrophages to the site of inflammation.

During the late-phase membrane attack response of the complement cascade, cleavage of C5 triggers the assembly of a membrane attack complex from the C5 to C9 proteins. The resulting complex creates a tube-like structure, which penetrates the microbial cell membrane allowing the passage of ions, small molecules, and water into the cell, causing the cell to ultimately burst. The multiple and complementary functions of the complement system make it an integral component of innate immunity and inflammation. It also serves as an essential bridge between the innate and humoral responses. Pathophysiologic manifestations associated with deficiencies of complement range from increased susceptibility to infection to inflammatory tissue and autoimmune disorders that are the result of impaired activated complement clearance.

SUMMARY CONCEPTS

The innate immune system is a complex system that works in an organized, rapid, yet nonspecific fashion as the body's first line of defense against invasion. It comprises the epithelial cells of the skin and mucous membranes; phagocytic cells such as the neutrophils, macrophages, and NK cells; and a series of plasma proteins including cytokines, chemokines, and the proteins of the complement system. These defenses exist before the body encounters an invading microorganism and are activated independent of the adaptive humoral response. The epithelial cells of the skin and mucous membranes block the entry of infectious agents and secrete antimicrobial enzymes, proteins, and peptides in an attempt to prevent microorganisms from invading the internal environment.

The phagocytes of the innate immune response engulf and digest infectious agents. They use PRRs, which are present on their membranes to recognize and bind broad

UNDERSTANDING ➡ The Complement System

The complement system provides one of the major effector mechanisms of both humoral and innate immunity. The system consists of a group of proteins (complement proteins C1 through C9) that are normally present in the plasma in an inactive form. Activation of the complement system is a highly regulated process, involving the sequential breakdown of the complement proteins to generate a cascade of cleavage products capable of proteolytic enzyme activity. This allows for tremendous amplification because each enzyme molecule activated by one step can generate multiple activated enzyme molecules at the next step. Complement activation is inhibited by proteins that are present on normal host cells; thus, its actions are limited to microbes and other antigens that lack these inhibitory proteins.

The reactions of the complement system can be divided into three phases: **(1)** the initial activation phase, **(2)** the early-step inflammatory responses, and **(3)** the late-step membrane attack responses.

1

Initial Activation Phase There are three pathways for recognizing microbes and activating the complement system: (1) the alternative pathway, which is activated on microbial cell surfaces in the absence of antibody and is a component of innate immunity; (2) the classical pathway, which is activated by certain types of antibodies bound to antigen and is part of humoral immunity; and (3) the lectin pathway, which is activated by a plasma lectin that binds to mannose on microbes and activates the classical system pathway in the absence of antibody.

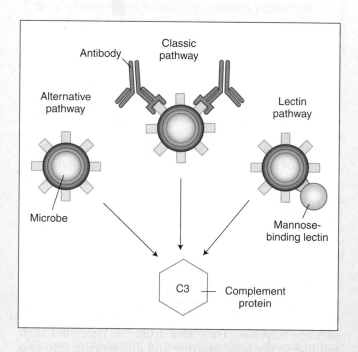

2

Early-Step Inflammatory Responses The central component of complement for all three pathways is the activation of the complement protein C3 and its enzymatic cleavage into a larger C3b fragment and a smaller C3a fragment. The smaller 3a fragment stimulates inflammation by acting as a chemoattractant for neutrophils. The larger 3b fragment becomes attached to the microbe and acts as an opsonin for phagocytosis. It also acts as an enzyme to cleave C5 into two components: a C5a fragment, which produces vasodilation and increases vascular permeability, and a C5b fragment, which leads to the late-step membrane attack responses.

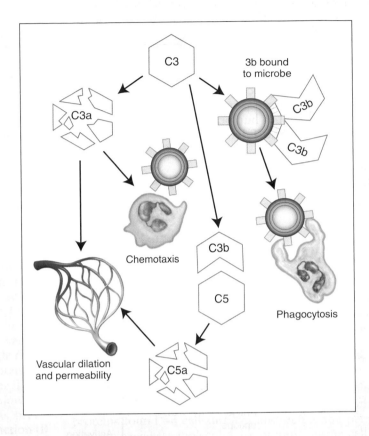

3

Late-Step Membrane Attack In the late-step responses, C3b binds to other complement proteins to form an enzyme that cleaves C5, generating C5a and C5b fragments. C5a stimulates the influx of neutrophils and the vascular phase of acute inflammation. The C5b fragment, which remains attached to the microbe, initiates the formation of a complex of complement proteins C6, C7, C8, and C9 into a membrane attack complex protein, or pore, that allows fluids and ions to enter and cause cell lysis.

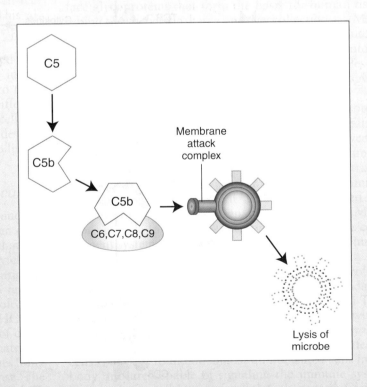

Regulation of the Adaptive Immune Response

In order for a host organism to remain healthy, the immune system must function properly. A weakened immune response may lead to immunodeficiency, but an inappropriate or excessive response can cause allergic reactions and autoimmune diseases. Therefore, the immune system must be capable of self-regulation. The process by which the body regulates itself is poorly understood but must involve all aspects of the innate and adaptive immune responses to be effective.

Each exposure to an antigen elicits a predictable response from the immune system. Once the immune system is activated, the response is amplified until it peaks and eventually subsides. This occurs because the body's normal immune responses are self-limiting. Once the antigen is destroyed and the action of chemical mediators terminated, the immune response ceases. It is believed that anti-inflammatory cytokines and regulatory T lymphocytes play a role in this process.[36]

Tolerance also plays a role in the self-regulation of the immune response. Tolerance is the ability of the immune system to react to foreign antigens but remain nonreactive to self-antigens. Tolerance to self-antigens protects the body from harmful autoimmune responses. This is exquisitely important in vital organs such as the brain, testes, ovaries, and eyes where immunologic damage could be lethal to the organism.

Many autoimmune diseases such as Hashimoto thyroiditis and insulin-dependent diabetes mellitus are caused by impairment in both B- and T-lymphocyte (specifically cytotoxic lymphocytes) functions resulting in direct cellular damage because the body's immune system is no longer capable of distinguishing "self" from "nonself."[37,38]

 SUMMARY CONCEPTS

Adaptive immunity comprises two distinct but interrelated processes: cell-mediated and humoral immunity. Together, they respond to foreign antigens, amplify and sustain immunologic responses, distinguish self from nonself, and confer "memory" so that a heightened response can be initiated on subsequent exposure to an organism. Antigens are usually substances foreign to the host that can stimulate an immune response. Antigens possess specific antigenic binding sites for the cells of the immune system known as epitopes. Epitopes allow the adaptive immune system to distinguish foreign antigens from normal cellular substances whose destruction would be detrimental to the organism. Adaptive immunity can be acquired actively or passively. Active immunity develops through immunization or by having a disease, whereas passive immunity develops when the host receives antibodies or immune cells from another source. An acquired immune response can improve with repeated exposure to an injected antigen or a natural infection.

The principal cells of the adaptive immune system are the B and T lymphocytes, APCs, and effector cells that are responsible for the elimination of antigens. The lymphocytes are produced and undergo maturation in the central lymphoid organs (bone marrow and thymus) and are subsequently stored in the peripheral lymphoid tissues. B lymphocytes differentiate into plasma cells that produce antibodies and provide for the elimination of microbes in the extracellular fluid (humoral immunity) as well as memory cells, which are responsible for the rapid immune response with repeat exposure. T lymphocytes differentiate into regulatory (helper T and T_{REGS}) and effector (cytotoxic T cells) cells. APCs consist of macrophages and DCs that process and present antigen peptides to CD4$^+$ helper T cells.

During cellular maturation, T lymphocytes express specific molecules on the cellular surfaces that distinguish between the different cell types and that help determine the cells' functionality. Regulatory CD4$^+$ helper T cells help to modulate the immune response and are essential for the differentiation of B cells into antibody-producing plasma cells and the differentiation of T lymphocytes into effector CD8$^+$ cytotoxic T cells. The CD8$^+$ cytotoxic cells eliminate intracellular microbes, such as viruses and other pathogens. Cells of both the innate and adaptive immune responses produce cytokines that influence adaptive immune responses. These cytokines function as communication molecules for the B and T lymphocytes, stimulate cellular proliferation and differentiation, and ensure the appropriate development of cytotoxic effector and memory cells.

People who are immunocompromised must be closely evaluated to determine the risk-to-benefit ratio when administering vaccines. Killed or inactive vaccines usually are safe, and booster may be required. For people who are immunocompromised and not associated with HIV or planned immunosuppression, such as congenital immunodeficiency, live virus vaccines are not generally administered. Immunosuppression affects B and/or T cells, causing a decreased or absent antibody response to vaccine. People who are HIV infected need evaluation and testing before live virus vaccines are administered.[39]

Developmental Aspects of the Immune System

Development of the immune system begins early in fetal life at approximately 5 to 6 weeks gestation when the fetal liver actively begins hematopoiesis. At about the same time (6 weeks gestation), the thymus arises from the third branchial arch, with the cortex arising from its ectodermal layer and the medulla from the endoderm.[40] Over the next 2 to 3 weeks, lymphoid cells initially migrate from the yolk sac and fetal liver and then from the bone marrow to colonize the fetal thymus.[40] Development of the secondary lymphoid organs (*i.e.*, spleen, lymph nodes, and mucosa-associated lymphoid tissues) begins soon after. The secondary lymphoid organs are rather small but well developed at birth and mature rapidly after exposure to microbes during the postnatal period. The thymus is the largest lymphoid tissue in the neonate relative to body size and normally reaches its mature weight by 1 year of age.

Transfer of Immunity from Mother to Infant

The neonate's immune system is functionally immature at birth so protection against infection and toxic substances occurs through transfer of maternal IgG antibodies. Maternal IgG antibodies readily cross the placenta during fetal development and remain functional in the newborn for the first few months of life, providing passive immunity until Ig production is well established in the newborn. IgG is the only class of Igs able to cross the placenta. Maternally transmitted IgG is effective against most microorganisms and viruses that a neonate encounters. Maternal vaccination may therefore offer fetal and neonatal passive immunity against common infections such as influenza or herpes zoster.[41] The largest amount of IgG crosses the placenta during the last weeks of pregnancy and is stored in fetal tissues. Infants born prematurely may be deficient in maternal antibodies and, therefore, more susceptible to infection. Because of transfer of IgG antibodies to the fetus, an infant born to a mother infected with HIV has a positive HIV antibody test result, although the child may not be infected with the virus.

Cord blood does not normally contain IgM or IgA. If present, these antibodies are of fetal origin and represent exposure to intrauterine infection because maternal IgM and IgA antibodies do not readily cross the placenta. Normally, the neonate begins producing IgM antibodies shortly after birth, as a result of exposure to the immense number of antigens normally found in the surrounding environment. However, this IgM is of lower binding affinity and effective against a limited range of antigens. It has also been demonstrated that premature infants can produce IgM as well as term infants. At approximately 6 days of age, the IgM rises sharply, and this rise continues until approximately 1 year of age, when the adult level is achieved.

Serum IgA normally is not present at birth but detected in the neonate approximately 13 days after birth. The levels of IgA increase during early childhood and reach between 6 and 7 years of age. Although maternal IgA is not transferred in utero, it is transferred to the breast-fed infant in colostrum. Because IgA antibodies are associated with mucosal members, these antibodies provide local immunity for the intestinal system during early life.

Immune Response in the Older Adult

As we age, the ability of the immune system to protect the body from pathogenic organisms and environmental toxins declines as a result of an overall decline in immune responsiveness. This results from changes in both cell-mediated and humoral immune responses. As a result, older adults are more susceptible to infections, have more evidence of autoimmune and immune complex disorders, and have a higher incidence of cancer than do younger people. In addition, the immune system of older adults is less likely to respond appropriately to immunization. As a result, older adults have a weakened response to vaccination. Older adults also frequently have many comorbid conditions that impair normal immune function and compromise the immune response.

The cause of the altered response in older adults is multifactorial. There is a continued decrease in the size of the thymus gland, which begins during puberty and affects overall T-cell production and function. The size of the thymus diminishes to 15% or less of its maximum size. There may also be a decrease in the number of the lymphocytes in the peripheral lymphoid tissue. The most common finding is a slight decrease in the proportion of T cells to other lymphocytes and a decrease in CD4+ and CD8+ cells.

Aging also produces qualitative changes in lymphocyte function. Lymphocytes seem to exhibit altered responses to antigen stimulation including unresponsiveness to activation. It appears that the CD4+ T lymphocyte is most severely affected because there is a decreased rate of synthesis of cytokines that stimulate the proliferation of lymphocytes and expression of the specific receptors that interact with the circulating cytokines. Specifically, IL-2, IL-4, and IL-12 levels decrease in older adults. Although actual B-cell function is compromised with age, the range of antigens that can be recognized by the B cells does not change.

SUMMARY CONCEPTS

Neonates are protected against antigens in early life as a result of passive transfer of maternal IgG antibodies through the placenta and IgA antibodies in colostrum and breast milk. Many changes occur with aging, but the exact mechanisms are not completely understood. However, the elderly population is more prone to infection and autoimmune disorders secondary to altered response in both innate and adaptive immune function.

CHAPTER 12

Disorders of the Immune Response, Including HIV/AIDS

HIV Infection in Pregnancy and in Infants and Children

Preventing Perinatal HIV Transmission
Diagnosis of HIV Infection in Children
Clinical Presentation of HIV Infection in Children

Learning Objectives

After completing this chapter, the learner will be able to meet the following objectives:

1. Identify the differences between primary and secondary immunodeficiency disorders.
2. Compare and contrast the pathology and clinical manifestations of humoral (B-cell), cellular (T-cell), and combined T- and B-cell immunodeficiency disorders.
3. Discuss the pathophysiology and clinical manifestations of complement disorders.
4. Discuss the pathophysiology of phagocytosis disorders.
5. Describe the adaptive immune responses that protect against microbial agents and hypersensitivity responses.
6. Discuss the immune response involved in the development of types I, II, III, and IV hypersensitivity reactions.
7. Describe the pathogenesis of common hypersensitivity reactions.
8. Discuss the rationale for matching of major histocompatibility complex or human leukocyte antigen types in organ transplantation.
9. Describe the mechanisms and manifestations of graft-versus-host disease.
10. Discuss the possible mechanisms and criteria for an autoimmune disease.
11. Describe the mechanisms of HIV transmission and relate them to the need for public awareness and concern regarding the spread of AIDS.
12. Describe the virus responsible for AIDS including the alterations in immune function that occur in persons with AIDS.
13. Relate the altered immune function in persons with HIV infection and AIDS to the development of opportunistic infections, malignant tumors, nervous system manifestations, wasting syndrome, and metabolic disorders.
14. Differentiate between the enzyme immunoassay (enzyme-linked immunosorbent assay) and Western blot antibody detection tests for HIV infection.
15. Compare the progress of HIV infection in infants and children with HIV infection in adults.

DISORDERS OF THE IMMUNE RESPONSE

The human immune system is a complex, multidimensional system designed to protect the host against invasion by foreign substances, microorganisms, and toxins.

In addition, it helps to protect against the proliferation of neoplastic cells and plays a key role in the process of inflammation and wound healing. Unfortunately, under certain circumstances, the immune system can become inefficient or hyperactive, causing the development of debilitating and/or life-threatening diseases. These disease processes can take the form of immunodeficiency disorders, allergic or hypersensitivity reactions, transplant rejection, and autoimmune disorders.

Immunodeficiency Disorders

Immunodeficiency is defined as an abnormality in one or more parts of the immune system that results in an increased susceptibility to disease states normally eliminated by a properly functioning immune response. Immunodeficiency syndromes can be classified as primary or secondary (acquired later in life). Primary immunodeficiency disorders are either congenital or inherited as sex-linked, autosomal dominant, or autosomal recessive traits. Secondary immunodeficiency disorders develop later in life because of other pathophysiologic states. The clinical manifestations and the impact on the client's day-to-day function are dependent upon the specific immunodeficiency disorder and the degree of immune system dysfunction. The various categories of immunodeficiency disorders are summarized in Chart 12-1.

The immune system is made up of two distinct but interrelated systems: the innate and adaptive immune systems. These two systems work in concert to protect the body from infection and disease. The innate immune system is the body's first line of defense against infection. It employs rapid yet nonspecific cellular and chemical responses. These include phagocytic leukocytes (*i.e.*, neutrophils, macrophages); natural killer (NK) cells; chemical mediators, such as chemokines and cytokines; and the complement system. The adaptive immune system differs from the innate immune system in its ability to exhibit "memory" for invading organisms and toxic substances. The adaptive immune response develops more slowly but with a great deal of specificity. The T and B lymphocytes of the adaptive immune system possess the ability to express their receptors (T cells) and produce immunoglobulins (Igs) (B cells) in billions of different combinations, which enables them to target billions of different epitopes, viruses, and microorganisms.

The ability of the adaptive immune system to function effectively is dependent upon the interaction of two distinct but intimately connected mechanisms, the humoral (B cell–mediated) and cell-mediated (T cell–mediated) responses. The humoral immune response relies upon the ability of B lymphocytes to produce antigen-specific Igs and "memory" cells. In contrast, the cell-mediated response relies upon the ability of the T lymphocytes to produce various cytokines, to present antigen to B lymphocytes for destruction, and, in the case of cytotoxic T cells, to kill cells infected with intracellular organisms.

Primary immunodeficiency diseases (PIDDs) are caused by genetic abnormalities of the immune system;

T, B, and NK cells in peripheral blood smears and a depressed T-cell response to antigen stimulation.[23]

Traditionally, bone marrow transplantation has been the treatment of choice in children with the most severe forms of T-cell immunodeficiency. However, in more recent years, immunologic restoration of the immune system through allogeneic hematopoietic stem cell transplantation (HSCT)[22] and gene therapy[24] is becoming increasingly popular for the treatment of specific T-cell disorders.

DiGeorge Syndrome

DiGeorge syndrome or velocardiofacial syndrome is an embryonic developmental defect associated with chromosome 22q11.2 deletion.[25,26] It occurs in approximately 1:4000 births. The incidence of this disorder is increasing because many of those now affected go on to give birth to affected children. The defect is thought to occur before the 12th week of gestation, when the thymus gland, parathyroid gland, and parts of the head, neck, and heart are developing. Children with DiGeorge syndrome present with a wide complex of defects including mild to moderate immunodeficiency resulting from a congenitally absent thymus, cardiac and renal anomalies, palatal abnormalities, hypoparathyroidism, skeletal defects, and developmental delays. Because of the presence of a limited number of thymic cells in aberrant locations, the severity of T-cell dysfunction ranges from no circulating T cells to normal counts The disorder affects both sexes.

When the thymus is not absent but is extremely small and located outside of the mediastinum, growth and development of the thymus may occur with normal stimulation of the immune system. The facial disorders can include hypertelorism (i.e., increased distance between the eyes); micrognathia (i.e., abnormally small jaw); low-set, posteriorly angulated ears with associated hearing loss; split uvula; a high-arched or cleft palate; and oropharyngeal and nasopharyngeal muscle weakness.[26] Renal abnormalities affect approximately one third of children with DiGeorge syndrome. Fortunately, renal dysplasia and **agenesis** are rare consequences requiring immediate dialysis. Hypocalcemia and tetany may develop within 24 hours of birth as a result of absent or hypoplastic parathyroid glands.

The immune system is affected in 75% of children with DiGeorge syndrome as a result of thymic hypoplasia.[26] Children with severe T-cell dysfunction are more prone to recurrent or chronic viral, fungal, and intracellular bacterial infections. Impaired helper T-cell function affects antigen presentation to B cells and subsequent antibody production. This phenomenon appears to be limited to children as there is no clinical evidence that adults have an increased risk of infection.

Treatment of DiGeorge syndrome is dependent upon the presenting symptoms. Cardiac anomalies are usually repaired shortly after birth. In children with true thymic **aplasia** and congenitally absent T cells, a thymus transplant or fully matched T-cell transplant is the treatment of choice to reconstitute T-cell immunity. As with any primary immunodeficiency, autoimmunity is a potential problem. Therefore, precautions must be taken during transplantation or transfusion therapy to prevent graft-versus-host disease (GVHD).

X-Linked Immunodeficiency with Hyper-IgM

The hyper–immunoglobulin M (HIGM) syndromes are a heterogeneous group of primary immunodeficiency disorders resulting from defective Ig class switch recombination during B-cell maturation leading to a deficiency in IgG, IgA, and IgE but elevated levels of IgM.[27] This X-linked disorder is found only in males. The disorder results from the inability of T cells to signal B cells to undergo isotype switching to IgG and IgA. Thus, they continue to express only the IgM subclass of Igs. In most cases, it is the result of a genetic mutation resulting in a CD40 ligand deficiency. Its primary cause is a defect in cell-mediated immunity.

Clinical manifestations of HIGM occur early in life with a median age of onset at less than 12 months.[28] Children usually present with recurrent sinopulmonary infections that may progress to bronchiectasis and pneumonia. In approximately 40% of cases, the presenting symptom is an opportunistic infection such as *Pneumocystis jiroveci* pneumonia (PJP).[29] Unfortunately, these children are at particular risk for the development of autoimmune disorders and malignancies of the biliary tree, intestine, and neuroendocrine system because of defects in CD40 signaling. Treatment is usually with Ig replacement and prophylactic antibiotic treatment.

Secondary Cell-Mediated Immunodeficiency Disorders

Secondary cell-mediated immunodeficiencies are more prevalent than primary deficiencies and are frequently associated with acute viral infections (e.g., measles virus, cytomegalovirus) and with certain malignancies such as Hodgkin disease and other lymphomas. Viral infections frequently impair cell immunity via direct infection of specific T-lymphocyte subpopulations (e.g., helper cells). Lymphotropic viruses such as human immunodeficiency virus (HIV) and human herpesvirus (HSV) type 6 selectively deplete the cell subtype that they invade, resulting in a concomitant loss of immunologic function associated with that subtype. People with malignancies can have impaired T-cell function because of either unregulated proliferation or depletion of a particular cell type. Some cases of T-cell immunodeficiency have no known etiology but are acquired later in life. **Idiopathic** CD4+ T-cell lymphocytopenia is a rare disorder characterized by a profound and persistent CD4+ T-cell defect that predisposes to the development of severe opportunistic infections in the absence of other immune defects.[30] Regardless of the etiology, people with secondary cell-mediated immune dysfunction may display an increased susceptibility to infections caused by normally harmless pathogens (i.e., opportunistic infections) or may be unable to mount delayed hypersensitivity reactions (i.e., **anergy**). People with anergy have a diminished or absent reaction to antigen even in the presence of known infection.

Combined T-Cell and B-Cell Immunodeficiencies

Combined T-cell and B-cell lymphocyte disorders manifest with defects in both the humoral and cell-mediated immune responses. Collectively, these disorders are known as combined immunodeficiency syndrome (CIDS), but they are a diverse group caused by mutations in a multitude of genes that influence lymphocyte development or response, including lymphocyte receptors, cytokines, or major histocompatibility complex (MHC) antigens, that could lead to combined immunodeficiency. The end result is a disruption in the communication pathways between the cells of the humoral and cell-mediated immune systems and failure of the adaptive immune response. The spectrum of disease resulting from combined immunodeficiency disorders (CIDs) ranges from mild to severe to, ultimately, fatal forms.

Severe Combined Immunodeficiency Disorders

SCIDs are a group of genetically diverse disorders characterized by profound deficiencies of T and B lymphocytes, and in some forms NK, with the subsequent loss of both humoral and cellular immunities.[22] The reported incidence of SCIDs is 1:100,000 live births, and they collectively account for approximately 20% of primary immunodeficiency disorders.[31] Affected infants are lymphopenic and lack T cells, which normally constitute 70% of the total circulating lymphocytes. They have a disease course that resembles that of acquired immunodeficiency syndrome (AIDS), with failure to thrive, chronic diarrhea, and the development of severe opportunistic infections. An SCID is usually fatal within the first 2 years of life, unless reconstitution of the immune system through bone marrow or HSCT can be accomplished. Early diagnosis is essential because the chances of successful treatment are better in infants who have not experienced severe opportunistic infections.[31]

X-linked mutations account for almost 45% of all cases as a result of defects in the common gamma chain of the cytokine receptor.[32] Impaired receptor function results in defective T-lymphocyte differentiation and production. Although the B-cell production is unaffected, antibody production is impaired because of a lack of T-cell help. Mutations inherited as autosomal recessive traits account for the majority of the remaining cases of SCID including mutations in the genes that code for *ADA* gene, Janus kinase 3 (*JAK3*) gene, the α chain of the interleukin-7 receptor (IL-7Rα chain [also known as CD127]), and recombination-activating genes 1 and 2 (*RAG1* and *RAG2*).[31] Many of these mutations result in defects that impair T-cell maturation including defects in cytokine receptor control of T-cell differentiation, antigen gene receptor arrangement on T and B cells, or any other component of T-cell antigen receptor function necessary for normal T-cell development.

Combined Immunodeficiency Disorders

CIDs are less severe than those categorized as SCIDs because they present with diminished, rather than absent, T-cell function and B-cell antibody production. Like SCID, the CIDs are a heterogeneous group of disorders with diverse genetic causes. They are often associated with other disorders such as AT and WAS.[33]

Like all primary immunodeficiencies, children with CID are prone to development of recurrent infections including pulmonary, skin, and urinary tract infections. They also have a higher incidence of chronic diarrhea and other gastrointestinal disorders, as well as gram-negative sepsis. Although they usually survive longer than do children with SCID, without treatment, they fail to thrive and often have a shortened life span.

Ataxia–Telangiectasia

AT is a rare autosomal recessive disorder caused by a gene mutation (ATM, ataxia–telangiectasia mutated) mapped to chromosome 11q22-23 with a worldwide prevalence estimated to be between 1 in 40,000 and 1 in 100,000 live births.[34] ATM is a large serine/threonine kinase that is involved in the cellular response to breakage in the double strand of the DNA helix. This multisystem disorder is characterized by neurodegeneration, primarily of the cerebellum, and oculocutaneous telangiectasia. Ataxia is the predominant neurodegenerative feature, which usually goes undiagnosed until the child begins to walk. It is associated with both cellular and humor immune deficiencies with decreased lymphocyte counts and ratio of CD4 helper T cells to CD8 suppressor T cells. Lymphopenia, hypogammaglobulinemia, and cell-mediated immune dysfunction results in recurrent sinopulmonary infections. People with this disorder have an increased risk of cancer and radiation sensitivity. The most common malignancies that occur with this condition are lymphoid in origin, but solid tumors of the kidney (Wilms tumor) are frequently reported.[34]

Cognitive development is normal early in the disease process but levels off during childhood and ceases by 10 years of age. The majority of people display Ig deficiencies in IgA, IgE, and IgG, with the IgG2 and IgG4 subclasses being most affected. Ninety-five percent of all affected children demonstrate elevated serum α-fetoprotein (AFP) levels.[34]

Wiskott–Aldrich Syndrome

Wiskott–Aldrich syndrome (WAS) is a severe, rare, and complex X-linked disorder characterized by the triad of thrombocytopenia, recurrent infections, and eczema, with an increased risk for the development of autoimmune disorders and lymphomas. The syndrome affects approximately one to four cases per 1,000,000 live male births and is caused by mutations in the WAS gene.35 For children lacking WAS protein (WASp) expression, life expectancy is approximately 15 years. WASp is a key regulator of actin assembly in all hematopoietic cells (including platelets) in response to signals arising at the cell membrane. Hemorrhage, ranging from mild to life threatening, is common and occurs in over 80% of cases. Abnormalities of humoral immunity include decreased serum levels of IgM and markedly elevated serum IgA and IgE concentrations. T-cell dysfunction is initially limited but increases over time resulting in greater susceptibility to infection and the development of malignancies of the mononuclear phagocytic system, including Hodgkin lymphoma and leukemia.[35,36]

Management of people with WAS focuses on treatment of eczema, control of infections, and management of bleeding episodes. Currently, the only definitive treatment is allogeneic HSCT , but this is associated with considerable risk of complications including death and transplant rejection.[37]

Disorders of the Complement System

The complement system is an integral part of the innate immune response and essential to the integrity of the immune system, including the adaptive immune response. Activation of the complement system occurs via one of three ways: the classic, lectin-mediated, or alternative pathways. Regardless of the pathway, activation of the complement system promotes chemotaxis, opsonization, and phagocytosis of invasive pathogens and bacteriolysis. Alterations in any component of the complement system can lead to enhanced susceptibility to infectious diseases and to the development of a host of autoimmune processes.

Primary Disorders of the Complement System

Primary disorders of the complement system can be transmitted as autosomal recessive, autosomal dominant, or autosomal codominant traits. In the case of codominance, heterozygotes usually have one functioning gene, and complement levels in most cases are sufficient to prevent disease. The majority of disorders associated with the complement system are the result of inappropriate activation and regulation of complement proteins, not necessarily deficiencies of complement proteins themselves.[38] In fact, protein deficiencies of the classic and alternative pathways are rarely seen. Protein deficiencies of the lectin pathway, although more common, are not a major cause of primary complement disorders.

Primary disorders of the complement system can involve one or more proteins, receptors, and/or control molecules at any point along the complement cascade. However, the clinical presentation is dependent upon the component affected. For example, defects in the classic pathway result in an increased of autoimmunity and infection with high-grade pathogens, whereas defects in the lectin pathway are associated with an increased risk of infection from unusual pathogens such as *Cryptosporidium* and *Aspergillus*.[39] Because all three pathways converge at the activation of C3, defects that impact C3 or late-acting proteins affect activation of complement by all three pathways and are associated with marked increases in infection with high-grade pathogens, including *Neisseria gonorrhoeae* and *N. meningitidis* infection, hemolytic uremic syndrome, and adult-onset macular degeneration.[40]

It is now known that the complement system plays a key role in the control of the adaptive immune response. Subjects deficient in complement proteins frequently have significant defects in the adaptive immune response. C1q, C3, and C4 deficiencies are associated with a diminished immune response especially to T cell–dependent antigens.[39] In addition, they have poor germinal center activity and poor immunologic memory. In the C1 subunit, C1q is essential for the binding of immune complexes and apoptotic cells, promoting their eventual removal from the circulation.[38] These people, therefore, have an increased risk of infection from encapsulated bacteria, particularly *S. pneumoniae*. In addition, they are at increased risk for the development of autoimmune disease processes, particularly systemic lupus erythematosus (SLE) and other forms of vasculitis.

Defects in the lectin pathway have just recently been defined to involve the essential protein mannose-binding lectin (MBL). MBL does not require antibody presentation for activation, as does C1 in the classic pathway. MBL possesses a central core and radiating arms with an intertwined, chained collagen structure capable of binding bacterial surface polysaccharides. A single-gene defect that is carried as an autosomal dominant trait results in improper winding of the MBL molecule and abnormally low plasma concentrations ($<2\ \mu g/mL$).[38]

The majority of the complement disorders are the result of defects in complement control receptors and molecules. Because tight regulation of C3 is essential to prevent host tissue damage, a host of substances and receptors play a role in the process. Deficiency or improper activation can cause significant disease despite normal circulating complement protein levels. Under normal circumstances, the binding of C3b to a target serves two functions, continuation of the complement cascade and opsonization. Factor H and factor I are essential for the inactivation of C3b in the plasma and on erythrocytes. Factor H is a cofactor for the cleavage of C3, and complete deficiencies are associated with glomerulonephritis, atypical hemolytic uremic syndrome (aHUS), age-related macular degeneration, and HELLP (hemolytic anemia, elevated liver enzymes, and low platelet count) syndrome during pregnancy.[41] Factor 1 is a cofactor for the cleavage of both C4 and C3. Complete deficiency is associated with low circulating C3 and opportunistic infection.[42]

Hereditary Angioneurotic Edema

Hereditary angioedema (HAE), a rare, life-threatening complement disorder that affects 1 in 10,000 to 1 in 150,000 persons, results from a quantitative (type I) or qualitative (type II) deficiency of C1-inhibitor (HAE-C1-INH).[43] HAE is inherited as an autosomal dominant trait that causes mutations in the SERPING1 gene located in the q12-q13.1 region of chromosome 11.[44] In the complement system, C1-INH normally inhibits activated C1r and C1s in the classic pathway as well as the early steps in the lectin pathway. It also functions as an inhibitor of the coagulation, fibrinolysis, and kinin-generating pathways through the inactivation of plasma kallikrein and factor XIIa. Deficiencies in C1-INH result in the uncontrolled release of various vasoactive substances that promote vascular permeability. The net result is the development of spontaneous episodes of deep localized tissue swelling in the subcutaneous tissues of the extremities, face, and torso or the submucosal tissues of the upper airway and gastrointestinal tracts.[44]

Laryngeal edema is a life-threatening manifestation that can lead to complete airway obstruction and death without intervention. Swelling of the structures of the gastrointestinal mucosa is associated with severe nausea, vomiting, and diarrhea. In some people, attacks may be preceded by the development of *erythema marginatum*, a macular, nonpruritic erythematous rash. HAE usually manifests during early childhood and progresses in severity into adolescence. Symptoms usually peak in 1.5 days and then resolve over the same time frame. Management of the disorder involves emergency management in cases of severe airway obstruction including emergency intubation or tracheotomy, C1-INH concentrate, bradykinin receptor B2 antagonists, or kallikrein inhibitor. Preventative treatment usually involves the avoidance of precipitating influences, the administration of attenuated androgens and antifibrinolytics, or C1-INH concentration.[45]

Secondary Disorders of the Complement System

Secondary complement deficiencies occur as a result of rapid activation or turnover of complement components in the face of normal complement levels as seen in immune complex disease. They are also seen in cases of chronic liver disease and malnutrition where complement protein production is negatively impacted. Regardless of the cause, the manifestations of secondary disorders are dependent upon the components of the complement pathways affected.

Disorders of Phagocytosis

The phagocytic system is composed primarily of polymorphonuclear leukocytes (*i.e.*, neutrophils and eosinophils) and mononuclear phagocytes (*i.e.*, circulating monocytes and tissue and fixed macrophages). These cells are primarily responsible for the removal of microorganisms, toxins, and cellular debris from the body. When activated by chemotactic factors, phagocytic cells migrate to the site of action and envelope the invading microorganisms or foreign substances. In addition, they produce microbicidal substances such as enzymes and metabolic by-products that kill or ingest pathogens. Following resolution of an infection process, phagocytic cells (*e.g.*, neutrophils) undergo programmed cell death or apoptosis, in order to prevent damage to host cells as a result of exposure to activated microbicidal proteases and chemotactic substances.[46] A defect in any of these functions or a reduction in the absolute number of available cells can disrupt the ability of phagocytic system to function effectively. People with phagocytic disorders are exquisitely susceptible to bacterial and fungal infections including *Candida*. However, the exact pathogen varies with the particular disease process. As with other alterations in immune function, defects in phagocytosis can be primary or secondary disorders.

Primary Disorders of Phagocytosis

Primary disorders of phagocytosis affect leukocyte adhesion (*e.g.*, leukocyte adhesion deficiency or LAD), microbicidal production and activity (*e.g.*, chronic granulomatous disease [CGD]), and the process of cellular degranulation (*e.g.*, Chédiak–Higashi syndrome [CHS]).

LADs are a group of rare genetic disorders (≤1: 1,000,000 births) that share a common defect in neutrophil adhesion. Currently, three distinct genetic mutations in chromosome 21q22.3 have been linked to the development of LAD, with LAD-1 being most common presenting with nonhealing ulcers and life-threatening bacterial infections. LAD-II results from a defect in fucose metabolism, which is responsible for the absence of fucosylated glycans on cell surface membranes and selectin-mediated adhesion. LAD-III appears to be the result of failed activation of several of the integrins necessary for CD18 expression.[47] mutations alter neutrophil CD18 expression resulting in defective chemotaxis, margination, and adherence. In addition, there is a decrease in NK cell and cytotoxic T-cell function.[48] During early stages of an infection, neutrophil adherence to postcapillary endothelium is weak because of rolling selectin interactions. As the immune response mounts, β-integrin interactions strengthen the adherence and allow neutrophils to migrate into surrounding tissues. Clinically relevant defects can occur at any point in this process.

CGD is one of the most common forms of primary phagocyte dysfunction affecting approximately 1: 200,000 births. It results in an increased susceptibility to both bacterial and fungal infections as well as the development of granulomatous lesions. CGD is characterized by defects in microbicidal oxidant production, specifically the superoxide-generating phagocyte oxidases known as *phox* that render affected individuals unable to phagocytize microorganisms. Six different subunits derived from nicotinamide adenine dinucleotide phosphate (NADPH) complex make up the *phox* oxidase molecule.[49] Each is found separately in the cytoplasm or in membrane vesicles in resting neutrophils. Upon neutrophil stimulation, these subunits normally come together to form active oxidases at the phagosome membranes, creating an intracellular environment capable of killing ingested microbes. In people with CGD, mutations exist in the genes that encode for essential components of the *phox* subunits that result in the production of inactive *phox*. Four different genetic forms of CGD exist with 75% of cases inherited as an X-linked trait (mutations in the gp91^{phox} subunit).[50] Therefore, the majority of cases are diagnosed in males.

Children with CGD are subject to chronic and acute infections including pneumonia, subcutaneous and organ abscesses, cellulitis, osteomyelitis, sepsis, and suppurative adenitis despite aggressive prophylactic and therapeutic antibiotic therapy.[51] These infections usually begin during the first 2 years of life. A wide range of fungi and bacteria are responsible for the infections including *S. aureus*, *Burkholderia cepacia*, *Burkholderia pseudomallei*, *Serratia marcescens*, *Escherichia coli*, *Candida albicans*, *Granulibacter bethesdensis*, and *Aspergillus* species. Chronic infection and inflammation result in the development of fibrotic granulomatous masses that may eventually require surgical excision or that cause end-organ damage. Cognitive defects are also associated with CGD, but the exact mechanism is unknown. Bone marrow transplantation is the only known cure for CGD. Supportive care includes the use of recombinant interferon-gamma and prophylactic antibiotic therapy.[50,51]

CHS is a rare (<500 cases) autosomal recessive disorder characterized by severe immunodeficiency, increased susceptibility to infection, bleeding tendency, partial oculocutaneous albinism, and progressive neurologic dysfunction.[52] Abnormally large, dysfunctional granules are readily seen in blood and bone marrow granulocytes and other cells including melanocytes, fibroblasts, endothelial cells, Schwann cells, and neurons. CHS is caused by mutations in a single gene located on chromosome 1q42-43, which encodes for the lysosomal trafficking regulator (LYST).[52] Affected cells exhibit defective chemotaxis, reduced mobilization and microtubular activity, and decreased bactericidal activity.

CHS manifests itself during infancy and early childhood, and few people survive into their teenage years. Sometime after the initial onset of infection, 50% to 85% of people enter into an "accelerated phase," which is characterized by lymphocytic infiltration of the major organs of the body.[53] Although the organisms responsible for the infections seen in CHS are usually bacterial, the trigger for the accelerated phase appears to be a reaction to a viral infection, probably with the Epstein–Barr virus (EBV). People with CHS are unable to clear the EBV infection, which leads to a state of constant lymphoproliferation, end-organ failure, and death. Prophylactic treatment of CHS is symptomatic and includes antibiotics but unfortunately does not prevent any of the complications from developing. Allogeneic hematopoietic cell transplantation continues to be the treatment of choice to restore hematologic and immunologic function, but does not prevent or reverse any of the other associated complications.[53]

Secondary Disorders of Phagocytosis

Secondary deficiencies of the phagocytic system can result from a multitude of disorders including leukemia, malnutrition, viral infections, or diabetes mellitus. People with diabetes mellitus are more prone to develop poor phagocytic function because of altered cellular chemotaxis. The exact mechanism of the dysfunction is not known, but it does not appear to be associated with age or the severity of the endocrine disorder. There is some evidence that phagocytic dysfunction is coinherited at a higher rate in people with diabetes. Drugs that impair or prevent inflammation and T-cell function, such as corticosteroids or cyclosporine, also alter phagocytic response through modulation of cytokines.

Stem Cell Transplantation

For most of the primary immunodeficiency disorders, HSCT from allogeneic human leukocyte antigen (HLA)-compatible sibling donors is the treatment of choice because it results in effective immunologic reconstitution and improved survival in approximately 90% of people.[54]

SUMMARY CONCEPTS

The immune response is a complex, multidimensional process that requires coordinated activities of both the innate and adaptive immune systems. Because of its complexity, it is not uncommon for one or more normal processes to become disrupted. An immunodeficiency is defined as an absolute or partial loss of the normal immune response that places a person at risk for the development of infection or malignancy. Disorders of the immune system can be classified as primary or secondary disorders. Primary disorders are inherited, as the underlying genetic defect is present as birth, whereas secondary disorders develop sometime later in life in response to another disease entity or condition. The extent to which any or all of these components are compromised dictates the severity of the immunodeficiency.

Immunodeficiency disorders can affect any component of the cellular or humoral immune response. B-lymphocytic or humoral immunodeficiency disorders can affect all circulating Igs, resulting in agammaglobulinemia, or target a single Ig (*e.g.*, IgA immunodeficiency). Defects in humoral immunity increase the risk of recurrent pyogenic infections but have limited impact on the defense against intracellular bacteria (mycobacteria), fungi, protozoa, and most viruses, except those that cause gastrointestinal infection. T-cell immunity is responsible for protection against fungal, protozoan, viral, and intracellular bacterial infections; for control of malignant cell proliferation; and for the coordination of the overall immune response. T-lymphocyte or cell-mediated immune disorders can present as selective T-cell immunodeficiency states or as combined T- and B-cell immunodeficiency disorders. Children born with SCID present with severe opportunistic infections and have a disease course that resembles AIDS. The majority of these children die before the age of 1 unless immune system reconstitution can be achieved through HSCT.

The complement system and phagocytic cells are integral components of innate immunity and can also be targeted in immunodeficiency disorders. The complement system plays a key role in promoting chemotaxis, opsonization, and phagocytosis of invasive pathogens. Deficiencies in complement proteins, control molecules, or receptors can lead to enhanced susceptibility to infectious diseases and autoimmune disorders, particularly SLE. People with phagocytic disorders are exquisitely susceptible to bacterial and fungal infections including *Candida*; however, the exact pathogen varies with the particular disease process. Primary disorders of phagocytosis include LAD disorders, degranulation abnormalities, and defects in microbicidal activity.

Hypersensitivity Disorders

Activation of the immune system normally results in the mobilization and coordination of T-cell and B-cell activity in order to protect the body from invading microorganisms and toxic substances. Unfortunately, this same system is capable of causing serious damage when it does not function as intended. Hypersensitivity is defined as an abnormal and excessive response of the activated immune system that causes injury and damage to host tissues. Disorders caused by immune responses are collectively referred to as *hypersensitivity reactions*. Hypersensitivity reactions are classified as one of four types: type I, IgE-mediated disorders; type II, antibody-mediated disorders; type III, complement-mediated immune disorders; and type IV, T cell–mediated disorders (Table 12-1). They differ with respect to the specific components of the immune response initiated, the onset of symptoms, and the eventual mechanism of injury.

Type I, Immediate Hypersensitivity Disorders

Type I hypersensitivity reactions are IgE-mediated reactions that develop rapidly upon exposure to an antigen. Type I hypersensitivity reactions represent the classic allergic response, and in this context, antigens are referred to as *allergens*. Environmental, medical, and pharmaceutical allergens are all capable of initiating a type I hypersensitivity reaction. Common allergens encountered include pollen proteins, house dust mites, animal dander, foods, household chemicals, and pharmaceutical agents like the antibiotic penicillin. Exposure to the allergen can be through inhalation, ingestion, injection, or skin contact. Depending on the portal of entry, type I reactions may be localized to a discrete area of the body (*e.g.*, contact dermatitis) or systemic causing significant disease (*e.g.*, asthma) and life-threatening anaphylaxis.[55-57]

Two types of cells play a key role in the development of a type I hypersensitivity reactions: type 2 helper T (T_2H) cells and mast cells or basophils. Two distinct subtypes of helper T cells (T_1H or T_2H) develop from activated CD4$^+$ helper T cells based upon the cytokines expressed by the antigen-presenting cells (APCs) at the site of activation. Macrophages and dendritic cells direct the maturation of CD4$^+$ helper T cells toward the T_1H subtype, whereas mast cells and T cells induce differentiation toward the T_2H subtype. The T_1H cells stimulate the differentiation of B cells into IgM- and IgG-producing plasma cells. The T_2H cells direct B lymphocytes to switch class and produce the IgE antibodies necessary for an allergic or hypersensitivity response. In addition, T_2H cytokines are responsible for the mobilization and activation of mast cells, basophils, and eosinophils, inducing inflammatory responses that are distinct from T_1H reactions.[56]

Mast cells, basophils, and eosinophils are essential to the development of type I hypersensitivity reactions. They are members of the *granulocyte* class of leukocytes because they contain granules rich in chemical mediators such as histamine and heparin. These mediators may be preformed or are enzymatically activated in response to T_2H signaling. Once they are released, they are capable of inducing a wide range of cellular responses. Mast cells and basophils are histologically similar and derived from CD34$^+$ progenitor cells.[58] However, basophils are confined to the bloodstream, and mast cells are distributed throughout the connective tissue, especially in areas beneath the skin and mucous membranes of the respiratory, gastrointestinal, and genitourinary tracts and adjacent to blood and lymph vessels.[58] This places the mast cells in close proximity to surfaces with frequent exposure to allergen. Mast cells in different parts of the body and even in a single site can have significant differences in mediator content and sensitivity to agents that produce mast cell degranulation.

Type I hypersensitivity reactions are dependent upon IgE-mediated activation of mast cells and basophils (Fig. 12-2). During the initial exposure to an antigen, allergen-specific IgE is produced as part of the normal humoral response and IgE to the high-affinity IgE receptors known as FcεRI, expressed on the surface of mast cells and basophils.[59,60] In contrast, lymphocytes, eosinophils, and platelets bind IgE via low-affinity FcεRII receptors.[61] On subsequent exposure to an allergen, the multimeric cross-linkages between IgE antibodies are formed creating a bridge between two IgE molecules. When IgE receptors aggregate, they induce a signal transduction that stimulates mast cell degranulation and release of vasoactive chemical mediators, the synthesis and secretion of platelet-activating factor (PAF) and leukotrienes, and the secretion of many growth factors, cytokines, and chemokines.[61]

Most type I hypersensitivity reactions such as bronchial asthma develop in two distinct and well-defined phases: (1) a primary or initial-phase response characterized by vasodilation, vascular leakage, and smooth muscle contraction and (2) a secondary or late-phase response characterized by more intense infiltration of tissues with eosinophils and other acute and chronic inflammatory cells as well as tissue destruction in the form of epithelial cell damage.

The primary or initial-phase response usually begins with 5 to 30 minutes of exposure to an allergen and subsides within 60 minutes. It is mediated by acute mast cell degranulation and the release of preformed and/or enzymatically activated mediators. These mediators include histamine, serotonin, acetylcholine, adenosine, chemotactic mediators, growth factors, and neutral proteases such as chymase and trypsin that lead to generation of kinins. Histamine is the most recognized mediator of type I hypersensitivity reactions. It is a potent vasoactive amine that increases nitric oxide production, relaxes vascular smooth muscle, increases the permeability of capillaries and venules, and causes smooth muscle contraction and bronchial constriction. Acetylcholine mimics many of the actions of histamine and produces bronchial smooth muscle contraction and dilation of small blood vessels via activation of the parasympathetic nervous system. The kinins are a group of potent inflammatory peptides that, once activated through enzymatic modification, produce vasodilation and smooth muscle contraction as well.

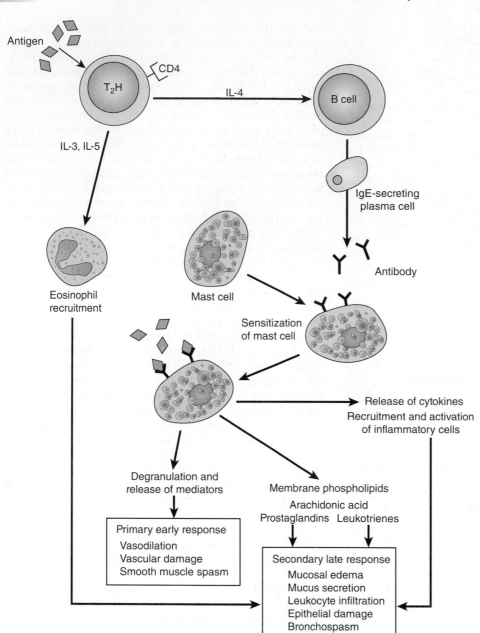

FIGURE 12-2. Type I, IgE-mediated hypersensitivity reaction. The stimulation of B-cell differentiation by an antigen-stimulated type 2 helper (T_2H) T cell leads to plasma cell production of IgE and mast cell sensitization. Subsequent binding of the antigen produces degranulation of the sensitized mast cell with release of preformed mediators that leads to a primary or early-phase response. T_2H T-cell recruitment of eosinophils, along with the release of cytokines and membrane phospholipids from the mast cell, leads to a secondary or late-phase response.

The secondary or late phase of the type I hypersensitivity response occurs 2 to 8 hours after resolution of the initial phase and can last for several days. In some cases, the late phase may be significantly prolonged or only partially resolved as in the case of uncontrolled bronchial asthma. It results from the action of lipid mediators and cytokines released from immune cells as part of the normal inflammatory process. The lipid mediators, which are derived from phospholipids found in mast cell membranes, are broken down to form arachidonic acid during the process of mast cell degranulation. Arachidonic acid is then utilized in the synthesis of leukotrienes and prostaglandins, which produce end-organ effects similar to histamine and acetylcholine, except that they have a longer onset and prolonged duration

of action. Mast cells also produce cytokines and chemotactic factors that promote migration of eosinophils and leukocytes to the site of allergen exposure, contributing to late-phase response.

It is important to point out that not all IgE-mediated reactions result in hypersensitivity or the development of disease. The IgE-mediated antibody response is a normal part of the immune response to parasitic infection. During the late phase of the response, IgE antibodies are directed against parasite larvae stimulating recruitment of large bodies of inflammatory cells including eosinophils and causing cell-mediated cytotoxicity. This type of type I hypersensitivity reaction is particularly important in developing countries where much of the population is infected with intestinal parasites.

Anaphylactic (Systemic) Reactions

Anaphylaxis is a catastrophic, systemic, life-threatening IgE-mediated hypersensitivity reaction associated with the widespread release of histamine into the systemic circulation that produces massive vasodilation, hypotension, arterial hypoxia, and airway edema.[62] It results from the presence of even minute quantities of allergen that are introduced into the body via the airway, skin, blood, or gastrointestinal mucosa. The level of severity, therefore, depends on the preexisting degree of sensitization and not with the quantity of exposure.

Clinical manifestations occur along a continuum in severity and can be graded on a scale of I to IV.[62] Grade I reactions are usually confined to the cutaneous and mucosal tissues manifesting as erythema and urticaria, with or without angioedema. Grade II reactions progress to include moderate multisystem signs such as hypotension, tachycardia, dyspnea, and gastrointestinal disturbances (e.g., nausea, vomiting, diarrhea, abdominal cramping from mucosal edema). Grade III reactions become life threatening because of the development of bronchospasm, cardiac dysrhythmias, and cardiac collapse. Once a hypersensitivity reaction reaches grade IV, cardiac arrest has occurred, and management is purely resuscitative in nature.

Preventing exposure to potential triggers that cause anaphylaxis is essential because any reaction can be life threatening. All people with potential for anaphylaxis should be advised to wear or carry a medical alert bracelet, necklace, or other identification to inform emergency personnel of the possibility of anaphylaxis. In addition, people with a history of anaphylaxis should be provided with preloaded epinephrine syringes and instructed in their use.

The initial management of anaphylaxis is dependent upon the stage at which a person presents but should always focus on withdrawal of the offending allergen, maintenance of a patent airway, establishment of appropriate intravenous access, volume resuscitation, and administration of epinephrine.[63] It is important to explain to all people with a potential for anaphylaxis that if they have a reaction and self-treat with epinephrine, it is essential for them to seek immediate professional help regardless of their initial response to self-treatment because reactions can reoccur.

Atopic (Local) Reactions

Local hypersensitivity reactions usually occur when the offending allergen is confined to a particular site of exposure. The term atopy is frequently used to describe these reactions and refers to a genetic predisposition to the development of immediate, type I IgE-mediated hypersensitivity reactions upon exposure to common environmental antigens such as pollens, food, or animal dander. Atopic reactions most commonly manifest as urticarial rash (hives), allergic rhinitis, atopic dermatitis, and bronchial asthma. People prone to atopy frequently develop reactions to more than one environmental allergen with symptoms present at different times throughout the year.

The incidence of immediate hypersensitivity reactions tends to be greater in people with a family history of **atopy**, yet the genetic basis for these disorders is not completely understood. Because of underlying genetic differences in people with type I hypersensitivity, the exact genome has been difficult to delineate. However, several chromosomal regions have been shown to contain gene sequences linked to the development of asthma and atopy, including the cytokine cluster on chromosome 5q, *interferon-γ (IFN-γ)* and STAT6 on 12q, and IL4R on 16p.[64] People with atopic allergic conditions tend to have high total serum and allergen-specific levels of IgE as well as increased numbers of eosinophils, basophils, and mast *cells*. Although the IgE-triggered response is likely a key factor in the pathophysiology of atopic allergic disorders, it is not the only factor and may not be responsible for the development of all forms of atopic dermatitis and asthma.

Allergic Rhinitis

Allergic rhinitis is a common hypersensitivity disorder of the upper respiratory tract that affects between 20% and 40% of the western population. Symptoms include rhinorrhea (runny nose), nasal obstruction, sneezing, nasal itching, and watery eyes (conjunctivitis).[65] The diagnosis of allergic rhinitis is made based upon the person's clinical presentation and a positive skin prick test or the presence of serum-specific IgE antibodies to aeroallergens. People with allergic rhinitis frequently present with other forms of atopy such as allergic asthma and **urticaria**.[66] Severe attacks may be accompanied by systemic malaise, fatigue, headache, and muscle soreness from sneezing. Fever is absent. The allergens associated with the development of allergic rhinitis are airborne and are therefore deposited directly onto the nasal mucosa. Typical allergens include pollens from ragweed, grasses, trees, and weeds; fungal spores; house dust mites; animal dander; and feathers.

Clinical manifestations are dependent upon the timing and severity of exposure. In people who are chronically exposed to allergens, symptoms can be present throughout the year. This form of atopy is known as *perennial rhinitis*. In contrast, people who present with symptoms only when exposed to high allergen counts, such as in the fall or spring, are said to have *seasonal allergic rhinitis*. Symptoms that become worse at night suggest a household allergen, and symptoms that disappear on weekends suggest occupational exposure.

The allergic response in allergic rhinitis is located specifically in the nasal mucosa. When aeroallergens are inhaled, they are deposited mainly on the nasal mucosa where they are presented to T cells by APCs. In the presence of cellular cytokines, B-cell class switching occurs, resulting in an increase in IgE production.[65,66] Once the allergen–IgE complex is formed, infiltration of the nasal mucosa by T_2H cells, mast cells, basophils, eosinophils, and Langerhans cells takes place, inducing a full cell-mediated immune response.

Treatment of allergic rhinitis focuses on the institution of avoidance measures and control of symptoms. Whenever possible, the offending allergen should be removed from the environment, or exposure should be kept to a minimum. Most symptoms can be controlled with over-the-counter antihistamines and topical nasal deconges-tants. Tolerance and rebound congestion may occur with chronic administration of topical nasal decongestants, so their use should be limited to less than 1 week. More severe symptoms may require prescription medication including topical nasal corticosteroids (*e.g.*, mometasone or *Nasonex*) and antihistamines (*e.g.*, azelastine hydrochloride). Mast cell stabilizers, such as intranasal cromolyn sodium, that prevent localized mast cell degranulation and release of intracellular mediators may be useful, especially when administered prophylactically. In people whose symptoms cannot be successfully controlled with these measures, a program of desensitization known as immunotherapy ("allergy shots") may be undertaken. Desensitization involves the frequent administration of progressively larger quantities of the offending antigen(s). The antigens stimulate production of high levels of IgG antibodies, which are capable of combining with the antigen and preventing activation of cell-bound IgE antibodies.

Food Allergies

Food allergy is very common in western countries around the world, often manifesting with life-threatening consequences. In fact, food-induced anaphylaxis is the leading cause of emergency room admissions, especially among children.[67] Currently, the prevalence rate of food allergy is between 3% and 6%, and, according to the Centers for Disease Control and Prevention (CDC), this represents an increase of 18% over the past decade.[67,68] and more common among children. The exact etiology of the increase in cases is unknown. Any food is capable of inducing a hypersensitivity reaction in susceptible people and occurs when specific food allergen comes in contact with IgE antibody present in the intestinal mucosa. The most commonly implicated foods include peanuts, tree nuts, and shellfish. In addition, milk is frequently implicated in children.[67,68] People with asthma, adolescents, and those with a personal or family history of food allergy are at increased risk of severe reactions.

The clinical manifestations of food allergy are dependent upon many factors including the amount of food ingested, the presence of an empty stomach, concurrent illness and medication, exercise, and the phase of the menstrual cycle.[67,68] Reactions may differ within a given person during different exposures, but the primary symptoms are seen in the skin, gastrointestinal tract, and respiratory system in approximately 80% of cases. The ability of a specific food to trigger a type I hypersensitivity reaction may be changed during the cooking process because heating can alter (denature) the protein structure of an allergen, so that it is no longer able to trigger the humoral response. Both acute reactions (hives and anaphylaxis) and chronic reactions (asthma, atopic dermatitis, and gastrointestinal disorders) to food allergens can occur.

Anaphylactic reactions to food allergens are common, and the presentation may differ between adults and children. Adults typically present with severe symptoms including cardiovascular collapse, whereas severe abdominal pain, hives, allergic rhinitis, conjunctivitis, and facial flushing are more common in children.[67,68] Within the pediatric population, wheezing and stridor are more common in preschoolers and older children, whereas hives and vomiting are usually seen in infants.[69] The majority of the reactions manifest within 1 hour of exposure, but delayed reactions are possible secondary to delayed absorption of the allergen. A rare form of anaphylaxis associated with food is known as *food-dependent exercise-induced anaphylaxis* (FDEIA). In FDEIA, both exercise and the food allergen are tolerated independently, and symptoms do not occur in the absence of exercise. The pathophysiology is not completely understood but seems to suggest that a pliable state of immunologic tolerance exists in susceptible people. Changes in plasma osmolality and pH, tissue enzyme activity, blood flow distribution, and gastrointestinal permeability may occur during exercise, which result in facilitated allergen recognition and binding.[70,71]

Diagnosis of food allergies relies upon a careful food history and provocative diet testing. Provocative testing involves the systematic elimination of suspected allergen(s) from the diet for a time to see if the symptoms disappear and then reintroducing the allergens(s) to the diet to determine if the symptoms reappear.

Treatment of food allergy focuses specifically on the avoidance of the offending allergen. However, this can be difficult due to inadvertent contamination with the allergen source. People with severe allergies or a history of anaphylaxis should be educated to carry an EpiPen and to seek emergency care immediately after exposure.

Type II, Antibody-Mediated Disorders

Type II (antibody-mediated) hypersensitivity or *cytotoxic hypersensitivity* reactions are mediated by IgG or IgM antibodies directed against target antigens on specific host cell surfaces or tissues. The antigens may be either intrinsic, that is, inherently part of the host cell, or extrinsic, that is, incorporated into the cell surface upon exposure to a foreign substance or infectious agent. Thus, the tissues that express the target antigens determine the clinical manifestations of type II hypersensitivity reactions. These antigens are known as *tissue-specific antigens*.[72] There are four general mechanisms by which type II hypersensitivity reactions can be propagated, but regardless of the pathway, it is always initiated by the binding of IgG or IgM antibody to tissue-specific antigens. These mechanisms include complement-activated cell destruction, antibody-mediated cell cytotoxicity, complement- and antibody-mediated inflammation, and antibody-dependent modulation of normal cell surface receptors[72] (Fig. 12-3).

Complement-Activated Cell Destruction

The destruction of target cells in type II hypersensitivity reactions can occur as a result of activation of the complement system via the classic pathway. First, formation of the membrane attack complex (MAC) by activation of C5–C9 allows the passage of ions, small molecules, and water into the cell, causing direct lysis of the cell.

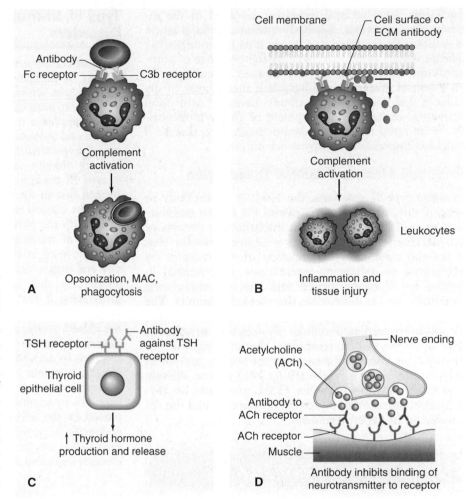

FIGURE 12-3. Type II, hypersensitivity reactions result from binding of antibodies to normal or altered surface antigens. (**A**) Opsonization and complement- or antibody receptor–mediated phagocytosis or cell lysis through membrane attack complex. (**B**) Complement- and antibody receptor–mediated inflammation resulting from recruitment and activation of inflammation-producing leukocytes (neutrophils and monocytes). (**C**) Antibody-mediated cellular dysfunction, in which antibody against the TSH receptor increases thyroid hormone production and (**D**) antibody to acetylcholine receptor inhibits receptor binding of the neurotransmitter in myasthenia gravis.

In addition, IgG and the complement fragment C3b act as opsonins by binding to receptors located on the cell surfaces of macrophages. This process activates the macrophages, which then destroys the target cells by phagocytosis. Thus, activation of the complement system produces a twofold response that culminates in cell destruction.

In people with AIHA, autoantibodies target epitopes located on red blood cells.[73] Erythrocytes coated with these autoantibodies are destroyed by phagocytes in the liver or spleen. Some, but not all, autoantibody types also induce phagocytosis and cell lysis via the complement system. The same process occurs in utero in the development of *erythroblastosis fetalis* or Rh incompatibility. Women who are Rh negative lack RhD antigen on their erythrocytes but produce anti-D antibodies. In the Rh-positive fetus, maternal anti-D antibodies will coat fetal red blood cells containing RhD, allowing them to be removed from the fetal circulation by macrophage- and monocyte-mediated phagocytosis.[74]

Antibody-Dependent Cell Cytotoxicity

Antibody-dependent cellular cytotoxicity (ADCC) incorporates components of both the innate and adaptive immune responses in the destruction of target cells but is not dependent upon activation or utilization of complement proteins. Rather, the mechanism relies upon the activity of nonspecific NK cells, but other cells such as macrophages and eosinophils have been implicated. The Fc fragment of the IgG antibody binds to an Fc receptor (FcγR) on the surface of the effector cell, and the variable fragment binds to the epitope on the target cell surface, causing release of chemotactic substances and destruction of the target cell.[75] ADCC is a common antiviral mechanism. It has been implicated in the development of several autoimmune disorders including *pemphigus vulgaris.*

Complement- and Antibody-Mediated Inflammation

When antigens that are normally expressed on vessel walls or that circulate in the plasma are deposited on the surface of endothelial cells or extracellular tissues, the manifestations are the result of localized inflammation as opposed to cell destruction. The presence of antibody in the tissues activates the complement cascade, resulting in the release of the activated complement proteins C3a and C5a, which in turn attracts neutrophils to the area and stimulates the deposition of complement protein C3b. Neutrophils will bind to the Fc antibody fragment or to C3b, but rather than destroying cells via phagocytosis, they undergo degranulation and release chemical mediators (enzyme and oxidases) involved in the inflammatory response. Antibody-mediated inflammation is responsible for the tissue injury seen in Goodpasture disease, which is characterized by the presence of autoantibodies against the α3NC1 domain of collagen IV, an essential protein in the basement membranes of the kidneys and lungs.[76] The antibody-mediated neutrophil activation causes the development of glomerulonephritis, acute renal failure, and hemorrhagic lung disease if immunosuppressive therapy is not initiated.

Antibody-Mediated Cellular Dysfunction

In some type II reactions, the binding of antibody to specific target cell receptors causes the cell to malfunction in some way, rather than initiating the process of cell destruction. The antibody–receptor complex that is formed modulates the function of the receptor by preventing or enhancing interactions with normal ligands, by replacing ligand and directly stimulating receptors, or by destroying the receptor entirely. The symptoms of type II hypersensitivity reactions caused by antibody-mediated cellular dysfunction are dependent upon the specific receptor(s) that are targeted. For example, in Graves disease, autoantibodies, known as *thyrotropin-binding inhibitory Ig*, bind to and activate thyroid-stimulating hormone (TSH) receptors on thyroid cells, stimulating thyroxine production and the development of hyperthyroidism.[77]

KEY POINTS

Allergic and Hypersensitivity Disorders

■ Type I hypersensitivity reactions are dependent upon IgE-mediated activation of mast cells and basophils and the subsequent release of chemical mediators of the inflammatory response.

■ Type II (antibody-mediated) hypersensitivity or *cytotoxic hypersensitivity* reactions are mediated by IgG or IgM antibodies directed against target antigens on specific host cell surfaces or tissues and result in complement-mediated phagocytosis and cellular injury.

■ Type III (immune complex) hypersensitivity is caused by the formation of antigen–antibody immune complexes in the bloodstream, which are subsequently deposited in vascular epithelium or extravascular tissues and which activate the complement system and induce a massive inflammatory response.

■ Type IV (cell-mediated) hypersensitivity involves tissue damage in which cell-mediated immune responses with sensitized T lymphocytes cause cell and tissue injury. Although all are T cell mediated, the pathophysiologic mechanisms and sensitized T-cell populations involved differ.

Type III, Immune Complex–Mediated Disorders

Immune complex allergic disorders are caused by the formation of antigen–antibody immune complexes in the bloodstream, which are later deposited in vascular epithelium or extravascular tissues (Fig. 12-4). The deposition of these complexes in the tissues activates the complement system and induces a massive inflammatory response. Like type II hypersensitivity reactions, IgG and IgM antibodies activate immune complex–mediated disorders. However, in type III reactions, the antibody–antigen complexes are formed first in the plasma and then deposited in the tissues. The clinical manifestations may therefore have little to do with the particular antigenic target but rather with the site of immune complex deposition. Immune complexes formed in the circulation can produce damage in any end-organ vessels including those feeding the renal glomerulus, skin, lung, and joint synovium. They can be generalized if the immune complexes are deposited in many organs or localized to a particular organ, such as the kidney, joints, or small blood vessels of the skin. Once deposited, the immune complexes elicit an inflammatory response by activating complement and generating chemotactic factors that recruit neutrophils and other cells of the inflammatory response. The activation of these inflammatory cells by immune complexes and complement, accompanied by the release of potent inflammatory mediators, is directly responsible for the injury. Type III reactions are responsible for the vasculitis seen in many autoimmune diseases including *SLE* and acute glomerulonephritis.

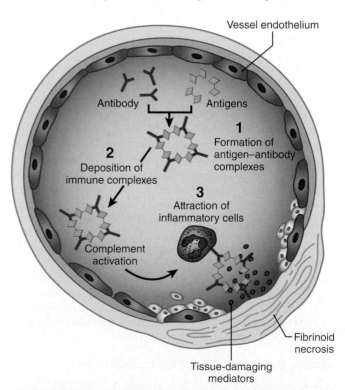

FIGURE 12-4. Type III, immune complex reactions involving complement-activating IgG or IgM Igs with (*1*) formation of blood-borne immune complexes that are (*2*) deposited in tissues. Complement activation at the site of immune complex deposition (*3*) leads to attraction of leukocytes that are responsible for vessel and tissue injury.

Systemic Immune Complex Disorders

Serum sickness is a clinical syndrome that results from the formation of insoluble antigen–antibody immune complexes in the presence of antigen excess and subsequent generalized deposition in target tissues such as blood vessels, joints, and the heart and kidneys. The deposited immune complexes activate the complement cascade, increase vascular permeability, and stimulate the recruitment of phagocytic cells. The net result is generalized tissue damage and edema. Clinical manifestations include rash, fever, generalized lymphadenopathy, and arthralgias, which usually begin approximately 1 to 2 weeks after the initial antigen exposure and subside upon withdrawal of the offending agent. In previously sensitized people, severe and life-threatening reactions have been reported. Serum sickness was first described in people receiving foreign serum, such as horse serum, for the treatment of diphtheria and scarlet fever. This antigen load was capable of stimulating the production of large quantities of immune complexes that were deposited in tissues causing activation of mast cells, monocytes, polymorphonuclear leukocyte, and platelets. Today, a variety of drugs including beta-lactam antibiotics and sulfonamides are capable of causing similar reactions.[78]

Treatment of serum sickness usually is directed toward removal of the sensitizing antigen and providing symptom relief. This may include aspirin for joint pain and antihistamines for **pruritus**. Epinephrine or systemic corticosteroids may be used for severe reactions.

Localized Immune Complex Reactions

The *Arthus reaction* is a localized immune complex reaction associated with discrete tissue necrosis, usually in the skin. It is caused by repeated local exposure to an antigen, where high levels of preformed circulating antibodies exist. Symptoms usually begin within 1 hour and peak within 6 to 12 hours of an exposure.[69] Lesions are typically red, raised, and inflamed. Ulcers may often form at the center of the lesions because of the release of inflammatory cytokines. The mechanism of the Arthus reaction is not completely understood but is believed to be the result of localized contact of injected antigen with circulating IgG antibody. This reaction is the prototypical model for the development of localized vasculitis associated with certain drug reactions in humans.

Type IV, Cell-Mediated Hypersensitivity Disorders

Type IV hypersensitivity reactions differ from type I to III hypersensitivity reactions in that they are cell-mediated and delayed, rather than antibody-mediated and immediate immune responses (Fig. 12-5). The cell-mediated immune response is normally the principal mechanism of defense against a variety of microorganisms, including intracellular pathogens such as *Mycobacterium tuberculosis* and viruses, as well as extracellular agents such as fungi, protozoa, and parasites. However, it can cause cell death and tissue injury in sensitized people

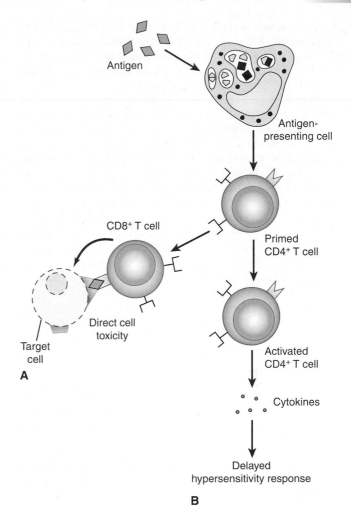

FIGURE 12-5. Type IV, cell-mediated hypersensitivity reactions, which include **(A)** direct cell-mediated cytotoxicity in which CD8$^+$ T cells kill the antigen-bearing target cells and **(B)** delayed-type hypersensitivity reactions in which presensitized CD4$^+$ cells release cell-damaging cytokines.

in response to topically administered chemical antigens (contact dermatitis) and systemic antigen exposure or as part of the autoimmune process.

Type IV hypersensitivity reactions are composed of a spectrum of disorders that range from mild to severe in clinical presentation. Although all are T cell mediated, the pathophysiologic mechanisms and sensitized T-cell populations involved differ. Because of the heterogeneity of delayed hypersensitivity reactions, current immunology experts subdivide type IV reactions into four distinct subtypes (IVa, IVb, IVc, and IVd) based upon the immune response, T-cell population, and pathologic characteristics involved.[79] In addition, depending upon the reaction, different T-cell subsets with different cytotoxic and regulatory functions can be activated at different stages of the disease process.

In type IVa hypersensitivity reactions (*e.g.*, eczema), the CD4$^+$-T$_1$H cells activate monocytes and macrophages through the secretion of large amounts of *IFN*-γ. Activated monocytes stimulate the production of complement-fixing antibodies and activate proinflammatory (*e.g.*, TNF-α and IL-12) and CD8⁺ responses.[72] Because type IVa responses require the synthesis of effector molecules, they can take up to 24 to 72 hours to develop, which is why they are called "delayed-type" hypersensitivity disorders.

Type IVb and IVd reactions are also considered to be delayed hypersensitivity reactions. Type IVb reactions (*e.g.*, *maculopapular exanthema and bullous exanthema*) are the result of T₂H cell activation and eosinophilic infiltration of the tissues. T₂H cells secrete the cytokines IL-4 and IL-5, which are necessary for activation of mast cell and eosinophilic responses. In addition, these cytokines deactivate macrophages and promote the production of IgE and IgG antibodies by the B lymphocytes. Type IVd reactions are very rare and involve the recruitment and activation of neutrophils by T lymphocytes that specifically secrete IL-8. The only disorder of this subtype is *acute generalized exanthematous pustulosis* (AGEP), which presents with neutrophil-filled sterile pustules of the skin, fever, and massive leukocytosis.[80]

Type IVc hypersensitivity reactions are cytotoxic responses mediated by CD4⁺ and CD8⁺ lymphocytes that secrete perforin and granzyme B.[81] Cytotoxic lymphocytes (CTLs) bind antigen fragments that are displayed on MHC molecules found on the surface of APCs. Peptides derived from cytosolic antigens (*e.g.*, viral) are presented by MHC class I molecules and activate CD8⁺ T cells, which kill any cell displaying the foreign antigen. Peptides derived from proteins degraded as a result of phagocytic ingestion (*e.g.*, bacteria) are presented on MHC class II molecules, which activate CD4⁺ T cells. Once activated in this manner, CD4⁺ T cells can be considered cytotoxic because they can activate other effector cells including cytotoxic CD8⁺, macrophages, and B lymphocytes.

In viral infections, cell damage is frequently the result of CTL responses rather than cytotoxic effects of the invading organism. While some viruses directly injure infected cells and are said to be cytopathic, other noncytopathic viruses do not. Because CTLs cannot distinguish between cytopathic and noncytopathic viruses, they destroy virtually all cells that are infected regardless of whether or not the virus is dangerous to the cell. In certain forms of hepatitis, for example, the destruction of liver cells is due to the host CTL response and not the virus.

Allergic Contact Dermatitis

Allergic contact dermatitis is a type IV hypersensitivity reaction associated with the activation of T₁H and T-helper lymphocytes. The inflammatory response takes place in two phases, sensitization and elicitation. It is usually confined to sites on the skin that have come in direct contact with a hapten (*e.g.*, cosmetics, hair dyes, metals, topical drugs, plant oils). During the sensitization phase, haptens are captured by dendritic cells, which then migrate to regional lymph nodes and stimulate T-cell production. In addition, local keratinocytes sense haptens and initiate and amplify the local immune response. Reexposure to the specific hapten results in rapid recruitment and activation of memory-specific T cells. The most common form of this condition is the dermatitis that follows an intimate encounter with poison ivy or poison oak antigens, although many other substances can trigger a reaction.

Clinical manifestations of contact dermatitis include an erythematous, papular, and vesicular rash that is associated with intense pruritus and weeping.[82] The affected area often becomes swollen and warm, with exudate formation and crusting. It is not uncommon for a secondary infection to develop. The location of the lesions often provides a clue about the antigen causing the disorder. However, with the same cases of contact dermatitis (*e.g.*, poison ivy), the allergen can be unknowingly spread from one part of the body to another. The severity of the reactions ranges from mild to intense, depending on the person and the allergen. Symptoms usually appear approximately 12 to 24 hours after exposure. Depending on the antigen and the duration of exposure, the reaction may last from days to weeks.

Diagnosis of contact dermatitis is made based upon the characteristics and distribution of the rash as well as the temporal relationship of exposure to the suspected allergen.[82] Patch tests can be performed to confirm the diagnosis. Treatment involves removal of the offending agent followed by application of topical preparations (*e.g.*, ointments, corticosteroid creams) to relieve symptomatic skin lesions and prevent secondary bacterial infections. Severe reactions may require the administration of systemic corticosteroid therapy.

Hypersensitivity Pneumonitis

Hypersensitivity pneumonitis, also known as extrinsic allergic alveolitis, is a form of inflammatory lung disease that results from an exaggerated immune response after exposure to a multitude of inhaled organic particles or related occupational antigens.[83] The exact pathophysiologic mechanism of hypersensitivity pneumonitis remains unclear, but evidence supports a role for both type III and type IV immune responses. People demonstrate both high levels of antigen-specific serum IgG levels and combined cellular infiltration and granuloma formation. T₁H cells appear to play a critical role in the development of the disease through the production and release of TNF, IFN-γ, IL-12, and IL-18 in lung tissue.[83] Symptoms, including labored breathing, dry cough, chills and fever, headache, and malaise, usually begin several hours after exposure and subside within hours after the sensitizing antigens are removed. However, long-term sequelae have been reported.

Diagnosis of hypersensitivity pneumonitis is based upon a history of exposure to possible antigens. Computed tomography scan of the chest demonstrates areas of lobar vascularity and the presence of centrilobular nodules. Removal of the offending agent and administration of oral corticosteroids are the only treatments available.

Latex Allergy

With the institution of universal precautions in the 1980s, the utilization of products containing natural rubber latex increased dramatically. Natural rubber latex is produced from the milky sap of the *Hevea brasiliensis* tree, and at least 13 allergenic proteins have been isolated from it to date, any one of which can illicit an allergic response in susceptible people.[84] In addition, it is a known component of over 40,000 products used in everyday life. As a result, latex allergy has emerged as a significant medical problem in westernized societies.

Although exposure to natural rubber latex is necessary for sensitization, other factors play a key role in the development of latex allergy. People with a history of atopic reactions, food allergies, and delayed hypersensitivity reactions are more likely to develop an allergic response to latex. The proteins found in latex are found in many naturally occurring substances including tree pollens, avocado, bananas, celery, and pears, so cross-sensitivity is possible.[84]

Exposure to latex may occur by a variety of mechanisms including contact with skin and mucous membranes, inhalation, contact with internal tissues, or through intravascular injection. The most severe reactions have resulted from latex proteins coming in contact with the mucous membranes of the mouth, vagina, urethra, or rectum.[85] Anaphylactic reactions have been caused by exposure of the internal organs to the surgeon's gloves during surgery.

Latex allergy can present as a type I IgE-mediated hypersensitivity reaction, type IV cell-mediated hypersensitivity reaction, or a combination of the two. Frequently, the exact pathophysiologic mechanism is unclear because the activation of the humoral and cell-mediated immune response is so intimately connected.

Type I, IgE-mediated hypersensitivity reactions develop in response to sensitization to one or more of the specific latex proteins. These reactions are immediate and often life threatening, occurring within minutes of exposure. Clinical manifestations range from mild to severe and include urticaria, wheezing, nasal congestion, coryza, rhinoconjunctivitis, bronchospasm, systemic hypotension, anaphylaxis, and cardiovascular collapse.

Type IV hypersensitivity reactions to latex gloves are the most common form of latex allergy seen. In this form of allergy, people usually develop a contact dermatitis to one of the chemical additives rather than the latex proteins within 48 to 96 hours of exposure. The contact dermatitis often affects the **dorsum** of the hands and is characterized by a vesicular, pruritic rash.

Diagnosis of latex allergy is based upon the person's history and the presence of symptoms after exposure to latex-containing products.[85] Definitive diagnosis is made through skin prick testing or intradermal injection of allergen and confirmed through latex-specific serum IgE immunoassays.[86]

Treatment of latex allergy consists mainly of avoidance measures and requires a great deal of education directed toward the latex-sensitive person and his/her family. People with severe type I IgE-mediated hypersensitivity reactions should be instructed to obtain and wear a medic alert bracelet or necklace. If type I reactions occur, they are treated with epinephrine, antihistamines (H1 and H2 blockers), and systemic corticosteroids in order to maintain airway patency and restore hemodynamic stability.[85]

SUMMARY CONCEPTS

Hypersensitivity reactions are exaggerated immunologic responses to environmental, food, or drug antigens that would not affect most of the population. There are four basic categories of hypersensitivity responses: (1) type I responses, which are mediated by the IgE class Igs and include anaphylactic shock, hay fever, and bronchial asthma; (2) type II responses, which involve complement-activated cell destruction (Rh incompatibility), ADCC, complement- and antibody-mediated inflammation (*e.g.,* Goodpasture disease), and antibody-mediated cell dysfunction (*e.g.,* Graves disease and myasthenia gravis); (3) type III, immune complex–mediated hypersensitivity disorders, which involve the formation and deposition of insoluble antigen–antibody complexes in blood vessels causing the development of vasculitis and organ damage as seen in SLE or acute glomerulonephritis, systemic immune complex disease (serum sickness), and local immune complex disease (Arthus reaction); and (4) type IV cell-mediated hypersensitivity reactions, which are subdivided into four different types based upon the T-cell population involved and the pathophysiologic response.

Transplantation Immunopathology

Traditionally, transplantation can be defined as the process of taking cells, tissues, or organs, called a *graft*, from one person and placing them into another person where they take over the normal function of the tissues replaced. Grafts transplanted from another person are known as *allografts*. In certain circumstances, grafts can be taken from one part of the body and transplanted in another part of the body in the same person. These grafts are referred to as *autografts*. The person who provided the graft is referred to as the *donor*, and the person who receives the graft is called either the *recipient* or the *host*. Tissue transplantation has become routine because of improved medical technology, but serious complications still occur. The most important of which is graft rejection mediated by the host's immune system.

In order for transplantation to be successful, it is essential for the host's immune system to recognize the graft as "self" rather than "nonself." It is the function of the T lymphocytes to respond to a limitless number of antigens while at the same time ignoring self-antigens expressed on tissues. The MHC molecules or *HLAs* expressed on the surface of cells enable the lymphocytes to do just this. Circulating B and T lymphocytes destroy cells that express unfamiliar peptide fragments on the MHC. Transplanted tissue can be categorized as an *autologous* graft (autograft) if the donor and recipient are the same person, *syngeneic* graft if the donor and recipient are identical twins, and *allogeneic* (or allograft) if the donor and recipient are unrelated but share similar HLA tissue expression. The HLA molecules that are recognized as foreign on allografts are called *alloantigens*. Donors of solid organ transplants can be living or dead (cadaver) and related or nonrelated (heterologous). The likelihood of rejection varies indirectly with the degree of HLA similarity that exists between the donor and recipient.

Mechanisms Involved in Transplant Rejection

The process of transplant rejection involves a complex but coordinated cell-mediated and antibody-mediated immune response. Although T lymphocytes have received the most attention as mediators of transplant rejection, it is now known that B cells, macrophages, eosinophils, and NK cells have a significant impact on the quality and the quantity of the rejection process. In fact, when T cell–depleting regimens are employed prior to transplantation, the importance of these cells in the rejection process becomes more evident.[87] Three classic forms of rejection exist: cell mediated, antibody mediated, and chronic rejection, although a mixed pattern of rejection can occur as well.

The most common form of acute allograft rejection is T cell mediated and known as *cellular rejection*. It is initiated by the presentation of donor alloantigens to host T lymphocytes by antigen-presenting dendritic cells and macrophages; APCs may come from recipient or donor tissue. When the APCs are donor in origin, T-lymphocyte activation is said to occur via the direct pathway. When the APCs are the recipient's innate cells, T-lymphocyte activation is said to be via the *indirect pathway*, which resembles the pathway normally involved in the recognition of foreign substances. Most of the alloantigen is presented in association with MHC I or II molecules, resulting in destruction of graft cells by CD8$^+$ cytotoxic T cells or the initiation of a delayed hypersensitivity reactions triggered by CD4$^+$ helper T cells.[88]

T cells of the recipient recognize allogeneic MHC molecules on the surface of APCs that have migrated to lymphoid tissue and on the graft itself. CD8$^+$ cells recognize class I MHC molecules and differentiate into mature CTLs, which directly kill the graft tissue as they would any foreign substance. CD4$^+$ helper T cells recognize class II MHC molecules and differentiate into T-helper effector cells, which secrete cytokines that influence almost all other cells of the immune response including B lymphocytes, cytotoxic T cells (CD8$^+$), macrophages, and NK cells. In addition, the cytokines cause increased vascular permeability and local accumulation and activation of macrophages and eventual graft injury. Although it was traditionally believed that T$_1$H helper cells mediated rejection and T$_2$H cells promoted tolerance, it is now known that T$_2$H helper cells alone can be responsible for graft rejection mediated via eosinophil activation.[88]

Antibody-mediated or humoral rejection is caused by B-lymphocyte proliferation and differentiation into plasma cells that produce donor-specific antibodies (DSAs). These antibodies may be preformed if the immune system was exposed pretransplantation, or they may be produced *de novo* following transplantation. B lymphocytes also play an antibody-independent role in graft rejection through the secretion of proinflammatory cytokines and chemokines and the participation in antigen presentation.[87] Antibody-mediated rejection can be hyperacute or acute in origin. *Hyperacute rejection* occurs almost immediately after vascular reperfusion to graft tissue occurs. Preformed antibodies against HLA antigens are deposited in the tissue endothelium and microvasculature where they activate the classic complement pathway causing tissue necrosis and graft injury.[88] Hyperacute rejection is considered a type III hypersensitivity response. *Acute antibody-mediated rejection* occurs within days to weeks after transplantation. The time frame is dependent upon whether or not the recipient received immunosuppressive therapy prior to transplantation. Previous exposure to the relevant HLA antigens is responsible, but unlike in hyperacute rejection, high circulating antibodies are not present at the time of transplantation.[89] Over a period of several days, high titers of complement-fixing antibodies are generated, which cause injury by several mechanisms, including complement-dependent cytotoxicity, inflammation, and ADCC. Regardless of the mechanism, the initial target of these antibodies in rejection appears to be the graft vasculature.

Chronic rejection involves immune-mediated inflammatory injury to a graft that occurs over a prolonged period. It is most often due to the inability to maintain adequate immunosuppression necessary to control residual circulating antigraft T lymphocytes or antibodies. Chronic rejection manifests itself with a progressive decline in tissue function usually as a result of vascular injury and impaired blood supply.[90] T lymphocytes and macrophages infiltrate the graft and set up a chronic immune response that causes cellular hypertrophy and subendothelial thickening. Antibody-mediated rejection may be responsible for chronic rejection in people with undetected low levels of preexisting or de novo DSAs. In renal transplantation, it is characterized by a gradual rise in serum creatinine over a period of 4 to 6 months.

Graft-Versus-Host Disease

GVHD is a major complication that most frequently occurs after allogeneic stem cell transplantation. There are three fundamental requirements for the development of GVHD:

1. The graft must contain cells that are immunologically competent.
2. The recipient's cells must express antigens that are not present on donor cells.
3. The recipient must be immunologically compromised and incapable of mounting an effective immune response.

Cases of GVHD have also been reported in other settings where tissues containing T lymphocytes, such as blood products, bone marrow, or solid organs (liver), are transplanted into people who are immunocompromised.[91]

GVHD occurs when donor T cells react to HLAs present on host cells. The incidence of acute GVHD directly correlates with the degree of mismatching between recipient and host HLA proteins. Class I HLA (A, B, and C) proteins are expressed on most nucleated cells in the body. Class II HLA proteins (DR, DQ, and DP) are mainly expressed on hemopoietic cells including B lymphocytes, dendritic cells, and monocytes. Class II HLA protein expression can also be stimulated on other cell types during inflammation and tissue injury. Therefore, donors and recipients are matched for class I HLA (A, B, and C) and class II CRB1 antigens in order to decrease the chance of rejection. However, even with tissue matching, 40% of HLA-identical graft recipients develop signs of system GVHD requiring treatment with high-dose steroids. It is believed that GVHD is the result of genetic differences encoded that encode for minor histocompatibility proteins.[91,92]

The development of GVHD involves a three-step process: (1) activation of recipient APCs; (2) activation, proliferation, differentiation, and migration of donor T lymphocytes; and (3) target tissue destruction. Prior to transplantation, host APCs are in a state of heightened activation as a result of the underlying disease process and HSCT preconditioning regimens. As a result, these cells exhibit amplified expression of adhesion molecules, MHC antigens, and costimulatory molecules. Following transplantation, donor T lymphocytes encounter these "heightened" APCs and activate both CD4$^+$ and CD8$^+$ T cells. The result is the stimulation of a complex cascade of cellular mediators and soluble inflammatory agents that amplify tissue injury and promote tissue destruction.

GVHD can be acute or chronic. Acute GVHD usually develops within the first 100 days of transplantation, whereas chronic GVHD occurs sometime after that. However, cases of late-onset acute GVHD have been reported, and in some cases, people present with features of both. Signs and symptoms usually develop first in the skin, coinciding with the engraftment of donor cells. People present with a pruritic, maculopapular rash that starts on the hands and feet but ultimately extends over the entire body. In severe cases, the skin can blister and ulcerations may develop. Gastrointestinal symptoms include nausea, anorexia, diarrhea, and abdominal pain. Gastrointestinal bleeding is an ominous sign as it indicates mucosal ulceration. Liver disease is common but is frequently hard to differentiate from liver involvement normally seen after transplantation. It can progress to the development of veno-occlusive disease, drug toxicity, viral infection, iron overload, extrahepatic biliary obstruction, sepsis, and coma. The severity of acute GVHD is determined based upon the involvement of the three primary target organs affected (skin, GI tract, and liver). Severe

GVHD is associated with a poor prognosis and a long-term survival rate of 5%.[91,92]

Chronic GVHD is a major late cause of death after high-dose myeloablative chemoradiotherapy. GVHD can progress to the acute form of the disease, recur sometime after resolution of an acute process, or develop *de novo*. The greatest risk factors for the development of chronic GVHD are advanced recipient age and a previous history of acute GVHD. Signs and symptoms of chronic GVHD are typical of an autoimmune process and can affect all major organ systems within the body.

Prevention of GVHD focuses on regimens that specifically deplete donor T lymphocytes. Immunosuppressive or anti-inflammatory drugs such as cyclosporine and tacrolimus or glucocorticoids can be used to block T-cell activation and the action of cytokines.[91,92]

 SUMMARY CONCEPTS

Transplantation can be defined as the process of taking cells, tissues, or organs, called a *graft*, from one person and placing them into another person where they take over the normal function of the tissues replaced. Although advances in medicine had dramatically improved the long-term survival following transplantation, rejection still exists as a major barrier to success. Rejection is the process by which the recipient's immune system recognizes the graft as foreign, mounts an immunologic response, and destroys it. Destruction of the cells or tissues of the graft can be cell mediated, antibody mediated, or a combination of both processes. Hyperacute antibody rejection occurs almost immediately after transplantation and is caused by existing recipient antibodies to graft antigens that initiate an immediate hypersensitivity reaction in the blood vessels of the graft. *Acute antibody-mediated rejection* occurs within days to weeks after transplantation. Previous exposure to the relevant HLA antigens is responsible, but unlike in hyperacute rejection, high circulating antibodies are not present at the time of transplantation. Chronic rejection occurs over a prolonged period and is caused by T cell–generated cytokines that stimulate fibrosis of graft tissue.

GVHD occurs when immunologically competent donor cells are transplanted into recipients who are immunologically compromised. Three basic requirements are necessary for GVHD to develop: (1) the donor cells must be immunologically competent, (2) the recipient tissue must bear antigens foreign to the donor cells, and (3) the recipient must be immunologically compromised so that it cannot destroy the transplanted cells.

Autoimmune Disease

Autoimmune diseases are a heterogenous group of disorders that occur when the body's immune system fails to differentiate "self" from "nonself" and mounts an immunologic response against host tissues. Autoimmune diseases can affect almost any cell type, tissue, or organ system. Some autoimmune disorders, such as Hashimoto thyroiditis, are tissue specific. Others, such as SLE, are systemic, affecting multiple organs and systems. Chart 12-2 lists some of the more common autoimmune diseases.

Immunologic Tolerance

A key feature of the immune system is its ability to differentiate between foreign antigens and self-antigens.

CHART 12-2

PROBABLE AUTOIMMUNE DISEASE*

Systemic
Mixed connective tissue disease
Polymyositis–dermatomyositis
Rheumatoid arthritis
Scleroderma
Sjögren syndrome
Systemic lupus erythematosus
Blood
Autoimmune hemolytic anemia
Autoimmune neutropenia and lymphopenia
Idiopathic thrombocytopenic purpura
Other Organs
Acute idiopathic polyneuritis
Atrophic gastritis and pernicious anemia
Autoimmune adrenalitis
Goodpasture syndrome
Hashimoto thyroiditis
Type 1 diabetes mellitus
Myasthenia gravis
Premature gonadal (ovarian) failure
Primary biliary cirrhosis
Sympathetic ophthalmia
Temporal arteritis
Thyrotoxicosis (Graves disease)
Crohn disease, ulcerative colitis

*Examples are not inclusive.

The capacity of the immune system to differentiate self from nonself is called *self-tolerance*. The development of self-tolerance relies upon two coordinated processes: *central tolerance*, the elimination of autoreactive lymphocytes during maturation in the central lymphoid tissues, and *peripheral tolerance*, the functional suppression of autoreactive lymphocytes in peripheral tissues that have escaped destruction in the thymus.[93] *Autoreactivity* is the process by which an organism acts against its own tissue.

B-Cell Tolerance

Under normal circumstances, circulating B lymphocytes do not produce antibodies against host tissues. B-cell antibody production is normally kept in check by the help of CD4$^+$ T-helper cells.[94] In addition, autoreactive B lymphocytes can be eliminated by apoptosis in the central lymphoid tissues, spleen, and peripheral lymph nodes, or they can be functionally inactivated in a process known as *anergy*. However, in many autoimmune diseases, the immune system loses its ability to recognize self and produces antibodies, also known as *autoantibodies*, against host tissues. For example, in Graves disease, hyperthyroidism is the result of autoantibody-induced hyperactivity of the TSH receptor (see Fig. 12-3).

T-Cell Tolerance

The primary mechanisms of T-cell tolerance involve a process of positive and negative selection of maturing lymphocytes (Fig. 12-6). When immature lymphocytes migrate into the thymus, the T-cell lineage undergoes TCR gene rearrangement at the α and β loci.[93] At this point, they can mature into either CD4$^+$ or CD8$^+$ cells and are considered to be double positive (CD4$^+$/8$^+$). After rearrangement, T cells with TCRs that respond appropriately to self-peptide–MHC complexes and possess little avidity for the antigen are signaled by the release of cytokines and chemokines to migrate into the thymic medulla and mature into CD4$^+$/8$^-$ and CD4$^-$/8$^+$ or single-positive lymphocytes. This is known as *positive selection*. In contrast, T cells with TCRs that possess high avidity for the self-peptide–MHC complex are directed to undergo apoptosis or programmed cell death. This is known as clonal deletion or *negative selection* and takes place in the thymic medulla as well. Although the processes governing the selection and maturation of T lymphocytes are extensive, autoreactive T cells can escape into the periphery, where peripheral mechanisms for the development of self-tolerance become important.

Several peripheral mechanisms are available to deal with autoreactive cells that escape central selection. One primary mechanism begins with the development of a specialized subpopulation of T lymphocytes. CD4$^+$CD25$^+$ regulator T cells are a subset of T lymphocytes produced in the thymus that regulate antigen-specific tolerance. These regulator T cells target and abolish the response

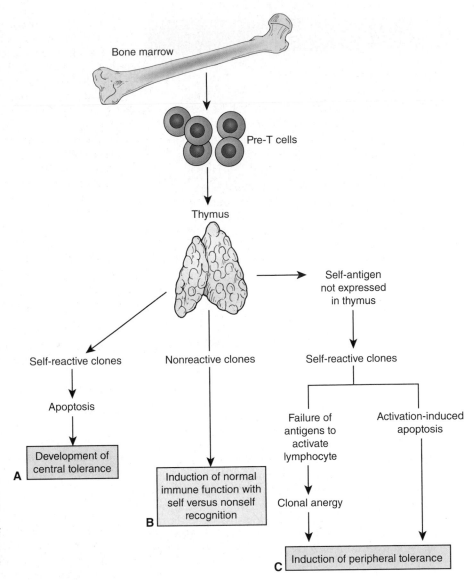

FIGURE 12-6. Development of immunologic tolerance. (**A**) Development of central tolerance with deletion of self-reactive T lymphocytes in the thymus. (**B**) Nonreactive lymphocytes with development of normal immune function. (**C**) Induction of peripheral tolerance in self-reactive cells that are not eliminated in the thymus.

of autoreactive T cells that have been released into the peripheral circulation by interrupting the production and release of IL-2. Regulatory T cells are also capable of inducing tolerance to foreign antigens by inhibiting activation and proliferation of naive CD4$^+$ T cells in response to antigen.[93]

The activity of autoreactive T cells can also be inhibited by local anatomic and physiologic factors. Some T cells are located in areas of the body where they fail to come in contact with their corresponding antigens (*e.g.*, blood–brain barrier), so they remain immunologically inactive. In other cases, autoreactive T cells encounter their corresponding antigens, but the costimulatory factors necessary for their activation are missing. The peripheral activation of T cells requires presentation of a peptide antigen in association with MHC molecules on the APCs as well as a set of secondary costimulatory factors. Because costimulatory signals are not strongly expressed on most normal tissues, the encounter of the autoreactive T cells with their specific target antigens

fails to initiate an immunologic response resulting in the development of anergy.

Another mechanism essential for the maintenance of functional tolerance involves the apoptotic death of autoreactive T cells when excessive or repeated TCR activation has occurred. This process is referred to as activation-induced cell death (AICD).[95] AICD is necessary in order to prevent activated T cells from inducing an autoimmune response. It is a normal process of the immune system designed to maintain internal homeostasis. AICD is mediated by the interaction between an apoptotic cell surface receptor (called FAS) that is present on the T cell and a soluble membrane messenger molecule known as the FAS ligand (FasL, CD95L). The FAS/FAS ligand bound activates the intracellular processes that result in programmed cell death. The expression of the FAS receptor is markedly increased on the cell surfaces of activated T cells. Therefore, expression of the FAS messenger molecule by the same cohort of activated autoreactive T cells can result in removal of the population from the circulation.

Mechanisms of Autoimmune Disease

Although it is clear that autoimmune disease results from a loss of self-tolerance, the exact mechanisms are largely unknown. Autoimmune diseases are a heterogeneous group of disorders, so a combination of both genetic and environmental factors plays a significant role. Gender may also be a factor because many autoimmune disorders such as SLE are predominantly seen in women, suggesting that female hormones like estrogens may play a role in the development of certain autoimmune diseases. Estrogen has been shown to have strong immunomodulatory effects including the stimulation of autoreactive B-lymphocyte antibody production, increased leukocyte adhesion to endothelial cells, and increased cytokine production.[96]

Heredity

Although the pathophysiology of autoimmune disease is multifactorial and complex, involving both environmental and genetic influences, it is known that heredity has a significant impact on the prevalence of these disorders. Autoimmune disorders are not inherited in the traditional fashion such as with a single-gene mutation. Rather, people with autoimmune disorders exhibit *susceptibility genes* that act in concert with environmental factors to increase a person's risk of developing the disease process.[97,98] In addition, many of these genes are shared between autoimmune disorders with similar underlying features. For example, type I IFN is a central mediator of the innate immune response stimulating monocyte maturation, plasma cell maturation and Ig class switching, and cytotoxic T-cell activity. People with SLE or systemic sclerosis (SSc) demonstrate defects in the IFN regulatory factor 5 (*IRF5*) gene, resulting in the abnormal transcription of IFN. In other cases, heritable changes occur as a result of changes in gene expression, rather than changes in DNA sequencing. This is termed *epigenetics*. This is the result of the methylation of deoxycytosine (dC) bases in cytosine–guanine DNA base pairs. As a result, the chromatin structure is altered in such a way that it cannot be accessed during the normal processes of DNA transcription and the functions encoded in the DNA sequence cease.

The high concordance rates in first-degree relatives and monozygotic twins provide strong evidence for the role of inheritance in autoimmune disorders. First-degree relatives have a relative risk of rheumatoid arthritis that is two to four times that of the general population. Studies of monozygotic and dizygotic twins indicate that rheumatoid arthritis is approximately 65% heritable with many affected people sharing alleles for the same anticyclic citrullinated peptide (anti-CCP) antibody. It is clear that autoimmunity does not develop in all people with genetic predisposition.[96] Therefore, other factors known as "triggering events" interact to precipitate the altered immune state. In most cases, the event or events that trigger the development of an autoimmune response are unknown, but in many cases, it appears that the "trigger" may be a viral infection, a chemical substance, or a self-antigen from a body tissue that has been hidden from the immune system during development and is suddenly expressed.

Environmental Factors

The role of environment in the development of autoimmune disease is complex. The incidence of some autoimmune diseases, such as type I diabetes mellitus, has increased in recent years faster than would be expected based upon genetic mechanisms alone, suggesting an increased impact of environmental factors in genetically susceptible people.[99] Environmental factors including viral infection, lack of exposure to maternal antibodies through breastfeeding, maternal smoking, and exposure to hazardous chemicals appear to be involved in the pathogenesis of autoimmune disorders, but their precise role in initiating the autoreactive response is largely unknown. Various factors work in concert resulting in the loss of self-tolerance including breakdown of T-cell anergy, release of sequestered antigens, molecular mimicry, and the development of superantigens.

Breakdown in T-Cell Anergy

Anergy is a state of reduced function, in which an immunocompetent, antigen-specific T cell is unable to respond to an appropriate stimulus. Anergy can develop if there is loss of normal costimulatory factors in the face of normal T-cell activation or from altered/chronic TCR stimulation. Primary CD4$^+$ and CD8$^+$ T cells' anergy is characterized by defective production of IFN-γ and TNF-α.[100] In addition, regulatory T cells control T-cell activation by failing to express T-cell stimulating inflammatory cytokines. Most normal tissues do not express costimulatory molecules and as a result are protected from circulating autoreactive T cells. However, if normal cells are induced to express costimulatory factors, then normal anergy is inhibited and autoimmunity can develop. This can occur after an infection or in situations where there is tissue necrosis and local inflammation.

Release of Sequestered Antigens

Under normal circumstances, the body does not produce antibodies against self-antigens. If self-antigens have been completely sequestered during T-cell development and reintroduced into the immune system, they are likely to be treated as foreign antigens. This has been documented in cases of autoimmune orchitis and autoimmune **uveitis** after systemic release of spermatozoa and ocular antigens.[101] Other times, self-antigens may change their structure and, once they come in contact with T cells, are no longer recognized as innate to the host. Once an autoimmune process has been initiated, it tends to become amplified and progress, sometimes with sporadic relapses and remissions. This occurs because the initial inflammatory process releases these altered self-antigens where they encounter the cells of the immune system. The result is continued activation of new lymphocytes that recognize the previously hidden epitopes.

Molecular Mimicry

Molecular mimicry is one theory that has been postulated to describe the mechanisms by which infectious agents or other foreign substances trigger an immune response against autoantigens. If a susceptible host is exposed to a foreign antigen that is immunologically similar to its own autoantigens (share epitopes), but which differs sufficiently to trigger an immune response, cross-reactivity between the two antigens and damage to host tissues can occur. For example, molecular mimicry has been used to explain the cardiac damage associated with acute rheumatic fever after infection with group A beta-hemolytic streptococci and the demyelinating injury in multiple sclerosis.[102] Not everyone exposed to this organism goes on to develop autoimmunity most likely due to differences in HLA expression.

Superantigens

Superantigens are a family of related substances, including staphylococcal and streptococcal exotoxins, that induce uncontrolled proliferation and activation of T lymphocytes, causing fever, shock, and death. Unlike antigens, superantigens bind as intact molecules to a wide variety of class II MHC molecules on APCs and then to the TCR on the variable region of the β-chain (TCR Vβ). Every superantigen is capable of binding a large subset of TCR Vβ domains and as a result activating up to 20% of all T cells.[103] Superantigens are involved in several diseases, including food poisoning and toxic shock syndrome.

Diagnosis and Treatment of Autoimmune Disease

The diagnosis of autoimmune disorders is not always easy due to overlapping presentations and nonspecific presentation. Diagnosis is made based upon evidence of autoimmunity as indicated by history as well as physical and serologic findings. Because the etiology of autoimmunity is multifactorial, it is unlikely that any one specific genetic testing alone will be able to determine a diagnosis with 100% certainty.[104]

The basis for most serologic assays is the demonstration of antibodies directed against tissue antigens or cellular components. The results of serologic testing are correlated with the physical findings during the diagnostic workup. For example, a child who presents with a chronic or acute history of fever, arthritis, and a macular rash and has high levels of antinuclear antibody has a probable diagnosis of SLE. The detection of autoantibodies in the laboratory usually is accomplished by one of three methods: indirect fluorescent antibody (IFA) assays, enzyme-linked immunosorbent assay (ELISA), or particle agglutination of some kind. Each technique relies upon the specificity of antibody for antigen. In the ELISA and IFA, the person's serum is diluted and allowed to react with an antigen-coated surface so that the antibody present in the sample can bind the antigen. The serum antibody is then linked to an enzyme or secondary antibody producing a visible reaction that allows the amount of antibody present to be quantified. Particle agglutination assays are much simpler because the binding of the person's antibody to antigen-coated particles causes a visible agglutination reaction, and a secondary reaction is not required.[104]

Treatment of autoimmune disorders is dependent upon the magnitude of the presenting manifestations and underlying mechanisms of the disease process. Because in many cases the pathophysiologic mechanisms are not always known, treatment may be purely symptomatic. Corticosteroids and immunosuppressive drugs are the mainstay of therapy directed at arresting or reversing the cellular damage caused by the autoimmune response. **Plasmapheresis** has been utilized in severe cases to remove autoreactive cells from the circulation.[105]

Recent therapies for the treatment of autoimmune disorders have focused on targeting the specific lymphocytes and cytokines involved in the autoimmune response; however the success has been variable.

SUMMARY CONCEPTS

Autoimmune disorders are caused by a loss of immunologic self-tolerance, which results in damage to body tissues. Autoimmune diseases are a heterogenous group of disorders and depending upon the target of the autoreactive lymphocytes can affect almost any cell or tissue of the body. The ability of the immune system to differentiate self from nonself is called *self-tolerance* and is normally maintained through central mechanisms that delete autoreactive lymphocytes before they come in contact with an autoantigen. Cells that escape deletion by central mechanisms may be suppressed or inactivated in the periphery. Defects in any of these mechanisms can be responsible for the development of autoimmune diseases.

T-cell activity is modulated through the expression of the HLA–MHC complex on cellular surfaces. Antigens are normally presented to TCRs in combination with MHC molecules. This interaction activates a variety of immune processes that culminate in destruction of the "foreign antigen." Disruption of any step in the antigen recognition process can result in the loss of self-tolerance including breakdown of T-cell anergy, release of sequestered antigens, molecular mimicry, and the development of superantigens. Diagnosis of autoimmune disease is made based upon evidence of autoimmunity as indicated by history as well as physical and serologic findings.

ACQUIRED IMMUNODEFICIENCY SYNDROME AND HUMAN IMMUNODEFICIENCY VIRUS

AIDS is a disease caused by infection with the HIV and is characterized by profound immunosuppression with associated opportunistic infections, malignancies, wasting, and central nervous system (CNS) degeneration. AIDS is considered a chronic illness today.

The AIDS Epidemic and Transmission of HIV Infection

According to the latest HIV surveillance report published by CDC, at the end of 2015, an estimated 1.1 million persons aged 13 and older were living with HIV infection in the United States, including an estimated 162,500 (15%) persons whose infections had not been diagnosed.[1,106-110]

Transmission of HIV Infection

HIV is a retrovirus that selectively attacks the CD4$^+$ T lymphocytes, the immune cells responsible for orchestrating and coordinating the immune response to infection. As a consequence, people with HIV infection have a deteriorating immune system and thus are more susceptible to severe infections with ordinarily harmless organisms.[111] The virus responsible for most HIV infection worldwide is called *HIV type 1* (HIV-1). A second type, *HIV type 2* (HIV-2), is endemic in many countries in West Africa but is rarely seen in other parts of the world. People with HIV-2 tend not to develop AIDS.[2,3]

HIV is transmitted from one person to another through sexual contact, through blood-to-blood contact, or perinatally. The CDC transmission categories of HIV for children include perinatal and other. The adult categories include male-to-male sexual contact, intravenous drug use, male-to-male sexual contact and intravenous drug use, heterosexual contact, and other.[3]

Several studies involving more than 1000 uninfected, nonsexual household contacts with persons with HIV infection (including siblings, parents, and children) have shown no evidence of casual transmission. Transmission can occur when infected blood, semen, or vaginal secretions from one person are deposited onto a mucous membrane or into the bloodstream of another person. Sexual contact is the most frequent mode of HIV transmission.[112] HIV is present in semen and vaginal fluids. There is a risk of transmitting HIV when these fluids come in contact with a part of the body that lets them enter the bloodstream. This includes the vaginal and anal mucosa, superficial lacerations, wounds, or sores on the skin. In most cities in the United States, sexual transmission of HIV is primarily related to vaginal or anal intercourse. However, the use of condoms is highly effective in preventing the transmission of HIV.

Because HIV is found in blood, the use of needles, syringes, and other drug injection paraphernalia is a direct route of transmission. Of the reported cases of AIDS in the United States, approximately 25% occurred among people who injected drugs.[112] Transfusions of whole blood, plasma, platelets, or blood cells before 1985 resulted in the transmission of HIV. Seventy to eighty percent of people with hemophilia who were treated with factor VIII supplements before 1985 became infected with HIV.[112] Since 1985, all blood donations in the United States have been screened for HIV, so this is no longer a transmission risk. Other blood products, such as gamma globulin or hepatitis B immune globulin, have not been implicated in the transmission of HIV.

Transmission from mother to infant is the most common way that children become infected with HIV. HIV may be transmitted from infected women to their offspring in utero, during labor and delivery, or through breastfeeding.[7] Ninety percent of infected children acquired the virus from their mother.

Occupational HIV infection among health care workers is uncommon. Universal Blood and Body Fluid Precautions should be used in encounters with all people in the health care setting because it should be assumed that any person may have a transmissible infection. Occupational risk of infection for health care workers most often is associated with percutaneous inoculation (i.e., needle stick) of blood from a person with HIV infection. Transmission is associated with the size of the needle, amount of blood present, depth of the injury, type of fluid contamination, stage of illness of the person, and viral load of the person.

People with other sexually transmitted diseases (STDs) are at increased risk for HIV infection. The risk of HIV transmission is increased in the presence of genital ulcerative STDs (i.e., syphilis, herpes simplex virus infection, and chancroid) and nonulcerative STDs (i.e., gonorrhea, chlamydial infection, and trichomoniasis). HIV increases the duration and recurrence of STD lesions, treatment failures, and atypical presentation of genital ulcerative diseases because of the suppression of the immune system.

The HIV-infected person is infectious even when no symptoms are present. The point at which an infected person converts from being negative for the presence of HIV antibodies in the blood to being positive is called *seroconversion*. Seroconversion typically occurs within 1 to 3 months after exposure to HIV but can take up to 6 months.[3] The time after infection and before seroconversion is known as the *window period*. During the window period, a person's HIV antibody test result will be negative. Rarely, infection can occur from transfused blood that was screened for HIV antibody and found negative because the donor was recently infected and still in the window period. Consequently, the U.S. FDA requires blood collection centers to screen potential donors through interviews designed to identify behaviors known to present a risk for HIV infection.

growing evidence of an association between HIV infection and other STDs. Infected individuals can transmit the virus to others before their own infections can be detected by antibody tests.

Pathophysiology and Clinical Course

Molecular and Biologic Features of HIV

HIV-1 is an enveloped member of the retroviruses specifically the subfamily of lentiviruses.[4] They can all produce slowly progressive fatal diseases that include wasting syndromes and CNS degeneration. Two genetically different but antigenically related forms of HIV, HIV-1 and HIV-2, have been isolated in people with AIDS. HIV-1 is the type most associated with AIDS in the United States, Europe, and Central Africa, whereas HIV-2 causes a similar disease principally in West Africa. HIV-2 appears to be transmitted in the same manner as HIV-1; it can also cause immunodeficiency as evidenced by a reduction in the number of CD4$^+$ T cells and the development of AIDS. Although the spectrum of disease for HIV-2 is similar to that of HIV-1, it spreads more slowly and causes disease more slowly than HIV-1. Specific tests are now available for HIV-2, and blood collected for transfusion is routinely screened for HIV-2. Because most people with HIV have HIV-1, the discussion focuses on HIV-1.

HIV infects a limited number of cell types in the body, including a subset of lymphocytes called CD4$^+$ T lymphocytes (also known as *T-helper cells* or *CD4$^+$ T cells*), macrophages, and dendritic cells.[10] The CD4$^+$ T cells are necessary for normal immune function. Among other functions, the CD4$^+$ T cell recognizes foreign antigens and helps activate antibody-producing B lymphocytes.[10] The CD4$^+$ T cells also orchestrate cell-mediated immunity, in which cytotoxic CD8$^+$ T cells and natural killer (NK) cells directly destroy virus-infected cells, tubercle bacilli, and foreign antigens. The phagocytic function of monocytes and macrophages is also influenced by CD4$^+$ T cells.

Like other retroviruses, HIV carries its genetic information in ribonucleic acid (RNA) rather than deoxyribonucleic acid (DNA). The HIV virion is spherical and contains an electron-dense core surrounded by a lipid envelope (Fig. 12-7). The virus core contains the major capsid protein p24, two copies of the genomic RNA, and three viral enzymes (protease, reverse transcriptase, and integrase). Because p24 is the most readily detected antigen, it is the target for the antibodies used in screening for HIV infection. The viral core is surrounded by a matrix protein called p17, which lies beneath the viral envelope. The viral envelope is studded with two viral glycoproteins, gp120 and gp41, which are critical for the infection of cells.

KEY POINTS

The AIDS Epidemic and Transmission of HIV

- AIDS is caused by the HIV.
- HIV is transmitted through blood, semen, vaginal fluids, and breast milk.
- People with HIV infection are infectious even when asymptomatic.

SUMMARY CONCEPTS

AIDS is an infectious disease of the immune system caused by HIV, a retrovirus that causes profound immunosuppression. The severity of the clinical disease and the absence of a cure or preventive vaccine have increased public awareness and concern. The greatest incidence of HIV in 2010 to 2015 has been in males and people between the age of 25 and 34 years.[1] HIV is transmitted from one person to another through sexual contact, through blood-to-blood contact, or perinatally. Transmission occurs when the infected blood, semen, or vaginal secretions from one person are deposited onto a mucous membrane or into the bloodstream of another person. The primary routes of transmission are through sexual intercourse, through intravenous drug use, and from mother to infant. Blood transfusions and other blood products continue to be routes of transmission in some underdeveloped countries. Occupational exposure in health care settings accounts for only a tiny percentage of HIV transmission. HIV infection is not transmitted through casual contact or by insect vectors. There is

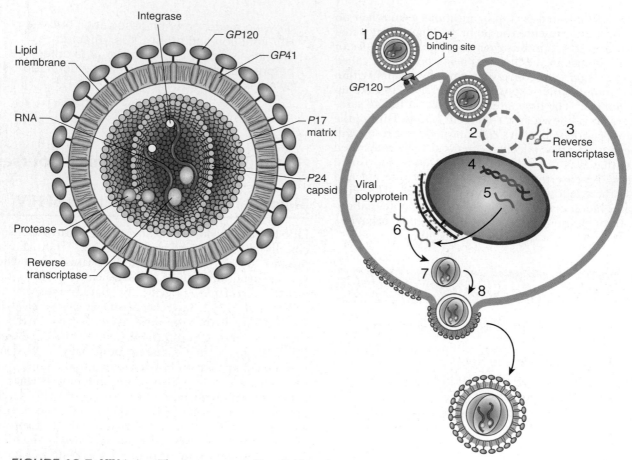

FIGURE 12-7. HIV-1 virus. The virus surrounded by a lipid envelope.

Replication of HIV is depicted in Figure 12-8. Each of these steps provides insights into the development of methods used for preventing or treating the infection. The *first step* involves the binding of the virus to the CD4$^+$ T cell. Once HIV has entered the bloodstream, it attaches to the surface of a CD4$^+$ T cell by binding to a CD4 receptor that has a high affinity for HIV. However, binding to the CD4 receptor is not sufficient for infection; the virus must also bind with other surface molecules that bind the gp120 and gp41 envelope glycoproteins. This process is known as *attachment*. The *second step* allows for the internalization of the virus. After attachment, the viral envelope peptides fuse to the CD4$^+$ T-cell membrane. Fusion results in an *uncoating* of the virus, allowing the contents of the viral core (the two single strands of viral RNA and the reverse transcriptase, integrase, and protease enzymes) to enter the host cell. The chemokine coreceptors are critical components of the HIV infection process.

The *third step* consists of DNA synthesis. In order for HIV to reproduce, it must change its RNA into DNA. It does this by using the *reverse transcriptase* enzyme. Reverse transcriptase makes a copy of the viral RNA and then in reverse makes another mirror-image copy. The result is double-stranded DNA that carries instructions for viral replication. The *fourth step* is called *integration*. During integration, the new DNA enters the nucleus

of the CD4$^+$ T cell and, with the help of the enzyme integrase, is inserted into the cell's original DNA. The *fifth step* involves *transcription* of the double-stranded viral DNA to form a single-stranded messenger RNA (mRNA) with the instructions for building new viruses. Transcription involves activation of the T cell and induction of host cell transcription factors such as nuclear factor-κB.[4] To finish, the cycle ribosomal RNA (rRNA) uses the instructions in the mRNA to create a chain of proteins and enzymes called a *polyprotein*. These polyproteins contain the components needed for the next stages in the construction of new viruses. The *seventh step* is called *cleavage*. During cleavage, the protease enzyme cuts the polyprotein chain into the individual proteins that will make up the new viruses. Finally, the proteins and viral RNA are assembled into new HIV viruses and released from the CD4$^+$ T cell.

Treatment of HIV/AIDS relies on the use of agents that interrupt steps of the HIV replication process. Currently, there are multiple drug classes of antiviral agents. The administration of highly active antiretroviral therapy (HAART), also referred to as combined antiretroviral therapy, typically comprising a combination of three to four antiviral agents, has become the current standard of care.[3]

HIV replication involves the killing of the CD4$^+$ T cell and the release of HIV copies into the bloodstream. These viral particles, or *virions*, invade other CD4$^+$ T cells,

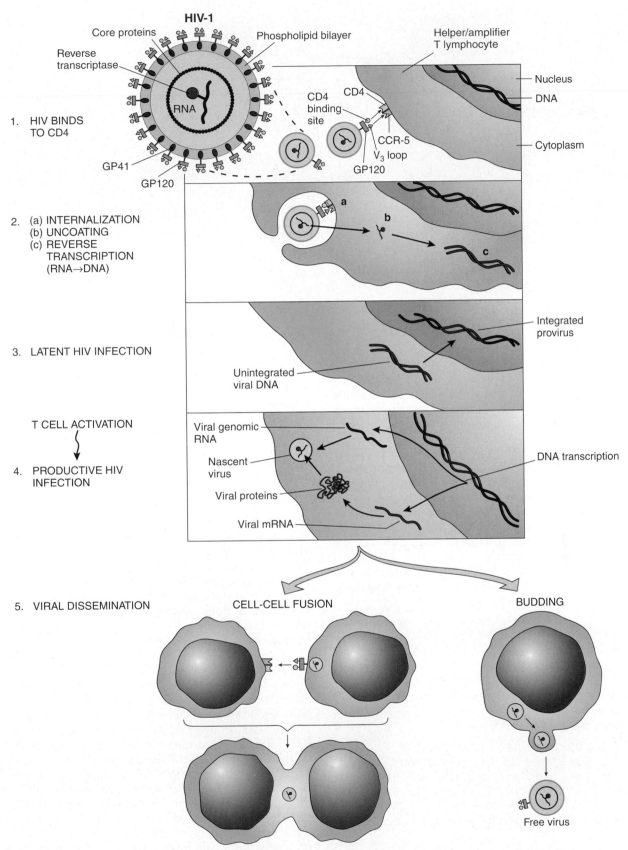

FIGURE 12-8. Life cycle of HIV-1 is a multistep process that includes (**A**) binding CD4 receptor in conjunction with chemokine receptor (*e.g.*, CCR5); (**B**) internalization, uncoating, and reverse transcription; (**C**) integration into host DNA as a provirus where it persists in a state of latency; (**D**) replication in concert with host T-cell activation; and (**E**) dissemination. (From Strayer D., Rubin R. (Eds.). (2015). *Rubin's clinicopathologic foundations of medicine* (7th ed., Fig. 4-23, p. 161). Philadelphia, PA: Lippincott Williams & Wilkins.)

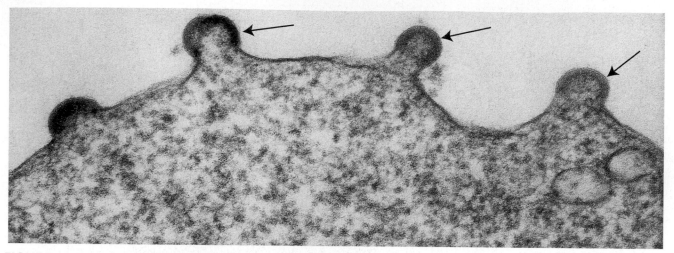

FIGURE 12-9. HIV-1 virions can be seen budding from infected cells (*arrows*). (From Strayer D., Rubin R. (Eds.). (2015). *Rubin's clinicopathologic foundations of medicine* (7th ed., Fig. 4-24, p. 162). Philadelphia, PA: Lippincott Williams & Wilkins.)

allowing the infection to progress (Fig. 12-9). Every day, millions of infected CD4$^+$ T cells are destroyed, releasing billions of viral particles into the bloodstream, but each day, nearly all the CD4$^+$ T cells are replaced and nearly all the viral particles are destroyed. The problem is that over the years, the CD4$^+$ T-cell count gradually decreases through this process, and the number of viruses detected in the blood of persons infected with HIV increases.[3]

Until the CD4$^+$ T-cell count falls to a very low level, a person infected with HIV can remain asymptomatic, although active viral replication is still taking place and serologic tests can identify antibodies to HIV.[12] These antibodies, unfortunately, do not convey protection against the virus. Although symptoms are not evident, the infection proceeds on a microbiologic level, including the invasion and selective destruction of CD4$^+$ T cells. The continual decline of CD4$^+$ T cells places the person with HIV at high risk for acquiring cancer or other infections.

KEY POINTS

Pathophysiology of HIV/AIDS

- The HIV is a retrovirus that destroys the body's immune system by taking over and destroying CD4$^+$ T cells.

- In the process of taking over the CD4$^+$ T cell, the virus attaches to receptors on the CD4$^+$ cell, fuses to and enters the cell, incorporates its RNA into the cell's DNA, and then uses the CD4$^+$ cell's DNA to reproduce large amounts of HIV, which are released into the blood.

- As the CD4$^+$ T-cell count decreases, the body becomes susceptible to opportunistic infections.

Phases of HIV Infection

The typical course of HIV infection is defined by three phases, which usually occur over a period of 8 to 12 years. The three phases are the primary infection phase, chronic asymptomatic or latency phase, and overt AIDS phase.[6]

Many persons, when they are initially infected with HIV, have an acute mononucleosis-like syndrome known as *primary infection* that can last for a few weeks. This acute phase may include fever, fatigue, myalgias, sore throat, night sweats, gastrointestinal problems, lymphadenopathy, maculopapular rash, and headache. During primary infection, there is an increase in viral replication, which leads to very high viral loads, sometimes greater than 1,000,000 copies/mL, and a decrease in the CD4$^+$ T-cell count. The signs and symptoms of primary HIV infection generally manifest about a month post HIV exposure but can show up quicker.[6] After several weeks, the immune system acts to control viral replication and reduces the viral load to a lower level, where it often remains for several years.

The primary phase is followed by a latent period during which the person has no signs or symptoms of illness. The median time of the latent period is about 10 years. During this time, the CD4$^+$ T-cell count falls gradually from the normal range of 800 to 1000 cells/μL to 200 cells/μL or lower. More recent data suggest that the CD4$^+$ T-cell decline may not fall in an even slope based on the level of HIV RNA levels and the factors related to variability in the decline in CD4$^+$ cells are under investigation. Some people experience swollen lymph nodes at this time. Persistent generalized lymphadenopathy (PGL) usually is defined as lymph nodes that are chronically swollen for more than 3 months in at least two locations, not including the groin. The lymph nodes may be sore or visible externally.

The third phase, overt AIDS, occurs when a person has a CD4$^+$ cell count of less than 200 cells/μL or an AIDS-defining illness.[16] Without antiretroviral therapy,

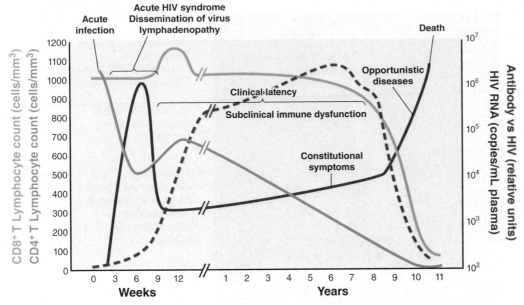

FIGURE 12-10. Generalized time course of HIV-1 infection. Important events in the development of HIV-1 infection are shown, including the clinical syndrome, virus loads, and CD4$^+$ and CD8$^+$ lymphocyte population dynamics over time. (From Strayer D., Rubin R. (Eds.). (2015). *Rubin's clinicopathologic foundations of medicine* (7th ed., Fig. 4-26, p. 164). Philadelphia, PA: Lippincott Williams & Wilkins.)

this phase can lead to death within 2 to 3 years or in some cases quicker. The risk of opportunistic infections and death increases significantly when the CD4$^+$ cell count falls below 200 cells/μL (Fig. 12-10).

Clinical Course

The clinical course of HIV varies from person to person. Most, 60% to 70% of those infected with HIV, develop AIDS 10 to 11 years after infection. These people are the *typical progressors*. Another 10% to 20% of those infected progress rapidly, with development of AIDS in less than 5 years, and are called *rapid progressors*. The final 5% to 15% are *slow progressors*, who do not progress to AIDS for more than 15 years.[7] There is a subset of slow progressors, called *long-term nonprogressors*, who account for 1% of all HIV infections. These people have been infected for at least 8 years, are antiretroviral naive, have high CD4$^+$ cell counts, and usually have very low viral loads. Among this group, there are some people who have spontaneous and sustained virologic suppression without the use of antiretroviral medications. This group of HIV-infected people is currently being investigated to assist in determining the immunologic and virologic interactions that allow those people to maintain virologic suppression of HIV.[7]

Severe immunodeficiencies and even death can occur if HIV goes untreated or undetected. Prophylactic antibiotics have reduced the cases of *P. jiroveci* (*P. carinii*) pneumonia; however, individuals with AIDS remain susceptible to *Legionella* infection. The most common gastrointestinal disorder associated with HIV/AIDS is diarrhea, occurring in 75% of cases. *Cryptosporidium*, *Isospora belli*, and *Giardia lamblia* are the most common protozoans;

Salmonella and *M. avium* are common bacterial causes. When the CD4 counts drop below 50 cells/mm,[3] colitis may occur. Nervous system complications include cryptococcal meningitis, cerebral toxoplasmosis, CNS lymphoma, and multifocal leukoencephalopathy due to JC virus. The most common skin disease is staphylococcus aureus causing bullous impetigo and ecthyma. Common skin disorders include chronic mucocutaneous herpes simplex and human papillomavirus (HPV). Malignancies associated with HIV/AIDS include Kaposi sarcoma (KS), a malignant neoplasm. Individuals under age 60 with KS are highly suspicious for HIV/AIDS. B-cell lymphoproliferative diseases, both congenital and acquired, exhibit generalized lymphadenopathy. B-cell proliferations or monoclonal B-cell lymphomas are associated with EBV. Opportunistic infections that occur with HIV are shown in Figure 12-11.[5]

Opportunistic Infections

Opportunistic infections begin to occur as the immune system becomes severely compromised. The number of CD4$^+$ T cells directly correlates with the risk of development of opportunistic infections. In addition, the baseline HIV RNA level contributes and serves as an independent risk factor.[113] Opportunistic infections involve common organisms that do not produce infection unless there is impaired immune function. Although a person with AIDS may live for many years after the first serious illness, as the immune system fails, these opportunistic illnesses become progressively more severe and difficult to treat.

Opportunistic infections are most often categorized by the type of organism (*e.g.*, fungal, protozoal, bacterial and mycobacterial, viral). Bacterial and mycobacterial opportunistic infections include bacterial pneumonia, salmonellosis, bartonellosis, *M. tuberculosis* (TB), and

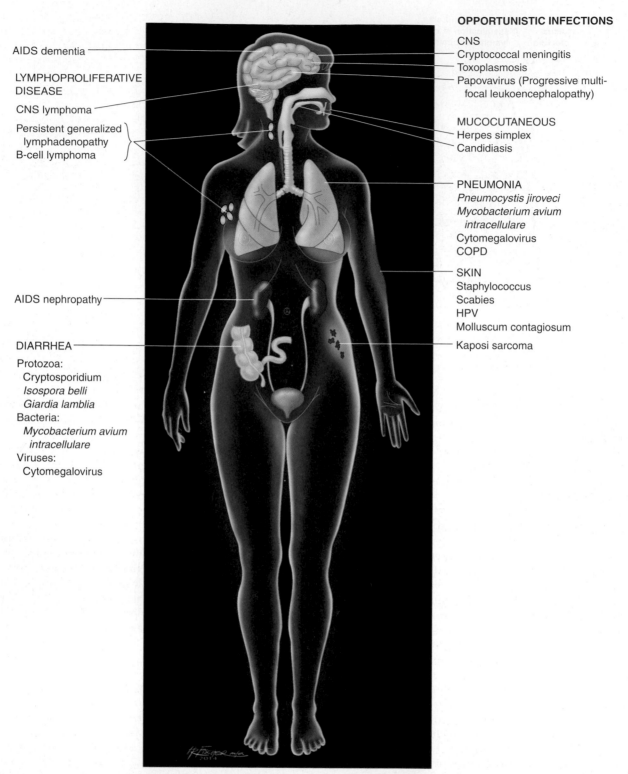

OPPORTUNISTIC INFECTIONS

AIDS dementia

LYMPHOPROLIFERATIVE DISEASE

CNS lymphoma

Persistent generalized lymphadenopathy
B-cell lymphoma

AIDS nephropathy

DIARRHEA

Protozoa:
 Cryptosporidium
 Isospora belli
 Giardia lamblia
Bacteria:
 Mycobacterium avium intracellulare
Viruses:
 Cytomegalovirus

CNS
Cryptococcal meningitis
Toxoplasmosis
Papovavirus (Progressive multifocal leukoencephalopathy)

MUCOCUTANEOUS
Herpes simplex
Candidiasis

PNEUMONIA
Pneumocystis jiroveci
Mycobacterium avium intracellulare
Cytomegalovirus
COPD

SKIN
Staphylococcus
Scabies
HPV
Molluscum contagiosum

Kaposi sarcoma

FIGURE 12-11. HIV-1–mediated destruction of the cellular immune system results in AIDS. The infectious and neoplastic complications of AIDS can affect practically every organ system. CNS, central nervous system; HPV, human papillomavirus. (From Strayer D., Rubin R. (Eds.). (2015). *Rubin's clinicopathologic foundations of medicine* (7th ed., Fig. 4-25, p. 163). Philadelphia, PA: Lippincott Williams & Wilkins.)

Mycobacterium avium–intracellulare complex (MAC). Fungal opportunistic infections include candidiasis, coccidioidomycosis, cryptococcosis, histoplasmosis, penicilliosis, and pneumocystosis. Protozoal opportunistic infections include cryptosporidiosis, microsporidiosis, isosporiasis, and toxoplasmosis. Viral infections include those caused by CMV, herpes simplex and zoster viruses, human papillomavirus (HPV), and JC virus, the causative agent of progressive multifocal leukoencephalopathy (PML).

SUMMARY CONCEPTS

HIV is a retrovirus that infects the body's CD4$^+$ T cells and macrophages. HIV genetic material becomes integrated into the host cell DNA, so new HIV can be made.

Manifestations of infection, such as acute mononucleosis-like symptoms, may occur shortly after infection, and this is followed by a latent phase that may last for many years. The end of the latent period is marked by the onset of opportunistic infections and cancers as the person is diagnosed with AIDS. The complications of these infections can manifest throughout the respiratory, gastrointestinal, and nervous systems and can include pneumonia, esophagitis, diarrhea, gastroenteritis, tumors, wasting syndrome, altered mental status, seizures, motor deficits, and metabolic disorders.

Prevention, Diagnosis, and Treatment

Prevention

Because there is no cure for HIV infection or AIDS, adopting risk-free or low-risk behavior is the best protection against the disease. Abstinence and long-term, mutually monogamous sexual relationships between two uninfected partners are the best ways to avoid HIV infection and other STDs. Correct and consistent use of latex condoms can provide protection from HIV by not allowing contact with semen or vaginal secretions during intercourse.

Avoiding recreational IV drug use and particularly avoiding the practice of using syringes that may have been used by another person are important for HIV prevention. Medical and public health authorities recommend that people who choose to inject drugs use a new sterile syringe for each injection or, if this is not possible, clean their syringes thoroughly with a household bleach mixture. Other substances that alter inhibitions can lead to risky sexual behavior and increase the risk of exposure to HIV. The addictive nature of many recreational drugs can lead to an increase in the frequency of unsafe sexual behavior and the number of partners as the user engages in sex in exchange for money or drugs. People concerned about their risk should be encouraged to get information and counseling and be tested to find out their infection status.

Anyone who is at continued risk for HIV infection should be tested at least annually. Those who are at high risk, including injection drug users and their partners, people who exchange sex for money or drugs, and anyone who has had more than one sex partner since the last HIV test, should be tested more frequently. The essential elements of any HIV prevention/counseling interaction include a personalized risk assessment and prevention plan. Education and behavioral interventions continue to be the mainstays of HIV prevention programs. Individual risk assessment and education regarding HIV transmission and possible prevention techniques or skills are delivered to persons in clinical settings and to those at high risk of infection in community settings. Community-wide education is provided in schools, the workplace, and the media. Training for professionals can have an impact on the spread of HIV and is an important element of prevention.

Diagnostic Methods

The diagnostic methods used for HIV infection include laboratory methods to determine infection and clinical methods to evaluate the progression of the disease. The most accurate and inexpensive method for identifying HIV infection is the HIV antibody test. The first commercial assays for HIV were introduced in 1985 to screen donated blood. Since then, use of antibody detection tests has been expanded to include evaluating persons at increased risk for HIV infection. The HIV antibody test procedure consists of screening with an *enzyme immunoassay* (EIA), also known as ELISA, followed by a confirmatory test, the *Western blot* assay, which is performed if the EIA is positive.[45] In light of the psychosocial issues related to HIV infection and AIDS, sensitivity and confidentiality must be maintained whenever testing is implemented.[8]

Polymerase chain reaction (PCR) is a technique for detecting HIV DNA. PCR detects the presence of the virus rather than the antibody to the virus, which the EIA and Western blot tests detect. PCR is useful in diagnosing HIV infection in infants born to infected mothers because these infants have their mothers' HIV antibody regardless of whether the children are infected. Because the amount of viral DNA in the HIV-infected cell is small compared with the amount of human DNA, direct detection of viral genetic material is difficult. PCR is a method for amplifying the viral DNA up to 1 million times or more to increase the probability of detection.

Treatment

There is no cure for HIV infection. The medications that are currently available to treat HIV infection decrease the amount of virus in the body, but they do not eradicate HIV. After HIV infection is confirmed, a baseline evaluation should be done. This evaluation should include a complete history and physical examination and baseline laboratory tests including a complete blood count (CBC) with differential. Routine follow-up care of a stable, asymptomatic person infected with HIV should include a history and physical examination along with CD4$^+$ cell count and viral load testing every 3 to 4 months.[112,114,115] People who are symptomatic may need to be seen more frequently.

81. Voskoboinik I., Whisstock J. C., Trapani J. A. (2015). Perforin and granzymes: Function, dysfunction and human pathology. *Nature Reviews Immunology* 15(6), 388–400.

82. Brasch J., Becker D., Aberer W., et al. (2014). Guideline contact dermatitis: S1-Guidelines of the German Contact Allergy Group (DKG) of the German Dermatology Society (DDG), the Information Network of Dermatological Clinics (IVDK), the German Society for Allergology and Clinical Immunology (DGAKI), the Working Group for Occupational and Environmental Dermatology (ABD) of the DDG, the Medical Association of German Allergologists (AeDA), the Professional Association of German Dermatologists (BVDD) and the DDG. *Allergo Journal International* 23(4), 126–138.

83. Spagnolo P., Rossi G., Cavazza A., et al. (2015). Hypersensitivity pneumonitis: A comprehensive review. *Journal of Investigational Allergology and Clinical Immunology* 25(4), 237–250; quiz follow 250.

84. Kelly K. J., Sussman G. N. (2017). Latex allergy: Where are we now and how did we get there? *The Journal of Allergy and Clinical Immunology. In Practice* 5(5), 1212–1216.

85. Kumar R. P. (2012). Latex allergy in clinical practice. *Indian Journal of Dermatology* 57(1), 66–70.

86. Wu M., McIntosh J., Liu J. (2016). Current prevalence rate of latex allergy: Why it remains a problem? *Journal of Occupational Health* 58(2), 138–144.

87. Moreau A., Varey E., Anegon I., et al. (2013). Effector mechanisms of rejection. *Cold Spring Harbor Perspectives in Medicine* 3(11), a015461.

88. Kant C. D., Akiyama Y., Tanaka K., et al. (2015). Both rejection and tolerance of allografts can occur in the absence of secondary lymphoid tissues. *Journal of Immunology* 194(3), 1364–1371.

89. Cai J., Qing X., Tan J., et al. (2013). Humoral theory of transplantation: Some hot topics. *British Medical Bulletin* 105, 139–155.

90. Lipshultz S. E., Chandar J. J., Rusconi P. G., et al. (2014). Issues in solid-organ transplantation in children: Translational research from bench to bedside. *Clinics (São Paulo, Brazil)* 69(Suppl 1), 55–72.

91. Nassereddine S., Rafei H., Elbahesh E., et al. (2017). Acute graft versus host disease: A comprehensive review. *Anticancer Research* 37(4), 1547–1555.

92. Zeiser R., Blazar B. R. (2017). Acute graft-versus-host disease – biologic process, prevention, and therapy. *New England Journal of Medicine* 377(22), 2167–2179.

93. Geenen V. (2017). History of the thymus: From an "accident of evolution" to the programming of immunological self-tolerance. *Medical Science (Paris)* 33(6–7), 653–663.

94. Chong A. S., Khiew S. H. (2017). Transplantation tolerance: Don't forget about the B cells. *Clinical and Experimental Immunology* 189(2), 171–180.

95. Sikora E. (2015). Activation-induced and damage-induced cell death in aging human T cells. *Mechanisms of Ageing and Development* 151, 85–92.

96. Rosenblum M. D., Remedios K. A., Abbas A. K. (2015). Mechanisms of human autoimmunity. *Journal of Clinical Investigation* 125(6), 2228–2233.

97. Costenbader K. H., Gay S., Alarcon-Riquelme M. E., et al. (2012). Genes, epigenetic regulation and environmental factors: Which is the most relevant in developing autoimmune diseases? *Autoimmunity Reviews* 11(8), 604–609.

98. Ceccarelli F., Agmon-Levin N., Perricone C. (2016). Genetic factors of autoimmune diseases. *Journal of Immunology Research* 2016, 3476023.

99. Eringsmark Regnell S., Lernmark A. (2013). The environment and the origins of islet autoimmunity and Type 1 diabetes. *Diabetic Medicine* 30(2), 155–160.

100. Crespo J., Sun H., Welling T. H., et al. (2013). T cell anergy, exhaustion, senescence, and stemness in the tumor microenvironment. *Current Opinion in Immunology* 25(2), 214–221.

101. Silva C. A., Cocuzza M., Carvalho J. F., et al. (2014). Diagnosis and classification of autoimmune orchitis. *Autoimmunity Reviews* 13(4–5), 431–434.

102. Cusick M. F., Libbey J. E., Fujinami R. S. (2012). Molecular mimicry as a mechanism of autoimmune disease. *Clinical Reviews in Allergy and Immunology* 42(1), 102–111.

103. Spaulding A. R., Salgado-Pabon W., Kohler P. L., et al. (2013). Staphylococcal and streptococcal superantigen exotoxins. *Clinical Microbiology Reviews* 26(3), 422–447.

104. Castro C., Gourley M. (2010). Diagnostic testing and interpretation of tests for autoimmunity. *Journal of Allergy and Clinical Immunology* 125(2 Suppl 2), S238–S247.

105. Rosenblum M. D., Gratz I. K., Paw J. S., et al. (2012). Treating human autoimmunity: Current practice and future prospects. *Science Translational Medicine* 4(125), 125sr121.

106. Centers for Disease Control and Prevention. (2018). Estimated HIV incidence and prevalence in the United States, 2010–2015. *HIV Surveillance Supplemental Report* 23(1)

107. Shaw G. M., Hunter E. (2012). HIV transmission. *Cold Spring Harbor Perspectives in Medicine* 2(11), a006965.

108. Maartens G., Celum C., Lewin S. R. (2014). HIV infection: Epidemiology, pathogenesis, treatment, and prevention. *Lancet* 384(9939), 258–271.

109. Centers for Disease Control and Prevention. (2016). *HIV Surveillance Report* 28.

110. Naif H. M. (2013). Pathogenesis of HIV infection. *Infectious Disease Reports* 5(Suppl 1), e6.

111. Marciano B. E., Huang C. Y., Joshi G., et al. (2014). BCG vaccination in patients with severe combined immunodeficiency: Complicastions, risks, and vaccination policies. *Journal of Allergy and Clinical Immunology* 133(4), 1134–1141.

112. Cihlar T., Fordyce M. (2016). Current status and prospects of HIV treatment. *Current Opinion in Virology* 18, 50–56.

113. Kutukculer N., Azarsiz E., Karaca N. E., et al. (2015). Fc gamma receptor polymorphisms in patients with transient hypogammaglobulinemia of infancy presenting with mild and severe infections. *Asian Pacific Journal of Allergy and Immunology* 33(4), 312–319.

114. Strayer D., Rubin R. (Eds.). (2015). *Rubin's clinicopathologic foundations of medicine* (7th ed.). Philadelphia, PA: Lippincott Williams & Wilkins.

115. Stevenson M. (2018). CROI 2018: Advances in basic science understanding of HIV. *Topics in Antiviral Medicine* 26(1), 17–21.

116. Centers for Disease Control and Prevention. (2014). National HIV testing day and new testing recommendations. *MMWR. Morbidity and Mortality Weekly Report* 63(25), 537.

117. Flynn P. M. (2018). A broader look at adolescents with perinatal HIV. [Online]. Available: https://www.nature.com/articles/d41586-018-04476-8?WT.ec_id=NATURE-20180426&utm_source=nature_etoc&utm_medium=email&utm_campaign=20180426&spMailingID=56487811&spUserID=MjA1NzcwMjE4MQS2&spJobID=1383950517&spReportId=MTM4Mzk1MDUxNwS2. Accessed May 14, 2018.

118. Center of Disease Control. (2018). Preventing mother-to-child transmission of HIV. [Online]. Available: https://aidsinfo.nih.gov/understanding-hiv-aids/fact-sheets/20/50/preventing-mother-to-child-transmission-of-hiv. Accessed May 14, 2018.

119. National Institutes of Health. (2017). Diagnosis of HIV infection in infants and children. [Online]. Available: https://aidsinfo.nih.gov/guidelines/html/2/pediatric-arv/55/diagnosis-of-hiv-infection-in-infants-and-children. Accessed May 14, 2018.

120. Rivera D. M., Steele R. W. (2017). Pediatric HIV infection clinical presentation. [Online]. Available: https://emedicine.medscape.com/article/965086-clinical#showall. Accessed May 14, 2018.

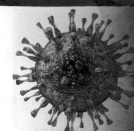

C H A P T E R 13

Organization and Control of Neural Function

Learning Objectives

**After completing this chapter, the learner
will be able to meet the following objectives:**

1. Distinguish between the functions of the neurons
   and neuroglial cells of the nervous system.
2. Describe the structure and function of the three
   parts of a neuron.
3. Describe the metabolic requirements of nervous
   tissue.
4. Describe the three phases of an action potential
   and relate the functional importance of ion
   channels to the different phases.
5. Characterize the role of excitatory and inhibitory
   postsynaptic potentials as they relate to spatial and
   temporal summation of membrane potentials.

UNDERSTANDING → Synaptic Transmission

Neurons communicate through chemical synapses via neurotransmitters. Chemical synapses consist of a presynapse, a synaptic cleft, and a postsynapse. This process relies on (1) synthesis and release of a neurotransmitter from a presynaptic neuron, (2) binding of a neurotransmitter to receptors in the postsynaptic neuron, and (3) neurotransmitter removal from the synapse.

1

Neurotransmitter Synthesis and Release. Neurotransmitters are synthesized in the presynaptic neuron and then stored in synaptic vesicles. Communication between the two neurons begins with a nerve impulse that stimulates the presynaptic neuron, followed by movement of the synaptic vesicles to the cell membrane and release of neurotransmitter into the synaptic cleft.

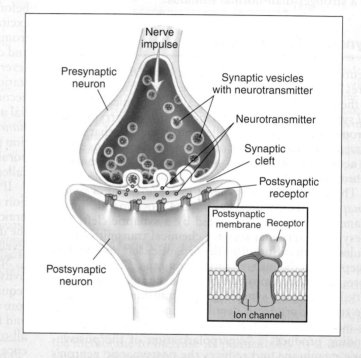

2

Receptor Binding. Once released from the presynaptic neuron, the neurotransmitter moves across the synaptic cleft and binds to receptors on the postsynaptic neuron. The action of a neurotransmitter is determined by the type of receptor to which it binds. Many presynaptic neurons also have receptors to which a neurotransmitter may bind. The presynaptic receptors function in a negative feedback manner to inhibit further release of the neurotransmitter.

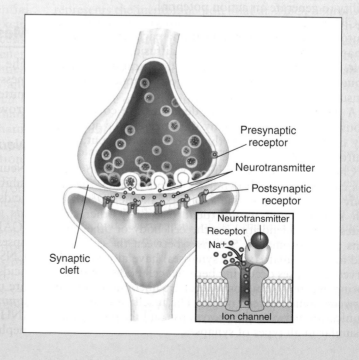

3 **Neurotransmitter Removal.**
Precise control of synaptic function relies on the rapid removal of the neurotransmitter from the synapse. A released neurotransmitter can (1) be taken back up into the neuron in a process called reuptake, (2) diffuse out of the synaptic cleft, or (3) be broken down by enzymes.

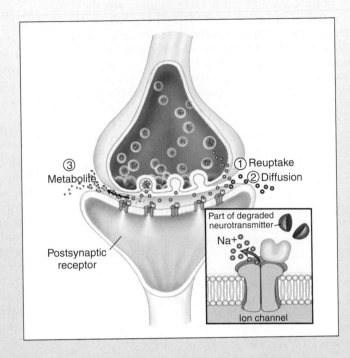

③ Metabolite
① Reuptake
② Diffusion
Postsynaptic receptor

Part of degraded neurotransmitter
Na+
Ion channel

Neurotransmitters are synthesized in the cytoplasm of the axon terminal. The synthesis of transmitters may require one or more enzyme-catalyzed steps. After synthesis, neurotransmitter molecules are stored in the axon terminal in tiny, membrane-bound sacs called *synaptic vesicles*. These vesicles protect the neurotransmitters from enzyme destruction in the nerve terminal. There may be thousands of vesicles in a single terminal, each vesicle containing 10,000 to 100,000 transmitter molecules. The arrival of an impulse at a nerve terminal causes the vesicles to move to the cell membrane and release their transmitter molecules into the synaptic space.

Neurotransmitters exert their actions through specific proteins, called *receptors*, embedded in the postsynaptic membrane. The interaction between a transmitter and receptor results in a specific physiologic response. The action of a transmitter is determined by the type and location of the receptor to which it binds. Receptors are named according to the type of neurotransmitter with which they interact (*e.g.*, a *cholinergic receptor* is a receptor that binds to acetylcholine).

Rapid removal of a transmitter is necessary to maintain precise control of neural transmission. A released transmitter can undergo one of these three processes:

1. It can be broken down into inactive substances by enzymes.
2. It can be taken back up into the presynaptic neuron in a process called *reuptake*.

3. It can diffuse into the intercellular fluid until its concentration is too low to influence postsynaptic excitability.

Neuromodulators

Other classes of messenger molecules, known as *neuromodulators*, may be released from axon terminals. Neuromodulators react with presynaptic or postsynaptic receptors to alter release of or response to neurotransmitters. Neuromodulators may act on postsynaptic receptors to produce longer-lasting changes in membrane excitability. This alters the action of neurotransmitters by enhancing or decreasing their effectiveness. By combining with autoreceptors on the presynaptic membrane, a transmitter can act as a neuromodulator to augment or inhibit further activity. In some nerves, a messenger molecule can have both transmitter and modulator functions.

Neurotrophic Factors

Neurotrophic or nerve growth factors are required to maintain the long-term survival of the postsynaptic cell and are secreted by axon terminals independent of action potentials. Trophic factors from target cells that enter the axon and are necessary for the long-term survival of presynaptic neurons also have been demonstrated. Target cell-to-neuron trophic factors likely aid in establishing specific neural connections during normal embryonic development.

SUMMARY CONCEPTS

Neurons are characterized by the ability to communicate with other cells through electrical signals called *action potentials*. Neuron cell membranes contain ion channels that are responsible for generating and propagating action potentials. Voltage-dependent gates that open and close with changes in the membrane potential guard these channels. Action potentials are divided into three parts—the resting phase, during which the membrane is polarized but no electrical activity occurs; the depolarization phase when sodium channels open, allowing rapid inflow of the ions to generate an electrical impulse; and the repolarization phase, during which the membrane is permeable to potassium ions, allowing for the efflux of potassium ions and return to resting.

Synapses are structures that permit communication between neurons. Two types of synapses have been identified—electrical and chemical. Electrical synapses consist of gap junctions between adjacent cells that allow action potentials to move rapidly from one cell to another. Chemical synapses involve special presynaptic and postsynaptic structures, separated by a synaptic cleft. They rely on chemical messengers, released from the presynaptic neuron, that cross the synaptic cleft and then interact with receptors on the postsynaptic neuron.

Neurotransmitters are chemical messengers that control neural function. They selectively cause excitation or inhibition of action potentials. Three major types of neurotransmitters are known—amino acids, neuropeptides, and monoamines. Neurotransmitters interact with cell membrane receptors to produce either excitatory or inhibitory actions. Neuromodulators are chemical messengers that react with membrane receptors to produce slower and longer-acting changes in membrane permeability. Neurotrophic or growth factors, also released from presynaptic terminals, are required to maintain the long-term survival of postsynaptic neurons.

Developmental Organization of the Nervous System

The organization of the nervous system can be described in terms of its development, in which newer functions and greater complexity resulted from the modification and enlargement of more primitive structures. Thus, the rostral or front end of the CNS became specialized, with the more ancient organization retained in the brain stem and spinal cord. The dominance of the front end of the CNS is reflected in what is termed a *hierarchy of control*: the forebrain has control over the brain stem, which has control over the spinal cord. As newer functions became concentrated at the **rostral** end, they also became more vulnerable. This is exemplified by the persistent vegetative state, which occurs when severe brain injury causes irreversible damage to higher cortical centers, whereas lower stem centers such as those that control breathing remain functional.

Embryonic Development

All body tissues and organs develop from the three embryonic layers (*i.e.*, ectoderm, mesoderm, and endoderm) that were present during the third week of embryonic life. The body is organized into the soma and viscera. The soma include all of the structures derived from the embryonic ectoderm, such as the epidermis of the skin and the CNS. Mesodermal connective tissues of the soma include the dermis of the skin, skeletal muscle, bone, and the outer lining of the body cavity (*i.e.*, **parietal** pleura and peritoneum). The nervous system innervates all somatic structures plus the internal structures making up the viscera. *Viscera* include the great vessels derived from the intermediate mesoderm, the urinary system, and the gonadal structures. It also includes the inner lining of the body cavities, such as the visceral pleura and peritoneum, and the mesodermal tissues that surround the gut and its derivative organs (*e.g.*, lungs, liver, and pancreas).

The nervous system appears at week 3 of embryonic development, which influences the development and organization of many other body systems. The organization of the nervous system retains many patterns established during embryonic life. The early pattern of segmental development in the embryo is presented as a framework for understanding the nervous system.

During the second week of development, embryonic tissue consists of two layers, the endoderm and the ectoderm. At the beginning of week 3, the ectoderm invaginates and migrates between the two layers, forming a third layer called the mesoderm (Fig. 13-6). Mesoderm along the midline of the embryo forms a specialized rod of embryonic tissue called the *notochord*. The notochord and mesoderm provide the induction signal for differentiating the overlying ectoderm and form a thickened structure called the *neural plate*, the primordium of the nervous system. Within the neural plate, an axial groove (or neural groove) develops and sinks into the mesoderm, allowing its walls to fuse across the top and form an ectodermal tube called the *neural tube*. This process, called *closure*, occurs during the third and fourth weeks of gestation and is vital to embryo survival.

During embryonic development, the neural tube develops into the CNS, whereas the notochord becomes the foundation around which the vertebral column develops. The surface ectoderm separates from the neural tube and fuses over the top to become the outer layer of

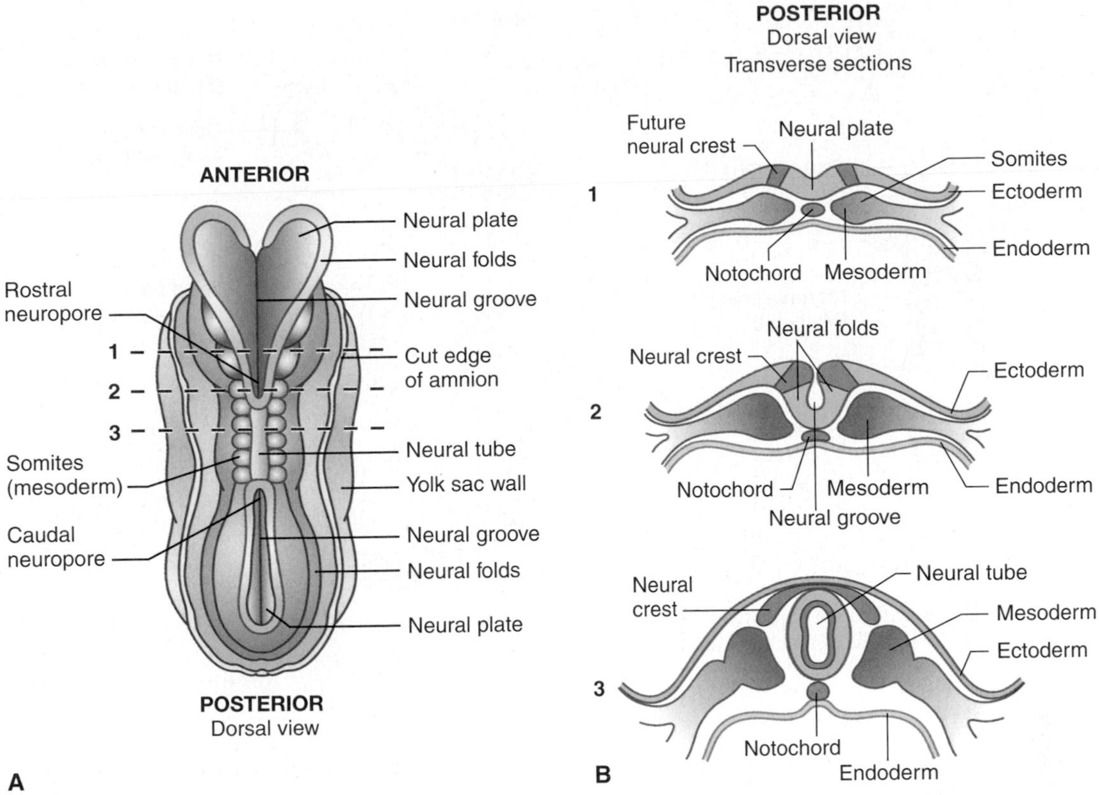

FIGURE 13-6. Folding of the neural tube. (**A**) Dorsal view of a six-somite embryo (22 to 23 days) showing the neural folds, neural groove, and fused neural tube. The anterior neuropore closes at about day 25 and the posterior neuropore at about day 27. (**B**) Three cross sections taken at the levels indicated in (**A**). The sections indicate where the neural tube is just beginning to form.

the skin. Initial closure of the neural tube begins at the cervical and high thoracic levels and zippers rostrally toward the **cephalic** end of the embryo and **caudally** toward the sacrum. Complete closure occurs around day 25 at the rostral-most end of the brain and around day 27 in the lumbosacral region.

As the neural tube closes, ectodermal cells called *neural crest cells* migrate away from the dorsal surface of the neural tube to become progenitors of the neurons and supporting cells of the PNS. Neural cell adhesion molecules decrease neural crest cell migration, and fibronectin molecules increase the formation of pathways to guide the neural crest cells. Some of these cells gather into clusters to form the *dorsal root ganglia* at the sides of each spinal cord segment and the *cranial ganglia* that are present in most brain segments. Neurons of these ganglia become afferent sensory neurons of the PNS. Other neural crest cells become pigment cells of the skin or contribute to meninges formation, structures of the face, and the peripheral ganglion cells of the autonomic nervous system (ANS), including those of the adrenal cortex.

During development, approximately 10 rostral segments of the embryonic neural tube undergo extensive modification to form the brain (Fig. 13-7). Three swellings, or primary vesicles, develop: prosencephalon, or forebrain from the first two segments; mesencephalon, or midbrain, from the third segment; and rhombencephalon, or hindbrain, from segments 4 to 10. The

brain stem is formed from modifications of the 10 rostral segments of the neural tube wall. Two pairs of outpouchings develop from the prosencephalon—the optic cup that becomes the optic nerve and retina, and the telencephalic vesicles that become cerebral hemispheres. Within the prosencephalon, the hollow central canal expands to become the CSF-filled first and second (lateral) ventricles. The remaining diencephalic portion of the neural tube develops into the thalamus and the hypothalamus. The neurohypophysis (posterior pituitary) grows as a midline ventral outgrowth at the junctions of segments 1 and 2. A dorsal outgrowth, the pineal body, develops between segments 2 and 3.

All brain segments, except segment 2, retain some portion of the basic segmental organization of the nervous system. The evolutionary development of the brain is reflected in the cranial- and upper cervical–paired segmental nerves. This reflects the original pattern of a segmented neural tube, each segment with multiple paired branches containing a group of component axons. One segment would have paired branches to body muscles, another set to visceral structures, and so on. The classic pattern of spinal nerve organization, which consists of a pair of dorsal and a pair of ventral roots, is a later evolutionary development that has not occurred in the cranial nerves (CNs). Consequently, the CNs, which are arbitrarily numbered 1 through 12, retain the ancient pattern, with more than one CN branching from a single segment. The truly segmental nerve pattern of the CNs

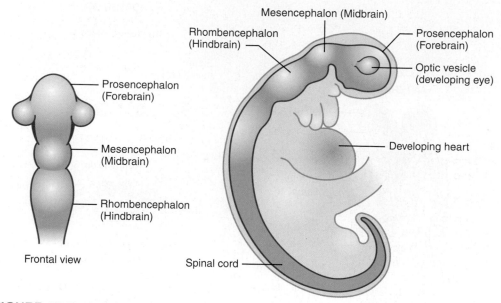

FIGURE 13-7. Frontal and lateral views of a 5-week-old embryo showing the brain vesicles and three embryonic divisions of the brain and brain stem.

is altered because all branches from segment 2 and most of the branches from segment 1 are missing. CN II, also called the *optic nerve*, is not a segmental nerve. It is a brain tract connecting the retina with the first forebrain segment from which it developed.

KEY POINTS

The Developmental Organization of the Nervous System

■ In the process of development, the basic organizational pattern is that of a longitudinal series of segments, each repeating the same basic fundamental organizational pattern: a body wall or soma containing the axial skeleton and a neural tube that develops into the nervous system.

■ As the nervous system develops, it becomes segmented, with a repeating pattern of afferent neuron axons forming the dorsal roots of each succeeding segmental nerve and the exiting efferent neurons forming the ventral roots of each succeeding segmental nerve.

Segmental Organization

Developmentally, the basic organizational pattern of the body is that of a longitudinal series of segments, each repeating a fundamental pattern. Although the early muscular, skeletal, vascular, and excretory systems and

the nerves that supply the somatic and visceral structures have the same segmental pattern, nervous system most clearly retains this organization in postnatal life. The CNS and its associated peripheral nerves consist of approximately 43 segments, 33 of which form the spinal cord and spinal nerves and the remaining 10 form the brain and its CNs.

Bilateral pairs of bundled nerve fibers, or roots—a ventral pair and a dorsal pair—accompany each segment of the CNS (Fig. 13-8). The paired dorsal roots connect

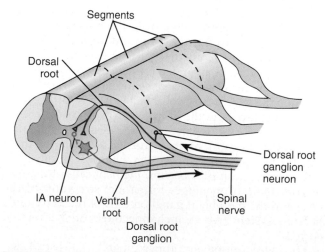

FIGURE 13-8. In this diagram of three segments of the spinal cord, three dorsal roots enter the dorsal lateral surface of the cord, and three ventral roots exit. The dorsal root ganglion contains dorsal root ganglion cells, whose axons bifurcate: one process enters the spinal cord in the dorsal root, and the other extends peripherally to supply the skin and muscle of the body. The ventral root is formed by axons from motoneurons in the spinal cord. IA, input association.

a pair of dorsal root ganglia and their corresponding CNS segment. The dorsal root ganglia contain many afferent nerve cell bodies, each having two axon-like processes—one that ends in a peripheral receptor and the other that enters the central neural segment. These axon-like processes that enter the central neural segment communicate with *input association* (IA) *neuron*s. Somatic afferent (SA) neurons transmit information from the soma to somatic IA (SIA) neurons, and visceral afferent (VA) neurons transmit information from the viscera to visceral IA (VIA) neurons. The paired ventral roots of each segment are bundles of axons that provide efferent output to effector sites.

On cross section, the embryonic neural tube can be divided into a central canal, or ventricle, containing CSF, and the wall of the tube. The latter develops into an inner gray portion, which is functionally divided into longitudinal columns of neurons called *cell columns*. These contain nerve cell bodies surrounded by a superficial white matter region containing the longitudinal tract systems of the CNS. These tract systems are composed of many nerve cell processes. The dorsal half, or *dorsal horn* of the gray matter, contains afferent neurons. The ventral portion, or *ventral horn*, contains efferent neurons that communicate by way of the ventral roots with effector cells of the body segment. Many CNS neurons develop axons that grow longitudinally as tract systems that communicate between adjacent and distal segments of the neural tube.

Cell Columns

The organizational structure of the nervous system can be described as a pattern in which functionally specific PNS and CNS neurons are repeated as parallel cell columns running lengthwise along the nervous system. In this pattern, afferent neurons, dorsal horn cells, and ventral horn cells are organized as a bilateral series of 11 cell columns.

The cell columns on each side can be further grouped according to their location in the PNS—four in the dorsal root ganglia that contain sensory neurons, four in the dorsal horn containing sensory IA neurons, and three in the ventral horn that contains motor neurons (Fig. 13-9).

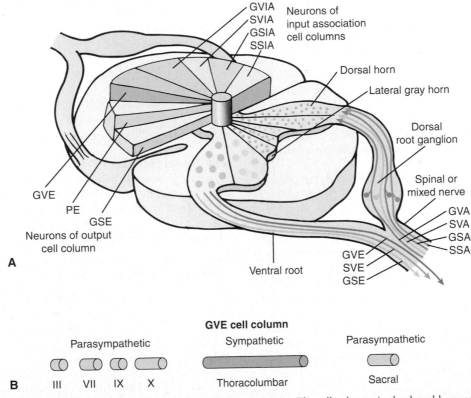

FIGURE 13-9. (A) Cell columns of the central nervous system. The cell columns in the dorsal horn contain input association (IA) neurons for the general visceral afferent (GVA), special visceral afferent (SVA), special sensory afferent (SSA), and general somatic afferent (GSA) neurons with cell bodies in the dorsal root ganglion. The cell columns in the ventral horn contain the general visceral efferent (GVE), pharyngeal efferent (PE), general visceral input association neurons (GVIA), specialized visceral input association neurons (SVIA), generalized somatic input association neurons (GSIA), specialized somatic input association neurons (SSIA) and general somite efferent (GSE) neurons, special visceral efferent (SVE) and their output association neurons. **(B)** Schematic of the GVE cell column showing both parasympathetic and sympathetic components. The column is not continuous but is interrupted in the brain stem because only the nuclei of cranial nerves III, VII, IX, and X contain preganglionic parasympathetic neurons. The column again is interrupted until levels T1 to L1 or L2, where the preganglionic neurons of the sympathetic portion are found in the lateral horn of the spinal cord. Another gap is evident until the sacral portion of the parasympathetic nervous system.

Each column of dorsal root ganglia projects to its column of IA neurons in the dorsal horn, which then distribute the afferent information to local reflex circuits and to rostral and elaborate segments of the CNS. The ventral horns contain output association (OA) neurons and lower motor neurons (LMNs). The LMNs provide the final circuitry for organizing efferent nerve activity.

Between the IA and OA neurons are networks of internuncial (interneuronal) neurons. Most of the billions of CNS cells in the spinal cord and brain gray matter are internuncial neurons.

Dorsal Horn Cell Columns

Four columns of afferent neurons in the dorsal root ganglia directly innervate four corresponding columns of IA neurons in the dorsal horn. These columns are categorized as special and general afferents: special SA, general SA, special VA, and general VA (see Fig. 13-9).

Special SA fibers are concerned with internal sensory information such as joint and tendon sensation. Neurons in the special SIA column cells relay information to local reflexes concerned with posture and movement, to the cerebellum, contributing to coordination of movement, and to the forebrain, contributing to experience. Afferents innervating the labyrinth and derived auditory end organs of the inner ear also belong to the special SA category.

General SAs innervate the skin and other somatic structures and respond to stimuli such as those that produce pressure or pain. General SIA column cells relay the sensory information to protective and other reflex circuits and project the information to the forebrain, where it is perceived as painful, warm, cold, and the like.

Special VA cells innervate specialized gut-related receptors, such as taste buds and olfactory mucosal receptors. Central processes communicate with special VIA column neurons that project to reflex circuits producing salivation, chewing, swallowing, and other responses. Forebrain projection fibers from these association cells provide sensations of taste and smell.

General VA neurons innervate visceral structures such as the gastrointestinal tract, urinary bladder, and heart and great vessels. They project to the general VIA column, which relays information to vital reflex circuits and sends information to the forebrain regarding visceral sensations such as stomach fullness, bladder pressure, and sexual experience.

Ventral Horn Cell Columns

The ventral horn contains three longitudinal cell columns—general visceral efferent, pharyngeal efferent, and general somatic efferent—each containing OA and efferent neurons (see Fig. 13-9). OA neurons coordinate and integrate the function of efferent motor neurons of their column.

General visceral efferent neurons transmit the efferent output of the ANS and are called *preganglionic neurons*. These neurons are structurally and functionally divided into sympathetic or parasympathetic nervous systems. Their axons project through segmental ventral roots to innervate smooth and cardiac muscle and glandular cells, most of which are in the viscera. In the viscera, three additional neural crest–derived cell columns are present on each side of the body. These become the postganglionic neurons of the ANS. In the sympathetic nervous system, the paravertebral ganglia and the prevertebral series of ganglia associated with the dorsal aorta represent the columns. For the parasympathetic system, these become the enteric **plexus** in the wall of the gut-derived organs and a series of ganglia in the head.

Pharyngeal efferent neurons innervate branchial arch skeletal muscles—the muscles of mastication and facial expression and muscles of the pharynx and larynx. Pharyngeal efferent neurons also innervate muscles responsible for moving the head.

The *general somatic efferent* neurons supply somite-derived muscles of the body and head, which include the skeletal muscles of the body and limbs, the tongue, and the extrinsic eye muscles. These efferent neurons transmit the commands of the CNS to peripheral effectors, the skeletal muscles. They are the "final common pathway neurons" in the sequence leading to motor activity. They are often called *LMNs* because they are under the control of higher levels of the CNS. LMNs have their cell bodies in the brain stem and spinal cord.

Peripheral Nerves

Peripheral nerves, including cranial and spinal nerves, contain afferent and efferent processes of more than one of the four afferent and three efferent cell columns. This provides the basis for assessing the function of any peripheral nerve (Table 13-1).

Longitudinal Tracts

The gray matter of the cell columns in the CNS is surrounded by bundles of myelinated axons and unmyelinated axons that travel longitudinally along the length of the neural axis. This white matter can be divided into three layers—inner, middle, and outer layer (Fig. 13-10). The inner layer, or *archilayer*, contains short fibers that project for a maximum of approximately five segments before reentering the gray matter. The middle layer, or *paleolayer*, projects to six or more segments. Archilayer and paleolayer fibers have many branches, or **collaterals**, that enter the gray matter of intervening segments. In the outer layer, or *neolayer*, large-diameter axons that

TABLE 13-1 The Segmental Nerves and Their Components

Segment and Nerve	Component	Innervation	Function
1. Forebrain			
I. Olfactory	SVA	Receptors in olfactory mucosa	Reflexes, olfaction (smell)
2. II. Optic nerve		Optic nerve and retina (part of brain system, not a peripheral nerve)	
3. Midbrain			
V. Trigeminal (V₁) ophthalmic division	SSA	Muscles: upper face: forehead, upper lid	Facial expression, proprioception
	GSA	Skin, subcutaneous tissue; conjunctiva; frontal/ethmoid sinuses	Somesthesia
			Reflexes (blink)
III. Oculomotor	GVE	Iris sphincter	Pupillary constriction
		Ciliary muscle	Accommodation
	GSE	Extrinsic eye muscles	Eye movement, lid movement
4. Pons			
V. Trigeminal (V₂) maxillary division	SSA	Muscles: facial expression	Proprioception
			Reflexes (sneeze), somesthesia
	GSA	Skin, oral mucosa, upper teeth, hard palate, maxillary sinus	
V. Trigeminal (V₃) mandibular division	SSA	Lower jaw, muscles: mastication	Proprioception, jaw jerk
	GSA	Skin, mucosa, teeth, anterior two thirds of the tongue	Reflexes, somesthesia
	PE	Muscles: mastication	Mastication: speech
		Tensor tympani	Protects the ear from loud sounds
		Tensor veli palatini	Tenses the soft palate
IV. Trochlear	GSE	Extrinsic eye muscle	Moves the eye down and in
5. Caudal Pons			
VIII. Vestibular, cochlear (vestibulocochlear)	SSA	Vestibular end organs	Reflexes, sense of head position
		Organ of Corti	Reflexes, hearing
VII. Facial nerve, intermedius portion	GSA	External auditory meatus	Somesthesia
	GVA	Nasopharynx	Gag reflex: sensation
	SVA	Taste buds of anterior two thirds of the tongue	Reflexes: gustation (taste)
	GVE	Nasopharynx	Mucus secretion, reflexes
		Lacrimal, sublingual, submandibular glands	Lacrimation, salivation
Facial nerve	PE	Muscles: facial expression, stapedius	Facial expression
			Protects the ear from loud sounds
VI. Abducens	GSE	Extrinsic eye muscle	Lateral eye deviation
6. Middle Medulla			
IX. Glossopharyngeal	SSA	Stylopharyngeus muscle	Proprioception
	GSA	Posterior external ear	Somesthesia
	SVA	Taste buds of posterior one third of the tongue	Gustation (taste)
	GVA	Oral pharynx	Gag reflex: sensation
	GVE	Parotid gland; pharyngeal mucosa	Salivary reflex: mucous secretion
	PE	Stylopharyngeus muscle	Assists swallowing
7–10. Caudal Medulla			
X. Vagus	SSA	Muscles: pharynx, larynx	Proprioception
	GSA	Posterior external ear	Somesthesia
	SVA	Taste buds, pharynx, larynx	Reflexes, gestation
	GVA	Visceral organs (esophagus to midtransverse colon, liver, pancreas, heart, lungs)	Reflexes, sensation
	GVE		Parasympathetic efferent
	PE	Visceral organs as above	Swallowing, phonation, emesis
		Muscles: pharynx, larynx	
XII. Hypoglossal	GSE	Muscles of the tongue	Tongue movement, reflexes

(continued)

TABLE 13-1 The Segmental Nerves and Their Components (*continued*)

Segment and Nerve	Component	Innervation	Function
Spinal Segments			
C1–C4 Upper Cervical	PE	Muscles: sternocleidomastoid, trapezius	Head, shoulder movement
XI. Spinal accessory nerve			
Spinal nerves	SSA	Muscles of the neck	Proprioception, DTRs
	GSA	Neck, back of the head	Somesthesia
	GSE	Neck muscles	Head, shoulder movement
C5–C8 Lower Cervical	SSA	Upper limb muscles	Proprioception, DTRs
	GSA	Upper limbs	Reflexes, somesthesia
	GSE	Upper limb muscles	Movement, posture
T1–L2 Thoracic, Upper Lumbar	SSA	Muscles: trunk, abdominal wall	Proprioception
	GSA	Trunk, abdominal wall	Reflexes, somesthesia
	GVA	All of viscera	Reflexes and sensation
	GVE	All of viscera	Sympathetic reflexes, vasomotor control, sweating, piloerection
	GSE	Muscles: trunk, abdominal wall, back	Movement, posture, respiration
L2–S1 Lower Lumbar, Upper Sacral	SSA	Lower limb muscles	Proprioception, DTRs
	GSA	Lower trunk, limbs, back	Reflexes, somesthesia
	GSE	Muscles: trunk, lower limbs, back	Movement, posture
S2–S4 Lower Sacral	SSA	Muscles: pelvis, perineum	Proprioception
	GSA	Pelvis, genitalia	Reflexes, somesthesia
	GVA	Hindgut, bladder, uterus	Reflexes, sensation
	GVE	Hindgut, visceral organs	Visceral reflexes, defecation, urination, erection
S5–Co2 Lower Sacral, Coccygeal	SSA	Perineal muscles	Proprioception
	GSA	Lower sacrum, anus	Reflexes, somesthesia
	GSE	Perineal muscles	Reflexes, posture

Afferent (sensory) components: GSA, general somatic afferent; GVA, general visceral afferent; SSA, special somatic afferent; SVA, special visceral afferent. Efferent (motor) components: DTRs, deep tendon reflexes; GSE, general somatic efferent; GVE, general visceral efferent (autonomic nervous system); PE, pharyngeal efferent.

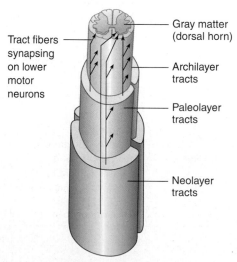

FIGURE 13-10. The three concentric subdivisions of the tract systems of the white matter. Migration of neurons into the archilayer converts it into the reticular formation of the white matter.

Tract fibers synapsing on lower motor neurons

Gray matter (dorsal horn)

Archilayer tracts

Paleolayer tracts

Neolayer tracts

can travel the entire length of the nervous system are found (Table 13-2). *Suprasegmental* is a term that refers to higher levels of the CNS, such as the brain stem and cerebrum, and structures above a given CNS segment. Paleolayer and neolayer fibers have suprasegmental projections.

The longitudinal layers are arranged in bundles, or fiber tracts, that contain axons that have the same destination, origin, and function (Fig. 13-11). These tracts are named systematically to reflect their origin and destination; the origin is named first, and the destination is named second.

The Inner Layer

Lying deep to the superficial gray matter, the inner layer of white matter contains the axons of neurons that connect neighboring segments of the nervous system. Axons of this layer permit motor neurons of several segments to work together as a functional unit. They also allow the afferent neurons of one segment to trigger reflexes that activate

TABLE 13-2 Characteristics of the Concentric Subdivisions of the Longitudinal Tracts in the White Matter of the Central Nervous System

Characteristics	Archilayer Tracts	Paleolayer Tracts	Neolayer Tracts
Segmental span	Intersegmental (<5 segments)	Suprasegmental (≥5 segments)	Suprasegmental
Number of synapses	Multisynaptic	Multisynaptic but fewer than archilayer tracts	Monosynaptic with target structures
Conduction velocity	Very slow	Fast	Fastest
Examples of functional systems	Flexor withdrawal reflex circuitry	Spinothalamic tracts	Corticospinal tracts

motor units in neighboring segments as well as in the same one. From the standpoint of evolutionary development, this is the oldest of the three layers, and it is sometimes called the *archilayer*. It is the first of the longitudinal layers to be functional and its circuitry may be limited to reflex types of movements, including reflex movements of the fetus that begin during the fifth month of intrauterine life.

The inner layer of the white matter differs from the other two layers in one important aspect. Many neurons in the embryonic gray matter migrate out into this layer, resulting in a rich mixture of neurons and local fibers called the *reticular formation*. The circuitry of most reflexes is contained in the reticular formation. In the brain stem, the reticular formation becomes large and contains major portions of vital reflexes, such as those controlling respiration, cardiovascular function, swallowing, and vomiting. A functional system called the *reticular activating system* operates in the lateral portions of the reticular formation of the medulla, pons, and especially the midbrain. Information derived from all sensory modalities, including those of the somesthetic, auditory, visual, and VA nerves, bombards the neurons of this system.

The reticular activating system has descending and ascending portions. The descending portion communicates with all spinal segmental levels through paleo-level reticulospinal tracts and serves to facilitate many cord-level reflexes. For example, it speeds reaction time and stabilizes postural reflexes. The ascending portion accelerates brain activity, particularly thalamic and cortical activity. This is reflected by the appearance of awake-type patterns of brain wave activity. Sudden stimuli result in protective and attentive postures and increased awareness.

The Middle Layer
The middle layer of the white matter contains most of the major fiber tract systems required for sensation and movement, including the ascending spinoreticular and spinothalamic tracts. This layer consists of larger-diameter and longer suprasegmental fibers, which ascend to the brain stem and are largely functional at birth. These tracts

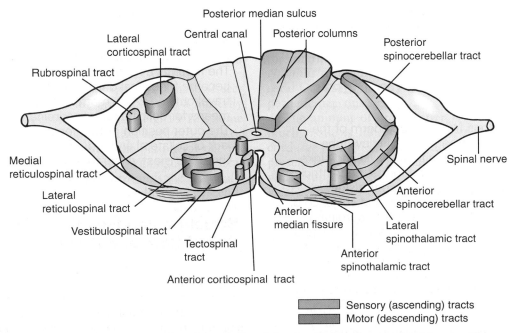

Sensory (ascending) tracts
Motor (descending) tracts

FIGURE 13-11. Transverse section of the spinal cord showing selected sensory and motor tracts. The tracts are bilateral but are indicated only on one half of the cord.

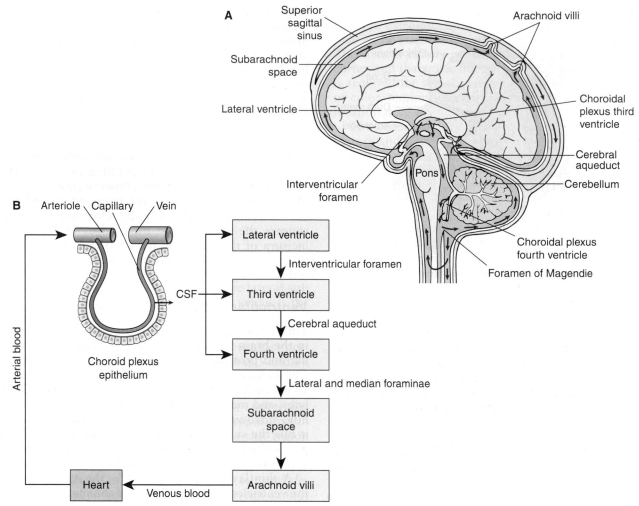

FIGURE 13-22. **(A)** The flow of cerebrospinal fluid (CSF) from the time of its formation from blood in the choroid plexuses until its return to the blood in the superior sagittal sinus. Plexuses in the lateral ventricles are not illustrated. **(B)** CSF is a blood filtrate produced by the choroid plexus epithelium that is found in each brain ventricle. The CSF from the lateral ventricles flows through the interventricular foramen (Monro) into the third ventricle. From the third ventricle, CSF is conveyed to the fourth ventricle via the cerebral aqueduct (Sylvius). Three openings, a midline foramen of Magendie and two lateral foramen (Luschka), pass the CSF into the subarachnoid space, where it is returned to the venous circulation through the arachnoid villi.

TABLE 13-3 Composition of Cerebrospinal Fluid Compared with Plasma

Substance	Plasma	Cerebrospinal Fluid
Protein (mg/dL)	6000.00	20.00
Na^+ (mEq/L)	135.00	131.00
Cl^- (mEq/L)	101.00	124.00
K^+ (mEq/L)	4.50	2.90
HCO_3^- (mEq/L)	25.00	24.00
pH	7.4	7.32
Glucose (mg/dL)	92.00	61.00

Reabsorption of CSF into the vascular system occurs along a pressure gradient. The normal CSF pressure is in the range of 60 to 180 mm H_2O.[7] The microstructure of the arachnoid villi is such that if the CSF pressure falls below approximately 50 mm H_2O, the passageways collapse, and reverse flow is blocked. Thus, the arachnoid villi function as one-way valves, permitting CSF outflow into the venous blood of the sagittal sinus but not allowing blood to pass into the arachnoid spaces.

Blood–Brain and Cerebrospinal Fluid–Brain Barriers

Maintenance of a chemically stable environment is essential to the function of the brain. In most regions of the body, extracellular fluid undergoes small fluctuations in pH and concentrations of hormones, amino acids, and potassium ions during routine daily activities. Similar fluctuations in the brain would result is uncontrolled neural activity: substances such as amino acids act as neurotransmitters, and ions such as potassium influence neural firing threshold. Two barriers, the blood–brain barrier and the CSF, maintain the stable chemical environment of the brain. Only water, carbon dioxide, and oxygen enter the brain with relative ease; the transport of other substances between the brain and the blood is slower and more controlled.

The blood–brain barrier depends on unique characteristics of brain capillaries. Endothelial cells of brain capillaries are joined by continuous tight junctions. In addition, most brain capillaries are surrounded by a basement membrane and by the processes of supporting cells of the brain, called *astrocytes* (Fig. 13-23). The blood–brain barrier permits passage of essential substances while excluding unwanted materials. Reverse transport systems remove materials from the brain. Large molecules, such as proteins and peptides, are largely excluded from crossing the blood–brain barrier. Acute cerebral lesions, such as trauma and infection, increase the permeability of the blood–brain barrier and alter brain concentrations of proteins, water, and electrolytes.

The blood–brain barrier prevents many drugs from entering the brain. Most highly water-soluble compounds are excluded from the brain, especially molecules with high ionic charge. In contrast, many lipid-soluble molecules cross the blood–brain barrier with ease. Some drugs, like alcohol, nicotine, and heroin, are highly lipid-soluble and therefore enter the brain readily. Substances that enter the capillary endothelium may be converted by metabolic processes to a chemical form incapable of moving into the brain.

The cerebral capillaries are much more permeable at birth than in adulthood, and the blood–brain barrier develops during the early years of life. In severely jaundiced infants, bilirubin can cross the immature blood–brain barrier, producing kernicterus and brain damage. In adults, the mature blood–brain barrier prevents bilirubin from entering the brain and the nervous system is spared.

The ependymal cells covering the choroid plexus are linked together by tight junctions, forming a blood–CSF barrier between the blood plasma and CSF. Water is transported through choroid epithelial cells by osmosis. Oxygen and carbon dioxide move into the CSF by diffusion, resulting in partial pressures roughly equal to those of plasma. The high sodium and low potassium of the CSF is actively regulated and kept relatively constant. Lipids and nonpeptide hormones diffuse through the barrier easily, but large molecules, such as proteins, peptides, many antibiotics, and other medications, do not normally get through. The choroid epithelium uses energy in the form of adenosine triphosphate to actively secrete many components into the CSF, including proteins, sodium ions, and several micronutrients such as vitamins C and B_6 (pyridoxine) and folate. Because the resultant CSF has a relatively high sodium content, the negatively charged chloride and bicarbonate diffuse into the CSF along an ionic gradient. The choroid cells also generate bicarbonate from carbon dioxide in the blood. This bicarbonate is important for regulating the pH of CSF.

Mechanisms exist that facilitate the transport of other molecules such as glucose without energy expenditure. Ammonia, a toxic metabolite of neuronal activity, is converted to glutamine by astrocytes. Glutamine moves by facilitated diffusion through the choroid epithelium into the plasma. Because the brain and spinal cord have no lymphatic channels, the CSF serves this function of removing toxic waste products from the CNS.

Several specific areas of the brain do not have a blood–CSF barrier. One such area is at the caudal end of the fourth ventricle (*i.e.*, area postrema), where specialized receptors for the CSF carbon dioxide level influence respiratory function. Another area is the walls of the third ventricle, which permit hypothalamic neurons to monitor blood glucose levels. Although most of the cells lining the third ventricle are ependymal cells, modified ependymal cells called *tanycytes* are also present. Processes of tanycytes extend through the glial lining of the third ventricle to terminate on blood vessels, neurons, or glial cells of the surrounding brain tissue.

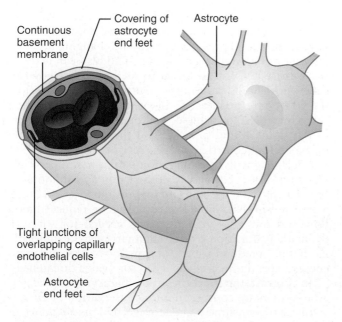

Continuous basement membrane

Covering of astrocyte end feet

Astrocyte

Tight junctions of overlapping capillary endothelial cells

Astrocyte end feet

FIGURE 13-23. The three components of the blood–brain barrier: the astrocyte and astrocyte end feet that encircle the capillary, the capillary basement membrane, and the tight junctions that join the overlapping capillary endothelial cells.

SUMMARY CONCEPTS

In the adult, the spinal cord is in the upper two thirds of the spinal canal of the vertebral column. Internally, the gray matter has the appearance of a butterfly or letter "H." The dorsal horns contain the IA neurons and receive afferent information from dorsal root and other connecting neurons.

The ventral horns contain the OA neurons and efferent LMNs that leave the cord by the ventral roots. Thirty-one pairs of spinal nerves (*i.e.*, 8 cervical, 12 thoracic, 5 lumbar, 5 sacral, and 1 coccygeal) are present. Each pair communicates with its corresponding body segments. The spinal nerves and the blood vessels that supply the spinal cord enter the spinal canal through an intervertebral foramen. After entering the foramen, they divide into two branches, or roots, one of which enters the dorsolateral surface of the cord (*i.e.*, dorsal root), carrying the axons of afferent neurons into the CNS. The other root leaves the ventrolateral surface of the cord (*i.e.*, ventral root), carrying the axons of efferent neurons into the periphery. These two roots fuse at the intervertebral foramen, forming the mixed spinal nerve.

A reflex provides a highly reliable relation between a stimulus and a motor response. Its anatomic basis consists of an afferent (sensory) neuron, the connection with CNS neurons that communicate with the effector (motor) neuron, and the effector neuron that innervates a muscle or organ. Reflexes allow the sensory pathway for an involuntary motor response to a stimulus.

The brain can be divided into three parts—the hindbrain, the midbrain, and the forebrain. The hindbrain, consisting of the medulla oblongata, pons, and cerebellum, contains the neuronal circuits for the eating, breathing, and locomotive functions required for survival. CNs III and IV arise from the midbrain, and CNs XII, XI, X, IX, VIII, VII, VI, and V are located in the hindbrain. The forebrain consists of the diencephalon and the telencephalon. The dorsal horn part of the diencephalon comprises the thalamus and subthalamus, and the ventral horn part is the hypothalamus. The cerebral hemispheres are lateral outgrowths of the diencephalon.

The cerebral hemispheres are divided into lobes—frontal, parietal, temporal, and occipital—named after the bones of the skull that cover them. The prefrontal premotor area and primary motor cortex are in the frontal lobe; the primary sensory cortex and somesthetic association area are in the parietal cortex; the primary auditory cortex and auditory association area are in the temporal lobe; and the primary visual cortex and association visual cortex are in the occipital lobe. The limbic system, which is involved in emotional experience and behaviors, is located in the medial cerebrum. Cortical areas are reciprocally connected with underlying thalamic nuclei through the internal capsule. Thalamic involvement is essential for normal forebrain function.

The brain is enclosed and protected by the dura, arachnoid, and pia mater. The CSF, in which the brain and spinal cord float, isolates them from minor and moderate trauma. CSF is secreted into the ventricles by the ependymal cells of the choroid plexus, circulates through the ventricular system, and is reabsorbed into the venous system through arachnoid villi. The CSF and blood–brain barrier protect the brain from substances in the blood that would disrupt brain function.

The Autonomic Nervous System

The ability to maintain homeostasis and perform the activities of daily living in an ever-changing physical environment is largely vested in the ANS. The ANS is involved in regulating, adjusting, and coordinating vital visceral functions such as blood pressure and blood flow, body temperature, respiration, digestion, metabolism, and elimination. It is strongly affected by emotional influences: blushing, pallor, palpitations of the heart, clammy hands, and dry mouth are several emotional expressions mediated through the ANS. Biofeedback and relaxation exercises have been used for modifying the subconscious functions of the ANS.

As with the somatic nervous system, the ANS is represented in both the CNS and the PNS. The efferent outflow from the ANS has two divisions—the sympathetic nervous system and the parasympathetic nervous system.[8] The two divisions of the ANS are viewed as having opposite and antagonistic actions. Exceptions are functions, such as sweating and regulation of arteriolar blood vessel diameter, which are controlled by the sympathetic nervous system.

The functions of the sympathetic nervous system include maintaining body temperature and adjusting blood vessels and blood pressure to meet the changing needs of the body. The sympathoadrenal system also can activate when there is a critical threat to the individual—the so-called fight-or-flight response. During a stress situation, the heart rate accelerates; blood pressure rises; blood sugar increases; bronchioles and pupils dilate; sphincters of the stomach and intestine and the internal sphincter of the urethra constrict; and the rate of secretion of exocrine glands involved in digestion diminishes. Emergency situations often require vasoconstriction and shunting of blood away from the skin and into the muscles and brain, a mechanism that, should a wound occur, reduces blood flow and preserves vital functions needed for survival. Sympathetic function is often summarized as "catabolic": its actions predominate during periods of pronounced energy expenditure, such as when survival is threatened.

In contrast, the functions of the parasympathetic nervous system are concerned with conservation of energy, resource replenishment and storage, and maintenance of organ function—the *rest–digest* response. This system slows heart rate, stimulates gastrointestinal function and related glandular secretion, promotes bowel and bladder elimination, and contracts the pupil, protecting the retina from excessive light during periods when visual function is not vital to survival.

The sympathetic and parasympathetic nervous systems are continually active. The *tone* of an effector organ or system can be increased or decreased and is usually regulated by a single division of the ANS (*e.g.*, vascular smooth muscle tone is controlled by the sympathetic nervous system). Increased sympathetic activity produces local vasoconstriction from increased vascular smooth muscle tone, and decreased activity results in vasodilation because of decreased tone. In structures such as the sinoatrial node and atrioventricular node of the heart, which are innervated by both divisions of the ANS, one division predominates in controlling tone. In this case, the parasympathetic nervous system exerts a braking effect on heart rate, and when parasympathetic outflow is withdrawn, the heart rate increases. The increase in heart rate that occurs with vagal withdrawal can be further augmented by sympathetic stimulation. Table 13-4 describes the responses of effector organs to sympathetic and parasympathetic impulses.

KEY POINTS

The Autonomic Nervous System
- The ANS is responsible for maintaining homeostatic functions of the body.
- The ANS has two divisions—sympathetic and parasympathetic. Although the two divisions function together, they are generally viewed as having opposite and antagonistic actions.

Autonomic Efferent Pathways

ANS outflow follows a two-neuron pathway. The first motor neuron, the *preganglionic neuron*, lies in the intermediolateral cell column of the spinal cord or its equivalent location in the brain stem. The second motor neuron, the *postganglionic neuron*, synapses with a preganglionic neuron in an autonomic ganglion in the PNS. The two divisions of the ANS differ as to location of preganglionic cell bodies, relative length of preganglionic fibers, the nature of their peripheral responses, and their preganglionic and postganglionic neurotransmitters (see Table 13-4). This two-neuron pathway and the interneurons in the autonomic ganglia that add further modulation to ANS function are distinctly different from arrangements in the somatic nervous system.

Most visceral organs are innervated by both sympathetic and parasympathetic fibers (Fig. 13-24). Exceptions include blood vessels and sweat glands that have input from only one division. Sympathetic actions, in which fibers are distributed throughout the body, tend to be more diffuse than parasympathetic actions, in which fibers are more localized. Preganglionic fibers of the sympathetic nervous system may traverse a considerable distance and pass through several ganglia before synapsing with postganglionic neurons, and their terminals contact many postganglionic fibers. The ratio of preganglionic to postganglionic cells may be up to 1:20. The parasympathetic nervous system, on the other hand, has its postganglionic neurons located near or in the target organ. Because the ratio of preganglionic to postganglionic communication is often 1:1, the effects of the parasympathetic nervous system are much more circumscribed.

Sympathetic Nervous System

The neurons of the sympathetic nervous system, also called the *thoracolumbar division* of the ANS, are located primarily in the intermediolateral cell column from T1 to L2.[8] These preganglionic neurons have short, largely myelinated axons. Postganglionic neurons are located in the paravertebral ganglia that lie on either side of the vertebral column or in prevertebral sympathetic ganglia such as the celiac ganglia. The sympathetic ganglia also contain neurons of the internuncial, short-axon type, similar to those associated with complex circuitry

TABLE 13-4 Characteristics of the Sympathetic and Parasympathetic Nervous Systems

Characteristic	Sympathetic Outflow	Parasympathetic Outflow
Location of preganglionic cell bodies	T1–T12, L1 and L2	CNs: III, VII (intermedius), IX, and X; sacral segments 2, 3, and 4
Relative length of preganglionic fibers	Short—to paravertebral chain of ganglia or to aortic prevertebral ganglia	Long—to ganglion cells near or in the innervated organ
General function	Catabolic—mobilizes resources in anticipation of challenge for survival (preparation for "fight-or-flight" response)	Anabolic—concerned with conservation, renewal, and storage of resources
Nature of peripheral response	Generalized	Localized
Transmitter between preganglionic terminals and postganglionic neurons	ACh	ACh
Transmitter of postganglionic neuron	ACh (sweat glands and skeletal muscle vasodilator fibers), norepinephrine (most synapses), norepinephrine and epinephrine (secreted by adrenal gland)	ACh

ACh, acetylcholine; CN, cranial nerve.

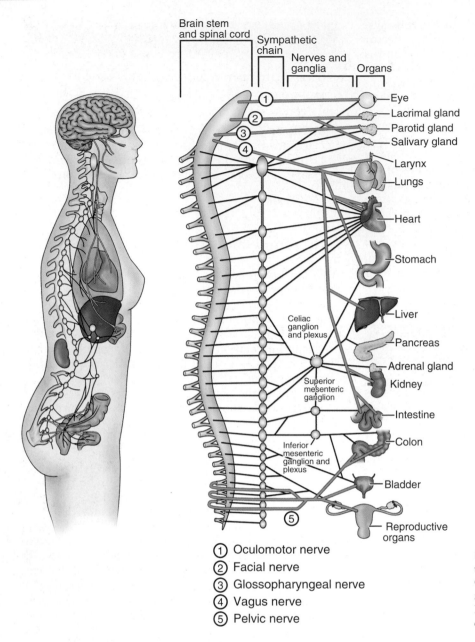

Brain stem
and spinal cord
Sympathetic
chain
Nerves and
ganglia
Organs

① Eye
② Lacrimal gland
③ Parotid gland
④ Salivary gland
Larynx
Lungs
Heart
Stomach
Celiac
ganglion
and plexus
Liver
Pancreas
Adrenal gland
Kidney
Superior
mesenteric
ganglion
Intestine
Colon
Inferior
mesenteric
ganglion and
plexus
Bladder
⑤
Reproductive
organs

① Oculomotor nerve
② Facial nerve
③ Glossopharyngeal nerve
④ Vagus nerve
⑤ Pelvic nerve

FIGURE 13-24. The anatomy of the autonomic nervous system. (From Hinkle J. L., Cheever K. H. (2018). *Brunner & Suddarth's textbook of medical-surgical nursing* (4th ed., Fig. 65-10, p. 1954). Philadelphia, PA: Lippincott Williams & Wilkins.)

in the brain and spinal cord. Many of these modulate preganglionic to postganglionic transmission.

The axons of the preganglionic neurons leave the spinal cord through the ventral roots of the spinal nerves (T1 to L2), enter the ventral primary rami, and leave the spinal nerve through white rami of the rami communicantes to reach the paravertebral ganglionic chain (Fig. 13-25). In the sympathetic chain of ganglia, preganglionic fibers may synapse with neurons of the ganglion they enter, pass up or down the chain and synapse with one or more ganglia, or pass through the chain and move outward through a splanchnic nerve to terminate in prevertebral ganglia scattered along the dorsal aorta and its branches.

Preganglionic fibers from the thoracic segments of the cord pass upward to form the cervical chain connecting the inferior, middle, and superior cervical sympathetic

ganglia with the rest of the sympathetic chain at lower levels. Postganglionic sympathetic axons of the cervical and lower lumbosacral chain ganglia spread further through nerve plexuses along continuations of the great arteries. Cranial structures, particularly blood vessels, are innervated by the spread of postganglionic axons along the external and internal carotid arteries into the face and the cranial cavity. The sympathetic fibers from T1 usually continue up the sympathetic chain into the head; those from T2 pass into the neck; those from T1 to T5 travel to the heart; those from T3, T4, T5, and T6 proceed to the thoracic viscera; those from T7, T8, T9, T10, and T11 pass to the abdominal viscera; and those from T12, L1, L2, and L3 pass to the kidneys and pelvic organs. Many preganglionic fibers from the fifth to the last thoracolumbar segments pass through the paravertebral ganglia to continue as the splanchnic nerves.

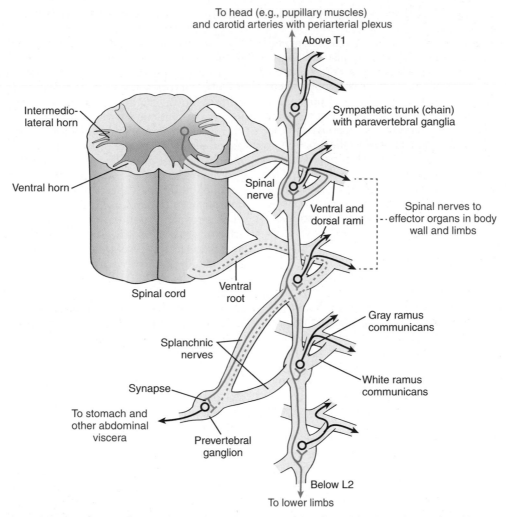

To head (e.g., pupillary muscles)
and carotid arteries with periarterial plexus

Above T1

Intermedio-
lateral horn

Sympathetic trunk (chain)
with paravertebral ganglia

Ventral horn

Spinal
nerve

Ventral and
dorsal rami

Spinal nerves to
effector organs in body
wall and limbs

Spinal cord

Ventral
root

Gray ramus
communicans

Splanchnic
nerves

White ramus
communicans

Synapse

To stomach and
other abdominal
viscera

Prevertebral
ganglion

Below L2

To lower limbs

FIGURE 13-25. Sympathetic pathways. Sympathetic preganglionic fibers (*blue*) leave the spinal cord by way of the ventral root of the spinal nerves, enter the ventral primary rami, and pass through the white rami to the prevertebral or paravertebral ganglia of the sympathetic chain, where they synapse with postganglionic neurons (*black*). Other preganglionic neurons (*orange dotted lines*) travel directly to their destination in the various effector organs.

Most of these fibers do not synapse until they reach the celiac or superior mesenteric ganglion; others pass to the adrenal medulla.

The adrenal medulla, which is part of the sympathetic nervous system, contains postganglionic sympathetic neurons that secrete sympathetic neurotransmitters into the bloodstream. Some postganglionic fibers, all of which are unmyelinated, exit the paravertebral ganglionic chain and reenter the segmental nerve through unmyelinated branches, called *gray rami*. These segmental nerves are then distributed to the body wall in spinal nerve branches. These innervate sweat glands, piloerector muscles, blood vessels of the skin and skeletal muscles, and the CNS itself.

Parasympathetic Nervous System

The preganglionic fibers of the parasympathetic nervous system, also called the *craniosacral division* of the ANS, originate in some segments of the brain stem and sacral segments of the spinal cord.[8] The midbrain outflow passes through CN III to the ciliary ganglion that lies in the orbit behind the eye; it supplies the pupillary sphincter and ciliary muscles that control lens thickness for accommodation. From the caudal pontine, outflow originates the preganglionic fibers of the intermedius component of the facial nerve CN VII. This outflow synapses in the submandibular ganglion, which sends postganglionic fibers to supply the submandibular and sublingual glands. In addition, preganglionic fibers are distributed to the pterygopalatine ganglia to synapse on postganglionic neurons that supply the lacrimal and nasal glands. Fibers in CN IX synapse in the otic ganglia, which supply the parotid salivary glands. The vagus nerve provides parasympathetic innervation for the heart, trachea, lungs, esophagus, stomach, small intestine, proximal half of the colon, liver, gallbladder, pancreas, kidneys, and upper portions of the ureters. The gastrointestinal tract has an intrinsic network of ganglionic cells located between the smooth muscle layers (the *enteric nervous system*), which controls local peristaltic and secretory functions. The enteric nervous system can be modified by ANS activity.

Sacral preganglionic axons leave the S2 to S4 segmental nerves by gathering into the pelvic nerves, also called the *nervi erigentes*. The pelvic nerves leave the sacral plexus on each side of the cord and distribute their peripheral fibers to the bladder, uterus, urethra, prostate, distal portion of the transverse colon, descending colon, and rectum. Sacral parasympathetic fibers also supply the venous outflow from the external genitalia to facilitate **erectile** function.

Except for CNs III, VII, and IX, which synapse in discrete ganglia, the long parasympathetic preganglionic fibers pass uninterrupted to short postganglionic fibers in organ walls. Here, postganglionic neurons send axons to modulate smooth muscle and glandular cell functions.

Central Integrative Pathways

General VA fibers accompany sympathetic and parasympathetic outflow into spinal nerves and CNs, bringing chemoreceptor, pressure, organ capsule stretch, and nociceptive information from organs to the brain stem, thoracolumbar cord, and sacral cord. Local reflex circuits relating VA and autonomic efferent activity are integrated into a hierarchic control system in the spinal cord and brain stem. Most visceral reflexes contain contributions from LMNs that innervate skeletal muscles as part of their response patterns.

The hypothalamus serves as the major control center for most autonomically mediated functions. The hypothalamus, with connections to the cerebral cortex, limbic system, and pituitary gland, is in a prime position to receive, integrate, and transmit information to other areas of the nervous system. Signals from the hypothalamus can affect almost all brain stem control centers. For example, stimulation of the posterior hypothalamus can cause the cardiovascular control centers to increase the arterial blood pressure to more than twice the normal. Other hypothalamic centers control body temperature and increase salivation and gastrointestinal activity.

Reflex adjustments of cardiovascular and respiratory function occur at the level of the brain stem. For example, increased blood pressure in the carotid sinus results in increased discharge from afferent fibers that travel by way of CN IX to cardiovascular centers in the brain stem. These centers increase the activity of descending efferent vagal fibers that slow heart rate, while inhibiting sympathetic fibers that increase heart rate and blood vessel tone. The ANS can change visceral function with rapidity and intensity: it can double the heart rate within 3 to 5 seconds. Bronchial smooth muscle tone is largely controlled by parasympathetic fibers carried in the vagus nerve, which produces mild to moderate constriction of the bronchioles.

Other important ANS reflexes are located at the level of the spinal cord. Spinal reflexes are modulated by input from higher centers. With loss of communication between higher centers and spinal reflexes (*i.e.*, in spinal cord injury), these reflexes function in an unregulated manner. This results in uncontrolled sweating, vasomotor instability, and reflex bowel and bladder function.

Autonomic Neurotransmission

The generation and transmission of impulses in the ANS occur in the same manner as in other neurons, with self-propagating action potentials and transmission of impulses across synapses and tissue junctions via transmitters. However, although somatic motor neurons divide into many branches, with each branch innervating a single muscle fiber, ANS postganglionic fibers form a diffuse neural plexus at the site of innervation. The membranes of many smooth muscle fibers are connected by conductive protoplasmic bridges (*gap junctions*) that permit rapid conduction through sheets of smooth muscle. Autonomic neurotransmitters released near a limited portion of these fibers provide a modulating function extending to many effector cells, as in the smooth muscle layers of the gut and bladder wall. Isolated smooth muscle cells may be individually innervated by the ANS, as with piloerector cells that elevate hair on the skin with cold exposure.

The main neurotransmitters of the ANS are acetylcholine and the catecholamines, epinephrine and norepinephrine (Fig. 13-26).[8] Acetylcholine is released at all preganglionic synapses of both sympathetic and parasympathetic nerve fibers and from postganglionic synapses of all parasympathetic nerve endings. It is also released at sympathetic nerve endings that innervate the sweat glands and cholinergic vasodilator fibers found in skeletal muscle. Norepinephrine is released at most sympathetic nerve endings. The adrenal medulla, which is a modified prevertebral sympathetic ganglion, produces epinephrine along with small amounts of norepinephrine. Dopamine, an intermediate compound in the synthesis of norepinephrine, also acts as a neurotransmitter. It is the principal inhibitory transmitter of internuncial neurons in the sympathetic ganglia. It also has vasodilator effects on renal, splanchnic, and coronary blood vessels when given intravenously and is sometimes used in the treatment of shock.

Acetylcholine and Cholinergic Receptors

Acetylcholine is synthesized in the cholinergic neurons from choline and acetyl coenzyme A (Fig. 13-27A). After acetylcholine is secreted by the cholinergic nerve endings, it is rapidly broken down by the enzyme acetylcholinesterase. The choline molecule is transported back into the nerve ending, where it is used again in the synthesis of acetylcholine.

Receptors that respond to acetylcholine are called *cholinergic receptors*. Two types of receptors are known—muscarinic and nicotinic. Muscarinic receptors are present on the targets of postganglionic fibers of the parasympathetic nervous system and on the sweat glands, which are innervated by the sympathetic nervous system. Nicotinic receptors are found in autonomic ganglia and skeletal muscle end plates. Acetylcholine is excitatory to most receptors, except those in the heart and lower esophagus where it is inhibitory. Atropine is an antimuscarinic drug that prevents the action of acetylcholine at muscarinic (but not nicotinic) receptor sites.

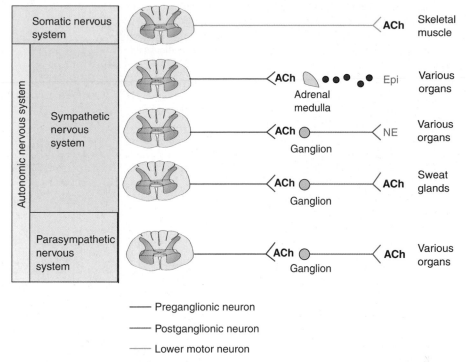

— Preganglionic neuron

— Postganglionic neuron

— Lower motor neuron

FIGURE 13-26. Comparison of neurotransmission in the somatic and autonomic nervous systems (ANS). In the somatic nervous system, all lower motor neurons release acetylcholine (ACh) as their neurotransmitter. In the ANS, both sympathetic and parasympathetic preganglionic neurons release ACh as their neurotransmitter. Parasympathetic postganglionic neurons release ACh at the site of organ innervation. Most postganglionic neurons of the sympathetic nervous system release norepinephrine (NE) at the site of organ innervation. The principal neurotransmitter released by the adrenal gland is epinephrine (Epi), which travels to the site of organ innervation through the bloodstream. The postganglionic neurons innervating the sweat gland are sympathetic fibers that use ACh as their neurotransmitter.

Catecholamines and Adrenergic Receptors

The catecholamines, which include norepinephrine, epinephrine, and dopamine, are synthesized from tyrosine in sympathetic nerve terminal endings (see Fig. 13-27B). Tyrosine is hydroxylated (*i.e.*, hydroxyl group added) to form DOPA, and DOPA is decarboxylated (*i.e.*, carboxyl group removed) to form dopamine. Dopamine in turn is hydroxylated to form norepinephrine. In the adrenal gland, norepinephrine is methylated (*i.e.*, methyl group added) to form epinephrine.

Each step in sympathetic neurotransmitter synthesis requires a different enzyme, and the type of neurotransmitter produced depends on the types of enzymes that are available. Epinephrine accounts for approximately 80% of catecholamines released from the adrenal gland. Epinephrine synthesis by the adrenal medulla is influenced by glucocorticoid secretion from the adrenal cortex. These hormones are transported through an intra-adrenal vascular network from the adrenal cortex to the adrenal medulla, where they cause the sympathetic neurons to increase their production of epinephrine through increased enzyme activity. Thus, any situation sufficiently stressful to evoke increased glucocorticoids also increases epinephrine levels. As catecholamines are synthesized, they are stored in vesicles, where the final step of norepinephrine synthesis occurs. The storage vesicles provide a means for concentrated storage of the catecholamines and protect neurotransmitters from the cytoplasmic enzymes that degrade them.

Besides neuronal synthesis, a second mechanism exists for the replenishment of norepinephrine in sympathetic nerve terminals: between 50% and 80% of norepinephrine released during an action potential is actively taken back up by the axon terminal. This stops action of the neurotransmitter and allows it to be reused. The remainder of the released catecholamines diffuse into surrounding tissue fluids or is degraded by two enzymes: catechol-*O*-methyltransferase, which is present in all tissues, and monoamine oxidase (MAO), which is found in the nerve endings. Some drugs, such as tricyclic antidepressants, are thought to increase the level of catecholamines at the site of nerve endings in the brain by blocking the reuptake process. Others, such as the MAO inhibitors, increase the levels of neurotransmitters by decreasing their enzymatic degradation.

Catecholamines can cause excitation or inhibition of smooth muscle contraction, depending on the site, dose, and type of receptor present. Norepinephrine has potent excitatory activity and low inhibitory activity. Epinephrine is potent as both an excitatory and an inhibitory agent.

In vascular smooth muscle, excitation of α receptors causes vasoconstriction, and excitation of β receptors causes vasodilation.[8] Endogenously and exogenously

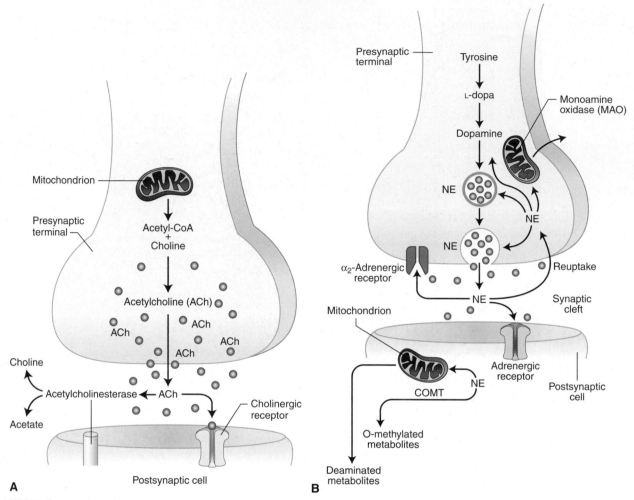

FIGURE 13-27. Schematic illustration of cholinergic parasympathetic (**A**) and noradrenergic sympathetic (**B**) neurotransmitter synthesis, release, receptor binding, neurotransmitter degradation, and metabolite transport back into the presynaptic neuron (acetylcholine) and reuptake (norepinephrine). CoA, coenzyme A; COMT, catechol-O-methyltransferase; NE, norepinephrine.

administered norepinephrine produces marked vasoconstriction of the blood vessels in the skin, kidneys, and splanchnic circulation that are supplied with α receptors. The β receptors are most prevalent in the heart, the blood vessels of skeletal muscle, and the bronchioles. Blood vessels in skeletal muscle have α and β receptors, and high levels of norepinephrine produce vasoconstriction; low levels produce vasodilation. The low levels are thought to have a diluting effect on norepinephrine levels in the arteries of these blood vessels so that the β effect predominates.

α-Adrenergic receptors have been further subdivided into α_1 and α_2 receptors and β-adrenergic receptors into β_1 and β_2 receptors. β_1-Adrenergic receptors are found primarily in the heart and can be selectively blocked by β_1 receptor–blocking drugs. β_2-Adrenergic receptors are found in the bronchioles and in other sites that have β-mediated functions. α_1-Adrenergic receptors are found primarily in postsynaptic effector sites; they mediate responses in vascular smooth muscle. α_2-Adrenergic receptors are mainly located presynaptically and can inhibit release of norepinephrine from sympathetic nerve terminals. α_2-Adrenergic receptors are abundant in the CNS and are thought to influence the central control of blood pressure.

The various classes of adrenergic receptors provide a mechanism by which the same neurotransmitter can have selective effects on different effector cells. This also permits neurotransmitters carried in the bloodstream to produce the same effects. The catecholamines produced in sympathetic nerve endings are called *endogenous neuromediators*. Sympathetic nerve endings also can be activated by *exogenous* forms of these neuromediators, which reach the bloodstream after being injected into the body or administered orally. These drugs mimic the action of neuromediators and have a **sympathomimetic** *action*. Other drugs can selectively block receptor sites and temporarily prevent the neurotransmitter from exerting its action.

SUMMARY CONCEPTS

The ANS is an efferent system that regulates, adjusts, and coordinates the visceral functions of the body and is divided into the sympathetic and parasympathetic systems. The outflow of the sympathetic and parasympathetic nervous systems follows a two-neuron pathway, which consists of a preganglionic neuron in the CNS and a postganglionic neuron outside the CNS. Sympathetic fibers leave the CNS at the thoracolumbar level, and the parasympathetic fibers leave at the craniosacral levels. The sympathetic and parasympathetic nervous systems can have opposing effects on visceral function—if one excites, the other inhibits. The hypothalamus serves as the major control center for most ANS functions; local reflex circuits relating VA and autonomic efferent activity are integrated in a hierarchic control system in the spinal cord and brain stem.

The main neurotransmitters for the ANS are acetylcholine and the catecholamines, epinephrine and norepinephrine. Acetylcholine is the transmitter for all preganglionic neurons, for postganglionic parasympathetic neurons, and for selected postganglionic sympathetic neurons. The catecholamines are the neurotransmitters for most postganglionic sympathetic neurons. Neurotransmitters exert their target action through specialized cell surface receptors—cholinergic receptors bind acetylcholine and adrenergic receptors bind the catecholamines. Cholinergic receptors are divided into nicotinic and muscarinic receptors, and adrenergic receptors are divided into α and β receptors. Different receptors for the same transmitter result in differences in response to the same transmitter. This arrangement also permits the use of pharmacologic agents that act at specific receptor types.

Review Exercises

1. An event such as cardiac arrest, which produces global ischemia of the brain, can produce a selective loss of recent memory and cognitive skills, whereas the more vegetative and life-sustaining functions such as breathing are preserved.
   A. Use principles related to the development of the nervous system and hierarchy of control to explain why.

2. Usually, spinal cord injury or disease produces both sensory and motor deficits. An exception is infection by the poliomyelitis virus, which produces weakness and paralysis without loss of sensation in the affected extremities.
   A. Explain, using information on the cell column organization of the spinal cord.

REFERENCES

1. Hammer G., McPhee S. (2013). *Pathophysiology of disease: An introduction to clinical medicine* (7th ed.). New York, NY: McGraw-Hill.
2. Waxman S. (2017). *Clinical neuroanatomy* (28th ed.). New York, NY: McGraw Hill Education.
3. Harlow D. E., Honce J. M., Miravalle A. A. (2013). Remyelination therapy in multiple sclerosis. *Frontiers in Neurology* 6, 1–13.
4. MacVicar B. A., Newman E. A. (2015). Astrocyte regulation of blood flow in the brain. *Cold Spring Harbor Perspectives in Biology* 7, 1–15.
5. Hickey J. (2013). *The clinical practice of neurological and neurosurgical nursing* (7th ed.). Philadelphia, PA: Lippincott Williams & Wilkins.
6. Tortora G., Derrickson B. (2017). *Principles of anatomy and physiology* (15th ed.). Hoboken, NJ: John Wiley & Sons.
7. Rowland L. P., Pedley T. A. (2015). *Merritt's neurology* (13th ed.). Philadelphia, PA: Lippincott Williams & Wilkins.
8. Bader M. K., Littlejohns L. R., Olson D. M. (2016). *AANN core curriculum for neuroscience nursing*. Chicago, IL: AANN.

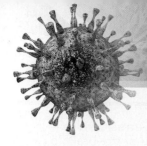

Somatosensory Function, Pain, Headache, and Temperature Regulation

Learning Objectives

After completing this chapter, the learner will be able to meet the following objectives:

1. Describe the organization of the somatosensory system in terms of first-, second-, and third-order neurons.
2. Summarize the structure and function of the dorsal root ganglion neurons in terms of sensory receptors, conduction velocities, and spinal cord projections.
3. Compare the tactile, thermal, and position sense modalities in terms of receptors, adequate stimuli, ascending pathways, and central integrative mechanisms.
4. Discuss the difference between Aδ- and C-fiber neurons in transmission of pain information.
5. Explain the transmission of pain signals with reference to the neospinothalamic, paleospinothalamic, and reticulospinal pathways, including the role of chemical mediators and factors that modulate pain transmission.
6. Define allodynia, hypoesthesia, **hyperesthesia**, paresthesias, hyperpathia, analgesia, and hypoalgesia and hyperalgesia.
7. Describe the cause, characteristics, and treatment of neuropathic pain, trigeminal neuralgia, postherpetic neuralgia, and complex regional pain syndrome.
8. Discuss the possible mechanisms of phantom limb pain.
9. Differentiate between the occurrence, manifestations, and treatment of

10. migraine headache, cluster headache, tension-type headache, and headache due to temporomandibular joint (TMJ) syndrome.
10. Cite the most common cause of TMJ pain.
11. Explain how pain response, assessment, and treatment may differ in children and older adults.
12. Differentiate between body core temperature and skin temperature.
13. Compare the differences between methods used for measuring body temperature.
14. Define the terms *conduction*, *radiation*, *convection*, and *evaporation* and relate them to the mechanisms for gain and loss of heat from the body.
15. Characterize the physiology of fever.
16. Differentiate between the physiologic mechanisms involved in fever and hyperthermia.
17. Compare the manifestations of mild, moderate, and severe hypothermia and relate them to changes in physiologic functioning that occur with decreased body temperature.
18. Describe the causes of heat loss and hypothermia in the newborn infant and in the person undergoing surgery.

The somatosensory component of the nervous system provides an awareness of body sensations such as touch, temperature, body position, and pain. The sensory receptors for somatosensory function consist of discrete nerve endings in body tissues. Two to three million sensory neurons deliver a steady stream of encoded information, most of which regulate reflex and automatic mechanisms.

Organization and Control of Somatosensory Function

The somatosensory system provides the central nervous system (CNS) with information on touch, temperature, body position, and pain. Sensory neurons can be divided into three types that vary in distribution and the type of sensation detected: general somatic, special somatic, and general visceral. *General somatic afferent neurons* have branches distributed throughout the body with distinct types of receptors for sensations, including pain, touch, and temperature.[1,2] *Special somatic afferent neurons* have receptors located primarily in muscles, tendons, and joints.[1,2] These receptors sense position and movement of the body. *General visceral afferent neurons* have receptors on various visceral structures that sense fullness and discomfort.[1,2]

Sensory Systems

Sensory systems can be conceptualized as a serial succession of neurons consisting of first-, second-, and third-order neurons. *First-order neurons* transmit sensory information from the periphery to the CNS. *Second-order neurons* communicate with various reflex

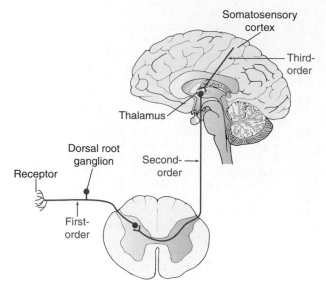

FIGURE 14-1. Arrangement of first-, second-, and third-order neurons of the somatosensory system.

networks and sensory pathways in the spinal cord and travel directly to the thalamus. *Third-order neurons* relay information from the thalamus to the cerebral cortex (Fig. 14-1).

These three primary levels of neural integration provide the organizing framework of the somatosensory system:

- The sensory units, which contain the sensory receptors
- The ascending pathways
- The central processing centers in the thalamus and cerebral cortex

Sensory information usually is relayed and processed in a cephalad (toward the head) direction by the three orders of neurons. Many interneurons process and modify the sensory information at the level of the second- and third-order neurons, and many more participate before movement responses occur. The number of participating neurons increases exponentially from the primary through the secondary and the secondary through the tertiary levels.

KEY POINTS

The Somatosensory System

- The somatosensory system relays information about four major modalities: touch, temperature, body position, and pain.

- Somatosensory information is sequentially transmitted: *first-order* neurons transmit information from sensory receptors to dorsal horn neurons; *second-order CNS association neurons* communicate with reflex circuits and transmit information to the thalamus; and *third-order neurons* forward information from the thalamus to the sensory cortex.

The Sensory Unit

The somatosensory experience arises from information provided by receptors distributed throughout the body. These receptors monitor stimulus discrimination, tactile sensation, thermal sensation, and position sensation.[1]

Somatosensory information from the limbs and trunk share a common class of sensory neurons called *dorsal root ganglion neurons*.[2] Somatosensory information from the face and cranial structures is transmitted by trigeminal sensory neurons, which function similar to the dorsal root ganglion neurons. The cell body of the dorsal root ganglion neuron, its peripheral branch (innervates an area of periphery), and its central axon (projects to the CNS) form what is called a *sensory unit*.

Fibers of the dorsal root ganglion neurons conduct impulses at rates ranging from 0.5 to 120 m/second.[1] There are three types of nerve fibers that transmit somatosensory information: type A, type B, and type C.[3] Type A fibers are myelinated and have the fastest rate of conduction. They convey cutaneous pressure and touch sensation, cold sensation, mechanical pain, and heat pain. Type B fibers are myelinated and transmit information from cutaneous and subcutaneous mechanoreceptors.[4] Unmyelinated type C fibers have the smallest diameter and slowest rate of conduction. They convey warm–hot sensation and mechanical and chemical as well as heat- and cold-induced pain sensation. A major problem in pain management is identifying the etiology of the pain. A neurometer can test the involvement of specific nerve fibers, allowing for a more comprehensive diagnosis of sensory function.[5]

Dermatomal Pattern of Dorsal Root Innervation

The somatosensory innervation of the body and head retains the basic segmental organizational pattern established during embryonic development. Thirty-three paired spinal nerves provide sensory and motor innervation of the body wall, the limbs, and the viscera. Sensory input to each spinal cord segment is provided by sensory neurons with cell bodies in the dorsal root ganglia.

The region of the body wall that is supplied by a single pair of dorsal root ganglia is called a **dermatome**. These dorsal root ganglion–innervated strips occur in a regular sequence moving upward from the second coccygeal segment through the cervical segments, reflecting the basic segmental organization of the body and the nervous system (Fig. 14-2). The cranial nerves that innervate the head send axons to equivalent nuclei in the brain stem. Neighboring dermatomes overlap sufficiently so that a loss of one dorsal root or root ganglion results in reduced but not total loss of sensory innervation (Fig. 14-3). Dermatome maps can help in interpreting the level and extent of sensory deficits caused by segmental nerve and spinal cord damage and can assist in determining the most effective pain management plan.

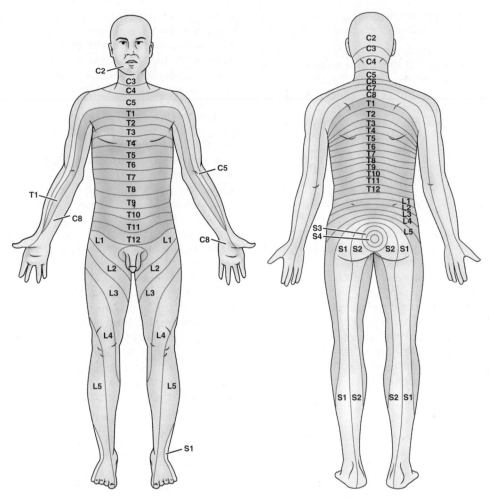

FIGURE 14-2. Dermatome distribution. (From Hinkle J. L., Cheever K. H. (2018). *Brunner & Suddarth's textbook of medical-surgical nursing* (14th ed., Fig. 65-9, p. 1953). Philadelphia, PA: Lippincott Williams & Wilkins.)

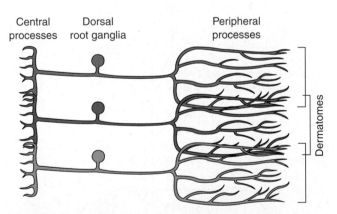

FIGURE 14-3. The dermatomes formed by the peripheral processes of adjacent spinal nerves overlap on the body surface. The central processes of these fibers also overlap in their spinal distribution.

Spinal Circuitry and Ascending Neural Pathways

On entry into the spinal cord, the central axons of the somatosensory neurons branch extensively and project to neurons in the spinal cord gray matter. Some branches are involved in local spinal cord reflexes and directly initiate motor reflexes. Two parallel pathways, the *discriminative pathway* and the *anterolateral pathway*, carry information from the spinal cord to the thalamic level of sensation. The discriminative pathway crosses at the base of the medulla, and the anterolateral pathway crosses within the first few segments of entering the spinal cord. These pathways relay information to the brain for three purposes: perception, arousal, and motor control. The advantages of having a two-pathway system include the following:

- Sensory information can be handled in two different ways.
- If one pathway is damaged, the other still can provide input.

The Discriminative Pathway

The discriminative pathway, also known as the dorsal column–medial lemniscal pathway, is used for the rapid transmission of sensory information.[1] It contains branches of primary afferent axons that travel up the ipsilateral (*i.e.*, same side) dorsal columns of the spinal cord white matter and synapse with somatosensory input association neurons in the medulla. The discriminative pathway uses three neurons to transmit information from a sensory receptor to the somatosensory strip of parietal cerebral cortex of the opposite (*i.e.*, contralateral) side of the brain:

1. The primary dorsal root ganglion neuron, which projects its central axon to the dorsal column nuclei.
2. The dorsal column neuron, which sends its axon through a rapid-conducting tract, called the *medial lemniscus*. It then crosses at the base of the medulla and travels to the thalamus on the opposite side of the brain, where basic sensation begins.
3. The thalamic neuron, which projects its axons through the somatosensory radiation to the primary sensory cortex (Fig. 14-4A).[1]

The medial lemniscus is joined by fibers from the sensory nucleus of the trigeminal nerve (cranial nerve V [CN V]) that supplies the face. Sensory information arriving at the sensory cortex by this route can be discretely localized and discriminated in terms of intensity.

The discriminative pathway relays precise information regarding spatial orientation. This is the only pathway taken by the sensations of muscle and joint movement, vibration, and delicate discriminative touch (*i.e.*, two-point discrimination). An important function of the discriminative pathway is to integrate the input from multiple receptors. Sensing the shape and size of an object in the absence of visualization, called *stereognosis*, requires precise information from muscle, tendon, and joint receptors. This complex interpretive perception requires function of both the discriminative system and the higher-order parietal association cortex. If the discriminative somatosensory pathway is functional but the parietal association cortex is damaged, the person can correctly describe the object but does not identify it. This deficit is called **astereognosis**.

The Anterolateral Pathway

The anterolateral pathways (anterior and lateral spinothalamic pathways) consist of bilateral, multisynaptic, slow-conducting tracts. These pathways transmit sensory information such as pain, thermal sensations, crude touch, and pressure that does not require discrete localization of signal source or fine discrimination of intensity. Anterolateral pathway fibers originate in the dorsal horns at the level of the segmental nerve where neurons enter the spinal cord. Within a few segments, the fibers cross in the anterior commissure to the opposite anterolateral pathway, where they ascend toward the brain. The spinothalamic tract fibers synapse with several nuclei in the thalamus and, en route, give off numerous branches that travel to the reticular activating system (RAS) of the brain stem. These projections provide the basis for increased wakefulness or awareness after strong somatosensory stimulation and for the generalized startle reaction that occurs with sudden and intense stimuli. They also stimulate autonomic nervous system responses

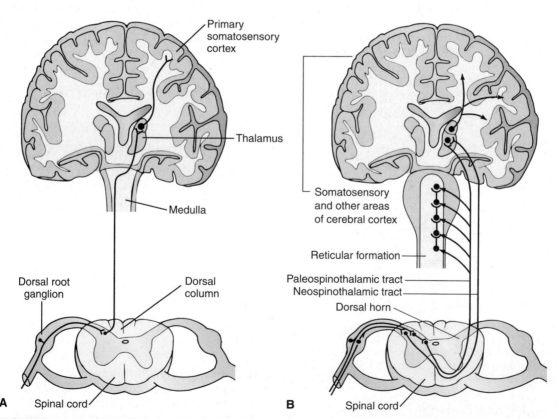

FIGURE 14-4. (**A**) Rapid-transmitting discriminative (dorsal column–medial lemniscal) pathway carrying axons mediating tactile sensation and proprioception. (**B**) Neospinothalamic and paleospinothalamic subdivisions of the anterolateral sensory pathway. The neurons of anterolateral pathways cross within the same segment as the cell body and ascend in the contralateral side of the spinal cord. The neospinothalamic tract travels mainly to thalamic nuclei that have third-order fibers projecting to the somatosensory cortex. The paleospinothalamic tract sends collaterals to the reticular formation and other structures, from which further fibers project to the thalamus.

such as a rise in heart rate and blood pressure, dilation of pupils, and activation of sweat glands.

There are two subdivisions in the anterolateral pathway—the *neospinothalamic tract* and the *paleospinothalamic tract* (Fig. 14-4B).[1] The neospinothalamic tract consists of a sequence of at least three neurons with long axons. It provides for rapid transmission of sensory information to the thalamus. The paleospinothalamic tract consists of bilateral, multisynaptic, slow-conducting tracts that transmit sensory signals that do not require discrete localization or discrimination of fine gradations in intensity. It also projects into the intralaminar nuclei of the thalamus, which have close connections with the limbic cortical systems. The circuitry gives touch its affective or emotional aspects, such as the peculiar pleasantness of the tickling and gentle rubbing of the kin.

Central Processing of Somatosensory Information

Perception involves awareness of the stimuli, localization and discrimination of characteristics, and interpretation of meaning. In the thalamus, the sensory information is roughly localized and perceived as a crude sense. The full localization, discrimination of the intensity, and interpretation of the meaning of the stimuli require processing by the somatosensory cortex.

The somatosensory cortex is located in the parietal lobe (Fig. 14-5). The strip of parietal cortex that borders the central sulcus is called the *primary somatosensory cortex* because it receives primary sensory information by direct projections from the thalamus. The *sensory homunculus* reflects the density of cortical neurons devoted to sensory input from corresponding peripheral areas. Most of the cortical surface is devoted to areas of the body such as the thumb, forefinger, lips, and tongue,

where fine touch and pressure discrimination are essential for normal function.

Parallel to and just behind the primary somatosensory cortex lie the somatosensory association areas, which are required to transform the raw material of sensation into meaningful learned perception. Most of the perceptive aspects of body sensation, or somesthesia, require the function of this parietal association cortex. The perceptive aspect, or meaningfulness, of a stimulus pattern involves the integration of present sensation with past learning.

Sensory Modalities

Somatosensory experience can be divided into *modalities,* including touch, heat, and pain, that require the function of sensory receptors and forebrain structures in the thalamus and cerebral cortex. Sensory experience also involves the ability to distinguish between levels of stimulation.

The receptive endings of afferent neurons are sensitive to physical and chemical energy and are usually highly tuned to be differentially sensitive to low levels of a particular energy type. Stimulating the ending with electric current or strong pressure also can result in action potentials. The amount of energy required, however, is much greater than it is for a change in temperature. Other afferent sensory terminals are most sensitive to slight indentations of the skin, and their signals are subjectively interpreted as touch. Cool versus warm, sharp versus dull pain, and delicate touch versus deep pressure are all based on different populations of afferent neurons or on central integration of simultaneous input from several differently tuned afferents.

When information from different primary afferents reaches the forebrain, where subjective experience occurs, the qualitative differences between warmth and touch are called *sensory modalities*. Although the information is relayed to the thalamus and cortex over separate pathways, the experience of a modality, such as cold versus warm, is uniquely subjective.

Stimulus Discrimination

The ability to discriminate the location of a somesthetic stimulus is called acuity and is based on the sensory field in a dermatome innervated by an afferent neuron. High acuity requires a high density of innervation by afferent neurons. For example, acuity is highest on the lips and cheek but lower on the arm or back. High acuity also requires a projection system that preserves distinctions between levels of activity in neighboring sensory fields. Receptors or receptive endings of primary afferent neurons differ as to the intensity at which they begin to fire. For instance, two-point discrimination can be assessed with the ends of an open paper clip. When placed on the lips, the person will readily detect two points of contact 5 mm apart. On the back, the ends of the paper clip must be moved farther apart before two points of contact can be detected.

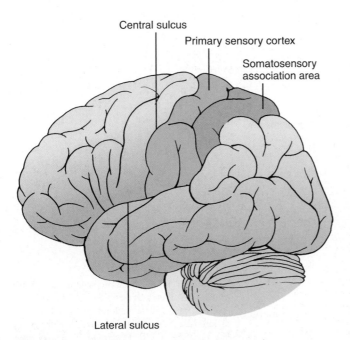

Central sulcus

Primary sensory cortex

Somatosensory association area

Lateral sulcus

FIGURE 14-5. Primary somatosensory cortex and somatosensory association area.

Tactile Sensation

The tactile system, which relays sensory information regarding touch, pressure, and vibration, is considered the basic somatosensory system. While loss of pain sensitivity may leave the person with no awareness of deficit, loss of the tactile system results in anesthesia of the involved area.

Touch sensation results from stimulation of tactile receptors in the skin and in tissues immediately beneath the skin, pressure from deformation of deeper tissues, and vibration from rapidly repetitive sensory signals. There are at least six types of specialized tactile receptors in the skin and deeper structures—free nerve endings, Meissner corpuscles, Merkel disks, Pacinian corpuscles, hair follicle end organs, and Ruffini end organs (Fig. 14-6).[1]

Free nerve endings are found in skin and other tissues to detect touch and pressure. *Meissner corpuscles* are elongated, encapsulated nerve endings present in nonhairy parts of the skin. They are abundant in the fingertips, lips, and other areas where the sense of touch is highly developed. *Merkel disks* are dome-shaped receptors found in the skin. In contrast to Meissner corpuscles, which adapt within a fraction of a second, Merkel disks transmit an initial strong signal that diminishes in strength but is slow in adapting. Meissner corpuscles are sensitive to the movement of very light objects over the skin surface and to low-frequency vibration. Merkel disks give steady-state signals that allow for continuous determination of touch against the skin.

The *Pacinian corpuscle* is located immediately beneath the skin and deep in the **fascial** tissues. It is stimulated by rapid movements of tissues and adapts within a few hundredths of a second and is important in detecting direct pressure changes and tissue vibration.[2] The *hair follicle end organ* consists of afferent unmyelinated fibers entwined around a hair follicle. These are rapidly adapting and detect movement on the surface of the body. *Ruffini end organs* are found in the skin and deeper structures, including joint capsules. They have multibranched encapsulated endings and little adaptive capacity. They are also important for signaling continuous states of **deformation**, such as heavy and continuous pressure, because they are sensitive to skin stretch.[2]

Almost all specialized touch receptors, such as Merkel disks, Meissner corpuscles, hair follicle end organs, Pacinian corpuscles, and Ruffini end organs, transmit their signals in large myelinated nerve fibers that have transmission velocities ranging from 30 to 70 m/second.[1] Most free nerve endings transmit signals by way of small myelinated fibers with conduction velocities of 5 to 30 m/second.[1]

The sensory information for tactile sensation enters the spinal cord through the dorsal roots of the spinal nerves. All tactile sensation that requires rapid transmission is transmitted through the discriminative pathway to the thalamus by way of the medial lemniscus. This includes touch sensation requiring a high degree of localization or fine gradations of intensity, vibratory sensation, and sensation that signals movement against the skin. Tactile sensation also uses the more primitive and crude anterolateral pathway. The afferent axons that carry tactile information up the dorsal columns have

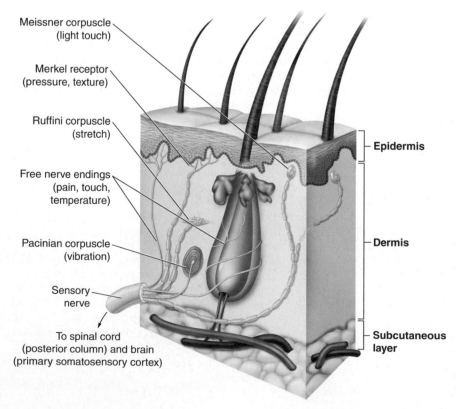

Meissner corpuscle (light touch)

Merkel receptor (pressure, texture)

Ruffini corpuscle (stretch)

Free nerve endings (pain, touch, temperature)

Pacinian corpuscle (vibration)

Sensory nerve

To spinal cord (posterior column) and brain (primary somatosensory cortex)

Epidermis

Dermis

Subcutaneous layer

FIGURE 14-6. Somatic sensory receptors in the skin. Free nerve endings, modified nerve endings, and specialized receptor cells detect different tactile stimuli. (From McConnell T. H., Hull K. L. (2011). *Human form, human function: Essentials of anatomy & physiology.* Philadelphia, PA: Lippincott Williams & Wilkins.)

many branches, and some of these synapse in the dorsal horn near the level of entry. Axons are projected up both sides of the anterolateral spinal cord to the thalamus. Few fibers travel directly to the thalamus—most synapse on reticular formation neurons that then send axons on toward the thalamus. The lateral nuclei of the thalamus contribute crude, poorly localized sensations from the opposite side of the body. From the thalamus, some projections travel to the somatosensory cortex, especially to the side opposite the stimulus.

Total destruction of the anterolateral pathway is rare. This crude alternative system is essential only when the discriminative pathway is damaged. Then, despite projection of the anterolateral system to somatosensory cortex, only a poorly localized, high-threshold sense of touch remains, causing loss in sense of joint and muscle movement, body position, and two-point discrimination.

Thermal Sensation

Thermal sensation is discriminated by three types of receptors: cold, warmth, and pain. Cold and warmth receptors are located immediately under the skin at discrete points. In some areas, there are more cold receptors than warmth receptors (*i.e.*, the lips have 15 to 25 cold receptors/cm^2, whereas a same-sized area of the finger has 3 to 5 cold receptors/cm^2).[1] Warmth receptors respond proportionately to increases in skin temperature between 32°C and 48°C and cold receptors to temperatures between 10°C and 40°C.[4] Thermal pain receptors are stimulated by extremes such as sensations of "freezing cold" (below 10°C) and "burning hot" (above 48°C).[4] Thermal receptors respond rapidly to sudden changes in temperature and then adapt over the next few minutes. They do not adapt completely, but continue to respond to steady states of temperature. For example, the sensation of heat one feels upon entering a hot water tub or of cold upon going outside on a cold day is the initial response to a change in temperature, followed by an adaptation in which one gets accustomed to but still feels the heat or cold as the receptors have not adapted completely.

Thermal afferents, with receptive thermal endings in the skin, send their central axons into the spinal cord dorsal horn. Thermal signals are then processed by second-order input association neurons, which activate projection neurons whose axons cross contralaterally and ascend in the multisynaptic, slow-conducting anterolateral system to the opposite side of the brain. Thalamic and cortical somatosensory regions for temperature are mixed with tactile sensibility.

Conduction of thermal information through peripheral nerves is slow compared with the rapid tactile afferents of the discriminative system. If a foot is placed in hot water, the tactile sensation occurs in advance of the burning sensations and local withdrawal reflexes will act before excessive heat is perceived. Local anesthetic agents block small-diameter afferents that carry thermal sensory information before they block large-diameter axons that carry discriminative touch information.

Position Sensation

Position sense refers to the sense of limb and body movement and position without vision. It is mediated by input from proprioceptive receptors (muscle spindle receptors and Golgi tendon organs) found primarily in muscles, tendons, and joint capsules. There are two submodalities of proprioception: the static component (limb position) and the dynamic aspects (**kinesthesia**). Both submodalities depend on constant transmission of information to the CNS regarding the degree of angulation of all joints and the rate of change in angulation. Stretch-sensitive receptors in the skin (Ruffini end organs, Pacinian corpuscles, and Merkel cells) also signal postural information, which are processed through the dorsal column–medial lemniscus pathway. They transmit signals from the periphery to the cerebral cortex via the thalamus. Lesions affecting the posterior column impair position sense. The vestibular system also plays an essential role in position sense.

Clinical Assessment of Somatosensory Function

A neurologic assessment of somatosensory function includes testing the spinal segmental nerves. A pinpoint pressed against the sole of the foot results in a withdrawal reflex. Complaint of pain confirms the functional integrity of afferent terminals in the skin; the pathway through peripheral nerves of the foot, leg, and thigh to S1 dorsal root ganglion; and through the dorsal root into the spinal cord segment. This confirms the function of somatosensory input association cells receiving this information and reflex circuitry of the cord segments (L5 to S2). Also, the lower motor neurons of the L4 to S1 ventral horn and their axons through the ventral roots can be considered intact and functional. The communication between the lower motor neuron and the muscle cells is functional, and these muscles have normal responsiveness and strength.

Testing is done at each segmental level, or dermatome, moving up from coccygeal through the high cervical levels to test the integrity of all spinal nerves. Similar dermatomes cover the face and scalp, and these, although innervated by cranial nerves, are tested in the same manner.

A normal withdrawal reflex rules out disorders of the peripheral nerve, dorsal root and ganglion, neuromuscular junction, and muscle. Reflex function indicates that many major descending CNS tracts are functioning within normal limits, and, if pinprick sensation and location are accurately reported, many ascending systems are functioning normally, as are basic intellect and speech.

Integrity of the discriminative dorsal column–medial lemniscus pathway versus the anterolateral tactile pathways is tested (with eyes closed) by brushing the skin with cotton, touching an area with one to two sharp points, touching corresponding body areas on each side concurrently or in random sequence, and passively bending the finger. If only the anterolateral pathway is functional, tactile threshold is markedly elevated, two-point discrimination and proprioception are missing, and the person has difficulty discriminating which side of the body received stimulation.

SUMMARY CONCEPTS

The somatosensory system provides an awareness of body sensations such as touch, temperature, position sense, and pain. There are three primary levels of neural integration: the sensory units, the ascending pathways, and the central processing centers. A sensory unit consists of a dorsal root ganglion neuron, its receptors, and its central axon that terminates in the dorsal horn of the spinal cord or medulla. The area innervated by the somatosensory afferent neurons of one set of dorsal root ganglia is a dermatome. Ascending pathways include the discriminative pathway, which crosses at the base of the medulla, and the anterolateral pathway, which crosses soon after entering the spinal cord. Perception involves centers in the thalamus and somatosensory cortex. In the thalamus, the sensory information is crudely localized and perceived. The full localization, discrimination of the intensity, and interpretation of the meaning of the stimuli require processing by the somatosensory cortex. The *sensory homunculus* reflects the density of cortical neurons devoted to sensory input from afferents in corresponding peripheral areas.

The tactile system relays sensations of touch, pressure, and vibration. It uses two anatomically separate pathways—the dorsal column discriminative pathway and the anterolateral pathway—to relay touch information to the opposite side of the forebrain. Delicate touch, vibration, position, and movement use the discriminative pathway to reach the thalamus, where third-order relay occurs to the primary somatosensory strip of the parietal cortex. Crude tactile sensation is carried by the bilateral, slow-conducting anterolateral pathway. Temperature sensations are the result of stimulation to thermal receptors of sensory units projecting to the thalamus and cortex through the anterolateral system on the opposite side of the body. Proprioception is the sense of limb and body movement and position without using vision and is processed through the rapid-transmitting dorsal column–medial lemniscus pathway. Testing of the ipsilateral dorsal column (discriminative touch) system or the contralateral temperature projection system permits diagnostic analysis of the level and extent of damage in the somatosensory pathways.

Pain

The International Association for the Study of Pain defines pain as an "unpleasant sensory and emotional experience associated with actual and potential tissue damage."[6] Pain is when a person reacts to a stimulus by removing the trigger causing the noxious stimulation.[1] Distress of pain is more heavily influenced by the reaction to pain than by actual pain intensity. Many factors can influence a person's reaction to pain, including anxiety, culture, and past experience.

Pain is a common symptom that varies in intensity and spares no age group. When severe, it can disrupt a person's behavior. Pain is the most common symptom for which people seek medical attention. Both acute and chronic pain are major health problems. Acute pain often results from injury, surgery, or invasive medical procedures. It also can be a presenting symptom for some infections. Chronic pain can be symptomatic of a wide range of health problems. Any pain persisting for more than 24 hours has been reported by an estimated 76.5 million Americans.[7]

The experience of pain depends on both sensory perception and stimulation. Perception of pain can be heavily influenced by the endogenous analgesia system that modulates the sensation of pain (*i.e.*, when injured soldiers do not perceive major injuries as painful until they leave the battlefield). Sensory stimulation refers to the processes by which a person experiences pain. Pain can be either nociceptive or neuropathic in origin.[8] The receptors for pain (nociceptors) are free nerve endings. When nociceptors are activated in response to actual or impending tissue injury, *nociceptive pain* is the consequence. *Neuropathic pain* arises from direct injury or dysfunction of the sensory axons of peripheral or central nerves.[9] Tissue and nerve injury can result in a wide range of symptoms. These include pain from noninjurious stimuli to the skin (*allodynia*), extreme sensitivity to pain (*hyperalgesia*), and the absence of pain from stimuli that normally would be painful (*analgesia*).[10] The latter, although not painful, can be extremely serious because the normally protective early warning system for tissue injury is absent.

Pain Theories

Traditionally, two theories were offered to explain the physiologic basis for the pain experience: specificity theory and pattern theory. *Specificity theory* regards pain as a separate sensory modality evoked by the activity of specific receptors that transmit information to forebrain regions where pain is experienced.[11] This theory predicts how painful a specific acute injury may be, but does not encompass how the pain feels or how the person has experienced pain in the past.[12] *Pattern theory* is a group of theories that propose pain receptors share pathways with other sensory modalities but different patterns of activity signal painful versus nonpainful stimuli.[11] For example, whereas light touch produces low-frequency firing, intense pressure produces pain through high-frequency firing of the same receptor. Both specificity and pattern theories focus on the neurophysiologic basis of pain, and both probably apply: specific nociceptive afferents have been identified, and if driven at a very high frequency, almost all afferent stimuli can be experienced as painful.

In 1965, *gate control theory* was proposed by Melzack and Wall who postulated the presence of neural gating mechanisms at the segmental spinal cord level to account for interactions between pain and other sensory modalities.[13] The original gate control theory proposed a spinal cord–level network of projection cells and internuncial neurons, forming a segmental-level gating mechanism that could block projection of pain information to the brain.

According to the gate control theory, the internuncial neurons involved are activated by large-diameter, faster-propagating fibers that carry tactile information. The firing of large-diameter touch fibers may block impulses from small-diameter pain fibers.[13] Pain therapists know that pain intensity can be temporarily reduced during active tactile stimulation: sweeping a soft brush over or near a painful area may result in pain reduction for several minutes to hours.

Pain modulation is now known to be more complex than what was originally proposed. Tactile information is transmitted by small- and large-diameter fibers. Major interactions between sensory modalities occur at several levels of the CNS rostral to the input segment. Locally applied stimuli that can block the experience of pain for prolonged periods has been difficult to explain on the basis of these theories. Other important factors include the effect of endogenous opioids and receptors at the segmental and brain stem level, descending feedback modulation, altered sensitivity, learning, and culture. Despite this, the Melzack and Wall theory sparked interest in pain and stimulated research and clinical activity related to pain-modulating systems.

Melzack developed the *neuromatrix theory* to tackle the brain's role and the multiple dimensions and determinants of pain.[14] This theory is useful in understanding chronic and phantom limb pain where there is no linear relationship between tissue injury and pain experience. It proposes that the brain contains a widely distributed neural network, the *body–self neuromatrix*, that contains somatosensory, limbic, and thalamocortical components. Genetic and sensory influences determine the architecture of an individual's neuromatrix that integrates multiple sources of input and yields the neurosignature pattern that evokes the sensory, affective, and cognitive dimensions of pain experience and behavior. These multiple sources include:

- Somatosensory inputs
- Other sensory inputs affecting interpretation of the situation
- Phasic and tonic inputs from the brain addressing such things as attention, expectation, culture, and personality
- Intrinsic neural inhibitory modulation
- Various components of stress regulation systems

The neuromatrix theory may open new areas of research, such as understanding the role cortisol plays in chronic pain, the effect estrogen has on pain mediated through the release of peripheral cytokines, and the reported increase in chronic pain that occurs with age.[14]

Pain Mechanisms and Pathways

Pain usually is viewed in the context of injury (*nocere* is Latin for "to injure"). Nociceptive stimuli may cause tissue damage, and the withdrawal reflex is used to determine when a stimulus is nociceptive. Stimuli used include pressure from a sharp object, electric current, or heat or cold applied to skin. At low levels of intensity, these noxious stimuli activate nociceptors, but are perceived as painful only when the intensity reaches a level where tissue damage may occur.

Nociceptive pathways are composed of first-, second-, and third-order neurons (Fig. 14-7). The receptive endings of first-order neurons detect stimuli that threaten the integrity of innervated tissues. Second-order neurons are located in the spinal cord and process nociceptive information. Third-order neurons project pain information to the brain. The thalamus and somatosensory cortex integrate and modulate pain as well as the person's subjective reaction to the experience.

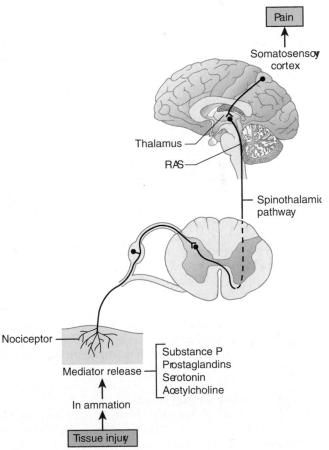

FIGURE 14-7. Mechanism of acute pain. Tissue injury leads to release of inflammatory mediators with subsequent nociceptor stimulation. Pain impulses are then transmitted to the dorsal horn of the spinal cord, where they make contract with second-order neurons that cross to the opposite side of the cord and ascend by the spinothalamic tract to the reticular activating system (RAS) and thalamus. The localization and meaning of pain occur at the level of the somatosensory cortex.

Pain Receptors and Mediators

Structurally, the receptive endings of the peripheral pain fibers are free nerve endings and are widely distributed in the skin, dental pulp, periosteum, meninges, and some internal organs. They translate noxious stimuli into action potentials that are transmitted by a dorsal root ganglion to the dorsal horn of the spinal cord.

Nociceptive action potentials are transmitted through myelinated Aδ fibers and unmyelinated C fibers. The larger Aδ fibers transmit impulses at 6 to 30 m/second.[1] The C fibers are the smallest of all peripheral nerve fibers and transmit impulses at 0.5 to 2.0 m/second.[1] Pain conducted by Aδ fibers (*fast pain*) is typically elicited by mechanical or thermal stimuli. C-fiber pain (*slow-wave pain*) is slower in onset and longer in duration and is elicited by chemical stimuli or persistent mechanical or thermal stimuli. The slow postexcitatory potentials generated in C fibers are responsible for central sensitization to chronic pain.

Stimulation of Nociceptors

Some nociceptors respond to one type of stimuli and others (*polymodal receptors*) respond to all three types of stimuli (mechanical, thermal, and chemical). Mechanical stimuli can arise from pressure applied to skin, violent contraction, or extreme stretch of muscle. Temperature extremes can also stimulate nociceptors. Chemical stimuli can arise from tissue trauma, ischemia, and inflammation. Chemical mediators are released from injured and inflamed tissues and stimulate nociceptors or sensitize them to the effects of nociceptive stimuli. This perpetuates the inflammatory responses that lead to the release of chemical agents that act as nociceptive stimuli or incites neurogenic reflexes that increase the response to the stimuli.[1] Adenosine triphosphate (ATP), acetylcholine, and platelets sensitize nociceptors through chemical agents such as prostaglandins. Aspirin and other nonsteroidal anti-inflammatory drugs (NSAIDs) block prostaglandin synthesis and are effective in controlling pain.

Nociceptive stimulation activates C fibers to cause *neurogenic inflammation*, which produces vasodilation and increased release of chemical mediators to which nociceptors respond.[1] The C-fiber mechanism is thought to be mediated by a dorsal root neuron reflex that produces retrograde transport and release of chemical mediators, which causes increasing inflammation of peripheral tissues. This reflex has implications for persistent pain and hyperalgesia.[9]

Mediators in the Spinal Cord

The transmission of impulses between the nociceptive neurons and the dorsal horn neurons is mediated by chemical neurotransmitters released from central nerve endings of nociceptive neurons. These neurotransmitters can be amino acids, amino acid derivatives, or low molecular weight peptides. The amino acid glutamate is a major excitatory transmitter released from central nerve endings of nociceptive neurons. Substance P, a neuropeptide, also is released in the dorsal horn by C fibers in response to nociceptive stimulation. While glutamate is confined to the synaptic terminal area, some neuropeptides can diffuse some distance because they are not inactivated by reuptake mechanisms. This may explain the excitability and unlocalized nature of many painful, persistent conditions. Neuropeptides appear to prolong and enhance the action of glutamate, and if released in large quantities or over extended periods, they can lead to secondary hyperalgesia in which second-order neurons are overly sensitive to low levels of noxious stimulation.[1]

KEY POINTS

Pain Sensation

■ The pathway for fast, sharply discriminated pain moves from the receptor to the spinal cord using myelinated Aδ fibers and from the spinal cord to thalamus using the neospinothalamic tract.

■ The pathway for slow, continuously conducted pain is transmitted to the spinal cord using unmyelinated C fibers and from the spinal cord to the thalamus using the more circuitous and slower-conducting paleospinothalamic tract.

Spinal Cord Circuitry and Pathways

On entering the spinal cord through the dorsal roots, the pain fibers bifurcate and ascend or descend one or two segments before synapsing with association neurons in the dorsal horn. The axons of association projection neurons cross through the anterior commissure to the opposite side and then ascend up in the neospinothalamic and paleospinothalamic pathways (Fig. 14-8).

The faster-conducting fibers in the neospinothalamic tract are associated with transmission of sharp-fast pain information to the thalamus. After synapsing in the thalamus, it continues to the contralateral parietal somatosensory area to provide the precise location of the pain.

The paleospinothalamic tract is a slower-conducting tract concerned with the diffuse, aching, and unpleasant sensations commonly associated with chronic and visceral pain. It travels through the small, unmyelinated C fibers, which also project up the contralateral anterolateral pathway to terminate in several thalamic regions, some of which project to the limbic system. It is associated with the emotional or affective–motivational aspects of pain. Spinoreticular fibers from this pathway project bilaterally to the reticular formation of the brain stem and facilitates avoidance reflexes at all levels. It also contributes to an increase in the electroencephalographic activity associated with alertness and indirectly influences hypothalamic functions such as increased heart rate and blood pressure. This may explain the arousal effects of certain pain stimuli.

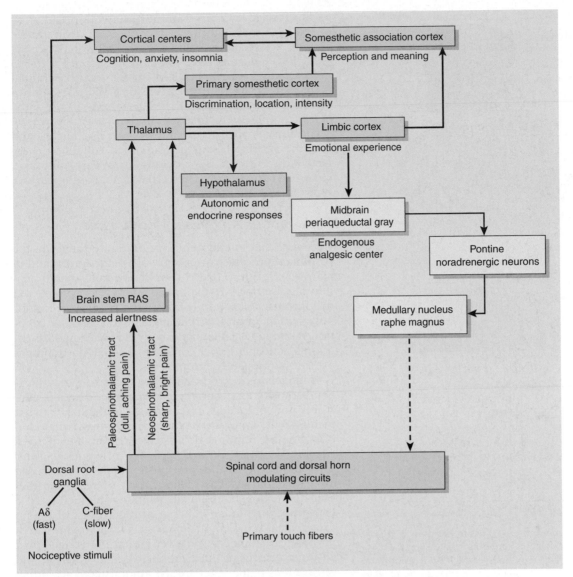

FIGURE 14-8. Primary pain pathways. The transmission of incoming nociceptive impulses is modulated by dorsal horn circuitry, which receives input from primary touch receptors and from descending pathways that involve the limbic cortical systems (orbital frontal cortex, amygdala, and hypothalamus), the periaqueductal endogenous analgesic center in the midbrain, pontine noradrenergic neurons, and the nucleus raphe magnus in the medulla. *Dashed lines* indicate inhibition or modulation of pain transmission by dorsal horn projection neurons. RAS, reticular activating system.

Dorsal horn (second-order) neurons are divided primarily into two types: wide dynamic range (WDR) neurons that respond to low-intensity stimuli and nociceptive-specific neurons that respond to noxious or nociceptive stimuli. WDR neurons respond more intensely when stimuli are increased to a noxious level. Aδ and C fibers respond more intensely with more severe damage to peripheral sensory afferents. When C fibers are repetitively stimulated (once per second), each stimulus produces a progressively increased response. This amplification has been called *windup* and may explain why pain sensation appears to increase with repeated stimulation. Windup and sensitization of dorsal horn neurons have implications for appropriate and early, or preemptive, pain therapy to avoid spinal cord neuron hypersensitivity or spontaneous firing.[4]

Brain Centers and Pain Perception

Injury information is carried from the spinal cord to brain centers in the thalamus where basic pain sensation occurs (Fig. 14-9). In the neospinothalamic system, interconnections between the lateral thalamus and somatosensory cortex add precision and meaning to pain sensation. The paleospinothalamic system projects from the intralaminar nuclei of the thalamus to large areas of limbic cortex and are associated with the mood-altering and attention-narrowing effect of pain. Magnetoencephalography has demonstrated cortical representation of pain: nociceptive Aδ afferent stimulation activates the contralateral primary somatosensory cortex, whereas C afferent stimulation activates the secondary somatosensory cortices and the anterior cingulate cortex.[15]

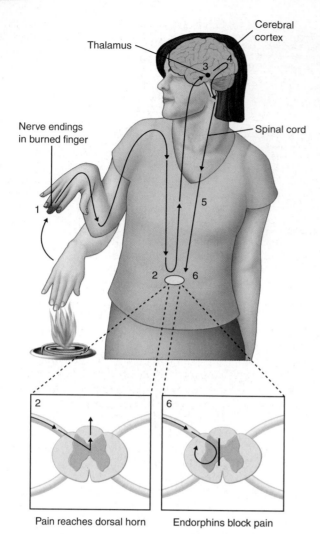

FIGURE 14-9. Pain transmission. (*1*) Pain begins as a message received by nerve endings, such as found in a burnt finger. (*2*) The release of substance P, bradykinin, and prostaglandins sensitize the nerve endings, which helps to transmit the pain from the site of injury toward the brain. (*3*) The pain signal then travels as an electrochemical impulse along the length of the nerve to the dorsal horn on the spinal cord, a region that receives signals from all over the body. (*4*) The spinal cord then sends the message to the thalamus, and then to the cortex. (*5*) Pain relief starts with signals from the brain that descend by way of the spinal cord, where (*6*) chemicals such as endorphin S are released in the dorsal horn to diminish the pain message. (From Jensen S. (2015). *Nursing health assessment: A best practice approach* (2nd ed., Fig. 6.1, p. 114). Philadelphia, PA: Lippincott Williams & Wilkins.)

Central Pathways for Pain Modulation

Neuroanatomic pathways arise in the midbrain and brain stem, descend to the spinal cord, and modulate ascending pain impulses. One such pathway begins in the *periaqueductal gray* (PAG) region in the midbrain. It was found that electrical stimulation of PAG regions produced a state of analgesia that lasted for many hours. Subsequently, opioid receptors were found to be highly concentrated in this and other regions of the CNS where electrical stimulation produced analgesia. Because of these findings, the PAG area of the midbrain often is referred to as the *analgesia system*.[1]

The PAG area receives input from widespread areas of the CNS and is intimately connected to the limbic system, which is associated with emotional experience. PAG neurons have axons that descend into the *nucleus raphe magnus* (NRM) of the rostral medulla. Axons of NRM neurons project to the dorsal horn of the spinal cord, where they terminate in the same layers as entering primary pain fibers (see Fig. 14-8). Serotonin is a neurotransmitter in NRM nuclei, and tricyclic antidepressant drugs, which enhance the effects of serotonin by blocking presynaptic uptake, have been found to be effective in managing certain types of chronic pain.[16]

Endogenous Analgesic Mechanisms

Opioid receptors and opioid peptides are found on the peripheral processes of primary afferent neurons and in many CNS regions (Fig. 14-9). Endogenous opioid peptide families include the enkephalins, endorphins, and dynorphins. Each family is derived from a precursor polypeptide and has a characteristic anatomic distribution. Although each family usually is located in different groups of neurons, occasionally more than one family is present in the same neuron.

Endogenous opioid peptides appear to function as neurotransmitters, but their significance in pain control is not completely understood. Although somewhat inconsistent, laboratory studies have found that opioid agonists inhibit calcium channels in dorsal root, trigeminal ganglion, and primary afferent neurons. This inhibition could prevent synaptic transmission of pain impulses. The identification of receptors that bind the endogenous opioid peptides has facilitated a more thorough understanding of the actions of opioid drugs, such as morphine. It also has facilitated research into the development of newer preparations, including 24-hour dispensing medications, dermal patches, and intravenous pumps that are self-administered according to perceived need.

Pain Threshold and Tolerance

Pain threshold and tolerance affect a person's response to a painful stimulus. *Pain threshold* is the point at which a stimulus is perceived as painful. *Pain tolerance* is the total pain experience and is defined as a lesser "response to a drug because of repeated drug administration."[17] Psychological, cultural, and environmental factors influence the amount of pain a person can tolerate. Separation and identification of the two aspects of pain pose fundamental problems for pain management.

Types of Pain

Pain can be classified according to duration (acute or chronic), location (cutaneous or deep and visceral), and site of referral. Classification based on associated medical diagnosis (*e.g.*, surgery, trauma, cancer) is also very useful in planning appropriate pain management interventions.

Acute and Chronic Pain

Pain research emphasizes differentiating acute and chronic pain. Diagnosis and therapy for each is distinctive; they differ in cause, function, mechanism, and psychological sequelae (Table 14-1)

Traditionally, the distinction between acute and chronic pain relies on a single continuum of time. Some conditions such as osteoarthritis exhibit dimensions of both acute and chronic pain.

Acute Pain

Acute pain is elicited by injury and activation of nociceptive stimuli at the site of local tissue damage.[1] It is generally of short duration and resolves with resolution of the pathology.[1] Acute pain alerts a person of actual or impending tissue damage. The location, radiation, intensity, duration, and factors that aggravate or relieve pain provide essential diagnostic clues.

Interventions that alleviate pain usually relieve concomitant problems such as anxiety and musculoskeletal spasms. Inadequately treated pain can provoke responses that alter circulation and tissue metabolism and increase sympathetic activity. Inadequately treated acute pain tends to decrease mobility and respiratory movements and may complicate or delay recovery.

Chronic Pain

Chronic pain persists longer than might be reasonably expected after an inciting event. It is sustained by both pathologically and physically remote factors from the originating cause. Chronic pain can continue for years. It may be unrelenting and severe, as with metastatic bone pain, or continuous with or without periods of escalation, as with some forms of back pain. Recurring episodes of acute pain are particularly problematic because they have characteristics of both acute and chronic pain (as in sickle cell crisis or migraine headaches).

Chronic pain is a leading cause of disability and usually serves no useful function. It imposes physiologic, psychological, familial, and economic stresses. Psychological and environmental influences may play an important role in the development of behaviors associated with chronic pain.

The biologic factors that influence chronic pain include peripheral, peripheral–central, and central mechanisms. Peripheral mechanisms result from persistent stimulation of nociceptors and are mostly involved with chronic musculoskeletal, visceral, and vascular disorders. Peripheral–central mechanisms are related to abnormal function of the peripheral and central portions of the somatosensory system, such as those resulting from partial or complete loss of descending inhibitory pathways or spontaneous firing of regenerated nerve fibers (as with causalgia and phantom limb pain). Central pain mechanisms are associated with CNS disease or injury and characterized by burning, aching, and other abnormal sensations (as with thalamic lesions, spinal cord injury, surgical interruption of pain pathways, and multiple sclerosis).

People with chronic pain may not exhibit behaviors often associated with acute pain. As pain becomes prolonged and continuous, autonomic nervous system responses decrease. Loss of appetite, sleep disturbances, and depression often are associated with chronic pain. Depression commonly is relieved once the pain is removed. The link between depression and decreased pain tolerance may be due to the manner by which both respond to changes in serotonergic and noradrenergic systems. Tricyclic antidepressants and other medications with serotonergic and noradrenergic effects have been shown to relieve a variety of chronic pain syndromes.[17]

Cutaneous and Deep Somatic Pain

Pain can be classified according to location. *Cutaneous pain* arises from superficial structures. It is a sharp pain with a burning quality that may be abrupt or slow in onset. It can be localized and may be distributed along the dermatomes. Because of an overlap of nerve fibers between the dermatomes, boundaries of pain frequently are not as clear-cut as dermatome diagrams indicate.

TABLE 14-1	Characteristics of Acute and Chronic Pain	
Characteristic	**Acute Pain**	**Chronic Pain**
Onset	Recent	Continuous or intermittent
Duration	Short (<6 months)	6 months or more
Autonomic responses	Consistent with sympathetic fight or flight response* Increased heart rate Increased stroke volume Increased blood pressure Increased pupillary dilation Increased muscle tension Decreased gut motility Decreased salivary flow (dry mouth)	Absence of autonomic responses
Psychological component	Associated anxiety	Increased irritability Associated depression Somatic preoccupation Withdrawal from outside interests Decreased strength of relationships
Other types of response		Decreased sleep Decreased libido Appetite changes

Responses are approximately proportional to intensity of the stimulus.

Deep somatic pain originates in deep body structures. It is more diffuse than cutaneous pain. Various stimuli, such as strong pressure on bone, muscle ischemia, and tissue damage, can produce deep somatic pain, which may radiate from the site of injury (as with a sprained ankle).

Visceral Pain

Visceral pain is one of the most common pains produced by disease. There is a low density of nociceptors in the viscera compared to the skin. There is functional divergence of visceral input within the CNS: many second-order neurons respond to a stimulus from a single visceral afferent. An important difference between surface pain and visceral pain is the type of damage that causes pain. Contractions, distention, or ischemia of visceral walls can induce severe pain. Visceral nociceptive afferents from the thorax and abdomen travel along the cranial and spinal nerve pathways of the autonomic nervous system.

Referred Pain

Referred pain is perceived at a site different from its point of origin but innervated by the same spinal segment. It is hypothesized that visceral and somatic afferent neurons converge on the same dorsal horn projection neurons (Fig. 14-10), making it difficult for the brain to correctly identify the source of pain. Pain that originates in the abdominal or thoracic viscera is diffuse and poorly localized and often perceived at a site far from the affected area. For example, the pain associated with myocardial infarction commonly is referred to the left arm, neck, and chest.

Referred pain may arise alone or concurrent with pain located at the origin of the noxious stimuli. This disconnect between pain location and painful stimuli location can make diagnosis difficult. Although the term *referred* usually is applied to pain that originates in the viscera and is experienced as if originating from the body wall, it may also be applied to pain that arises from somatic structures. Understanding pain referral is critical in diagnosing illness. The typical pattern of pain referral can be derived from our understanding that the afferent neurons from visceral or deep somatic tissue enter the spinal cord at the same level as the afferent neurons from the cutaneous areas to which the pain is referred (Fig. 14-11).

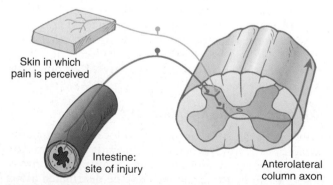

FIGURE 14-10. Convergence of cutaneous and visceral inputs onto the same second-order projection neuron in the dorsal horn of the spinal cord. Although virtually all visceral inputs converge with cutaneous inputs, most cutaneous inputs do not converge with other sensory inputs.

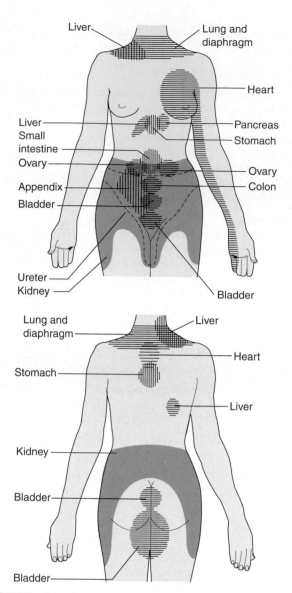

FIGURE 14-11. Areas of referred pain. (**Top**) Anterior view. (**Bottom**) Posterior view.

Sites of referred pain are determined embryologically: visceral and somatic structures share the same site for entry of sensory information into the CNS. For example, a person with peritonitis (inflammation of the peritoneum lining the central part of the diaphragm) may complain of shoulder pain. In the embryo, the diaphragm originates in the neck, and its central portion is innervated by the phrenic nerve, which enters the cord at the level of the third to fifth segments (C3 to C5). The diaphragm descends to its adult position between the thoracic and abdominal cavities while maintaining its embryonic pattern of innervation. Thus, fibers that enter the spinal cord at the C3 to C5 levels carry information from both the neck area and the diaphragm, and the diaphragmatic pain is interpreted by the forebrain as originating in the shoulder or neck area.

Although the visceral pleura, pericardium, and peritoneum are said to be relatively free of pain fibers, the parietal pleura, pericardium, and peritoneum do react to nociceptive stimuli. Visceral inflammation can involve parietal and somatic structures, which may give rise to diffuse local or referred pain. For example, when the parietal peritoneum is irritated from appendicitis, it may give rise to pain in the lower right quadrant, evoking pain referred to the umbilical area.

Muscle spasm, or *guarding*, occurs when somatic structures are involved. Guarding is a protective reflex rigidity that may cause blood vessel compression and give rise to the pain of muscle ischemia, causing local and referred pain.

KEY POINTS

Types of Pain

■ Pain can be classified according to duration, location, and site of referral.

■ Acute pain is a self-limiting pain that lasts less than 6 months.

■ Chronic pain is persistent pain that lasts longer than 6 months, lacks the autonomic and somatic responses associated with acute pain, and is accompanied by loss of appetite, sleep disturbances, depression, and other debilitating responses.

Assessment of Pain

Careful assessment assists clinicians in diagnosing, managing, and relieving pain. Assessment includes such things as the nature, severity, location, and radiation of the pain. Eliminating the cause is preferable to simply treating the symptoms of pain. A history often provides information about triggering factors and the site of nociceptive stimuli. A pain history should include:

■ Pain onset
■ Description, localization, radiation, intensity, quality, and pattern of the pain
■ Anything that relieves or exacerbates it
■ The person's personal reaction to the pain

Various methods have been developed to quantify pain based on the person's report, including numeric pain intensity, visual analog, and verbal descriptor scales. Most pain questionnaires assess a single aspect of pain such as pain intensity. A *numeric pain intensity* scale asks people to select which number best represents the intensity of their pain, where 0 represents no pain and 10 represents the most intense pain imaginable. A *visual analog* scale is a straight line, often 10 cm in length, with a word description (*e.g.*, "no pain" and "the most intense pain imaginable") at each of the ends of the line representing the continuum of pain intensity. The response can be quantified by measuring the line to determine the distance of the mark, measured in millimeters, from the "no pain" end of the line. *Verbal descriptor* scales consist of several numerically ranked choices of words such as none = 0, slight = 1, mild = 2, moderate = 3, and severe = 4. The word chosen is used to determine the numeric representation of pain severity on an ordinal scale.

Management of Pain

The therapeutic approaches to managing acute and chronic pain differ markedly. In acute pain, therapy is directed at providing pain relief by interrupting the nociceptive stimulus. Because the pain resolves as the injured tissues heal, long-term therapy usually is not needed. Chronic pain management is more complex and is based on multiple considerations, including life expectancy.

Managing Acute Pain

Acute pain should be aggressively managed and pain medication provided before it becomes severe. This allows the person to be comfortable and to assume a greater role in directing his or her own care. Health care workers may be reluctant to provide adequate relief for acute pain due to fear of addiction. However, addiction to opioid medications is thought to be virtually nonexistent when prescribed for acute pain. Usually, less medication is needed when the drug is given before the pain becomes severe and the pain pathways become sensitized.

Managing Chronic Pain

Management of chronic pain requires early attempts to prevent pain and adequate therapy for acute bouts of pain. Specific treatment depends on the cause of the pain, the natural history of the underlying health problem, and the life expectancy of the person. If the illness causing the pain cannot be cured, then noncurative methods of pain control become the cornerstone of treatment. Treatment methods can include neural blockade, electrical modalities (*e.g.*, transcutaneous electrical nerve stimulation [TENS]), physical therapy, cognitive–behavioral interventions, and nonnarcotic and narcotic medications. Nonnarcotic medications such as tricyclic antidepressants, antiepileptic medications, and NSAIDs serve as useful adjuncts to opioids for the treatment of chronic pain. Chronic pain is best handled by a multidisciplinary team that includes specialists in areas such as anesthesiology, nursing, physical therapy, social services, and surgery. Cancer is a common cause of chronic pain, and the World Health Organization has created an analgesic ladder for cancer pain that assists clinicians in choosing the appropriate analgesic.[18]

Nonpharmacologic Pain Management

There are a number of nonpharmacologic methods of pain control that are often used with analgesics, including cognitive–behavioral interventions, physical agents, and electroanalgesia.

Cognitive–Behavioral Interventions
Cognitive–behavioral interventions include relaxation, distraction, cognitive reappraisal, imagery, meditation, and biofeedback. If the person is having surgery or a painful procedure, it is ideal to teach these techniques before the pain begins. If the person is already in severe pain, the use of cognitive–behavioral interventions should be based on the person's ability to master the technique as well as his or her response to the intervention. For example, it may be a more appropriate adjunct to analgesics

for a terminally ill person in severe pain to use self-selected relaxing music rather than trying to teach that person an intervention requiring more attention. Prescribed analgesics should not be denied to people because they appear to be coping with their pain without medication. Appropriate assessment is needed to determine the level of pain and what other interventions may be needed.

Relaxation is one of the best-evaluated cognitive–behavioral approaches to pain relief. Relatively simple strategies, such as slow, rhythmic breathing and brief jaw relaxation procedures, have been successful in decreasing self-reported pain and analgesic use.

Distraction (*i.e.*, focusing attention on stimuli other than painful stimuli or negative emotions) does not eliminate pain, but can make it more tolerable. It may serve as sensory shielding whereby attention to pain is sacrificed to pay attention to other stimuli. Examples include counting, repeating poems, and engaging in activities that require concentration. *Cognitive reappraisal* is a form of self-distraction or cognitive control in which people focus their attention on the positive aspects of the experience and away from their pain. Individuals using distraction may not appear to be in severe pain.

Imagery consists of using one's imagination to develop a mental picture. In pain management, therapeutic guided imagery (*i.e.*, goal-directed imaging) is used. It can be used alone or in conjunction with other cognitive–behavioral interventions to develop sensory images that may decrease the perceived intensity of pain. Therapeutic guided imagery can also be used to lessen anxiety and reduce muscle tension. Also *meditation* can be used, but requires practice and the ability to concentrate.

Biofeedback provides feedback to a person about the status of a body function (*e.g.*, temperature, temporal artery pulsation, blood pressure, or muscle tension). It involves a process of learning designed to make the person aware of certain functions in order to modify them at a conscious level. Interest in biofeedback increased with the possibility of use modality in the management of migraine and tension headaches or for other pain that has a muscle tension component.

Physical Agents

Heat and cold are physical agents that are used to provide pain relief. The choice of physical agent depends on the type of pain being treated and, in many cases, personal preference. *Heat* dilates blood vessels and increases local blood flow. It can also influence transmission of pain impulses and increase collagen extensibility. Increased circulation can reduce the level of nociceptive stimulation by reducing local ischemia caused by muscle spasm or tension, increase removal of metabolites and inflammatory mediators that act as nociceptive stimuli, and help reduce swelling and relieve pressure on local nociceptive endings. The heat sensation is carried to the posterior horn of the spinal cord and may exert its effect by modulating pain transmission. It may also trigger the release of endogenous opioids. Heat also alters the viscosity of collagen fibers in ligaments, tendons, and joint structures so that they are more easily extended and can be stretched further before the nociceptive endings are stimulated. Thus, heat often is applied before therapy aimed at stretching joint structures and increasing range of motion. When excessive heat is used, the heat itself becomes a noxious stimulus, which results in actual or impending tissue damage and pain. In certain conditions, the use of heat is controversial, and in conditions where increased blood flow or metabolism would be detrimental, the use of heat is contraindicated.

Like heat, the application of *cold* may produce a dramatic reduction in pain. Cold exerts its effect through circulatory and neural mechanisms. The initial response to local application of cold is local vasoconstriction, followed by alternating periods of vasodilation and vasoconstriction during which the body determines a normal level of blood flow to prevent local tissue damage. Vasoconstriction is caused by local stimulation of sympathetic fibers and direct cooling of blood vessels, and **hyperemia** by local autoregulatory mechanisms. In acute injury, cold is used to produce vasoconstriction and prevent extravasation of blood into the tissues. Pain relief results from decreased swelling and decreased stimulation of nociceptive endings. The vasodilation that follows can be useful in removing substances that stimulate nociceptive endings.

Cold also can have a dramatic effect on pain that results from the spasm-induced accumulation of metabolites in muscle. Cold may reduce afferent activity reaching the posterior horn of the spinal cord by modulating sensory input. Cold is a noxious stimulus and may influence the release of endogenous opioids from the PAG. Cold packs should be flexible to conform to body parts easily, adequately wrapped to protect the skin, and applied for 15 to 20 minutes at a time.

Stimulus-Induced Analgesia

Stimulus-induced analgesia is one of the oldest known methods of pain relief. Electrical stimulation methods of pain relief include TENS, electrical acupuncture, and neurostimulation. TENS is the transmission of electrical energy across the surface of the skin to peripheral nerve fibers. TENS units are convenient, easily transported, and relatively economical to use.

The system usually consists of three parts: a pair of electrodes, lead wires, and a stimulator. The electrical stimulation is delivered in a pulsed waveform that can vary the amplitude, width, and rate. An understanding of physiologic pathways and pain mechanisms determine electrode placement. They may be placed on either side of a painful area, over an affected dermatome, over an affected peripheral nerve where it is most superficial, or over a nerve trunk (electrodes commonly are placed medial and lateral to the incision when treating postoperative pain).

There probably is no single explanation for the physiologic effects of TENS. TENS has the advantage that it is noninvasive, easily regulated by the person or health professional, and effective in some forms of acute and chronic pain. Its use can be taught before surgery, possibly reducing postoperative analgesic medication and preventing development of persistent pain.

Acupuncture

Acupuncture involves introducing needles into specific points on the surface of the body to relieve pain. Palpation is also sometimes used. Acupuncture is widely available in pain clinics despite the lack of large, high-quality, randomized studies on the effects of acupuncture.

Neurostimulation

Neurostimulation delivers low-voltage electrical stimulation to the spinal cord or targeted peripheral nerve to block the sensation of pain. Melzack and Wall (gate theory) proposed that neurostimulation activates the body's pain-inhibiting system. For a totally implantable system, the power source (battery) and lead(s) are surgically implanted.

Pharmacologic Treatment

An analgesic drug acts on the nervous system to decrease or eliminate pain without inducing loss of consciousness. Analgesic drugs do not cure the underlying cause, but appropriate use may prevent acute pain from progressing to chronic pain. Analgesic drugs enable a person to achieve mobility after surgery, when exercises such as coughing and deep breathing may be required.

The ideal analgesic would be effective, nonaddictive, and inexpensive, and it would produce minimal adverse effects and not affect the person's level of consciousness. Although long-term treatment with opioids can result in opioid tolerance and physical dependence, this should not be confused with addiction. The unique needs and circumstances presented by each person in pain must be addressed to achieve satisfactory pain management. The use of analgesics is only one aspect of a comprehensive pain management program with acute pain, and even more so with chronic pain.

Nonnarcotic Analgesics

Nonnarcotic oral analgesic medications include aspirin, other NSAIDs, and acetaminophen. Aspirin (acetylsalicylic acid) blocks transmission of pain impulses. It has antipyretic and anti-inflammatory properties. Aspirin and other NSAIDs inhibit the action of cyclooxygenase (COX) enzymes, which mediate biosynthesis of prostaglandins. NSAIDs also decrease the sensitivity of blood vessels to bradykinin and histamine, affect cytokine production by T lymphocytes, reverse vasodilation, and decrease the release of inflammatory mediators from granulocytes, mast cells, and basophils.[17] Acetaminophen is an alternative to NSAIDs. Although usually considered equivalent to aspirin as an analgesic and antipyretic agent, it lacks anti-inflammatory properties.

Opioid Analgesics

The term *opioid* or *narcotic* is used to refer to a group of medications, natural or synthetic, which has morphine-like actions.[17] The older term *opiate* was used to designate drugs derived from opium—morphine, codeine, and other semisynthetic congeners of morphine. Opioids are used for relief of short-term pain and for long-term use in conditions such as cancer pain. There is strong evidence that opioids given routinely before the pain starts (preemptive analgesia in surgery) or becomes extreme are far more effective than those administered in a sporadic manner. People treated in this manner seem to require fewer doses and are able to resume regular activities sooner.

The opioid analgesics are characterized by their interaction with opioid receptors, including mu (μ, for "morphine"), delta (δ), and kappa (κ) receptors.[17] Morphine and most opioids used clinically exert their effects through the μ receptor. Kappa receptor opioids are effective analgesics but have troublesome side effects, and the clinical impact of delta receptor opioids has been negligible.

The mu receptors modulate both the therapeutic effect of analgesia and the adverse side effects of respiratory depression, **miosis**, reduced gastrointestinal motility (causing constipation), feelings of well-being or euphoria, and physical dependence. Mu receptors are found at presynaptic and postsynaptic sites in the spinal dorsal horn and in the ascending pathways of the brain stem, thalamus, and cortex as well as the descending inhibitory system that modulates pain at the spinal cord. Their spinal location has been used clinically by injection, infusion, or implantable intrathecal device (pump), which provides regional anesthesia while minimizing the adverse side effects that occur with systemically administered drugs. Mu receptors are also found in peripheral sensory neurons after inflammation, which supports the clinical use of locally applied opioids (*e.g.*, intraarticular instillation of opioids after knee surgery).

Adjuvant Analgesics

Adjuvant analgesics include medications such as tricyclic antidepressants, antiepileptic medications, and neuroleptic anxiolytic agents. The pain suppression system has nonendorphin synapses, raising the possibility that potent, centrally acting, nonopiate medications may relieve pain. Serotonin also plays an important role in producing analgesia. The tricyclic antidepressant medications that block removal of serotonin from the synaptic cleft produce pain relief in some people, which is useful in some chronic painful conditions (*i.e.*, postherpetic neuralgia).[16,17]

Certain antiepileptic medications, such as carbamazepine and gabapentin, have analgesic effects in some pain conditions. These medications, which suppress spontaneous neuronal firing, are useful in the management of pain that occurs after nerve injury (neuropathic pain), including diabetic neuropathy and chronic regional pain syndrome. Other agents, such as corticosteroids, may be used to decrease inflammation and the nociceptive stimuli responsible for pain.[17]

Surgical Intervention

If surgery removes the problem causing the pain, it can be curative. Surgery can also be used for symptom management. Surgery for severe, intractable pain of peripheral or central origin has met with some success. Surgery can remove the cause or block the transmission of intractable pain from phantom limb pain, severe neuralgia, inoperable cancer of certain types, and causalgia.

SUMMARY CONCEPTS

Pain is an elusive and complex phenomenon; it is a symptom common to many illnesses. It is a highly individualized experience shaped by a person's previous life experiences and is difficult to measure. Scientifically, pain is viewed within the context of **nociception**. Nociceptors are receptive nerve endings that respond to noxious stimuli (mechanical, thermal, and chemical). Nociceptive neurons transmit impulses to dorsal horn neurons using chemical neurotransmitters. The neospinothalamic and paleospinothalamic pathways are used to transmit pain information to the brain. Several neuroanatomic pathways and endogenous opioid peptides modulate pain in the CNS.

Pain can be classified according to duration, location, and referral as well as associated medical diagnoses. Acute pain is self-limiting pain that ends when the injured tissue heals, whereas chronic pain lasts much longer than the healing time for the underlying cause of the pain. Pain can arise from cutaneous, deep somatic, or visceral locations. Referred pain is pain perceived at a site different from its origin. Pain threshold, pain tolerance, and other factors affect a person's reaction to pain.

Treatment modalities for pain include the use of physiologic, cognitive, and behavioral measures; heat and cold; stimulation-induced analgesic methods; and pharmacologic agents. Even with chronic pain, the most effective approach is early treatment or prevention. Success in pain assessment and management is achieved with an interdisciplinary approach.

Alterations in Pain Sensitivity and Special Types of Pain

Alterations in Pain Sensitivity

Sensitivity to and perception of pain vary among people and in the same person under different conditions and in different parts of the body. Irritation, mild hypoxia, and mild compression of a peripheral nerve often result in hyperexcitability of the sensory nerve fibers or cell bodies. This is experienced as an unpleasant hypersensitivity (*i.e.*, hyperesthesia) or an increased painfulness (*i.e.*, hyperalgesia). Primary hyperalgesia describes pain sensitivity that occurs directly in damaged tissues. Secondary hyperalgesia occurs in the surrounding uninjured tissue. Possible causes of hyperalgesia include increased sensitivity to noxious stimuli, a decrease in nociceptor threshold, an increase in pain produced by suprathreshold stimuli, and the windup phenomenon.[19]

Hyperpathia is a syndrome in which the sensory threshold is raised, but when it is reached, continued stimulation, especially if repetitive, results in a prolonged and unpleasant experience. This pain can be explosive and radiates through a peripheral nerve distribution. It is associated with pathologic changes in peripheral nerves. Spontaneous, unpleasant sensations called *paresthesias* occur with more severe irritation. The general term *dysesthesia* is given to distortions of somesthetic sensation that typically accompany partial loss of sensory innervation.

Severe pathologic processes can result in reduced or lost tactile (*e.g.*, *hypoesthesia*, *anesthesia*), temperature (*e.g.*, *hypothermia*, *athermia*), and pain sensation (*i.e.*, *hypoalgesia*). *Analgesia* is the absence of pain or pain relief without loss of consciousness. Congenital indifference is when transmission of nerve impulses appears normal but sensation of painful stimuli at higher levels appears absent. Congenital insensitivity is when a peripheral nerve defect exists such that transmission of painful nerve impulses does not result in pain perception. People who lack pain perception are at risk of tissue damage because pain is not serving its protective function.[20]

Allodynia is the phenomenon of pain that follows a nonnoxious stimulus to apparently normal skin. It can result from increased responsiveness within the spinal cord (central sensitization) or reduced threshold for nociceptor activation (peripheral sensitization). Allodynia can involve *trigger points*, which are highly localized points on the skin or mucous membrane that produce immediate intense pain when stimulated by light tactile stimulation. Myofascial trigger points are foci of extreme tenderness found in muscles and can be responsible for pain projected to sites remote from the points of tenderness. Trigger points are widely distributed in the back of the head and neck, and in the lumbar and thoracic regions. They cause reproducible myofascial pain syndromes in specific muscles and are major source of pain at chronic pain treatment centers.

Special Types of Pain

Neuropathic Pain

Neuropathic pain is caused by a problem with the neurologic system. When peripheral nerves are affected by injury or disease, it can lead to unusual and intractable sensory disturbances. Features that point to neuropathic processes as a cause of pain include widespread pain that is otherwise unexplainable and evidence of sensory deficit. Neuropathic pain is distinguished from other pain conditions where the pain stimulus begins in nonneuronal tissues.

Conditions that lead to neuropathic pain can be categorized according to the extent of peripheral nerve involvement. Damage to peripheral nerves in a single area include nerve entrapment, nerve compression from a tumor mass, and various neuralgias. Damage to peripheral nerves in a wide area include diabetes mellitus, long-term alcohol use, and hypothyroidism. Diabetes often causes a length-dependent neuropathy (longest axons in a peripheral nerve are most vulnerable). Injury to a nerve also can lead to a multisymptom, multisystem syndrome called *complex regional pain syndrome*. Nerve damage associated with amputation is believed to be a cause phantom limb pain.

Neuropathic pain can vary with the extent and location of disease or injury. There may be allodynia or pain that is stabbing, jabbing, burning, or shooting, which may be persistent or intermittent. The diagnosis depends on the mode of onset, distribution of abnormal sensations, quality of the pain, and other relevant medical conditions. Injury to peripheral nerves sometimes results in pain that persists beyond the time required for the tissues to heal. Peripheral pathologic processes and neural plasticity are the working hypotheses to explain persistent neuropathic pain.

Treatment methods include measures aimed at restoring or preventing further nerve damage and the palliation of pain. Although many adjuvant analgesics are used for neuropathic pain, control is often difficult. The initial approach is to try drugs in sequence and then in combination with nonpharmacologic interventions. Adjuvant analgesic treatments can be divided into two classes: neuropathic and bone pain. Often, neuropathic pain is treated with tricyclic antidepressants, antiepileptics, local anesthetics, and α_2-adrenergic agonists and bone pain is treated with glucocorticoids, bisphosphonates, osteoclast inhibitors, and skeletal muscle relaxants.[16]

Poor pain control or side effects may lead to use of other medications. Opioids can be used, but concerns about side effects and possibility of addiction must be considered. The use of long-acting opioids with a plan for breakthrough pain is desired to address the typically continuous nature of neuropathic pain. Nonpharmacologic therapies are used for neurogenic pain, including electrical stimulation of the peripheral nerve or spinal cord (used in radiculopathies and neuralgias).

Neuralgia

Neuralgia is characterized by severe, brief, often repetitive attacks of lightning-like or throbbing pain. It occurs along the distribution of a spinal or cranial nerve and usually is precipitated by stimulation of the cutaneous region supplied by that nerve.

Trigeminal Neuralgia

Trigeminal neuralgia, or *tic douloureux*, is one of the most common and severe neuralgias. It is characterized by recurring, sudden onset of sharp, stabbing, pains without numbness in one or more nerve branches of CN V.[3] The pathophysiology of trigeminal neuralgia is thought to be caused by demyelination of axons in the ganglion, root, and nerve.[16]

Treatment of trigeminal neuralgia includes pharmacologic and surgical modalities. Other interventions include avoidance of precipitating factors and eye injury because of irritation, provision for adequate nutrition, and avoidance of social isolation. Carbamazepine (Tegretol), an antiepileptic drug, is recognized as a first-line agent for the treatment of trigeminal neuralgia.[16] Surgical release of vessels, dural structures, or scar tissue surrounding the semilunar ganglion or root in the middle cranial fossa often eliminates the symptoms.

Postherpetic Neuralgia

Herpes zoster (*shingles*) is caused by the same herpes virus (varicella-zoster virus) that causes chickenpox. It is thought to represent a localized recurrent infection by the varicella-zoster virus that has remained latent in the dorsal root ganglia.[16] Reactivation of viral replication is associated with a decline in cellular immunity. The probability of developing herpes zoster increases after the age of 60.[16]

During the acute attack of herpes zoster, the reactivated virus travels from the affected sensory ganglia and peripheral nerve to the skin of the corresponding dermatomes, causing a unilateral localized vesicular eruption and hyperpathia. In the acute infection, proportionately more of the large nerve fibers are destroyed. Regenerated fibers appear to have smaller diameters. Because there is a relative loss of large fibers with age, older adults are particularly prone to pain because of the shift in the proportion of large- to small-diameter nerve fibers. People with postherpetic neuralgia may experience constant pain ("burning, aching, throbbing"), intermittent pain ("stabbing, shooting"), and stimulus-evoked pain (allodynia).

Early treatment of shingles with antiviral drugs such as acyclovir or valacyclovir that inhibit herpes virus DNA replication may reduce the severity of herpes zoster. Initially, postherpetic neuralgia can be treated with a topical anesthetic agent, lidocaine–prilocaine cream or 5% lidocaine gel. A tricyclic antidepressant medication, such as amitriptyline or desipramine, may be used for pain relief. Regional nerve blockade has been used with limited success. A live attenuated herpes zoster vaccine (Zostavax) for adults over 60 years of age offers approximately 60% protection against herpes zoster and postherpetic neuralgia.[16]

Phantom Limb Pain

Phantom limb pain, a type of neurologic pain, follows amputation of a limb or part of a limb. The pain can start out as tingling, squeezing, or heaviness, followed by burning, cramping, or shooting pain.[21] It may disappear spontaneously or persist for many years. Multiple theories attempt to explain the causes of phantom pain including damage of regenerating nerves, spontaneous firing of spinal cord neurons with abnormal sensory input, and the pain actually arises in the brain itself. Treatment has been accomplished using sympathetic blocks, TENS of the large myelinated afferents innervating the area, hypnosis, and relaxation training.

SUMMARY CONCEPTS

Pain may occur with or without an adequate stimulus or may be absent in the presence of an adequate stimulus. There may be analgesia (absence of pain), hyperalgesia (increased sensitivity to pain), hypoalgesia (a decreased sensitivity to painful stimuli), hyperpathia (an unpleasant and prolonged response to pain), hyperesthesia (an abnormal increase in sensitivity to sensation), hypoesthesia (an abnormal decrease in sensitivity to sensations), paresthesia (abnormal touch sensation such as tingling or "pins and needles" in the absence of external stimuli), or allodynia (pain produced by stimuli that do not normally cause pain).

Neuropathic pain may be due to trauma or disease of neurons in a focal area or in a more global distribution. Neuralgia is characterized by severe, brief, often repetitive attacks of lightning-like or throbbing pain that occurs along the distribution of a spinal or cranial nerve and usually is precipitated by stimulation of the cutaneous region supplied by that nerve. Trigeminal neuralgia is one of the most common and severe neuralgias. It is manifested by facial tics or spasms. Postherpetic neuralgia is a chronic pain that can occur after shingles—an infection of the dorsal root ganglia and corresponding areas of innervation by the varicella-zoster virus. Phantom limb pain, a neurologic pain, can occur after amputation of a limb or part of a limb.

Headache and Associated Pain

Headache

Over 18 million Americans visit their health care provider because of a headache annually.[16] Although head and facial pain have characteristics that distinguish them from other pain disorders, they also share many of the same features.

Headache is caused by several conditions. Some represent primary disorders and others occur secondary to disease conditions in which head pain is a symptom. The most common types of primary or chronic headaches are migraine headache, tension-type headache, cluster headache, and chronic daily headache (CDH). Although most causes of secondary headache are benign, some are indications of serious disorders such as meningitis, brain tumor, or cerebral aneurysm. Other times a person may experience a headache post head trauma. Research suggests that people with mild traumatic brain injury (TBI) have more problems with headache than those with moderate or severe TBI.[22] The sudden onset of a severe, intractable headache in an otherwise healthy person is more likely related to a serious intracranial disorder, such as subarachnoid hemorrhage or meningitis, than to a chronic headache disorder. Headaches that disturb sleep, exertional headaches, and headaches accompanied by neurologic symptoms such as drowsiness, visual or limb disturbances, or altered mental status also are suggestive of underlying intracranial lesions or other pathologic processes. Other red flags for secondary headache disorder include a fundamental change or progression in headache pattern, or a new headache in people with cancer or immunosuppression, in pregnancy, or in people over the age of 50.[23,24] Older adults need a comprehensive assessment of any headache if they have not had prior headaches.[25]

The diagnosis and classification of headaches requires a comprehensive history and physical examination to exclude secondary causes. The history should include factors that precipitate headache, such as foods, missed meals, medications, alcohol use, and the menstrual period. A headache diary in which the person records his or her headaches and concurrent or antecedent events may be helpful in identifying factors that contribute to headache onset.

In 2013, the International Headache Society (IHS) published the third edition of *The International Classification of Headache Disorders* (ICHD-3).[24] The classification system is divided into as follows: (1) primary headaches, (2) secondary headaches, and (3) painful cranial neuropathies, other facial pains, and other headaches.[24]

Migraine Headache

Migraine headaches affect 38 million people in the United States. Migraine headaches tend to run in families and may be inherited as an autosomal dominant trait with incomplete penetrance.

Etiology and Pathogenesis

The pathophysiologic mechanisms of the pain associated with migraine headaches remain poorly understood. It is well established that the CN V becomes activated during a migraine.[26] Stimulation of CN V sensory fibers may lead to the release of neuropeptides, causing painful neurogenic inflammation within the meningeal vasculature, or neurogenic vasodilation of meningeal blood vessels may contribute to inflammatory processes. Supporting the neurogenic basis for migraine is the presence of premonitory symptoms before the headache begins: the presence of **focal** neurologic disturbances cannot be explained by cerebral blood flow.[27]

Hormonal variations, particularly in estrogen levels, play a role in the pattern of migraine attacks. For many women, migraine headaches coincide with their menstrual periods. Dietary substances, such as monosodium glutamate, aged cheese, and chocolate, also may precipitate migraine headaches. The actual triggers for migraine are the chemicals in the food, not allergens.

Clinical Manifestations

The ICHD-3 classifies migraine headaches into migraines without aura and migraines with aura.[24] Migraine without aura is a pulsatile, throbbing, unilateral headache that typically lasts 1 to 2 days and is aggravated by routine physical activity. It is accompanied by nausea and vomiting and sensitivity to light and sound. Visual disturbances commonly occur and consist of hallucinations such as stars, sparks, and flashes of light. Migraine with aura has similar symptoms, but with the addition of reversible visual symptoms, including positive features (*e.g.*, flickering lights, spots, or lines) or negative features (*e.g.*, loss of vision); fully reversible sensory symptoms, including positive features (*e.g.*, feeling of pins or needles) or negative features (*e.g.*, numbness); and fully reversible speech disturbances or neurologic symptoms that precede the headache.[24] The aura typically develops over 5 to 20 minutes and lasts from 5 minutes to an hour. A small percentage of people with migraine experience an aura before an attack, but many without aura have prodromal symptoms, such as fatigue and irritability, that precede the attack by hours or days.[26]

Other ICHD-3 migraine headache subtypes are chronic migraine, complications of migraine, probable migraine, and episodic syndromes that may be associated with migraine.[24] Retinal migraines are rare and characterized by recurrent attacks of fully reversible scintillations (*e.g.*, sparks or flashes of light), scotomata (*e.g.*, visual blind spots), or blindness affecting one eye, followed within an hour by migrainous headache. Chronic migraine is classified as a headache meeting the criteria for migraine that is present on 15 or more days per month for 3 months or more, in the absence of medication overuse. Migrainous infarction is an uncommon occurrence in which typical aura symptom(s) persist beyond 1 hour and neuroimaging confirms ischemic infarction. Strictly applied, these criteria distinguish this disorder from stroke, which must be excluded.[24]

Migraine headache can present as a mixed headache, including symptoms typically associated with tension-type headache, sinus headache, or CDH. These *transformed migraines* are difficult to classify. Although nasal symptoms are not one of the diagnostic criteria for migraine, they frequently accompany migraine. Sinus pain may indicate a headache due to sinus inflammation or migraine.

Before puberty, migraine headaches are equally distributed between the sexes. The diagnostic criterion for migraine in children is the presence of recurrent headaches separated by pain-free periods. Diagnosis is generally based on the child experiencing three of the following: abdominal pain, nausea or vomiting, throbbing headache, unilateral location, associated aura, relief during sleep, and a positive family history. Symptoms vary widely among children, from those that interrupt activities to those that are detectable only by direct questioning. A common feature of migraine in children is intense nausea and vomiting. Vomiting may be associated with abdominal pain and fever and thus may be confused with other conditions. Because headaches in children can be a symptom of other serious disorders, it is important that other causes of headache be ruled out.

Treatment

The treatment of migraine headaches includes preventive and abortive nonpharmacologic and pharmacologic treatment. Nonpharmacologic treatment includes the avoidance of migraine triggers, such as foods or smells that precipitate an attack. Many people with migraines benefit from maintaining regular eating and sleeping habits and controlling stress. During an attack, many people find it helpful to retire to a quiet, darkened room until the symptoms subside. Pharmacologic treatment involves both abortive therapy for acute attacks and preventive therapy. First-line agents for acute symptoms include acetylsalicylic acid; acetaminophen, acetylsalicylic acid, and caffeine combinations; NSAIDs; serotonin ($5\text{-}HT_1$) receptor agonists; ergotamine derivatives; and antiemetic medications.[16,27] Nonoral routes of administration may be preferred in people who develop severe pain rapidly or on awakening, or with severe nausea and vomiting. Frequent use of abortive headache medications may cause rebound headache.

Preventive pharmacologic treatment may be necessary if migraine headaches become disabling, if they occur more than two or three times a month, if abortive treatment is being used more than two times a week, or if the person has hemiplegic migraine, migraine with prolonged aura, or migrainous infarction.[16,27] In most cases, preventive treatment must be taken daily for months to years. First-line agents include β-adrenergic blocking medications, antidepressants, and antiepileptic medications.[16] Discontinuation of preventive therapy should be gradual. Other effective medications are available, but they can have serious side effects (*i.e.*, $5\text{-}HT_1$ receptor agonists increase risk of coronary vasospasm and should be avoided in coronary artery disease).

Cluster Headache

Cluster headaches are relatively uncommon headaches that occur more frequently in men than in women and typically begin in the third decade of life.[28] They tend to occur in clusters over weeks or months, followed by a headache-free remission period. Cluster headache is a type of primary neurovascular headache that typically includes severe, unrelenting, unilateral pain.

Etiology and Pathogenesis

The underlying pathophysiologic mechanisms of cluster headaches are not completely known, although an autosomal dominant gene may play a role in the pathogenesis. The most likely pathophysiologic mechanisms include the interplay of vascular, neurogenic, metabolic, and humoral factors. Activation of the trigeminovascular system and the cranial autonomic parasympathetic reflexes may explain the pain and autonomic symptoms. The regulating centers in the anterior hypothalamus are implicated from observations of circadian biologic changes and neuroendocrine disturbances. Magnetic resonance imaging has demonstrated dilated intracranial arteries on the painful side, perhaps due to a defect in sympathetic perivascular innervation.

Clinical Manifestations

The pain associated with cluster headache is of rapid onset and peaks in approximately 10 to 15 minutes, lasting for 15 to 180 minutes. Pain behind the eye radiates to the ipsilateral trigeminal nerve. The headache is associated with restlessness, conjunctival redness, lacrimation on one side, nasal congestion, rhinorrhea, forehead and facial sweating, miosis, ptosis, and eyelid edema.

Treatment

The most effective treatments for cluster headache act quickly. Oxygen inhalation may be indicated for home use. Prophylactic medications for cluster headaches include verapamil, lithium carbonate, corticosteroids, and sodium valproate.[27]

Tension-Type Headache

Tension-type headache is the most common type of headache and is usually not sufficiently severe that it interferes with daily activities.

Etiology and Pathogenesis

The exact mechanisms of tension-type headache are not known. Tension-type headaches may result from sustained tension of the muscles of the scalp and neck or by migraine headaches transformed gradually into chronic tension-type headache. They may also be caused by oromandibular dysfunction, stress, anxiety, depression, or overuse of analgesics or caffeine.

Clinical Manifestations

Tension-type headaches frequently are described as dull, aching, diffuse, nondescript headaches, occurring in a hatband distribution around the head, and not associated with nausea or vomiting or worsened by activity. They can be infrequent, episodic, or chronic.

Treatment

Tension-type headaches often are more responsive to nonpharmacologic techniques, such as biofeedback, massage, acupuncture, and physical therapy, than other types of headache. A combination of range-of-motion exercises, relaxation, and posture improvement may be helpful.

The medications of choice for acute treatment of tension-type headaches are analgesics, including acetylsalicylic acid, acetaminophen, and NSAIDs.[16,27] These agents should be used cautiously as rebound headaches can develop when the medications are taken regularly.

Chronic Daily Headache

The term *chronic daily headache* is used to refer to headaches that occur 15 days or more a month, for greater than 3 months.[27] Little is known about the prevalence and incidence of CDH. Diagnostic criteria for CDH are not provided in the IHS classification system.

Etiology and Pathogenesis

The cause of CDH is unknown, although there are several hypotheses. They include transformed migraine headache, evolved tension-type headache, new daily persistent headache, and posttraumatic headache. Although overuse of symptomatic medications has been related to CDH, there is a group of people in whom CDH is unrelated to excessive use of medications.

Clinical Manifestations

In many people, CDH retains certain characteristics of migraine, whereas in others, it resembles chronic tension-type headache. CDH may be associated with chronic and episodic tension-type headache. New daily persistent headache may have a rapid onset, with no history of migraine, tension-type headache, trauma, or psychological stress.

Treatment

Treatment may include both pharmacologic and behavioral interventions. Nonpharmacologic techniques include biofeedback, massage, acupuncture, relaxation, imagery, and physical therapy. Reduction or elimination of medication, including caffeine, may be helpful.

Temporomandibular Joint Pain

A common cause of head pain is temporomandibular joint (TMJ) syndrome. It is usually caused by an imbalance in joint movement because of poor bite, bruxism, or joint problems.[27] The pain is usually referred and commonly presents as facial muscle pain, headache, neck ache, or earache. Pain is aggravated by jaw function. These headaches are common in all ages and can cause chronic pain problems.

Treatment of TMJ pain is aimed at correcting the problem. The initial therapy for TMJ should be directed toward relief of pain and improvement in function. Pain relief often can be achieved with use of the NSAIDs. Muscle relaxants may be used when muscle spasm is a problem.

SUMMARY CONCEPTS

Head pain is a common disorder that is caused by several conditions. Some headaches represent primary disorders and others occur secondary to another disease state. Primary headache disorders include migraine headache, tension-type headache, cluster headache, and CDH. Although most causes of secondary headache are benign, some are indications of serious disorders such as meningitis, brain tumor, or cerebral aneurysm. TMJ syndrome is a major cause of headaches. It is usually caused by an imbalance in joint movement because of poor bite, teeth grinding, or joint problems such as inflammation, trauma, and degenerative changes.

Pain in Children and Older Adults

Pain frequently is underrecognized and undertreated in both children and older adults. Common obstacles to adequate pain management include concerns of analgesia on respiratory status and opioid addiction. Additional concerns for these populations include difficulty of assessing the location and intensity of pain in cognitively immature or cognitively impaired individuals.[19]

Pain in Children

Responsiveness to painful stimuli begins in the neonatal period. Pain pathways, cortical and subcortical centers, and neurochemical responses associated with pain transmission are functional by the last trimester of pregnancy. Neonates perceive pain as demonstrated by their integrated physiologic response to nociceptive stimuli. Dorsal horn neurons in neonates have a wider receptive field and lower excitatory threshold than those in older children.

Pain response evolves with the maturation of cognitive and developmental processes. Children feel pain, accurately report pain, and remember pain. This is evidenced in children with cancer, whose distress during painful procedures increases over time without intervention, and in neonates who demonstrate withdrawal responses to a heel stick after repeated episodes.

Pain Assessment

Ongoing assessment of the presence of pain and response to treatment is essential.[16] Self-report is usually the most reliable estimate of pain. With children of 8 years of age or older, numeric scales and word graphic scales can be used. With children 3 to 8 years of age, scales with faces of children or cartoon faces can be used to obtain a report of pain. Another supplementary strategy for assessing a child's pain is to use a body outline and

ask the child to indicate where the pain is located. Care must be taken in assessing children's reports of pain as they may be influenced by factors including age, anxiety and fear levels, and parental presence. Some physiologic measures, such as heart rate, are convenient to measure and respond rapidly to brief nociceptive stimuli, but they are nonspecific. Relying on indicators of sympathetic nervous system activity and behaviors can also be problematic because they can be caused by things other than pain and they do not always accompany pain, particularly chronic pain.

Pain Management

Pain management in children falls into two categories: pharmacologic and nonpharmacologic. Pharmacologic interventions include many of the analgesics used in adults, which can be used safely and effectively in children and adolescents. It is critical to determine that the medication has been approved for use with children and that it is dosed according to weight and physiologic development. Age-related differences in physiologic functioning affect drug action. Neonates and infants have decreased levels of the hepatic enzymes needed for metabolism of many analgesics. These hepatic enzymes increase to adult levels in the first few months of life. The renal excretion of drugs depends on renal blood flow, glomerular filtration rate, and tubular secretion, all of which are decreased in neonates, particularly premature neonates.

The overriding principle in all pediatric pain management is to treat each child's pain on an individual basis and to match the analgesic agent with the cause and level of pain. A second principle involves maintaining the balance such that pain relief is obtained with as little opioid and sedation as possible. One strategy is to time the administration of analgesia so that a steady blood level is achieved and, as much as possible, pain is prevented. This requires that the child receive analgesia on a regular dosing schedule, not "as needed." Most drugs are packaged for adult use, and dose calculations and serial dilutions may predispose to medication errors.

Nonpharmacologic strategies can be very effective in reducing the overall amount of pain and analgesia used. In addition, some nonpharmacologic strategies can reduce anxiety and increase the child's level of self-control during pain. Children can be taught simple distraction techniques such as application of heat and cold. Other nonpharmacologic techniques can be taught to provide psychological preparation for a painful procedure or surgery. These include positive self-talk, imagery, play therapy, modeling, and rehearsal. The nonpharmacologic interventions must be developmentally appropriate, and if possible, the child and parent should be taught these techniques when the child is not in pain so that it is easier to practice the technique.

Pain in Older Adults

The prevalence of pain in the general population increases with age. Some apparent age-related differences may be due to differences in willingness to report pain rather than actual differences in pain. It is important for the provider to ask specific questions to older adults regarding their pain in order to elicit the correct information so best management of the pain can be given.[29]

Pain Assessment

When possible, a person's report of pain is the gold standard, but behavioral signs of pain should also be considered. Accurately diagnosing pain in an individual with many health problems or a decline in cognitive function can be challenging. The Assessment for Discomfort in Dementia Protocol includes behavioral criteria for assessing pain and recommended interventions.[30]

Pain Management

When prescribing pain management in older patients, the cause of pain, concurrent therapies, the person's health, and mental status must all be considered. Risk of adverse events is higher in older populations, and nonpharmacologic options are usually less costly and cause fewer side effects.

Relaxation techniques, massage, and biofeedback may be useful nonpharmacologic interventions. Physical therapy and occupational therapy, including the use of braces or splints, changes in biomechanics, and exercise, have been shown to promote pain relief.

Although efficacy is important, cost and safety must also be considered. Safety issues that must be considered among older adults include changes in drug metabolism, disease comorbidity, and polypharmacy. Older adults may have physiologic changes that affect the pharmacokinetics of medications prescribed, including decreased blood flow to organs, delayed gastric motility, reduced kidney function, and decreased albumin related to poor nutrition.[17] Adding analgesics to a complex medication regimen is even more likely to cause drug interactions and complicate compliance in older adults. However, this should not preclude the appropriate use of analgesic drugs to achieve pain relief. Nonopioids are generally the first line of therapy for mild to moderate pain, and acetaminophen is usually the first choice because it is relatively safe for older adults.[16] Opioids are used for more severe pain and for palliative care. Adjuvant analgesics are effectively used for treatment of pain in older adults. An assessment tool to evaluate the level of pain and effectiveness of treatment is essential, along with monitoring for side effects.

SUMMARY CONCEPTS

Children experience and remember pain, and young children are able to accurately and reliably report pain. Recognition of this has changed the clinical practice of health professionals involved in the assessment of children's pain. Pharmacologic and nonpharmacologic pain management interventions have been shown

to be effective in children. Nonpharmacologic techniques must be based on the developmental level of the child and are taught to both children and parents.

Pain is a common symptom in older adults. Assessment, diagnosis, and treatment of pain in older adults can be complicated. Older adults may be reluctant or cognitively unable to report their pain. Diagnosis and treatment can be complicated by comorbidities and age-related changes in cognitive and physiologic function.

 Body Temperature Regulation

Most biochemical processes in the body are affected by changes in temperature. Metabolic processes speed up or slow down depending on whether the body temperature is rising or falling. *Core body temperature* normally is maintained within a range of 36.0°C to 37.5°C (97.0°F to 99.5°F).[31] Within this range, there are individual differences. For example, core temperature of most females increases approximately 0.5°C to 1.0°C during the postovulation phase of their menstrual cycle.[31] There are diurnal variations. Internal core temperatures reach their highest point between 3:00 and 6:00 PM and their lowest point between 3:00 and 6:00 AM (Fig. 14-12).[31]

Body temperature reflects the difference between heat production and heat loss and varies with exercise and environmental temperature. Exercise can increase metabolic heat production by 10-fold, and thermoregulatory responses such as sweating prevent body temperature from rising dangerously high.[31] Shivering increases metabolic heat production and can offset the increased heat loss resulting from cold ambient conditions. Properly protected and hydrated, the body can function in environmental conditions from −50°C (−58°F) to +50°C (122°F). The failure to adequately manage heat production and/or loss results in devastating consequences. Ice crystals can form in tissues exposed to very cold and damp ambient temperatures, and, at the other extreme, very high temperatures (+45°C [113°F]) cause proteins to coagulate and/or aggregate. As will be discussed later

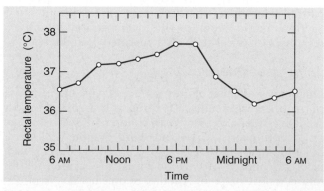

FIGURE 14-12. Normal diurnal variations in body temperature.

in this chapter, much smaller, systemic changes in body temperature can be equally devastating, leading to tissue damage, organ failure, coma, and even death.[32]

KEY POINTS

Thermoregulation

- Core body temperature is a reflection of the balance between heat gain and heat loss by the body. Metabolic processes produce heat, which must be dissipated.

- The hypothalamus is the thermal control center for the body; it receives information from peripheral and central thermoreceptors and compares that information with its set point.

- An increase in core temperature results from vasoconstriction and shivering, and a decrease in temperature results from vasodilation and sweating.

Most of the body's heat is produced by the deeper core tissues, which are insulated from the environment and protected against heat loss by an outer shell of subcutaneous tissues and skin (Fig. 14-13). In a warm environment, blood flow is increased, allowing for greater dissipation of heat. In a cold environment, the vessels supplying blood flow to the skin and underlying tissues constrict, which helps to minimize the loss of core heat for the body. The subcutaneous fat layer contributes to the insulation value of the outer shell because of its thickness and because it conducts heat only about one third as effectively as other tissues.

Temperatures differ in various parts of the body. The rectal temperature is a measure of core temperature and is considered the most accurate parameter.[1] Rectal temperatures usually range from 37.3°C (99.1°F) to 37.6°C (99.6°F). Core temperatures may also be obtained from the esophagus using a flexible thermometer or from a pulmonary artery catheter. Pulmonary artery and esophageal temperatures closely reflect the temperatures of the heart and thoracic organs.

 Concept Mastery Alert

The pulmonary artery catheter is the preferred measurement when body temperatures are changing rapidly and need to be followed reliably on an acutely ill person in an intensive care setting.

The oral temperature, taken sublingually, is usually 0.2°C (0.36°F) to 0.51°C (0.9°F) lower than the rectal temperature, but closely follows changes in core temperature. The axillary temperature also can be used to estimate core temperature, but the parts of the axillary fossa must be pressed closely together for an extended period (5 to 10 minutes for a glass thermometer) because this method requires considerable heat to accumulate before the final temperature is reached.

Ear-based thermometry uses an infrared sensor to measure blood flow from the carotid artery at the tympanic membrane and is considered to directly reflect core temperature.[33] It is popular because of its ease and speed of measurement, acceptability to people, and cost savings in the personnel time. However, there is continuing debate regarding the accuracy of this method.[34]

Core body and skin temperatures are sensed and integrated by thermoregulatory regions in the hypothalamus and other brain structures (*i.e.*, thalamus and cerebral cortex). Temperature-sensitive ion channels (thermo-TRPs) present in peripheral and central sensory neurons are activated by innocuous (warm and cool) and noxious (hot and cold) stimuli.[35] Peripheral temperature signals are initiated by changes in local membrane potentials and transmitted to the brain through dorsal root ganglia.[35] The *set point* of the hypothalamic thermoregulatory center is the ideal core temperature for the individual, helping regulate the temperature of the body core within the normal range of 36.0°C (96.8°F) to 37.5°C (99.5°F). When body temperature begins to rise above the set point, the hypothalamus signals the central and peripheral nervous systems to initiate heat-dissipating behaviors. When the temperature falls below the set point, signals from the hypothalamus elicit behaviors that increase heat conservation and production. Core temperatures above 41°C (105.8°F) or below

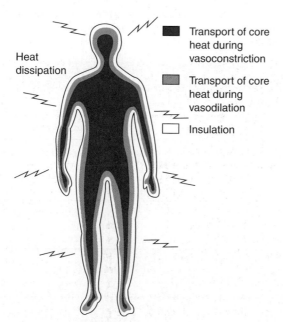

FIGURE 14-13. Control of heat loss. Body heat is produced in the deeper core tissues of the body, which is insulated by the subcutaneous tissues and skin to protect against heat loss. During vasodilation, circulating blood transports heat to the skin surface, where it dissipates into the surrounding environment. Vasoconstriction decreases the transport of core heat to the skin surface, and vasodilation increases transport.

34°C (93.2°F) indicate impairment in the body's thermoregulation. Responses that produce, conserve, and dissipate heat are described in Table 14-2. Spinal cord injuries at T6 or above can impair temperature regulation because the hypothalamic thermoregulatory centers can no longer control skin blood flow and sweating.

In addition to reflexive and automatic thermoregulatory mechanisms, humans engage in voluntary behaviors to regulate body temperature based on the conscious sensation of being too hot or too cold. These include the selection of proper clothing and regulation of environmental temperature through heating systems and air conditioning. Body positions that hold the extremities close to the body prevent heat loss and are commonly assumed in cold weather.

Mechanisms of Heat Production

Metabolism is the body's main source of heat production or thermogenesis. Many factors impact the metabolic rate, including:

- Metabolic rate of each cell
- Factor that may increase basal metabolic rate (BMR), such as that caused by muscle activity
- Extra metabolism caused by hormones, such as thyroxine, growth hormone, or testosterone
- Any extra metabolism caused by the sympathetic nervous system stimulation on cells
- Extra metabolism caused by increased cellular chemical activity
- Thermogenic effect of food digestion, absorption, or storage[1]

There is a 0.55°C (1°F) increase in body temperature for every 7% increase in metabolism. The sympathetic neurotransmitters, epinephrine and norepinephrine, which are released when an increase in body temperature is needed, act at the cellular level to shift body metabolism to heat production. This may be why fever produces feelings of weakness and fatigue. Thyroid hormone increases cellular metabolism but usually requires several weeks to reach maximal effectiveness.

Fine involuntary actions such as shivering and chattering of the teeth can produce a threefold to fivefold increase in body temperature. *Shivering* is initiated by impulses from the hypothalamus, resulting in an increase in body temperature and increased use of oxygen.[36]

Shivering starts with a general increase in muscle tone, followed by oscillating rhythmic tremors involving the spinal-level reflex that controls muscle tone. Physical exertion increases body temperature. Muscles convert most of the energy in the fuels they consume into heat. With strenuous exercise, more than three fourths of the increased metabolism resulting from muscle activity appears as heat within the body; the remainder appears as mechanical work.[37]

Mechanisms of Heat Loss

Most of the body's heat losses occur at the skin surface. There are numerous arteriovenous (AV) **anastomoses** under the skin surface that allow blood to move from the arterial to the venous system.[3] These AV anastomoses are like the radiators in a heating system. When the **shunts** are open, body heat is freely dissipated to the skin and surrounding environment; when the shunts are closed, heat is retained in the body. Blood flow in the AV anastomoses is controlled almost exclusively by the sympathetic nervous system in response to changes in core and environmental temperature. Contraction of the *pilomotor muscles*, which raises skin hairs and produces

---

TABLE 14-2 Heat Gain and Heat Loss Responses Used in Regulation of Body Temperature

Heat Gain		Heat Loss	
Body Response	**Mechanism of Action**	**Body Response**	**Mechanism of Action**
Vasoconstriction of the superficial blood vessels	Confines blood flow to the inner core of the body, with the skin and subcutaneous tissues acting as insulation to prevent loss of core heat	Dilatation of the superficial blood vessels	Delivers blood containing core heat to the periphery where it is dissipated through radiation, conduction, and convection
Contraction of the pilomotor muscles that surround the hairs on the skin	Reduces the heat loss surface of the skin	Sweating	Increases heat loss through evaporation
Assumption of the huddle position with the extremities held close to the body	Reduces the area for heat loss		
Shivering	Increases heat production by the muscles		
Increased production of epinephrine	Increases the heat production associated with metabolism		
Increased production of thyroid hormone	Is a long-term mechanism that increases metabolism and heat production		

goose bumps, also aids in heat conservation by reducing the surface area available for heat loss.

Heat is lost from the body through radiation, conduction, and convection from the skin surface; through the evaporation of sweat and insensible perspiration; through the exhalation of air that has been warmed and humidified; and through heat lost in urine and feces. Of these mechanisms, only heat losses that occur at the skin surface are directly under hypothalamic control.

Radiation

Radiation is the transfer of heat through air or a vacuum. Heat from the sun is carried by radiation. Environmental temperature must be less than body temperature for heat loss to occur. A nude person at room temperature loses approximately 60% of their body heat by radiation.[1]

Conduction

Conduction is the direct transfer of heat from one molecule to another. Blood conducts heat from the inner core of the body to the skin surface. A small amount of body heat is lost via conduction to a cooler surface. Cooling blankets or mattresses used for reducing fever rely on conduction of heat from the skin to the cool mattress. Heat can be conducted from the external environment to the body surface. For instance, body temperature may rise slightly after a hot bath.

Due to its high specific heat, water absorbs greater amounts of heat than air. Loss of body heat can be life-threatening in situations of cold water immersion or cold exposure in damp clothing.

The conduction of heat to the body's surface is influenced by blood volume. In hot weather, the body increases blood volume to dissipate heat. Mild ankle swelling during hot weather provides evidence of blood volume expansion. Exposure to cold produces a cold diuresis and a reduction in blood volume as a means of controlling the transfer of heat to the body's surface.[38]

Convection

Convection is heat transfer through the circulation of air currents. Normally, a layer of warm air remains near the body's surface. Convection causes continual removal of this layer and replaces it with air from the surrounding environment. The wind-chill factor often included in weather reports combines the effect of convection due to wind with the still-air temperature.

Evaporation

Evaporation uses body heat to convert water on the skin to water vapor. Water that diffuses through the skin independent of sweating is called *insensible perspiration* and these losses are greatest in a dry environment. Sweating occurs through the sweat glands and is controlled by the sympathetic nervous system, mediated by acetylcholine. This is unlike other sympathetically mediated functions in which the catecholamines serve as mediators. The impact of this is that anticholinergic drugs, such as atropine, can interfere with heat loss by interrupting sweating.

Evaporative heat losses involve insensible perspiration and sweating, with 0.58 cal lost for each gram of water evaporated.[1] When body temperature is greater than atmospheric temperature, heat is lost through radiation. When the temperature of the surrounding environment becomes greater than skin temperature, evaporation is the only way through which the body can get rid of heat. Any condition that prevents evaporative heat losses causes the body temperature to rise.

SUMMARY CONCEPTS

Core body temperature is normally maintained within a range of 36.0°C to 37.5°C (97.0°F to 99.5°F). Core body and skin temperatures are sensed and integrated by thermoregulatory regions in the hypothalamus and other brain structures that function to modify heat production and heat loss. Metabolic processes that occur within deeper core structures (*i.e.*, muscles and viscera) of the body produce most of the body's heat. Sympathetic neurotransmitters and thyroid hormone act at the cellular level to shift body metabolism to heat production. Shivering and chattering of the teeth use heat liberated from involuntary muscle movements to increase the body temperature. Most of the body's heat losses occur at the skin surface as heat from the blood moves through the skin and into the surrounding environment. Heat is lost from the skin through radiation, conduction, convection, and evaporation of perspiration and sweat. Contraction of the *pilomotor muscles* of the skin aids in heat conservation by reducing the surface area available for heat loss.

Increased Body Temperature

Fever and hyperthermia describe conditions in which body temperature is higher than the normal range. Fever is due to an upward displacement of the set point of the thermoregulatory center in the hypothalamus. In hyperthermia, the set point is unchanged, but the mechanisms that control body temperature are ineffective in maintaining body temperature within a normal range during situations when heat production outpaces the ability of the body to dissipate that heat.

Fever

Fever, or *pyrexia*, describes an elevation in body temperature that is caused by an upward displacement of the thermostatic set point of the hypothalamic thermoregulatory center. Temperature is one of the most frequent physiologic responses to be monitored during illness.

Mechanisms

Many proteins, breakdown products of proteins, and certain other substances released from bacterial cell membranes can cause the set point to rise. Fever is resolved when the condition that caused the increase is removed. Fevers that are regulated by the hypothalamus usually do not rise above 41°C (105.8°F). Temperatures above this level are usually the result of superimposed activity, such as convulsions, hyperthermic states, or direct impairment of the temperature control center.

Pyrogens are exogenous or endogenous substances that produce fever. *Exogenous pyrogens* are from outside the body and include bacterial products, bacterial toxins, or whole microorganisms. Exogenous pyrogens induce host cells to produce fever-producing mediators called *endogenous pyrogens*. When bacteria or breakdown products of bacteria are present in blood or tissues, phagocytic cells of the immune system engulf them, digest the bacterial products, and release pyrogenic cytokines into the bloodstream for transport to the hypothalamus, where they exert their action.[3] These cytokines induce prostaglandin E_2 (PGE_2).[31]

At this point, PGE_2 binds to receptors in the hypothalamus to induce increases in the thermostatic set point. The hypothalamus then initiates shivering and vasoconstriction that raise the body's core temperature to the new set point, and fever is established.

In addition to their fever-producing actions, endogenous pyrogens mediate a number of other responses. For example, IL-1 and TNF-α are inflammatory mediators that produce other signs of inflammation such as leukocytosis, anorexia, and malaise. Noninfectious disorders such as myocardial infarction, pulmonary emboli, or the trauma of surgery may produce injured cells that incite the production of endogenous pyrogens. Malignant cells of leukemia and Hodgkin disease secrete chemical mediators that function as endogenous pyrogens.

A fever that has its origin in the CNS is sometimes referred to as a *neurogenic fever*. It is usually caused by damage to the hypothalamus because of CNS trauma, intracerebral bleeding, or an increase in intracranial pressure. Neurogenic fever is characterized by a high temperature that is resistant to antipyretic therapy and is not associated with sweating.

Purpose

The purpose of fever is not completely understood, but it is a valuable index to health status. Fever below 40°C (104°F) is likely not harmful; in fact, animal studies demonstrate a survival advantage in infected members with fever compared with animals unable to produce a fever. Small elevations in temperature, such as those that occur with fever, enhance immune function by T lymphocyte proliferation.[3] Many microbial agents that cause infection grow best at normal body temperatures, and their growth is inhibited by temperatures in the fever range.

A mild fever may be negative in many situations, such as in older adults, because it causes more of a demand for oxygen. For every elevated 1°C of temperature, the BMR increases by 7%, causing increased work for the heart. Fever can also produce confusion, tachycardia, and tachypnea. Cell damage can occur at temperatures greater than 42.2°C (108°F), and this can ultimately cause life-threatening acidosis, hypoxia, and hyperkalemia.[38]

Patterns

The patterns of temperature change in people with fever vary[32] (Fig. 14-14). An *intermittent fever* is one in which temperature returns to normal at least once every 24 hours. In a *remittent fever*, the temperature does not return to normal and varies a few degrees in either direction. In a *sustained* or *continuous fever*, the temperature remains above normal with minimal variations (usually <0.55°C or 1°F). In *recurrent* or *relapsing fever*, there is one or more episodes of fever, each as long as several days, with one or more days of normal temperature between episodes.

Most people respond to an increase in temperature with an appropriate increase in heart rate. A rise in temperature unaccompanied by the anticipated change in heart rate can provide useful information about the cause of the fever: a heart rate slower than anticipated can occur with Legionnaire disease and drug fever and a heart rate more rapid than anticipated can be symptomatic of hyperthyroidism and pulmonary emboli.

Clinical Manifestations

The physiologic behaviors that occur during fever development are divided into four successive stages: prodrome, chill (during which temperature rises), flush, and defervescence (Fig. 14-15).

During the *first* or *prodromal* period, there are nonspecific complaints such as mild headache and fatigue, general malaise, and fleeting aches and pains. During the *second stage* or *chill*, there is the sensation of being chilled and the onset of generalized shaking (rigors), despite temperature rising. Vasoconstriction and piloerection usually precede the onset of shivering. The skin is pale and there is a drive to conserve body heat. Once the body temperature reaches the new set point, the shivering ceases and a sensation of warmth develops. At this point, the *third stage* or *flush* begins, during which

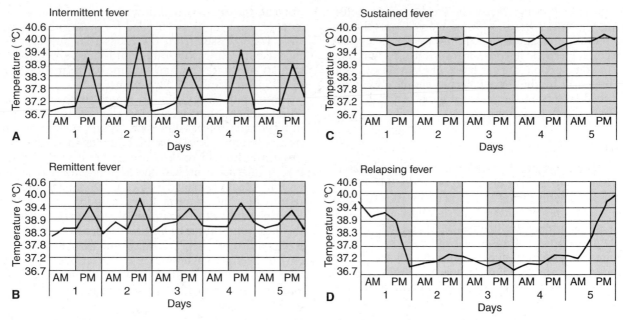

FIGURE 14-14. Schematic representation of fever patterns: (**A**) intermittent, (**B**) remittent, (**C**) sustained, and (**D**) recurrent or relapsing.

cutaneous vasodilation occurs and the skin becomes warm and flushed. The *fourth*, or *defervescence*, stage of the febrile response is marked by the initiation of sweating. Not all people proceed through the four stages of fever development.

Common clinical manifestations of fever are anorexia, myalgia, arthralgia, and fatigue and are worsened when the temperature rises rapidly or exceeds 39.5°C (103.1°F). Respiration increases, and the heart rate usually is elevated. Dehydration occurs because of sweating and the increased vapor losses because of the rapid respiratory rate. Many fever symptoms are related to increases in metabolic rate and oxygen demands and use of body proteins as an energy source. Prolonged fever increases breakdown of endogenous fat stores, resulting in metabolic acidosis.

Headache is a common accompaniment of fever and is thought to result from the vasodilation of cerebral vessels occurring with fever. **Delirium** is possible when the temperature exceeds 40°C (104°F). Confusion and delirium may follow only moderate elevations in temperature in older adults. Pulmonary function may

FIGURE 14-15. Mechanisms of fever. (*1*) Release of prostaglandin E$_2$ (PGE$_2$) or fever-producing cytokines from inflammatory cells; (*2*) resetting of the thermostatic set point in the hypothalamus to a higher level (prodrome); (*3*) generation of hypothalamus-mediated responses that raise body temperature (chill); (*4*) development of fever with elevation of body to new thermostatic set point; and (*5*) production of temperature-lowering responses (flush and defervescence) and return of body temperature to a lower level.

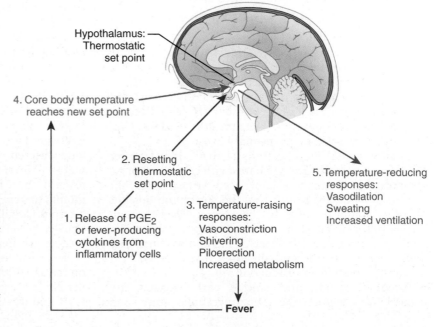

prove to be a limiting factor in the hypermetabolism that accompanies fever in older persons. Confusion, incoordination, and agitation commonly reflect cerebral hypoxemia. Herpetic lesions, or fever blisters, which develop in some people during fever, are caused by a separate infection by the type 1 herpes simplex virus that established latency in the regional ganglia and is reactivated by a rise in body temperature.

Diagnosis

A prolonged fever for which the cause is difficult to ascertain is referred to as *fever of unknown origin* (FUO). FUO is defined as a temperature elevation of 38.3°C (101°F) or higher that is present for 3 weeks or longer and includes 1 week of comprehensive diagnostic testing that does not identify a diagnosis.[27] Causes of FUO include malignancies; infections such as human immunodeficiency virus, tuberculosis, or abscessed infections; and drug fever. Malignancies are important causes of FUO in the elderly. Cirrhosis of the liver is another cause of FUO.

Recurrent or periodic fevers may occur in predictable intervals or without any discernible time pattern. They may be associated with no discernible cause or as presenting symptom of several serious illnesses. Familial Mediterranean fever, an autosomal recessive disease, is characterized by an early age of onset (<20 years) of acute episodic bouts of peritonitis and high fever with an average duration of less than 2 days. Pleuritis, pericarditis, and arthritis may be present. The primary chronic complication is the presence of serum antibodies that can result in kidney or heart failure. Other conditions with recurrent fevers at irregular intervals include repeated viral or bacterial infections, parasitic and fungal infections, and some inflammatory conditions, such as lupus erythematosus or Crohn disease. The clinical challenge is in the differential diagnosis of periodic or recurrent fever. A thorough history and physical examination are required to rule out the more serious medical conditions that present initially with fever.

Treatment

Fever treatment focuses on modifications to increase heat transfer from the internal to the external environment, support of the hypermetabolic state that accompanies fever, protection of vulnerable body organs and systems, and treatment of the cause of the fever. Because fever is a disease symptom, it suggests the need for diagnosis and treatment of the primary cause.

Environmental modifications facilitate heat transfer away from the body. Sponge baths with cool water or an alcohol solution can increase evaporative heat losses, but caution is necessary to not cool the person too quickly. More profound cooling can be accomplished through the use of forced air blankets or a cooling mattress. Care must be taken so that the cooling method does not produce vasoconstriction and shivering that decrease heat loss and increase heat production.

Adequate fluids and simple carbohydrates are needed to support the hypermetabolic state and prevent the tissue breakdown characteristic of fever. Replacement fluids are needed for sweating and insensible water losses from the lungs that accompany an increase in respiratory rate. Fluids are needed to maintain an adequate vascular volume for heat transport to the skin surface.

Antipyretic drugs, such as aspirin, ibuprofen, and acetaminophen, often are used to alleviate the discomforts of fever and protect vulnerable organs, such as the brain, from extreme elevations in body temperature. These drugs are thought to reset the set point of the temperature-regulating center in the hypothalamus to a lower level by blocking the activity of COX, an enzyme that is required for the conversion of arachidonic acid to PGE_2. Routine administration of antipyretics may not decrease the duration of fever or illness.[36,39] Because of the risk of Reye syndrome, the CDC, FDA, and the American Academy of Pediatrics Committee on Infectious Diseases advise against the use of aspirin and other salicylates in children with influenza or chickenpox.

Fever in Children

Fever occurs frequently in infants and young children. Infants and young children have decreased immunologic function and are more commonly infected with virulent organisms. The mechanisms for controlling temperature are not as well developed in infants as they are in older children and adults. Infants with fever may not appear ill, but this does not imply an absence of disease. In infants under 3 months, a mild elevation in temperature can indicate serious infection.

The majority of febrile children have an underlying infection. Common causes are infections of the respiratory system, gastrointestinal tract, urinary tract, or CNS. The epidemiology of serious bacterial disease has changed dramatically with the introduction of the *Haemophilus influenzae* and *Streptococcus pneumoniae* vaccines in developed countries. *Haemophilus influenzae* type b has been nearly eliminated, and the incidence of pneumococcal disease caused by vaccine and cross-reactive vaccine serotypes has declined substantially. Fever in infants and children can be classified as low or high risk depending on the probability of the infection progressing to **bacteremia** or meningitis and signs of toxicity. Infants under 28 days with a fever should be considered to have a bacterial infection that can cause bacteremia or meningitis. Signs of toxicity include lethargy, poor feeding, hypoventilation, and **cyanosis**. A white blood cell count with differential and blood cultures usually is taken in high-risk infants and children to determine the cause of fever. A chest radiograph should be obtained in febrile infants under 3 months of age with at least one sign of a respiratory illness.[27] Febrile children under 1 year and females between 1 and 2 years of age should be considered at risk for a urinary tract infection.[27]

Treatment of a fever without a known source depends on the age of the child. High-risk infants and infants under 28 days are often hospitalized for evaluation of their fever and treatment.[27]

Fever in Older Adults

In the elderly, slight elevations in temperature may indicate serious infection or disease, most often caused by bacteria. The elderly often have a lower baseline temperature, and increases in temperature during an infection may fail to reach a level equated with significant fever.[27,40] The circadian pattern of temperature variation often are altered in the elderly. Fever in the elderly increases the immunologic response, but it is generally weaker compared to younger people.[40]

Older adults with serious infections may have an absent or blunted febrile response, perhaps due to disturbances in temperature sensing by the hypothalamic thermoregulatory center, alterations in endogenous pyrogens release, and the failure to elicit responses such as vasoconstriction of skin vessels, increased heat production, and shivering that increase body temperature.

Absence of fever may delay diagnosis and treatment. Therefore, it is important to perform a thorough history and physical examination focusing on other signs of infection and sepsis, including unexplained changes in functional capacity, mental status, strength, and weight loss.

Another factor that may delay recognition of fever in older adults is the method of temperature measurement. Rectal and tympanic membrane methods are likely more effective in detecting fever in the elderly. This is because conditions such as mouth breathing, tongue tremors, and agitation often make it difficult to obtain accurate oral temperatures in older adults.

Hyperthermia

Hyperthermia is an increase in body temperature that occurs without a change in the set point of the hypothalamic thermoregulatory center. It occurs when the thermoregulatory mechanisms are overwhelmed by heat production, excessive environmental heat, or impaired dissipation of heat.[40] It includes (in order of increasing severity) heat cramps, heat exhaustion, and heatstroke. Hyperthermia also may occur as the result of a drug reaction.

If muscle exertion is continued for long periods in warm weather, excessive heat loads are generated. Adequate circulatory function is essential for heat dissipation, so the elderly and those with cardiovascular disease are at increased risk for hyperthermia. Drugs that increase muscle tone and metabolism or reduce heat loss can impair thermoregulation. Infants and small children left in a closed car in hot weather are at risk for hyperthermia.

The best approach to heat-related disorders is prevention, primarily by avoiding activity in hot environments, increasing fluid intake, and wearing appropriate clothing. The ability to tolerate a hot environment depends on both temperature and humidity. High relative humidity retards heat loss through sweating and evaporation and decreases the body's cooling ability. The *heat index* is the temperature that the body senses when both the temperature and humidity are combined.

Heat Cramps

Heat cramps are slow, painful, skeletal muscle cramps and spasms lasting 1 to 3 minutes. Muscles are tender and the skin usually is moist. Cramping results from salt depletion when fluid losses from heavy sweating are replaced by water alone. Body temperature may be normal or slightly elevated. There almost always is a history of vigorous activity preceding the onset of symptoms.

Heat Exhaustion

Heat exhaustion is related to a gradual loss of salt and water, usually after prolonged exertion in a hot environment. Symptoms may include thirst, fatigue, nausea, oliguria, gastrointestinal flulike symptoms, giddiness, and delirium. Hyperventilation may contribute to heat cramps and tetany by causing respiratory alkalosis. The skin is moist, rectal temperature is 37.8°C (100°F) to 40°C (104°F), and heart rate is elevated. Signs of heat cramps may accompany heat exhaustion.

Heatstroke

Heatstroke is a failure of thermoregulatory mechanisms resulting in excessive increases in body temperature—a core temperature greater than 40°C (104°F); hot, dry skin; absence of sweating; and possible CNS abnormalities such as delirium, convulsions, and loss of consciousness.[41] The risk of developing heatstroke in response to heat stress is increased in conditions and with drugs that impair vasodilation and sweating.[41]

The pathophysiology of heatstroke is thought to result from the effect of heat on body cells and release of cytokines from heat-stressed endothelial cells, leukocytes, and epithelial cells. Local and systemic inflammatory responses together may result in acute respiratory distress syndrome, acute renal failure, disseminated intravascular coagulation, and multiorgan disorders.

Heatstroke symptoms include tachycardia, hyperventilation, dizziness, weakness, nausea and vomiting,

Vasoconstriction can be profound, heart rate is accelerated, and stroke volume is increased. Blood pressure increases slightly, and hyperventilation is common. Urinary flow increases prior to a fall in temperature. Dehydration and increased hematocrit may develop within hours, augmented by an extracellular to intracellular water shift.

In moderate hypothermia, shivering gradually decreases and the muscles become rigid. Heart rate and stroke volume decrease and blood pressure and metabolic rate fall. Oxygen consumption and carbon dioxide production decrease. Decreased carbon dioxide decreases respiratory rate. Decreases in mentation, cough reflex, and respiratory tract secretions may lead to difficulty in clearing secretions and aspiration. A gradual decline in heart rate and cardiac output occurs as hypothermia progresses. Blood pressure initially rises and then gradually falls. There is increased risk of dysrhythmia and ventricular fibrillation is a major cause of death in hypothermia.

Carbohydrate metabolism and insulin activity are decreased resulting in hyperglycemia relative to the cooling. Cold-induced loss of cell membrane integrity allows intravascular fluids to move into the skin, giving it a puffy appearance. Acid–base disorders occur at temperatures below 25°C (77°F) unless adequate ventilation is maintained. Extracellular sodium and potassium concentrations decrease and chloride levels increase. There is a temporary loss of plasma from the circulation along with increased blood viscosity due to trapping in the small vessels and skin.

Diagnosis and Treatment

Oral temperatures are inaccurate during hypothermia due to severe vasoconstriction and sluggish blood flow. Electronic thermometers with flexible probes are available for measuring rectal, bladder, and esophageal temperatures. A thermometer that registers 25°C (77°F) or an electrical thermistor probe is needed to monitor temperatures in hypothermia. Treatment consists of rewarming, support of vital functions, and the prevention and treatment of complications.

Therapeutic Hypothermia

Controlled hypothermia may be used after brain injury and during certain surgeries to decrease inflammation and brain metabolism. It is helpful for people who have had cardiac arrest because of ventricular fibrillation as measured by neurologic outcomes.[47] Intraoperatively, people are kept hypothermic between 82.4°F and 89.6°F to decrease metabolic demands and prevent ischemic injury.[45] Myocardial ischemia is prevented by injecting cold cardioplegia solution at 39.2°F into the aortic root under pressure.[45] This solution is composed of potassium, which causes asystole and hypothermia to protect the myocardium.[45] To maintain myocardial hypothermia, an iced normal saline slush is administered topically. There are, however, some potential complications to cold cardioplegia, such as ventricular dysrhythmias, decreased cerebral blood flow, and postoperative myocardial depression.[45]

After the surgery is complete, warmed blood is perfused to people who were hypothermic during surgery. Rewarming has to be performed slowly and attempts to prevent shivering and severe vasoconstriction are made.[45] If there is a bleeding problem postoperatively, restoration of body temperature needs to be done as quickly and as safely as possible. Using hypothermia in certain situations such as TBI, cardiac arrest, increased intracranial pressure and spinal cord injury remains controversial.[47]

 SUMMARY CONCEPTS

Hypothermia is a potentially life-threatening disorder in which the body's core temperature drops below 35°C (95°F). Accidental hypothermia can develop in otherwise healthy people in the course of accidental exposure and in older adults or disabled people with impaired perception of or response to cold. Alcoholism, cardiovascular disease, malnutrition, and hypothyroidism contribute to the risk of hypothermia. Hypothermia is also a common occurrence in newborn infants, particularly those born prematurely, and in people undergoing an operation. The greatest effect of hypothermia is a decrease in the metabolic rate, leading to a decrease in carbon dioxide production and respiratory rate. Clinical manifestations of hypothermia include poor coordination, stumbling, slurred speech, irrationality, poor judgment, amnesia, hallucinations, blueness and puffiness of the skin, dilation of the pupils, decreased respiratory rate, weak and irregular pulse, stupor, and coma. Treatment of hypothermia includes passive or active rewarming, support of vital functions, and the prevention and treatment of complications.

Review Exercises

1. A 25-year-old man is admitted to the emergency department with acute abdominal pain that began in the epigastric area and has now shifted to the lower right quadrant of the abdomen. There is localized tenderness and guarding or spasm of the muscle over the area. His heart rate and blood pressure are elevated, and his skin is moist and cool from perspiring. He is given a tentative diagnosis of appendicitis and referred for surgical consultation.

   A. Describe the origin of the pain stimuli and the neural pathways involved in the pain that this man is experiencing.

B. Explain the neural mechanisms involved in the spasm of the overlying abdominal muscles.

C. What is the significance of his cool, moist skin and increased heart rate and blood pressure?

2. A 65-year-old woman with breast cancer is receiving hospice care in her home. She is currently receiving a long-acting opioid analgesic supplemented with a short-acting combination opioid and nonnarcotic medication for breakthrough pain.

A. Explain the difference between the mechanisms and treatment of acute and chronic pain.

B. Describe the action of opioid drugs in the treatment of pain.

C. Define the terms tolerance and cross-tolerance as they refer to the use of opioids for treatment of pain.

D. Describe the common side effects associated with the use of opioid drugs to relieve pain in persons with cancer.

3. A 42-year-old woman presents with sudden, stabbing-type facial pain that arises near the right side of her mouth and then shoots toward the right ear, eye, and nostril. She is holding her hand to protect her face because the pain is "triggered by touch, movement, and drafts." Her initial diagnosis is trigeminal neuralgia.

A. Explain the distribution and mechanisms of the pain, particularly the triggering of the pain by stimuli applied to the skin.

B. What are the possible treatment methods for this woman?

4. A 21-year-old woman presents to the student health center with complaints of a throbbing pain on the left side of her head, nausea and vomiting, and extreme sensitivity to light, noise, and head movement. She also tells you she had a similar headache 3 months ago that lasted for 2 days and states that she thinks she is developing migraine headaches like her mother. She is concerned because she has been unable to attend classes and has exams next week.

A. Are this woman's history and symptoms consistent with migraine headaches? Explain.

B. Use the distribution of the trigeminal nerve and the concept of neurogenic inflammation to explain this woman's symptoms.

5. A 72-year-old man presents to the emergency department after a fall with a complaint of the "worst headache ever experienced." He is able to answer your questions with increasing difficulty.

A. Differentiate primary headache from secondary headache.

B. Given the information that you have, what type of headache do you suspect, and why?

6. A 3-year-old child is seen in a pediatric clinic with a temperature of 39°C (102.2°F). Her skin is warm and flushed, her pulse is 120 beats/minute, and her respirations are shallow and rapid at 32 breaths/minute. Her mother states that her daughter has complained of a sore throat and has refused to drink or take medications to bring her temperature down.

A. Explain the physiologic mechanisms of fever generation.

B. Are the warm and flushed skin, rapid heart rate, and increased respirations consistent with this level of fever?

C. After receiving an appropriate dose of acetaminophen, the child begins to sweat, and the temperature drops to 37.2°C (98.9°F). Explain the physiologic mechanisms responsible for the drop in temperature.

7. A 25-year-old man was brought to the emergency department after having been found unconscious in a snow bank. The outdoor temperature at the time he was discovered was −23.3°C (−10°F). His car, which was stalled a short distance away, contained liquor bottles, suggesting that he had been drinking. His temperature on admission was 29.8°C (85.6°F). His heart rate was 40 beats/minute and his respirations were 18 breaths/minute and shallow. His skin was cool, his muscles rigid, and his digits blue.

A. What factors might have contributed to this man's state of hypothermia?

B. Is this man able to engage in physiologic behaviors to control loss of body heat?

C. Given the two methods that are available for taking this man's temperature (oral or rectal), which would be more accurate? Explain.

D. What precautions should be considered when deciding on a method for rewarming this man?

REFERENCES

1. Guyton A., Hall J. E. (2016). *Textbook of medical physiology* (13th ed.). Philadelphia, PA: Elsevier Saunders.
2. Ross M. H., Pawlina W. (2016). *Histology: A text and atlas with correlated cell and molecular biology* (7th ed.). Philadelphia, PA: Lippincott Williams & Wilkins.
3. Rowland L., Pedley T. (Eds.). (2015). *Merritt's neurology* (13th ed.). Philadelphia, PA: Lippincott Williams & Wilkins.
4. Tortora G., Derrickson B. (2014). *Principles of anatomy & physiology* (14th ed.). Hoboken, NJ: John Wiley & Sons.
5. Quaghebeur J., Wyndaele J. (2015). A review of techniques used for evaluating lower urinary tract symptoms and the level of quality of life in patients with chronic pelvic pain syndrome. *Itch & Pain* 2, 1–6.
6. International Association for the Study of Pain. (1994). Definition of pain. [Online]. Available: https://www.iasp-pain.org/Taxonomy#Pain. Accessed December 23, 2017.

7. The American Academy of Pain Medicine. (2018). Highlights from the National Center for Health Statistics Report: Health, United States, 2006, Special Feature on Pain. [Online]. Available: http://www.painmed.org/PatientCenter/Facts_on_Pain.aspx#incidence. Accessed March 16, 2018.

8. Falk S., Dickenson A. (2014). Pain and nociception: Mechanisms of cancer-induced bone pain. *Journal of Clinical Oncology* 32, 1647–1654.

9. Cohan S. P., Mao J. (2014). Neuropathic pain: Mechanisms and their clinical implications. *British Medical Journal* 348, 1–12.

10. Shaygan M., Boger A., Kroner-Herwig B. (2014). Neuropathic sensory symptoms: Association with pain and psychological factors. *Neuropsychiatric Disease and Treatment* 10, 897–906.

11. Moayedi M., Davis K. D. (2013). Theories of pain: From specificity to gate control. *Journal of Neurophysiology* 109, 5–12.

12. Prescott S. A., Ma Q., Koninck Y. (2014). Normal and abnormal coding of painful sensations. *National Neuroscience* 17(2), 183–191.

13. Melzack R., Wall P. D. (1965). Pain mechanisms: A new theory. *Science* 150, 971–979.

14. Melzack R. (1999). From the gate to the neuromatrix. *Pain* 6(Suppl), S121–S126.

15. Gopalakrishnan R., Burgess R. C., Plow E. B., et al. (2014). A magnetoencephalography study of multi-modal processing of pain anticipation in primary sensory cortices. *Neuroscience* 304, 176–189.

16. Dunphy L. M., Winland-Brown J., Porter B., et al. (2015). *Primary care: The art and science of advanced practice nursing* (4th ed.). Philadelphia, PA: FA Davis.

17. Lehne R. A. (2015). *Pharmacology for nursing care* (9th ed.). St. Louis, MO: Elsevier.

18. Carlson C. L. (2016). Effectiveness of the World Health Organization cancer pain relief guidelines: An integrative review. *Journal of Pain Research* 9, 515–534.

19. Jensen S. (2015). *Nursing health assessment: A best practice approach* (2nd ed.). Philadelphia, PA: Lippincott Williams & Wilkins.

20. Kumaz R., Asci M., Balta O., et al. (2017). Congenital insensitivity to pain syndrome accompanied by neglected orthopedic traumas and complications. *Archive of Clinical Cases* 4(1), 27–33.

21. McCormick Z., Chang-Chien G., Marshall B., et al. (2014). Phantom limb pain: A systematic neuroanatomical-based review of pharmacologic treatment. *Pain Medicine* 15, 292–305.

22. D'Onofrio F., Russo A., Conte F., et al. (2014). Post-traumatic headaches: An epidemiological overview. *Neurological Science* 35(Suppl 1), S203–S206.

23. Chaudhry P., Friedman D. I. (2015). Neuroimaging in secondary headache disorders. *Current Pain and Headache Reports* 19, 1–11.

24. Olesen J., Bendtsen L., Dodick D., et al. (2013). The international classification of headache disorders (3rd ed. beta version). *Cephalalgia* 33(9), 629–808.

25. Hershey L., Bednarczyk E. (2013). Treatment of headache in the elderly. *Current Treatment Options in Neurology* 15, 56–62.

26. Noseda R., Burstein R. (2013). Migraine pathophysiology: Anatomy of the trigeminovascular pathway and associated neurological symptoms, CSD, sensitization and modulation of pain. *Pain* 154(Suppl 1), 1–21.

27. Goroll A. H., Mulley A. G. (2014). *Primary care medicine: Office evaluation and management of the adult patient* (7th ed.). Philadelphia, PA: Lippincott Williams & Wilkins.

28. Weaver-Agostoni J. (2013). Cluster headache. *American Family Physician* 88(2), 122–128.

29. Hadjistavropoulos T., Herr K., Prkachim K. M., et al. (2014). Pain assessment in elderly adults with dementia. *The Lancet* 13, 1–13.

30. Achterberg W., Pieper M. J., van Dalen-Kok A. H., et al. (2013). Pain management in patients with dementia. *Clinical Interventions in Aging* 8, 1471–1482.

31. Boron Q. F., Boulpaep E. L. (2016). *Medical physiology* (3rd ed.). Philadelphia, PA: Elsevier.

32. Andreoli T. E., Benjamin I. J., Griggs R. C., et al. (2015). *Andreoli and Carpenter's cecil essentials of medicine* (9th ed.). Philadelphia, PA: Elsevier.

33. Gasim G., Musa I., Abdien M., et al. (2013). Accuracy of tympanic temperature measurement using an infrared tympanic membrane thermometer. *BioMed Central Research Notes* 6, 1–5.

34. Pak S., Lee H., Kwack M., et al. (2014). Systematic review and meta-analysis of the diagnostic accuracy of an infrared tympanic thermometer for use with adults. *International Journal of Nursing* 1(2), 115–134.

35. Auliciems A. (2014). Thermal sensation and cell adaptability. *International Journal of Biometeorology* 58, 325–335.

36. Golembiewski J. (2015). Pharmacological management of perioperative shivering. *Journal of PeriAnesthesia Nursing* 30(4), 357–359.

37. Flouris D., Schlader Z. J. (2015). Human behavioral thermoregulation during exercise in the heat. *Scandinavian Journal of Medical Science of Sports* 25(Suppl 1), 52–64.

38. Rubin R., Strayer D. (Eds.). (2015). *Rubin's pathology: Clinicopathologic foundations of medicine* (7th ed.). Philadelphia, PA: Lippincott Williams & Wilkins.

39. Egi M., Makino S., Mizobuchi, S. (2018). Management of fever in critically ill patients with infection. *Journal of Emergency Critical Care Medicine* 2(10), 1–6.

40. Outzen M. (2009). Management of fever in older adults. *Journal of Gerontological Nursing* 35(5), 17–23.

41. Pryor R., Roth R., Suyama J., et al. (2015). Exertional heat illness: Emerging concepts and advances in prehospital care. *Prehospital Disaster Medicine* 30(3), 297–305.

42. Ferreira C., Costa T., Marques A. V. (2015). Diffuse alveolar haemorrhage secondary to propylthiouracil-induced vasculitis. *British Medical Journal Case Report*. doi:10.1136/bcr-2014-208289.

43. Rosenberg H., Pollock N., Shiemann A., et al. (2015). Malignant hyperthermia: A review. *Orphanet Journal of Rare Disease* 10, 1–19.

44. Davis C. (2017). Hypothermia. [Online]. Available: https://www.emedicinehealth.com/hypothermia/article_em.htm#what_is_hypothermia. Accessed April 22, 2019.

45. Plitnick K., Biehle K. J., Meinken C. (2015). Shivering suppression in therapeutic hypothermia. *Nursing 2015 Critical Care* 10(5), 22–26.

46. Morton M. G., Fontaine D. K. (2017). *Critical care nursing: A holistic approach* (11th ed.). Philadelphia, PA: Lippincott Williams & Wilkins.

47. Alvis-Miranda H. R., Alcala-Cerra G., Rubiano A. M., et al. (2014). Therapeutic hypothermia in brain trauma injury: Controversies. *Romanian Neurosurgery* 3, 259–268.

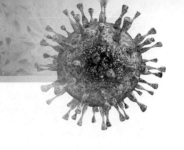

CHAPTER **15**

Disorders of Motor Function

Learning Objectives

After completing this chapter, the learner will be able to meet the following objectives:

1. Define a *motor unit* and characterize its mechanism of controlling skeletal muscle movement.
2. Indicate between the functions of the primary, premotor, and supplemental motor cortices.
3. Compare upper motor neuron (UMN) and lower motor neuron (LMN) lesions on spinal cord stretch reflex function and muscle tone.
4. Define *peripheral nervous system* and describe the characteristics of peripheral nerves.
5. Compare the cause and manifestations of peripheral mononeuropathies with polyneuropathies.
6. Relate the functions of the cerebellum to production of vestibulocerebellar ataxia, decomposition of movement, and cerebellar tremor.
7. Describe the functional organization of the basal ganglia and communication pathways with the thalamus and cerebral cortex.
8. Relate the pathologic UMN and LMN changes that occur in amyotrophic lateral sclerosis to the manifestations of the disease.

9. Explain the significance of demyelination and plaque formation in multiple sclerosis.
10. State the effects of spinal cord injury on ventilation and communication, the autonomic nervous system; cardiovascular function; sensorimotor function; and bowel, bladder, and sexual functions..

Skeletal muscles are required for smooth, purposeful, and coordinated movement. Purposeless and disruptive movements can be as disabling as absence of movement. This chapter provides an introduction to the organization and control of motor function, followed by a discussion of disorders of motor function, including muscular dystrophy and disorders of the neuromuscular junction (NMJ), peripheral nerves, basal ganglia and cerebellum, and upper motor neurons (UMNs).

KEY POINTS

Motor Systems

- Motor systems require UMNs that project from the motor cortex to the brain stem or spinal cord, where they directly or indirectly innervate the lower motor neurons (LMNs) of the contracting muscles; sensory feedback from the involved muscles that is continuously relayed to the cerebellum, basal ganglia, and sensory cortex; and a functioning NMJ that links nervous system activity with muscle contraction.

- The pyramidal motor system originating in the motor cortex provides control of delicate muscle movement and the extrapyramidal system originating in the basal ganglia provides the background for the more crude, supportive movement patterns.

- The efficiency of movement by the motor system depends on a background of muscle tone provided by the stretch reflex and vestibular system input to maintain stable postural support.

Organization and Control of Motor Function

Motor function requires movement and maintenance of posture.[1] The neuromuscular system consists of the motor unit (motor neuron and the muscle fibers it innervates); the spinal cord, which contains the basic reflex circuitry for posture and movement; and the descending pathways from brain stem circuits, the cerebellum, basal ganglia, and the motor cortex.

Organization of Movement

Motor systems are organized in a functional hierarchy (Fig. 15-1). The lowest level occurs at the spinal cord, which contains the reflex circuitry needed to coordinate motor units for planned movement. Above the spinal cord is the brain stem, and then the cerebellum and basal ganglia—structures that modify the actions of the brain stem systems. Overseeing supraspinal structures are motor centers in the cerebral cortex. The highest level of function, which occurs at the level of the frontal cortex, is concerned with purpose and planning.

The Spinal Cord

The spinal cord has neuronal circuits that mediate reflexes and automatic rhythmic movements. Similar circuits governing reflexes of the face and mouth are located in the brain stem. Most reflexes are polysynaptic, involving one or more interposed interneurons. Interneurons and motor neurons also receive input from descending axons. Supraspinal signals can modify reflex responses to peripheral stimuli and can coordinate movements through these interneurons.

The Brain Stem

The brain stem contains two descending systems—the medial and lateral pathways (Fig. 15-2). The medial pathways provide basic postural control systems that cortical motor

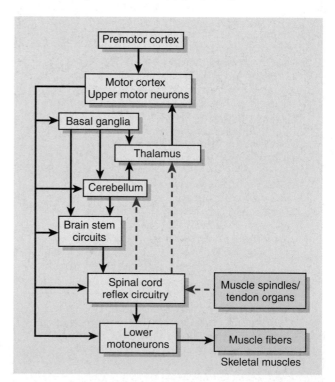

FIGURE 15-1. The motor control system. The final common pathway transmits all central nervous system commands to the skeletal muscles. This path is influenced by sensory input from the muscle spindles and tendon organs (*dashed lines*) and descending signals from the cerebral cortex and brain stem. The cerebellum and basal ganglia influence the motor function indirectly, using brain stem and cortical pathways.

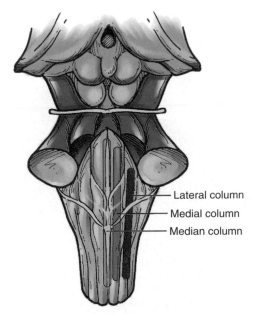

FIGURE 15-2. The median, medial, and lateral columns of the reticular formation. (From Hickey J. V. (2014). *The clinical practice of neurological and neurosurgical nursing* (7th ed.). Philadelphia, PA: Wolters Kluwer.)

areas use to organize highly differentiated movements. Medial pathway tracts descend in the ipsilateral ventral columns of the spinal cord and terminate in interneurons that influence motor neurons of axial and proximal muscles, which are responsible for postural reflexes.

Lateral brain stem pathways mediate goal-directed movements. They terminate on interneurons in the dorsolateral part of the spinal gray matter and thus influence the motor neurons that control distal muscles of the limbs. These descending pathways modify the activity of extensor and flexor motor neurons to produce complex motor movements such as walking and running.

The Motor Cortex

The cortex represents the highest level of motor function. The primary, premotor, and supplementary motor cortices located in the posterior part of the frontal lobe initiate and control precise, skillful, and intentional movements of the distal and especially flexor muscles of the limbs and speech apparatus[2] (Fig. 15-3). These motor areas receive information directly from the thalamus and somatosensory cortex and indirectly from the cerebellum and basal ganglia.

The primary motor cortex (the *motor strip*) is situated on the rostral surface and adjacent portions of the

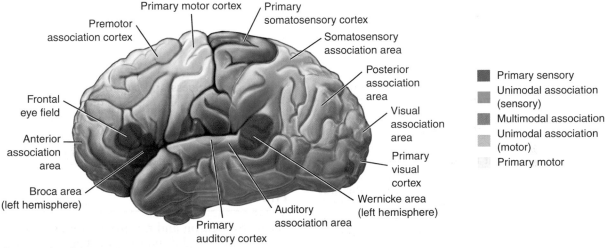

A Functional areas

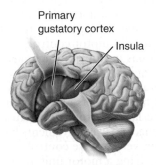

B The gustatory cortex and insula

FIGURE 15-3. **(A)** Functional areas of the cerebrum. Primary sensory areas of the cerebrum receive sensory information from many sources. The motor association cortex organizes movements, and the primary motor cortex sends commands to individual muscles. **(B)** By pulling back the parietal and temporal lobes, the gustatory cortex and insula are visible. (From McConnell T. H., Hull K. L. (2011). *Human form human function: Essentials of anatomy and physiology* (p. 297). Philadelphia, PA: Lippincott Williams & Wilkins.)

of neurologic conditions. Stretch reflexes may be hypoactive or absent in cases of peripheral nerve damage or ventral horn injury. They are hyperactive when lesions of the corticospinal tract (*e.g.*, spinal cord injury [SCI]) reduce or disrupt the inhibitory effect of the brain on the spinal cord.

Muscle spindles consist of a group of miniature skeletal muscle fibers (*intrafusal fibers*) encased in a connective tissue capsule and attached to the extrafusal fibers of a skeletal muscle. Intrafusal muscle fibers function as stretch receptors. When a skeletal muscle is stretched, the spindle and its intrafusal fibers are stretched, increasing afferent nerve fiber firing. Afferent axons enter the spinal cord through several branches of the dorsal root. Some branches end in the segment of entry, others ascend to adjacent segments, and still others ascend in the dorsal column to the medulla. Segmental branches make connections that pass to the anterior gray matter of the spinal cord and establish monosynaptic contact with LMNs that have motor units in the muscle containing the spindle receptor. This produces opposing muscle contraction. A segmental branch of the same neuron innervates an internuncial neuron that is inhibitory to motor units of antagonistic muscle groups. This disynaptic inhibitory pathway is the basis for the reciprocal activity of agonist and antagonist muscles (*i.e.*, when an agonist muscle is stretched, antagonists relax). Reciprocal innervation is useful for stretch reflex and voluntary movements. Relaxation of the antagonist muscle enhances speed and efficiency.[2]

Ascending fibers from the stretch reflex provide information about muscle length to the cerebellum and cerebral cortex. When a skeletal muscle lengthens or shortens against tension, gamma motor neurons provide a feedback mechanism such that spindle fiber length is adjusted to match the length of the extrafusal muscle fiber. Descending fibers synapse with and activate both alpha and gamma motor neurons so that the sensitivity of spindle fibers is coordinated with muscle movement.

Central control over gamma motor neurons also permits changes in muscle tone in anticipation of changes in muscle force. The CNS, through its coordinated control of the muscle's alpha and the spindle's gamma motor neurons, can suppress the stretch reflex. This occurs during centrally programmed movements that require a muscle to produce a full range of unopposed motion. Without this programmed adjustability, any movement is immediately opposed and prevented.

Motor Pathways

The primary motor cortex contains many layers of pyramid-shaped output neurons that

- Transmit to the premotor and somatosensory areas on same side of the cortex
- Transmit to the opposite side of the cortex
- Descend to subcortical structures such as the basal ganglia and thalamus

Large pyramidal cells located in the fifth layer transmit to the brain stem and spinal cord. These UMN axons travel through the subcortical white matter and internal capsule to the brain stem, through the ventral pons, and to the ventral surface of the medulla, where they form a *pyramid*. About 90% of corticospinal axons cross the midline at the junction of the medulla and cervical spinal

cord to form the lateral corticospinal tract in the lateral white matter of the spinal cord, which extends throughout the spinal cord.[4] The 10% of uncrossed fibers travel down the ventral column, mainly to cervical levels, where they cross and innervate contralateral LMNs.[4]

Motor tracts are classified into the pyramidal (direct) or extrapyramidal (indirect) pathways. The pyramidal pathway consists of motor pathways from the motor cortex and terminating in the corticobulbar fibers in the brain stem and the corticospinal fibers in the spinal cord. Other fibers from the cortex and basal ganglia project to the brain stem reticular formation and reticulospinal pathways to LMNs of proximal and extensor muscles. These fibers do not decussate in the pyramids, hence the name *extrapyramidal system*. Disorders of the pyramidal tracts (*e.g.*, stroke) are characterized by **spasticity** and paralysis. Disorders of the extrapyramidal tracts (*e.g.*, Parkinson disease [PD]) result in involuntary movements, rigidity, and immobility without paralysis.

Assessment of Motor Function

Assessing the motor system should include assessment of body position, involuntary movements, muscle characteristics (strength, size, and tone), spinal reflexes, and coordination.[5]

Body Position and Involuntary Movements

Observe the body position of the person when moving and at rest. Continually observe for involuntary movements and note the location, quality, rate, and rhythm of the movements.

Muscle Characteristics

Muscle Strength

Moving each extremity against gravity and resistance tests strength. Abnormalities in the motor pathway can produce impaired strength or muscle weakness. Paralysis is the loss of movement, and **paresis** is the incomplete loss of strength. Pattern of weakness may help localize the lesion.

- *Monoparesis* or *monoplegia*: destruction of pyramidal UMN innervation of one limb
- *Hemiparesis* or *hemiplegia*: destruction of pyramidal UMN innervation of both limbs on one side
- *Diparesis* or *diplegia* or *paraparesis* or *paraplegia*: destruction of pyramidal UMN innervation of both upper or lower limbs
- *Tetraparesis* or *tetraplegia*, also called *quadriparesis* or *quadriplegia*: destruction of pyramidal UMN innervation of all four limbs

Paresis or paralysis can be further designated as of UMN or LMN origin. UMN lesions typically affect the extensors in the upper extremities and the flexors in the lower extremities. In LMN or peripheral nerve disorders, the weakness is predominantly in the distal limb, whereas in muscle disorders, proximal limb function may be affected sooner than distal limb function.

Muscle Size

Muscle size may help localize the lesion or provide helpful hints to the pathology. Muscular atrophy, or loss of bulk, usually results from LMN lesions or muscle diseases. Hypertrophy is an increase in muscle bulk with a proportionate increase in strength. Pseudohypertrophy, as with Duchenne muscular dystrophy (DMD), is an increase in bulk without an increase in strength.

Fasciculations are visible twitching movements of muscle fibers under the skin. They are caused by spontaneous contractions of all the muscle fibers in a motor unit because of hyperexcitability of the cell body and its motor neuron, and suggest LMN disease.

Muscle Tone

Muscle tone is the normal state of muscle tension and can be palpated at rest and during passive stretching. The joints are put through the normal range of motion (**flexion and extension**) by the examiner. Disorders of skeletal muscle tone are characteristic of many nervous system lesions. Interruption of the stretch reflex pathway at any point from the peripheral nerve, NMJ, spinal cord, or corticospinal system can result in disturbances of muscle tone.

Muscle tone abnormalities may be described as hypotonia (less than normal), flaccidity (absent), or hypertonia, rigidity, spasticity, or tetany (all indicating higher-than-normal tone). Typically, UMN lesions produce increased tone, whereas LMN lesions produce decreased tone. Increased resistance that varies and is worse at the extremes of the range of motion is *spasticity*. Resistance that becomes worse throughout the range in both directions is *rigidity*. Decreased resistance suggests LMN disease or acute stages of SCI. Floppiness indicates hypotonic or flaccid muscles.

Spinal Reflex Activity

Testing deep tendon reflexes (see Understanding the Stretch Reflex and Muscle Tone) can provide information about the CNS status. Hyperactive reflexes suggest an UMN disorder. *Clonus* is the rhythmic contraction and relaxation of a limb caused by suddenly stretching a muscle and maintaining it in the stretched position. It is seen in the hypertonia of spasticity associated with UMN lesions such as SCI. *Hyporeflexia* suggests an LMN lesion. The distribution of abnormality in the reflexes is also helpful in determining the location of the lesion. For example, hyperreflexia in both lower extremities would suggest a lesion in the spinal cord, whereas hyperreflexia on one side of the body would suggest a lesion in the UMN along the motor pathway.

Coordination of Movement

Muscle movement coordination requires four areas of the nervous system to function together: the motor system for muscle strength, the cerebellar system for rhythmic movement and steady posture, the vestibular system for posture and balance, and the sensory system for position sense.

In cerebellar disease, movements are slow, irregular, clumsy, unsteady, and inappropriately varying in their speed, force, and direction. *Dysdiadochokinesia* is the failure to accurately perform rapid alternating movements. Ataxia describes a wide-based, unsteady gait. *Dysmetria* describes inaccuracies of movements leading to a failure to reach a specified target. A test for dysmetria is to have the person touch the examiner's finger and then alternately touch his or her finger. To test for position sense, ask the person to touch the examiner's finger with an outstretched arm and finger, first with eyes open and then closed.

Consistent deviation to one side, which is worse with the eyes closed, suggests cerebellar or vestibular disease.

Chorea (abnormal writhing movements), *dystonia* (abnormal, simultaneous contractions of agonist and antagonist muscles, leading to abnormal postures), tremor (rhythmic movements of a body part), *bradykinesia* (slowness of movements), and **myoclonus** (involuntary jerking) indicate abnormalities in the basal ganglia, although the exact localization may be difficult to determine.

SUMMARY CONCEPTS

Motor function requires movement and maintenance of posture. The system consists of LMNs, located in the ventral horn of the spinal cord, and the group of muscle fibers it innervates; spinal cord circuitry and reflexes; and UMNs that project from the motor cortex to the opposite side of the medulla, where they cross the midline to form the lateral corticospinal tract in the spinal cord. The primary, premotor, and supplementary motor cortices provide the voluntary control of motor function, which is directed by the motor cortex. The primary motor cortex is responsible for movement execution, the premotor cortex for generating a movement plan, and the supplemental motor cortex for rehearsing the motor sequences of a movement. Motor systems are organized in a functional hierarchy of, from bottom to top, the spinal cord, brain stem, and motor cortex, each with circuits that can contribute to the organization and regulation of complex motor responses.

Control of muscle function requires reflex circuitry that monitors the functional status of the muscle fibers on a moment-by-moment basis and the excitation of the muscle by LMNs in the spinal cord. The muscle spindles of the stretch reflex monitor and correct for changes in muscle length when extrafusal fibers are shortened or lengthened.

Assessments of muscle strength, size, tone, reflexes, patterns of motor movement, and posture allow for localization of disorders of motor function. Paresis (weakness) and paralysis (loss of muscle movement) reflect a loss of muscle strength. UMN lesions may produce spastic paralysis and LMN lesions, flaccid paralysis. Changes in muscle size are characterized by a loss of muscle mass (atrophy) or an increase in muscle mass (hypertrophy). Muscle tone is maintained through function of the spinal cord stretch reflex, and higher centers monitor and buffer UMN innervation of the LMNs. Hypotonia or flaccidity is a condition of less-than-normal muscle tone, and hypertonia or spasticity is a condition of excessive tone. Abnormal and uncoordinated movements and postures are suggestive of a cerebellar or basal ganglia pathologic process.

UNDERSTANDING ➔ The Stretch Reflex and Muscle Tone

The stretch reflex can be divided into three steps: **(1)** activation of the stretch receptors, **(2)** integration of the reflex in the spinal cord, and **(3)** regulation of reflex sensitivity by higher centers in the brain. Testing the knee-jerk reflex provides a means of assessing that reflex.

1 **Stretch Reflex Receptors.** Skeletal muscle is composed of extrafusal fibers, which control muscle movement, and intrafusal fibers, which control muscle tone. Intrafusal fibers are encapsulated in sheaths, forming a spindle that runs parallel to extrafusal fibers. Intrafusal fibers are innervated by a large Ia sensory nerve fiber, which encircles the central non-contractile part of the fiber to form the *annulospiral ending*. Because the spindles are parallel to the extrafusal muscle fibers, stretching extrafusal fibers also stretches the spindle fibers and stimulates the receptive endings of the Ia afferent neuron.

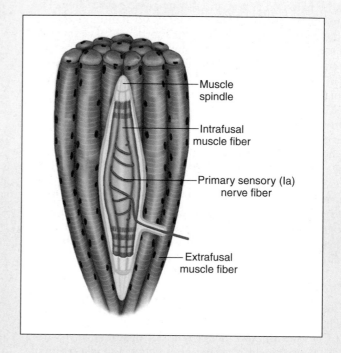

2 **Spinal Reflex Centers.** Afferent impulses from the Ia sensory fiber of the muscle spindle travel to the spinal cord, where they synapse with alpha motor neurons of the stretched muscle to form a *monosynaptic reflex arc*: one synapse separates the primary sensory input from the motor neuron output. The reflex muscle contraction that follows resists further stretching of the muscle. Simultaneously, impulses providing information on muscle length are transmitted to higher centers in the brain. The coordinated activity of all the monosynaptic reflexes supplying the extrafusal fibers in a skeletal muscle provides the muscle tone needed for organized movement.

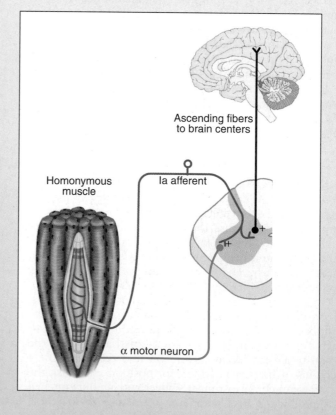

3 **Brain Center Connections.**
The sensitivity of a spinal reflex is adjusted by higher centers in the brain. Extrafusal muscle fibers are supplied with large alpha motor neurons, which produce muscle contraction. Intrafusal muscle fibers are supplied with smaller gamma motor neurons, which control the sensitivity of the stretch reflex. Motor pathways synapse with both alpha and gamma motor neurons, and impulses are sent simultaneously to the large extrafusal fibers and to the intrafusal fibers to maintain muscle spindle tension (and sensitivity) during muscle contraction.

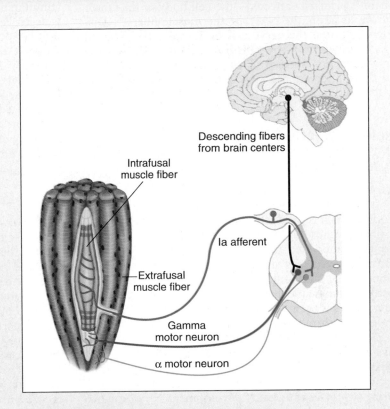

4 **The Knee-Jerk Reflex.** The knee-jerk reflex tests the stretch reflex arc in the quadriceps muscle. Stretching of extrafusal fibers by tapping with a reflex hammer lengthens the intrafusal fibers and increases firing of the type Ia afferent neuron. Impulses from the Ia fiber enter the dorsal horn of the spinal cord and make monosynaptic contact with the ventral horn alpha motor neuron that supplies the extrafusal fibers in the quadriceps muscle. The resultant contraction of the quadriceps muscle causes the knee jerk. These muscle reflexes are *deep tendon reflexes*, which can be checked at the wrists, elbows, knees, and ankles to assess stretch reflexes at different spinal cord segments.

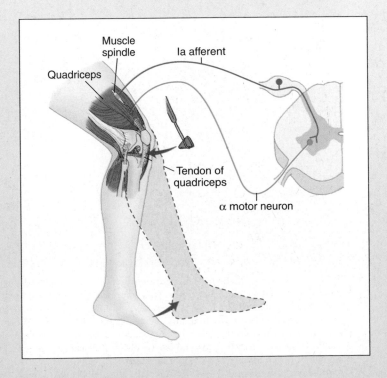

Disorders of the Motor Unit

Most motor unit diseases cause weakness and atrophy of skeletal muscles and vary depending on which component is primarily affected—the cell body of the motor neuron, its axon, the NMJ, or the muscle fibers.[6,7] Disorders affecting the nerve cell body are often referred to as *lower motor neuron disorders*. Those affecting the nerve axon are referred to as *peripheral neuropathies*, and those affecting the muscle fibers are referred to as *myopathies*.

Skeletal Muscle Disorders

Muscle Atrophy

Maintenance of muscle strength requires frequent movements against resistance. Reduced use results in muscle atrophy, which is a reduction in the diameter of the muscle fibers because of loss of protein filaments.[7] When a normally innervated muscle is not used for long periods, the muscle cells shrink in diameter, and although the muscle cells do not die, they lose much of their contractile proteins and become weakened. This is *disuse atrophy*, and it occurs with conditions such as immobilization and chronic illness. It is likely that not all skeletal muscle atrophy is the same, as different signaling pathways manage skeletal muscle protein turnover.[8]

Extreme muscle atrophy is present in disorders that deprive muscles of innervation (*denervation atrophy*). During early embryonic development, outgrowing skeletal nerves innervate partially mature muscle cells. Muscle cells that are not innervated do not mature and eventually die. In this process, randomly contracting muscle cells become enslaved by innervating neurons, and from then on, the muscle cell contracts only when stimulated by that neuron. If the LMN dies or its axon is destroyed, the skeletal muscle cell begins to have temporary spontaneous contractions, called *fibrillations*. In contrast to fasciculations, fibrillations are not visible clinically and can be detected only by electromyography (EMG). The muscle begins to lose its contractile proteins, and, after several months, if not reinnervated, is replaced by fibrous connective tissue, making rehabilitation difficult. Atrophy of denervation may be delayed by electrically stimulating the muscle periodically while waiting to determine if the damaged nerve fiber regenerates.

Muscular Dystrophy

Muscular dystrophy is a term applied to genetic disorders that produce progressive deterioration of skeletal muscles because of mixed muscle cell hypertrophy, atrophy, and necrosis. They are primary diseases of muscle tissue and probably do not involve the nervous system. As the muscle undergoes necrosis, fat and connective tissue replace the muscle fibers (*pseudohypertrophy*), which increases muscle size and results in muscle weakness (Fig. 15-6). The muscle weakness is insidious in onset but continually progressive, varying with the type of disorder.

The most common form of the disease is DMD, which occurs once in every 3500 live male births.[9] DMD is a

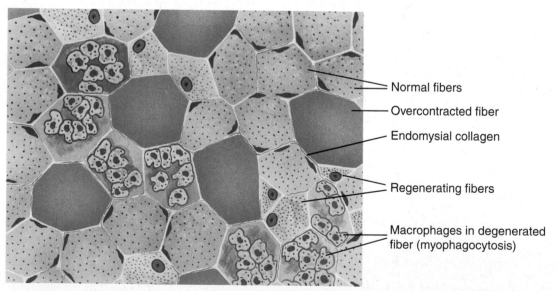

FIGURE 15-6. Duchenne muscular dystrophy. The pathologic changes in skeletal muscle. Some fibers are slightly larger and darker than normal. These represent overcontracted segments of sarcoplasm situated between degenerated segments. Other fibers are packed with macrophages that remove degenerated sarcoplasm. Other fibers are smaller than normal and have granular sarcoplasm. These fibers have enlarged, vesicular nuclei with prominent nucleoli and represent regenerating fibers. Developing endomysial fibrosis is represented by the deposition of collagen around individual muscle fibers. The changes are those of a chronic, active noninflammatory myopathy. (From Strayer D. S., Rubin E., Saffitz J. E., et al. (Eds.). (2015). *Rubin's pathology: Clinicopathologic foundations of medicine* (7th ed., Chapter 31). Philadelphia, PA: Lippincott Williams & Wilkins.)

Labels in figure:
- Normal fibers
- Overcontracted fiber
- Endomysial collagen
- Regenerating fibers
- Macrophages in degenerated fiber (myophagocytosis)

recessive, single-gene defect on the X chromosome, transmitted from mother to male offspring. A spontaneous form may occur in females. *Becker muscular dystrophy* is also X-linked but manifests later in childhood or adolescence and has a slower course of progression.

Etiology and Pathogenesis

DMD is caused by mutations in a gene located on the short arm of the X chromosome that codes for *dystrophin*. Dystrophin is a large cytoplasmic protein on the inner surface of the sarcolemma or muscle fiber membrane. Dystrophin molecules are concentrated at the Z bands of the muscle, where they form a strong link between actin filaments of the intracellular contractile apparatus and the extracellular connective tissue matrix.[6,7] Abnormalities in the dystrophin-associated protein complex likely compromise sarcolemma integrity, especially with sustained contractions. This disrupted integrity may be responsible for the increased fragility of dystrophic muscle, excessive influx of calcium ions, and release of soluble muscle enzymes such as creatine kinase into the serum. The degenerative process consists of necrosis of muscle fibers, accompanied by repair and regeneration, and progressive fibrosis. The degenerative process eventually outpaces the regenerative capacity of the muscle, causing a gradual replacement of muscle fibers by fibrofatty connective tissue. The end stage is characterized by almost complete loss of skeletal muscle fibers, with relative sparing of intrafusal fibers of the muscle spindles.[7]

Clinical Manifestations

Signs of muscle weakness manifested by frequent falling usually become evident at 2 to 3 years of age. The postural muscles of the hips and shoulders are usually the first to be affected, followed by pseudohypertrophy of the calf muscles. Imbalances between agonist and antagonist muscles lead to abnormal postures and the development of contractures and joint immobility. Scoliosis is common. Function of distal muscles usually is preserved enough to continue to use eating utensils and a keyboard. Function of extraocular muscles also is well preserved, as is the function of smooth muscle controlling bladder and bowel activity. Incontinence is an uncommon and late event. Respiratory muscle involvement results in weak and ineffective cough, frequent respiratory infections, and decreasing respiratory reserve. Cardiac muscle is affected, and cardiomyopathy is a common feature of the disease. The severity of cardiac involvement does not necessarily correlate with skeletal muscle weakness and ranges from fatal cardiomyopathy to adequate cardiac function until the terminal stages of the disease. Death from respiratory and cardiac muscle involvement usually occurs in young adulthood.

Diagnosis

Important diagnostic data for this disease include observation of voluntary movements and a complete family history. Serum levels of creatine kinase, which leaks from damaged muscle fibers, can assist the diagnosis. Muscle biopsy, which shows a mixture of muscle cell degeneration and regeneration and fat and scar tissue replacement, is diagnostic of the disorder. Echocardiography, electrocardiography, and chest radiography assess cardiac function. A specific molecular genetic diagnosis is possible by demonstrating defective dystrophin via immunohistochemical staining of sections of muscle biopsy tissue or by polymerase chain reaction analysis of genomic DNA derived from leukocytes. DNA analysis may also be used to establish carrier status in female relatives at risk, such as sisters and cousins.

Treatment

There is no known cure for DMD. Disease management is directed toward maintaining ambulation and preventing deformities via passive stretching, correct or counterposturing, and splints. Precautions should be taken to avoid respiratory infections.

Disorders of the Neuromuscular Junction

The NMJ serves as a synapse between a motor neuron and a skeletal muscle fiber. It consists of the axon terminals of a motor neuron and a specialized region of the muscle membrane called the motor *end-plate*. Transmission of impulses at the NMJ is mediated by *acetylcholine* (ACh) release from the axon terminals, which binds to nicotinic ACh receptors (nAChR) at the motor end-plate to cause muscle contraction (Fig. 15-7). ACh is active in the NMJ only for the time it takes to generate an action potential in the innervated muscle cell. In the synaptic space are large quantities of the enzyme *acetylcholinesterase* (AChE), which destroy ACh a few milliseconds after it has been released. The rapid inactivation of ACh allows repeated muscle contractions and gradations of contractile force.

Drug- and Toxin-Induced Disorders

Drugs can alter neuromuscular function by changing the release, inactivation, or receptor binding of ACh. A drug that acts on the postjunctional membrane of the motor end-plate to prevent the depolarizing effect of the neurotransmitter is curare. Curare-type drugs block the neuromuscular transmission and relax musculature during surgical procedures. Physostigmine and neostigmine inhibit the action of AChE and allow ACh to accumulate in the NMJ and prolong its action.[10] These drugs are used in the treatment of myasthenia gravis.

Neurotoxins from the botulism organism (*Clostridium botulinum*) produce paralysis by blocking ACh release.[7] Clostridia are anaerobic, gram-positive, spore-forming bacilli found worldwide in soils, marine and freshwater sediments, and in the intestines of many animals.[7] Spores can be dormant, are resistant to heat, and germinate in low-acidity and low-nitrate environments. Ingestion of spores leads to toxin synthesis and absorption of the toxins from the intestinal tract. Wound botulism occurs through colonization of wounds with *C. botulinum*.[7] Infant botulism occurs through infant ingestion of *C. botulinum* spores.[11] An infant's immature

Axonal Degeneration

Axonal degeneration is caused by primary injury to a neuronal cell body or its axon. Damage to the axon may be due to either a focal event at a point along the length of the nerve or a more generalized abnormality affecting the neuronal cell body.

Damage to a peripheral nerve axon results in degenerative changes, followed by breakdown of the myelin sheath and Schwann cells. In distal axonal degeneration, the proximal axon and neuronal cell body, which synthesizes the material required for nourishing and maintaining the axon, remain intact. In neuropathies and crushing injuries in which the endoneurial tube remains intact, the fiber will grow within the tube to its original target (Fig. 15-8). It can take weeks or months for the fiber to reach its target organ. More time is required for Schwann cells to form new myelin segments and for the axon to recover its original diameter and conduction velocity.

Regeneration of a nerve fiber in the peripheral nervous system depends on many factors. If a nerve fiber is destroyed close to the cell body, the nerve cell will likely die. If it does, it will not be replaced. If there is a crushing injury, partial or often full recovery of function occurs. If there is cutting-type trauma, connective scar tissue forms rapidly at the wound site. Only the rapidly regenerating axonal branches are able to get through to the intact distal endoneurial tubes. Neuropathies involving the cell body are less common, and there is little potential for recovery of function because death of the neuronal cells precludes axonal regeneration.

Mononeuropathies

Mononeuropathies usually are caused by localized conditions such as trauma, compression, or infection that affect a single spinal nerve, plexus, or peripheral nerve trunk. Fractured bones may lacerate or compress nerves. Tight tourniquets may injure nerves or produce ischemic injury. Infections may affect a single segmental afferent nerve distribution. Recovery of nerve function usually is complete after compression lesions and incomplete or faulty after nerve transection.

Carpal Tunnel Syndrome

Carpal tunnel syndrome is a common compression-type mononeuropathy.[7] It is caused by compression of the median nerve as it travels with the flexor tendons through a canal made by the carpal bones and transverse carpal ligament. It can be caused by a variety of conditions that produce a reduction in the capacity of the carpal tunnel or an increase in the volume of the tunnel contents. Most cases of carpal tunnel syndrome are due to repetitive use of the wrist.

Clinical Manifestations. Carpal tunnel syndrome is characterized by pain, paresthesia, and numbness of the thumb and first two and one-half digits of the hand; pain in the wrist and hand, which worsens at night; atrophy of the abductor pollicis muscle; and weakness in precision grip. These abnormalities may contribute to clumsiness of fine motor activity.

Diagnosis and Treatment. Diagnosis is based on sensory disturbances confined to median nerve distribution and a positive Tinel or Phalen sign.[15] The *Tinel sign* is a tingling sensation radiating into the palm elicited by light percussion over the median nerve at the wrist. The *Phalen maneuver* is performed by having the person hold the wrist in complete flexion for a minute. If numbness and paresthesia along the median nerve are reproduced or exaggerated, the test result is considered to be positive. EMG and nerve conduction studies can confirm the diagnosis and exclude other causes.

Treatment includes avoidance of movements that cause nerve compression, nighttime splinting, and anti-inflammatory medications. Measures to decrease causative repetitive movements should be initiated. When splinting is ineffective, corticosteroids may be injected into the carpal tunnel to reduce inflammation and swelling. Surgical intervention consists of operative division of the volar carpal ligaments as a means of relieving pressure on the median nerve.

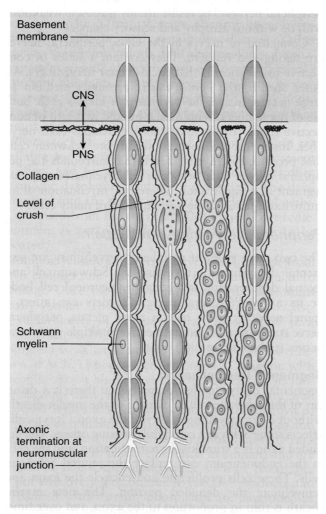

FIGURE 15-8. Sequential stages in efferent axon degeneration and regeneration within its endoneurial tube, after peripheral nerve crush injury. CNS, central nervous system; PNS, peripheral nervous system.

Polyneuropathies

Polyneuropathies involve demyelination or axonal degeneration of multiple peripheral nerves that leads to symmetric sensory, motor, or mixed sensorimotor deficits. The longest axons are involved first, with symptoms beginning in the distal part of the extremities. If the autonomic nervous system is involved, there may be postural hypotension, constipation, and impotence. Polyneuropathies can result from immune mechanisms (*e.g.*, Guillain–Barré syndrome), toxic agents (*e.g.*, arsenic, lead, alcohol), and metabolic diseases (*e.g.*, diabetes mellitus, uremia). Different causes affect axons of different diameters and neuron classes to different degrees.

Guillain–Barré Syndrome

Guillain–Barré syndrome is an acute immune-mediated polyneuropathy.[16] There are several indices of the disorder, including pure motor axonal degeneration and axonal degeneration of both motor and sensory nerves.[7] It is caused by infiltration of mononuclear cells around the capillaries of peripheral neurons, edema of the endoneurial compartment, and demyelination of ventral spinal roots. The cause likely has an immune component. Most people report having had an acute, influenza-like illness before the onset of symptoms. About one third of people with Guillain–Barré syndrome have antibodies against nerve gangliosides.

Clinical Manifestations. Progressive ascending muscle weakness of the limbs, producing a symmetric flaccid paralysis, characterizes the disorder. Symptoms of paresthesia and numbness often accompany loss of motor function. A ventilator is required if paralysis involves respiratory muscles. Autonomic nervous system involvement that causes postural hypotension, arrhythmias, facial flushing, abnormalities of sweating, and urinary retention is common. Pain is a common feature. Guillain–Barré syndrome may have a rapid development of ventilatory failure and autonomic disturbances or it may present as a slow, insidious process. Cranial nerve involvement may occur resulting in facial, oculomotor, or bulbar weakness. Severity and duration of Guillain–Barré syndrome can range from mild weakness with spontaneous recovery to developing tetraplegic and ventilator dependence with no signs of recovery for several months or longer.[17]

Treatment. Treatment includes support of vital functions and prevention of complications such as skin breakdown and thrombophlebitis. Treatment is most effective if initiated early.[17] Plasmapheresis and high-dose intravenous immunoglobulin therapy are treatment mainstays.

Back Pain

Low back pain or strain affects almost 70% of people at least once in their lifetime.[15] It affects males and females equally, with onset between the ages of 30 and 50.[16] Risk factors include heavy lifting, smoking, obesity, and depressive symptoms.[18] Although acute low back pain resolves within 3 to 6 weeks in most people, recurrences are common.[15]

Back pain can result from many interrelated problems involving spinal structures and spinal nerve roots. People with low back pain frequently experience musculoligamentous injuries and age-related degenerative changes in the intervertebral disks and facet joints. Other causes include disk herniation, which is a herniated nucleus pulposus and spinal stenosis, which is characterized by narrowing of the central canal, typically from hypertrophic degenerative changes.[15]

Diagnosis includes a thorough history, physical, and neurologic examination. MRI or radiography is not generally recommended early in the course of low back pain. The diagnostic challenge is to identify people who require further evaluation for more serious problems.

Treatment of back pain consists of analgesic medications, muscle relaxants, and instruction in the correct mechanics for lifting and methods of protecting the back.[15] Pain relief is usually nonsteroidal anti-inflammatory drugs, other analgesics, and muscle relaxants. Comorbidities include sleep disorders, which should also be managed by the provider.[19]

Herniated Intervertebral Disk

Intervertebral disks are a critical component of the load-bearing structures of the spinal column. They consist of a gelatinous center (the *nucleus pulposus*), which is encircled by a strong collar of fibrocartilage (the *annulus fibrosus*).[2] The disk absorbs shock, changes shape, and allows movement. The nucleus pulposus can be squeezed out of place and herniate through the annulus fibrosus, a condition referred to as a *herniated, ruptured,* or *slipped disk* (Fig. 15-9A and B).

Etiology and Pathogenesis

The intervertebral disk can dysfunction due to trauma, aging, or degenerative disorders of the spine. Trauma can result from activities such as lifting while in the flexed position or simply suppressing a sneeze. With age, the gelatinous center of the disk dries and loses elasticity, causing it to fray and tear. Degenerative processes such as osteoarthritis or ankylosing spondylitis predispose to malalignment of the vertebral column.

The cervical and lumbar regions are the most flexible areas of the spine and are often involved in disk herniations. Usually, herniation occurs at lower lumbar spine levels where the mass is being supported and bending is the greatest. Most lumbar herniations occur at L4 or L5 to S1. Most cervical herniations occur at C6 to C7 and C5 to C6. Nucleus pulposus protrusion usually occurs posteriorly, toward the intervertebral foramen and its contained spinal nerve root (Fig. 15-9B).

When the injury is in the lumbar area, only the nerve fibers of the cauda equina are involved. Because these elongated dorsal and ventral roots contain endoneurial tubes of connective tissue, regeneration of the nerve fibers is likely. Several weeks or months are required for full recovery because of the distance to the innervated muscle or skin of the lower limbs.

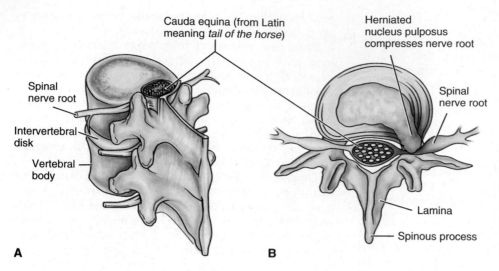

Cauda equina (from Latin meaning *tail of the horse*)

Spinal nerve root

Intervertebral disk

Vertebral body

A

Herniated nucleus pulposus compresses nerve root

Spinal nerve root

Lamina

Spinous process

B

FIGURE 15-9. (A) Normal lumbar spine vertebrae, intervertebral disks, and spinal nerve root. (B) Ruptured vertebral disk. (From Hinkle J. L., Cheever K. H. (2014). *Brunner & Suddarth's textbook of medical-surgical nursing* (13th ed., p. 2074). Philadelphia, PA: Lippincott Williams & Wilkins.)

Clinical Manifestations. Symptoms are localized to the area of the body innervated by the nerve roots and include both motor and sensory manifestations (Fig. 15-10). Pain is the first, most common symptom. The nerve roots of L4, L5, S1, S2, and S3 give rise to back pain that spreads down the back of the leg and over the sole of the foot. Pain may increase with normal activities such as coughing, straining, stooping, and walking. Major weakness is rare. The most common sensory deficits from spinal nerve root compression are paresthesias and numbness, particularly of the leg and foot. A herniated disk must be differentiated from other causes of acute back pain.

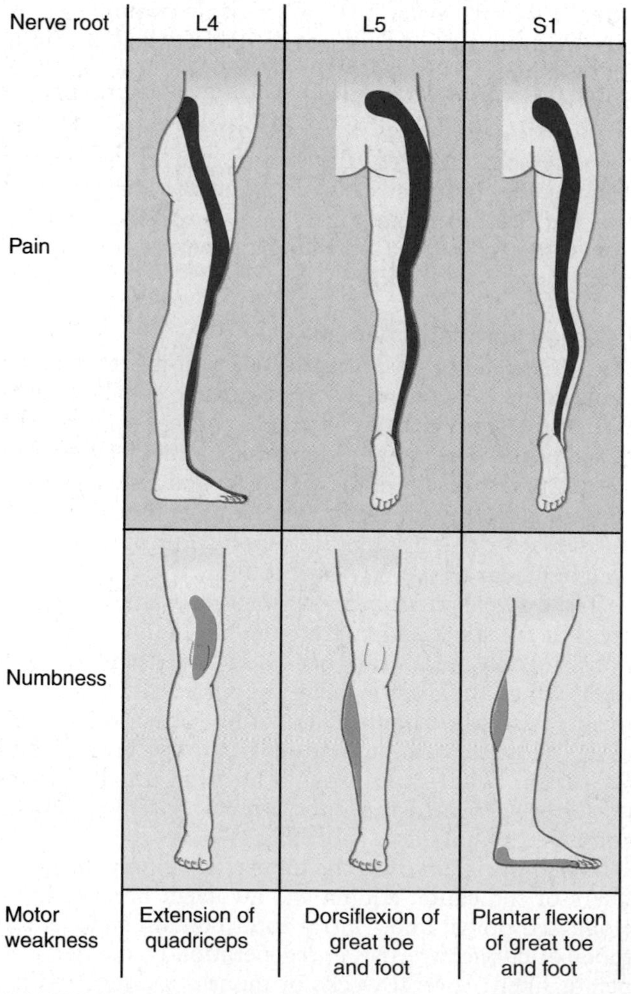

Diagnosis

Diagnosis includes history and physical and neurological examination. The straight-leg test is done in the supine position and is performed by passively raising the person's leg or by extending the knee while the person sits with both hip and knee flexed at 90 degrees. This test applies traction along the nerve root, which exacerbates pain if the nerve root is acutely inflamed. Normally, the leg can be raised about 90 degrees without causing discomfort of the hamstring muscles. The test is positive if pain is produced when the leg is raised to 60 degrees or less.[15] Other methods include radiographs of the back, MRI, computed tomography (CT), and CT myelography.

Treatment

Treatment usually consists of analgesic medications and education on how to protect the back. Pain relief can be provided using nonsteroidal anti-inflammatory drugs, and short-term use of opioid pain medications may be required. Muscle relaxants may be used on a short-term basis. For initial treatment, guidelines suggest nonpharmacologic treatment, including superficial heat, massage, acupuncture, or spinal manipulation. Nonpharmacologic treatment of chronic low back pain may also include exercise, tai chi, yoga, progressive relaxation, cognitive behavioral therapy, or spinal manipulation.[20] Surgical treatment may be indicated if there is herniation, consistent pain, or neurologic deficit that has failed to respond to conservative therapy.

Back Pain Emergencies

Acute back pain is usually a non-life-threatening condition, but for a few people, it can be a manifestation of serious pathology. Vascular catastrophes, malignancy,

Nerve root	L4	L5	S1
Pain			
Numbness			
Motor weakness	Extension of quadriceps	Dorsiflexion of great toe and foot	Plantar flexion of great toe and foot

FIGURE 15-10. Dermatomes of the leg (L1 through S5) where pain and numbness would be experienced with spinal root irritation.

spinal cord compression syndromes, and infectious processes may all present as acute back pain.

Clinical findings, commonly referred to as *red flags*, which indicate the possibility of more serious disease include gradual onset of pain; age under 20 years or over 50 years; thoracic back pain; history of trauma, fever, chills, night sweats, immunosuppression, or malignancy; unintentional weight loss; bacteremia; and history of intravenous drug use.[15]

Gradual onset of pain may indicate malignancy or infection. Back pain that begins before 20 years of age suggests congenital or developmental disorders, and new pain in people over 50 years of age may be due to an aortic aneurysm, malignancy, or compression fracture. Pain that is aggravated by lying down suggests malignancy or infection; pain that improves with sitting or slight flexion of the spine suggests the presence of spinal stenosis. Reports of neurologic symptoms such as paresthesia, motor weakness, urinary or fecal incontinence, or gait abnormalities require additional diagnostic tests to rule out spinal cord compression.

SUMMARY CONCEPTS

The motor unit consists of the LMN, the NMJ, and the skeletal muscle that the nerve innervates. Disorders of the neuromuscular unit include muscular dystrophy and myasthenia gravis. *Muscular dystrophy* describes several disorders that produce progressive deterioration of skeletal muscle followed by fibrofatty tissue replacement. One form, DMD, is inherited as an X-linked trait and transmitted by the mother to her male offspring. Myasthenia gravis is a disorder of the NMJ resulting from a deficiency of functional AChR, which causes weakness of the skeletal muscles. Because the disease affects the NMJ, there is no loss of sensory function. The most common manifestations are weakness of the eye muscles, with ptosis and diplopia.

Peripheral nerve disorders involve motor and sensory neurons outside the CNS. There are two main types of peripheral nerve injury based on target of the insult: segmental demyelination involving the Schwann cell and axonal degeneration involving the nerve axon or cell body. Peripheral nerve disorders include mononeuropathies, involving a single spinal nerve, plexus, or peripheral nerve, and polyneuropathies that involve demyelination or axonal degeneration of multiple peripheral nerves that leads to symmetric sensory, motor, or mixed sensorimotor deficits. Carpal tunnel syndrome, a mononeuropathy, is caused by compression of the median nerve that passes through the carpal tunnel in the wrist. Guillain–Barré syndrome is a subacute polyneuropathy that causes progressive ascending motor, sensory, and autonomic nervous system manifestations. Respiratory involvement necessitates mechanical ventilation.

Acute back pain is commonly due to muscle strain; treatment focuses on improving activity tolerance. A herniated intervertebral disk is characterized by protrusion of the nucleus pulposus into the spinal canal with irritation or compression of the nerve root. Usually, herniation occurs at the lower levels of the lumbar and sacral (L4 or L5 to S1) and cervical (C6 to C7 and C5 to C6) regions of the spine. The symptoms of a herniated disk are localized to the area of the body innervated by the affected nerve roots and include pain and both motor and sensory signs.

Disorders of the Cerebellum and Basal Ganglia

Disorders of the Cerebellum

The cerebellum is located in the posterior fossa and attached to the pons, medulla, and midbrain by the three paired cerebellar peduncles.[2,7] The cerebellum is especially vital during rapid muscular activities such as running, typing, and talking. Loss of cerebellar function can result in total incoordination of these functions even though paralysis does not ensue.

The functions of the cerebellum are integrated into connected afferent and efferent pathways throughout the brain. The *corticopontocerebellar* afferent pathway originates in the motor and premotor cortices and the somatosensory cortex. Other important afferent pathways link the cerebellum to input from the basal ganglia, muscle and joint tension information from the stretch receptors, visual input from the eyes, and balance and equilibrium sensation from the vestibular system in the inner ear. There are three general efferent pathways leading out of the cerebellum:

- *Vestibulocerebellar pathway:* functions in close association with the brain stem vestibular nuclei to maintain equilibrium and posture
- *Spinocerebellar pathway:* provides the circuitry for coordinating the movements of the distal portions of the limbs, especially the hands and fingers
- *Cerebrocerebellar pathway:* transmits output information in the upward direction to the brain, functioning in a feedback manner with the motor and somatosensory systems to coordinate sequential body and limb movements

Cerebellum-Associated Movement Disorders

Cerebellar dysfunction can be grouped into vestibulocerebellar disorders, cerebellar ataxia, and cerebellar tremor. These occur on the side of cerebellar damage and are caused by congenital defect, vascular accident, or growing tumor. Visual monitoring of movement cannot compensate for cerebellar defects, and the abnormalities occur whether the eyes are open or closed.

Damage to the cerebellar area associated with the vestibular system leads to difficulty or inability to maintain a steady posture of the trunk. This unsteadiness of the trunk (*truncal ataxia*) can be so severe that standing is not possible. The ability to fix the eyes on a target also can be affected. Constant conjugate readjustment of eye position, called nystagmus, results and makes reading extremely difficult, especially when the eyes are deviated toward the side of cerebellar damage.

Cerebellar ataxia and tremor are different aspects of defects in smooth, continuously correcting functions. Cerebellar dystaxia or ataxia is characterized by a decomposition of movement, with each component of a movement occurring separately instead of a smooth action. Ethanol affects cerebellar function and people who are inebriated often walk with a staggering and unsteady gait. Rapid alternating movements are jerky and performed slowly. Reaching to touch a target results in the finger or toe moving jerkily toward the target, missing, correcting in the other direction, and worsening as the target is approached. This is called *over- and underreaching* or *dysmetria*. Multiple sclerosis (MS) is the most common cause of cerebellar ataxia.[21] Acute postinfectious cerebellar ataxia can occur with a prior history of varicella in preschool children.[22]

Cerebellar tremor results from the inability to maintain ongoing fixation of a body part and to make smooth, continuous corrections in the movement trajectory; overcorrection occurs, first in one direction and then the other. Often, tremor of an arm or leg can be detected during the beginning of an intended movement (*intention tremor*). It is possible to assess cerebellar function as it relates to tremor by asking a person to touch one heel to the opposite knee, to gently move the toes along the back of the opposite shin, or to touch the nose with a finger.

Cerebellar function also can affect the motor skills of chewing and swallowing (dysphagia) and speech (dysarthria). Speech requires smooth control of respiratory muscles and coordinated control of the laryngeal, lip, and tongue muscles. Cerebellar dysarthria is characterized by slow, slurred speech of varying loudness. Speech therapy can provide rehabilitation, including slowing the rate of speech and compensating with less-affected muscles.

Disorders of the Basal Ganglia

The basal ganglia are a group of subcortical nuclei that are essential in movement control. They function in the organization of inherited and highly learned and automatic movement programs, especially those affecting the trunk and proximal limbs. The basal ganglia are important in starting, stopping, and monitoring movements ordered and executed by the cortex, especially relatively slow and sustained, or stereotyped, movements such as arm-swinging during walking. They help to regulate the intensity of these movements, and inhibit antagonistic or unnecessary movements. The basal ganglia are also involved in cognitive and perceptual functions.

The structural components of the basal ganglia include the caudate nucleus, putamen, and globus pallidus.[2] They are located lateral and caudal to the thalamus. The caudate and putamen form the *striatum*, and the putamen and globus pallidus form the *lentiform nucleus*. The *substantia nigra* of the midbrain *and subthalamic nucleus* of the diencephalon are also part of the basal ganglia[2] (Fig. 15-11). The dorsal part of the substantia nigra contains dopaminergic cells that are rich in the black pigment *melanin*, hence the name *substantia nigra*. Axons of the substantia nigra form the *nigrostriatal pathway*, which supplies dopamine to the striatum. The subthalamic nucleus lies below the thalamus and above the anterior portion of the substantia nigra. The glutaminergic cells of this nucleus are the only excitatory projections to the basal ganglia.

Several thalamic nuclei are associated with the basal ganglia. Each region of the cerebral cortex is interconnected with specific ventral thalamic nuclei. The cortex-to-thalamus and thalamus-to-cortex feedback circuitries are excitatory and, if unmodulated, produce hyperactivity of the cortical area, causing stiffness and rigidity of the face, body, and limbs, and, if alternating, a continuous tremor. Thalamic excitability is modulated through inhibition by the basal ganglia. Discrete inhibitory cortex-to-basal ganglia and thalamus-to-cortex loops modulate the function of all cerebral cortex regions.

The basal ganglia have input structures that receive afferent information, internal circuits that connect

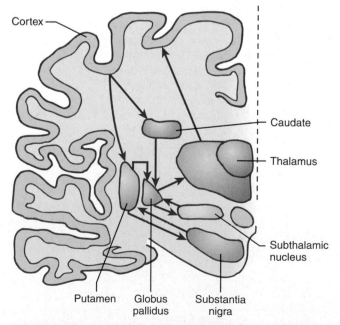

FIGURE 15-11. Structures and basal neural circuitry of the basal ganglia.

various basal ganglia nuclei, and output structures that deliver information to other brain centers. The striatum is the major input structure for the basal ganglia. All principal pathways for executing learned movements pass through the striatum.

Internal circuits within the basal ganglia balance and integrate information. For example, the *striatonigral pathway* sends GABA-ergic projections from the striatum to the substantia nigra, and the *nigrostriatal pathway* sends dopaminergic axons from the substantia nigra back to the striatum. PD is a deficiency in these dopaminergic neurons. The function of the striatum also involves local cholinergic interneurons. The destruction of these interneurons is thought to be related to the choreiform movements of Huntington disease.

The output functions of the basal ganglia are mainly inhibitory. The output nuclei of the basal ganglia, the globus pallidus and the substantia nigra, tonically inhibit their target nuclei in the thalamus. The basal ganglia also monitor sensory information coming into the brain and apply it to information stored in memory.

This cognitive control of motor activities determines within seconds which movement patterns will be needed. The caudate nucleus receives input from the association areas of the brain and plays a major role in the cognitive control of motor activity.

Basal Ganglia–Associated Movement Disorders

Basal ganglia disorders are a group of motor disturbances defined by tremor and involuntary movements, changes in posture and muscle tone, and poverty and slowness of movement. They include tremors and tics, hypokinetic disorders, and hyperkinetic disorders[1] (Table 15-1).

Hypokinetic and hyperkinetic disorders can be explained by pathology in the striatal direct and indirect pathways that link the basal ganglia with the thalamocortical motor circuit. Overactivity of the indirect pathway results in hypokinetic disorders such as PD. Underactivity of the indirect pathway results in hyperkinetic disorders such as chorea and **ballismus**.

Parkinson Disease

PD is a degenerative disorder of basal ganglia function that results in variable combinations of tremor, rigidity, **akinesia**/bradykinesia, and postural changes. PD is characterized by progressive destruction of the nigrostriatal pathway and reduction in striatal dopamine. The prevalence of PD in the United States is estimated at 1.0% of the population over 65 years of age.[15] The mean onset of PD is 57 years of age, with approximately 60,000 new cases being diagnosed annually.

The clinical syndrome arising from degenerative changes in basal ganglia function is referred to as *parkinsonism*. PD is also known as *idiopathic parkinsonism*. Parkinsonism can also develop as a postencephalitic syndrome, a side effect of antipsychotic drugs that block dopamine receptors, a toxic reaction to a chemical

TABLE 15-1 Characteristics of Basal Ganglia–Associated Movement Disorders

Movement Disorder	Characteristics
Tremor	Involuntary, oscillating contractions of opposing muscle groups around a joint Usually fairly uniform in frequency and amplitude Can occur as resting tremors and postural tremors, which occur when the part is maintained in a stable position
Hypokinetic disorders	Slowness in initiating movement and reduced range and force of the movement (bradykinesia)
Chorea	Irregular wriggling and writhing movements Accentuated by movement and by environmental stimulation; they often interfere with normal movement patterns May be grimacing movements of the face, raising the eyebrows, rolling of the eyes, and curling, protrusion, withdrawal of the tongue In the limbs, the movements largely are distal. There may be piano playing–type movements with alternating extension and flexion of the fingers
Athetosis	Continuous, wormlike, twisting, and turning motions of the joints of a limb or the body
Ballismus	Violent, sweeping, flinging motions, especially of the limbs on one side of the body (hemiballismus)
Dystonia	Abnormal maintenance of a posture resulting from a twisting, turning movement of the limbs, neck, or trunk Often the result of simultaneous contraction of agonist and antagonist muscles Can result in grotesque and twisted postures
Dyskinesias	Bizarre wriggling and writhing movements Frequently involve the face, mouth, jaw, and tongue, causing grimacing, pursing of the lips, or protrusion of the tongue Limbs affected less often Tardive dyskinesia is an untoward reaction that can develop with long-term use of some antipsychotic medications

agent, or an outcome of severe carbon monoxide poisoning. Symptoms of parkinsonism can occur with damage to the nigrostriatal pathway, as in cerebral vascular disease, brain tumors, repeated head trauma, or a degenerative neurologic disease.

The primary brain abnormality in PD is the degeneration of the pigmented nigrostriatal dopamine neurons.[15] (Fig. 15-12). Some residual nerve cells are atrophic, and few contain *Lewy bodies*, which are spherical, eosinophilic cytoplasmic inclusions. Lewy bodies are produced

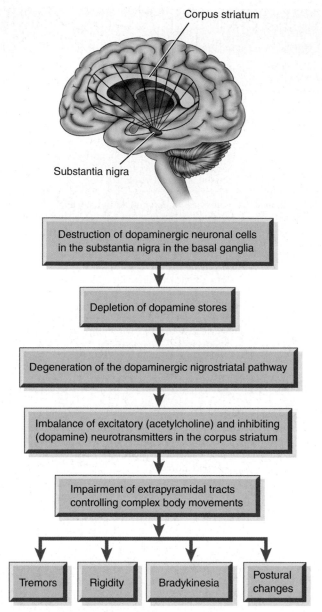

FIGURE 15-12. Pathophysiology of Parkinson disease. The nuclei in the substantia nigra project fibers to the corpus striatum. The nerve fibers carry dopamine to the corpus striatum. The loss of dopamine nerve cells from the brain's substantia nigra is thought to be responsible for the symptoms of parkinsonism. (From Hinkle J. L., Cheever K. H. (2014). *Brunner & Suddarth's textbook of medical-surgical nursing* (13th ed., p. 2063). Philadelphia, PA: Lippincott Williams & Wilkins.)

inside degenerated neurons in many people with PD or parkinsonism.[15]

Etiology and Pathogenesis

It is believed that PD is caused by an interaction of environmental and genetic factors. Several pathologic processes (*e.g.*, oxidative stress and mitochondrial disorders) that might lead to degeneration have been identified. Some environmental factors have also been identified, including contact with specific agricultural pesticides and rural living with private wells, especially if the area has been sprayed with herbicides and pesticides. Smoking cigarettes and drinking coffee are linked to a lower risk of PD.[23] Multiple genes illustrate there are different types of PD: the recessive form causes a milder set of symptoms compared to the dominant form, which resembles the more complex and severe form of PD with Lewy bodies.[24] Alpha-synuclein is one of the major components of the Lewy bodies.[7,24] Mutations in a gene coding the protein *parkin* is associated with an autosomal recessive, early-onset form of PD. The parkin protein acts as an enzyme in the ubiquitin-conjugating system that targets defective and abnormally folded proteins for destruction. Loss of normal parkin function is postulated to cause abnormal proteins to aggregate and cause neurodegenerative changes.[7] Several new diagnostic tools are available regarding genomic, proteomic, transcriptomic, lipidomic, and metabolomic molecules and signaling pathways.[24] There are also syndromes that can cause parkinsonism but not idiopathic PD such as 1-methyl-4-phenyl-1,2,3,6-tetrahydropyridine–induced parkinsonism, postinfectious parkinsonism, striatonigral degeneration, and progressive supranuclear palsy where the common finding is loss of pigmented dopaminergic neurons in the substantia nigra.[7]

Clinical Manifestations

Tremor is the most visible manifestation of the disorder and affects mainly the hands and feet; head, neck, face, lips, and tongue; or jaw. It is characterized by rhythmic, alternating flexion and contraction movements (4 to 6 beats/minute) that resemble rolling a pill between the thumb and forefinger. The tremor is initially unilateral, occurs when the limb is supported and at rest, and disappears with movement and sleep. The tremor eventually progresses bilaterally.

Rigidity is the resistance to movement of flexors and extensors throughout the full range of motion. It is most evident during passive joint movement and involves jerky, ratchet-like movements that require considerable energy to perform. Flexion contractions may develop due to rigidity. As with tremor, rigidity usually begins unilaterally but progresses bilaterally.

Bradykinesia is the slowness in initiating and performing movements and difficulty with sudden, unexpected stopping of voluntary movements. Unconscious associative movements occur in disconnected steps rather than in a smooth, coordinated manner. People with bradykinesia may freeze in place while walking and feel as if their feet are glued to the floor, especially when moving through a doorway or preparing to turn. When walking, they lean forward and take small, shuffling steps without swinging their arms, and have difficulty changing their stride. People with advanced-stage parkinsonism are at risk of falls, fluctuations in motor function, neuropsychiatric disorders, and sleep disorders. Loss of postural reflexes predisposes to falling, often backward. Emotional and voluntary facial movements become limited and slow with progression, and facial expression becomes stiff and masklike. There is loss of the blinking reflex and a failure to express emotion. The tongue, palate, and throat muscles become rigid, and the person may drool because of difficulty in moving and swallowing saliva. Speech becomes slow and monotonous, without modulation, and poorly articulated.

Because the basal ganglia also influence the autonomic nervous system, people with PD often have excessive and uncontrolled sweating, sebaceous gland secretion, and salivation. Autonomic symptoms, such as lacrimation, dysphagia, orthostatic hypotension, thermal regulation, constipation, impotence, and urinary incontinence, may be present, especially late in the disease.

Cognitive dysfunction may also be an important feature in PD. Severe dementia is seen in about 20% of people with PD. Deficits in visuospatial discrimination, frontal lobe executive function, and memory retrieval are typical of the cognitive dysfunction seen in people with PD. Deficits in executive functioning may be among the earliest signs of cognitive decline, as evidenced by difficulty in planning, starting, and carrying out tasks. Dementia is usually a late manifestation of the disease, and the rate of decline is slow compared with Alzheimer disease.

Treatment

PD treatment must be highly individualized. Treatment only manages the symptoms; there is no treatment that will fully prevent disease progression.[15] Nonpharmacologic interventions include group support, education, daily exercise, and adequate nutrition. Botulinum toxin injections may be used in the treatment of dystonias such as eyelid spasm and limb dystonias that frequently are associated with PD. People with parkinsonism other than idiopathic PD usually do not respond significantly to medications developed for PD.

Pharmacologic treatment usually is determined by the severity of symptoms. Drugs that improve the function of the dopaminergic system include those that increase dopamine levels (levodopa), stimulate dopamine receptors (dopamine receptor agonists), or retard breakdown of dopamine (monoamine oxidase inhibitors). Because dopamine transmission is disrupted in PD, there is a preponderance of cholinergic activity, which may be treated with anticholinergic drugs.[25]

Dopamine does not cross the blood–brain barrier. Levodopa, a precursor of dopamine, crosses the blood–brain barrier, and remains the most effective drug for treatment. Levodopa is absorbed from the intestinal tract, crosses the blood–brain barrier, and is converted to dopamine by centrally acting dopa decarboxylase. When levodopa (a decarboxylase inhibitor) is given in with carbidopa, the peripheral metabolism of levodopa is reduced, plasma levels of levodopa are increased and its half-life is longer, more levodopa is available for entry into the brain, and a smaller dose is needed.[25] A later adverse effect of levodopa is the *on–off phenomenon*, in which frequent, abrupt, and unpredictable fluctuations in motor performance occur during the day. These fluctuations include *on* periods without dyskinesia, *on* periods with dyskinesia, and *off* periods with bradykinesia. Some fluctuations reflect the timing of drug administration, in which case the *on* response coincides with peak drug levels and the *off* response with low drug levels.

Treatment with dopamine agonists directly stimulates dopamine receptors.[25] The dopamine agonist rotigotine is supplied transdermally, while apomorphine can be given intravenously. Bromocriptine, pramipexole, and ropinirole can be used as initial or adjunctive therapy and can be given in combination with carbidopa/levodopa. Selegiline and rasagiline are monoamine oxidase type B inhibitors that inhibit the metabolic breakdown of dopamine and may be used as adjunctive treatment to reduce mild on–off fluctuations of people who are receiving levodopa.[15]

Anticholinergic drugs are thought to restore a *balance* between reduced dopamine and uninhibited cholinergic neurons in the striatum. Anticholinergic drugs lessen the tremors and rigidity and afford some improvement of function. However, their potency seems to decrease over time, and increasing the dosage increases side effects such as blurred vision, dry mouth, bowel and bladder problems, cognitive dysfunction, and hallucinations.[15]

Surgical treatment for PD is limited to thalamotomy and pallidotomy, in which part of the thalamus or globus pallidus is destroyed using an electrical stimulator or supercooled tip of a metal probe. Brain mapping is done during the surgery to identify and prevent injury to sensory and motor tracts. Thalamotomy and pallidotomy are generally confined to one side of the brain because of adverse effects associated with bilateral lesioning procedures.

Deep brain stimulation, which involves implantation of electrodes into the subthalamic nuclei or the pars interna of the globus pallidus, is performed more frequently for treatment of PD in the United States because it is nondestructive and reversible.[15] The electrodes are connected to a surgically implanted impulse generator that delivers electrical simulation to block abnormal nerve activity that causes tremor and abnormal motor activity. The stimulation is programmed to control the symptoms, and the parameters can be changed over time as the disease progresses. Deep brain stimulation is used for people with PD who respond to levodopa but experience side effects associated with it. It is not a cure, but serves to increase the duration of the *on* periods, may allow for a reduction in medication dosages, and improves function.

SUMMARY CONCEPTS

Alterations in coordination and abnormal muscle movements result from disorders of the cerebellum and basal ganglia. The functions of the cerebellum, which are vital during rapid muscular movements, use afferent input from various sources, including the stretch receptors, proprioceptors, tactile receptors in the skin, visual input, and vestibular system. Cerebellar disorders include vestibulocerebellar dysfunction, cerebellar ataxia, and cerebellar tremor.

The basal ganglia organize basic movement patterns into complex patterns, contributing gracefulness to cortically initiated and controlled skilled movements. Basal ganglia disorders are characterized by involuntary movements, alterations in muscle tone, and disturbances in posture. These disorders include tremor, tics, hemiballismus, chorea, **athetosis**, dystonias, and dyskinesias.

Parkinsonism, a disorder of the basal ganglia, is characterized by destruction of the nigrostriatal pathway, with a subsequent reduction in striatal concentrations of dopamine. This results in an imbalance between the inhibition and excitation. The disorder is manifested by resting tremor, increased muscle tonus and rigidity, slowness of movement, gait disturbances, and impaired autonomic postural responses. The disease usually is slowly progressive over several decades. The tremor often begins in one or both hands and then becomes generalized. Postural changes and gait disturbances continue to become more pronounced, resulting in significant disability.

Upper Motor Neuron Disorders

UMN disorders involve neurons that are fully contained within the CNS. They include the motor neurons arising in the motor areas of the cortex and their fibers as they project to the spinal cord. Amyotrophic lateral sclerosis (ALS) is a mixed UMN and LMN disorder. Disorders that affect UMNs include MS and SCI.

Amyotrophic Lateral Sclerosis

ALS, also known as *Lou Gehrig disease*, is a devastating neurologic disorder that selectively affects motor function. It has an annual incidence of 1 per 100,000 people.[7] ALS primarily affects people in their fifties, and males develop the disease nearly twice as often as females.

ALS affects the LMNs of the spinal cord; the motor nuclei of the brain stem, particularly the hypoglossal nuclei; and the UMNs of the cerebral cortex.[7] The disease is more extensive in the distal parts of the affected tracts rather than the proximal parts, suggesting that affected neurons first undergo degeneration at their distal terminals, and the disease proceeds until the parent nerve cell dies. A remarkable feature of ALS is that the entire sensory system, the regulatory mechanisms of control and coordination of movement, and the intellect remain intact. Neurons for ocular motility and parasympathetic neurons in the sacral spinal cord also are spared.

Death of LMNs leads to denervation, shrinkage of musculature, and muscle fiber atrophy (*amyotrophy*). The loss of nerve fibers in *lateral* columns of the white matter of the spinal cord and fibrillary gliosis impart a firmness or *sclerosis* to this CNS tissue.

Etiology and Pathogenesis

The cause of LMN and UMN destruction in ALS is uncertain. Five percent of cases are familial and the rest are believed to be sporadic.[7] The gene for a subset of familial ALS is superoxide dismutase 1 (*SOD1*) on chromosome 21.[7] Neurofilament proteins used for axonal transport are destroyed with ALS. Another suggested mechanism of pathogenesis is exotoxic injury through activation of glutamate-gated ion channels, which are distinguished by their sensitivity to N-methyl-D-aspartic acid. Although autoimmunity has been suggested as a cause of ALS, the disease does not respond to immunosuppressant agents.

Clinical Manifestations

The symptoms of ALS may be due to UMN or LMN involvement. Manifestations of UMN lesions include weakness, spasticity or stiffness, and impaired fine motor control.[7] Dysphagia, dysarthria, and dysphonia may result from brain stem LMN involvement or from dysfunction of UMNs descending to the brain stem. Manifestations of LMN lesions include fasciculations, weakness, muscle atrophy, and hyporeflexia.[7] Muscle cramps involving the distal legs often are an early symptom. The most common clinical presentation is slowly progressive weakness and atrophy in distal muscles of one upper extremity, followed by regional spread of clinical weakness. Eventually, UMNs and LMNs involving multiple limbs and the head are affected. In more advanced stages, muscles of the palate, pharynx, tongue, neck, and shoulders are involved, causing impairment of chewing, swallowing, and speech. Dysphagia with recurrent aspiration and weakness of the respiratory muscles produces the most significant acute complications of the disease. Death usually results from involvement of cranial nerves and respiratory musculature.

Treatment

Currently, there is no cure for ALS. Management is challenging and requires a multidisciplinary team. Management of symptoms, nutritional status, and respiratory muscle weakness allow people with ALS to live longer. Riluzole decreases glutamate accumulation and prolongs survival.[26] Clinical trials focus on exercise programs, nutritional interventions, transplanted stem cells, and antisense therapy.[26]

Multiple Sclerosis

MS is the inflammation and destruction of mostly the CNS myelin.[16,27] The peripheral nervous system is spared, and there is usually no evidence of an associated systemic disease. MS affects 400,000 people in the United States.[28] Age of onset is between 20 and 30 years, with females affected twice as frequently as males.[15] MS results in significant functional disability.

Etiology

MS occurs more commonly in people of Northern European ancestry and is uncommon in Asia, Africa, and northern South America.[28] MS is more common in northern latitudes, perhaps due to the selective migration of people with a susceptible genetic background to these regions.[28]

A person with MS has a 10% to 20% chance of having a family member with MS.[28] The risk without any family history is 1/1000.[7] People with the human leukocyte antigen HLA-DR2 haplotype are at higher risk for MS.[29]

Pathogenesis

MS is likely an immune-mediated disorder occurring in genetically susceptible people. The target antigen has not been identified, but data suggest an immune response to a CNS protein.

MS lesions consist of hard, sharp-edged, demyelinated patches that are visible throughout the white matter and occasionally in the gray matter of the CNS[7] (Fig. 15-13). These lesions, which represent the result of acute myelin breakdown, are called *plaques*. Plaques have a predilection for optic nerves, periventricular white matter, brain stem, cerebellum, and spinal cord white matter.[7] In an active plaque, there is evidence of ongoing myelin breakdown. The lesions contain small amounts of myelin basic proteins and increased amounts of proteolytic enzymes, macrophages, lymphocytes, and plasma cells.

Oligodendrocytes are decreased in number and may be absent, especially in older lesions. Acute, subacute, and chronic lesions often are seen at multiple sites throughout the CNS.

MRI has shown that the lesions of MS may occur in two stages:

1. A first stage that involves the sequential development of small inflammatory lesions
2. A second stage during which the lesions extend and consolidate and when demyelination and gliosis (scar formation) occur

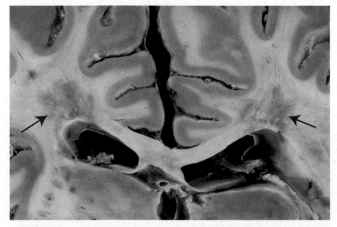

FIGURE 15-13. Multiple sclerosis. This fresh coronal section shows darker hues of the somewhat irregular periventricular plaques (*arrows*) reflecting the loss of myelin, which imparts the normal glistening white appearance of white matter. (From Strayer D. S., Rubin E., Saffitz J. E., et al. (Eds.). (2015). *Rubin's pathology: Clinicopathologic foundations of medicine* (7th ed., Chapter 32). Philadelphia, PA: Lippincott Williams & Wilkins.)

It is not known whether the inflammatory process, present during the first stage, is directed against myelin or against the oligodendrocytes that produce myelin.

Clinical Manifestations and Course

MS pathophysiology involves the demyelination of nerve fibers in the white matter of the brain, spinal cord, and optic nerve. CNS myelin is formed by oligodendrocytes, chiefly those lying among the nerve fibers. The properties of the myelin sheath—high electrical resistance and low capacitance—permit it to function as an electrical insulator. Demyelinated nerve fibers display conduction abnormalities ranging from decreased velocity to conduction blocks. The interruption of neural conduction in demyelinated nerves is manifested by symptoms that depend on the location and extent of the lesion. Areas commonly affected by MS are the optic nerve (visual field), corticobulbar tracts (speech, swallowing), corticospinal tracts (muscle strength), cerebellar tracts (gait, coordination), spinocerebellar tracts (balance), medial longitudinal fasciculus (conjugate gaze function), and posterior cell columns of the spinal cord (position, vibratory sensation). Typically, an otherwise healthy person presents with an acute or subacute episode of paresthesias, optic neuritis, diplopia, or specific types of gaze paralysis.

Paresthesias are evidenced as numbness, tingling, burning sensations, or pressure on the face or extremities, with symptoms ranging from annoying to severe. Pain from spasticity may be alleviated by certain stretching exercises. Other common symptoms are abnormal gait, bladder and sexual dysfunction, vertigo, nystagmus, fatigue, and speech disturbance. These usually last for days to weeks and completely or partially resolve. After a period of relatively normal function, new symptoms appear. Psychological manifestations, such as mood swings, may represent an emotional reaction to the disease or involvement of the cerebral cortex white matter. Depression, euphoria, inattentiveness, apathy, forgetfulness, and loss of memory may occur. Fatigue is a common problem and is a generalized low-energy feeling not related to depression and different from weakness. Fatigue has a harmful impact on activities of daily living and sustained physical activity. Interventions such as spacing activities and setting priorities often are helpful.

The course of the disease may fall into one of four categories. The *relapsing–remitting* form of the disease is characterized by episodes of acute worsening with recovery and a stable course between relapses. *Secondary progressive disease* involves gradual neurologic deterioration with or without superimposed acute relapses in a person with previous relapsing–remitting disease. *Primary progressive disease* is characterized by nearly continuous neurologic deterioration from onset of symptoms. The *progressive relapsing* category of disease involves gradual neurologic deterioration from the onset of symptoms but with subsequent superimposed relapses.[7,15]

Diagnosis

MS diagnosis is based on established clinical and laboratory criteria. There is no one definitive diagnostic test.

A definite diagnosis of MS requires evidence of one of the following patterns:

- Two or more episodes of exacerbation separated by 1 month or more and lasting more than 24 hours, with subsequent recovery
- A clinical history of clearly defined exacerbations and remissions, with or without complete recovery, followed by progression of symptoms over a period of at least 6 months
- Slow and stepwise progression of signs and symptoms over a period of at least 6 months[15]

Primary progressive MS may be suggested by a progressive course that lasts over 6 months. A person who has not had a relapse or progression of symptoms is described as having stable MS.

MRI studies can detect lesions and measure size when CT scans appear normal. Many new areas of myelin abnormality are asymptomatic. Serial MRI studies can be done to detect asymptomatic lesions, monitor existing lesions, and evaluate the effectiveness of treatment. Although MRI can provide evidence of disseminated lesions, normal findings do not exclude the diagnosis. Electrophysiologic evaluations and CT scans may assist in identifying and documenting lesions.

A large percentage of people with MS have elevated immunoglobulin G (IgG) levels in the cerebrospinal fluid (CSF), and some have oligoclonal patterns even with normal IgG levels. Total protein or lymphocyte levels may be mildly elevated in the CSF. These test results can be altered in a variety of inflammatory neurologic disorders and are not specific for MS.

Treatment

Most treatment measures for MS are directed at modifying the course and managing the primary symptoms. People who are minimally affected by the disorder require no specific treatment and are encouraged to maintain a healthy lifestyle, including good nutrition and adequate rest and relaxation. Physical therapy may help maintain muscle tone. Excessive fatigue, physical deterioration, emotional stress, viral infections, and extremes of environmental temperature may precipitate an exacerbation of the disease and must be avoided.

Pharmacologic agents used for MS management fall into three categories: (1) those used to treat acute attacks or initial demyelinating episodes, (2) those used to modify the course of the disease, and (3) those used to treat symptoms of the disorder.

Corticosteroids are the main treatment for acute attacks of MS. They are thought to reduce the inflammation, improve nerve conduction, and have immunologic effects. Long-term administration does not appear to alter the disease course and can have harmful side effects. Plasmapheresis and intravenous immunoglobulin have also proven beneficial in some cases.

Agents used to modify the course of the disease include interferon beta, glatiramer acetate, and mitoxantrone that have shown some benefit in reducing exacerbations in people with relapsing–remitting MS. Interferon beta is a cytokine that acts as an immune enhancer. It is injected

and is usually well tolerated. The most common side effects are flulike symptoms for 24 to 48 hours after each injection, which usually subside after 2 to 3 months of treatment. Glatiramer acetate is a synthetic polypeptide that simulates parts of the myelin basic protein. It seems to block myelin-damaging T cells by acting as a myelin decoy. The drug is injected daily subcutaneously.[16]

Mitoxantrone is an antineoplastic agent that prevents the ligation of DNA strands and thus delays the cell cycle progression and has immunomodulatory properties. Acute drug side effects include nausea and alopecia. A humanized monoclonal antibody that suppresses leukocyte entry into the CNS, natalizumab, is approved for relapsing–remitting MS.[25]

Medications for managing the chronic problems associated with MS are dantrolene, baclofen, or diazepam for spasticity; cholinergic drugs for bladder problems; and antidepressant drugs for depression. A high-fiber diet is recommended to ameliorate constipation.

Vertebral and Spinal Cord Injury

SCI is damage to the neural elements of the spinal cord. Most SCI occur in the 29- to 42-year age group.[30] In the United States, there are 282,000 people with SCI.[30] The most common cause is motor vehicle crash, followed by falls, violence (primarily gunshot wounds), and recreational sporting activities.[30] Life expectancy for people with SCI continues to increase, but is below life expectancy for those without SCI. Mortality rates are significantly higher during the first year after injury, particularly for people who are severely injured.[30]

Most SCIs involve damage to the vertebral column or supporting ligaments and to the spinal cord. Because of extensive tract systems that connect sensory afferent neurons and LMNs with high brain centers, SCIs commonly involve both sensory and motor function. Although this section focuses on traumatic SCI, much of the content is applicable to SCI caused by other disorders.

Injury to the Vertebral Column

Injuries to the vertebral column include fractures, dislocations, and **subluxations**. A fracture can occur at any part of the bony vertebrae, causing fragmentation of bone. It most often involves the pedicle, lamina, or facets. Dislocation or subluxation injury displaces vertebral bodies, with one overriding another and misalignment of the vertebral column. Damage to the ligaments or bony vertebrae may make the spine unstable. In an unstable spine, unguarded movement of the spinal column can impinge on the spinal canal, causing compression or overstretching of neural tissue.

Most SCI injuries occur due to writhing movements and a compressive force. Flexion injuries occur when forward bending of the spinal column exceeds normal movement limits. Typical flexion injuries result when the head is struck from behind. Extension injuries occur with excessive forced bending of the spine backward. A typical extension injury involves a fall in which the chin or face is the point of impact, causing hyperextension of the neck.

Concept Mastery Alert

Injuries of flexion and extension occur more commonly in the cervical spine (C4 to C6) than in any other area. Limitations imposed by the ribs, spinous processes, and joint capsules in the thoracic and lumbar spine make this area less flexible and less susceptible to flexion and extension injuries than the cervical spine.

A compression injury, causing the vertebral bones to shatter, squash, or even burst, occurs when there is spinal loading from a high-velocity blow to the top of the head, such as a diving injury (Fig. 15-14A). Compression injuries may occur when the vertebrae are weakened by conditions such as osteoporosis and bone metastasis. Axial rotation injuries can produce highly unstable injuries. Maximal axial rotation occurs in the cervical region, especially between C1 and C2, and at the lumbosacral joint (Fig. 15-14B). Coupling of vertebral motions is common in injury when two or more individual motions occur (*e.g.*, lateral bending and axial rotation).

Acute Spinal Cord Injury

SCI involves damage to the neural elements of the spinal cord, which may result from direct trauma from penetrating wounds or indirect injury resulting from vertebral fractures, fracture–dislocations, or subluxations of the spine. The spinal cord may be contused at and around the site of injury, causing it to swell. Loss of blood flow to the cord may result in infarction.

Sudden, complete transection of the spinal cord results in complete loss of motor, sensory, reflex, and autonomic function below the level of injury (*spinal shock*). It is characterized by flaccid paralysis with loss of tendon reflexes and absence of somatic and visceral sensations below the level of injury, and loss of bowel and bladder function. Loss of systemic sympathetic vasomotor tone may result in vasodilation, increased venous capacity, and hypotension. These occur regardless of whether the level of the lesion will produce spastic (UMN) or flaccid (LMN) paralysis. Spinal shock may last for hours to weeks. If reflex function returns by the time the person reaches the hospital, the neuromuscular changes are likely reversible. In people in whom the loss of reflexes persists, hypotension and bradycardia may become critical but manageable problems. In general, the higher the level of injury (*i.e.*, T6 and above), the greater is the effect.

Pathophysiology

The pathophysiology of acute SCI can be divided into two types: primary and secondary.[2] *Primary neurologic injury* occurs at the time of injury and is irreversible. It is characterized by small hemorrhages in the gray matter, followed by edematous changes in the white matter that lead to necrosis of neural tissue. This injury results from the forces of compression, stretch, and shear associated with fracture or compression of the spinal vertebrae, dislocation of vertebrae, and **contusions**. Penetrating injuries produce lacerations and direct trauma to the cord and may occur with or without spinal column damage. Lacerations occur when there is cutting or tearing of the spinal cord, which injures nerve tissue and causes bleeding and edema.

Secondary injuries follow the primary injury and promote the spread of injury. Vascular lesions can lead to ischemia, increased vascular permeability, and edema. Blood flow may be further compromised by spinal shock that results from a loss of vasomotor tone and neural reflexes below the level of injury. The release of vasoactive substances from the wound tissue causes vasospasm and impedes blood flow in the microcirculation, producing further necrosis of blood vessels and neurons. The release of proteolytic and lipolytic enzymes from injured cells causes delayed swelling, demyelination, and necrosis in the neural tissue in the spinal cord.

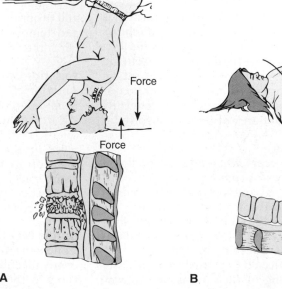

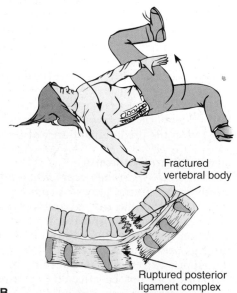

FIGURE 15-14. **(A)** Compression vertebral fracture secondary to axial loading as occurs when a person falls from a height and lands on the buttocks. **(B)** Rotational injury, in which there is concurrent fracture and tearing of the posterior ligamentous complex, is caused by extreme lateral flexion or twisting of the head or neck. (From Morton P. G., Fontaine D. K. (2018). *Critical care nursing: A holistic approach* (11th ed., p. 941). Philadelphia, PA: Lippincott Williams & Wilkins.)

A   B

Treatment

Management of acute SCI aims to reduce the neurologic deficit and prevent additional loss of function. Most traumatic injuries to the spinal column mandate measures such as immobilization or limiting the movement of people at risk for, or with known, SCI. People with multiple trauma or head injury are automatically treated for a cervical cord injury until ruled out with imaging.

In unstable injuries of the cervical spine, cervical traction improves or restores spinal alignment, decompresses neural structures, and facilitates recovery. Fractures and dislocations of thoracic and lumbar vertebrae may be stabilized by restricting the person to bed rest. Gunshot or stab wounds of the spinal column may not produce instability and may not require immobilization.

The goal of early surgical intervention for an unstable spine is to provide internal skeletal stabilization so that early mobilization and rehabilitation can occur. One of the more important aspects of early SCI care is the prevention and treatment of spinal or systemic shock and the hypoxia associated with compromised respiration. The cord must be perfused to prevent hypoxia.

Types and Classification of Spinal Cord Injury

Alterations in body function that result from SCI depend on the level of injury and the amount of cord involvement. *Tetraplegia*, sometimes referred to as *quadriplegia*, is the impairment or loss of motor and/or sensory function after damage to neural structures in the cervical segments of the spinal cord.[31] It results in impairment of function in the arms, trunk, legs, and pelvic organs. *Paraplegia* refers to impairment or loss of motor and/or sensory function in the thoracic, lumbar, or sacral segments of the spinal cord from damage of neural elements in the spinal canal. Arm functioning is spared, but depending on the level of injury, functioning of the trunk, legs, and pelvic organs may be impaired. Paraplegia includes conus medullaris and cauda equina injuries.

Complete cord injuries can result from severance of the cord, disruption of nerve fibers, or interruption of blood supply to that segment, resulting in complete destruction of neural tissue and UMN or LMN paralysis. With complete injuries, no motor or sensory function is preserved in segments S4 to S6. *Incomplete cord injuries* imply residual motor or sensory function below the level of injury. The prognosis for return of function is better in an incomplete injury because of preservation of axonal function. Incomplete injuries can be organized into certain patterns or *syndromes* that occur more frequently and reflect the predominant area of the cord involved.

Central Cord Syndrome

Central cord syndrome occurs when injury is predominantly in the central gray or white matter of the cord[33] (Fig. 15-15). Some axonal transmission may remain intact because corticospinal tract fibers controlling the arms are located more centrally and fibers controlling the legs are located more laterally. Motor function of the upper extremities is affected, but the lower extremities may not be affected (or affected to a lesser degree) with some sparing of sacral sensation. Bowel, bladder, and sexual functions usually are affected and

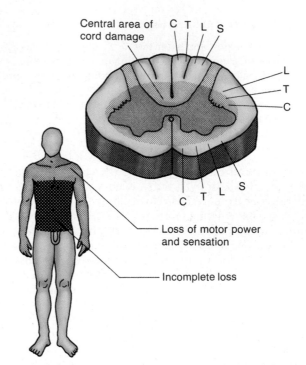

FIGURE 15-15. Central cord syndrome. A cross-section of the cord shows central damage and the associated motor and sensory loss (C, cervical; L, lumbar; S, sacral; T, thoracic.) (From Hickey J. V. (2014). *The clinical practice of neurological and neurosurgical nursing* (7th ed., first figure in Chart 17-2, p. 398). Philadelphia, PA: Lippincott Williams & Wilkins.)

may parallel the degree of lower extremity involvement. This syndrome occurs almost exclusively in the cervical cord (UMN lesion with spastic paralysis). Central cord damage is frequent in older adults with narrowing or stenotic changes in the spinal canal related to arthritis. Damage also may occur with congenital stenosis.

Brown–Séquard Syndrome

A condition called *Brown–Séquard syndrome* results from damage to a hemisection of the anterior and posterior cord[33] (Fig. 15-16). The effect is an ipsilateral loss of voluntary motor function from the corticospinal tract and proprioception loss with a contralateral loss of pain and temperature sensation from the lateral spinothalamic tracts for all levels below the lesion.

Anterior Cord Syndrome

Anterior cord syndrome usually is caused by damage from infarction of the anterior spinal artery, resulting in damage to the anterior two thirds of the cord[1] (Fig. 15-17). Deficits include loss of motor function provided by the corticospinal tracts and loss of pain and temperature sensation provided by the lateral spinothalamic tracts. The posterior third of the cord is mostly unaffected, preserving the dorsal column axons that convey position, vibration, and touch sensation.

Conus Medullaris and Cauda Equina Syndromes

Conus medullaris syndrome involves damage to the conus medullaris or the sacral cord and lumbar nerve roots in the neural canal. Functional deficits result in flaccid bowel and bladder and altered sexual function.

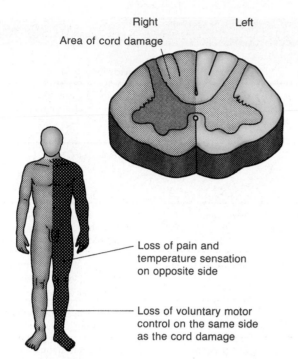

Right　　　　Left

Area of cord damage

Loss of pain and temperature sensation on opposite side

Loss of voluntary motor control on the same side as the cord damage

FIGURE 15-16. Brown–Séquard syndrome. Cord damage and associated motor and sensory loss are illustrated. (From Hickey J. V. (2014). *The clinical practice of neurological and neurosurgical nursing* (7th ed., third figure in Chart 17-2, p. 399). Philadelphia, PA: Lippincott Williams & Wilkins.)

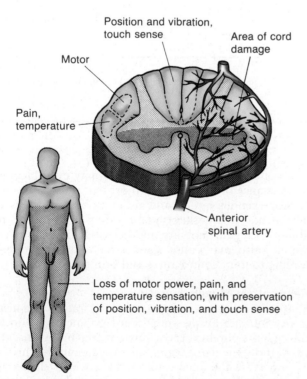

Position and vibration, touch sense

Motor

Area of cord damage

Pain, temperature

Anterior spinal artery

Loss of motor power, pain, and temperature sensation, with preservation of position, vibration, and touch sense

FIGURE 15-17. Anterior cord syndrome. Cord damage and associated motor and sensory loss are illustrated. (From Hickey J. V. (2014). *The clinical practice of neurological and neurosurgical nursing* (7th ed., second figure in Chart 17-2, p. 398). Philadelphia, PA: Lippincott Williams & Wilkins.)

Sacral segments occasionally show preserved reflexes if only the conus is affected. Motor function in the legs and feet may be impaired without significant sensory impairment. Cauda equina syndrome occurs when damage to the lumbosacral nerve roots in the spinal canal results in LMN and sensory neuron damage. Functional deficits present as patterns of asymmetric flaccid paralysis, sensory impairment, and severe, asymmetric pain. Emergent surgery is indicated for cauda equina syndrome.

Disruption of Somatosensory and Skeletal Muscle Function

Functional abilities after SCI are subject to degrees of somatosensory and skeletal muscle function loss and altered reflex activity based on level injury and extent of damage (Table 15-2).

Motor and Somatosensory Function

Motor function in cervical injuries ranges from complete dependence to independence with or without assistive devices. The functional levels of cervical injury are related to C5, C6, C7, or C8 innervation. At the C5 level, deltoid and biceps function is spared, allowing full head, neck, and diaphragm control with good shoulder strength and elbow flexion. At the C6 level, wrist dorsiflexion by the wrist extensors is functional, allowing tenodesis (natural bending and flexion of fingers when the wrist is extended and bent backward). Tenodesis can be used to pick up objects when finger movement is absent. A functional C7 injury allows full elbow flexion and extension, wrist plantar flexion, and some finger control. At the C8 level, finger flexion is added.

T1 and T12 injuries allow full upper extremity control with limited to full control of intercostal and trunk muscles and balance. Injury at the T1 level allows full fine motor control of the fingers. The level of injury usually is determined by sensory level testing.

Functional capacity in the L1 through L5 nerve innervations allows hip flexion, hip abduction (L1 to L3), knees movement (L2 to L5), and ankle dorsiflexion (L4 to L5). Sacral (S1 to S5) innervation allows for full leg, foot, and ankle control and innervation of perineal musculature for bowel, bladder, and sexual functions.

Reflex Activity

Spinal cord reflexes are fully integrated in the spinal cord and can function independent of input from higher centers. Altered spinal reflex activity after SCI is determined by the level of injury and whether UMNs or LMNs are affected. With UMN injuries at T12 and above, the cord reflexes remain intact, but communication pathways with higher centers are interrupted. This results in spasticity of involved skeletal muscle groups and of smooth and skeletal muscles that control bowel, bladder, and sexual functions. In LMN injuries at T12 or below, the reflex circuitry has been damaged at the level of the spinal cord or spinal nerve, resulting in decreased or absent reflex function. LMN injuries cause flaccid paralysis of involved skeletal muscle groups and the smooth and skeletal muscles that control bowel, bladder, and sexual functions. However, injuries near the T12 level may result in mixed UMN and LMN deficits.

TABLE 15-2 Functional Abilities by Level of Cord Injury

Injury Level	Segmental Sensorimotor Function	Dressing, Eating	Elimination	Mobility*
C1	Little or no sensation or control of head and neck; no diaphragm control; requires continuous ventilation	Dependent	Dependent	Limited. Voice-controlled or sip-n-puff electric wheelchair
C2–C3	Head and neck sensation; some neck control; independent of mechanical ventilation for short periods	Dependent	Dependent	Same as for C1
C4	Good head and neck sensation and motor control; some shoulder elevation; diaphragm movement	Dependent; may be able to eat with adaptive sling	Dependent	Limited to voice-, mouth-, head-, chin-, or shoulder-controlled electric wheelchair
C5	Full head and neck control; shoulder strength; elbow flexion	Independent with assistance	Maximal assistance	Electric or modified manual wheelchair; needs transfer assistance
C6	Fully innervated shoulder; wrist extension or dorsiflexion	Independent or with minimal assistance	Independent or with minimal assistance	Independent in transfers and wheelchair
C7–C8	Full elbow extension; wrist plantar flexion; some finger control	Independent	Independent	Independent; manual wheelchair
T1–T5	Full hand and finger control; use of intercostal and thoracic muscles	Independent	Independent	Independent; manual wheelchair
T6–T10	Abdominal muscle control; partial to good balance with trunk muscles	Independent	Independent	Independent; manual wheelchair
T11–L5	Hip flexors, hip abductors (L1–L3), knee extension (L2–L4), knee flexion, and ankle dorsiflexion (L4–L5)	Independent	Independent	Short distance to full ambulation with assistance
S1–S5	Full leg, foot, and ankle control; innervation of perineal muscles for bowel, bladder, and sexual functions (S2–S4)	Independent	Normal to impaired bowel and bladder function	Ambulate independently with or without assistance

Assistance refers to adaptive.

After the period of spinal shock in an UMN injury, isolated spinal reflex activity and muscle tone that are not under the control of higher centers return. This may result in hypertonia and spasticity of skeletal muscles below the level of injury.[33] The antigravity muscles, the flexors of the arms and extensors of the legs, are predominantly affected. The stimuli for reflex muscle spasm arise from somatic and visceral afferent pathways that enter the cord below the level of injury. Common stimuli are muscle stretching, bladder infections or stones, fistulas, bowel distention or impaction, pressure areas or irritation of the skin, and infections. Because stimuli that precipitate spasms vary from person to person, careful assessment is necessary to identify the factors that precipitate spasm. Passive range-of-motion exercises to stretch the spastic muscles help to prevent spasm induced by muscle stretching, such as occurs with a change in body position.

Spasticity is not detrimental and may even facilitate maintenance of muscle tone to prevent muscle wasting, improve venous return, and aid in mobility. Spasms are detrimental when they impair safety and reduce the ability to regain mobility and activities of daily living. Spasms also may cause trauma to bones and tissues, leading to joint contractures and skin breakdown.

Respiratory Muscle Function

Ventilation requires innervation of expiratory and inspiratory muscles by the spinal cord. Segments C3 to C5 through the phrenic nerves innervate the main muscle of ventilation, the diaphragm. Spinal segments T1 through T7 innervate the intercostal muscles, which elevate the rib cage and are needed for coughing and deep breathing. The major muscles of expiration are the abdominal muscles, which receive their innervation from levels T6 to T12.

Although the ability to inhale and exhale may be preserved, functional deficits in ventilation are most apparent in the ability to oxygenate tissues, eliminate carbon dioxide, and mobilize secretions. Cord injuries involving C1 to C3 result in a lack of respiratory effort, and people who are affected require assisted ventilation. Although a C3 to C5 injury allows partial or full diaphragmatic function, ventilation is diminished because of loss of intercostal muscle function, resulting in shallow breaths and a weak cough. Below the C5 level, the ability to take a deep breath and cough is less impaired. Maintenance therapy consists of muscle training to strengthen muscles for endurance and mobilization of secretions. Speaking is compromised with assisted ventilation and ensuring adequate communication of needs is essential.

Disruption of Autonomic Nervous System Function

If there is an SCI, all autonomic nerve function below the injury site will be stopped. Because of their sites of exit, the cranial nerves are unaffected. Depending on the level of injury, the spinal reflexes that control autonomic nervous system function are isolated from the rest of the CNS. Afferent sensory input and efferent motor output are unaffected. Lacking are the regulation and integration of reflex function by centers in the brain and brain stem. This results in autonomic reflexes that are uncontrolled below but relatively controlled above the level of injury.

The higher the level of injury and the greater the surface area affected, the more profound the effects on circulation and thermoregulation. People with injury at or above the T6 level experience problems in regulating vasomotor tone. Those with injuries below T6 usually have sufficient sympathetic function to maintain adequate vasomotor function. The level of injury and corresponding problems vary among people, and some dysfunctions may be seen at levels below T6. With lower lumbar and sacral injuries, sympathetic function remains essentially unaltered.

Vasovagal Response
The vagus nerve (cranial nerve X), which is unaffected in SCI, normally exerts a continuous inhibitory effect on heart rate. Vagal stimulation that causes a marked bradycardia is called the *vasovagal response*. Visceral afferent input to the vagal centers in the brain stem of people with tetraplegia or high-level paraplegia can produce marked bradycardia when unchecked by a dysfunctional sympathetic nervous system. Severe bradycardia and even asystole can result when deep endotracheal suctioning or rapid position change elicits the vasovagal response. Preventive measures, such as hyperoxygenation before, during, and after suctioning, are advised. Rapid position changes should be avoided or anticipated, and anticholinergic drugs should be immediately available to counteract severe episodes of bradycardia.

Autonomic Dysreflexia
Autonomic dysreflexia, also known as *autonomic hyperreflexia*, represents an acute episode of exaggerated sympathetic reflex responses in people with injuries at T6 and above, in which CNS control of spinal reflexes is lost (Fig. 15-18). It does not occur until spinal shock has resolved and autonomic reflexes return, most often within the first 6 months after injury. It is most unpredictable during the first year after injury, but can occur throughout the person's lifetime.

Autonomic dysreflexia is characterized by mild to severe hypertension, skin pallor, and the piloerector response. Because baroreceptor function and parasympathetic control of heart rate travel by way of the cranial nerves, these responses remain intact. Continued hypertension produces a baroreflex-mediated vagal slowing of the heart rate to bradycardic levels. There is an accompanying baroreflex-mediated vasodilation, with flushed skin and profuse sweating above the level of injury, headache ranging from dull to severe, nasal stuffiness, and feelings of anxiety. A person may experience one, several, or all of the symptoms with each episode.

Stimuli initiating the dysreflexic response include visceral distention (full bladder or rectum), stimulation of pain receptors (pressure ulcers, ingrown toenails, dressing changes, and medical procedures), and visceral contractions (ejaculation, bladder spasms, or uterine contractions).

Autonomic dysreflexia is a clinical emergency: convulsions, loss of consciousness, and death can occur. Treatment includes monitoring blood pressure while correcting the initiating stimulus. The person should be placed upright and all support binders should be removed to promote venous pooling of blood and reduce venous return, thereby decreasing blood pressure. If the stimuli have been removed or cannot be identified and the upright position is established but the blood pressure remains elevated, drugs can block autonomic function. Prevention of stimuli that trigger dysreflexic events is advocated.

Postural Hypotension
Postural, or orthostatic, hypotension can occur with injuries at T4 to T6 and above and is due to the interruption of sympathetic outflow to blood vessels in the extremities and abdomen. Pooling of blood, along with gravitational forces, impairs venous return to the heart, and cardiac output is decreased when in an upright position. Signs of orthostatic hypotension include dizziness, pallor, excessive sweating above the level of the lesion, blurred vision, and possibly fainting. Postural hypotension is prevented by slow changes in position and measures to promote venous return.

Disruption of Bladder, Bowel, and Sexual Functions

Loss of bladder function results from disruption of neural pathways between the bladder and the reflex voiding center at the S2 to S4 level (*i.e.*, an LMN lesion) or between the reflex voiding center and higher brain centers for communication and coordinated sphincter control (*i.e.*, a UMN lesion). People with UMN lesions or spastic bladders lack awareness of bladder filling and voluntary control of voiding. In LMN lesions or flaccid bladder dysfunction, lack of awareness of filling and

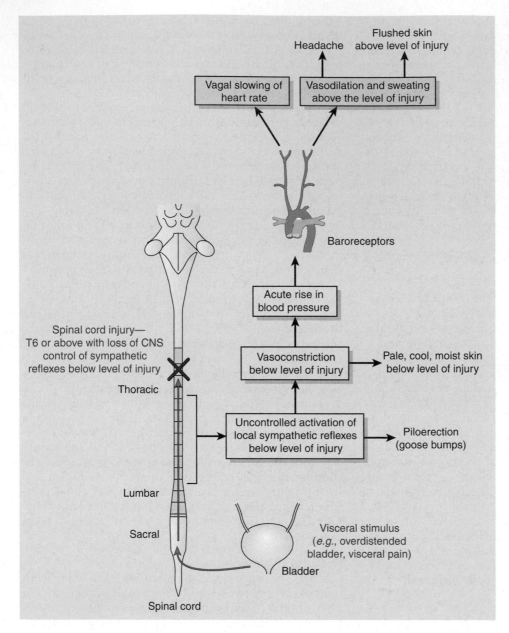

FIGURE 15-18. Mechanisms of autonomic dysreflexia.

lack of bladder tone render the person unable to void voluntarily or involuntarily.

Bowel elimination involves the enteric and autonomic nervous systems and the CNS. People with SCI above S2 to S4 develop spastic functioning of the **defecation** reflex and loss of voluntary control of the external anal sphincter. SCI at the S2 to S4 level causes flaccid functioning of the defecation reflex and loss of anal sphincter tone. While the enteric nervous system innervation, without the defecation reflex, peristaltic movements are ineffective in evacuating stool.

Sexual function is also mediated by the S2 to S4 segments. The genital sexual response in SCI (erection in males, vaginal lubrication in females) may be initiated by mental or touch stimuli, depending on the level of injury. The T11 to L2 cord segments are the psychogenic sexual response area where autonomic nerve pathways in communication with the forebrain leave the cord and innervate the genitalia. The S2 to S4 cord segments are the sexual-touch reflex center. In T10 or higher injuries, reflex sexual response to genital touch may occur but a sexual response to mental stimuli (T11 to L2) does not because spinal lesion blocks the pathway. In an injury at T12 or below, the sexual reflex center may be damaged, and there may be no response to touch.

In males, the lack of erectile ability or inability to experience penile sensations or orgasm is not a reliable indicator of fertility, which should be evaluated by an expert. In females, fertility is parallel to menses. Usually, it is delayed 3 to 5 months after injury.

Disruption of Other Functions

Temperature Regulation

The central mechanisms for thermoregulation are in the hypothalamus. In response to cold, the hypothalamus stimulates vasoconstrictor responses in peripheral blood vessels, particularly in the skin, decreasing loss of body heat. Heat production results from increased metabolism, voluntary activity or shivering. To reduce heat, hypothalamus-stimulated mechanisms produce vasodilation of skin blood vessels to dissipate heat and sweating to increase evaporative heat losses.

SCI disrupts communication between the thermoregulatory centers and the sympathetic effector responses below the level of injury. Higher levels of injury produce greater disturbances in thermoregulation. In tetraplegia and high paraplegia, there are few defenses against temperature changes, and body temperature tends to assume the temperature of the external environment, a condition known as *poikilothermy*. People with lower-level injuries have various degrees of thermoregulation. Disturbances in thermoregulation are chronic and may cause continual loss of body heat. Treatment consists of education in the adjustment of clothing and awareness of how environmental temperatures affect the person's ability to accommodate to these changes.

Deep Vein Thrombosis and Edema

People with SCI are at high risk for deep vein thrombosis (DVT) and pulmonary embolism. The high DVT risk in acute SCI is due to immobility, decreased vasomotor tone below the level of injury, and hypercoagulability and stasis of blood flow. Local pain is often absent due to sensory deficits. Thus, a regular schedule of visual inspection for local signs of DVT is important. Testing of people at high risk for DVT includes plethysmography and duplex ultrasonography.

Dependent edema is also common with SCI. Edema development is related to decreased peripheral vascular resistance, decreased muscle tone in the paralyzed limbs, and immobility that causes increased venous pressure and abnormal pooling of blood in the abdomen, lower limbs, and upper extremities. Positioning to minimize gravitational forces or by using compression devices that encourage venous return usually relieves edema in the dependent body parts.

Skin Integrity

The skin surface is innervated by nerves organized into dermatomes. The sympathetic nervous system, through control of vasomotor and sweat gland activity, provides adequate circulation, excretion of body fluids, and temperature regulation. The lack of sensory warning mechanisms and voluntary motor ability below the level of injury, coupled with circulatory changes, places a person with SCI at major risk for disruption of skin integrity. Significant factors associated with disruption of skin integrity are pressure, shearing forces, and localized trauma and irritation. Relieving pressure, allowing adequate circulation to the skin, and skin inspection are primary ways to maintain skin integrity. Skin breakdown is the most preventable of SCI complications.

Future Directions in Repair of the Injured Spinal Cord

Strategies for repairing an injured spinal cord focus on promoting regrowth of nerve tracts, using nerve growth–stimulating factors or molecules that suppress inhibitors of neuronal extension; bridging spinal cord lesions with scaffolds impregnated with nerve growth factors to promote axon growth and reduce barriers caused by scar tissue; repairing damaged myelin and restoring nerve conductivity in the lesion area; and promoting compensatory growth of spared, intact nerve fibers above and below the level of injury. Although these strategies may not allow for complete repair, even small successes may be useful for someone with SCI.

 SUMMARY CONCEPTS

ALS is a progressive, devastating disorder that selectively affects motor function. It affects LMNs in the spinal cord and UMNs in the brain stem and cerebral cortex. MS is a slowly progressive demyelinating disease of the CNS. The most common symptoms are paresthesias, optic neuritis, and motor weakness. The disease is usually characterized by exacerbations and remissions. Initially, near-normal function returns between exacerbations.

SCI is a disabling condition commonly caused by motor vehicle accidents, falls, and sports injuries. Dysfunctions of the nervous system after SCI comprise various degrees of sensorimotor loss and altered reflex activity based on the level of injury and extent of damage. The physical problems of SCI include spinal shock; ventilation and communication problems; autonomic nervous system dysfunction that predisposes to the vasovagal response, autonomic hyperreflexia, impaired body temperature regulation, and postural hypotension; impaired muscle pump and venous innervation leading to edema and risk for DVT; altered sensorimotor integrity that contributes to uncontrolled muscle spasms, altered pain responses, and threats to skin integrity; alterations in bowel and bladder elimination; and impaired sexual function.

Review Exercises

1. A 32-year-old woman presents with complaints of drooping eyelids, difficulty chewing and swallowing, and weakness of her arms and legs that is less severe in the morning but becomes worse as the day progresses. She complains that climbing stairs and lifting objects are becoming increasingly difficult. Clinical examination confirms weakness of the eyelid and jaw muscles. She is told that she may have myasthenia gravis and is scheduled for a blood test to assess for antibodies.

   A. Explain the pathogenesis of this woman's symptoms as it relates to myasthenia gravis.
   B. Explain how information from the antibody blood test can be used to assist in the diagnosis of the disorder.
   C. Explain the rationale for avoiding the use of aminoglycoside antibiotics for treatment of infections in this woman.

2. A 66-year-old man complains of right-hand tremor at rest that interferes with his various graphic design creations. He also complains of dragging his left leg when walking, being unsteady when turning, and a stooped over posture. Upon examination, he is found to also have mild rigidity in all limbs, flat facies, hypophonia, and impaired rapid alternating movements. Based on his clinical presentation, he is diagnosed with Parkinson disease.

   A. How would you go about helping him to outline the role of the cerebellum and basal ganglia in performing the motor movements associated with these maneuvers?

3. A 20-year-old man suffered an SCI at the C2 to C3 level as the result of a motorcycle accident.

   A. Explain the effects of this man's injury on ventilation and communication; sensorimotor function; autonomic nervous system function; bowel, bladder, and sexual functions; and temperature regulation.
   B. Autonomic dysreflexia, which is a threat to people with SCI at T6 or above, is manifested by hypertension, often to extreme levels, and bradycardia; constriction of skin vessels below the level of injury; and severe headache and nasal stuffiness. Explain the origin of the elevated blood pressure and bradycardia. The condition does not occur until after shock has resolved and usually occurs only in people with injuries at T6 and above. Explain.

REFERENCES

1. Patton K., Thibodeau G. (2016). *Anatomy & physiology* (9th ed., p. 333). Philadelphia, PA: Elsevier.
2. Hall J. E. (2016). *Guyton and Hall textbook of medical physiology* (13th ed.). Philadelphia, PA: Elsevier.
3. Penfield W., Rasmussen T. (1950). *The cerebral cortex of man.* New York, NY: Macmillan.
4. Tortora G., Derrickson B. (2017). *Principles of anatomy & physiology* (15th ed.). New York, NY: John Wiley.
5. Bickley L. S., Szilagyi P. G. (2013). *Bates' guide to physical examination and history taking* (11th ed., pp. 708–718). Philadelphia, PA: Lippincott Williams & Wilkins.
6. Anthony D. P., Anthony D. C. (2015). Peripheral nerve and skeletal muscle. In Kumar V., Abbas A. K., Fausto N. (Eds.), *Robbins and Cotran pathologic basis of disease* (9th ed., pp. 1227–1250). Philadelphia, PA: Elsevier.
7. Strayer D. S., Rubin E., Saffitz J. E., et al. (Eds.). (2015). *Rubin's pathology: Clinicopathologic foundations of medicine* (7th ed.). Philadelphia, PA: Lippincott Williams & Wilkins.
8. Malavaki C. J., Sakkas G. K., Mitrou G. I., et al. (2015). Skeletal muscle atrophy: Disease-induced mechanisms may mask disuse atrophy. *Journal of Muscle Research and Cell Motility* 36(6), 405–421.
9. Louis E., Mayer S. A., Rowland L. P. (Eds.). (2015). *Merritt's neurology.* Philadelphia, PA: Wolters Kluwer.
10. Katzung B., Trevor A. (2015). *Basic and clinical pharmacology* (13th ed.). New York, NY: Lange Medical Books/McGraw-Hill.
11. Rosow L. K., Strober J. B. (2015). Infantile botulism: Review and clinical update. *Pediatric Neurology* 52(5), 487–492.
12. King A. M., Aaron C. K. (2015). Organophosphate and carbamate poisoning. *Emergency Medicine Clinics of North America* 33, 133–151.
13. Cavalcante P., Galbardi B., Franzi S., et al. (2016). Increased expression of toll-like receptors 7 and 9 in myasthenia gravis thymus characterized by active Epstein-Barr virus infection. *Immunobiology* 221(4), 516–527.
14. Della Marina A., Trippe H., Lutz S., et al. (2014). Juvenile myasthenia gravis: Recommendations for diagnostic approaches and treatment. *Neuropediatrics* 45(2), 75–83.
15. Dunphy L. M., Windland-Brown J. E., Porter B. O., et al. (2015). *Primary care: The art and science of advanced practice nursing* (4th ed.). Philadelphia, PA: FA Davis.
16. Ansar V., Valadi N. (2015). Guillain-Barré syndrome. *Primary Care; Clinics in Office Practice* 42(2), 189–193.
17. Willison H. J., Jacobs B. C., van Doorn P. A. (2016). Guillain–Barré syndrome. *Lancet* 388, 717–727.
18. Maher C., Underwood M., Buchbinder R. (2017). Non-specific low back pain. *Lancet* 389, 736–747.
19. Bahouq H., Allali F., Rkain H., et al. (2013). Prevalence and severity of insomnia in chronic low back pain patients. *Rheumatology International* 33, 1277–1281.
20. Oaseem A., Wilt T. J., McLean R. M., et al. (2017). Noninvasive treatments for acute, subacute, and chronic low back pain: A clinical practice guideline from the American College of Physicians. *Annals of Internal Medicine* 166, 514–530.
21. Wilkins A. (2017). Cerebellar dysfunction in multiple sclerosis. *Frontiers in Neurology* 8, 1–6.
22. Sivaswamy L. (2014). Approach to acute ataxia in childhood: Diagnosis and evaluation. *Pediatric Annals* 43(4), 153–159.
23. Derkinderen P., Shannon K., Brundin P. (2014). Gut feelings about smoking and coffee in Parkinson's disease. *Movement Disorders* 29(18), 976–979.
24. Miller D. B., O'Callaghan J. P. (2015). Biomarkers of Parkinson's disease: Present and future. *Metabolism* 64(301), S40–S46.

25. Lehne R. A. (2013). *Pharmacology for nursing care* (8th ed.). Philadelphia, PA: Elsevier.
26. Gordon P. H. (2013). Amyotrophic lateral sclerosis: An update for 2013 clinical features, pathophysiology, management and therapeutic trials. *Aging and Disease* 4(5), 295–310.
27. Hickey J. V. (2014). *The clinical practice of neurological and neurosurgical nursing* (7th ed.). Philadelphia, PA: Wolters Kluwer.
28. Bader M. K., Littlejohns L. R., Olson D. M. (2016). *AANN core curriculum for neuroscience nursing.* Chicago, IL: AANN.
29. Sawcer S., Franklin R. J., Ban M. (2014). Multiple sclerosis genetics. *Lancet Neurology* 13, 700–709.
30. National Spinal Cord Injury Statistical Center. (2016). *Facts and figures at a glance.* Birmingham, AL: University of Alabama at Birmingham.
31. Hurlbert R. J., Hadley M. N., Walters B. C., et al. (2013). Pharmacological therapy for acute spinal cord injury. *Neurosurgery* 72(3), 93–105.
32. Bonner S., Smith C. (2013). Initial management of acute spinal cord injury. *Continuing Education in Anesthesia, Critical Care, & Pain* 13(6), 224–231.
33. Morton P. G., Fontaine D. K. (2018). *Critical care nursing: A holistic approach* (11th ed.). Philadelphia, PA: Lippincott Williams & Wilkins.

Disorders of Brain Function

Learning Objectives

After completing this chapter, the learner will be able to meet the following objectives:

1. Identify the levels of consciousness and their characteristics.
2. Describe the determinants of intracranial pressure (ICP) and compensatory mechanisms used to prevent ICP.
3. Discuss cytotoxic and vasogenic cerebral edema.
4. Describe the effects of primary and secondary brain injuries.
5. Summarize the different types of hematomas that can occur in the brain.
6. Identify focal versus diffuse brain injuries.
7. Identify the major vessels in the cerebral circulation.
8. Describe the autoregulation of cerebral blood flow.
9. Summarize the pathologies of ischemic and hemorrhagic stroke.
10. Discuss the assessment and management of meningitis.
11. Describe the symptoms of encephalitis.
12. Identify the classification of major brain tumors.
13. Describe the general clinical manifestations of brain tumors.
14. Discuss the causes of seizures.
15. Describe the origin of seizure activity in focal and generalized seizures and compare the manifestations of a focal seizure with generalized seizure.

The brain is susceptible to injury by trauma, ischemia, tumors, degenerative processes, and metabolic derangements. Brain injuries can be categorized as traumatic or nontraumatic and can cause changes in consciousness, cognition, motor, and sensory function. Brain damage can result from the ischemia, excitatory amino acids, edema, and increased intracranial pressure (ICP).

Manifestations and Mechanisms of Brain Injury

The brain is protected from external forces by the rigid skull and the cushioning cerebrospinal fluid (CSF). Metabolic stability is maintained by regulatory mechanisms including the blood–brain barrier and autoregulatory mechanisms for its blood supply. The brain remains vulnerable to injury by trauma, ischemia, tumors, degenerative processes, and metabolic derangements.

Manifestations of Brain Injury

Brain injury is manifested by changes in the level of consciousness and alterations in cognitive, motor, and sensory function. Focal brain injury causes focal neurologic deficits that may or may not alter consciousness. Global brain injury usually results in altered levels of consciousness, ranging from inattention to stupor or coma.

The cerebral hemispheres are the most susceptible to damage. As structures in the diencephalon, midbrain, pons, and medulla are affected, signs related to pupillary and eye movement reflexes, motor function, and respiration become evident (Table 16-1). Hemodynamic and respiratory instability are the last signs to occur because their regulatory centers are low in the medulla.

With progressive neurologic deterioration, the person's neurologic capabilities deteriorate in a stepwise fashion.

Similarly, as neurologic function returns, there appears to be a stepwise progress to higher levels of consciousness. Deterioration of brain function from supratentorial lesions follows a rostral-to-caudal stepwise progression, because the brain initially compensates for injury and then decompensates with loss of autoregulation and cerebral perfusion. Infratentorial (brain stem) lesions may lead to an early, sometimes abrupt disturbance in consciousness without orderly rostrocaudal progression of neurologic signs.

Altered Levels of Consciousness

Brain injury and disease can lead to altered levels of consciousness. Consciousness is the state of awareness of self and environment and of being able to orient to new stimuli.[1] It is divided into (1) arousal and wakefulness and (2) content and cognition.[2] Arousal and wakefulness require function of both cerebral hemispheres and an intact reticular activating system (RAS). The content and cognition aspects of consciousness are determined by a functioning cerebral cortex.

Anatomic and Physiologic Basis of Consciousness

The reticular formation constitutes the central core of the brain stem, extending from the medulla through the pons to the midbrain, that is continuous caudally with the spinal cord and rostrally with the subthalamus, the hypothalamus, and the thalamus (Fig. 16-1).[2] Fibers from the RAS also project to the autonomic nervous system and motor systems. The hypothalamus plays a predominant role in maintaining homeostasis through integration of somatic, visceral, and endocrine functions. Inputs from the reticular formation, vestibulospinal projections, and other motor systems are integrated to provide a continuously adapting background of muscle tone and posture to facilitate voluntary motor actions. Reticular formation neurons that function in the regulation of cardiovascular, respiratory, and other visceral

TABLE 16-1 Key Signs in Rostral-to-Caudal Progression of Brain Lesions	
Level of Brain Injury	**Key Clinical Signs**
Diencephalon	Impaired consciousness; small, reactive pupils; intact oculocephalic response; abnormal flexion posturing; Cheyne–Stokes respirations
Midbrain	Coma; fixed, midsize pupils; impaired oculocephalic response; central neurogenic hyperventilation; extension posturing
Pons	Coma; fixed, miotic (small) pupils; dysconjugate gaze; impaired oculovestibular response; loss of corneal reflex; hemiparesis/quadriparesis; extension posturing; apneustic respirations
Medulla	Coma, fixed pupils, flaccidity, loss of gag and cough reflexes, ataxic/apneic respirations

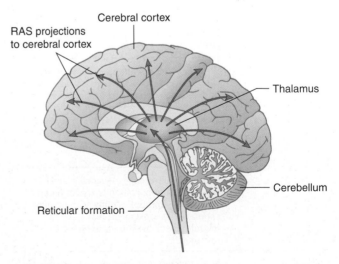

FIGURE 16-1. The brain stem reticular formation and reticular activating system (RAS). Ascending sensory tracts send axon collateral fibers to the reticular formation. These give rise to fibers synapsing in the nonspecific nuclei of the thalamus. From there, the nonspecific thalamic projections influence widespread areas of the cerebral cortex and limbic system.

functions are intermingled with those that maintain other reticular formation functions.

The ascending RAS transmits activating information to the cerebral cortex. It activates the hypothalamic and limbic structures that regulate emotional and behavioral responses, and exerts facilitatory effects on cortical neurons. Without cortical activation, a person is less reactive to environmental stimuli, and the level of consciousness is reduced.

The pathways for the ascending RAS travel from the medulla through the midbrain, and lesions of the brain stem can interrupt RAS activity, leading to altered levels of consciousness and coma. Any deficit in the level of consciousness indicates direct injury either to the RAS or to both cerebral hemispheres concurrently. Brain injuries that affect a hemisphere unilaterally and spare the RAS, such as cerebral infarction, usually do not cause impaired consciousness.

Levels of Consciousness

A person who is fully conscious is totally aware of her or his surroundings and is able to react to stimuli in the environment.[1] Levels of consciousness exist on a continuum that includes consciousness, confusion, lethargy, obtundation, stupor, and coma (Table 16-2).

Early signs of reduced consciousness are inattention, mild confusion, disorientation, and blunted responsiveness. The person experiencing delirium becomes inattentive and lethargic or agitated. They may progress to

TABLE 16-2 Descending Levels of Consciousness and Their Characteristics

Level of Consciousness	Characteristics
Full consciousness	Awake, alert, and oriented to time, place, and person; comprehends spoken and written word and is able to express ideas
Confusion	Disoriented to time, place, or person; memory difficulty; difficulty following commands
Lethargy	Oriented to time, place, and person; very slow in mental processes, motor activity, and speech; responds to pain appropriately
Obtundation	Responds verbally with a word; arousable with stimulation; responds appropriately to painful stimuli; follows simple commands; appears very drowsy
Stupor	Unresponsive except to vigorous and repeated stimuli; responds appropriately to painful stimuli; lies quiet with minimal spontaneous movement; may have incomprehensible sounds and/or eye opening
Coma	Does not respond appropriately to stimuli; sleeplike state with eyes closed; does not make any verbal sounds

Data from Hickey J. V. (2014). The clinical practice of neurological and neurosurgical nursing *(7th ed.). Philadelphia, PA: Lippincott Williams & Wilkins.*

TABLE 16-3 The Glasgow Coma Scale

Test	Score*
Eye Opening (E)	
Spontaneous	4
To speech	3
To painful stimuli	2
No response	1
Motor Response (M)	
Obeys commands	6
Localizes pain	5
Normal flexion (withdrawal)	4
Abnormal flexion (decorticate)	3
Extension (decerebrate)	2
No response	1
Verbal Response (V)	
Oriented	5
Confused conversation	4
Inappropriate words	3
Incomprehensible sounds	2
No response	1

*GCS score = E + M + V. Best possible score = 15; worst possible score = 3. From Teasdale G., Jennett B. (1974). Assessment of coma and impaired consciousness. A practical scale. Lancet 304(7872), 81–84. Copyright © 1974 Elsevier. With permission.

become obtunded and may respond only to vigorous or noxious stimuli.

The Glasgow Coma Scale provides an organized method to assess level of consciousness. This scale is for easy use as a bedside assessment for impaired consciousness in people with brain injury[3,4] (Table 16-3). Numbered scores are given to responses of eye opening and verbal and motor responses. The total score is the sum of the best response in each category.

KEY POINTS

Brain Injury and Levels of Consciousness

■ Consciousness is a global function that depends on a diffuse neural network that includes both cerebral hemispheres and activity of the RAS. Impaired consciousness implies diffuse brain injury to both cerebral hemispheres simultaneously or the RAS at any level. In contrast, local brain injury causes focal neurologic deficit but does not disrupt consciousness.

Other Manifestations of Deteriorating Brain Function

The initial neurologic evaluation of a person with brain injury includes checking pupil size and reaction to light, abnormal flexion or extension posturing, and altered patterns of respiration.

Pupillary Reflexes and Eye Movements

Although pupils may initially respond to light, they become nonreactive and dilated as brain function deteriorates. Bilateral loss of pupillary light response suggests brain stem lesion. Unilateral loss of pupillary light response suggests optic or oculomotor pathway lesion. The oculocephalic reflex can determine if the brain stem centers for eye movement are intact (Fig. 16-2).

If the oculocephalic reflex is inconclusive, and if there are no contraindications, the oculovestibular reflex may be used to elicit nystagmus.

Abnormal Flexion and Extension Posturing

With early onset of unconsciousness, there is some purposeful movement in response to pain. As coma progresses, noxious stimuli can initiate rigidity and abnormal (decorticate and decerebrate) postures if motor tracts are interrupted at specific levels.[2] Decerebrate (extensor) posturing results from increased muscle excitability (see Fig. 16-3A). There is rigidity of arms with palms turned away from the body and with stiffly extended legs and plantar flexion of the feet. This occurs with rostral-to-caudal deterioration, when diencephalon lesions involve the midbrain and upper brain stem. Decorticate posturing is the flexion of arms, wrists, and fingers, with **adduction** of the upper extremities, internal rotation, and plantar flexion of the lower extremities (see Fig. 16-3B). Decorticate posturing results from lesions of the cerebral hemisphere or internal capsule. Both decerebrate and decorticate posturing are poor prognostic signs.

Respiratory Responses

Early respiratory changes include yawning and sighing, with progression to Cheyne–Stokes breathing. With progression of injury continuing to the midbrain, respirations change to central neurogenic hyperventilation, in which respirations may exceed 40 breaths/minute because of uninhibited stimulation of inspiratory and expiratory centers. With medullary involvement, respirations become ataxic (*i.e.*, uncoordinated and irregular). Apnea may occur due to a lack of responsiveness to carbon dioxide stimulation. Complete ventilatory assistance is often required.

Brain Death

Brain death is defined as the irreversible loss of function of the brain, including the brain stem.[5] Some conditions such as drug and metabolic intoxication can cause

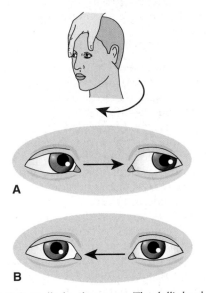

FIGURE 16-2. Doll's head response. The *doll's head eye response* demonstrates the always-present vestibular static reflexes without forebrain interference or suppression. Severe damage to the forebrain or to the brain stem rostral to the pons often results in loss of rostral control of these static vestibular reflexes. If the person's head is moved from side to side or up and down, the eyes will move in conjugate gaze to the opposite side (**A**), much like those of a doll with counterweighted eyes. If the doll's head phenomenon is observed, brain stem function at the level of the pons is considered intact (in a person who is comatose). In the person who is unconscious without intact brain stem function and vestibular static reflexes, the eyes stay in midposition (fixed) or turn in the same direction (**B**) as the head is turned.

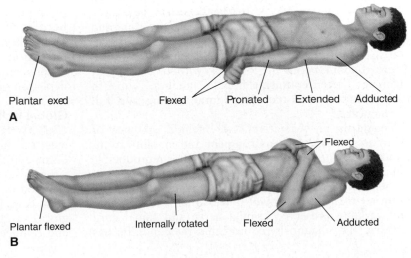

FIGURE 16-3. Abnormal posturing. (**A**) Decerebrate posturing. In decerebrate rigidity, the upper arms are held at the sides with elbows, wrists, and fingers flexed. The legs are extended and internally rotated. The feet are plantar flexed. (**B**) Decorticate posturing. In decorticate rigidity, the jaws are clenched and neck extended. The arms are adducted and stiffly extended at the elbows with the forearms pronated and the wrists and fingers flexed. (From Hickey J. V. (2014). *The clinical practice of neurological and neurosurgical nursing* (7th ed., p. 173). Philadelphia, PA: Lippincott Williams & Wilkins.)

cessation of brain functions that is completely reversible, even when they produce clinical cessation of brain functions and electroencephalogram (EEG) silence. This needs to be excluded before declaring a person brain dead.

The definition of death is continually reexamined.[5] The parameters set by the Quality of Standards Subcommittee of the American Academy of Neurology in 2010 state that "brain death is the absence of clinical brain function when the proximate cause is known and demonstrably irreversible."[5] Complex–spontaneous motor movements and false-positive triggering of the ventilator may occur in people who are brain dead. It is safe to determine apnea with the apneic oxygenation diffusion, but there is insufficient evidence for the comparative safety of techniques used for apnea testing. Longer periods of observation of absent brain activity are required if in children and in cases of drug and neuromuscular diseases such as myasthenia gravis, hypothermia, and shock. Medical circumstances may require the use of confirmatory tests.

Medical documentation should include: cause and irreversibility of the condition, absence of brain stem reflexes and motor responses to pain, absence of respiration with a pressure of carbon dioxide (PCO_2) of 60 mm Hg or more, and results from confirmatory tests. Apnea is confirmed after ventilation with pure oxygen 10 minutes before withdrawal from the ventilator, followed by passive flow of oxygen. This allows the PCO_2 to rise to 60 mm Hg after a 10-minute period of apnea, without hazardously lowering the oxygen content of the blood. If respiratory reflexes are intact, hypercarbia that develops should stimulate ventilatory effort within 30 seconds. Spontaneous breathing efforts indicate brain stem functioning. Confirmatory tests of brain death include conventional angiography, transcranial Doppler ultrasonography, technetium-99m hexamethylpropyleneamine oxime brain scan, somatosensory evoked potentials, and EEG.

Persistent Vegetative State

Advances in the care of people with brain injury have resulted in the survival of many people who previously may have died. Unfortunately, most people in prolonged coma who survive evolve to the *persistent vegetative state*, characterized by loss of all cognitive functions and unawareness of self and surroundings. Reflex and vegetative functions remain, including sleep–wake cycles.[6] There is spontaneous eye opening without concurrent awareness, often confusing hopeful families. People in the vegetative state require nonoral feeding and full nursing care.

Diagnosis of vegetative state includes absence of awareness of self and environment and inability to interact with others; absence of sustained or reproducible voluntary behavioral responses; lack of language comprehension; sufficiently preserved hypothalamic and brain stem function; bowel and bladder incontinence; and variably preserved cranial nerve and spinal cord reflexes.[6] The diagnosis requires that the condition has

continued for at least 1 month. The minimally conscious state has been defined as a state of arousal similar to persistent vegetative state, but with the distinction of the objective presence of some awareness.[7]

Mechanisms of Brain Injury

Injury to brain tissue can be due to trauma, tumors, stroke, metabolic derangements, and degenerative disorders. Brain damage involves several common pathways, including the effects of ischemia, excitatory amino acid injury, cerebral edema, and injury because of ICP. The mechanisms of injury are often interrelated.

Hypoxic and Ischemic Injury

The energy requirements of the brain are provided mainly by adenosine triphosphate (ATP). It is essential that cerebral circulation deliver oxygen in high concentrations to facilitate metabolism of glucose and generate ATP. The brain is 2% of the body's weight but it receives 15% of the resting cardiac output and accounts for 20% of the oxygen consumption.[8,9]

Hypoxia is deprivation of oxygen with maintained blood flow, whereas ischemia is reduced or interrupted blood flow. Hypoxia interferes with delivery of oxygen, whereas ischemia interferes with oxygen and glucose delivery and metabolic waste removal. Hypoxia may be due to reduced atmospheric pressure, carbon monoxide poisoning, severe anemia, and failure to oxygenate the blood. Hypoxia results in decreased oxygen levels and produces a generalized depressant effect on the brain. Neurons are capable of anaerobic metabolism and are tolerant of pure hypoxia. It produces euphoria, listlessness, drowsiness, and impaired problem solving. Unconsciousness and seizures may occur when hypoxia is sudden and severe (*i.e.*, **anoxia**), but the effects on brain function seldom are seen because it rapidly leads to cardiac arrest and ischemia.

Cerebral ischemia can be focal, as in stroke, or global, as in cardiac arrest. In global ischemia, blood flow to the entire brain is compromised. In focal ischemia, only a region of the brain is underperfused. Collateral circulation provides blood flow to uninvolved brain areas during focal ischemia and may provide substrates to the borders of the ischemic region to maintain a low level of metabolic activity, preserving membrane integrity. Interruption in the delivery of glucose in anaerobic conditions may cause additional lactic acid production and depletion of ATP stores.[8]

Global Ischemia

Global ischemia occurs when blood flow is inadequate to meet the metabolic needs of the brain. Unconsciousness occurs within seconds of severe global ischemia, resulting either from complete cessation or from marked decrease in blood flow. If cerebral circulation is restored immediately, consciousness is regained quickly. Energy sources, glucose and glycogen, are exhausted in 2 to 4 minutes, and cellular ATP stores are depleted in 4 to 5 minutes;

50% to 75% of the total energy requirement of neuronal tissue is spent on maintenance of ionic gradients across the cell membrane, resulting in fluxes of sodium, potassium, and calcium ions.[10] Excessive influx of sodium results in neuronal and interstitial edema. The influx of calcium initiates a cascade of events, including release of intracellular and nuclear enzymes that cause cell destruction. When ischemia is sufficiently severe or prolonged, infarction or death of all the cellular elements of the brain occurs. Even if blood flow is restored, if ischemic thresholds for injury are exceeded, permanent cell death ensues. Furthermore, reperfusion of injured tissues can lead to secondary brain injury through the delivery of inflammatory cells and toxic by-products, including excitatory amino acids. Such reperfusion injury compounds initial ischemic damage.

The pattern of global ischemia reflects the arrangement of cerebral vessels and the sensitivity of specific tissues to oxygen deprivation[11] (Fig. 16-4). Selective neuronal sensitivity to a lack of oxygen is apparent in cerebellar Purkinje cells and hippocampal neurons in the Sommer sector, where cell death occurs earliest after global ischemia. The anatomic arrangement of the cerebral blood vessels results in two types of injury: watershed infarcts and laminar necrosis.

Watershed infarcts are concentrated in vulnerable border zones (*watershed zones*) between overlapping territories supplied by the middle, anterior, and posterior cerebral arteries. During events such as severe hypotension, these distal territories have profoundly reduced blood flow, predisposing to focal ischemia and infarction of brain tissues. Global ischemia can thus result in focal infarcts in the border zones between major vascular territories. In contrast, the pattern of infarction in primarily focal ischemia is within a vascular territory. Laminar necrosis refers to short, serpiginous segments of necrosis that occur within and parallel to the cerebral cortex, in areas supplied by the penetrating arteries. Cortical gray matter receives its major blood supply through short penetrating arteries that emerge from larger vessels in the pia mater and repeatedly branch, forming a rich capillary network. An abrupt loss of arterial blood pressure markedly diminishes flow through these capillary channels. Because the third cortical layer is most sensitive to ischemia, the necrosis is laminar and is most severe in this layer.

If the period of nonflow or low flow is minimal, the neurologic damage usually is minimal to nonexistent. When the period is extensive or resuscitation is lengthy, the early neurologic clinical picture is that of coma; fixed, dilated pupils; and abnormal motor posturing. If the person survives, there may be gradual improvement in neurologic status, although permanent cognitive and focal deficits usually persist and can prevent a return to preischemic levels of functioning.

An exception to this is when a person, especially a child, is submerged in cold water for longer than 30 minutes.[12] Hypothermia develops and reduces the cerebral metabolic requirements for oxygen, minimizes intracellular acidosis, and lessens the effects of excitotoxic by-products. Recovery can be rapid, and resuscitation efforts should not be discontinued precipitously.

Treatment of global cerebral ischemia varies with the underlying cause. General goals are aimed at providing oxygen and decreasing the metabolic needs of brain tissue during the nonflow state. Hemodynamic support to restore systemic and cerebral perfusion is required. Respiratory support including mechanical ventilation and supplemental oxygen may be needed. Methods to decrease brain temperature in order to decrease brain metabolism are effective in certain people after cardiac arrest.[13] Normovolemic hemodilution may be used to overcome sludging of cerebral blood flow during reperfusion. Because hypoglycemia and hyperglycemia affect outcomes in people with global ischemia, blood glucose should be maintained around 140 mg/dL.[14]

Excitotoxic Brain Injury

The final common pathway for neuronal injury and death is triggered by excessive activity of excitatory neurotransmitters and the receptor-mediated effects (excitotoxicity supratentorial).[15] Neurologic conditions involved in excitotoxic injury range from acute insults such as stroke, hypoglycemic injury, and trauma to degenerative disorders such as Huntington disease.

Glutamate is the principal excitatory neurotransmitter in the brain and is responsible for many higher-order functions, including memory, cognition, movement, and sensation.[15] Extracellular glutamate concentrations are tightly regulated, with excess amounts actively transported into astrocytes and neurons. Glutamate action often involves receptor-operated ion channels. One subtype, the *N*-methyl-D-aspartate (NMDA) receptor, has been implicated in causing central nervous system (CNS) injury.[15] This NMDA receptor opens a channel that permits calcium and sodium ions to enter the cell

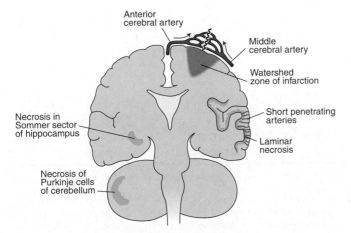

FIGURE 16-4. Consequences of global ischemia. A global insult induces lesions that reflect the vascular architecture (watershed infarcts, laminar necrosis) and the sensitivity of individual neuronal systems (pyramidal cells of the Sommer section, Purkinje cells). (Courtesy of Dimitri Karetnikov, artist.) (From Strayer D. S., Rubin E. (Eds.). (2015). *Rubin's pathology: Clinicopathologic foundations of medicine* (Fig. 32-23, p. 1427). Philadelphia, PA: Lippincott Williams & Wilkins.)

and allows potassium ions to exit, resulting in prolonged (seconds) action potentials.

During prolonged ischemia, glutamate transport mechanisms become immobilized, causing extracellular glutamate to accumulate. Intracellular glutamate is also released from the damaged cells. Glutamate excess drives uncontrolled opening of NMDA receptor–operated channels, producing an increase in intracellular calcium, which leads to a series of calcium-mediated processes called the *calcium cascade* (Fig. 16-5), including the release of intracellular enzymes that cause protein breakdown, free radical formation, lipid peroxidation, fragmentation of deoxyribonucleic acid, mitochondrial injury, nuclear breakdown, and eventually cell death.

Acute glutamate toxicity may be reversible if the excess glutamate can be removed or if its effects can be blocked before the full cascade progresses. *Neuroprotectant drugs* interfere with the calcium cascade and thus reduce brain cell injury. Other strategies being explored include drugs that inhibit synthesis or release of excitatory amino acid transmitters, block NMDA receptors, stabilize the membrane potential to prevent initiation of the calcium cascade using lidocaine and certain barbiturates, and block certain intracellular proteases, endonucleases, and lipases that are known to be cytotoxic.[15] The drug riluzole, which acts presynaptically to inhibit glutamate release, is used in the treatment of amyotrophic lateral sclerosis (see Chapter 15).

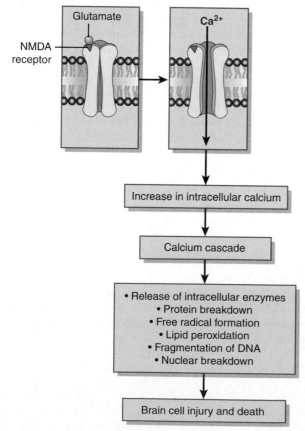

FIGURE 16-5. The role of the glutamate NMDA receptor in brain cell injury. DNA, deoxyribonucleic acid; NMDA, N-methyl-D-aspartate.

Increased Intracranial Pressure

The brain is enclosed in the rigid confines of the skull, or cranium, making it susceptible to increases in ICP. Excessive ICP can obstruct cerebral blood flow, destroy brain cells, displace brain tissue (as in herniation), and otherwise damage delicate brain structures (Table 16-5).

The cranial cavity contains blood (~10%), brain tissue (~80%), and CSF (~10%) (Fig. 16-6).[2] Each of these three volumes contributes to the ICP, which normally is maintained between 0 and 15 mm Hg when measured in the lateral ventricles. The volumes of each of these components can vary slightly without causing marked changes in ICP because small increases in one component can be compensated for by a decrease in the volume of one or both of the other components. This dynamic equilibrium is called the *Monro–Kellie hypothesis*.[2] Abnormal variation in intracranial volume with subsequent changes in ICP can be caused by a volume change in any of the intracranial components. For example, an increase in tissue volume can result from a brain tumor, edema, or bleeding. An increase in blood volume can result from vasodilation of cerebral vessels or obstruction of venous outflow. An increase in CSF can result from excess production, decreased absorption, or obstructed circulation.[2]

Although tissue volume is relatively restricted in its ability to undergo change, CSF and blood volume are able to compensate for changes in ICP. Initial increases in ICP are buffered by a translocation of CSF to the spinal subarachnoid space and increased CSF reabsorption. The blood compartment is limited by the small amount of blood in the cerebral circulation, most of which is contained in the low-pressure venous system. As the volume-buffering capacity of this compartment becomes exhausted, venous pressure increases, and cerebral blood volume and ICP rise. Cerebral blood flow is also highly controlled by autoregulatory mechanisms, which affect its compensatory capacity. Conditions such as ischemia and elevated partial PCO_2 in the blood produce a compensatory vasodilation of cerebral blood vessels. Decreased PCO_2 has the opposite effect, so hyperventilation, which decreases PCO_2 levels, may be used in the treatment of ICP.

TABLE 16-4 Early and Late Signs of Increased Intracranial Pressure

Signs	Early Sign	Late Sign
Level of consciousness	Decreased alertness to drowsy	Stupor or coma
Pupil size and reaction to light	Small and sluggish reaction	Large and nonreactive
Motor function	Hemiparesis	Hemiplegia
Vital signs	No change	Hypertension, widened pulse pressure, bradycardia, abnormal respiratory patterns
Other signs	Headache, slurred speech	Vomiting

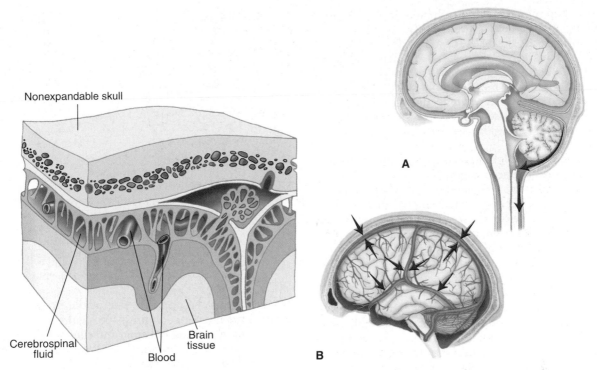

Nonexpandable skull

Cerebrospinal fluid

Blood

Brain tissue

A

B

FIGURE 16-6. Three compartments contained within the rigid confines of the skull—the brain tissue and interstitial fluid (80%), the blood (10%), and the cerebrospinal fluid (10%). The CSF (**A**) can be displaced from the ventricles and cerebral subarachnoid space to the spinal subarachnoid space, and it can also undergo increased absorption or decreased production. Because most of the blood in the cranial cavity is contained in the low-pressure venous system, venous compression (**B**) serves as a means of displacing blood volume.

The impact of increases in blood, brain tissue, or CSF volumes on ICP varies among people and depends on the amount of increase, effectiveness of compensatory mechanisms, and compliance of brain tissue.[2] Compliance is the brain's ability to maintain ICP during changes in intracranial volume. Compliance (C) is the ratio of change (Δ) in volume (V) to change in pressure (P): $C = \Delta V/\Delta P$. The effects of changes in intracranial volume and compliance on ICP can be illustrated on a graph (Fig. 16-7). This demonstrates the effect on ICP of adding volume to the intracranial cavity. From points A to B, the compensatory mechanisms are adequate, compliance is high, and ICP remains relatively constant. At point B, the ICP is relatively normal, but the compensatory mechanisms have reached their limits, compliance is decreased, and ICP begins to rise. From points C to D, the compensatory mechanisms have been exceeded, and ICP rises significantly with each increase in volume as compliance is lost.

An increase in intracranial volume will have little effect on ICP as long as compliance is high. Compliance is influenced by the amount of volume increase, the time frame for accommodation, and the size of the compartments. For example, small volume increments over long periods of time can be accommodated more easily than a comparable amount over a short time.

The cerebral perfusion pressure (CPP), which is the difference between mean arterial pressure (MAP) and ICP (CPP = MAP − ICP), is the pressure gradient driving blood flow to the brain.[9,16] Normal CPP ranges

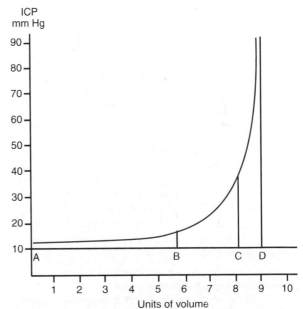

ICP mm Hg

FIGURE 16-7. The dynamic effects of changes in intracranial volume and compliance (which represents the ratio of change (Δ) in volume (V) to change in pressure (P): $C = \Delta V/\Delta P$) on ICP can be illustrated on a graph with the volume represented on the horizontal axis and ICP on the vertical axis. The shape of the curve demonstrates the effect on ICP of adding volume to the intracranial cavity. From points A to B, the compensatory mechanisms are adequate, compliance is high, and the ICP remains relatively constant as volume is added to the intracranial cavity. At point B, the ICP is relatively normal, but the compensatory mechanisms have reached their limits, compliance is decreased, and ICP begins to rise with each change in volume. From points C to D, the compensatory mechanisms have been exceeded, and ICP rises significantly with each increase in volume as compliance is lost. ICP, intracranial pressure.

from 70 to 100 mm Hg. Brain ischemia develops below 40 mm Hg.[2] When the pressure in the cranial cavity approaches or exceeds the MAP, tissue perfusion becomes inadequate, cellular hypoxia results, and neuronal death may occur. A decrease in the level of consciousness is one of the earliest and most reliable signs of increased ICP. Continued cellular hypoxia leads to general neurologic deterioration. Consciousness may deteriorate from alertness through confusion, lethargy, obtundation, stupor, and coma.

The *Cushing reflex* is triggered by ischemia of the vasomotor center in the brain stem. Neurons here respond to ischemia with a marked increase in MAP in an attempt to increase CPP, and a widening of pulse pressure and reflex slowing of heart rate. These three signs (*i.e.*, hypertension, bradycardia, and widened pulse pressure) are important but late indicators of increased ICP.[17]

Brain Herniation

The brain is protected by the skull and supporting septa, the falx cerebri and the tentorium cerebelli, that divide the intracranial cavity into fossae or compartments that protect against excess movement. The falx cerebri is a sickle-shaped septum that separates the two hemispheres. The tentorium cerebelli divides the cranial cavity into anterior and posterior fossae. Extending posteriorly into the center of the tentorium is a large semicircular opening called the *incisura* or *tentorial notch*. The temporal lobe rests on the tentorial incisura, and the midbrain occupies the anterior portion of the tentorial notch. The cerebellum is closely opposed to the dorsum of the midbrain and fills the posterior part of the notch. The oculomotor nerve (CN III) emerges from the mediolateral surface of each peduncle just caudal to the tentorium.

Brain herniation represents a displacement of brain tissue under the falx cerebri or through the tentorial notch or incisura of the tentorium cerebelli (Fig. 16-8). It occurs when an elevated ICP in one brain compartment causes displacement of the cerebral tissue toward an area of lower ICP. Different types of herniation syndromes are based on the area of the brain that has herniated and the structure under which it has been pushed. They commonly are divided into supratentorial and infratentorial herniations, based on whether they are located above or below the tentorium.

Supratentorial Herniations

Three major patterns of supratentorial herniation are cingulate, central transtentorial, and uncal transtentorial (Table 16-5). Cingulate herniation poses the least serious threat in terms of clinical outcomes.[2] Transtentorial herniations result in an uncal syndrome and a central syndrome. Clinically, these display distinct patterns early in their course, but both merge in a similar pattern once they begin to involve the midbrain level and below (brain stem structures).

Cingulate herniation is the displacement of the cingulate gyrus and hemisphere beneath the sharp edges of the

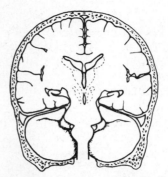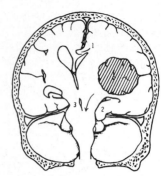

FIGURE 16-8. Patterns of herniation. Normal brain (**left**), supratentorial herniations (**right**). (*1*) Herniation of cingulate gyrus under the falx cerebri. (*2*) Herniation of the temporal lobe into the tentorial notch. (*3*) Downward displacement of the brain stem through the notch. (From Hickey J. V. (2014). *The clinical practice of neurological and neurosurgical nursing* (7th ed., p. 1427). Philadelphia, PA: Lippincott Williams & Wilkins.)

falx cerebri to the opposite side of the brain. Displacement of the falx can compress the local brain tissue and blood supply, causing ischemia and edema, which further increase ICP levels. Unilateral or bilateral leg weakness is an early sign of impending cingulate herniation.

Central transtentorial herniations involve the downward displacement of cerebral hemispheres, basal ganglia, diencephalon, and midbrain through the tentorial incisura. The diencephalon may be compressed against the midbrain with such force that edema and hemorrhage result. It may be associated with uncal or lateral herniation. In the early diencephalic stage, there is clouding of consciousness, bilaterally small pupils (2 mm in

TABLE 16-5 Key Structures and Clinical Signs of Cingulate, Central, and Uncal Herniations

Herniation Syndrome	Key Structures Involved	Key Clinical Signs
Cingulate	Anterior cerebral artery	Leg weakness
Central transtentorial	Reticular activating system	Altered level of consciousness
	Corticospinal tract	Decorticate posturing
		Rostral–caudal deterioration
Uncal	Cerebral peduncle	Hemiparesis
	Oculomotor nerve	Ipsilateral pupil dilation
	Posterior cerebral artery	Visual field loss
	Cerebellar tonsil	Respiratory arrest
	Respiratory center	

diameter) with full range of constriction, and motor responses to pain that are purposeful or semipurposeful and often asymmetric. Clouding of consciousness, an early sign of central herniations, is caused by pressure on the RAS. With progression to the late diencephalic stage, painful stimulation results in decorticate posturing, which may be asymmetric (Fig. 16-3B), and there are ebbs and flows of respirations with periods of apnea (Cheyne–Stokes respirations). With midbrain involvement, pupils are fixed and midsize (5 mm in diameter), and reflex adduction of the eyes is impaired; pain elicits decerebrate posturing (Fig. 16-3B); and respirations change to neurogenic hyperventilation, with excess of 40 breaths/minute due to uninhibited stimulation of inspiratory and expiratory centers. Involvement of the lower pons and upper medulla produces fixed, midpoint (3- to 5-mm) pupils with loss of reflex abduction and adduction of the eyes, and absence of motor responses or only leg flexion on painful stimuli. Once the area of herniation has progressed into the midbrain and brain stem, the process is generally irreversible and the prognosis poor.[2]

Uncal herniation occurs when a lateral mass pushes the brain tissue centrally and forces the medial aspect of the temporal lobe, containing the uncus and hippocampal gyrus, under the edge of the tentorial incisura, into the posterior fossa. The diencephalon and midbrain are compressed and displaced laterally to the opposite side of the tentorium. CN III (oculomotor nerve) and the posterior cerebral artery are often caught between the uncus and the tentorium. CN III controls pupillary constriction and entrapment causes ipsilateral pupillary dilation, which may be an early sign of uncal herniation. Consciousness may be unimpaired because RAS has not yet been affected but deterioration is rapid once any signs of herniation or compression appear.

As uncal herniations progress, compression of descending motor pathways results in changes in motor strength and coordination of voluntary movements. Initial changes may occur ipsilateral to the side of damage due to compression of contralateral cerebral peduncles. This may result in a false localizing sign of hemiparesis on the same side as CN III. As the condition progresses, bilateral positive Babinski responses and respiratory changes occur. Decorticate and decerebrate posturing may develop, followed by dilated, fixed pupils, flaccidity, and respiratory arrest.

Infratentorial Herniation

Infratentorial herniation results from increased pressure in the infratentorial compartment. Because it is likely to involve the lower brain stem centers that control vital cardiopulmonary functions, it often progresses rapidly and can cause death. Herniation may occur superiorly through the tentorial incisura or inferiorly through the foramen magnum.

Upward displacement of brain tissue can block the aqueduct of Sylvius, leading to hydrocephalus and coma. Downward displacement of the midbrain through the tentorial notch or the cerebellar tonsils through the foramen magnum can interfere with medullary functioning and cause cardiac or respiratory arrest. With preexisting ICP elevations, herniation may occur when the pressure is released from below (*i.e.*, lumbar puncture). If CSF cannot leave the ventricles, volume expands, and fluid is displaced downward through the tentorial notch. Thus, expansion ceases all function at a given level as destruction progresses rostral-to-caudal. The result is brain stem ischemia and hemorrhage extending from the diencephalon to the pons. If the lesion expands rapidly, displacement and obstruction occur quickly, leading to irreversible infarction and hemorrhage.

Cerebral Edema

Cerebral edema occurs with an increase in water and sodium content, causing an increase in brain volume.[18] *Vasogenic edema* occurs when fluid escapes into the extracellular fluid that surrounds brain cells, whereas *cytotoxic edema* involves the swelling of brain cells themselves.[8] The impact of brain edema depends on the compensatory mechanisms and extent of swelling.

Vasogenic Edema

Vasogenic edema occurs with conditions that impair blood–brain barrier function and allow transfer of water and protein from the vascular into the interstitial space. It occurs with tumors, prolonged ischemia, hemorrhage, brain injury, and infectious processes. Vasogenic edema occurs primarily in the white matter of the brain, possibly because it is more compliant than gray matter. Vasogenic edema can displace a cerebral hemisphere and can be responsible for various types of herniation. The functional manifestations of vasogenic edema include focal neurologic deficits, disturbances in consciousness, and severe intracranial hypertension.

Cytotoxic Edema

Cytotoxic edema occurs in hypo-osmotic states such as water intoxication or severe ischemia that impair sodium–potassium pump function. Ischemia also results in the inadequate removal of anaerobic metabolic end products such as lactic acid, producing extracellular acidosis. Altered osmotic conditions result in water entry and cell swelling. If blood flow is reduced for extended periods or to extremely low levels for a few minutes, cellular edema can cause cell membrane rupture, allowing escape of intracellular contents into surrounding extracellular fluid and damaging neighboring cells. Major changes in cerebral function, such as stupor and coma, occur. The edema associated with ischemia may produce cerebral infarction with brain tissue necrosis.

Treatment

Cerebral edema does not necessarily disrupt brain function unless it increases ICP. Localized edema surrounding a brain tumor or abscess rapidly improves with glucocorticoid therapy, but these drugs are not effective for cerebral infarction, intracranial hemorrhage (ICH), subarachnoid hemorrhage (SAH), or traumatic brain injury (TBI) edema. Osmotherapy may be useful in the acute phase of vasogenic and cytotoxic edema.

Hydrocephalus

Enlargement of the CSF compartment occurs with hydrocephalus, which is an abnormal increase in CSF volume in any part of the ventricular system. It is caused by decreased absorption of CSF and obstruction of CSF flow, and can be noncommunicating or communicating.

Noncommunicating hydrocephalus occurs when obstruction in the ventricular system prevents CSF from reaching the arachnoid villi. CSF flow can be obstructed by congenital malformations, tumors encroaching on the ventricular system, and inflammation or hemorrhage. The ependyma is especially sensitive to viral infections, particularly during embryonic development; ependymitis is believed to be the cause of congenital aqueductal stenosis.[11]

Communicating hydrocephalus is caused by impaired reabsorption of CSF from the arachnoid villi into the venous system. Decreased absorption can result from a blocked CSF pathway to the arachnoid villi or failure of the villi to transfer CSF to the venous system. It can occur if too few villi are formed, if postinfective scarring occludes them, or if villi are obstructed with fragments of blood or infectious debris. Choroid plexus adenomas can cause CSF overproduction.

Similar pathologic patterns occur with noncommunicating and communicating hydrocephalus. Cerebral hemispheres are enlarged and the ventricular system beyond the obstruction is dilated. Sulci become effaced and shallow and white matter is reduced in volume. Presence and extent of ICP are determined by fluid accumulation and type of hydrocephalus, the age at onset, and the rapidity and extent of pressure rise. Computed tomography (CT) and magnetic resonance imaging (MRI) scans diagnose hydrocephalus. Usual treatment is a shunting procedure, which provides an alternative route for CSF return to the circulation.

When hydrocephalus develops in utero or before the cranial sutures have fused in infancy, the ventricles expand beyond the point of obstruction, the cranial sutures separate, the head expands, and there is bulging of the fontanelles. Because the skull is able to expand, signs of increased ICP may be absent and intelligence spared. Seizures, weakness, and uncoordinated movement are common, and in severe cases, optic nerve atrophy leads to blindness. Surgical placement of a shunt diverts excess CSF, preventing extreme enlargement of the head and neurologic deficits.

Cranial sutures are fully fused in adults. Slowly developing hydrocephalus is unlikely to increase ICP, but it may produce progressive dementia and gait changes, as in normal-pressure hydrocephalus (*pseudotumor cerebri*) in the elderly. Acute-onset hydrocephalus in adults is marked by symptoms of increased ICP, including headache, vomiting, and papilledema or lateral rectus palsy from pressure on the cranial nerves. If obstruction is not relieved, progression to herniation ensues. Treatment includes surgical decompression and shunting.

SUMMARY CONCEPTS

Brain injury is manifested by changes in the level of consciousness and alterations in motor, sensory, and cognitive function. Consciousness is a state of awareness of self and environment. It exists on a continuum from normal wakefulness and sleep to states of stupor and coma. In progressive brain injury, the onset of coma may follow a rostral-to-caudal progression with changes in levels of consciousness, respiratory activity, pupillary and oculovestibular reflexes, and muscle tone occurring as the diencephalon through the medulla is affected.

Brain death is the irreversible loss of function of the brain, including that of the brain stem. Clinical examination must disclose at least the absence of responsiveness, brain stem reflexes, and respiratory effort. The vegetative state is characterized by loss of all cognitive functions and the unawareness of self and surroundings, whereas reflex and vegetative functions remain intact.

Many agents cause brain damage through common pathways, including hypoxia or ischemia, accumulation of excitatory neurotransmitters, increased ICP, and cerebral edema. Hypoxia or ischemia can have deleterious effects on the brain. Focal ischemia causes localized brain injury, as in stroke. Global ischemia, as in cardiac arrest, occurs when blood flow to the entire brain is inadequate, causing global deficits such as altered mental status.

Traumatic Brain Injury

Although the skull affords protection to the CNS from external forces, it is a potential source of injury from internal forces. The internal skull surface can induce traumatic and ischemic injuries when tissues increase in volume (swelling or bleeding) or shift (swelling or mechanical trauma). Skull fractures can compress sections of the nervous system and cause penetrating wounds.

TBI is the leading cause of death and disability among people under 24 years of age. The main causes of TBI are motor vehicle crashes, falls, and assaults. The most common cause of fatal head injuries is motor vehicle crashes involving vehicles and pedestrians.[16]

TBI can involve the scalp, skull, meninges, or brain. A linear skull fracture is a break in the continuity of bone. A comminuted skull fracture refers to a splintered or multiple fracture line. When bone fragments are embedded into the brain tissue, the fracture is said to be depressed. A basilar skull fracture is a fracture of the bones that form the base of the skull.

Radiologic examination usually confirms the presence and extent of a skull fracture and is important due to possible damage to underlying tissues. The ethmoid cribriform plate is the most fragile portion of the neurocranium and is shattered in basal skull fractures. A frequent complication of basilar skull fractures is leakage of CSF from the nose or ear; this occurs due to the proximity of the base of the skull to the nose and ears. This break in protection of the brain becomes a probable source of infection of the meninges or of brain substance. There may be subconjunctival hemorrhage of the eye or periorbital **ecchymosis**. Skull fractures can damage the cranial nerves (I, II, III, VII, and VIII) as they exit.

Primary and Secondary Brain Injuries

The effects of traumatic head injuries can be divided into *primary injuries*, in which damage is caused by impact, and *secondary injuries*, in which damage results from the subsequent brain swelling, infection, or cerebral hypoxia.

Primary brain injuries include focal (*e.g.*, contusion, laceration, hemorrhage) and diffuse (*e.g.*, concussion, diffuse axonal injury) injuries. Secondary brain injuries are diffuse or multifocal, including edema, infection, and hypoxic brain damage. When mechanical forces cause excess movement, a contusion, coup–contrecoup injury, can occur. Because the brain floats freely in the CSF, blunt force to the head accelerates the brain within the skull and decelerates abruptly upon hitting the inner skull surfaces (Fig. 16-9). The direct contusion of the brain at the site of external force is a *coup* injury; the rebound injury on the opposite side of the brain is the *contrecoup* injury. As the brain strikes the rough surface of the cranial vault, brain tissue, blood vessels, nerve tracts, and other structures are bruised and torn, resulting in contusions and hematomas.

The most common cause of secondary brain injury is ischemia. It can result from the hypoxia and hypotension that occur during resuscitation or from impairment of regulatory mechanisms by which cerebrovascular responses maintain an adequate blood flow and oxygen supply.[19]

Secondary injuries depend on the extent of damage caused by the primary injury. In mild brain injury, there may be momentary loss of consciousness without noticeable neurologic symptoms or residual damage, except for possible residual amnesia. Microscopic changes may be detected within hours of injury, but brain imaging is negative. Concussion is a transient dysfunction caused by some mechanical force to the brain.[16] Recovery usually takes place within 24 hours, but mild symptoms, such as headache, irritability, insomnia, and poor concentration and memory, may persist for months. This is *postconcussion syndrome*. Memory loss usually includes an interval of time preceding (retrograde amnesia) and after (anterograde amnesia) the accident. Duration of retrograde amnesia correlates with the severity of brain injury. Cognitive complaints are subjective and may be regarded as having psychological origin. Postconcussion syndrome can have a significant effect on daily activities and return to employment. People with postconcussion syndrome may need cognitive retraining, medications, or psychological support.

In moderate brain injury, many small hemorrhages and swelling of brain tissue occur. These contusions can be visualized on CT scan and often are distributed along the rough, irregular inner surface of the brain. They are

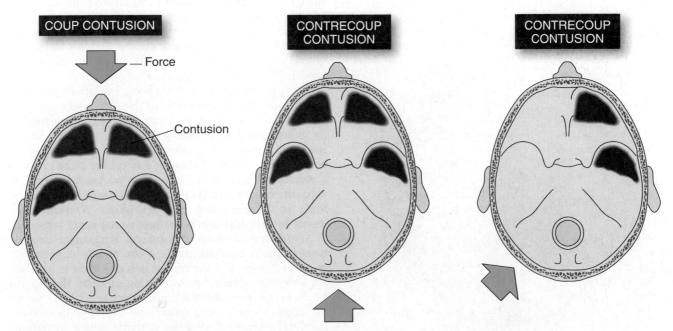

FIGURE 16-9. Biomechanics of cerebral contusion. The cerebral hemispheres float in the cerebrospinal fluid. Rapid deceleration or acceleration of the skull causes the cortex to impact forcefully into the anterior and middle fossa. The position of a contusion is determined by the direction of the force and the intracranial anatomy. (From Strayer D. S., Rubin E. (Eds.). (2015). *Rubin's pathology: Clinicopathologic foundations of medicine* (7th ed., Fig. 32-18, p. 1423). Philadelphia, PA: Wolters Kluwer.)

more likely to occur in the frontal or temporal lobes, resulting in cognitive and motor deficits. Moderate brain injury has a period of unconsciousness and may be associated with focal manifestations such as hemiparesis, aphasia, and cranial nerve palsy.

Severe brain injury involves extensive primary and secondary injury to the brain structures. The primary injury is instantaneous and irreversible, resulting from shearing and pressure forces that cause diffuse axonal injury, disruption of blood vessels, and tissue damage. Contusions and intracerebral, subdural, epidural hemorrhage and SAH are often evident on CT scan. It often is accompanied by severe neurologic deficits such as coma, hemiplegia, and elevated ICP. Severe brain injuries often occur with injury to other body parts such as the neck, extremities, chest, and abdomen.

Hematomas

Hematomas result from vascular injury and bleeding. Bleeding can occur in any of several compartments, including the epidural, subdural, intracerebral, and subarachnoid spaces.

Epidural Hematoma

Epidural hematomas usually are caused by head injury in which the temporal area of the skull is fractured. An epidural hematoma develops between the inner table of the bones of the skull and the dura (Fig. 16-10). It usually results from a tear in an artery, most often the middle

meningeal, usually in association with a skull fracture.[8] Because bleeding is arterial in origin, rapid expansion of the hematoma compresses the brain. Epidural hematoma is more common at younger ages because the dura is less firmly attached to the skull surface; as a consequence, the dura can be easily separated from the inner surface of the skull, allowing the hematoma to grow.

Typically, a person with an epidural hematoma has a history of head injury and a brief period of unconsciousness followed by a lucid period in which consciousness is regained, followed by rapid progression to unconsciousness. The lucid interval does not always occur but is of great diagnostic value. With rapidly developing unconsciousness, focal symptoms relate to the area of the brain involved and can include ipsilateral pupil dilation and contralateral hemiparesis from uncal herniation. Prognosis is excellent if the hematoma is removed before loss of consciousness. If it is not removed, the condition progresses, with increased ICP, tentorial herniation, and death.

Subdural Hematoma

A subdural hematoma develops in the area between the dura and the arachnoid and usually is the result of a tear in the small bridging veins that connect veins on the surface of the cortex to dural sinuses. The bridging veins pass from the pial vessels through the CSF-filled subarachnoid space, penetrate the arachnoid and the dura, and empty into the intradural sinuses.[11] These veins are readily snapped when the brain moves suddenly in relation to the skull (Fig. 16-11).

The venous source of bleeding in a subdural hematoma develops more slowly than the arterial bleeding in an epidural hematoma. Subdural hematomas are acute, subacute, or chronic, based on the approximate time before the appearance of symptoms. Symptoms of acute hematoma appear up to 48 hours after the injury. Symptoms of subacute hematoma appear 2 to 14 days after injury. Symptoms of chronic subdural hematoma appear several weeks after the injury.

Acute subdural hematomas progress rapidly and have a high mortality rate because of the severe secondary injuries related to edema and increased ICP. High mortality is associated with uncontrolled ICP increase, loss of consciousness, extension posturing, and delay in surgical hematoma removal. Clinically, it is similar to an epidural hematoma, except there usually is no lucid interval. In subacute hematoma, there may be a period of improvement in consciousness and neurologic symptoms followed by deterioration if the hematoma is not removed.

Symptoms of chronic subdural hematoma develop weeks after a head injury, and the person may not remember having had the injury. It is common in alcoholics and older adults because brain atrophy shrinks the brain away from the dura and stretches fragile bridging veins. These veins rupture and blood seeps into the subdural space. Fibroblastic activity causes hematoma to become encapsulated. The sanguineous fluid in this encapsulated area has high osmotic pressure and draws in fluid from the surrounding subarachnoid space; the mass expands, exerting pressure on the cranial contents. In some instances, the most prominent symptom is a

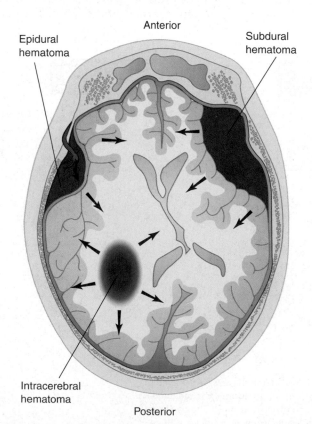

FIGURE 16-10. Location of epidural, subdural, and intracerebral hematomas.

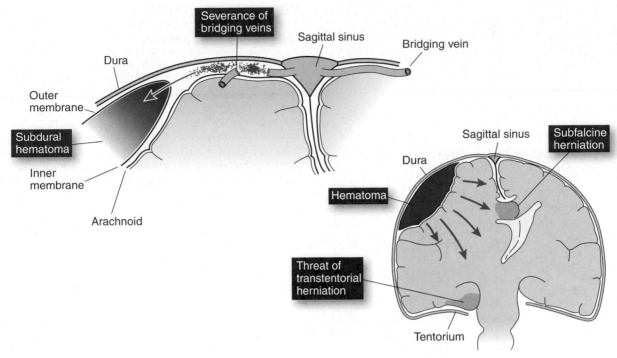

FIGURE 16-11. Mechanism of bleeding in subdural hematoma. (Courtesy of Dmitri Karetnikov, artist.) (From Strayer D. S., Rubin E. (Eds.). (2015). *Rubin's pathology: Clinicopathologic foundations of medicine* (7th ed., p. 1463). Philadelphia, PA: Wolters Kluwer.)

decreasing level of consciousness indicated by drowsiness, confusion, headache, and apathy.

Traumatic Intracerebral Hematomas

Traumatic intracerebral hematomas may be single or multiple. They can occur in any lobe of the brain but are most common in the frontal or temporal lobes, related to the bony prominences on the inner skull surface (Fig. 16-12). They may occur in association with the severe motion that the brain undergoes during head injury, or a contusion can coalesce into a hematoma. Intracerebral hematomas occur more frequently in older adults and alcoholics, whose cerebral vessels are more friable.

The signs and symptoms depend on its size and location. Signs of increased ICP can be manifested if the hematoma is large and encroaching on vital structures. A hematoma in the temporal lobe can be dangerous because of the potential for lateral herniation.

Treatment can be medical or surgical. Surgery to evacuate the clot is indicated for a large hematoma with a rapidly deteriorating condition. Surgery may not be needed in someone who is neurologically stable despite neurologic deficits; the hematoma may resolve like a contusion.

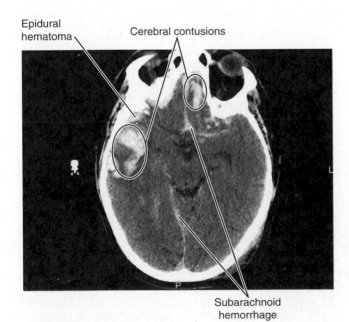
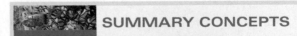

FIGURE 16-12. Computed tomography scan of the brain in traumatic brain imaging, showing hemorrhagic cerebral contusions in right temporal and bifrontal lobes, subarachnoid hemorrhage, and epidural hematoma.

SUMMARY CONCEPTS

The effects of TBI can be divided into primary and secondary injuries. Primary injuries result from direct impact, resulting in skull fracture, concussion, or contusion. In secondary injuries, damage results from the subsequent brain swelling; epidural, subdural, or intracerebral hematoma formation; infection; cerebral hypoxia; and ischemia. Even if there is no break in the skull, a blow to the head can cause severe and diffuse brain damage. Such closed injuries vary in severity and can be classified as focal or diffuse. Diffuse injuries include concussion and diffuse axonal injury. Focal injuries include contusion, laceration, and hemorrhage.

Cerebrovascular Disease

Cerebrovascular disease encompasses a number of disorders involving vessels in the cerebral circulation. These disorders include transient ischemic attacks (TIAs) and stroke.

Cerebral Circulation

Cerebral Blood Vessels

The blood flow to the brain is supplied by two internal carotid arteries anteriorly and vertebral arteries posteriorly (Fig. 16-13A). The internal carotid artery, a terminal branch of the common carotid artery, branches into several arteries: ophthalmic, posterior communicating, anterior choroidal, anterior cerebral, and middle cerebral (see Fig. 16-13B). Most of the blood in the internal carotid arteries is distributed through the anterior and middle cerebral arteries. The anterior cerebral arteries supply the medial surface of the frontal and parietal lobes and the anterior half of the thalamus, the corpus striatum, part of the corpus callosum, and the anterior limb of the internal capsule. The genu and posterior limb

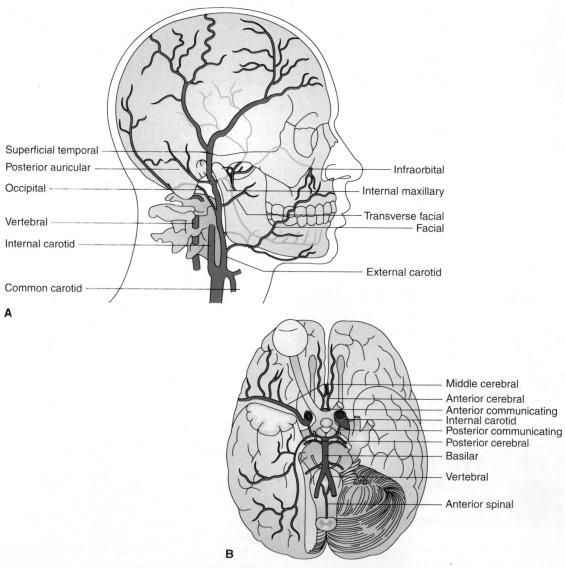

FIGURE 16-13. Cerebral circulation. (**A**) Branches of the right external carotid artery. The internal carotid artery ascends to the base of the brain. The right vertebral artery is also shown as it ascends through the transverse foramen of the cervical vertebrae. (**B**) The cerebral arterial circle (circle of Willis).

of the internal capsule and medial globus pallidus are fed by the anterior choroidal branch of the internal carotid artery. The middle cerebral artery passes laterally, supplying the lateral basal ganglia and the insula, and then emerges on the lateral cortical surface, supplying the inferior frontal gyrus, the motor and premotor frontal cortex concerned with delicate face and hand control. It is the major vascular source for the language cortices (frontal and superior temporal), the primary and association auditory cortex (superior temporal gyrus), and the primary and association somatosensory cortex for the face and hand (postcentral gyrus, parietal). The middle cerebral artery is a continuation of the internal carotid; emboli of the internal carotid most frequently become lodged in branches of the middle cerebral artery. Ischemia of these areas results in damage to the fine manipulative skills of the face and upper limbs and to receptive and expressive communication functions.

Two vertebral arteries arise from the subclavian artery, enter the foramina at the level of the sixth cervical vertebra, continue upward through the foramina, and enter the skull through the foramen magnum and unite to form the basilar artery, which terminates in the posterior cerebral arteries. Branches of the basilar and vertebral arteries supply the medulla, pons, cerebellum, midbrain, and caudal part of the diencephalon. The posterior cerebral arteries supply the occipital and inferior regions of the temporal lobes and the thalamus.

The distal branches of the internal carotid and vertebral arteries communicate at the base of the brain through the circle of Willis, an **anastomosis** of arteries that provides continuous circulation of blood flow even if a vessel is disrupted (see Fig. 16-13B). For instance, occlusion of a middle cerebral artery may have limited consequence if anterior and posterior communicating arteries are open, allowing collateral flow from ipsilateral posterior cerebral and opposite carotid arteries.

The cerebral circulation is drained by the deep cerebral and the superficial venous systems that empty into the dural venous sinuses. The deep system is well protected. These vessels connect to the sagittal sinuses in the falx cerebri by bridging veins. They travel through the subarachnoid space and penetrate the arachnoid and dura to reach the dural venous sinuses. This system of sinuses returns blood to the heart primarily through the internal jugular veins. Alternate routes for venous flow also exist: venous blood may exit through the emissary veins that pass through the skull and through veins that traverse various foramina to empty into extracranial veins.

The intracranial venous system has no valves. Direction of flow depends on gravity or relative pressure in the venous sinuses compared with the extracranial veins. Increases in intrathoracic pressure, as with coughing or the Valsalva maneuver (exhaling against a closed glottis), produce rises in venous pressure that is reflected back into the internal jugular veins and the dural sinuses.

Regulation of Cerebral Blood Flow

Blood flow to the brain is approximately 750 mL/minute or one sixth of the resting cardiac output.[17] Regulation of blood flow to the brain is controlled largely by autoregulatory or local mechanisms that respond to the metabolic needs of the brain. Cerebral autoregulation is the ability of the brain to maintain constant blood flow despite changes in systemic arterial pressure. This allows the cerebral cortex to adjust blood flow locally to satisfy its metabolic needs. Autoregulation is efficient within an MAP of approximately 60 to 140 mm Hg.[17] Although total cerebral blood flow remains stable with changes in cardiac output and arterial blood pressure, regional blood flow may vary markedly in response to local changes in metabolism. If blood pressure falls below 60 mm Hg, cerebral blood flow becomes severely compromised, and if it rises above the upper limit of autoregulation, blood flow increases rapidly and overstretches the cerebral vessels. In hypertension, this autoregulatory range shifts to higher MAP levels.

Carbon dioxide, hydrogen ion, and oxygen concentration affect cerebral blood flow. Increased carbon dioxide provides a potent stimulus for vasodilation—doubling PCO_2 in the blood doubles cerebral blood flow. Increased hydrogen ion concentrations also increase cerebral blood flow to wash away the neurally depressive acidic materials.[17] Profound extracellular acidosis induces vasomotor paralysis, and cerebral blood flow may depend entirely on systemic arterial blood pressure. Decreased oxygen concentration also increases cerebral blood flow.

 Concept Mastery Alert

Decreased oxygen saturation increases cerebral blood flow, as does an increased carbon dioxide level. Both of these factors result in less oxygen for the cells of the brain. The body attempts to compensate by increasing blood flow to the area.

The deep cerebral blood vessels appear to be completely controlled by autoregulation, whereas the superficial and major cerebral blood vessels are innervated by the sympathetic nervous system. Local regulatory and autoregulatory mechanisms override the effects of sympathetic stimulation, but sympathetic control of cerebral blood pressure is important when local mechanisms fail.[17] For example, arterial pressure rises during strenuous exercise and the sympathetic nervous system will constrict large and intermediate-sized superficial blood vessels to protect smaller, easily damaged vessels. Sympathetic reflexes may cause vasospasm in the intermediate and large arteries in some types of brain damage, such as that caused by rupture of a cerebral aneurysm.

Stroke

Stroke is acute focal neurologic deficit from a vascular disorder that injures brain tissue. Stroke is a leading cause of mortality and morbidity in the United States. Each year, 795,000 Americans are afflicted with stroke; many survivors have some degree of neurologic impairment.[20] Eighty-seven percent of all strokes are ischemic strokes, caused by an interruption of blood flow in a cerebral vessel.[20] Thirteen percent of all strokes are hemorrhagic strokes (10% intracerebral hemorrhage, 3% SAH).[20] A hemorrhagic stroke usually is from a blood vessel rupture caused by hypertension, aneurysm, or arteriovenous malformation and has a much higher fatality rate than ischemic strokes.

Etiology

Risk factors for stroke include age, sex, race, prior stroke, family history, hypertension, smoking, diabetes mellitus, cardiac disease, hypercholesterolemia, and hypercoagulopathy.[21] Incidence of stroke increases with age: stroke incidence rates in males are higher than in females at younger ages, but not at older ages. Because females live longer than males, yearly more females die of stroke. Blood pressure is a powerful determinant of stroke risk.[21] Heart disease, particularly atrial fibrillation and conditions that encourage clot formation on the heart wall or valve leaflets or paradoxical embolisms through right-to-left shunting, increases the risk of cardioembolic stroke. Blood disorders (polycythemia, sickle cell) increase the risk of clot formation in cerebral vessels.

Behavioral risk factors include obesity, physical inactivity, and oral contraceptive use.[21] In addition, increased risk of stroke is associated with hormone replacement therapy, heavy alcohol consumption, and drugs of abuse including cocaine, amphetamines, and heroin.[21,22]

Elimination or control of risk factors for stroke is essential to prevent cerebral ischemia from cerebral atherosclerosis. Primary prevention of stroke by early detection and treatment of modifiable risk factors offers significant advantages over waiting until a serious event occurs.

Ischemic Stroke

Ischemic strokes are caused by cerebrovascular obstruction by thrombosis or emboli (Fig. 16-14). Ischemic stroke is classified by mechanism and frequency: 20% large artery thrombosis (atherosclerotic disease), 25% small penetrating artery thrombosis disease (**lacunar stroke**), 20% cardiogenic embolism, 30% cryptogenic stroke (undetermined cause), and 5% other.[2]

Ischemic Penumbra in Evolving Stroke

During the evolution of a stroke, there usually is a core of dead or dying cells, surrounded by an ischemic band of minimally perfused cells called the *penumbra* (border zone). Brain cells of the penumbra receive marginal blood flow, their metabolic activities are impaired, but the structural integrity of the cell is maintained.[15] Survival of the penumbra cells depends on timely return of adequate circulation, volume of toxic products released by neighboring dying cells, degree of edema, and alterations in local blood flow. If the toxic products result in additional cell death, the border zone of dead or dying tissue enlarges, and the volume of ischemic tissue increases.

Transient Ischemic Attacks

TIA reflects a temporary disturbance in focal cerebral blood flow that reverses before infarction occurs. Causes of TIAs are similar to ischemic stroke and include atherosclerotic disease of cerebral vessels and emboli. TIAs may provide warning of impending stroke. There is a high risk of early stroke after TIA: 10% to 15% have a stroke within 3 months, with 50% occurring in 48 hours.[23] Diagnosis of TIA before a stroke may permit intervention to prevent a future stroke.

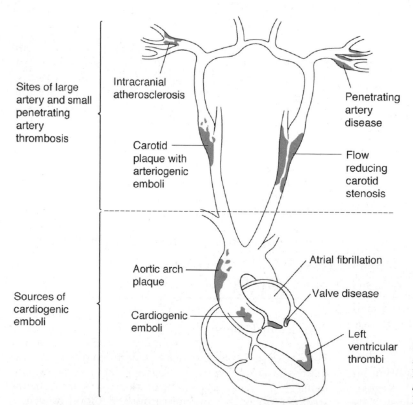

Sites of large artery and small penetrating artery thrombosis

Intracranial atherosclerosis

Carotid plaque with arteriogenic emboli

Penetrating artery disease

Flow reducing carotid stenosis

Sources of cardiogenic emboli

Aortic arch plaque

Cardiogenic emboli

Atrial fibrillation

Valve disease

Left ventricular thrombi

FIGURE 16-14. The most frequent sites of arterial and cardiac abnormalities causing ischemic stroke. (From Hickey J. V. (2014). *The clinical practice of neurological and neurosurgical nursing* (7th ed., p. 531). Philadelphia, PA: Lippincott Williams & Wilkins.)

Thrombotic Stroke

Thrombi are the most common cause of ischemic strokes, usually occurring in atherosclerotic blood vessels. In the cerebral circulation, atherosclerotic plaques are commonly found at arterial bifurcations and the larger vessels of the brain. Cerebral infarction can result from acute local thrombosis and occlusion at the site of chronic atherosclerosis, with or without embolization of the plaque material distally, or from critical perfusion failure distal to a stenosis (watershed). These infarcts often affect the cortex, causing aphasia or neglect, visual field defects, or transient monocular blindness (amaurosis fugax). In most cases of stroke, a single cerebral artery and its territories are affected. Usually, thrombotic strokes are seen in older people and frequently are accompanied by evidence of atherosclerotic heart or peripheral arterial disease.

Lacunar Stroke

Lacunar infarcts are small (1.5- to 2-cm) to very small (3- to 4-mm) infarcts located in the single deep penetrating arteries supplying the internal capsule, basal ganglia, or brain stem. They result from occlusion of the smaller penetrating branches of large cerebral arteries, commonly the middle cerebral and posterior cerebral arteries. When healing, lacunar infarcts leave behind small cavities, or *lacunae*. Because of their size and location, lacunar infarcts usually do not cause cortical deficits like aphasia or apraxia. Instead, they produce *lacunar syndromes* such as pure motor hemiplegia, pure sensory hemiplegia, and dysarthria with the clumsy hand syndrome. CT or MRI may show several lacunae and diffuse white matter changes associated with dementia.

Embolic Stroke

Although most cerebral emboli originate from a thrombus in the left heart, they may originate in an atherosclerotic plaque in the carotid arteries. The embolus travels quickly to the brain and becomes lodged in a smaller artery through which it cannot pass. The most frequent site of embolic strokes is the middle cerebral artery, reflecting its position as the carotid artery terminus. Embolic stroke usually has a sudden onset with immediate deficit.

Various cardiac conditions increase the risk of emboli formation that produces embolic stroke, including rheumatic heart disease, atrial fibrillation, recent myocardial infarction, ventricular aneurysm, mobile aortic arch atheroma, and bacterial endocarditis.

Hemorrhagic Stroke

The most frequently fatal stroke results from spontaneous rupture of a cerebral blood vessel.[24–26] The resulting intracerebral hemorrhage can cause focal hematoma, edema, compression of the brain contents, or spasm of adjacent blood vessels. Common risk factors are advancing age and hypertension. Aneurysms and arteriovenous malformations can cause sudden hemorrhage. A cerebral hemorrhage occurs suddenly, usually when the person is active. Vomiting commonly occurs initially, and headache often occurs. Focal symptoms depend on which vessel is involved. Hemorrhage into the basal ganglia results in contralateral hemiplegia, with initial flaccidity progressing to spasticity. The hemorrhage and resultant edema exert great pressure on the brain, and the clinical course progresses rapidly to coma and frequently to death.

Aneurysmal Subarachnoid Hemorrhage

Aneurysmal SAH is a hemorrhagic stroke caused by rupture of a cerebral aneurysm. Resulting bleeding into the subarachnoid space can flood into the basal cistern, ventricles, and spinal subarachnoid space.[8,11,27] An aneurysm is a bulge at the site of localized weakness in the wall of an arterial vessel. Most cerebral aneurysms are small saccular aneurysms called *berry aneurysms* that occur in the anterior circulation and are found at bifurcations and other junctions of vessels including the circle of Willis (Fig. 16-15). They are thought to arise from a congenital defect in the media of the involved vessel. Incidence is higher in polycystic kidney disease, fibromuscular dysplasia, coarctation of the aorta, and brain arteriovenous malformations.[8,11] Other causes of cerebral aneurysms are atherosclerosis, hypertension, and bacterial infection.

Rupture of a cerebral aneurysm results in SAH. Probability of rupture increases with aneurysm size.[27] Environmental factors such as cigarette smoking, hypertension, and excessive alcohol intake appear to be major risk factors for aneurysmal SAH.[27,28] Intracranial aneurysms are rare in children; the mean age for SAH is approximately 50 years. Mortality and morbidity rates with aneurysmal SAH are high. Only one third of people recover without major disability.[28]

Clinical Manifestations. Symptoms of cerebral aneurysms can be divided into two phases: those presenting before and those presenting after rupture and bleeding. Most small aneurysms are asymptomatic. Intact aneurysms frequently are found at autopsy as an incidental finding.[8] Ten percent to 20% of people with SAH have a history of atypical headaches occurring days to weeks

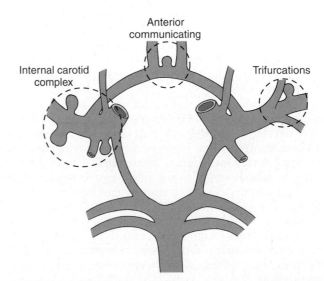

FIGURE 16-15. Common sites of berry aneurysms.

before the hemorrhage, suggesting the presence of a small leak.[27,28] These headaches are characterized by sudden onset, often accompanied by nausea, vomiting, and dizziness. Onset of subarachnoid aneurysmal rupture often is heralded by a sudden and severe headache.[27,28] If the bleeding is severe, the headache may be accompanied by collapse and loss of consciousness. Other manifestations include signs of meningeal irritation such as nuchal rigidity (neck stiffness) and photophobia; cranial nerve deficits, especially CN II, and sometimes III and IV (diplopia and blurred vision); stroke syndromes (focal motor and sensory deficits); cerebral edema and increased ICP; and pituitary dysfunction (diabetes insipidus and hyponatremia). Hypertension, a frequent finding, and cardiac arrhythmias result from massive release of catecholamines triggered by the SAH.

Diagnosis. Diagnosis of SAH and intracranial aneurysms is made by clinical presentation, noncontrast CT scan, lumbar puncture if CT is normal and suspicion of SAH is strong, and angiography.[27,28] Conventional catheter angiography is the definitive diagnostic tool for detecting the aneurysm. Magnetic resonance angiography (MRA) is noninvasive but is less sensitive. Helical (spiral) computed tomography angiography (CTA) requires intravenous contrast, but can be used in people after aneurysmal clipping, when use of MRI may be contraindicated.

Treatment. The treatment course depends on the extent of neurologic deficit. The best outcomes are achieved when the aneurysm is secured early and prevention of complications initiated.[28–30] People with mild to no neurologic deficits may undergo cerebral arteriography and early surgery within 24 to 72 hours. Surgery involves craniotomy and inserting a clip tightened around the neck of the aneurysm, which offers protection from rebleeding. Endovascular coiling is an alternative to surgery, particularly in inaccessible aneurysms or those who are poor surgical candidates. Complications of aneurysmal rupture include rebleeding, vasospasm with cerebral ischemia, hydrocephalus, hypothalamic dysfunction, and seizure activity. Rebleeding and vasospasm are the most serious and most difficult to treat. Rebleeding, which has its highest incidence on the first day after the initial rupture, results in further and usually catastrophic neurologic deficits.

Vasospasm is difficult to treat and is associated with a high incidence of morbidity and mortality. The condition develops within 3 to 10 days (peak, 7 days) after aneurysm rupture and involves a focal narrowing of the cerebral artery or arteries. Neurologic status deteriorates as blood supply to the brain in the region of the spasm is decreased, which usually can be differentiated from the rapid deterioration seen in rebleeding. Vasospasm is treated by attempting to improve CPP through vasoactive drugs or intravenous fluids to achieve euvolemia. Endovascular techniques include intraarterial vasodilators and mechanical dilation of vessels with balloon angioplasty.

Another complication of aneurysm rupture is development of hydrocephalus caused by plugging arachnoid villi with products from lysis of blood in the subarachnoid space. Hydrocephalus is diagnosed by serial CT scans showing increasing ventricle size and by signs of increased ICP. Ventriculostomy, lumbar drain, or ventriculoperitoneal shunt may be used to decrease the ICP.

Arteriovenous Malformations

Arteriovenous malformations are a tangle of abnormal arteries and veins linked by fistula(s).[2] These networks lack a capillary bed, and the small arteries have a deficient muscularis layer. Arteriovenous malformations are thought to arise from failure in development of the capillary network in the embryonic brain. As the brain grows, the malformation forms a tangled collection of thin-walled vessels that shunt blood directly from arterial to venous circulation. Arteriovenous malformations typically present before 40 years of age and affect males and females equally. Rupture of vessels causing hemorrhagic stroke accounts for approximately 1% of all strokes.[2]

Pathophysiology. There are two major hemodynamic effects of arteriovenous malformations. First, blood goes from a high-pressure arterial system to a low-pressure venous system without the buffering of the capillary network, predisposing venous channels to rupture and hemorrhage. Second, elevated arterial and venous pressures divert blood from surrounding tissue, impairing tissue perfusion.

Clinical Manifestations. The major clinical manifestations of arteriovenous malformations are intracerebral hemorrhage and SAH, seizures, headache, and progressive neurologic deficits. Headaches often are severe, described as throbbing and synchronous with their heartbeat. Other, focal symptoms depend on the location of the lesion and include visual symptoms, hemiparesis, mental deterioration, and speech deficits.

Diagnosis and Treatment. Definitive diagnosis often is made through cerebral angiography. Treatments include surgical excision, endovascular occlusion, radiosurgery, and conservative treatment.[2] Each of these methods is accompanied by a risk of complications. If the arteriovenous malformation is accessible, surgical excision usually is the treatment of choice.

Clinical Manifestations of Stroke

The specific manifestations of stroke or TIA are determined by the cerebral artery affected, the area of brain tissue supplied by the vessel, and the collateral circulation. Symptoms of stroke/TIA are sudden in onset, focal, and usually one sided. Common symptoms are a facial droop, arm weakness, and slurred speech. Other frequent stroke symptoms are unilateral numbness, vision loss in one eye or to one side, language disturbance, and sudden, unexplained imbalance or ataxia. TIA symptoms resolve spontaneously, usually within minutes, although the underlying mechanisms are the same as for stroke. Generally, carotid ischemia causes monocular visual loss or aphasia (dominant hemisphere) or hemineglect (nondominant hemisphere), contralateral sensory or motor loss, or other discrete cortical signs such as apraxia and agnosia. Vertebrobasilar ischemia induces ataxia, diplopia, **hemianopia**, vertigo, cranial nerve deficits, contralateral hemiplegia, sensory deficits, and arousal defects. Discrete subsets of these vascular syndromes usually occur, depending on which branches are blocked (Table 16-6).

Stroke-Related Motor Deficits

Motor deficits are most common, followed by deficits of language, sensation, and cognition. After a stroke affects the corticospinal tract, there is profound weakness on the contralateral side. Subcortical lesions of the corticospinal tracts cause equal weakness of the face, arm, and leg. In 6 to 8 weeks, the initial weakness and flaccidity is replaced by hyperreflexia and spasticity. Spasticity involves increased muscle tone and usually an element of weakness. Flexor muscles usually are more affected in the upper extremities and extensor muscles are more affected in the lower extremities. There is a tendency toward foot drop; outward rotation and **circumduction** of the leg with gait; flexion at the wrist, elbow, and fingers; lower facial paresis; slurred speech; Babinski sign; and dependent edema in the affected extremities. A slight corticospinal lesion may be indicated only by clumsiness in carrying out fine coordinated movements rather than obvious weakness. Passive range-of-motion exercises help to maintain joint function and prevent edema, shoulder subluxation, and muscle atrophy and may help to reestablish motor patterns. If no voluntary movement appears within a few months, significant function usually will not return.

Stroke-Related Dysarthria and Aphasia

Dysarthria is the imperfect **articulation** of speech sounds or changes in voice pitch or quality. It results from a stroke affecting muscles of the pharynx, palate, tongue, lips, or mouth and does not relate to speech content. *Aphasia* encompasses varying inabilities to comprehend, integrate, and express language. Aphasia may be localized to the dominant cerebral cortex or thalamus. In children, language dominance can shift to the unaffected hemisphere and transient language deficits after stroke. Middle cerebral artery stroke is the most common aphasia-producing stroke.

Aphasia can be receptive or expressive, or as fluent or nonfluent. Fluency is defined by the rate of speech: *fluent* denoting many words and *nonfluent* few words. Expressive or nonfluent aphasia is characterized by an inability to easily communicate spontaneously or translate thoughts or ideas into meaningful speech or writing. Speech production is effortful, halting, and often may be poorly articulated because of a concurrent dysarthria. The person may utter or write a few words, especially ones with emotional overlay. Comprehension is normal and the person seems aware of the deficits but is unable to correct them, often leading to frustration, anger, and depression.

TABLE 16-6 Signs and Symptoms of Stroke by Involved Cerebral Artery

Cerebral Artery	Brain Area Involved	Signs and Symptoms*
Anterior cerebral	Infarction of the medial aspect of one frontal lobe if lesion is distal to communicating artery; bilateral frontal infarction if flow in other anterior cerebral artery is inadequate	Paralysis of contralateral foot or leg; impaired gait; paresis of contralateral arm; contralateral sensory loss over toes, foot, and leg; problems making decisions or performing acts voluntarily; lack of spontaneity, easily distracted; slowness of thought; aphasia depends on the hemisphere involved; urinary incontinence; cognitive and affective disorders
Middle cerebral	Massive infarction of most of lateral hemisphere and deeper structures of the frontal, parietal, and temporal lobes; internal capsule; basal ganglia	Contralateral hemiplegia (face and arm); contralateral sensory impairment; aphasia; homonymous hemianopia; altered consciousness (confusion to coma); inability to turn eyes toward paralyzed side; denial of paralyzed side or limb (hemiattention); possible acalculia, alexia, finger agnosia, and left–right confusion; vasomotor paresis and instability
Posterior cerebral	Occipital lobe; anterior and medial portion of temporal lobe	Homonymous hemianopia and other visual defects such as color blindness, loss of central vision, and visual hallucinations; memory deficits, perseveration (repeated performance of same verbal or motor response)
	Thalamus involvement	Loss of all sensory modalities; spontaneous pain; intentional tremor; mild hemiparesis; aphasia
	Cerebral peduncle involvement	Oculomotor nerve palsy with contralateral hemiplegia
Basilar and vertebral	Cerebellum and brain stem	Visual disturbance such as diplopia, dystaxia, vertigo, dysphagia, dysphonia

*Depend on the hemisphere involved and adequacy of collaterals.

Fluent speech requires little or no effort, is articulate, and is of increased quantity. *Fluent* refers only to the ease and rate of output and does not relate to the content of speech or the ability of the person to comprehend what is being said. *Wernicke aphasia* is an inability to comprehend the speech of others or written material. Lesions of the posterior superior temporal or lower parietal lobe are associated with receptive, fluent aphasia. *Anomic aphasia* is a difficulty with finding singular words. *Conduction aphasia* is impaired repetition and speech riddled with letter substitutions, despite good comprehension and fluency. Conduction aphasia results from destruction of the fiber system under the insula that connects the Wernicke and Broca areas.

Stroke-Related Cognitive and Other Deficits

One distinct cognitive syndrome is hemineglect or hemi-inattention. Usually caused by strokes affecting the nondominant hemisphere, hemineglect is the inability to attend and react to stimuli from the contralateral side. People may not visually track or reach to the neglected side. They may neglect limbs, despite normal motor function, and may not shave, wash, or comb that side. Such people are unaware of this deficit (*anosognosia*). Other cognitive deficits include apraxia, agnosia, memory loss, behavioral syndromes, and depression. Sensory deficits (numbness, tingling paresthesias, or distorted sensations such as dysesthesia and neuropathic pain) affect the body contralateral to the lesion. Visual disturbances from stroke are diverse, but most common are hemianopia from a lesion of the optic radiations or monocular blindness from occlusion of the ipsilateral central retinal artery, a branch of the internal carotid.

Diagnosis and Treatment of Stroke

Diagnosis

A careful history, including previous TIAs, time of onset, specific focal symptoms (to determine likely vascular territory), and any coexisting diseases can help determine the type of stroke. Diagnostic evaluation should determine the presence of ischemia or hemorrhage, identify the stroke or TIA mechanism, characterize the severity of deficits, and unmask the presence of risk factors.

Brain imaging documents brain infarction; vascular imaging reveals anatomy and pathologic processes of related blood vessels. CT scans are necessary in the acute setting for identifying hemorrhage but are insensitive to ischemia within 24 hours and to any brain stem or small infarcts. MRI is superior for imaging ischemic lesions and differentiating nonstroke pathologic processes. MRI techniques such as perfusion- and diffusion-weighted imaging (DWI) can reveal cerebral ischemia immediately after onset and identify areas of potentially reversible damage (*i.e.*, penumbra). MR DWI is used in settings of emergency stroke evaluation to rapidly identify the area and volume of ischemia, identifying candidates for emergency treatments.

Vascular imaging is accomplished with CTA, MRA, catheter-based *conventional* arteriography, and ultrasonography. All except ultrasonography demonstrate the site of vascular abnormality (intracranial, extracranial) and visualize most intracranial vascular areas. MRA is noninvasive and widely available, but less sensitive and specific than CTA or catheter angiography. CTA is noninvasive and detailed, but is limited in availability and requires iodinated contrast, which is nephrotoxic. Catheter angiography allows visualization of collateral flow patterns but is invasive and requires significant contrast doses. CTA and MRA have largely replaced angiography for screening vascular lesions. Ultrasonographic techniques allow quick bedside assessment of the carotid bifurcation or of flow velocities in the cerebral circulation.

Treatment

Salvaging brain tissue, preventing secondary stroke, and minimizing long-term disability are the treatment goals for an acute ischemic stroke. Stroke care has shifted from the nearest hospital to certified *stroke centers*. Certification establishes that a hospital can manage people with stroke with appropriate care from emergency treatments, through inpatient stay, and rehabilitation.

Stroke care begins with emergency treatments aimed at reversing the evolving ischemic brain injury. There is a window during which ischemic but viable brain tissue can be salvaged. Reperfusion techniques and neuroprotective strategies are used in the early treatment of ischemic stroke. Reperfusion techniques include thrombolytic drugs (intravenous or intraarterial), catheter-directed mechanical clot disruption, and augmentation of CPP during acute stroke.

The only agent approved by the US Food and Drug Administration for the treatment of acute ischemic stroke is tissue plasminogen activator (tPA). A subcommittee of the Stroke Council of the American Heart Association has developed guidelines, which recommend that in suspected stroke, diagnosis of hemorrhagic stroke be excluded via CT before thrombolytic therapy, which must be given within 3 hours of onset of symptoms. The major risk of treatment with thrombolytic agents is ICH. A number of conditions, including therapeutic levels of oral anticoagulant medications, history of gastrointestinal or urinary tract bleeding in the previous 21 days, prior stroke or head injury within 3 months, major surgery in the past 14 days, and a blood pressure greater than 185/110 mm Hg, are considered contraindications to intravenous thrombolytic therapy.[14] A longer time window for treatment with tPA has been tested formally and should be administered to eligible people who can be treated in the time period of 3 to 4.5 hours after stroke.[31]

Emerging treatments for ischemic stroke include catheter-based methods to allow recanalization of a visualized cerebral clot with intraarterial techniques. The specialist may mechanically disrupt the clot, deliver thrombolytic drug intraarterially at the clot surface, or stent intracranial vessels to restore flow. Person selection is stringent for these invasive methods, but people can be treated past the 3-hour time window for intravenous tPA. These methods require experienced interventional angiography teams and remain limited to tertiary care centers. Other experimental treatments include neuro-protection with drugs that limit the calcium cascade (see Fig. 16-5) and treatments like hypothermia to decrease brain metabolic demands in ischemia.

Poststroke treatment aims to prevent recurrent stroke and medical complications and promote fullest possible recovery of function. Risk of stroke recurrence is highest in the first week after stroke or TIA, so early implementation of antiplatelet agents in most cases, or warfarin in cardioembolic stroke, is imperative. Long-term stroke recurrence is most effectively prevented with reduction of risk factors, primarily hypertension, diabetes, smoking, and hyperlipidemia. In carotid territory stroke with carotid stenosis, revascularization with surgery or stenting should be considered. Early hospital care requires careful prevention of aspiration, deep vein thrombosis, and falls. Recovery is maximized with early and aggressive rehabilitation efforts that include the rehabilitation team and the family. The successful treatment of stroke depends on education of the public, paramedics, and health care professionals about the need for early diagnosis and treatment, and for risk factor reduction and prevention. Prevention is key; treat stroke symptoms as an emergency. Effective procedures may preserve brain function and prevent disability.

SUMMARY CONCEPTS

A stroke is an acute focal neurologic deficit caused by a vascular disorder that injures brain tissue. It is the fifth leading cause of death in the United States and a major cause of disability. Ischemic stroke, which is the most common type of stroke, is caused by cerebrovascular obstruction by a thrombus or emboli. Hemorrhagic stroke, which is associated with greater morbidity and mortality, is caused by the rupture of a blood vessel and bleeding into the brain.

One form of hemorrhagic stroke, known as aneurysmal SAH, results from a ruptured cerebral aneurysm. Presenting symptoms include worst headache of life, nuchal rigidity, photophobia, and nausea. Complications include rebleeding, vasospasm, and hydrocephalus.

Arteriovenous malformations are congenital abnormal communications between arterial and venous channels that result from failure in development of the capillary network in the embryonic brain. The vessels in the arteriovenous malformations may enlarge to form a space-occupying lesion, become weak and predisposed to bleeding, and divert blood away from other parts of the brain; they can cause brain hemorrhage, seizures, headache, and neurologic deficits.

The acute manifestations of stroke depend on the location of the blood vessel that is involved and can include motor, sensory, language, speech, and cognitive disorders. Early diagnosis and treatment with thrombolytic agents can prevent disabling brain injury from ischemic stroke. Treatment of long-term neurologic deficits from stroke is primarily symptomatic, involving the combined efforts of the health care team, the person who has had stroke, and the family.

Infections and Neoplasms

Infections

CNS infections are classified according to the structure involved: meninges (meningitis), brain parenchyma (encephalitis), spinal cord (myelitis), and brain and spinal cord (encephalomyelitis).

Infections also may be classified by the type of invading organism, including bacterial, viral, fungal, or other. In general, pathogens enter the CNS through the bloodstream by crossing the blood–brain barrier or by direct invasion through skull fracture or a bullet hole or, rarely, by contamination during surgery or lumbar puncture.

Meningitis

Meningitis is an inflammation of the pia mater, the arachnoid, and the CSF-filled subarachnoid space. Inflammation spreads rapidly because of CSF circulation around the brain and spinal cord. Inflammation usually is caused by an infection, but chemical meningitis can occur. Two types of acute infectious meningitis are acute purulent meningitis (usually bacterial) and acute lymphocytic (usually viral) meningitis.[8] Factors responsible for severity include virulence factors of the pathogen, host factors, brain edema, and permanent neurologic sequelae.

Bacterial Meningitis

Most cases of bacterial meningitis are caused by *Streptococcus pneumoniae* (pneumococcus) or *Neisseria meningitidis* (meningococcus), except in neonates (usually group B streptococci).[32] Other pathogens that cause infection are gram-negative bacilli and *Listeria monocytogenes*.

Epidemics of meningococcal meningitis occur when people reside in close contact. The very young and the old are at highest risk for pneumococcal meningitis. Risk factors associated with contracting meningitis include head trauma with basilar skull fractures, otitis media, sinusitis or mastoiditis, neurosurgery, dermal sinus tracts, systemic sepsis, or immunocompromise.

Pathophysiology. In the pathophysiologic process of bacterial meningitis, the bacteria replicate and undergo lysis in the CSF, releasing endotoxins or cell wall fragments. These initiate release of inflammatory mediators, which permits pathogens, neutrophils, and albumin to move across the capillary wall into the CSF. As the pathogens enter the subarachnoid space, they cause inflammation and a cloudy, purulent exudate. Thrombophlebitis of bridging veins and dural sinuses or obliteration of arterioles by inflammation may develop, causing vascular congestion and infarction in the surrounding tissues. The meninges thicken and adhesions form, which may impinge on cranial nerves, giving rise to cranial nerve palsies, or may impair CSF outflow, causing hydrocephalus.

Clinical Manifestations. Common symptoms of acute bacterial meningitis are fever and chills; headache; stiff neck; back, abdominal, and extremity pain; and nausea and vomiting.[9] Other signs include seizures, cranial nerve palsies, and focal cerebral signs. Meningococcal meningitis causes a petechial rash with palpable purpura in most people. The petechiae vary from pinhead to large ecchymoses, or areas of skin gangrene. Other types of meningitis also may produce a petechial rash. People infected with *Haemophilus influenzae* or *S. pneumoniae* may present with difficulty in arousal and seizures, and those with *N. meningitidis* infection may present with delirium or coma.[33] The development of brain edema, hydrocephalus, or increased cerebral blood flow can increase ICP.

Meningeal signs (*e.g.*, photophobia and nuchal rigidity) also may be present. The Kernig sign is resistance to knee extension while the person is lying with the hip flexed at a right angle. The Brudzinski sign is when flexion of the neck induces flexion of the hip and knee. These postures reflect resistance to painful stretching of inflamed meninges from the lumbar level to the head. Cranial nerve damage and hydrocephalus may occur as complications of pyogenic meningitis.

Diagnosis. Diagnosis is based on history, physical examination, and laboratory data. Lumbar puncture showing a cloudy, purulent CSF under increased pressure is necessary for accurate diagnosis. CSF contains large numbers of polymorphonuclear neutrophils (up to 90,000/mm^3), increased protein content, and reduced sugar content. Bacteria can be visualized and cultured. Previous antibiotic use limits culture sensitivities, in which case latex agglutination or polymerase chain reaction testing for *N. meningitidis*, *H. influenzae*, and *Listeria* species can be used. Complications associated with lumbar puncture include life-threatening cerebral herniation, and people who are at risk (*i.e.*, immunocompromised, a seizure within a week, papilledema, or specific neurologic abnormalities) should have a CT scan before the procedure.

Treatment. Treatment includes urgent antibiotics while diagnostic testing ensues.[2,9,18,33] Delay in antimicrobial therapy can result in poor outcomes.[3,33] Initial antibiotics include broad-spectrum coverage with a third-generation cephalosporin, vancomycin, and ampicillin. Adjustment of antibiotics is driven by results of CSF cultures. Effective antibiotics produce lysis of the pathogen, which produces inflammatory mediators that may exacerbate the abnormalities of the blood–brain barrier. To suppress this inflammation, adjunctive corticosteroid therapy is increasingly administered with or just before the first dose of antibiotics.[2,9,18,32]

People who have been exposed to someone with meningococcal meningitis should be treated prophylactically with antibiotics.[32] Effective polysaccharide vaccines are available to protect against meningococcal groups A, C, Y, and W-135. Vaccines are recommended for military recruits and college students, who are at increased risk for invasive meningococcal disease.

Viral Meningitis

Viral meningitis is similar to bacterial meningitis, but the course is less severe and CSF findings are markedly different. There are lymphocytes in the fluid, the protein content is only moderately elevated, and the sugar content usually is normal. The acute viral meningitides are self-limited and usually require only symptomatic treatment, except for herpes simplex virus (HSV) type 2, which responds to intravenous acyclovir. Viral meningitis can be caused by many viruses, most often enteroviruses, including coxsackievirus, poliovirus, and echovirus. Others include Epstein–Barr virus, mumps virus, HSV, and West Nile virus. Although often the virus cannot be identified, newer assays may allow for rapid identification of viral ribonucleic acid in CSF.

Encephalitis

Encephalitis is a generalized infection of the brain or spinal cord parenchyma, usually due to a virus. Encephalitis may also be caused by bacteria, fungi, and other organisms. The mode of transmission may be a mosquito bite (arbovirus), a rabid animal (rabies virus), or ingestion (poliovirus). Common causes in the United States are HSV and West Nile virus. Less frequent causes are toxic substances such as ingested lead and vaccines for measles and mumps.

Pathology of encephalitis includes local necrotizing hemorrhage, which becomes generalized, with prominent edema. There is progressive degeneration of nerve cell bodies. Histology may reveal specific characteristics: poliovirus destroys cells of the anterior horn of the spinal cord.

Encephalitis is characterized by fever, headache, and nuchal rigidity. People also experience neurologic disturbances, such as lethargy, disorientation, seizures, focal paralysis, delirium, and coma. Diagnosis is made by clinical history, presenting symptoms, and traditional CSF studies.

Brain Tumors

Primary brain tumors account for 2% of cancer deaths. The American Cancer Society estimates 23,820 new cases and over 17,760 deaths from brain and other nervous system cancers in 2019.[34] Metastases to the brain develop in 10% to 15% of people with cancer.[9] In children, primary brain tumors are second only to leukemia, and mortality rate approaches 30%.[34,35]

Types of Tumors

For most neoplasms, *malignant* describes the tumor's lack of cell differentiation, invasive nature, and ability to metastasize. In the brain, a well-differentiated and histologically benign tumor may grow and cause death because of its location. Benign tumors infiltrate the normal brain tissue, preventing total resection and allowing for tumor recurrence. Classification of brain tumors is based on histopathologic characteristics. The World Health Organization classification system is widely used.[2,9]

Brain tumors can be divided into: (1) primary intracranial tumors of neuroepithelial tissue, (2) primary intracranial tumors that originate in the skull cavity but are not derived from the brain tissue itself, and (3) metastatic tumors.[11]

Collectively, neoplasms of astrocytic origin are the most common type of primary brain tumor in adults, followed by primary CNS lymphoma.

Glial Tumors

Glial tumors are divided into astrocytic and oligodendroglial. Astrocytic tumors can be subdivided into fibrillary (infiltrating) astrocytic tumors and pilocytic astrocytomas.

Fibrillary or diffuse astrocytomas account for 80% of adult primary brain tumors. They are most common in middle age, with peak incidence of anaplastic astrocytomas occurring in the sixth decade. Although usually found in the cerebral hemispheres, they can also occur in the cerebellum, brain stem, or spinal cord. Astrocytomas of the cerebral hemispheres commonly are divided into three grades of increasing pathologic anaplasia and rapidity of progression: well-differentiated lesions (*astrocytomas*); intermediate-grade tumors (*anaplastic astrocytomas*); and the least differentiated and most aggressive glioma (*glioblastoma multiforme*). Clinically, infiltrating astrocytic tumors present with symptoms of increased ICP or focal abnormalities related to their position.

Pilocytic astrocytomas are characterized by their cellular appearance and benign behavior. Typically, they occur in children and young adults and are located in the cerebellum, but also can be found in the walls of the third ventricle, the optic chiasm and nerves, and the cerebral hemispheres. Prognosis is better for surgically resectable tumors, such as those in the cerebellar cortex, than for less accessible tumors, such as those involving the hypothalamus or brain stem.

Oligodendrogliomas are tumors of the oligodendrocytes or their precursors, or with histologic features representing both oligodendrocytes and astrocytes. They represent 5% to 20% of glial tumors and are most common in middle life.[36] Prognosis is less predictable than for people with infiltrating astrocytomas. It depends on the histologic grade of the tumor, its location, and recognition of molecular features that can be linked to chemosensitivity.[36] Oligodendroglial tumors are prone to spontaneous hemorrhage owing to their delicate vasculature.

Ependymomas

Ependymomas are derived from the single layer of epithelium that lines the ventricles and spinal canal. They are more common in children and affect the ventricle lining. They constitute 12% of all adult CNS tumors and commonly affect the spinal cord.[36] Clinical features depend on location: intracranial tumors are often associated with hydrocephalus and increased ICP.

Meningiomas

Meningiomas develop from the meningothelial cells of the arachnoid and are outside the brain. Onset is usually in the middle or later years of life and constitute 35% of primary brain tumors in this age group.[36] They are slow-growing, well-circumscribed, often highly vascular tumors. They usually are benign, and complete removal is possible if it does not involve vital structures.

Primary Central Nervous System Lymphomas

Primary CNS lymphoma accounts for 4% of all CNS tumors. These deep, periventricular, and diffuse tumors are common in immunocompromised people and are associated with Epstein–Barr virus. Most are malignant, and recurrence is common despite treatment. Behavioral and cognitive changes, hemiparesis, and aphasia are common symptoms. Visual field deficits occur in 20% of people.[36] Biopsy is usually performed, and then the lymphoma is treated with chemotherapy.

Etiology

High-dose irradiation increases the risk of gliomas, meningiomas, and nerve sheath tumors. Acquired immune suppression also increases the risk of primary CNS lymphoma. Other environmental risk factors and occupational exposures have not been convincingly demonstrated to increase the risk of brain tumors.[18] Several genetic syndromes increase the risk of brain tumors like neurofibromatosis type 1 and 2, Li–Fraumeni syndrome, tuberous sclerosis, von Hippel–Lindau syndrome, and Burkitt syndrome.[18]

Clinical Manifestations

Intracranial tumors give rise to focal disturbances in brain function, which occur because of brain compression, tumor infiltration, disturbances in blood flow, and brain edema and increased ICP.

Tumors may be located intra-axially (*i.e.*, within brain tissue) or extra-axially (*i.e.*, outside brain tissue, but within the cranium). Disturbances in brain function are greatest with fast-growing, infiltrative, intra-axial tumors because of compression, infiltration, and necrosis. Extra-axial tumors, such as meningiomas, may reach a large size without producing signs and symptoms. Cysts may form in tumors and contribute to brain compression. General symptoms include headache, nausea, vomiting, mental changes, papilledema, visual disturbances, alterations in sensory and motor function, and seizures. Brain tumors cause a generalized increase in ICP when they reach sufficient size or produce edema. Cerebral edema usually is of the vasogenic type, which develops around tumors and is characterized by increased brain water and expanded extracellular fluid. Tumors can also obstruct CSF flow in ventricular cavities and produce hydrocephalic dilation of the proximal ventricles and atrophy of the cerebral hemispheres. With very slow-growing tumors, complete compensation of ventricular volumes can occur, but with rapidly growing tumors, increased ICP is an early sign. Depending on the location, brain displacement and herniation of the uncus or cerebellum may occur.

Headache that accompanies brain tumors results from compression or distortion of pain-sensitive dural or vascular structures. It may be felt on the same side of the head as the tumor, but more commonly is diffuse. In the early stages, the headache is mild and occurs in the morning on awakening and improves with head elevation. The headache becomes more constant as the tumor enlarges and often is worsened by coughing, bending, or sudden movements of the head.

Vomiting occurs with or without nausea, may be projectile, and is a common symptom of increased ICP and brain stem compression. Papilledema (edema of the optic disk) results from increased ICP and obstruction of the CSF pathways. It is associated with decreased visual acuity, diplopia, and deficits in the visual fields. Visual defects associated with papilledema often are the reason people with brain tumor seek medical care.

People with brain tumors often are irritable initially and later become quiet and apathetic. They may become forgetful, seem preoccupied, and appear to be psychologically depressed. Because of the mental changes, a psychiatric consultation may be sought before a diagnosis is made.

Focal symptoms are determined by the location. Frontal lobe tumors may grow to a large size, increase ICP, and cause signs of generalized brain dysfunction before focal signs are recognized. Tumors that impinge on the visual system cause visual loss or visual field defects before developing generalized signs. Temporal lobe tumors often produce seizures as their first symptom. Smell or hearing hallucinations and déjà vu phenomena are common focal manifestations of temporal lobe tumors. Brain stem tumors often produce upper and lower motor neuron signs that occur with or without involvement of sensory or motor tracts. Cerebellar tumors often cause ataxia of gait.

Diagnosis and Treatment

Diagnosis of brain tumors is mainly done with MRI. Gadolinium-enhanced MRI is the test of choice for identifying and localizing the presence and extent of tumor involvement. Diagnostic maneuvers that suggest a possible tumor and indicate the need for MRI include physical and neurologic examinations and visual field and funduscopic examination. Cerebral angiography can visualize the tumor's vascular supply, which is important when planning surgery. Positron emission tomography characterizes the metabolic properties of the tumor, which is useful in planning treatment.[18] MRA and CTA can distinguish vascular masses from tumors.

The general methods for the treatment of brain tumors are surgery, irradiation, and chemotherapy. Surgery is part of the initial management of all brain tumors; it establishes the diagnosis and achieves tumor removal in many cases. The degree of removal may be limited by the location of the tumor and its invasiveness. Stereotactic surgery uses three-dimensional coordinates and CT and MRI to localize a brain lesion precisely. Ultrasonographic technology localizes and removes tumors. The ultrasonic aspirator combines a vibrating head with suction and permits atraumatic removal of tumors from cranial nerves and important cortical areas. Intraoperative monitoring of evoked potentials is an important adjunct to some types of surgery. Evoked potentials can monitor auditory, visual, speech, or motor responses during surgery done under local anesthesia.

Most malignant brain tumors respond to external irradiation. Irradiation can increase longevity and can allay symptoms when tumors recur. Treatment dose depends on the tumor's histologic type, radioresponsiveness, and anatomic site and on the level of tolerance of the surrounding tissue. Radiation therapy is avoided in children younger than 2 years because of the long-term effects, which include developmental delay, panhypopituitarism, and secondary tumors.

Chemotherapy for brain tumors is somewhat limited by the blood–brain barrier, but can be an adjunct to surgery and radiation therapy. Agents can be administered intravenously, intraarterially, intrathecally, or intraventricularly and is standard of care for high-grade gliomas.[9]

 SUMMARY CONCEPTS

CNS infections may be classified according to the structures involved or the organism causing the infection. Damage may predispose to hydrocephalus, seizures, or other neurologic defects.

Brain tumors account for 2% of all cancer deaths and are the second most common type of cancer in children. Tumors from other parts of the body often metastasize to the brain. Primary brain tumors can arise from any structure in the cranial cavity. Most begin in brain tissue, but the pituitary, the pineal region, and the meninges also are sites of tumor development. Brain tumors cause focal disturbances in brain function and increased ICP. The clinical manifestations of brain tumor depend on the size and location of the tumor. General signs and symptoms include headache, nausea, vomiting, mental changes, papilledema, visual disturbances, alterations in motor and sensory function, and seizures. Diagnostic tests include physical examination, visual field testing and funduscopic examination, CT scans, MRI studies, brain scans, and cerebral angiography. Treatment includes surgery, radiation therapy, and chemotherapy.

Seizure Disorders

A seizure represents the abnormal behavior caused by an electrical discharge from neurons. A seizure is a discrete clinical event with associated symptoms that vary according to the site of abnormality. Manifestations generally include sensory, motor, autonomic, or psychic phenomena. Americans have a 10% chance of experiencing a seizure in their lifetime.[9] Seizure activity is commonly encountered in pediatric neurology, and among adults its incidence is exceeded only by cerebrovascular disorders. The first seizure episode usually occurs before 20 years of age. After 20 years, a seizure is often caused by structural change, trauma, tumor, or stroke.

Seizures may occur during all serious illnesses or injuries affecting the brain including metabolic derangements, infections, tumors, drug abuse, vascular lesions, congenital deformities, and brain injury. A seizure is a single event of abnormal discharge that results in an abrupt, altered state of function.[2] Epilepsy is a chronic disorder of recurrent seizures.[2]

KEY POINTS

Seizures

- Focal seizures begin in a specific area of the cerebral hemisphere. Focal seizures are without impairment of consciousness (aware) or with impaired consciousness (impaired awareness).
- Generalized seizures begin simultaneously in both cerebral hemispheres. They include unconsciousness and involve varying bilateral degrees of symmetric motor responses without localization to one hemisphere. These seizures are divided into motor and nonmotor.

Etiology

Seizures may be caused by alterations in cell membrane permeability or ion distribution across cell membranes. Another cause may be decreased inhibition or structural changes that alter the excitability. Neurotransmitter imbalances have been proposed as causes. Certain epilepsy syndromes have been linked to specific genetic mutations causing ion channel defects.[37]

Classification

The International Classification of Epileptic Seizures determines seizure type by clinical symptoms and EEG activity. It divides seizures into two broad categories:

- Focal onset, in which the seizure begins in a specific or focal area of one cerebral hemisphere
- Generalized onset, which begins simultaneously in both cerebral hemispheres[38] (Chart 16-1)

CHART 16-1

CLASSIFICATION OF SEIZURES

Focal Onset
- Without impairment of consciousness or awareness (aware)
- With impairment of consciousness or awareness (impaired awareness)

Motor Onset
- Automatisms
- Atonic
- Clonic
- Epileptic spasms
- Hyperkinetic
- Myoclonic
- Tonic

Nonmotor Onset
- Autonomic
- Behavior arrest
- Cognitive
- Emotional
- Sensory

Generalized Onset
Motor
- Tonic–clonic
- Clonic
- Tonic
- Myoclonic
- Myoclonic–tonic–clonic
- Myoclonic–tonic
- Atonic
- Epileptic spasms

Nonmotor (absence)
- Typical
- Atypical
- Myoclonic
- Eyelid myoclonia

Unknown Onset
Motor
- Tonic–clonic
Epileptic spasm
Nonmotor
- Behavior arrest

From Fisher R. S., Cross J. H., French J. A., et al. (2017). Operational classification of seizure types by the International League Against Epilepsy. Epilepsia 58(4), 522–530. Copyright © 2017 International League Against Epilepsy. Reprinted by permission of John Wiley & Sons, Inc.

The purpose of this chapter is to present both the pathophysiology of common psychiatric disorders, also referred to as mental illness, and disorders of memory and cognition. These disorders are characterized by imbalances of thought, mood, and/or behaviors, which interfere with people's ability to function. The *Diagnostic and Statistical Manual of Mental Disorders*, Fifth Edition (*DSM-5*) is an evidence-based manual recognizing 297 different diagnoses of mental illness.[1] Please consult the *DSM-5* for specific criteria for each disorder discussed in this chapter. There is a 17.9% prevalence of mental illness among US adults,[2] highlighting the need for a clear understanding of these disorders and appropriate evidence-based treatments.

Psychiatric Disorders

Incidence and Prevalence

Mental health affects how well our brain and body function, how we handle stress, and how we relate to others, and it also affects our ability to work and enjoy life. Mental illness is common among Americans, with one in five experiencing the consequences of a psychiatric disorder in any given year. One in 25 adults lives with serious mental illness, such as schizophrenia, bipolar disorder, or major depression. Children are not exempt. Fifty percent of all chronic mental illness begins before age 14 years, and 75% begins by age 24 years.[3] Importantly, 30% of people with a physical disorder have a coexisting psychiatric disorder.[4] Fifty percent of people with a substance use disorder (SUD) have a coexisting psychiatric disorder.[2,3]

The Diagnosis of Psychiatric Disorders

Psychiatric diagnoses are made using the *DSM-5*.[1] These disorders consist of symptom categories or syndromes of observable traits often occurring together. A different international coding system developed by the World Health Organization, the *International Statistical Classification of Diseases and Related Health Problems* (*ICD-10*), corresponds with some of the *DSM-5* codes.[5] Psychopathology is determined by symptoms relying on subjective judgments, based on social norms. Neuroimaging and other diagnostic tests are generally performed to rule out neurologic or medical conditions, which may be causing symptoms but are generally not diagnostic of the psychiatric disorder.

Understanding Psychiatric Disorders

There is increasing evidence that psychiatric disorders can be caused by multiple causes: biologic, psychological, and environmental conditions or a combination of these factors. Biologic factors consist of genetics, infections, brain defects or injury, poor nutrition, exposure to toxins, or abnormalities in fetal development. Psychological factors include stress, early loss of a parent, or neglect. Environmental factors may involve dysfunctional family dynamics, cultural expectations, and substance use.

The Role of Genetics

Epigenetics, the study of heritable changes in gene expression not involving changes to the underlying deoxyribonucleic acid (DNA) sequence, involves a change in phenotype without a change in genotype, which affects how cells read genes without changing the DNA. Endophenotype is a term used to describe specific phenotypes with a clear genetic connection to psychiatric illness. Research using endophenotypes suggests that multiple pathways contribute to psychiatric diagnosis.[6–11]

The Stress–Diathesis Theory

The stress–diathesis model of psychiatric disorders evolved from a recognition that genetics (diathesis) and environment (stress) both contribute to the development of psychiatric disorders.[10] Large-scale epidemiologic and case-control studies suggest that trauma because of a variety of reasons underlies a wide range of psychiatric disorders as well as medical illness.[12] The body's response and the long-term consequences of a disturbing event depend on a multitude of factors, such as age, developmental stage, coping skills, support system, cognitive deficits, preexisting neural physiology, and the nature of the trauma.[13]

The incidence of mental health problems such as obesity, sexually transmitted diseases, alcoholism, severe and persistent mental illness, psychosis, substance abuse, eating disorders, anxiety, and depression has been significantly and positively correlated with what is termed adverse childhood experiences (ACE). Prospective studies involving ACE confirm that those with episodes of maternal neglect, and physical and sexual abuse were almost three times as likely to experience major depression by their early 30s. These study participants were at risk for high inflammation levels (high-sensitivity C-reactive protein level >3 mg/L) and clustering of metabolic risk biomarkers (obesity, high blood pressure, high total cholesterol, low high-density lipoprotein cholesterol, high glycated hemoglobin, and low maximum oxygen consumption levels). These physiologic changes predispose a person to develop cardiovascular disease, doubling the risk of heart disease.[14] Long-term emotional, immune, and metabolic changes result from exposure to adverse psychosocial experiences in childhood.

Researchers have found that the key pathway for these physiologic changes is the complex bodily reactions to the stress response. Trauma is different from stress. Trauma refers to events leaving a person helpless. Stress refers to a state of burdened response to outside stressors, resulting in deterioration and dysfunction. Stress responses are beneficial in mobilizing the body for action, but prolonged activation of the stress response, particularly in early childhood, leads to profound long-term physical changes. Early adversity has been found to alter the DNA in the brain through a process called methylation. Methyl groups affix genes that govern the production of stress hormone receptors in the brain, preventing the brain from regulating its response to stress. Research evidence suggests exposure to stress can induce long-lasting changes in DNA methylation and its relationship to the pathogenesis of some psychiatric disorders.[6,15]

Parental nurturing can mediate this epigenetic response. In the absence of nurturing, children have difficulties with attention and following directions. As teenagers, they are more likely to engage in high-risk behavior and, as adults, show increased aggression, impulsive behavior, weakened cognition, and an inability to discriminate between real and imagined threats. Traumatic events and prolonged stress are thought to underlie or contribute to a wide range of psychiatric disorders and medical problems.[16]

Information Processing

Information processing systems are distributed throughout the brain and display synchronized oscillations. This synchronization allows for the creation of neural temporal maps; thus, perception, memory, cognition, emotion, language, and sensations result from the interactions between these systems of neural networks.

Neuroplasticity is the capacity of the nervous system to change its structure and function in response to biologic, psychological, and environmental events. Psychopathology is thought to result when there is a dysregulation disrupting the integration of neural networks and plasticity. The more intense the arousal of the amygdala, the stronger the memory imprint, and the less likely the experience is processed. Neuronal circuits connect the amygdala to the prefrontal lobe in the cortex, serving as the translator of the emotion so amygdala activation can be modulated.[17–19]

Perception is the final stage of information processing. Perception consists of the input of sensory information from the outside world and the processing of this information into meaning. All sensory information from the external world is transmitted to the thalamus and then projected to the somatosensory cortex and prefrontal association area. The prefrontal association area keeps track of where information has been put in long-term memory and is responsible for retrieving and then integrating memories with sensory input for decision making. It is the conscious awareness of sensory stimuli that results in behavioral responses to the sensation. For people with trauma, brain injury, or degenerative changes, information processing and cognitive function may be impaired.[18,19]

Neurochemicals

Neurochemicals and neurohormones play key roles in mediating endocrine and behavioral responses to stress. These messenger substances are made of amino acids and include hormones in the endocrine system, neurotransmitters in the autonomic nervous system, immune cells, and neuropeptides. Genes are turned off and on by these messenger molecules, with more than 300 messenger molecules identified. Neurotransmitters, important in the development and treatment of psychiatric disorders, are acetylcholine (ACh), dopamine (DA), glutamate, γ-aminobutyric acid (GABA), norepinephrine (NE), epinephrine, and serotonin (5-HT). Neurotransmission involves several discrete steps including synthesis, storage and release, binding to receptors on the postsynaptic membrane, and removal of the transmitter from the synaptic cleft.[19,20]

An outline of selected neurochemical response patterns in stress and potential psychiatric disorders is included in Table 18-1.[18–20]

TABLE 18-1 Neurochemicals and Possible Disorders of Thought, Emotion, and Memory

Neurochemicals	Proposed Action	Brain Region	Psychiatric Disorder
Acetylcholine	Excitatory or inhibitory Learning and memory	Basal ganglia Motor cortex	Neurocognitive disorders (NCDs)
Dopamine	Involuntary motor movement Mood states Reward systems Judgment	Substantia nigra Ventral segmental area of midbrain	Schizophrenia Mood disorders Anxiety disorders Substance use disorders NCDs
Norepinephrine and epinephrine	Learning and memory Reward systems	Sympathetic nervous system	Mood disorders Anxiety disorder
Serotonin	Appetite, sleep, and mood Hallucinations Pain perception	Raphe nucleus in the brain stem	Schizophrenia Mood disorders Anxiety disorders NCDs

(continued)

TABLE 18-1 Neurochemicals and Possible Disorders of Thought, Emotion, and Memory (*continued*)

Neurochemicals	Proposed Action	Brain Region	Psychiatric Disorder
Amino acids γ-Aminobutyric acid, glutamate, aspartate, and glycine	Inhibits excitability of neurons	Throughout brain	Schizophrenia Mood disorders Anxiety disorders Substance use disorders NCDs
Corticotropin-releasing hormone	Activates fear behaviors Increases motor activity	Hypothalamic–pituitary–adrenal axis	Mood disorders
Cortisol	Mobilizes energy Increases arousal	Hypothalamus	Mood disorders
DHEA	Neuroprotective Positive mood effect	Hypothalamus	Mood disorders
Enkephalins	Nociception	Central nervous system	Substance use disorders

DHEA, dehydroepiandrosterone.

Neurohormonal factors mediate behavioral responses to stress. There is considerable evidence that the regulation of corticotropin-releasing hormone (CRH) and the hypothalamic–pituitary–adrenal (HPA) axis is essential for adaptation to stress, and traumatic experiences early in life are particularly disruptive to these systems. Elevation of CRH because of trauma early in life may cause long-term pathophysiologic changes.[21]

Memory

Memory can be classified as immediate, recent, or remote.[19] Immediate memory is typically confined to remembering information for a period of several seconds to minutes. It is thought memories involve implicit information with respect to the ability to pay attention. Recent memory encompasses remembering something from minutes to days, whereas long-term memory, which lasts for years, is generally thought to result from actual structural changes in the synapses. Brain structures critical to the formation of memories include the amygdala, the hippocampus, the prefrontal cortex, and the cerebellum.[19]

Memory is stored in neural networks across the brain, and these connections are linked together and organized around associated emotions, thoughts, images, and sensations. These interconnected biochemical and neuronal networks serve as templates for future experiences depending on how the memory was perceived and stored in the brain. Pathways of neurons are shaped by experience and continually revised by new and ongoing experiences depending on plasticity of the specific brain structure.

Behavior is altered by environmental cues processed through learning and memory. Learning changes the pattern of receptors in the information network. There are two forms of memory: implicit memory, which is largely unconscious and includes somatic, motor, emotional, and procedural memories, and explicit memory, which is involved with processing the factual knowledge of people, places, and things and its meaning. People with psychiatric disorders not only experience specific cortical dysfunctions but may have trouble in the proposed pathways for learning and memory.

Thought processes involve a pattern of stimuli from many parts of the nervous system at the same time and in a definite sequence. Each thought requires simultaneous input from portions of the cerebral cortex, the thalamus, the limbic system, and the reticular formation in the brain stem. The prefrontal association cortex processes information from many areas of the brain, is necessary to achieve thinking, and can keep track of bits of information and recall them simultaneously from working memory. This allows planning, goal setting, and problem solving. Thoughts are expressed in the form of language through the functions of the left hemisphere, the Broca area in the frontal lobe for word formation, and the Wernicke area in the temporal lobe for language comprehension.[19] Figure 18-1 illustrates the four lobes of the cerebral cortex.

One of the most important structures in the brain processing memory is the hippocampus. This structure of the brain is not fully developed until between 16 and 18 months of age. It is here, deep in the limbic brain, where information from the neocortex is processed, transmitted, and integrated.[22] The hippocampus is important for explicit memory, reality testing, and inhibition of the amygdala. Research has found the size of the amygdala and hippocampus is significantly reduced for those who have been significantly traumatized.[17] The excessive stimulation of the amygdala interferes with hippocampal functioning, so the ability to accurately describe the traumatic experience is impaired.

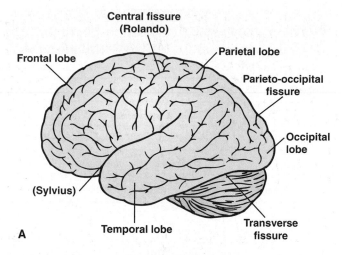

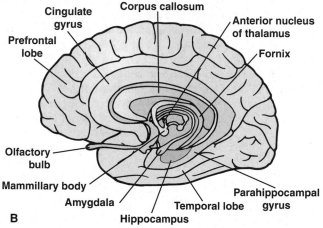

FIGURE 18-1. (**A**) Lateral aspects of the cerebral hemispheres, including the frontal, temporal, parietal, and occipital lobes. (**B**) The structure of the limbic cortex, which includes the limbic cortex (cingulate gyrus, parahippocampal gyrus, hippocampus) and associated subcortical structures (thalamus, hypothalamus, amygdala).

This inability to integrate the traumatic memory into a coherent narrative may leave a person with images and sensations without the words, and/or there may only be a somatic memory of the experience. The decreased functioning and size of the hippocampus is thought to result in behavioral disinhibition and an inability to learn from experience.

Another important structure with respect to memory is the cerebellum, the largest structure in the brain. The cerebellum is activated when information processing and semantic memory occur. The cerebellum is important in memory because it allows for attention to be shifted rapidly, accurately, smoothly, and efficiently.[23] Figure 18-2 illustrates brain structures important for memory and information processing.

SUMMARY CONCEPTS

Because the brain integrates the processes of learning, memory, and emotions, symptoms may be somatic, cognitive, and/or emotional impairment or a combination of all these dimensions. People with psychiatric disorders and brain injuries often experience difficulty in the proposed pathways for learning and memory. These difficulties are likely to influence behavior and can result in significant problems in daily living and functioning in relationships and work. An increased understanding of the complex interactions among the different parts of the brain will assist in the development of more effective psychotherapies and more efficacious use of psychotropic drugs.

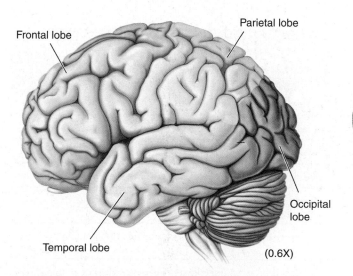

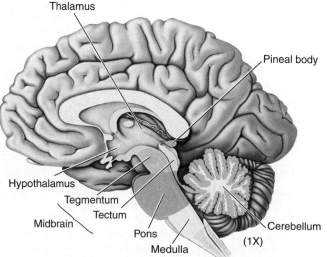

FIGURE 18-2. Lateral (**left**) and medial (**right**) surfaces of the brain. (From Bear M. F., Connors B. W., Paradiso M. A. (2016). *Neuroscience: Exploring the brain* (4th ed., pp. 223, 225). Philadelphia, PA: Wolters Kluwer.)

Types of Psychiatric Disorders

Schizophrenia

Schizophrenia is a chronic debilitating psychotic disorder affecting 1% of the population and results in marked impairment in functioning.[3,24] Schizophrenia affects a person's thoughts, feelings, perceptions, and overall behavior while interfering with filtering of stimuli from the environment. The onset of the disorder typically occurs between the ages of 16 and 30. The prevalence of schizophrenia is greater in men throughout most of adulthood but is equal to women by the age of 50 or 60 years. Proposed risk factors for schizophrenia include childhood trauma, malnutrition, long-term cannabis use, vitamin D deficiency, migrant status, older fathers, prenatal famine, retroviruses, chronic amphetamine use, obstetric complications, poverty, and other psychosocial disorders.[25] Another risk factor is having a close relative with schizophrenia. In fact, first-degree relatives of a person with schizophrenia have a 10-fold greater prevalence of the illness than the population at large.[25,26]

Schizophrenia spectrum and psychotic disorders are characterized by symptoms such as delusions, hallucinations or false perceptions, psychosis resulting in a break with reality, disjointed behaviors and speech, limited emotions, and impaired ability to reason and problem solve, along with social dysfunction. The criteria for schizophrenia require two or more psychotic manifestations that last 6 months before diagnosis is made.[27]

Clinical Manifestations

Characteristics of schizophrenia include *positive* and *negative symptoms* reflecting the presence of abnormal behaviors. *Positive* or *psychotic symptoms* include:

- Incomprehensible speech
- Hallucinations
- Delusions
- Grossly disorganized or catatonic behavior

Frequently, people with schizophrenia lose the ability to sort and interpret incoming stimuli, which impairs their ability to respond appropriately to the environment. An enhancement or a blunting of the senses is very common in the early stages of schizophrenia. Sounds may be experienced as louder and more intrusive; colors may be brighter and sharper. Sensory overload owing to a loss of the ability to screen external sensory stimuli occurs. Some people with schizophrenia have a blunted response to pain. Examples of altered speech patterns reflecting positive schizophrenia symptoms are included in Table 18-2.[18,19]

Hallucinations and *delusions* are *hallmarks of schizophrenia* and may be related to the inability to filter, interpret, and respond appropriately to stimuli. Auditory hallucinations are especially common. Auditory hallucinations range from simple repetitive sounds to many voices speaking at once. Sometimes, the voices are pleasant, but often, they accuse and curse. When visual hallucinations occur, they are usually in conjunction with auditory hallucinations.[18,28]

TABLE 18-2 Positive Symptoms of Schizophrenia Reflecting Altered Speech Patterns in Schizophrenia

Speech Pattern	Description
Neologisms	Using invented words
Derailment	Loose associations
Tangentiality	Inability to stick to the original point
Incoherence	Loss of logical connections
Word salad	Groups of disconnected words

Delusions are false ideas that cannot be corrected by reason. They range from simply believing people are watching them (ideas of reference) to beliefs they are being punished and/or manipulated by others (delusions of paranoia). Delusions of being a historical figure also are common and are called grandiose delusions. Sometimes, the delusions include a belief the affected person can control others with his or her thoughts.[18]

The *negative symptoms* of schizophrenia reflect the absence of normal social and interpersonal behaviors. Examples of these negative behaviors are included in Table 18-3.[18,19] *Negative symptoms* are the most difficult to treat and often are severe and persistent between acute episodes of illness.[9] Another component of the negative symptoms of schizophrenia is referred to as *disorganized behavior*. In addition to agitation or aggression, other specific disorganized behavior may occur and is included in Table 18-4.[18,19]

Neurophysiology of Symptoms

The complete set of pathogenic mechanisms underlying schizophrenia is not clear. Research suggests that changes in the dysregulation of the DA and serotonergic system[22,28] and other neurotransmitter changes such as decreased glutamate activity through dysfunction of its

TABLE 18-3 Negative Symptoms of Schizophrenia Reflecting Absence of Normal Social and Interpersonal Behaviors

Behavior	Description
Alogia	Tendency to speak very little
Avolition	Lack of motivation for goal-oriented activity
Apathy	Lack of interest or concern
Affective flattening	Lack of emotional expression
Inappropriate affect	Affect does not match the situation
Anhedonia	Inability to experience pleasure in things ordinarily pleasurable

TABLE 18-4 Negative Symptoms of Schizophrenia Reflecting Disorganized Behavior

Behavior	Description
Catatonic excitement	Hyperactive, purposeless activity with abnormal movements such as grimacing or posturing
Echopraxia	Imitation of another person's movement
Regressed behavior	Go back to behavior of another time
Stereotypy	Repetitive, idiosyncratic movements
Hypervigilance	Enhanced state of sensory stimulation
Waxy flexibility	Posture held in odd fixed position for extended periods of time

N-methyl-D-aspartate (NMDA) receptor play a role.[29] Many of the symptoms of impaired cognition seen in schizophrenia are thought to be tied to deficits in GABA. Lower production of this amino acid has been found in the dorsolateral prefrontal cortex and may be a consequence of messenger ribonucleic acid dysfunction.[29] Neuroimaging suggests several functional abnormalities occur in schizophrenia. These include excessive loss of cortical gray matter, abnormal cortical thinning, reduced numbers of synaptic structures on neurons, reduced dendritic spine density of pyramidal neurons in the prefrontal cortex, and arrested migration of hippocampal neurons. Enlargement of the lateral and third ventricles; a reduction in frontal lobe, temporal lobe, and amygdala; and diminished neuronal content in the thalamus have also been noted.[28,30-32] Interestingly, genetically identical twins are only 50% concordant for developing schizophrenia, suggesting 50% of the variance is attributed to environmental or other nongenetic contributions.[6]

Treatment

Schizophrenia is considered a chronic illness with remissions and exacerbations. Goals of treatment for schizophrenia are to induce a remission, prevent a recurrence, and improve behavioral, cognitive, and psychosocial functions. Early intervention programs are associated with a better treatment response.[32] The goal is *recovery*. According to the Substance Abuse and Mental Health Services Administration, four dimensions supporting mental health recovery include health, home, purpose, and community.[33] Treatment in the community is preferred. However, hospitalization may be indicated if a person is a danger to self or others, is unable to provide basic care for self, or refuses to eat or drink.

Pharmacologic treatment with antipsychotics is often helpful with the positive symptoms of schizophrenia. Both typical and atypical antipsychotic drugs address these positive symptoms. The negative symptoms of schizophrenia respond more favorably to the atypical antipsychotic drugs. Evidence supports psychosocial

interventions.[18,34] Family members may need assistance in learning about the illness and the best ways to support each other and their family member with schizophrenia.

Mood Disorders

Mood disorders are relatively common, but only half of those who need treatment are diagnosed and treated. The *DSM-5* section on mood disorders includes depression and bipolar disorders.[1] The 12-month prevalence of mood disorders in the United States is 9.5%, with 45% of these cases classified as severe. Mood disorder rates are higher among people living in or near poverty.[35,36]

Depressive Disorders

The *DSM-5* recognizes eight types of depressive disorders.[1] Prevalence of depression is higher in people from families with a history of mood disorders than in the population at large. The prevalence of major depression among women is double that in men.[36] Data suggest that major depressive episodes (MDEs) occur in 6.7% of adults yearly and 12.8% of adolescents.[2,3] In all age groups, MDEs have increased. Depression can vary in intensity and often is recurrent. The average onset of depression is in the mid-30s. The age of onset of depression has been decreasing, with increasing MDE in ages 18 to 25 years.[37] The earlier and more frequent the onset of symptoms, the more likely it is medications will be required for symptom relief. Depression in older adults often appears with an element of confusion and often is left untreated. A first episode of depression occurring after 65 years of age can be a precursor to neurocognitive disorder (NCD) and should precipitate both assessment and treatment of the depression, as well as a complete evaluation for NCDs. Early intervention often greatly slows progression, allowing the older adult to maintain independence and quality of life.[37]

Major Depressive Disorder
People with major depressive disorder (MDD) experience loss of interest in previously enjoyed activities and resist attempts to engage them in such activities. Recurring thoughts of suicide, lack of appetite, inability to concentrate, difficulty or complete inability to make decisions, and feelings of worthlessness are common. Lack of energy, decreased motor skills, substance abuse, and a range of sleep disturbances from insomnia to oversleep can be characteristic. The criteria for diagnosis include the presence of symptoms most of the day nearly every day for a minimum of 2 weeks that interfere with activities such as work or functioning. Depression has various subclassifications distinguished by symptom patterns.[38]

Persistent Depressive Disorders (Dysthymia)
Dysthymia is a chronic but mild state of depression lasting at least 2 years. There is a roller-coaster presentation in which the person may move from major to less severe depression,[39] often feeling sad. At least two of the following must also be present: altered sleep pattern (too much or not enough), fatigue, altered eating patterns (lack of appetite or overeating), inability to concentrate,

www.drugabuse.gov/news-events/nida-notes/2017/03/impacts-drugs-neurotransmission. Accessed April 30, 2019.

78. Wingo T., Nesil T., Choi J.-S., et al. (2016). Novelty seeking and drug addiction in humans and animals: From behavior to molecules. *Journal of Neuroimmune Pharmacology* 11(3), 456. doi:10.1007/s11481-015-9636-7.

79. Bodnar R. (2016). Endogenous opiates and behavior. *Peptides* 75, 18–70. doi:10.1016/j.peptides.2015.10.009.

80. Wackernah R., Minnick M., Clapp P. (2014). Alcohol use disorder: Pathophysiology, effects, and pharmacologic options for treatment. *Substance Abuse and Rehabilitation* 5, 1–12. doi:10.2147/SAR.S37907.

81. U.S. Department of Health and Human Services. (2016). *Facing addiction in America: The surgeon general's report on alcohol, drugs, and health*. Washington, DC: US Department of Health and Human Services.

82. Teicher M., Samson J. (2016). Annual research review: Enduring neurobiological effects of childhood abuse and neglect. *Journal of Child Psychology & Psychiatry* 57(3), 241–266. doi:10/1111/jcpp.12507.

83. Shrivastava A., Desousa A. (2016). Resilience: A psychobiological construct for psychiatric disorders. *Indian Journal of Psychiatry* 58(1), 38. doi:10.4103/0019-5545.174365.

84. Smits L., van Harten A. C., Pijnenburg Y. A., et al. (2015). Trajectories of cognitive decline in different types of dementia. *Psychological Medicine* 45(5), 1051–1059. doi:10.1017/S0033291714002153.

85. Harada C., Natelson Love M. C., Triebel K. L., et al. (2013). Normal cognitive aging. *Clinics in Geriatric Medicine* 29(4), 737–752. doi:10.1016/j.cger.2013.07.002.

86. Smith C., Cotter V. (2016). Age related changes. In Boltz M., Capezuti E., Fulmer T., et al. (Eds.), *Evidence based geriatric protocols for best practice* (pp. 23–41). New York, NY: Springer.

87. Alzheimer's Association. (2017). What is dementia? [Online]. Available: http://www.alz.org/what-is-dementia.asp. Accessed April 30, 2019.

88. Alzheimer's Association. (2011). In brief for healthcare professionals: New Diagnostic Criteria and guidelines for Alzheimer's disease. [Online]. https://www.alz.org/research/for_researchers/diagnostic-criteria-guidelines

89. Alzheimer's Association. (n.d.). In brief for healthcare professionals: Differentiating dementias. [Online]. Available: https://www.alz.org/health-care-professionals/documents/InBrief_Issue7_Final.pdf. Accessed April 30, 2019.

90. Alzheimer's Association. (2019). 2019 Alzheimer's disease facts and figures. *Alzheimer's and Dementia* 15(3), 321–387.

91. Adamis D., Rooney S., Meagher D., et al. (2015). A comparison of delirium diagnosis in elderly medical inpatients using the CAM, DRS-R98, DSM-IV and DSM-5 criteria. *International Psychogeriatrics* 27(6), 883–889. doi:10.1017/S1041610214002853.

92. Arvanitakis Z., Capuano A. W., Leurgans S. E., et al. (2016). Articles: Relation of cerebral vessel disease to Alzheimer's disease dementia and cognitive function in elderly people: A cross-sectional study. *Lancet Neurology* 15(9), 934–943. doi:10.1016/S1474-4422(16)30029-1.

93. Ramesh K., Hemachandra R. (2016). Therapeutics of neurotransmitters in Alzheimer's disease. *Journal of Alzheimer's Disease* 57(4), 1049–1069. doi:10.3233/JAD-161118.

94. Liu P., Fleete M. S., Jing Y., et al. (2014). Altered arginine metabolism in Alzheimer's disease brains. *Neurobiology of Aging* 35(9), 1992–2003. doi:10.1016/j.neurobiolaging.2014.03.013.

95. Sanabria-Castro A., Alvarado-Echeverría I., Monge-Bonilla C. (2017). Molecular pathogenesis of Alzheimer's disease: An update. *Annals of Neurosciences* 24(1), 46–54. doi:10.1159/000464422.

96. Villemagne V., Doré V., Bourgeat P., et al. (2017). Aβ-amyloid and Tau imaging in dementia. *Seminars in Nuclear Medicine* 47, 75–88. doi:10.1053/j.semnuclmed.2016.09.006.

97. Alzheimer's Association. (2017). What we know today about Alzheimer's: The search for Alzheimer's causes and risk factors. Alzheimer's Research Center. [Online]. Available: http://www.alz.org/research/science/alzheimers_disease_causes.asp. Accessed April 30, 2019.

98. Cai Y., An S., Kim S. (2015). Mutations in presenilin 2 and its implications in Alzheimer's disease and other dementia-associated disorders. *Clinical Interventions in Aging* 10, 1163–1172. doi:10.2147/CIAS85808.

99. Lee J., Lee A. J., Dang L. H., et al. (2017). Candidate gene analysis for Alzheimer's disease in adults with Down syndrome. *Neurobiology of Aging* 56, 150–158. doi:10.1016/j.neurobiolaging.2017.04.018.

100. Hamlett E., Goetzl E. J., Ledreux A., et al. (2017). Neuronal exosomes reveal Alzheimer's disease biomarkers in Down syndrome. *Alzheimer's & Dementia: Journal of the Alzheimer's Association* 13(5), 541–549. doi:10.1016/j.jalz.2016.08.012.

101. Walter C., Edwards N. E., Griggs R., et al. (2014). Differentiating Alzheimer's disease, Lewy body, and Parkinson dementia using DSM-5. *Journal for Nurse Practitioners* 10(4), 262–270. doi:10/1016/jnurpra.2014.01.002.

102. Thomas K., Baier R., Kosar C., et al. (2017). Individualized music program is associated with improved outcomes for U.S. nursing home residents with dementia. *American Journal of Geriatric Psychiatry* 25(9), 931–938. doi:10.1016/jagp2017.04.008.

103. Long E. (2017). Innovative approach to managing behavioral and psychological dementia. *Journal for Nurse Practitioners* 13(7), 475–481. doi:10.1016.j/nurpra.2017.05.003.

104. Amstadter A., Maes H. H., Sheerin C. M., et al. (2016). The relationship between genetic and environmental influences on resilience and on common internalizing and externalizing psychiatric disorders. *Social Psychiatry and Psychiatric Epidemiology* 51(5), 669–678. doi:10.1007/s00127-015-1163-6.

105. Alzheimer's Association. (2017). Health care professionals and Alzheimer's: Differential diagnosis of vascular dementia. [Online]. Available: https://www.alz.org/professionals/healthcare-professionals/dementia-diagnosis/differential-diagnosis/differential_diagnosis_of_vascular_dementia. Accessed April 30, 2019.

106. Centers for Disease Control and Prevention. (2015). *Report to congress on traumatic brain injury in the United States: Epidemiology and rehabilitation*. Atlanta, GA: National Center for Injury Prevention and Control; Division of Unintentional Injury Prevention.

107. Aarsland D. (2015). Epidemiology of dementia associated with Parkinson's disease. In Emre M. (Ed.), *Cognitive impairment and dementia in Parkinson's disease* (pp. 5–16). Oxford, UK: Oxford University Press.

108. Alzheimer's Association. (2017). Frontotemporal dementia. [Online]. Available: http://www.alz.org/dementia/fronto-temporal-dementia-ftd-symptoms.asp#types. Accessed April 30, 2019.

109. Scaber J., Talbot K. (2016). What is the role of TDP-43 in C9orf72-related amyotrophic lateral sclerosis and frontotemporal dementia? *Brain: A Journal of Neurology* 139(12), 3057–3059. doi:10.1093/brain/aww264.

110. World Health Organization. (2017). Genomic resource centre: Genes and human disease. [Online]. Available: http://

www.who.int/genomics/public/geneticdiseases/en/index2.html. Accessed April 30, 2019.

111. Cepeda C., Murphy K. P., Parent M., et al. (2014). The role of dopamine in Huntington's disease. *Progress in Brain Research* 211, 235–254. doi:10.1016/B978-0-444-63425-2.00010-6.

112. Saylor D., Dickens A. M., Sacktor N., et al. (2016). HIV-associated neurocognitive disorder—Pathogenesis and prospects for treatment. *Neurology* 12(4), 234–248. doi:10.1038/nrneurol.2016.27.

113. Hartney E. (2017). What is mild neurocognitive disorder due to substance/medication use? [Online]. Available: https://www.verywellmind.com/medication-or-substance-induced-neurocognitive-disorder-4144778. Accessed February 22, 2018.

114. Rawat P.J., Pinto C., Dave M., et al. (2016). Neuropathology in neuropsychiatric disorders secondary to alcohol misuse. In Preedy V. (Ed.), *Neuropathology of drug addictions and substance misuse* (pp. 627–636). London, UK: Elsevier.

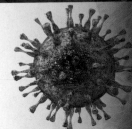
C H A P T E R 19

Disorders of Visual Function

Learning Objectives

After completing this chapter, the learner will be able to meet the following objectives:

1. Describe the cause of eyelid weakness.
2. Compare *entropion* and *ectropion*.
3. Compare marginal blepharitis, a hordeolum, and a chalazion regarding causes and manifestations.
4. Compare symptoms associated with red eye caused by conjunctivitis, corneal irritation, and acute glaucoma.
5. Characterize the manifestations, treatment, and possible complications of bacterial, *Acanthamoeba*, and herpes keratitis.
6. Describe tests used in assessing the pupillary reflex including indications of abnormal pupillary reflexes.
7. Describe how the formation and outflow of aqueous humor from the eye are related to the development of glaucoma.
8. Compare open-angle and angle-closure glaucoma in terms of pathology, symptomatology, diagnosis, and treatment.
9. Explain why glaucoma leads to blindness.
10. Describe changes in eye structure that occur with nearsighted and farsighted vision.
11. Describe changes in lens structure, risk factors, and visual changes associated with cataract.
12. Cite the manifestations and long-term visual effects of papilledema.
13. Describe the pathogenesis of background and proliferative diabetic retinopathies and their mechanisms of visual impairment.
14. Explain the pathology and visual changes associated with macular degeneration.
15. Characterize what is meant by a *visual field defect*.
16. Define the terms *hemianopia*, *quadrantanopia*, *heteronymous hemianopia*, and *homonymous hemianopia* and relate them to disorders of the optic pathways.
17. Describe visual defects associated with disorders of the visual cortex and visual association areas.
18. Describe the function and innervation of the extraocular muscles.
19. Explain the difference between paralytic and nonparalytic strabismus.
20. Define *amblyopia* and explain its pathogenesis.

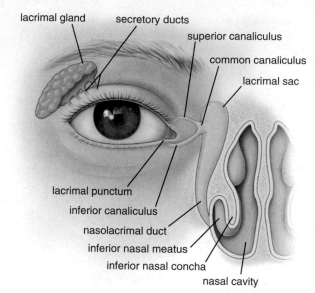

FIGURE 19-1. Schematic diagram of the eye and lacrimal apparatus. (From Pawlina W. (2016). *Histology: A text and atlas: With correlated cell and molecular biology* (7th ed., p. 923, Fig. 24.18). Philadelphia, PA: Wolters Kluwer.)

humor and retina (retinopathy and macular degeneration), optic pathways and visual cortex, and extraocular muscles and eye movement. The optic globe, commonly called the *eyeball*, is a remarkably mobile, nearly spherical structure contained in a pyramid-shaped cavity of the skull called the *orbit*. The eyeball occupies only the anterior one fifth of the orbit. The remainder is filled with muscles, nerves, the lacrimal gland, and adipose tissue that support the normal position of the optic globe. Exposed surfaces of the eyes are protected by the eyelids, which are mucous membrane–lined skin flaps that provide a means for shutting out most light. Tears bathe the anterior surface of the eye. They prevent friction between it and the lid, maintain hydration of the cornea, and protect the eye from infection and irritation by foreign objects. Figure 19-1 illustrates the eyelid and lacrimal apparatus.

Disorders of the Accessory Structures of the Eye

Three distinct layers form the wall of the eyeball—the sclera or outer supporting layer, the uvea or middle vascular layer, and the retina, which is composed of the neuronal retinal layer and the outer pigmented layer (see Fig. 19-2). The outer layer of the eyeball consists of a tough, opaque, white fibrous layer called the *sclera*. It is strong yet elastic and maintains the shape of the globe. The sclera is continuous with the cornea anteriorly and with the cranial dural sheath that surrounds and protects the optic nerve posteriorly. The choroid (uvea) predominantly provides vascular support of the retina, whereas the retina is the neurosensory tissue that provides the sensory input for sight.

The World Health Organization (WHO) reports that 161 million people worldwide are visually impaired: 124 million have low vision, and 37 million are blind.[1] An additional 153 million have visual impairment due to uncorrected refractive errors (nearsightedness, farsightedness, or astigmatism).[1] In 2017, the World Health Assembly stated that more than 90% of the world's visually impaired people live in low- and middle-income countries.[1] The WHO is a founding partner of Vision 2020 and is working to eliminate the main causes of avoidable blindness by the year 2020.[1]

Alterations in vision can result from disorders of the eyelids and optic globe (conjunctiva, cornea, and uvea), intraocular pressure (glaucoma), lens (cataract), vitreous

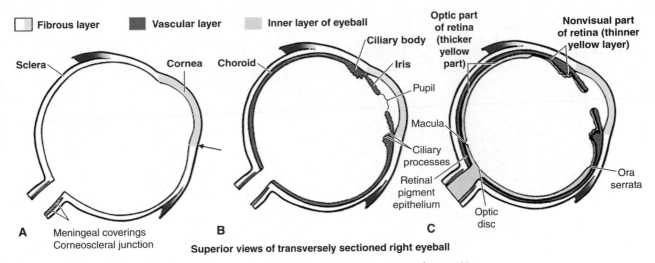

FIGURE 19-2. The layers of the eye. The wall of the eyeball is organized in three separate layers: (**A**) an outer fibrous layer, (**B**) a middle vascular layer, and (**C**) an inner photosensitive layer, the retina. (From Moore K. L., Agur A. M., Dalley A. F. (2015). *Essential clinical anatomy* (5th ed., p. 522, Fig. 7.26). Philadelphia, PA: Wolters Kluwer/Lippincott Williams & Wilkins.)

KEY POINTS

Vision

- Vision is a special sensory function that incorporates the visual receptor functions of the eyeball, the optic nerve, and optic pathways that carry and distribute sensory information from the optic globe to the central nervous system (CNS) via photoreceptors in the retina and the primary and visual association cortices that translate the sensory signals into visual images.

- Binocular vision depends on the coordination of three pairs of extraocular nerves that provide for the conjugate eye movements, with optical axes of the two eyes maintained parallel with one another as the eyes rotate in their sockets.

Disorders of the Eyelids

The upper and lower eyelids, the *palpebrae*, are modified folds of skin with associated muscle and cartilaginous plates that protect the eyeball. The palpebral fissure is the oval opening between the upper and lower eyelids. At the corners of the eye, where the upper and lower lids meet, is an angle called the *canthus*. The lateral canthus is the outer, or temporal, angle, and the medial canthus is the inner, or nasal, angle. In each lid, a tarsus, or plate of dense connective tissue, gives the lid its shape (Fig. 19-3). Each tarsus contains modified sebaceous glands, called *meibomian glands*, the ducts of which open onto the eyelid margins. Sebaceous secretions of the meibomian glands enable airtight closure of the lids and prevent rapid evaporation of tears.

Two striated muscles, the levator palpebrae superioris and the orbicularis oculi, provide for movement of the eyelids. The levator palpebrae superioris, innervated by the oculomotor nerve (cranial nerve [CN] III), serves to raise the upper lid. Encircling the eye is the orbicularis oculi muscle, which is supplied by the facial nerve (CN VII). When this muscle contracts, it closes the eyelids. Between the nose and medial angle of the eye is the medial palpebral ligament, which connects to the medial margin of the orbit (see Fig. 19-3). A similar palpebral ligament attaches to the lateral margin of the orbit. The orbicularis oculi nerve inserts into the medial palpebral ligament that passes through each eyelid and inserts into the lateral palpebral junction. The four recti and two oblique muscles provide for movement of the eyeball.

Eyelid Weakness

Drooping of the eyelid is called *ptosis*. Figure 19-4 illustrates ptosis with Horner syndrome. It can result from weakness of the levator muscle that elevates the upper lid in conjunction with the unopposed action of the orbicularis oculi that forcefully closes the eyelids. Weakness of the orbicularis oculi causes an open eyelid, but not ptosis. Neurologic causes of eyelid weakness include damage to the innervating cranial nerves or to the nerves' central nuclei in the midbrain and the caudal pons.

Normally, the edges of the eyelids, or palpebrae, are in such a position that the palpebral conjunctiva that lines the eyelids is not exposed and the eyelashes do not rub against the cornea. Turning in of the lid margin is called *entropion*. It is usually caused by scarring of the palpebral conjunctiva or degeneration of the fascial attachments to the lower lid that occurs with aging. Corneal irritation may occur as the eyelashes turn inward. *Ectropion* refers to eversion of the lower lid margin and is the most frequent bilateral lid condition. It is caused by relaxation of the orbicularis oculi muscle because of CN VII weakness or the aging process.[2] Ectropion causes tearing and ocular irritation and may lead to inflammation of the cornea.

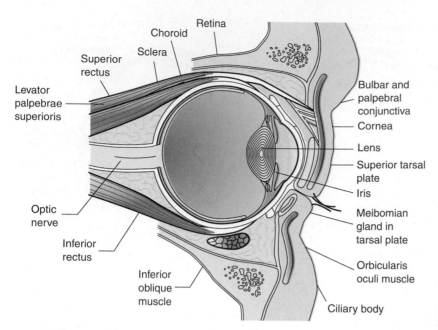

FIGURE 19-3. The eye and its appendages: anterior view.

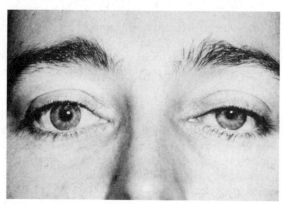

FIGURE 19-4. Ptosis in Horner syndrome—there is mild unilateral ptosis, anisocoria with smaller pupil on side of ptosis. (From Miller N. R., Newman N. J., Biousse V., et al. (Eds.). (2016). *Walsh and Hoyt's clinical neuro-ophthalmology: The essentials* (3rd ed., p. 431). Philadelphia, PA: Lippincott Williams & Wilkins.)

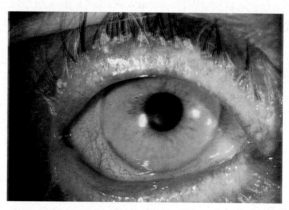

FIGURE 19-5. Blepharitis—inflammation of margin of eyelid. (From Jensen S. (2015). *Nursing health assessment: A best practice approach* (2nd ed., p. 341). Philadelphia, PA: Lippincott Williams & Wilkins.)

Entropion and ectropion can be treated surgically. Contraction of the resulting scar tissue usually draws the lid up to its normal position.

Eyelid Inflammation

Blepharitis is a common chronic bilateral inflammation involving the lashes and lid margins (Fig. 19-5). Two main types of anterior blepharitis occur—inflammatory and infectious. The inflammatory form is usually associated with seborrhea (*i.e.,* dandruff) of the scalp or brows. Infectious blepharitis may be caused by *Staphylococcus epidermidis* or *Staphylococcus aureus*, in which case the lesions are often ulcerative. The main symptoms of anterior blepharitis are irritation, burning, redness, and itching of the eyelid margins. Treatment includes careful cleaning with a damp applicator to remove the scales. When the disorder is associated with a microbial infection, an antibiotic (ointment or drops) is prescribed.[3]

Posterior blepharitis is inflammation of the eyelids that involves the meibomian glands. It may result from a bacterial infection, particularly with staphylococci, or dysfunction of the meibomian glands, in which there is a strong association with acne rosacea.[3] The meibomian glands and their orifices are inflamed, with dilation of the glands, plugging of the orifices, and abnormal secretions. The tears may be frothy and abnormally greasy from the meibomian secretions. Treatment of posterior blepharitis is determined by associated conjunctival and corneal changes. Initial therapies can include warm compresses and lid massage. Systemic antibiotic therapy can be prescribed, guided by results of bacterial cultures.[3]

A *hordeolum*, or *stye*, is usually caused by an infection of the meibomian gland or other structures of the eyelid margin. The infection is usually caused by *S. aureus*. Symptoms include pain, redness, and swelling. Applying warm, moist compresses to the site assists in treatment. A referral to an ophthalmologist may be required if the infection does not resolve after 2 to 3 days.[3]

A *chalazion* is a focal chronic inflammation developing when the meibomian gland becomes obstructed. A small, painless nodule develops on the tarsus. Treatment consists of warm, moist compresses. Referral to an ophthalmologist may be necessary if the nodule does not resolve. Antibiotics are not given because this is not an infectious process.[3]

Disorders of the Lacrimal System

The lacrimal system includes the major lacrimal gland, which produces the tears; the puncta, canaliculi, and tear sac, which collect the tears; and the nasolacrimal duct, which empties the tears into the nasal cavity. The lacrimal gland lies in the orbit, superior and lateral to the eyeball (see Fig. 19-1). Approximately 12 small ducts connect the lacrimal gland to the superior conjunctival fornix. Tears contain approximately 98% water, 1.5% sodium chloride, and small amounts of potassium, albumin, and glucose. The function of tears is to provide a smooth optical surface by abolishing minute surface irregularities. Tears also wet and protect the delicate surface of the cornea and conjunctiva. They flush and remove irritating substances and microorganisms and provide the cornea with necessary nutrient substances. Tears also contain lysozymes and immunoglobulin A (IgA), IgG, and IgE, which synergistically act to protect against infection. Although IgA predominates, IgE concentrations are increased in some allergic conditions.

Dry Eyes

Dry eye is a multifactorial disease characterized by unstable tear film causing a variety of symptoms and/or visual impairment, potentially accompanied by ocular surface damage.[4]

The thin film of tears that covers the cornea is essential in preventing drying and damage of the outer layer of the cornea as well as providing immune protection. This tear film is composed of three layers:

1. An outer lipid layer, which is derived from the meibomian glands and which limits evaporative loss
2. An intermediate aqueous layer, secreted by the lacrimal glands
3. An inner mucin layer, which overlies the cornea and epithelial cells[5]

Dry eye symptoms are common and can be divided into two categories: aqueous-deficient and evaporative.[5] The aqueous-deficient category is associated with autoimmune diseases and disorders. The evaporative category has a variety of causes, but the most common is related to an obstruction of meibomian gland opening. Other causes include poor eyelid closure, infrequent blinking, and contact lens wear.[5] People may complain that the eyes feel gritty. There may be pain or burning, light sensitivity, redness, or itching. Occasionally, vision may be blurred.[5] Artificial tears are commonly used for relief of symptoms. Persistent discomfort requires an evaluation by a health care provider.[5]

Dacryocystitis

Dacryocystitis is an inflammation and infection of the lacrimal sac and occurs secondary to an anatomic obstruction (dacryostenosis) of the tear duct (nasolacrimal duct). The symptoms include tearing and discharge, pain, swelling, and tenderness. The treatment includes application of warm compresses and topical and oral antibiotic therapy.

In infants, dacryostenosis is usually caused by failure of the nasolacrimal ducts to open spontaneously before birth. Treatment requires surgery.[6]

SUMMARY CONCEPTS

The eyelids serve to protect the eye. Ptosis refers to drooping of the upper lid, which is caused by injury to CN III. Entropion, which refers to turning in of the upper eyelid and eyelashes, is discomforting and causes corneal irritation. Ectropion, or eversion of the lower eyelid, causes tearing and may lead to corneal inflammation. Marginal blepharitis is the most common disorder of the eyelids. It commonly is caused by a staphylococcal infection or seborrhea.

The lacrimal system includes the major lacrimal gland, which produces the tears; the puncta and tear sac, which collect the tears; and the nasolacrimal duct, which empties the tears into the nasal cavity. Tears protect the cornea from drying and irritation. Impaired tear production or conditions that prevent blinking and the spread of tears produce drying of the eyes and predispose them to corneal irritation and injury. Dacryocystitis is an inflammation caused by an infection of the lacrimal sac.

Disorders of the Conjunctiva, Cornea, and Uveal Tract

Disorders of the Conjunctiva

The conjunctiva is a delicate mucous membrane that lines the anterior surface of both eyelids as the *palpebral conjunctiva* and folds back over the anterior surface of the optic globe as the *ocular* or *bulbar conjunctiva*.[7] The ocular conjunctiva covers only the sclera or white portion of the optic globe, not the cornea. When both eyes are closed, the conjunctiva lines the closed conjunctival sac. Although the conjunctiva protects the eye, its main function is the production of a lubricating mucus that bathes the eye and keeps it moist.

Conjunctivitis, or inflammation of the conjunctiva (*i.e.*, red or pink eye), is one of the most common forms of eye disease. It may result from bacterial or viral infection, allergens, chemical agents, physical irritants, or radiant energy. Depending on the cause, conjunctivitis can vary in severity from a mild hyperemia (redness) with tearing to severe conjunctivitis with purulent drainage. The conjunctiva is extremely sensitive to irritation and inflammation.

Clinical manifestations of conjunctivitis include a foreign body sensation, a scratching or burning sensation, itching, and photophobia. Severe pain suggests corneal rather than conjunctival disease. A discharge, or exudate, may be present. It is usually watery when the conjunctivitis is caused by allergy, a foreign body, or viral infection and mucopurulent in the presence of bacterial or fungal infection. A characteristic of many forms of conjunctivitis is papillary hypertrophy. This occurs because the palpebral conjunctiva is bound to the tarsus by fine fibrils. As a result, inflammation that develops between the fibrils causes the conjunctiva to be elevated in mounds called **papillae**. When the papillae are small, the conjunctiva has a smooth, velvety appearance. Red papillary conjunctivitis suggests bacterial or chlamydial conjunctivitis. In allergic conjunctivitis, the papillae often become flat-topped, polygonal, and milky in color and have a cobblestone appearance.

The diagnosis of conjunctivitis is based on history, physical examination, and microscopic and culture studies to identify the cause. In contrast to corneal lesions and acute glaucoma, both of which cause red eye, conjunctivitis produces infection (*i.e.*, enlargement and redness) of the peripheral conjunctival blood vessels rather than those radiating around the corneal limbus. Conjunctivitis also produces only mild discomfort compared with the moderate to severe discomfort associated with corneal lesions or the severe and deep pain associated with acute glaucoma. Infectious forms of conjunctivitis are usually bilateral and may involve other family members and associates. Unilateral disease suggests sources of irritation such as foreign bodies or chemical irritation.

Allergic Conjunctivitis

Allergic conjunctivitis encompasses a spectrum of conjunctival conditions usually characterized by itching. The most common of these is seasonal allergic rhinoconjunctivitis, or hay fever. Seasonal allergic conjunctivitis is an IgE-mediated hypersensitivity reaction precipitated by small airborne allergens such as pollens.[3] It typically causes bilateral tearing, itching, and redness of the eyes (Fig. 19-6).

The treatment of seasonal allergic rhinoconjunctivitis includes allergen avoidance and the use of cold compresses and eye washes with tear substitute. Allergic conjunctivitis also has been successfully treated with oral second-generation, nonsedating antihistamines.[3]

Infectious Conjunctivitis

Causes of infectious conjunctivitis include bacteria, viruses, gonorrhea, herpes, and chlamydia. Infections may spread from areas adjacent to the conjunctiva or may be blood-borne, such as in measles or chickenpox. Newborns can contract conjunctivitis during the birth process.

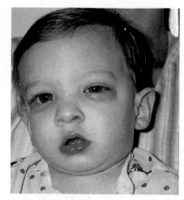

FIGURE 19-6. Allergic conjunctivitis—usually bilateral and common in people with allergic conditions. (From Jensen S. (2015). *Nursing health assessment: A best practice approach* (2nd ed., p. 341). Philadelphia, PA: Lippincott Williams & Wilkins.)

Bacterial Conjunctivitis

Bacterial conjunctivitis may present as a hyperacute, acute, or chronic infection. *Hyperacute conjunctivitis* is a severe, sight-threatening ocular infection most commonly caused by *Neisseria gonorrhoeae* and less commonly caused by *Neisseria meningitidis*. In newborns, *N. gonorrhoeae is the cause of the most serious type of conjunctivitis.*[3] In adults and adolescents, infection occurs through autoinoculation from infected genitalia. The infection has an abrupt onset and is characterized by a copious amount of yellow-green drainage. The symptoms, which typically are progressive, include conjunctival redness; chemosis (swelling around the cornea); lid swelling; and tender, swollen preauricular lymph nodes (Fig. 19-7). Gonococcal ocular infections left untreated result in corneal ulceration with ultimate perforation and sometimes permanent loss of vision. Diagnostic methods include immediate Gram staining of ocular specimens and special cultures for *Neisseria* species. Treatment includes systemic antibiotics supplemented with ocular antibiotics.[3]

Acute bacterial conjunctivitis typically presents with burning, tearing, and mucopurulent or purulent discharge. Common agents of bacterial conjunctivitis are *Streptococcus pneumoniae*, *S. aureus*, and *Haemophilus*

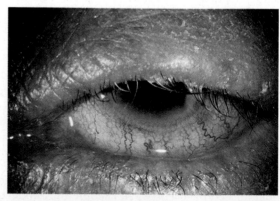

FIGURE 19-7. Bacterial conjunctivitis—usually purulent discharge and infected conjunctiva. (From Jensen S. (2015). *Nursing health assessment: A best practice approach* (2nd ed., p. 341). Philadelphia, PA: Lippincott Williams & Wilkins.)

influenzae in adults. In children, *Moraxella catarrhalis* is also common.[3] Infection normally begins in one eye and within 24 to 48 hours spreads to the unaffected eye. Drainage may be green, white, or yellow. Treatment may include local application of antibiotic drops or ointment.

Viral Conjunctivitis

Etiologic agents of viral conjunctivitis include adenoviruses, herpesviruses, and enteroviruses. One of the most common causes of viral conjunctivitis is infection with adenovirus.[3] The infection, which causes generalized conjunctival hyperemia, copious tearing, and minimal exudate, is usually associated with an upper respiratory tract infection (Fig. 19-8). Children are affected more often than are adults.

Swimming pools contaminated because of inadequate chlorination are common sources of infection.[3] Symptoms will resolve over time with the use of cool compresses and artificial tears. Topical antibiotics may be given if a secondary infection is present. Topical antivirals are not recommended.[3]

Chlamydial Conjunctivitis

There are two types of chlamydial eye infections:

- Trachoma, which includes serotypes A through C, causing chronic keratoconjunctivitis. According to the WHO, it is the leading cause of preventable blindness. It is rare in the United States and Europe, whereas it is commonly found in developing countries.[3,8]
- Inclusion conjunctivitis, which is associated with serotypes D through K. It is a common, sexually transmitted infection in adolescents and adults and can be transmitted to vaginally delivered infants.[3]

Sexually transmitted eye infections should be evaluated and treated promptly by a health care provider.

Disorders of the Cornea

At the anterior part of the eyeball, the outer covering of the eye is modified to form the transparent cornea, which bulges anteriorly from its junction with the sclera (Fig. 19-9). A major part of the refraction of light rays

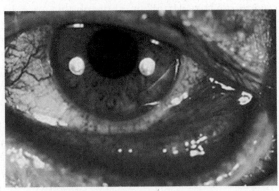

FIGURE 19-8. Viral conjunctivitis—usually clear discharge, which may be accompanied by sinus congestion and rhinorrhea. (From Jensen S. (2015). *Nursing health assessment: A best practice approach* (2nd ed., p. 341). Philadelphia, PA: Lippincott Williams & Wilkins.)

and focusing of vision occurs in the cornea. Three layers of tissue form the cornea:

1. An extremely thin outer epithelial layer, which is continuous with the bulbar conjunctiva
2. A middle layer called the *substantia propria* or *stroma*
3. An inner endothelial layer, which lies next to the aqueous humor of the anterior chamber[9]

The substantia propria is composed of regularly arranged collagen bundles embedded in a mucopolysaccharide matrix that makes the substantia propria transparent, which is necessary for light transmission. Hydration within a limited range is necessary to maintain the spacing of the collagen fibers and transparency. The three layers of the cornea are separated by two important basement membranes: the Bowman and Descemet membranes. The *Bowman membrane*, which lies between the corneal epithelium and stoma, acts as a barrier to infection. It does not regenerate. If damaged, an opaque scar forms that can impair vision. The *Descemet membrane*, which lies between the corneal endothelium and stroma, has a feltlike appearance and consists of interwoven fibers and pores. Unlike the Bowman membrane, it regenerates readily after injury.

The cornea is avascular and obtains its nutrient and oxygen supply by diffusion from blood vessels of the adjacent sclera, from the aqueous humor at its deep surface, and from tears. The corneal epithelium is heavily innervated by sensory neurons (trigeminal nerve [CN V], ophthalmic division [CN V_1]). Epithelial damage causes discomfort that ranges from a foreign body sensation and burning of the eyes to severe, incapacitating pain. Reflex lacrimation is common.

Disorders of the cornea include trauma, inflammation and infection, abnormal corneal deposits, and degenerative processes such as arcus senilis. Diagnosis of corneal disorders is based on history of trauma, medication use, and signs and symptoms associated with corneal irritation and disease.[9] Fluorescein staining can be used to outline an ulcerated area. The biomicroscope (slit lamp) is used for proper examination of the cornea. In cases of an infectious etiology, scrapings from the ulcer are obtained for staining and culture studies.

Corneal Trauma

The integrity of the epithelium and the endothelium is necessary to maintain hydration of the cornea within a limited range. Damage to either structure leads to edema and loss of transparency. Among the causes of corneal edema is prolonged wearing of contact lenses, which can deprive the epithelium of oxygen, disrupting its integrity. Corneal edema also occurs after a sudden rise in intraocular pressure. With corneal edema, the cornea appears dull, uneven, and hazy. In addition, visual acuity decreases and iridescent vision (*i.e.*, rainbows around lights) occurs.

Trauma that causes abrasions of the cornea can be extremely painful, but if minor, the abrasions usually heal in a few days. The epithelial layer can regenerate, and small defects heal without scarring. If the stroma is damaged, healing occurs more slowly, and the danger of infection is increased. Injuries to the Bowman membrane and the stromal layer heal with scar formation that impairs the transmission of light.

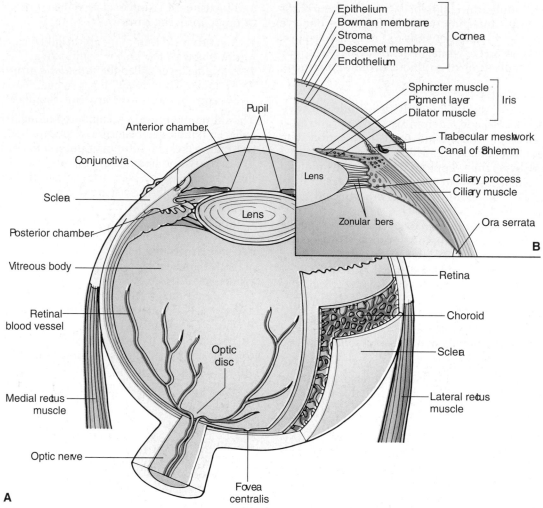

FIGURE 19-9. (A) Transverse section of the eyeball. (B) Enlargement of the anterior and posterior chambers of the eye, showing the layers of the cornea, the structures of the iris, aqueous drainage system (trabecular meshwork, canal of Schlemm), and the ciliary process and ciliary muscle.

Keratitis

Keratitis refers to inflammation of the cornea, which can result in partial or total loss of vision. Infectious sources include bacteria, viruses, fungi, and amoebae. Noninfectious causes include eye trauma, chemical exposure, and ultraviolet exposure. Contact lens wear is a major risk factor for infectious keratitis.[10] Symptoms of keratitis can include pain, photophobia, conjunctival hyperemia (redness), and corneal cloudiness with stromal involvement.[11] Immediate evaluation and treatment by a health care provider should be sought.

Herpes Simplex Keratitis

Herpes simplex virus (HSV) keratitis is the leading cause of corneal scarring and opacity causing blindness worldwide.[12] Most cases are caused by HSV type 1, the cause of labial or lip infections. However, in neonatal infections acquired during passage through the birth canal, approximately 80% are caused by HSV type 2 (the cause of genital herpes). The disease can occur as

a primary or recurrent infection.[13] After the initial primary infection, the virus may persist in a latent state in the trigeminal ganglion and possibly in the cornea without causing signs of infection.

Recurrent infection may be precipitated by various poorly understood, stress-related factors that reactivate the virus. Involvement is usually unilateral. The first symptoms are irritation, photophobia, and tearing. Some reduction in vision may occur when the lesion affects the central part of the cornea. Because corneal anesthesia occurs early in the disease, the symptoms may be minimal, and the person may delay seeking medical care. A history of fever blisters or other herpetic infection is often noted, but corneal lesions may be the only sign of recurrent herpes infection. Most typically, the corneal lesion involves the epithelium and has a typical branching pattern. These epithelial lesions heal without scarring. Herpetic lesions that involve the stromal layer of the cornea produce increasingly severe corneal opacities. The treatment of HSV keratitis focuses on eliminating viral replication in the cornea while minimizing the damaging effects of the inflammatory process. Topical antiviral agents are used to promote healing.[14,15] Oral antiviral agents have not been studied in comparative trials for efficacy, and resistance is increasing. The use of topical corticosteroids is contraindicated.[14,15]

Varicella Zoster Ophthalmicus

Herpes zoster or shingles is a relatively common infection caused by herpesvirus type 3, the same virus that causes varicella (chickenpox). It occurs when the varicella virus, which has remained dormant in the neurosensory ganglia since the primary infection, is reactivated. Herpes zoster ophthalmicus, which represents 10% to 25% of all cases of herpes zoster, occurs when reactivation of the latent virus occurs in the ganglia of the ophthalmic division of the trigeminal nerve.[9,13] Immunocompromised people, particularly those with human immunodeficiency virus infection, are at higher risk for developing herpes zoster ophthalmicus than are those with a normally functioning immune system.

Herpes zoster ophthalmicus usually presents with malaise, fever, headache, and burning and itching of the periorbital area followed by ocular eruption in a day or two. The rash, which is initially vesicular, becomes pustular and then crusting. Involvement of the tip of the nose and lid margins indicates a high likelihood of ocular involvement. Ocular signs include conjunctivitis, keratitis, and anterior uveitis, often with elevated intraocular pressure. People with corneal disease present with varying degrees of decreased vision, pain, and sensitivity to light.

Treatment includes the use of high-dose oral antiviral drugs.

Acanthamoeba Keratitis

Acanthamoeba is a free-living protozoan in contaminated water frequented by travelers. *Acanthamoeba* keratitis is a rare but serious and sight-threatening complication of exposure from continuous wearing of soft contact lenses, either extended wear or those worn overnight beyond doctor-recommended periods, or when poor disinfection techniques are used. It also may occur in non–contact lens wearers after exposure to contaminated water or soil. It is characterized by pain that is disproportionate to the clinical manifestations, redness of the eye, and photophobia. The disorder commonly is misdiagnosed as herpes keratitis or fungal keratitis. Diagnosis is confirmed by fluorescein staining of the eye.[16] Corneal biopsies with cultures may be indicated. To preserve vision, an immediate referral to a health care provider is required.[17–19]

Abnormal Corneal Deposits

The cornea frequently is the site for deposition of abnormal metabolic products. In hypercalcemia, calcium salts can precipitate in the cornea, producing a cloudy band keratopathy. Cystine crystals are deposited in cystinosis, cholesterol esters in hypercholesterolemia, and a golden ring of copper (*i.e.*, Kayser–Fleischer ring) in hepatolenticular degeneration due to Wilson disease. Pharmacologic agents, such as chloroquine, can result in crystal deposits in the cornea.

Arcus senilis is an extremely common, bilateral, benign corneal degeneration that may occur at any age but is more common in the elderly. It consists of a grayish-white infiltrate, approximately 2 mm wide, that occurs at the periphery of the cornea. It may represent an extracellular lipid infiltration and commonly is associated with hyperlipidemia. Arcus senilis does not produce visual symptoms, and there is no treatment necessary for this finding in older adults.

Corneal Transplantation

Over 40,000 corneal transplants are performed in the United States yearly.[20] Unlike kidney or heart transplantation procedures, which are associated with considerable risk of rejection of the transplanted organ, corneal transplants entail minimal danger of rejection. However, corneas that have been subjected to burns or that are unhealthy lose their "immune-privileged" status and become susceptible to graft rejection.[8]

Disorders of the Uveal Tract

The middle vascular layer, or uveal tract, is an incomplete ball with gaps at the pupil and the optic nerve. The pigmented uveal tract has three distinct regions: the choroid, ciliary body, and the iris. Several mutations affect the pigment of the uveal tract, including albinism. *Albinism* is a genetic (autosomal recessive trait) deficiency of tyrosinase, the enzyme needed for the synthesis of melanin by the melanocytes. Affected people have white hair, pink skin, and light blue eyes. In these people, excessive light penetrates the unpigmented iris and choroid and, to some extent, the anterior sclera. Their photoreceptors are flooded with excess light, and visual acuity is markedly reduced. Excess stimulation of the photoreceptors at normal or high illumination levels is experienced as painful photophobia.

Uveitis

Inflammation of the entire uveal tract, which supports the lens and neural components of the eye, is called uveitis. Uveitis is caused by infectious (virus, bacteria, fungi, or parasite) or noninfectious (autoimmune, malignant, or idiopathic) agents. One type of noninfectious etiology, autoimmune, results from an inflammatory disorder of ocular tissue with clinical features in common and an immunologically based cause. A serious consequence of uveitis can be the involvement of the underlying retina. Parasitic invasion of the choroid can result in local atrophic changes that usually involve the retina; examples include toxoplasmosis and histoplasmosis. Metastatic uveal tumors from malignancies such as breast, lung, and colon cancers have been documented. Primary uveal lymphoma is not common but occurs and requires radiation treatment.[9,21]

likely to develop in eyes with preexisting shallow anterior chambers. An acute attack is often precipitated by pupillary dilation, which causes the iris to thicken, thus blocking the circulation between the posterior and anterior chambers.[25-27] It is seen more commonly in people of Asian or Inuit (Eskimo) descent and in people with hypermetropic eyes. This defect is exaggerated by the anterior displacement of the peripheral iris that occurs in older adults because of the increase in lens thickness that occurs with aging.

Clinical Manifestations

Symptoms of acute angle-closure glaucoma are related to sudden, intermittent increases in intraocular pressure. Administration of topical pharmacologic agents such as atropine drops and some systemic oral medications can cause pupillary dilation (**mydriasis**) and precipitate an acute episode of increased intraocular pressure in people with the potential for angle-closure glaucoma. Attacks of increased intraocular pressure are manifested by ocular pain and blurred or iridescent vision caused by corneal edema.[23,26,27] The pupil may be enlarged and fixed. Symptoms are often spontaneously relieved by sleep and conditions that promote pupillary constriction. With repeated or prolonged attacks, the eye becomes reddened, and edema of the cornea may develop, giving the cornea a hazy appearance. A unilateral, often excruciating, headache is common. Nausea and vomiting may occur, causing the headache to be confused with migraine.

Because of the dangers of vision loss, those with narrow anterior chambers should be warned about the significance of blurred vision, halos, and ocular pain. Sometimes, decreased visual acuity and an unreactive pupil may be the only clues to angle-closure glaucoma in older adults.

Diagnosis and Treatment

The depth of the anterior chamber can be evaluated by side/shadow illumination or by a technique called *gonioscopy*. Gonioscopy uses a special contact lens and mirrors or prisms to view and measure the angle of the anterior chamber. The side/shadow illumination method uses only a penlight. The light source is held at the temporal side of the eye and directed horizontally across the iris. In people with a normal-sized anterior chamber, the light passes through the chamber to illuminate both halves of the iris. In people with a narrow anterior chamber, only the half of the iris adjacent to the light source is illuminated, whereas a shadow is cast on the half of the iris opposite the light source.

Acute angle-closure glaucoma is an ophthalmic emergency. Treatment is initially directed at reducing the intraocular pressure, usually with pharmacologic agents. Once the intraocular pressure is under control, a laser peripheral iridotomy is performed to create a permanent opening between the anterior and posterior chambers, allowing the aqueous humor to bypass the pupillary block. The anatomic abnormalities responsible for angle-closure glaucoma are usually bilateral, and prophylactic surgery is often performed on the other eye.

Congenital and Infantile Glaucoma

There are several types of childhood glaucoma that can be a primary or secondary disorder, including congenital glaucoma that is present at birth and infantile glaucoma that develops during the first 2 to 3 years of life.

Etiology and Pathophysiology

Congenital glaucoma is caused by a disorder in which the anterior chamber retains its fetal configuration, with aberrant trabecular meshwork extending to the root of the iris, or is covered by a membrane. In general, it has a much poorer prognosis than infantile glaucoma. Primary infantile glaucoma occurs in approximately 1 in 10,000 live births but accounts for 2% to 15% of people in institutions for the blind.[26,28] It is bilateral in 65% to 80% of cases and occurs more commonly in boys than in girls. About 10% of cases have a familial origin, and the rest are either sporadic or possibly multifactorial with reduced penetrance.[26,28] The familial cases are usually transmitted as an autosomal dominant trait with potentially high penetrance. Recent studies suggest a mutation in chromosome 2 that plays an important role in the metabolism of molecules that are used in signaling pathways during the terminal stages of anterior chamber development.[28]

Clinical Manifestations and Treatment

The earliest symptoms of congenital or infantile glaucoma are excessive tearing and photophobia. Affected infants tend to be fussy, have poor eating habits, and rub their eyes frequently. Diffuse edema of the cornea usually occurs, giving the eye a grayish-white appearance. Chronic elevation of the intraocular pressure before the age of 3 years causes enlargement of the entire optic globe. Early surgical treatment is necessary to prevent blindness.[28]

SUMMARY CONCEPTS

Glaucoma is a leading cause of blindness worldwide. It is characterized by conditions that cause an increase in intraocular pressure and that, if untreated, can lead to atrophy of the optic disc and progressive blindness. Glaucoma results from overproduction or impeded outflow of aqueous humor from the anterior chamber of the eye.

There are two types of glaucoma: open-angle and angle-closure. Open-angle glaucoma is caused by microscopic obstruction of the trabecular meshwork. Open-angle glaucoma is usually asymptomatic, and considerable loss of the visual field often occurs before medical treatment is sought. Routine screening by applanation tonometry provides one of the best means for early detection of glaucoma before vision loss has occurred. Angle-closure glaucoma is caused by a narrow anterior chamber and blockage of the outflow channels at the angle formed by the iris and the cornea. This occurs when the iris becomes thickened during pupillary dilation. Congenital glaucoma is caused by a disorder in which the anterior chamber retains its fetal configuration, with aberrant trabecular meshwork extending to the root of the iris, or is covered by a membrane. Early surgical treatment is necessary to prevent blindness.

Disorders of the Lens and Lens Function

The function of the eye is to transform light energy into nerve signals that can be transmitted to the cerebral cortex for interpretation. Optically, the eye is similar to a camera. It contains a lens system that focuses an inverted image, an aperture (*i.e.*, the pupil) for controlling light exposure, and a retina that corresponds to the film and records the image.

Disorders of Refraction and Accommodation

The lens is an avascular, transparent, biconvex body, the posterior side of which is more convex than the anterior side. A thin, highly elastic lens capsule is attached to the surrounding ciliary body by delicate suspensory radial ligaments called *zonules*, which hold the lens in place (see Fig. 19-9). The tough elastic sclera, in providing for a change in lens shape, acts as a bow, and the zonule and the lens capsule act as the bowstring. The suspensory ligaments and lens capsule are normally under tension, causing the lens to have a flattened shape for distant vision. Contraction of the muscle fibers of the ciliary body narrows the diameter of the ciliary body, relaxes the fibers of the suspensory ligaments, and allows the lens to relax to a more convex shape for near vision.

When light passes from one medium to another, its velocity is decreased or increased, and the direction of light transmission is changed. This change in direction of light rays is called *refraction*. When light rays pass through the center of a lens, their direction is not changed. However, other rays passing peripherally through a lens are bent (Fig. 19-11A). The refractive power of a lens is usually described as the distance (in meters) from its surface to the point at which the rays come into focus (*i.e.*, focal length). Usually, this is reported as the reciprocal of this distance (*i.e.*, **diopters**).[22]

In the eye, the major refraction of light begins at the convex corneal surface. Further refraction occurs as light moves from the posterior corneal surface to the aqueous humor, from the aqueous humor to the anterior lens surface, from the anterior lens surface to the

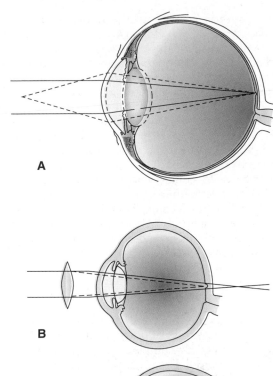

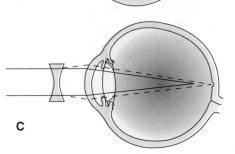

FIGURE 19-11. (A) Accommodation. The *solid lines* represent rays of light from a distant object, and the *dotted lines* represent rays from a near object. The lens is flatter for the former and more convex for the latter. In each case, the rays of light are brought to a focus on the retina. (B) Hyperopia corrected by a biconvex lens, shown by the *dashed lines*. (C) Myopia corrected by a biconcave lens, shown by the *dashed lines*.

posterior lens surface, and from the posterior lens surface to the vitreous humor.

Disorders of Refraction

A perfectly shaped optic globe and cornea result in optimal visual acuity, producing a sharp image in focus at all points on the retinal surface in the posterior part, or **fundus**, of the eye. Unfortunately, individual differences in formation and growth of the eyeball and cornea frequently result in inappropriate focal image formation. If the anteroposterior dimension of the eyeball is too short, the image is theoretically focused posterior to (behind) the retina. This is called *hyperopia* or *farsightedness*. In such cases, the accommodative changes of the lens can bring distant images into focus, but near images become blurred. Hyperopia (Fig. 19-11B) is corrected by appropriate convex surface lenses. If the anteroposterior dimension of the eyeball is too long, the focus point for an infinitely distant target is anterior to the retina. This condition is called *myopia* or *nearsightedness* (Fig. 19-11C). People with myopia can see close objects without problems because accommodative changes in their lens bring near objects into focus, but distant objects are blurred. Myopia can be corrected with an appropriate concave surface lens. Refractive corneal surgeries such as laser in situ keratomileusis, photorefractive keratectomy, and radial keratotomy can be performed to correct the corneal curvature to create accurate optical focus.[29,30]

Refractive defects of the corneal surface do not permit the formation of a sharp image. Nonuniform curvature of the refractive medium with regard to the horizontal and vertical planes is called *astigmatism*. Astigmatism is usually the result of an asymmetric bowing of the cornea, but it can result from defects in the cornea, lens, or the retina. Lens correction is available to sharpen focus in case of such refractive error.

Disorders of Accommodation

Because the retina is at a fixed distance from the lens, adjustability in the refractive power of the lens is needed so that a clear image is maintained as gaze is shifted from a far to a near object. The process by which the refractive power of the lens is increased, and the diverging light rays are bent more sharply, is called accommodation. Accommodation is the convergence of the eyes and pupillary constriction that results from thickening of the lens through contraction of the ciliary muscle. Contraction of the ciliary muscles is controlled mainly by the parasympathetic fibers of the oculomotor CN III. In near vision, pupillary constriction (*i.e.*, miosis) improves the clarity of the retinal image. This must be balanced against the resultant decrease in light intensity reaching the retina. During changes from near to far vision, pupillary dilation partially compensates for the reduced size of the retinal image by increasing the light entering the pupil. A third component of accommodation involves the reflex narrowing of the palpebral opening during near vision and widening during far vision.

Paralysis of the ciliary muscle, with loss of accommodation, is called *cycloplegia*.[31,32] Lens shape is totally controlled by the pretectal region and the parasympathetic pathways through the oculomotor nerve to the ciliary muscle. Accommodation is lost with destruction of this pathway.

The term **"presbyopia"** refers to a decrease in accommodation that occurs because of aging. The lens consists of transparent fibers arranged in concentric layers, of which the external layers are the newest and softest. No loss of lens fibers occurs with aging; instead, additional fibers are added to the outermost portion of the lens. As the lens ages, it thickens, and its fibers become less elastic, so that the range of focus or accommodation is diminished to the point where reading glasses become necessary for near vision.

Cataracts

A cataract is a lens opacity that interferes with the transmission of light to the retina. It has been estimated that 18 million people in the world are visually disabled because of cataracts.[31,33] Cataracts are the most common cause of age-related visual loss in the world. They are found in approximately 50% of those between 65 and 74 years of age and in 70% of those older than 75 years.[1] Cataract surgery is the most common surgical procedure covered by Medicare, with more than 1 million procedures performed annually. More than 95% of people undergoing cataract surgery experience visual improvement if there is no ocular comorbidity.[31,33,34]

Causes and Types of Cataracts

The cause of cataract development is thought to be multifactorial, with different factors being associated with different types of opacities. The pathogenesis of cataracts is not completely understood. Several risk factors have been proposed, including the effects of aging, genetic influences, environmental and metabolic influences, drugs, and injury.[35,36] Metabolically induced cataracts are caused by disorders of carbohydrate metabolism (diabetes) or inborn errors of metabolism. Long-term exposure to sunlight (ultraviolet B radiation) and heavy smoking have been associated with increased risk of cataract formation.[35] Occasionally, cataracts occur as a developmental defect (*i.e.*, congenital cataracts) or secondary to trauma or diseases.[32,35]

Cataracts can result from several drugs. Corticosteroid drugs have been implicated as causative agents in cataract formation. Both systemic and inhaled corticosteroids have been cited as risk factors.[34] Other drugs associated with cataracts include the phenothiazines, amiodarone, and strong miotic ophthalmic drugs such as phospholine iodide.[36] Frequent examination of lens transparency should accompany the use of these and any other medications with potential cataract-forming effects.

Traumatic Cataract

Traumatic cataracts are usually caused by foreign body injury to the lens or blunt trauma to the eye. Foreign body injury that interrupts the lens capsule allows aqueous and vitreous humor to enter the lens and initiate cataract formation. Other causes of traumatic cataract are overexposure to heat or to ionizing radiation.

Congenital Cataract

A congenital cataract is one that is present at birth. Among the causes of congenital cataracts are genetic defects, toxic environmental agents, and viruses such as rubella. Cataracts and other developmental defects of the ocular apparatus depend on the total dose of the agent and the embryonic stage at the time of exposure. During the last trimester of fetal life, genetically or environmentally influenced malformation of the superficial lens fibers can occur. Congenital lens opacities may occur in children of mothers with diabetes.[35] Most congenital cataracts are not progressive and are not dense enough to cause significant visual impairment. However, if the cataracts are bilateral and the opacity is significant, lens extraction should be done on one eye by the age of 2 months to permit the development of vision (see later section on amblyopia). If the surgery is successful, the contralateral lens should be removed soon after.

Senile Cataract

Cataracts are the most common cause of age-related vision loss in the world.[35] With normal aging, the nucleus and the cortex of the lens enlarge as new fibers are formed in the cortical zones of the lens. In the nucleus, the old fibers become more compressed and dehydrated. Metabolic changes occur and lens proteins become more insoluble, and concentrations of calcium, sodium, potassium, and phosphate increase. During the early stages of cataract formation, a yellow pigment and vacuoles accumulate in the lens fibers. The unfolding of protein molecules, cross-linking of sulfhydryl groups, and conversion of soluble to insoluble proteins lead to the loss of lens transparency. The onset is gradual, and the only symptoms are increasingly blurred vision and visual distortion.

Clinical Manifestations

The manifestations of cataract depend on the extent of opacity and whether the defect is bilateral or unilateral. With the exception of traumatic or congenital cataract, most cataracts are bilateral. Visual acuity for far and near objects decreases. Dilation of the pupil in dim light improves vision. In addition to decreased visual acuity, cataracts tend to cause light entering the eye to be scattered, thereby producing glare or the abnormal presence of light in the visual field.

Diagnosis and Treatment

Diagnosis of cataract is based on ophthalmoscopic examination and the degree of visual impairment on the Snellen vision test. On ophthalmoscopic examination, cataracts may appear as a gross opacity filling the pupillary aperture or as an opacity silhouetted against the red background of the fundus. There is no effective medical treatment for cataract. Strong bifocals, magnification, appropriate lighting, and visual aids may be used as the cataract progresses. Surgery is the only treatment for correcting cataract-related vision loss. Surgery usually involves lens extraction and intraocular lens implantation.[36] Phacoemulsification involves ultrasonic fragmentation of the lens into fine pieces, which then are aspirated from the eye.

One of the greatest advances in cataract surgery has been the development of reliable intraocular implants. Monofocal intraocular lenses that correct for distance vision are available, and eyeglasses may be needed for near vision, although this has been addressed by the recent introduction of multifocal intraocular lenses.

 SUMMARY CONCEPTS

The lens is a biconvex, avascular, colorless, and almost transparent structure suspended behind the iris. The shape of the lens is controlled by the ciliary muscle, which contracts and relaxes the zonule fibers, thus changing the tension on the lens capsule and altering the focus of the lens. Refraction, which refers to the ability to focus an object on the retina, depends on the size and shape of the eyeball and the cornea and on the focusing ability of the lens. Errors in refraction occur when the visual image is not focused on the retina because of individual differences in the size or shape of the eyeball or cornea. In hyperopia, or farsightedness, the image theoretically falls behind the retina. In myopia, or nearsightedness, the image falls in front of the retina. Accommodation is the process by which a clear image is maintained as the gaze is shifted from a far to a near object. It is associated with convergence of the eyes and pupillary constriction, and thickening of the lens results from contraction of the ciliary muscle. Presbyopia is a change in the lens that occurs because of aging such that the lens becomes thicker and less able to change shape and accommodate for near vision.

A cataract is a lens opacity. It can occur as the result of congenital influences, metabolic disturbances, infection, injury, and aging. The most common type of cataract is senile cataract that occurs with aging. The treatment for a totally opaque or mature cataract is surgical extraction. An intraocular lens implant may be inserted during the surgical procedure to replace the removed lens; otherwise, thick convex lenses or contact lenses are used to compensate for the loss of lens function.

Disorders of the Vitreous and Retina

The posterior segment, comprising five sixths of the eyeball, contains the transparent vitreous humor and the neural retina. The innermost layer of the eyeball, the fundus, is visualized through the pupil with an ophthalmoscope.

Disorders of the Vitreous

Vitreous humor (*i.e.*, vitreous body) is a colorless, **amorphous** biologic gel that fills the posterior cavity of the eye (see Fig. 19-2). It consists of approximately 99% water, some salts, glycoproteins, proteoglycans, and dispersed collagen fibrils. The vitreous is attached to the ciliary body and the peripheral retina in the region of the ora serrata and to the periphery of the optic disc.

Disease, aging, and injury can disturb the factors that maintain the water of the vitreous humor in suspension, causing liquefaction of the gel to occur. With the loss of gel structure, fine fibers, membranes, and cellular debris develop. When this occurs, floaters (images) can often be noticed as these substances move within the vitreous cavity during head movement. In disease, blood vessels may grow from the surface of the retina or optic disc onto the posterior surface of the vitreous, and blood may fill the vitreous cavity.

In a procedure called a *vitrectomy*, the removal and replacement of the vitreous with a balanced saline solution can restore sight in some people with vitreous opacities resulting from hemorrhage or vitreoretinal membrane formations that cause legal blindness. Using this procedure, a small probe with a cutting tip is used to remove the opaque vitreous and membranes. The procedure is difficult and requires complex instrumentation. It is of no value if the retina is not functional.

Disorders of the Retina

The function of the retina is to receive visual images, partially analyze them, and transmit this modified information to the brain.[37] It is composed of two layers: the inner neural retina that contains the photoreceptors and an outer melanin-containing layer that rests on, and is firmly attached to, the choriocapillaris, the capillary layer of the choroid. A non–light-sensitive portion of the retina, along with the retinal pigment epithelium, continues anteriorly to form the posterior surface of the iris. A wavy border called the *ora serrata* exists at the junction between the light-sensitive and the non–light-sensitive retinas. Separating the vascular portion of the choroid from pigmented cells of the retina is a thin layer of elastic tissue, the *Bruch membrane*, which contains collagen fibrils in its superficial and deep portions. Cells of the pigmented layer receive their nourishment by diffusion from the choriocapillaris.

Disorders of the retina and its function include derangements of the pigment epithelium (*e.g.*, retinitis pigmentosa), ischemic conditions caused by disorders of the retinal blood supply, disorders of the retinal vessels such as retinopathies that cause hemorrhage and the development of opacities, separation of the pigment and sensory layers of the retina (*i.e.*, retinal detachment), abnormalities of the Bruch membrane and choroid (*e.g.*, macular degeneration), and malignant tumors of the nuclear layer of the retina (*i.e.*, retinoblastoma). Because the retina has no pain fibers, most diseases of the retina are painless and do not cause redness of the eye.

The Neural Retina

The neural retina is composed of three layers of neurons: a posterior layer of photoreceptors, a middle layer of bipolar cells, and an inner layer of ganglion cells that communicate with the photoreceptors (Fig. 19-12). A pattern of light on the retina falls on a massive array of photoreceptors. These photoreceptors synapse with bipolar and other interneurons before action potentials in ganglion cells relay the message to specific regions of the brain and the brain stem associated with vision. For rods, this microcircuitry involves the convergence of signals from many rods on a single ganglion cell. This arrangement maximizes spatial summation and the detection of stimulated (light vs. dark) receptors. The interneurons, composed of horizontal and amacrine cells, have cell bodies in the bipolar layer, and they play an important role in modulating retinal function. A superficial marginal layer contains the axons of the ganglion cells as they collect and leave the eye through the optic nerve. These fibers lie beside the vitreous humor. Light must pass through the transparent inner layers of the sensory retina before it reaches the photoreceptors.

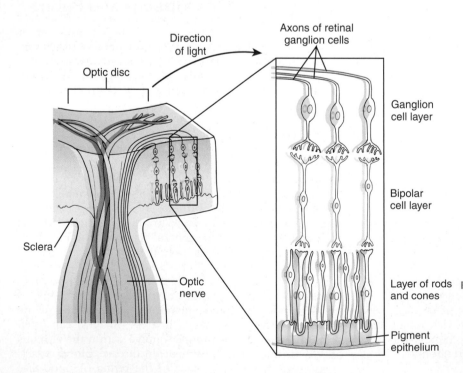

FIGURE 19-12. Organization of the human retina. The optic pathway begins with photoreceptors (rods and cones) in the retina. The responses of the photoreceptors are transmitted by the bipolar cells to the ganglion cell layer of the retina.

Photoreceptors

Two types of photoreceptors are present in the retina: rods, capable of black–white discrimination, and cones, capable of color discrimination. Both types of photoreceptors are thin, elongated, mitochondria-filled cells with a single, highly modified cilium (Fig. 19-13). The cilium has a short base, or inner segment, and a highly modified outer segment. The plasma membrane of the outer segment is tightly folded to form membranous discs (rods) or conical shapes (cones) containing visual pigment. These discs are continuously synthesized at the base of the outer segment and shed at the distal end. Discarded membranes are phagocytized by the retinal pigment cells. If this phagocytosis is disrupted, as in retinitis pigmentosa, the sensory retina degenerates.

Rods

Rod-based vision is particularly sensitive to detecting light, especially moving light stimuli, at the expense of clear pattern discrimination. Rod vision is particularly adapted for night and low-level illumination.

Cones and Color Sensitivity

Cone receptors that are selectively sensitive to different wavelengths of light provide the basis for color vision. Three types of cones, or cone–color systems, respond to the blue, green, and red portions of the visible electromagnetic spectrum. The color a person perceives depends on which set of cones or combination of sets of cones is stimulated in a given image.

Cones do not have the dark adaptation capability of rods. Consequently, the dark-adapted eye is a rod receptor eye with only black–gray–white discrimination (scotopic or **night vision**). The light-adapted eye (*photopic vision*) adds the capacity for color discrimination. Rhodopsin has its maximum sensitivity in the blue–green region of the electromagnetic spectrum.

Macula and Fovea

An area approximately 1.5 mm in diameter near the center of the retina, called the *macula lutea* (*i.e.*, "yellow spot"), is especially adapted for acute and detailed vision.[37] This area is composed entirely of cones. In the central portion of the macula, the **fovea** *centralis* (foveola), the blood vessels, and innermost layers are displaced to one side instead of resting on top of the cones (Fig. 19-14). This allows light to pass unimpeded to the cones without passing through several layers of the retina.

Color Blindness

Color blindness is inherited as an X-linked deficiency of a specific type of retinal photoreceptor. The most common abnormality is red–green color blindness. The deficiency is usually partial but can be complete. Rarely are two of the color mechanisms missing; when this occurs, usually red and green are missing. Complete lack of color discrimination is rare. For such people, the world is experienced entirely as black, gray, and white.

Retinitis Pigmentosa

Retinitis pigmentosa represents a group of hereditary diseases that cause slow degenerative changes in the retinal photoreceptors. The disease can be inherited as autosomal dominant (20% to 30%) and autosomal recessive (10% to 15%). The remaining percent is X-link associated. There are over 100 gene mutations associated with retinitis pigmentosa.[38] Nonocular diseases can be associated with retinitis pigmentosa such as Usher syndrome, Refsum disease, and Bardet–Biedl syndrome.[38]

In cases known as rod–cone dystrophy, a number of characteristic clinical symptoms including night blindness and bilateral symmetric loss of midperipheral fields occur. With progression, cone photoreceptor cells are also affected and day vision and central visual acuity are compromised. The rate of visual failure is variable.[38]

Disorders of Retinal Blood Supply

The blood supply for the retina is derived from two sources: the choriocapillaris (*i.e.*, the capillary layer of the choroid) and branches of the central retinal artery (Fig. 19-15). Oxygen and other nutritional substances needed by the retina and its component parts (pigment cells, rods, and cones) are supplied by diffusion from blood vessels in the choroid. Because the choriocapillaris provides the only blood supply for the fovea centralis (*i.e.*, foveola), detachment of this part of the sensory retina from the pigment epithelium causes irreparable visual loss.

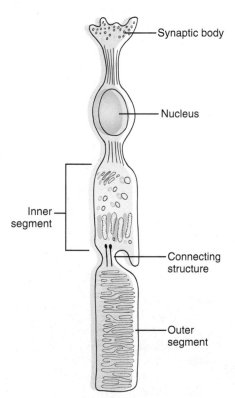

FIGURE 19-13. Retinal rod, showing its component parts and the distribution of its organelles. Its outer segment contains the discs (rods). The connecting structure joins the outer and inner segments. The inner segment contains the mitochondria, the ribosomal endoplasmic reticulum, the free ribosomes, and the Golgi saccules. The synaptic body is the site where the photoreceptor synapses with other nerve cells.

Labels in figure: Synaptic body; Nucleus; Inner segment; Connecting structure; Outer segment

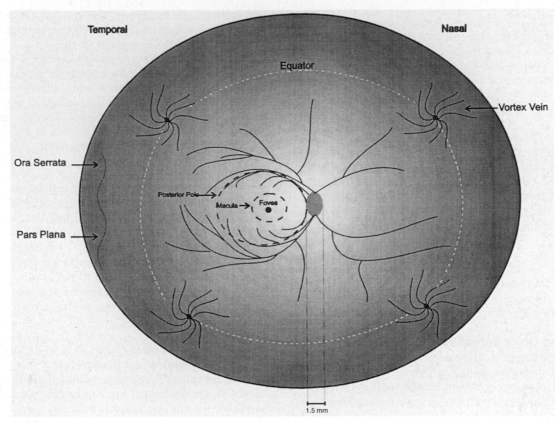

FIGURE 19-14. Anatomy of retina as viewed by funduscopic examination. (From Miller N. R., Newman N. J., Biousse V., et al. (Eds.). (2008). *Walsh and Hoyt's clinical neuro-ophthalmology: The essentials* (2nd ed., p. 43). Philadelphia, PA: Lippincott Williams & Wilkins.)

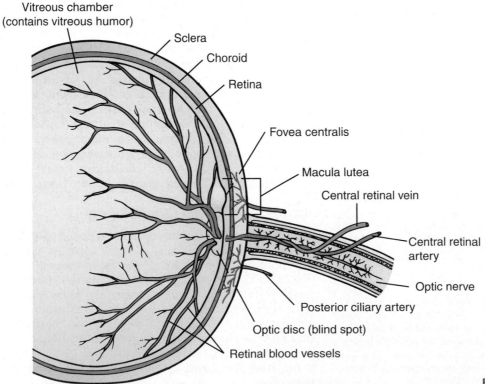

FIGURE 19-15. Retinal circulation.

The bipolar, horizontal, amacrine, and ganglion cells and the ganglion cell axons that gather at the optic disc are supplied by branches of the retinal artery.[37] The central artery of the retina is a branch of the ophthalmic artery. It enters the globe through the optic disc. Branches of this artery radiate over the entire retina, except the central fovea, which is surrounded by, but is not crossed by, arterial branches. The central artery of the retina is an end artery, meaning that it does not anastomose with other arteries. This is critical because an infarct in this artery will totally deprive distal structures of their vascular supply. Retinal veins follow a distribution parallel to the arterial branches and carry venous blood to the central vein of the retina, which exits the back of the eye through the optic disc.

Funduscopic examination of the eye with an ophthalmoscope provides an opportunity to examine the retinal blood vessels and other aspects of the retina (Fig. 19-16).

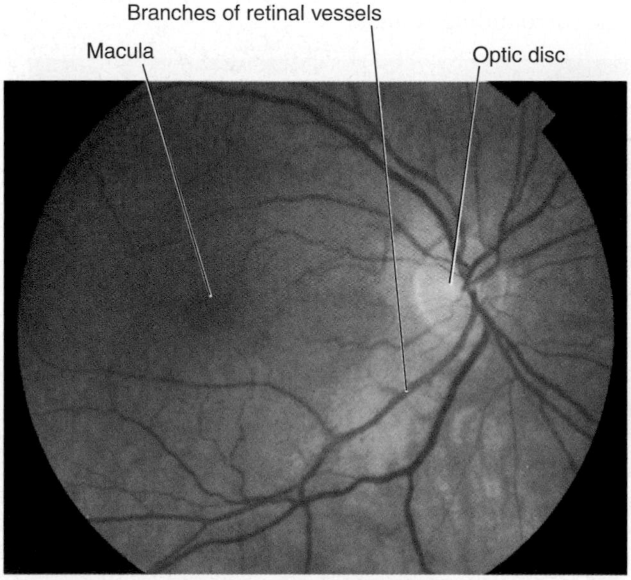

Because the retina is an embryonic outgrowth of the brain and the blood vessels are to a considerable extent representative of brain blood vessels, the ophthalmoscopic examination of the fundus of the eye permits the study and diagnosis of metabolic and vascular diseases of the brain as well as pathologic processes that are specific to the retina.

Ischemia of the retina occurs during general circulatory collapse. If a person survives cardiopulmonary arrest, for instance, permanently decreased visual acuity can occur as a result of edema and the ischemic death of retinal neurons.[37] Intermittent retinal ischemia can accompany internal carotid or common carotid stenosis. *Amaurosis fugax* is characterized by transient episodes of monocular visual loss lasting 5 to 10 minutes.[39]

Papilledema

The central retinal artery enters the eye through the optic papilla in the center of the optic nerve. An accompanying vein exits alongside the same path. The entrance and exit of the central retinal artery and vein running through the tough scleral tissue at the optic papilla can be compromised by any condition causing persistent increased intracranial pressure. The most common of these conditions are cerebral tumors, subdural hematomas, hydrocephalus, and malignant hypertension.

Usually, the thin-walled, low-pressure veins are the first to collapse, with the consequent backup and slowing of arterial blood flow. Under these conditions, capillary permeability increases and leakage of fluid results in edema of the optic papilla, called *papilledema* (Fig. 19-17).

Retinopathies

Disorders of the retinal vessels can result in microaneurysms, neovascularization, hemorrhage, and formation of retinal opacities. *Microaneurysms* are outpouchings of the retinal vasculature. On ophthalmoscopic

Branches of retinal vessels

Macula

Optic disc

FIGURE 19-16. Funduscopic image of normal retina. (From Moore K. L., Dalley A. F., Agur A. M. R. (2018). *Clinically oriented anatomy* (8th ed., p. 905, Fig. 8.52). Philadelphia, PA: Wolters Kluwer.)

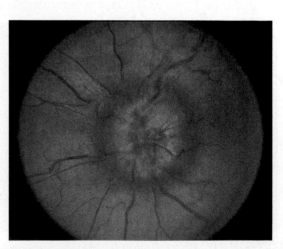

FIGURE 19-17. Chronic papilledema. The optic nerve head is congested and protrudes anteriorly toward the interior of the eye. It has blurred margins, and vessels within it are poorly seen. (From Klintworth G. K. (2015). The eye. In Rubin R., Strayer D. E. (Eds.), *Rubin's pathology: Clinicopathologic foundations of medicine* (7th ed., p. 1518, Fig. 33-15). Philadelphia, PA: Lippincott Williams & Wilkins.)

examination, they appear as minute, unchanging red dots associated with blood vessels. These microaneurysms tend to leak plasma, resulting in localized edema that gives the retina a hazy appearance. Microaneurysms can be identified with certainty using fluorescein angiography; the fluorescein dye is injected intravenously, and the retinal vessels subsequently are photographed using a special ophthalmoscope and fundus camera. The microaneurysms may bleed, but areas of hemorrhage and edema tend to clear spontaneously. However, they reduce visual acuity if they encroach on the macula and cause degeneration before they are absorbed.

Neovascularization involves the formation of new blood vessels. They can develop from the choriocapillaris, extending between the pigment layer and the sensory layer, or from the retinal veins, extending between the sensory retina and the vitreous cavity and sometimes into the vitreous. These new blood vessels are fragile, leak protein, and are likely to bleed. Neovascularization occurs in many conditions that impair retinal blood flow, including stasis because of hyperviscosity of blood or decreased flow, vascular occlusion, sickle cell disease, sarcoidosis, diabetes mellitus, and retinopathy of prematurity.[39-41]

Hemorrhage can be preretinal, intraretinal, or subretinal. *Preretinal hemorrhages* occur between the retina and the vitreous. These hemorrhages are usually large because the blood vessels are only loosely restricted; they may be associated with a subarachnoid or subdural hemorrhage and are usually regarded as a serious manifestation of the disorder. They usually reabsorb without complications unless they penetrate into the vitreous. *Intraretinal hemorrhages* occur because of abnormalities of the retinal vessels, diseases of the blood, increased pressure in the retinal vessels, or vitreous traction on the vessels. Systemic causes include diabetes mellitus, hypertension, and blood dyscrasias. *Subretinal hemorrhages* are those that develop between the choroid and pigment layer of the retina. A common cause of subretinal hemorrhage is neovascularization. Photocoagulation may be used to treat microaneurysms and neovascularization.

Light normally passes through the transparent inner portions of the sensory retina before reaching the photoreceptors. *Opacities* such as hemorrhages, exudate, cotton wool spots, edema, and tissue proliferation can produce a localized loss of transparency observable with an ophthalmoscope. Exudates are opacities resulting from inflammatory processes. The development of exudates often results in the destruction of the underlying retinal pigment and choroid layer. Deposits are localized opacities consisting of lipid-laden macrophages or accumulated cellular debris. Cotton wool spots are retinal opacities with hazy, irregular outlines. They occur in the nerve fiber layer and contain cell organelles. Cotton wool patches are associated with retinal trauma, severe anemia, papilledema, and diabetic retinopathy.

Diabetic Retinopathy

Diabetic retinopathy is the most common cause of blindness in the industrialized countries of the world. It ranks first as the cause of newly reported cases of blindness in people between the ages of 20 and 74 years.[39,42] Advances in treatment have greatly reduced the risk of blindness from diabetes, but because diabetes is so common, retinopathy remains an important cause of visual impairment.

Diabetic retinopathy can be divided into two types: *nonproliferative* (i.e., background) and *proliferative*.[40-42] Background or nonproliferative retinopathy is confined to the retina. It involves engorgement of the retinal veins, thickening of the capillary endothelial basement membrane, and development of capillary microaneurysms (Fig. 19-18A). Small intraretinal hemorrhages may develop and microinfarcts may cause cotton wool spots and leakage of exudates. A sensation of glare (because of the scattering of light) is a common complaint. The most common cause of decreased vision in people with background retinopathy is macular edema. The edema is caused primarily by the breakdown of the inner blood–retina barrier at the level of the capillary endothelium, allowing leakage of fluid and plasma constituents into the surrounding retina.

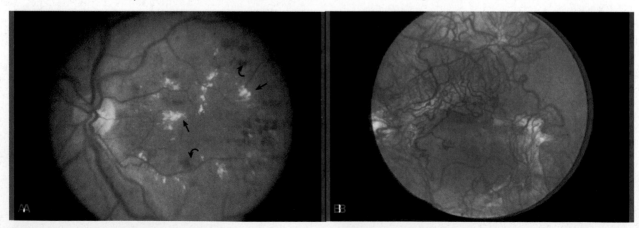

FIGURE 19-18. Diabetic retinopathy. **(A)** Ocular fundus of a person with background diabetic retinopathy. Several yellowish "hard" exudates (*straight arrows*) and several relatively small retinal hemorrhages (*curved arrows*) are present. **(B)** A vascular frond (top half) has extended anteriorly to the retina in the eye with proliferative diabetic retinopathy. (From Klintworth G. K. (2015). The eye. In Rubin R., Strayer D. E. (Eds.), *Rubin's pathology: Clinicopathologic foundations of medicine* (7th ed., p. 1514, Fig. 33-10A and B). Philadelphia, PA: Lippincott Williams & Wilkins.)

Proliferative diabetic retinopathy represents a more severe retinal change than background retinopathy (Fig. 19-18B). It is characterized by formation of new, fragile blood vessels (*i.e.*, neovascularization) at the disc and elsewhere in the retina. These vessels grow in front of the retina along the posterior surface of the vitreous or into the vitreous. They threaten vision in two ways. First, because they are abnormal, they often bleed easily, leaking blood into the vitreous cavity and decreasing visual acuity. Second, the blood vessels attach firmly to the retinal surface and posterior surface of the vitreous, such that normal movement of the vitreous may exert a pull on the retina, causing retinal detachment and progressive blindness. Because proliferative diabetic retinopathy is likely to be asymptomatic, it must be identified early, before bleeding occurs and obscures the view of the fundus or leads to fibrosis and retinal detachment.

The cause of diabetic retinopathy is uncertain.[40,43] Chronically elevated levels of blood glucose contribute to the development and progression of retinopathy as well as other complications of diabetes. Hypertension is also thought to increase the risk of the development and progression of diabetic retinopathy. In addition to chronic hyperglycemia and hypertension, several studies have indicated the association of diabetic exudative retinopathy with hypercholesteremia and combined inflammatory mediators on the retinal microvasculature.[44]

Preventing diabetic retinopathy from developing or progressing is considered the best approach to preserving vision. Growing evidence suggests that careful control of blood glucose levels in people with diabetes mellitus may retard the onset and progression of retinopathy. There also is a need for intensive management of hypertension and hyperlipidemia, both of which have been shown to increase the risk of diabetic retinopathy in people with diabetes.[42]

Photocoagulation using an argon laser provides the major direct treatment modality for diabetic retinopathy.[40,41] Because laser photocoagulation destroys the proliferating vessels and the ischemic retina, it reduces the stimulus for further neovascularization. Vitrectomy has proved effective in removing vitreous hemorrhage and severing vitreoretinal membranes that develop.

Hypertensive Retinopathy

As with other blood vessels in the body, the retinal vessels undergo changes in response to chronically elevated blood pressure. In the initial, vasoconstrictor stage, there is vasospasm and an increase in retinal arterial tone because of local autoregulatory mechanisms. On ophthalmoscopy, this stage is represented by a general narrowing of the retinal arterioles. Persistently elevated blood pressure results in the compensatory thickening of arteriolar walls, which effectively reduces capillary perfusion pressure. With severe, uncontrolled hypertension, there is disruption of the blood–retina barrier, necrosis of smooth muscle and endothelial cells, exudation of blood and lipids, and retinal ischemia. These changes are manifested in the retina by microaneurysms, intraretinal hemorrhages, hard exudates, and cotton wool spots. Swelling of the optic disc may occur at this stage and usually indicates severely elevated blood pressure (malignant hypertension). Older adults often have more rigid vessels that are unable to respond to the same degree as those in younger people.

Studies have shown that signs of hypertensive retinopathy regress with control of blood pressure.[44] There is also evidence that advanced signs of hypertensive retinopathy (*e.g.*, retinal hemorrhages, microaneurysms, and cotton wool spots) predict death from stroke independent of elevated blood pressure and other risk factors.[44] People with these signs may benefit from close monitoring of cerebrovascular risk and intensive measures to reduce the risk.

Retinal Detachment

Retinal detachment involves the separation of the neurosensory retina from the pigment epithelium (Fig. 19-19). It occurs when traction on the inner sensory layer or a tear in this layer allows fluid, usually vitreous, to accumulate between the two layers.[37,45] There are four types of retinal detachments: exudative, traction, rhegmatogenous, and combined traction/rhegmatogenous.[45–47]

Exudative (or serous) *retinal detachment* results from the accumulation of serous or hemorrhagic fluid in the subretinal space due to severe hypertension, inflammation, or neoplastic effusions. It usually resolves with successful treatment of the underlying disease and without visual impairment. *Traction retinal attachment* occurs with mechanical forces on the retina, usually mediated by fibrotic tissue, resulting from previous hemorrhage (*e.g.*, from diabetic retinopathy), injury, infection, or inflammation. Intraocular surgery such as cataract extraction may produce traction on the peripheral retina that causes eventual detachment months or even years after surgery. Correction of traction retinal detachment requires disengaging scar tissue from the retinal surface, and vision outcomes are often poor.

Rhegmatogenous detachment (*rhegma* is the Greek for "rent" or "hole") is the most common type of retinal detachment. The vitreous is a hydrated gel whose structure is maintained by a collagenous and mucopolysaccharide matrix. As people age, this macromolecular network begins to liquefy and collapse. As this occurs, the vitreous shrinks and partly separates from the retinal surface, a condition known as *posterior vitreous detachment* (see Fig. 19-19). Rhegmatogenous detachment occurs when the liquid vitreous enters the subretinal space through the retinal tear. Detachment of the neural retina from the retinal pigment layer separates the receptors from their major blood supply, the choroid. If retinal detachment continues for some time, permanent destruction and blindness of that part of the retina occur.

Etiology and Pathophysiology

Risk factors for retinal detachment can include but are not limited to advancing age, myopia, previous eye surgeries, intraocular tumors, and diabetes. Approximately one in four people between the ages of 61 and 70 years develops a posterior vitreous detachment. In about 10% to 15% of these people, a retinal tear or hole forms as

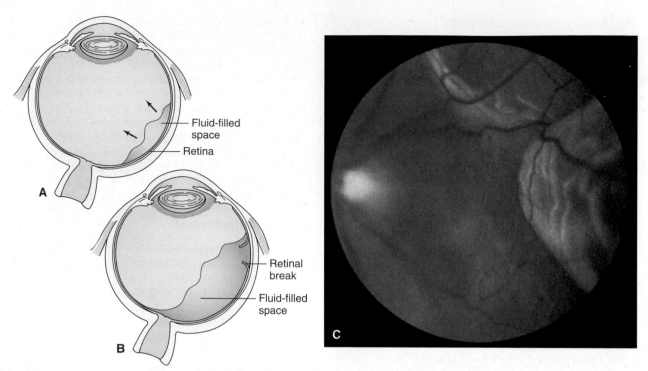

FIGURE 19-19. Retinal detachment. (**A**) Changes in the vitreous structure cause it to shrink and separate from the retina, causing posterior vitreous detachment; (**B**) sustained fluid collection and tractional forces cause the retina to tear (rhegmatogenous retinal detachment). (**C**) Ophthalmoscopic photograph of retinal detachment. (From Moore K. L., Dalley A. F., Agur A. M. R. (2018). *Clinically oriented anatomy* (8th ed., p. 918, Fig. B8.25). Philadelphia, PA: Lippincott Williams & Wilkins.)

the vitreous pulls away from the retina, especially in the periphery where the retina is thinner.[37,45] People with high grades of myopia may have abnormalities in the peripheral retina that predispose to sudden detachment. In moderate to severe myopia or nearsightedness, the axial (anteroposterior) length of the eye is increased, resulting in an egg-shaped globe. As a result, there is greater vitreoretinal traction, and posterior vitreous detachment may occur at a younger age than in people without myopia. Also, the retina tends to be thinner and more prone to formation of a hole or tear. Other, less common risk factors include a family history of retinal detachment, a history of congenital eye disease (glaucoma, cataracts), and hereditary vitreopathies with abnormal vitreous gel.

Clinical Manifestations and Diagnosis

The primary symptom of retinal detachment consists of painless changes in vision. Commonly, flashing lights or sparks, followed by small floaters or spots in the field of vision, occur as the vitreous pulls away from the posterior pole of the eye. As detachment progresses, the person perceives a shadow or dark curtain progressing across the visual field. Because the process begins in the periphery and spreads circumferentially and posteriorly, initial visual disturbances may involve only one quadrant of the visual field. Large peripheral detachments may occur without involvement of the macula, so that visual acuity remains unaffected. An altered red reflex can be associated with retinal detachment.[45]

Diagnosis is based on a history of visual disturbances (*e.g.*, presence of floaters, luminous rays, or light flashes) and the ophthalmoscopic appearance of the retina. The direct (handheld) ophthalmoscope is useful in detecting an altered red reflex sometimes associated with retinal detachment. However, because the view is narrow, a negative examination with direct ophthalmoscopy cannot exclude the diagnosis of retinal detachment. Ophthalmologists and optometrists use indirect examination techniques that greatly enhance visualization of the peripheral retina.[45]

Treatment

Because there is a variable interval between a retinal break and retinal detachment, treatment methods focus on early detection and prevention of further vitreous detachment and retinal tear formation. Symptomatic retinal breaks are usually treated with laser or cryotherapy to seal the retinal tears so that the vitreous can no longer leak into the subretinal space.[37,45–47]

Macular Degeneration

Macular degeneration is characterized by degenerative changes in the central portion of the retina (the macula) that result primarily in loss of central vision. Age-related macular degeneration (AMD) is the most common cause of reduced vision and legal blindness worldwide.[48,49] Risk factors include age over 50 years, female sex, white race, cigarette smoking, nutritional factors, cardiovascular diseases, and genes that are implicated in the regulation of lipid pathways.[48–52]

There are two types of AMD: an atrophic nonexudative or "dry" form and an exudative or "wet" form.

Although both types are progressive, they differ in terms of manifestations, prognosis, and management. Although most people with AMD manifest nonproliferative changes only, those who experience severe vision loss do so from the development of the exudative form of the disease.

Clinical Manifestations and Diagnosis

Nonexudative AMD is characterized by various degrees of atrophy and degeneration of the outer retina, Bruch membrane, and the choriocapillaris. It does not involve leakage of blood or serum. Therefore, it is called *dry AMD* (Fig. 19-20). On ophthalmoscopic examination, there are visible changes in the retinal pigmentary epithelium and pale yellow spots, called *drusen*, which may occur individually or in groups throughout the macula. Histopathologically, most drusen contain remnants of materials representative of focal detachment of the pigment epithelium. With time, the drusen enlarge, coalesce, and increase in number. The level of associated visual impairment is variable and may be minimal. Most people with macular drusen do not experience significant loss of central vision, and the atrophic changes may stabilize or progress slowly. However, people with the nonexudative form of AMD need to be followed closely because the exudative stage may develop suddenly, at any time. Careful monitoring for metamorphopsia, or distorted vision of straight lines, can aid in the early detection of retinal damage.

The exudative or "wet form" of macular degeneration is characterized by the formation of a choroidal neovascular membrane that separates the pigmented epithelium from the neuroretina. These new blood vessels have weaker walls than normal and are prone to leakage. The leakage of serous or hemorrhagic fluid into the subretinal space causes separation of the pigmented epithelium from the neurosensory retina. Over time, the subretinal hemorrhages organize to form scar tissue, causing death of the underlying retinal tissue and loss of all visual function in the corresponding macular area (see Fig. 19-20). The early stages of subretinal neovascularization may be difficult to detect with an ophthalmoscope. Therefore, there is a need to be alert for recent or sudden changes in central vision, blurred vision, or scotomata in people with evidence of AMD.

Although some subretinal neovascular membranes may regress spontaneously, the natural course of exudative macular degeneration is toward irreversible loss of central vision. People with late-stage disease often find it difficult to see at long distances (*e.g.*, in driving), do close work (*e.g.*, reading), see faces clearly, or distinguish colors. However, they may not be severely incapacitated because the peripheral retinal function usually remains intact. With the use of low-vision aids, many of them are able to continue many of their normal activities.

Treatment

Effective therapies for exudative or wet-type macular degeneration include thermal laser photocoagulation, photodynamic therapy, intravitreal and periocular corticosteroid injections, and intravitreal injections of vascular endothelial growth factor (VEGF) inhibitors. Currently, there is no established effective treatment for the dry form of macular degeneration, and most current therapies and new investigational treatments are directed at choroidal (or subretinal) neovascularization.[52,53]

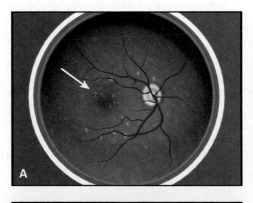

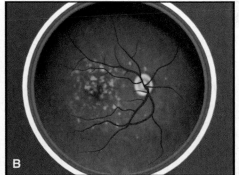

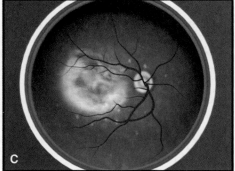

FIGURE 19-20. Funduscopic view of different states of AMD. (**A**) Early intermediate AMD (*white arrow*), (**B**) intermediate AMD, and (**C**) advanced AMD with fibrosis. AMD, age-related macular degeneration. (From the National Eye Institute, National Institutes of Health.)

Tobacco smoking is consistently identified as a preventable AMD risk. Therefore, elimination of tobacco smoking should be one of the first therapeutic recommendations. Preventative recommendations also include dietary supplementation with antioxidants and minerals such as vitamin E (α-tocopherol), vitamin C (ascorbic acid), zinc, and β-carotene for people at risk for developing macular degeneration and for slowing the progression of AMD in people with the disease.[52,53]

Retinoblastoma

Retinoblastoma is the most common intraocular malignant neoplasm of children, affecting 1 in 20,000.[54] The tumor occurs most frequently in children younger than 2 years and may even be found at birth. Retinoblastomas are related to inherited or acquired mutations in the retinoblastoma (Rb) tumor suppressor gene, located on the long arm of chromosome 13. If untreated, almost all children die of intracranial extension and disseminated disease. However, new diagnostic and treatment methods allow for a high rate of cure (93% survival in the United States).[54,55]

Clinical Manifestations

Leukocoria (i.e., cat's-eye reflex, white reflex, or white pupil) is the most common presenting sign and is often noticed by the family; light entering the eye commonly reflects a yellowish-white color similar to that of the membranous covering of a cat's eye (Fig. 19-21). Strabismus (squint) is the second most common sign.[56] Red, tearing, and painful eyes are a late sign of the disorder. Limited or poor vision is also a late sign. Most retinoblastomas occur sporadically and are unilateral. Up to 25% of sporadic retinoblastomas and most inherited forms of the disorder are bilateral.

Diagnosis and Treatment

Diagnostic measures for the detection of retinoblastoma are usually prompted by abnormal results of an eye examination in the hospital nursery or health care provider's office. All children with a family history of retinoblastoma should be screened soon after birth. Screening should be repeated every 4 to 6 weeks until 1 year of age and then every 2 to 3 months until 3 years of age.[55,56] Congenital cataracts are an important cause of childhood leukocoria and should be ruled out. A definitive diagnosis usually requires ophthalmoscopic examination under general anesthesia by an ophthalmologist to obtain complete visualization of both eyes, which facilitates photographing and mapping of the tumors. CT or MRI scans are used to evaluate the extent of intraocular disease and extraocular spread.

The goals of treatment are primarily to save the child's life and secondarily to save the eye. Treatment options include laser thermotherapy, cryotherapy, chemotherapy, and enucleation (removal of the eye). Advances in genetics have enabled emerging therapies such as intravitreal chemotherapy and tumor hypoxia; the goal of both is preserving the globe (eyeball).[57–59]

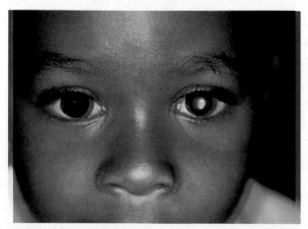

FIGURE 19-21. The white pupil reflex (leukocoria) in the left eye of a child with intraocular retinoblastoma. (From Klintworth G. K. (2015). The eye. In Rubin R., Strayer D. E. (Eds.), *Rubin's pathology: Clinicopathologic foundations of medicine* (7th ed., p. 1523, Fig. 33-22A). Philadelphia, PA: Lippincott Williams & Wilkins.)

SUMMARY CONCEPTS

The neural retina covers the inner aspect of the posterior two thirds of the eyeball and is continuous with the optic nerve. It contains the neural receptors for vision, and it is here that light energy of different frequencies and intensities is converted to graded local potentials, which then are converted to action potentials and transmitted to visual centers in the brain. The photoreceptors normally shed portions of their outer segments. Cells in the pigment epithelium phagocytize these segments. Failure of phagocytosis, as occurs in one form of retinitis pigmentosa, results in degeneration of the pigment layer and blindness.

The retina receives its blood from two sources: the choriocapillaris, which supplies the pigment layer and the outer portion of the sensory retina adjacent to the choroid, and the branches of the retinal artery, which supply the inner half of the retina. Retinal blood vessels are normally apparent through the ophthalmoscope. Neovascularization involves the formation of new, fragile blood vessels that leak protein and are likely to bleed. Although the cause of neovascularization is uncertain, research links the process with a VEGF produced by the lining of blood vessels. Hypoxia is a key regulator of VEGF-induced retinal neovascularization.

Disorders of retinal vessels can result from many local and systemic disorders, including diabetes mellitus and hypertension. They cause vision loss through changes that result in hemorrhage, production of opacities, and separation of the pigment epithelium and sensory retina. Retinal detachment involves separation of the sensory receptors from their blood supply; it causes blindness unless reattachment is accomplished promptly. Macular degeneration is characterized by loss of central vision due to destructive changes of the macula of the retina. There are two types of AMD: a nonexudative "dry form" that causes atrophy and degeneration of the outer retina and an exudative "wet form" that results in formation of a choroidal neovascular membrane with vessels that leak blood and serum and predispose to separation of the pigmented epithelium from the neuroretina. Although there are currently no effective therapies for the dry form of AMD, effective treatment for the wet form includes photodynamic therapy, laser photocoagulation, and intravitreal injection of corticosteroids and VEGF inhibitors.

Retinoblastoma is an intraocular malignant neoplasm of children (most often those younger than 2 years) that is caused by inherited or acquired mutations in the retinoblastoma (*Rb*) tumor suppressor gene. The most common presenting sign is leukocoria (white reflex or white pupil), with strabismus being the second most common sign. With new diagnostic and treatment methods, nearly 95% of retinoblastomas are cured in the United States.

Disorders of Neural Pathways and Cortical Centers

Full visual function requires the normally developed brain-related functions of photoreception and the pupillary reflex. These functions depend on the integrity of all optic pathways, including retinal circuitry and the pathway from the optic nerve to the visual cortex and other visual regions of the brain and brain stem.

Optic Pathways

Visual information is carried to the brain by axons of the retinal ganglion cells, which form the optic nerve. Surrounded by pia mater, cerebrospinal fluid, arachnoid, and the dura mater, the optic nerve represents an outgrowth of the brain rather than a peripheral nerve. The optic nerve extends from the back of the optic globe through the orbit and the optic foramen, into the middle cranial fossa, and onto the optic chiasm at the base of the brain[54] (Fig. 19-22). Axons from the nasal portion of the retina remain medial, and those from the temporal retina remain lateral in the optic nerve.

The two optic nerves meet and fuse in the optic chiasm, beyond which they are continued as the optic tracts. In the optic chiasm, axons from the nasal retina of each eye cross to the opposite side and join with the axons of the temporal retina of the contralateral eye to form the optic tracts. Thus, one optic tract contains fibers from both eyes that transmit information from the same visual hemifield (half-field).

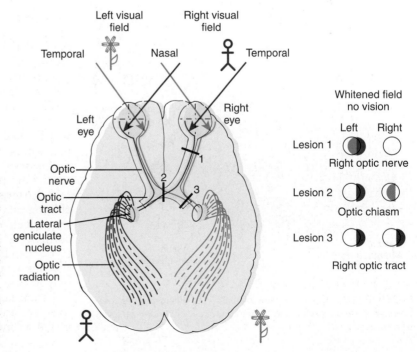

FIGURE 19-22. Diagram of optic pathways. The *red lines* indicate the right visual field and the *blue lines* the left visual field. Note the crossing of fibers from the medial half of each retina at the optic chiasm. Lesion 1 (right optic nerve) produces unilateral blindness. Lesion 2 (optic chiasm) may involve only those fibers that originate in the nasal half of each retina and cross to the opposite side in the optic chiasm; visual loss involves the temporal half of each field (bitemporal hemianopia). Lesion 3 (right optic tract) interrupts fibers (and vision) originating on the same side of both eyes (homonymous) with loss of vision from half of each field (hemianopia).

Visual Cortex

The primary visual cortex (area 17) surrounds the calcarine fissure, which lies in the occipital lobe. It is at this level that visual sensation is first experienced (Fig. 19-23). Immediately surrounding area 17 are the visual association cortices (areas 18 and 19) and several other association cortices. These association cortices, with their thalamic nuclei, must be functional to add meaningfulness to visual perception.

Circuitry in the primary visual cortex and the visual association areas is extremely discrete with respect to the location of retinal stimulation. For example, specific neurons respond to the particular orientation of a moving edge, specific colors, or familiar shapes. This elaborate organization of the visual cortex, with its functionally separate and multiple representations of the same visual field, provides the major basis for visual sensation and perception. Because of this discrete circuitry, lesions of the visual cortex must be large to be detected clinically.

Visual Fields

The *visual field* refers to the area that is visible during fixation of vision in one direction. Because visual system deficits are often expressed as visual field deficits rather than as direct measures of neural function, the terminology for normal and abnormal visual characteristics usually is based on visual field orientation.

Most of the visual field is *binocular* or seen by both eyes. This binocular field is subdivided into central and peripheral portions. Central portions of the retina provide high visual acuity and correspond to the field focused on the central fovea; the peripheral and surrounding portion provides the capacity to detect objects, particularly moving objects. Beyond the visual field shared by both eyes, the left lateral periphery of the visual field is seen exclusively by the left nasal retina, and the right peripheral field is seen by the right nasal retina.

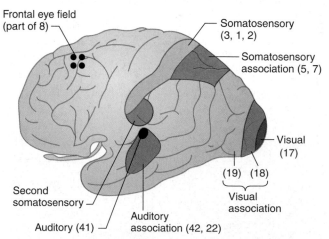

Frontal eye field (part of 8)

Somatosensory (3, 1, 2)

Somatosensory association (5, 7)

Visual (17)

(19) (18)

Visual association

Second somatosensory

Auditory (41)

Auditory association (42, 22)

FIGURE 19-23. Lateral view of the cortex illustrating the location of the visual, visual association, auditory, and auditory association areas.

As with a camera, the simple lens system of the eye inverts the image of the external world on each retina. In addition, the right and left sides of the visual field also are reversed. The right binocular visual field is seen by the left retinal halves of each eye—the nasal half of the right eye and the temporal half of the left eye.

Once the level of the retina is reached, the nervous system plays a consistent role. The upper half of the visual field is received by the lower half of the retinas of both eyes. Representations of this upper half of the field are carried in the lower half of each optic nerve: They synapse in the lower half of the lateral geniculate nucleus (LGN) of each side of the brain (see Fig. 19-18). Neurons in this part of the LGN send their axons through the inferior half of the optic radiation, looping into the temporal lobe to terminate in the lower half of the primary visual cortex on each side of the brain.

Because of the lateral separation of the two eyes, each eye contributes a different image of the world to the visual field. This is called *binocular disparity*. Disparity between the laterally displaced images seen by the two eyes provides a powerful source of three-dimensional depth perception for objects within a distance of 30 m. Beyond that distance, binocular disparity becomes insignificant: Depth perception is based on other cues (*e.g.,* the superimposition of the image of near objects over that of far objects and the faster movement of near objects than of far objects).

Visual Field Defects

Visual field defects result from damage to the retina, optic pathways, or the visual cortex. Perimetry or visual field testing, in which the limits of the visual field of each eye are measured and plotted in an arc, is used to identify defects and determine the location of lesions.

Disorders of the Optic Pathways

Localized damage to the optic tracts, LGN, optic radiation, or primary visual cortex affects corresponding parts of the visual fields of both eyes (see Fig. 19-18). Examination of visual system function is of particular importance because lesions at various points along the pathway have characteristic symptoms that assist in the localization of the lesion.

Among the disorders that can interrupt the optic pathway are vascular lesions, trauma, and tumors. For example, normal visual system function depends on adequate perfusion of the ophthalmic artery and its branches; the central artery of the retina; the anterior and middle cerebral arteries, which supply the intracranial optic nerve, chiasm, and optic tracts; and the posterior cerebral artery, which supplies the LGN, optic radiation, and visual cortex. The adequacy of posterior cerebral artery function depends on that of the vertebral and basilar arteries that supply the brain stem. Vascular insufficiency in any one of these arterial systems can seriously affect vision.

Visual field defects of each eye and of the two eyes together are useful in localizing lesions affecting the system. Blindness in one eye is called *anopia*. If half of the visual field for one eye is lost, the defect is called hemianopia, and if a quarter of the field is lost, it is called *quadrantanopia*. Enlarging pituitary tumors can produce longitudinal damage through the optic chiasm, with loss of the medial fibers of the optic nerve representing both nasal retinas and both temporal visual half-fields. The loss of different half-fields in the two eyes is called a *heteronymous loss*, and the abnormality is called *heteronymous hemianopia*. Destruction of one or both lateral halves of the chiasm is common with multiple aneurysms of the circle of Willis. In this condition, the function of one or both temporal retinas is lost, and the nasal fields of one or both eyes are lost. The loss of the temporal fields (nasal retina) of both eyes is called *bitemporal heteronymous anopia*. With both eyes open, the person with bilateral defects still has the full binocular visual field.

Loss of the optic tract, LGN, full optic radiation, or complete visual cortex on one side results in loss of the corresponding visual half-fields in each eye. *Homonymous* means "the same" for both eyes. In left-side lesions, the right visual field is lost for each eye and is called *complete right homonymous hemianopia*. Partial injury to the left optic tract, LGN, or optic radiation can result in the loss of a quarter of the visual field in both eyes. This is called *homonymous quadrantanopia*, and depending on the lesion, it can involve the upper (superior) or lower (inferior) fields. Because the optic radiation fibers for the superior quarter of the visual field traverse the temporal lobe, superior quadrantanopia is more common.

Disorders of the Visual Cortex

Discrete damage to the binocular portion of the primary visual cortex also can result in scotomata in the corresponding visual fields. The central high-acuity portion of the visual field is located at the occipital pole. If the visual loss is in the central high-acuity part of the field, severe loss of visual acuity and pattern discrimination occur. Mechanical trauma to the cortex results in firing of neurons, experienced as flashes of light or "seeing stars." Destruction of the polar visual cortex causes severe loss of visual acuity and pattern discrimination. Such damage is permanent and cannot be corrected with lenses.

The bilateral loss of the entire primary visual cortex, called *cortical blindness*, eliminates all visual experience. Crude analysis of visual stimulation at reflex levels, such as eye-orienting and head-orienting responses to bright moving lights, pupillary reflexes, and blinking at sudden bright lights, may be retained even though vision has been lost. Extensive damage to the visual association cortex (areas 18 and 19) that surrounds an intact primary visual cortex results in a loss of the learned meaningfulness of visual images (*i.e.*, visual agnosia). The person can see the patterns of color, shapes, and movement, but no longer can recognize formerly meaningful stimuli. Familiar objects can be described but not named or reacted to meaningfully. However, if other sensory modalities, such as hearing and touch, can be applied, full recognition occurs. This disorder represents a problem of recognition rather than intellect.

Testing of Visual Fields

Crude testing of the binocular visual field and the visual field of each individual eye (*i.e.*, monocular vision) can be accomplished without specialized equipment. In the confrontation method, the examiner stands or sits in front of the person to be tested and instructs the person to focus with one eye closed on the examiner's nose while random presentations of finger quantities are presented roughly 3 feet from the observer in each of the four major field quadrants to assess for the awareness of the finger quantities.[60] In a kinetic assessment of the expansiveness of the gross visual field, an object such as a penlight is moved from the center toward the periphery of the person's visual field and from the periphery toward the center, and the person is instructed to report the presence or absence of the object. By moving the object through the vertical, horizontal, and oblique aspects of the visual field, a crude estimate can be made of the visual field. Large field defects can be estimated by the confrontation method, and it may be the only way for testing young children and uncooperative adults.

SUMMARY CONCEPTS

Visual information is carried to the brain by axons of the retinal ganglion cells that form the optic nerve. The two optic nerves meet and fuse in the optic chiasm. The axons of each nasal retina cross in the chiasm and join the uncrossed fibers of the temporal retina of the opposite eye to form the optic tracts. The fibers of each optic tract then synapse in the LGN and, from there, travel by way of the optic radiations to the primary visual cortex in the calcarine area of the occipital lobe. Damage to the visual association cortex can result in the phenomenon of seeing an object without the ability to recognize it (*i.e.*, visual agnosia). Optic pathway or visual cortex damage leads to visual field defects that can be identified through visual field testing. Perimetry, which maps the sensitivity contours of the visual field, can be used to determine the presence, size, and shape of smaller holes, or scotomata, in the visual field of an eye.

Disorders of Eye Movement

For complete visual function, it is necessary that the two eyes focus on the same fixation point, that the image of the object falls simultaneously on the fovea of each eye, and that the retinal and CNS visual mechanisms are functional. It is through these mechanisms that an object is simultaneously imaged on the fovea of both eyes and perceived as a single image. Strabismus and amblyopia are two disorders that affect this highly integrated system.

Extraocular Eye Muscles and Their Innervation

Three pairs of extraocular muscles—the superior and inferior recti, the medial and lateral recti, and the superior and inferior obliques—control the movement of each eye (Fig. 19-24). The four rectus muscles are named according to where they insert into the sclera on the medial, lateral, inferior, and superior surfaces of each eye. The two oblique muscles insert on the lateral posterior quadrant of the eyeball—the superior oblique on the upper surface and the inferior oblique on the lower. Each of the three sets of muscles in each eye is reciprocally innervated so that one muscle relaxes when the other contracts. Reciprocal contraction of the medial and lateral recti moves the eye from side to side (adduction and abduction); the superior and inferior recti move the eye up and down (elevation and depression). The oblique muscles rotate (intorsion and extorsion) the eye around its optic axis. A seventh muscle, the levator palpebrae superioris, elevates the upper lid.

The extraocular muscles are innervated by three cranial nerves. The abducens nerve (CN VI) innervates the lateral rectus, the trochlear nerve (CN IV) innervates the superior oblique, and the oculomotor nerve (CN III) innervates the remaining four muscles (Table 19-1). The CN VI (abducens) nucleus, in the caudal pons, innervates the lateral rectus muscle, which rotates the ipsilateral (same side) eye laterally (abduction). Partial or complete damage to this nerve results in weakness or complete paralysis of the muscle. Medial gaze is normal, but the affected eye fails to rotate laterally with an attempted gaze toward the affected side, a condition called *medial strabismus*. The CN IV (trochlear) nucleus, at the junction of the pons and midbrain, innervates the contralateral or opposite side superior oblique muscle, which rotates the top of the globe inward toward the nose, a movement called *intorsion*. In combination with other muscles, it also contributes strength to movement of the innervated eye downward and inward.

The CN III (oculomotor) nucleus, which extends through a considerable part of the midbrain, contains clusters of lower motor neurons for each of the five eye muscles it innervates: inferior rectus, superior rectus, inferior oblique, medial rectus, and levator palpebrae superioris. The medial rectus, superior rectus, and inferior

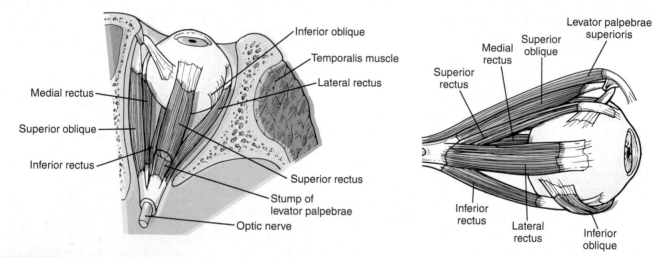

FIGURE 19-24 Extraocular muscles of the right eye.

Muscle*	Innervation	Primary	Secondary	Tertiary
MR: medial rectus	III	Adduction		
LR: lateral rectus	VI	Abduction		
SR: superior rectus	III	Elevation	Intorsion	Adduction
IR: inferior rectus	III	Depression	Extorsion	Adduction
SO: superior oblique	IV	Intorsion	Depression	Abduction
IO: inferior oblique	III	Extorsion	Elevation	Abduction

TABLE 19-1 Eye in Primary Position: Extrinsic Ocular Muscle Actions

*In the schema of the functional roles of the six extraocular muscles, the major directional force applied by each muscle is indicated on the top. These muscles are arranged in functionally opposing pairs per eye and in parallel opposing pairs for conjugate movements of the two eyes. The numbers associated with each muscle indicate the cranial nerve innervation: 3, oculomotor (III) cranial nerve; 4, trochlear (IV) cranial nerve; 6, abducens (VI) cranial nerve.

rectus rotate the eye in the directions shown in Table 19-1. The action of the inferior rectus is antagonistic to the superior rectus. Because of its plane of attachment to the globe, the inferior oblique rotates the eye in the frontal plane (*i.e.*, torsion), pulling the top of the eye laterally (*i.e.*, *extorsion*). CN III also innervates the levator palpebrae superioris muscle that elevates the upper eyelid and is involved in vertical gaze eye movements. As the eyes rotate upward, the upper eyelid is reflexively retracted, and in the downward gaze, it is lowered, restricting exposure of the conjunctiva to air and reducing the effects of drying.

Communication between the eye muscle nuclei of each side of the brain occurs primarily through the posterior commissure at the rostral end of the midbrain. Longitudinal communication among the three nuclei occurs along a fiber tract called the *medial longitudinal fasciculus* (MLF), which extends from the midbrain to the upper part of the spinal cord. Each pair of eye muscles is reciprocally innervated, by the MLF or other associated pathways, so that as one muscle contracts, the other relaxes. These MLF-linked communication paths are vulnerable to damage in the caudal midbrain and pons. Damage to the pontine MLF on one side of the brain results in loss of this linkage, such that lateral deviation of the ipsilateral eye is no longer linked to adduction on the contralateral side. If the MLF is damaged bilaterally, the linkage is lost for lateral gaze in either direction.

Eye Movements and Gaze

Conjugate movements are those in which the optical axes of the two eyes are kept parallel, sharing the same visual field. *Gaze* refers to the act of looking steadily in one direction. Eye movements can be categorized into smooth pursuit movements, saccadic movements, optic tremor, and vergence movements. Although the conjugate reflexes are essential to efficient visual function during head movement or target movement, their circuitry is so deeply embedded in CNS function that they are present and can be elicited when the eyes are closed, during sleep, and in deep coma, and they function normally and accurately in congenitally blind people.

Strabismus

Strabismus, or squint, refers to any abnormality of eye coordination or alignment that results in loss of binocular vision. When images from the same spots in visual space do not fall on corresponding points of the two retinas, diplopia, or double vision, occurs. Strabismus affects approximately 4% of children younger than 6 years.[61,62] Because 30% to 50% of these children sustain

permanent secondary loss of vision, or amblyopia, if the condition is left untreated, early diagnosis and treatment are essential.

In standard terminology, the disorders of eye movement are described according to the direction of movement. *Esotropia* refers to medial (inward) deviation, *exotropia* to lateral (outward) deviation, *hypertropia* to upward deviation, *hypotropia* to downward deviation, and *cyclotropia* to torsional deviation. The term *concomitance* refers to equal deviation in all directions of gaze. A nonconcomitant strabismus is one that varies with the direction of gaze. Strabismus may be divided into nonparalytic (concomitant) forms, in which there is no primary muscle impairment, and paralytic (nonconcomitant) forms, in which there is weakness or paralysis of one or more of the extraocular muscles. Strabismus is called *intermittent*, or *periodic*, when there are periods in which the eyes are parallel. It is monocular when the same eye always deviates and the opposite eye fixates. Figure 19-25 illustrates abnormalities in eye movement associated with esotropia and exotropia.

Nonparalytic Strabismus

Nonparalytic esotropia is the most common type of strabismus. The individual ocular muscles have no obvious defect, and the amount of deviation is constant or relatively constant in the various directions of gaze. With persistent deviation, secondary abnormalities may develop because of overactivity or underactivity of the extraocular muscles in some fields of gaze.

The disorder may be nonaccommodative, accommodative, or a combination of the two. Infantile esotropia is the most common cause of nonaccommodative strabismus. It occurs in the first 6 months of life, with large-angle deviations, in an otherwise developmentally and neurologically normal infant. Eye movements are full, and the child often uses each eye independently to alter fixation (cross-fixation). The cause of the disorder is unclear. Research suggests that idiopathic strabismus may have a genetic basis; siblings often present with similar disorders.

Accommodative strabismus is caused by disorders such as uncorrected hyperopia of a significant degree, in which the esotropia occurs with accommodation that is undertaken to focus clearly. Onset of this type of esotropia characteristically occurs between 18 months and 4 years of age because accommodation is not well developed until that time. The disorder most often is monocular but may be alternating.

Paralytic Strabismus

Paralytic strabismus results from paresis (*i.e.*, weakness) or plegia (*i.e.*, paralysis) of one or more of the extraocular muscles. When the normal eye fixates, the affected eye is in the position of primary deviation. In the case of esotropia, there is weakness of one of the lateral rectus muscles, usually due to a disorder of the abducens nerve (CN VI). When the affected eye fixates, the unaffected eye is in a position of secondary deviation. The secondary deviation of the unaffected eye is greater than the primary deviation of the affected eye. This is because

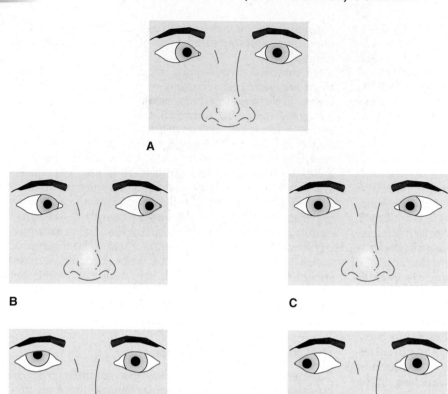

FIGURE 19-25. (A–E) Paralytic strabismus associated with paralysis of the right lateral rectus muscle: **(A)** primary position with right esotropia of the eyes (looking straight ahead), **(B)** left gaze with no deviation, and **(C)** right gaze with left esotropia. **(D)** Primary position of the eyes with weakness of the right inferior rectus and right hypertropia. **(E)** Primary position of the eyes with weakness of the right medial rectus and right exotropia.

the affected eye requires an excess of innervational impulse to maintain fixation; the excess impulses also are distributed to the unaffected eye, causing overaction of its muscles.[62,63]

Paralytic strabismus is uncommon in children but accounts for nearly all cases of adult strabismus. It can be caused by infiltrative processes (*e.g.*, Graves disease), myasthenia gravis, stroke, and direct optical trauma. The pathway of the oculomotor, trochlear, and abducens nerves through the cavernous sinus and the back of the orbit makes them vulnerable to basal skull fracture and tumors of the cavernous sinus or orbit. In infants, paralytic strabismus can be caused by birth injuries affecting the extraocular muscles or the cranial nerves supplying these muscles. In general, paralytic strabismus in an older child or adult does not produce amblyopia, and binocular vision can be maintained when the strabismus is corrected. Most adult strabismus represents deterioration of childhood strabismus, which can occur even decades after good ocular alignment.

Treatment

Treatment of strabismus is directed toward the development of normal visual acuity, correction of the deviation, and superimposition of the retinal images to provide binocular vision. Early and adequate treatment is crucial because a delay in or lack of treatment can lead to amblyopia and permanent loss of vision. In addition to its effects on visual function, strabismus can have an adverse impact on interpersonal relationships, self-image, schoolwork, and participation in extracurricular activities. Children begin to develop negative attitudes toward classmates with strabismus.

Treatment includes both surgical and nonsurgical methods. Infantile esotropia is usually treated surgically by weakening the medial rectus muscle on each eye while the infant is under general anesthesia. Surgery in children with esotropia should be done as early as possible to preserve stereoscopic acuity. Early surgical treatment also appears to result in better outcomes than later intervention. Recurrent strabismus is common with infantile esotropia, and multiple surgeries are often required.[63,64]

Nonsurgical treatment includes glasses, occlusive patching, and eye exercises (*i.e.*, pleoptics). Glasses are often used in the treatment of accommodative esotropia that occurs with hypermetropia (farsightedness). Because accommodation is linked with convergence, focusing drives the eyes inward, producing esotropia. Intermittent exotropia is commonly treated with patching, use of overminus glasses, and eye exercises. Although no appreciable deviation is present when the child with intermittent strabismus sees near objects, the deviation becomes obvious when the child views distant objects or is fatigued. Patching for 1 to 2 hours daily for several months works by preventing, rather than treating, suppression of an eye. Patching is most effective in infants, and the efficacy is limited in children older than 3 years. The use of overminus glasses stimulates accommodative convergences, which contracts the exotropic drift. Vision therapy involves exercises to stimulate convergence (*e.g.*, focusing on reading distance targets up to 30 minutes several times a day) and techniques to train the visual system to recognize the suppressed images. Surgical treatment of intermittent exotropia is indicted when conservative methods fail to correct the deviation. Early treatment of children with intermittent exotropia is not as crucial as it is for those with constant deviations because stereopsis can still develop.

Another form of treatment involves the injection of botulinum toxin type A (Botox) into the extraocular muscle to produce a dose-dependent paralysis of that extraocular muscle.[65] Paralysis of the muscle shifts the eye into the field of action of the antagonist muscle. During the time the eye is deviated, the paralyzed muscle is stretched, whereas the antagonistic muscle is contracted. Usually, two or more injections of the drug are necessary to obtain a lasting effect.

Amblyopia

Amblyopia, sometimes called *lazy eye*, describes a decrease in visual acuity resulting from abnormal visual development in infancy or early childhood. The vision loss ranges from mild (worse than 20/25) to severe (legal blindness, 20/200 or worse).[61,62] It is the leading cause of visual impairment, affecting 1% to 4% of the population. With early detection and treatment, most cases of amblyopia are reversible and the most severe forms of the condition can be prevented.

Etiology and Pathophysiology

Normal development of the thalamic and cortical circuitry necessary for binocular visual perception requires simultaneous binocular use of each fovea during a critical period early in life (0 to 5 years). Amblyopia can result from visual deprivation (*e.g.*, cataracts, ptosis) or abnormal binocular interactions (*e.g.*, strabismus, anisometropia) during visual immaturity. In infants with unilateral cataracts that are dense, central, and larger than 2 mm in diameter, this time is before 2 months of age.[66] In conditions causing abnormal binocular interactions, one image is suppressed to provide clearer vision. In esotropia, vision of the deviated eye is suppressed to prevent diplopia. A similar situation exists in anisometropia, in which the refractive indexes of the two eyes are different. Although the eyes are correctly aligned, they are unable to focus together, and the image of one eye is suppressed.

Treatment

The reversibility of amblyopia depends on the maturity of the visual system at the time of onset and the duration of the abnormal experience. Occasionally in strabismus, some people alternate eye fixation and do not experience deep amblyopia or diplopia. With late adolescent or adult onset, this habit pattern must be unlearned after correction. Amblyopia is remarkably responsive to treatment if the treatment is initiated early in life. Thus, all infants and young children should be evaluated for visual conditions that could lead to amblyopia.

The treatment of children with the potential for development of amblyopia must be instituted well before the age of 6 years to avoid the suppression phenomenon. Surgery for congenital cataracts and ptosis should be done early. Severe refractive errors should be corrected. In children with strabismus, the alternate blocking of the vision in one eye and then the other forces the child to use both eyes for form discrimination. The duration of occlusion of vision in the good eye must be short (2 to 5 hours/day) and closely monitored, or deprivation amblyopia can develop in the good eye as well. Although amblyopia is not likely to occur after 8 or 9 years of age, some plasticity in central circuitry is evident even in adulthood. For example, after refractive correction for long-standing astigmatism in adults, visual acuity improves slowly, requiring several months to reach normal levels.

Eye Examination in Infants and Children

Early detection and prompt treatment of ocular disorders in children are important to prevent amblyopia and lifelong visual impairment. The American Academy of Pediatrics in association with the American Association of Certified Orthoptists, American Association of Pediatric Ophthalmology and Strabismus, and American Academy of Ophthalmology recommends that all newborn infants be examined in the nursery for structural abnormalities and have a red reflex test performed to check for abnormalities in the back of the eye (posterior segment) and opacities in the visual axis, such as cataracts or corneal opacity.[63,64] An infant with an abnormal red reflex requires immediate referral to an eye care specialist. Visual examinations should then be performed on all well-child visits. These should include age-appropriate evaluation of visual acuity, ocular alignment, and ocular media clarity (cataracts, tumors).

SUMMARY CONCEPTS

Binocular vision depends on the extraocular muscles and their innervating cranial nerves to move the eye up and down and rotate it around its optical axis. For full visual function, it is necessary that the two eyes point toward the same fixation point and the two images become fused. Binocular fusion is controlled by ocular reflex mechanisms that adjust the orientation of each eye to produce a single image. The term *conjugate gaze* refers to the use of both eyes to look steadily in one direction. During conjugate eye movements, the optical axes of the two eyes are maintained parallel with each other as the eyes rotate upward, downward, or side to side in their sockets.

Strabismus refers to abnormalities in the coordination of eye movements, with loss of binocular eye alignment. This inability to focus a visual image on corresponding parts of the two retinas results in diplopia. Esotropia refers to medial deviation, exotropia to lateral deviation, hypertropia to upward deviation, hypotropia to downward deviation, and cyclotropia to torsional deviation. Paralytic strabismus is caused by weakness or paralysis of the extraocular muscles, whereas nonparalytic strabismus results from the inappropriate length or insertion of the extraocular muscles or from accommodation disorders.

Amblyopia (*i.e.*, lazy eye) is a decrease in visual acuity resulting from abnormal visual development in infancy and early childhood. It results from inadequately developed CNS circuitry because of visual deprivation (*e.g.*, cataracts) or abnormal binocular interactions (*e.g.*, strabismus) during visual immaturity.

Review Exercises

1. The mother of a 3-year-old boy notices that his left eye is red and watering when she picks him up from day care. He keeps rubbing his eye as if it itches. The next morning, however, she notices that both eyes are red, swollen, and watering. Being concerned, she takes him to the pediatrician in the morning and is told that he has "pink eye." She is told that the infection should go away by itself.

   A. What part of the eye is involved?
   B. What type of conjunctivitis do you think this child has: bacterial, viral, or allergic?
   C. Why didn't the pediatrician order an antibiotic?
   D. Is the condition contagious? What measures should she take to prevent its spread?

2. During a routine eye examination to get new glasses because she had been having difficulty with her distant vision, a 75-year-old woman is told that she is developing cataracts.

   A. What type of visual changes occurs as the result of a cataract?
   B. What can the woman do to prevent the cataracts from getting worse?
   C. What treatment may she eventually need?

3. A 50-year-old woman is told by her "eye doctor" that her intraocular pressure is slightly elevated and that although there is no evidence of damage to her eyes now, she is at risk for developing glaucoma and should have regular eye examinations.

   A. Describe the physiologic mechanisms involved in the regulation of intraocular pressure.
   B. What are the risk factors for developing glaucoma?
   C. Explain how an increase in intraocular pressure produces its damaging effects.

4. The parents of a newborn infant have been told that their son has congenital cataracts in both eyes and will require cataract surgery to prevent loss of sight.

   A. Explain why the infant is at risk for losing his sight if the cataracts are not removed.
   B. When should this procedure be done to prevent loss of vision?

REFERENCES

1. World Health Organization. (2017). Blindness and visual impairment. [Online]. Available: www.WHO.int. Accessed July 1, 2017.
2. Michels K. S., Czyz C. N., Cahill K. V., et al. (2014). Age-matched, case-controlled comparison of clinical indicators for development of entropion and ectropion. *Journal of Ophthalmology* 2014, 231487. doi:10.1155/2014/.
3. Uphold C. R., Graham M. V. (2013). *Clinical guidelines in family practice* (pp. 301–302, 304–307). North Miami Beach, FL: Barmarrae Books, Inc.
4. Tsubota K., Yokoi N., Shimazaki J., et al. (2016). New perspectives on dry eye definition and diagnosis: A consensus report by the Asia Dry Eye Society. *The Ocular Surface* 15(1), 65–67.
5. Goldberg R., Banta J. (2013). Dry eye syndrome. In Buttarom T., Trybulski J., Baily P., et al. (Eds.), *Primary care a collaborative practice* (pp. 333–335). St. Louis, MO: Elsevier Mosby.
6. Kossler A., Banta J. (2013). Nasolacrimal duct obstruction and dacryocystitis. In Buttarom T., Trybulski J., Baily P., et al. (Eds.), *Primary care a collaborative practice* (pp. 335–336). St. Louis, MO: Elsevier Mosby.
7. Gilbard J. P. (2009). Dry eye and blepharitis: Approaching the patient with chronic eye irritation. *Geriatrics* 64(6), 22–26.
8. World Health Organization. (2017). Trachoma. [Online]. Available: www.WHO.int. Accessed July 4, 2017.
9. Riordan-Eva P. (2011). Anatomy and embryology of the eye. In Riordan-Eva P., Cunningham E. T. (Eds.), *Vaughan & Asbury's general ophthalmology* (18th ed., pp. 1–26). New York, NY: McGraw-Hill.
10. Collier S., Gronostaj M., MacGurn, A. K., et al. (2014). Estimated burden of keratitis. [Online]. Available: www.cdc.gov. Accessed July 5, 2017.
11. Weiss M., Banta J. (2013). Evaluation and management of eye disorders. In Buttarom T., Trybulski J., Baily P., et al. (Eds.), *Primary care a collaborative practice* (p. 320). St. Louis, MO: Elsevier Mosby.

12. Farooq A. V., Shukla D. (2012). Herpes simplex epithelial and stromal keratitis: An epidemiologic update. *Survey of Ophthalmology* 57(5), 448–462. doi:10.1016/j.survophthal.2012.01.005.

13. Biswell R. (2011). Cornea. In Riordan-Eva P., Cunningham E. T. (Eds.), *Vaughan & Asbury's general ophthalmology* (18th ed., pp. 120–144). New York, NY: McGraw-Hill.

14. Guess S., Stone D., Chodosh J. (2007). Evidence-based treatment of herpes simplex virus keratitis: A systematic review. *The Ocular Surface Journal* 15(3), 240–250.

15. Piret J., Boivin G. (2016). Antiviral resistance in herpes simplex virus and varicella-zoster virus infections: Diagnosis and management. *Current Opinion Infectious Disease* 29(6), 654–662.

16. Kumar R., Cruzat A., Hamrah P. (2010). Current state of in vivo confocal microscopy in management of microbial keratitis. *Seminars in Ophthalmology* 25(5–6), 166–170.

17. Ikeda Y., Miyazaki D., Yakura K., et al. (2012). Assessment of real-time polymerase chain reaction detection of acanthamoeba and prognosis determinants of acanthamoeba keratitis. *Ophthalmology* 119(6), 1111–1119.

18. Seal D. (2003). Acanthamoeba keratitis update-incidence, molecular epidemiology and new drugs for treatment. *Eye Journal* 17(8), 893–905.

19. Iovieno A., Gore D., Carnt N., et al. (2014). Acanthamoeba sclerokeratitis: Epidemiology, clinical features and treatment outcomes. *Ophthalmology* 121(12), 2340–2347.

20. National Eye Institute. (2017). Corneal transplantation. [Online]. Available: https://www.nei.nih.gov. Accessed July 8, 2017.

21. Caspi R. (2010). A look at autoimmunity and inflammation in the eye. *Journal of Clinical Investigation* 120(9), 3073–3083.

22. Tham Y., Li X., Wong T., et al. (2014). Global prevalence of glaucoma and projections of glaucoma burden through 2040: A systematic review and meta-analysis. *Ophthalmology* 121(11), 2081–2090.

23. Salmon J. (2011). Glaucoma. In Riordan-Eva P., Cunningham E. T. (Eds.), *Vaughan & Asbury's general ophthalmology* (18th ed., pp. 22–237). New York, NY: McGraw-Hill.

24. Fernandez-Bahamonde J., Roman-Rodriguez C., Fernandez-Ruiz M. (2011). Central corneal thickness as a predictor of visual field loss in primary open angle glaucoma for a Hispanic population. *Seminars in Ophthalmology* 26(1), 28–32.

25. Prum B., Rosenberg L., Gedde S. J., et al. (2016). Primary open-angle glaucoma preferred practice pattern guidelines. *Ophthalmology* 123(1), 41–111.

26. Tarongoy P., Ho C., Walton D. (2009). Angle closure glaucoma: The role of the lens in the pathogenesis prevention and treatment. *Survey of Ophthalmology* 54(2), 211–225.

27. Lai J., Gangwani R. (2012). Medication induced acute angle closure attack. *Hong Kong Medical Journal* 18(2), 139–145.

28. Mandal A., Chakrabarti D. (2011). Update on congenital glaucoma. *Indian Journal of Ophthalmology* 59(Suppl), 148–157.

29. Riordan-Eva P. (2011). Optics and refractions. In Riordan-Eva P., Cunningham E. T. (Eds.), *Vaughan & Asbury's general ophthalmology* (18th ed., pp. 396–411). New York, NY: McGraw-Hill.

30. Messmer J. (2010). LASIK: A primer for family physicians. *American Family Physician* 81(1), 42–47.

31. Krantz E., Cruickshanks K., Klein B., et al. (2010). Measuring refraction in adults in epidemiological studies. *Archives of Ophthalmology* 128(1), 88–92.

32. Harper R., Shock J. (2011). Lens. In Riordan-Eva P., Cunningham E. (Eds.), *Vaughan & Asbury's general ophthalmology* (18th ed., pp. 174–181). New York, NY: McGraw-Hill.

33. Townsend J., Banta J. (2013). Cataracts. In Buttaro T., Trybulski J., Bailey P., et al. (Eds.), *Primary care: A collaborative practice* (4th ed. pp. 322–324). St. Louis, MO: Elsevier Mosby.

34. Vizzeri G., Weinreb R. (2010). Cataract surgery and glaucoma. *Current Opinion in Ophthalmology* 21(1), 20–24.

35. Pringle E., Graham E. (2011). Ocular disorders associated with systemic disease. In Riordan-Eva P., Cunningham E. T. (Eds.), *Vaughan & Asbury's general ophthalmology* (18th ed., pp. 314–346). New York, NY: McGraw-Hill.

36. Riordan-Eva P. (2011). Disorders of the eyes and lids. In McPhee S., Papadakis M. (Eds.), *Current medical diagnosis and treatment* (50th ed., pp. 166–197). New York, NY: McGraw-Hill.

37. Fletcher E., Chong N., Augsburger J., et al. (2011). Retina. In Riordan-Eva P., Cunningham E. T. (Eds.), *Vaughan & Asbury's general ophthalmology* (18th ed., pp. 190–221). New York, NY: McGraw-Hill.

38. Genetics Home Reference. (2017). Retinitis Pigmentosa. [Online]. Available: https://ghr.nlm.nih.gov. Accessed July 12, 2017.

39. Beran D., Murphy-Lavoie H. (2009). Acute, painless vision loss. *Journal of the Louisiana State Medical Society* 161(4), 214–216, 218–223.

40. Fante R., Durairaj V., Oliver S. (2010). Diabetic retinopathy: An update on treatment. *The American Journal of Medicine* 123(3), 213–216.

41. Zhang X., Saaddine J., Chou C., et al. (2010). Prevalence of diabetic retinopathy in the United States, 2005-2008. *Journal of the American Medical Association* 304(6), 649–656.

42. The ACCORD Study Group and ACCORD Eye Study Group. (2010). Effects of medical therapies on retinopathy progression in type 2 diabetes. *New England Journal of Medicine* 363, 233–244.

43. Heng L., Comyn O., Peto C., et al. (2013). Diabetic retinopathy: Pathogenesis, clinical grading, management and future developments. *Diabetic Medicine* 30(6), 640–650.

44. Cuspidi C., Negri F., Giudici V., et al. (2009). Retinal changes and cardiac remodeling in systemic hypertension. *Therapeutic Advances in Cardiovascular Disease* 3(3), 205–214.

45. D'Amico D. (2008). Primary retinal detachment. *New England Journal of Medicine* 359(22), 2346–2354.

46. Sun Q., Sun T., Xu Y., et al. (2012). Primary vitrectomy verses scleral buckling for the treatment of rhegmatogenous retinal detachment: A meta-analysis of randomized controlled clinical trials. *Current Eye Research* 37(6), 492–499.

47. Hatef E., Sena D., Fallano K., et al. (2015). Pneumatic retinopexy verses scleral buckle for repairing simple rhegmatogenous retinal detachments. *Cochrane Database of Systematic Review* (5), CD008350. [Online]. Available: www.cochranelibrary.com. Accessed July 14, 2017.

48. Kokotas H., Grigoriadou M., Petersen M. (2011). Age-related macular degeneration: Genetic and clinical findings. *Clinical Chemistry and Laboratory Medicine* 49(4), 601–616.

49. Klein R., Myers C., Klein B. (2014). Vasodilator, blood pressure-lowering medications, and age-related macular degeneration: The Beaver Dam Eye Study. *Ophthalmology* 121(8), 1604–1611.

50. Chiang A., Regillo C. (2011). Preferred therapies for neovascular age-related macular degeneration. *Current Opinion in Ophthalmology* 22(3), 199–204.

51. Jonasson F., Fisher D., Eiriksdottir G., et al. (2014). Five-year incidence, progression, and risk factors for age-related macular degeneration: The age, gene/environment susceptibility study. *Ophthalmology* 121(9), 1766–1772.

52. Lim L., Mitchell P., Seddon J., et al. (2012). Age-related macular degeneration. *Lancet* 379(9827), 1728–1738.

53. Yehoshua Z., Rosenfeld P., Albini T. (2011). Current clinical trials in dry AMD and the definition of appropriate clinical outcome measures. *Seminars in Ophthalmology* 26(3), 167–180.

54. Klintworth G. (2008). The eye. In Rubin R., Strayer D. (Eds.), *Rubin's pathology: Clinicopathologic foundations of medicine* (5th ed., pp. 1265–1266). Philadelphia, PA: Lippincott Williams & Wilkins.

55. Li J., Coats D., Fung D., et al. (2010). The detection of simulated retinoblastoma by using red-reflex testing. *Pediatrics* 126(1), 202–207.

56. Kembhavi S., Sable N., Vora T., et al. (2011). Leukocoria: All that's white is not retinoblastoma. *Journal of Clinical Oncology* 29(19), 586–587.

57. Nale P. (2011). Early recognition of recurrence key to successfully treating retinoblastoma. *Ocular Surgery News* 29(10), 18.

58. Smith S., Smith B. (2013). Evaluating the risk of extraocular tumor spread following intravitreal injection therapy for retinoblastoma: A systematic review. *British Journal of Ophthalmology* 97(10), 1231–1236.

59. Villegas V., Hess D., Wildner A., et al. (2013). Retinoblastoma. *Current Opinions in Ophthalmology* 24(6), 581–588.

60. Kerr N., Chew S., Eady E., et al. (2010). Diagnostic accuracy of confrontation visual field test. *Neurology* 74(15), 1184–1190.

61. Motley W., Asbury T. (2004). Strabismus. In Riordan-Eva P., Cunningham E. T. (Eds.), *Vaughan & Asbury's general ophthalmology* (18th ed., pp. 238–258). New York, NY: McGraw-Hill.

62. Granet D., Khayali S. (2011). Amblyopia and strabismus. *Pediatric Annals* 40(2), 89–94.

63. Minnal V., Rosenberg J. (2011). Refractive surgery: A treatment for and a cause of strabismus. *Current Opinion in Ophthalmology* 22(4), 222–225.

64. Wang L., Nelson L. (2010). One muscle strabismus surgery. *Current Opinion in Ophthalmology* 21(5), 335–340.

65. Rowe F., Noonan C. (2017). Botulinum toxin for the treatment of strabismus. *Cochrane Database of Systematic Reviews* 3. [Online]. Available: onlinelibrary.wiley.com. Accessed July 29, 2017.

66. Hered R. (2011). Effective vision screening of young children in the pediatric office. *Pediatric Annals* 40(2), 76–82.

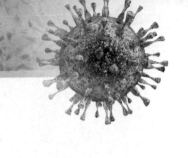

CHAPTER **20**

Disorders of Hearing and Vestibular Function

Learning Objectives

After completing this chapter, the learner will be able to meet the following objectives:

1. Relate the functions of the eustachian tube to the development of middle ear problems, including acute otitis media and otitis media with effusion.
2. Describe the disease process associated with otosclerosis and relate it to progressive conductive hearing loss.
3. Differentiate between conductive, sensorineural, and mixed hearing loss and name the common causes of each.
4. Explain the function of the vestibular system with respect to postural reflexes and maintaining a stable visual field despite marked changes in head position.
5. Compare the manifestations and pathologic processes associated with benign paroxysmal positional vertigo and Ménière disease.
6. Distinguish the characteristics of peripheral and central vestibular disorders.

The ear is a sensory organ of hearing and vestibular equilibrium consisting of three parts: the external, middle, and inner ear. The external and middle ears are designed to capture and transmit sound waves to the inner ear while amplifying sound. The inner ear, which is fluid-filled, contains structures necessary for hearing and balance. The fluid in the inner ear conducts and transmits sound waves and vibrations. Acute otitis media (AOM), or inflammation of the middle ear, is a leading cause of primary care visits and the number one reason for antimicrobial prescriptions for children. Hearing loss is one of the most common disabilities experienced by people in the United States, particularly among older adults. It is also a cause of impaired language development in children. Vertigo, a disorder of vestibular function, is also

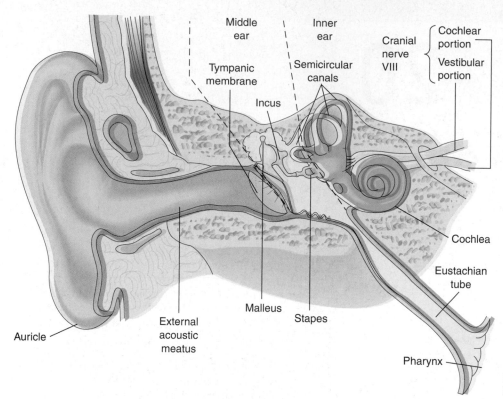

FIGURE 20-1. External, middle, and internal subdivisions of the ear.

a common cause of disability among older adults. This chapter is divided into two parts: the first part focuses on disorders of the ear and auditory function and the second part on disorders of the inner ear and vestibular function.

Disorders of the Auditory System

Disorders of the External Ear

The external ear consists of the auricle and the external acoustic meatus(Fig. 20-1). The auricle, or pinna, which collects sound, is composed of cartilage that is covered by a thin skin and very fine hair.[1] The rim, or helix, is somewhat thicker, and the fleshy earlobe lacks surrounding cartilage. The funnel shape of the auricle concentrates high-frequency sound into the ear canal.

The external acoustic meatus, or ear canal, is approximately 2.5-cm long in adults.[1] In infants and young children, the canal is relatively shorter, so extra care must be taken when inspecting it with an otoscope. A thin layer of skin containing fine hairs, sebaceous glands, and ceruminous glands lines the ear canal. These glands produce cerumen, or earwax, which has certain antimicrobial properties and is thought to serve a protective function.

Branches of the trigeminal nerve (cranial nerve [CN] V) innervate the anterior portion of the auricle and external part of the ear canal. The posterior portions of the auricle and the wall of the ear canal are innervated by auricular branches of the facial (CN VII), glossopharyngeal (CN IX), and vagus (CN X) nerves. Because of the vagal innervation, the insertion of a speculum or

an otoscope into the external ear canal can stimulate coughing or vomiting reflexes.

The tympanic membrane, approximately 1 cm in diameter, is a thin, semitransparent membrane that separates the external ear from the middle ear.[1] The tympanic membrane is covered with thin skin externally and the mucous membrane of the middle ear internally. The tympanic membrane vibrates when audible sound waves enter the external auditory canal. Movements of the membrane are transmitted through the middle ear to the inner ear.

When viewed through an otoscope, the tympanic membrane appears as a shallow, oval cone pointing inward toward its apex the umbo, and other structures can be seen in Figure 20-2. The function of the external ear is disturbed when sound transmission is obstructed by impacted cerumen, inflammation (i.e., otitis externa [OE]), or drainage from the external ear (otorrhea).

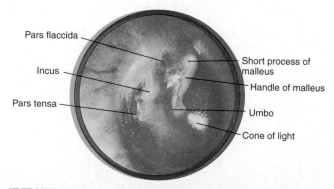

FIGURE 20-2 Bony landmarks of the tympanic membrane. (From Bickley L. S. (2017). *Bates' guide to physical examination and history taking* (12th ed., Figure 7-40). Philadelphia, PA: Wolters Kluwer.)

Impacted Cerumen

Cerumen, or earwax, is a protective secretion produced by the sebaceous and ceruminous glands of the skin that lines the ear canal. Although cerumen is beneficial in cleaning, protecting, and lubricating the ear, the cerumen can accumulate and narrow the canal causing reversible conductive hearing loss.[2]

Impacted cerumen usually produces no symptoms unless it hardens and touches the tympanic membrane or the canal becomes irritated by a buildup of hardened cerumen. Clinical manifestations may include pain, itching, and a sensation of fullness. As the canal becomes completely occluded, a person may experience a feeling of fullness, a conductive hearing loss, vertigo, and tinnitus (i.e., ringing in the ears).[2]

Removal of cerumen is only indicated when visualization of the ear canal and tympanic membrane is necessary. In most cases, cerumen can be removed by manual extraction using a curette or gentle irrigation using a bulb syringe and warm tap water. Consideration must be given to conditions such as an immunocompromised state, diabetes mellitus, and radiation to the head and neck.[2] Cerumen that has become hardened or impacted can be softened by instillation of a few drops of a ceruminolytic agent, a compound that disintegrates earwax.[2]

Otitis Externa

OE, also called swimmer's ear, involves inflammation of the external ear that can vary in severity. It can be caused by infectious agents, irritation, or allergic reactions. OE is a common disease that affects all age groups.[3] OE is more prevalent in hot and humid conditions, and peak incidence occurs in children aged 7 to 12 years.

Etiology

Predisposing factors include swimming, trauma to the canal caused by cleaning or scratching, cerumen buildup, hearing aid use, and allergies or skin conditions such as eczema and seborrhea. Bacterial infections are the cause of 91% of acute OE cases. The most common bacterial pathogens are gram-negative rods (*Pseudomonas aeruginosa*, *Proteus* species) and fungi (*Aspergillus*) that grow in the presence of excess moisture.[3]

Clinical Manifestations and Treatment

OE commonly occurs in the summer and is manifested by itching, redness, tenderness, discharge, impaired hearing, and narrowing of the ear canal because of swelling. Inflammation of the pinna or canal makes movement of the ear painful. There may be watery or purulent drainage and intermittent hearing loss.[4]

Treatment usually includes the use of eardrops containing an appropriate antimicrobial or antifungal agent. For bacterial infections, a corticosteroid solution may be combined with an antimicrobial to reduce inflammation. Protection of the ear from additional moisture (i.e., use of earplugs) and avoidance of trauma from scratching with cotton-tipped applicators and other devices are important.[4]

Disorders of the Middle Ear and Eustachian Tube

The middle ear is an air-filled space inside the temporal bone, which contains three tiny bones called *ossicles*. These bones are the *malleus (hammer)*, *incus*, *(anvil)*, and *stapes (stirrup)*[1] (Fig. 20-1). The middle ear begins as a thin, translucent membrane called the *tympanic membrane*. The tympanic membrane appears pearly gray to light pink with peripheral blood vessels. The tympanic membrane is attached to the temporal bone by a fibrous border called the *annulus*. The malleus holds the tympanic membrane slightly inward, which causes the oval membrane to be slightly concave. The concave shape creates a "cone of light" when light is reflected on the tympanic membrane.

The translucency of the membrane allows visualization of the middle ear, which includes the malleus: The *umbo* is the tip of the malleus that meets the membrane, the *manubrium (handle of malleus)* is attached to the membrane, and the short process of the malleus is another landmark of the tympanic membrane.[1] The middle ear is connected to the nasopharynx by the *eustachian tube*. The walls of the eustachian tube are typically collapsed and valvelike, opening only during swallowing, chewing, and yawning or when expansion is forced.[1] The malleus (hammer), incus, (anvil), and stapes (stirrup) are connected by synovial joints and are covered with the epithelial lining of the cavity.[1] The ossicles move when sound waves reach the tympanic membrane, transmitting sound from the external ear canal to the inner ear.[1] The head of the malleus communicates with the incus, which communicates with the stapes. The stapes attaches to the *oval window*, which vibrates from sound, separates the inner and middle ear, and is in contact with the inner ear fluid. Lying inferior to the oval window, the *round window* communicates with the inner ear and acts as a valve by bulging outward when fluid pressure increases in the inner ear.[1]

KEY POINTS

Disorders of the Middle Ear

■ The middle ear is a small, air-filled compartment in the temporal bone. It is separated from the outer ear by the tympanic membrane; communication between the nasopharynx and the middle ear occurs through the eustachian tube and tiny bony ossicles that span the middle ear transmit sound to the sensory receptors in the inner ear.

■ Otitis media (OM) refers to inflammation of the middle ear. It can represent an AOM, which has an abrupt onset and is usually related to bacterial infection, or otitis media with effusion (OME), which is associated with fluid in the middle ear without the manifestations of infection and does not usually require treatment with antimicrobial agents.

Eustachian Tube Dysfunction

The eustachian tube extends from the middle ear to the nasopharynx and allows air or secretions to enter or leave the middle ear cavity (Fig. 20-1). The eustachian tube serves the following three basic functions:

1. Equalization of pressure on both sides of the tympanic membrane
2. Protection of the middle ear from excessively loud sound, abrupt changes in pressure, and nasopharyngeal secretions
3. Drainage of middle ear secretions into the nasopharynx

The nasopharyngeal entrance to the eustachian tube, which usually is closed, is opened by the action of the trigeminal (CN V)–innervated *tensor veli palatini muscle*. Opening of the eustachian tube, which normally occurs with swallowing and yawning reflexes, allows for equalization of pressure in the middle ear with that of the atmosphere. This equalization of pressure ensures that sound transmission is not reduced and rupture does not result from sudden changes in external pressure, as occurs during plane travel.[5]

The eustachian tube is lined with a mucous membrane that continues into the pharynx. Infections from the nasopharynx can travel to the middle ear, causing AOM (discussed later in this chapter). Toward the nasopharynx, the eustachian tube is lined by columnar epithelium with mucus-secreting cells. Expansion of mucus-secreting cells is thought to contribute to the mucoid secretions that develop during certain types of OM.[5]

Abnormalities in eustachian tube function are important factors in the development of middle ear infections. There are two important types of eustachian tube dysfunction: abnormal patency and obstruction. The *abnormally patent tube* does not close or does not close completely. In infants and children with an abnormally patent tube, air and secretions often are pushed into the eustachian tube during crying and nose blowing. The eustachian tubes of children are short and positioned nearly horizontal, allowing air and secretions from the pharynx to move to the middle ear.[5]

Obstruction of the eustachian tube can be functional or mechanical. *Functional obstruction* results from the persistent collapse of the eustachian tube because of a lack of tubal stiffness or poor function of the tensor veli palatini muscle that controls the opening of the eustachian tube. This condition is common in young children because the amount and rigidity of the cartilage supporting the eustachian tube are less than in older children and adults. Changes in the craniofacial base also reduce the efficiency of the tensor muscle. In addition, craniofacial disorders, such as a cleft palate, alter the attachment of the tensor muscle, producing functional obstruction of the eustachian tube.

Mechanical obstruction results from internal obstruction or external compression of the eustachian tube. Ethnic differences in the structure of the palate may increase the likelihood of obstruction. The most common internal obstruction is caused by swelling and secretions resulting from allergy and viral respiratory infections.

External compression by prominent or enlarged adenoidal tissue surrounding the opening of the eustachian tube may make drainage less effective. Tumors also may obstruct drainage. With obstruction, air in the middle ear is absorbed, causing a negative pressure and the passage of watery capillary fluid into the middle ear.

Barotrauma

Barotrauma is ear pain or damage resulting from rapid changes in air pressure or imbalances between the middle ear and the atmosphere. It occurs most often when there is a sudden change in atmospheric pressure, such as during rapid airplane or sea-level descent, when the air must move through the eustachian tube to equalize pressure in the middle ear. If the eustachian tube is completely or even partially blocked by infection, swelling, or inflammation from a common cold or allergy, air is prevented from moving in and out of the middle ear. Pain, hearing loss, bruising to the tympanic membrane, or even rupture of the tympanic membrane (Fig. 20-3) can result from the differing pressures.[6]

Acute negative middle ear pressure that persists is treated with decongestants and attempts at autoinflation with yawning, swallowing, or chewing gum. More severe hearing loss or discomfort may require that the person consult an otolaryngologist.

Barotrauma often results in the perforation of the tympanic membrane if exposed to concussive forces such as a direct blow or an explosion (Fig. 20-3). Traumatic perforations must be assessed for signs of injury to other structures on the middle or inner ear. Symptoms such as hearing loss, vertigo, nystagmus, or possible leakage of cerebrospinal fluid warrant urgent consultation by an otolaryngologist.

Otitis Media

OM refers to inflammation of the middle ear without reference to etiology or pathogenesis. The term OM is broad and includes conditions caused by bacterial and viral processes. *Acute otitis media* (AOM) is an acute bacterial or viral infection in the middle ear[6] (Fig. 20-4). It usually has an abrupt onset of signs and symptoms related to middle ear inflammation, such as otalgia and fever, and an accompanying upper respiratory infection. *OME*, or serous OM, refers to the presence of fluid in the middle ear without signs and symptoms of acute ear infection. OME can develop spontaneously because of poor eustachian tube function, accompany a viral upper respiratory tract infection, or occur as a prelude or a sequela to AOM.[6]

Risk Factors

Although AOM may occur in any age group, it is most frequently diagnosed in children between the ages of 3 months and 3 years. Smoking in the household is a significant risk factor for AOM. Other risk factors include prematurity, daycare attendance, having an unimmunized status, bottle-feeding, feeding in the supine position, being overweight or obese, having a family history of OM, being of the male gender, and sharing a

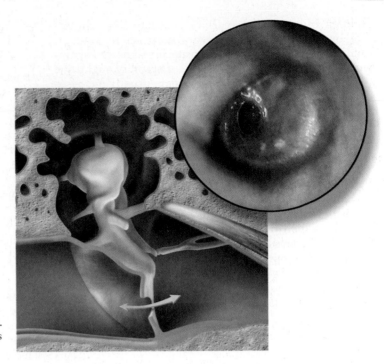

FIGURE 20-3. Perforation of the tympanic membrane. (From Anatomical Chart Company, Middle Ear Conditions chart.)

bedroom. AOM is more frequent in children with craniofacial anomalies or congenital syndromes associated with craniofacial anomalies.[6]

The most important factor that contributes to AOM is believed to be a dysfunction of the eustachian tube that allows reflux of fluid and bacteria into the middle ear space from the nasopharynx. Structural immaturity contributes to the increased risk of AOM in infants and young children:

- The eustachian tube is shorter, more horizontal, and wider in this age group than in older children and adults.
- Infection can spread more easily through the eustachian canal of infants who spend most of their day in the supine position.

Bottle-fed infants have a higher incidence of AOM than breast-fed infants, probably because they are held in a more horizontal position during feeding, and swallowing while in the horizontal position facilitates the reflux

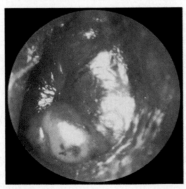

FIGURE 20-4. Acute otitis media of the right ear. (From Jensen S. (2015). *Nursing health assessment: A best practice approach* (2nd ed., p. 370). Philadelphia, PA: Lippincott Williams & Wilkins.)

of milk into the middle ear.[7] Breast-feeding also provides for the transfer of protective maternal antibodies to the infant.

Etiology

The etiology of AOM may be of either bacterial or viral origin. The mucosal lining of the middle ear is continuous with the eustachian tube and nasopharynx, and most middle ear infections enter through the eustachian tube (Fig. 20-1). Respiratory syncytial virus and influenza are the viruses most responsible for the increased incidence rate of AOM in children during late winter and early spring. Respiratory viruses may infect the middle ear mucosa, either alone or in combination with bacteria. Although a virus is usually the initial causative agent in the development of AOM, bacteria may proliferate in the fluid of the middle ear. Most cases of AOM follow an uncomplicated upper respiratory tract infection that has been present for several days. *Streptococcus pneumoniae*, *Haemophilus influenzae*, *Moraxella catarrhalis*, and *Streptococcus pyogenes* (group A streptococci) are the most common infecting bacterial organisms responsible for the development of AOM.

Clinical Manifestations

AOM is characterized by the following key criteria:

- Acute onset of otalgia (or pulling of the ears in an infant) that may interfere with sleep and/or activity
- Fever (>39°C)
- Irritability
- Otorrhea
- Hearing loss
- Evidence of middle ear inflammation
- Middle ear effusion (decreases mobility of the tympanic membrane)

Children older than 3 years of age may have rhinorrhea, or runny nose, vomiting, and diarrhea. In contrast, younger children often have nonspecific signs and symptoms that manifest as ear tugging, irritability, nighttime awakening, and poor feeding. Ear pain usually increases as the effusion accumulates behind the tympanic membrane. Perforation of the tympanic membrane may occur acutely, allowing purulent material from the eustachian tube to drain into the external auditory canal. This may prevent spread of the infection into the temporal bone or intracranial cavity. Healing of the tympanic membrane usually follows resolution of the middle ear infection.

As mentioned earlier in this chapter, OME is a condition in which the tympanic membrane is intact and there is an accumulation of fluid in the middle ear without signs or symptoms of infection. The duration of the effusion may range from less than 3 weeks to more than 3 months. Although often asymptomatic and afebrile, clinical findings of OME include[7]:

- Complaint of intermittent ear pain
- Sensation of fullness in the ear
- Complaint of hearing loss
- Dizziness
- Decreased tympanic membrane mobility
- Visible air–fluid level with or without bubble

Many cases of OME resolve spontaneously, but some experience recurrent OME. Persistent middle ear fluid from OME results in decreased motility of the tympanic membrane and serves as a barrier to sound conduction.

Diagnosis

Distinguishing between AOM and OME is often straightforward, but each condition may evolve into the other without any clearly differentiating physical findings. Because of the increasing antimicrobial resistance, distinguishing between AOM and OME has become increasingly important.

Both AOM without otorrhea (drainage from the ear) and OME are accompanied by otoscopic signs of middle ear effusion (MME), namely, the presence of at least two or three abnormalities:

- White- or yellow-appearing tympanic membrane (may be seen in either AOM or OME)
- Tympanic membrane that appears amber (usually seen in OME)
- Opacification of tympanic membrane other than scarring (may be seen in either)
- Decreased or absent motility of tympanic membrane (may be seen in either)

With OME, the tympanic membrane is often cloudy with distinct impairment of mobility, and an air–fluid level or bubble may be visible in the middle ear.

A definitive diagnosis of AOM requires the following[7]:

- History of acute onset of signs and symptoms
- The presence of MME confirmed by bulging of tympanic membrane, limited or absent mobility by pneumatic otoscopy, air–fluid level behind tympanic membrane, and or otorrhea

- Signs and symptoms of middle ear inflammation confirmed by erythema of tympanic membrane or onset of pain

Pneumatic otoscopy is the most efficient way to make the diagnosis and should be used to either make or confirm the diagnosis. The use of the pneumatic otoscope allows the introduction of air into the ear canal for the purpose of determining tympanic membrane mobility. The movement of the tympanic membrane is decreased in some cases of AOM and absent in chronic middle ear infection. The diagnosis of AOM can also be confirmed using tympanometry. *Tympanometry* is helpful in detecting effusion in the middle ear or high negative middle ear pressure. Tympanocentesis (puncture of the tympanic membrane with a needle) may be done to relieve pain from an effusion or to obtain a specimen of middle ear fluid for culture and sensitivity testing.

Treatment

The treatment of OM focuses on symptom control and management of the underlying pathologic process. A number of options for pain management are available, including the local application of heat or cold, distraction, and use of weight- and age-appropriate analgesic medications such as acetaminophen, ibuprofen, and naproxen. Myringotomy (incision of the tympanic membrane), performed by an otolaryngologist, can be used for relief of pressure in the person who is in severe pain.

Most cases of OME resolve spontaneously within a 3-week to 3-month period. The management options for this duration include observation, detailed charting to include location (unilateral or bilateral), the description of fluid, and any associated symptoms. Other management options include conducting hearing tests and identifying people at risk for speech, language, or learning delays. There is no evidence that decongestants, antibiotics, and nasal steroids are of any benefit in the management of OME.[6]

Complications of Otitis Media

The complications of OM include hearing loss, adhesive OM, cholesteatoma, mastoiditis, and intracranial complications such as otologic meningitis. Hearing loss, which is a common complication of OM, usually is conductive and temporary based on the duration of the effusion. Hearing loss that is associated with fluid collection usually resolves when the effusion clears. Permanent hearing loss may occur as the result of damage to the tympanic membrane or other middle ear structures. Cases of sensorineural hearing loss are rare. Children younger than 3 years of age with recurrent OME are at increased risk of impaired language development. Persistent and episodic conductive hearing loss in children may impair their cognitive, linguistic, and emotional development.[6]

Cholesteatoma is usually the result of a chronic ear infection and involves the formation of an epidermal cyst of the middle ear or mastoid.[6] The cyst, which can be small (approximately 2 mm in diameter) or large (approximately 4 cm in diameter), consists of desquamated debris from the keratinizing, squamous epithelial lining of the middle ear.[7] Surrounding structures can be destroyed by the growth of the cholesteatoma. The cysts can be congenital, primary acquired, or secondary acquired. Research indicates the formation may be related to the inflammatory process, TM perforation, or the collection of desquamated tissue in the middle ear.[7] Cholesteatomas commonly appear whitish or pearl-like in color. Symptoms commonly include painless drainage from the ear and hearing loss. Treatment involves surgery to remove the cholesteatomatous material.

Mastoiditis is a suppurative infection of the mastoid cells.[7] Mastoiditis can develop as the result of chronic middle ear infection. The mucoperiosteal lining of the mastoid air cells becomes inflamed, resulting in swelling and obstruction from mastoid drainage.[6] Treatment of AOM with antimicrobial medication does not eliminate the occurrence of mastoiditis. The incidence of mastoiditis isn't known, but its prevalence has decreased since the introduction of modern antibiotics.[7] Although uncommon, mastoiditis can be life threatening. It is most common during childhood, specifically between the ages of 6 and 13 months.[7] Clinical manifestations include[6]:

- Chronic or concurrent AOM
- Fever
- Otalgia
- Persistent OM
- Swelling in the supra-auricular or postauricular area

Mastoiditis, suspected or confirmed, warrants immediate referral to the closest surgical hospital. Intracranial complications are uncommon since the advent of antimicrobial therapy. Although rare, these complications can develop when the infection spreads through vascular channels or by direct extension. These complications are seen more often with chronic suppurative OM and mastoiditis. They include otogenic meningitis, brain abscess, lateral sinus thrombophlebitis or thrombosis, labyrinthitis, and facial nerve paralysis. Any child who develops persistent headache, tinnitus, stiff neck, or visual or other neurologic symptoms should be investigated for possible intracranial complications.

Otosclerosis

Otosclerosis is a disease of the bone of the otic capsule that causes the formation of new spongy bone around the stapes and oval window.[6] The newly formed bone causes the stapes to become fixed or immobile, resulting in conductive hearing loss. In most cases, the condition is hereditary and follows an autosomal dominant pattern of inheritance. It most commonly affects Caucasian females. Although otosclerosis may begin at any time in life, it typically appears during adolescence and progresses during early adulthood. Pregnancy seems to accelerate the disease. Generally, both ears are affected, but the rate of hearing loss is not symmetric.[1]

Pressure of otosclerotic bone on middle ear structures or the vestibulocochlear nerve (CN VIII) may contribute to the development of tinnitus, sensorineural hearing loss, and vertigo.[6] Because bone conduction is maintained, persons with otosclerosis may be able to use the telephone but have difficulty in carrying on face-to-face conversations.[1]

The treatment of otosclerosis can be medical or surgical. A hearing aid may allow a person with conductive hearing loss to hear and interact with others. To slow bone resorption and overgrowth, sodium fluoride may be recommended. Surgical treatment involves a stapedectomy and reconstruction of the middle ear (stapedotomy). During a stapedectomy, the diseased stapes is removed using a microsurgical technique. A prosthesis is inserted, with one end connecting to the incus and the other inserted into the oval window. During a stapedotomy, a small hole is created in the footplate of the stapes and a wire or ribbon is inserted. Surgical intervention is usually successful at restoring hearing.[6]

Disorders of the Inner Ear

The inner ear is composed of intricate channels that facilitate hearing and position sense. Structurally, it consists of an outer bony labyrinth located in the otic capsule of the petrous part of the temporal bone and an inner membranous labyrinth. The membranous labyrinth lies in the bony labyrinth and consists of a complex system of sacs and ducts (*i.e.*, semicircular ducts). The bony labyrinth, which occupies a space with a diameter less than 1.5 cm, is a series of cavities (the cochlea, vestibule, and semicircular canals)[8] (Fig. 20-5). The receptors for hearing are contained in the cochlea and those for head position sense are contained in the semicircular ducts, the utricle, and the saccule. The vestibule is the central egg-shaped cavity of the bony labyrinth that lies posterior to the cochlea and anterior to the semicircular canals. It contains the utricle and saccule and parts of the balancing apparatus (vestibular labyrinth). The vestibule features the oval window on its lateral wall, occupied by the base of the stapes.

The cochlea is the shell-shaped part of the bony labyrinth that contains the inner membranous cochlear duct, the part of the inner ear concerned with hearing. The spiral canal of the cochlea, which is shaped like a snail shell, begins at the vestibule and winds around a central core of spongy bone called the *modiolus*. The modiolus contains canals for blood vessels and for distribution of the cochlear nerve. The cochlea consists of three tubes coiled side by side:

1. The *scala vestibuli*
2. The *scala media*
3. The *scala tympani*

The vestibular membrane, also known as *Reissner membrane*, separates the scala vestibuli and scala media from each other. The basilar membrane separates the scala tympani from the scala media. On the surface of the basilar membrane lies the spiral organ of Corti, which contains a series of electromechanically sensitive cells, the *hair cells*. They are the receptive organs that generate nerve impulses in response to sound vibrations.

The endolymph and perilymph are the two types of fluids in the inner ear. The scala vestibuli and scala

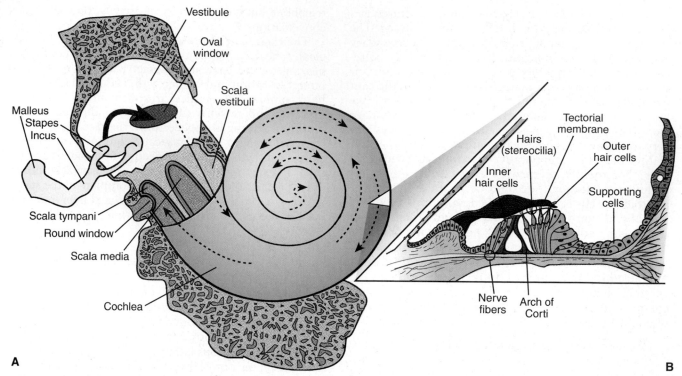

A

B

FIGURE 20-5. The cochlea and the organ of Corti. **(A)** The pea-sized, snail-shaped cochlea is a coiled system and the hearing portion of the inner ear. **(B)** An enlargement of a cross-section of the organ of Corti, showing the relationships among the hair cells and the membranes. Hair cells in the organ of Corti transduce fluid movement into neural signals. (From Rhoades R. A., Bell D. A. (2018). *Medical physiology* (5th ed., Figure 4.18, p. 72). Philadelphia, PA: Wolters Kluwer.)

tympani communicate directly with the subarachnoid space around the brain, so the perilymph is similar to cerebrospinal fluid.[8] The endolymph that fills the scala media is an entirely different fluid; it is secreted by the stria vascularis on the outer wall of the scala media (Fig. 20-6). The perilymph that fills the scala vestibuli and scala tympani has a high sodium (Na^+) concentration, whereas the endolymph that fills the scala media has a high potassium (K^+) content. This is significant because there is a direct current resting membrane potential of about +80 mV that exists between the endolymph and perilymph, with positivity inside the scala media and negativity outside the scala media. This difference in polarity causes a current, called the *endolymphatic potential*, and is generated by a continual exchange of K^+ ions into the scala media by Na^+/K^+ adenosine triphosphatase pumps in the stria vascularis. This current is believed to sensitize the hair cells of the organ of Corti, increasing their ability to respond to the slightest sound.

Unlike light, which can be transmitted through a vacuum, sound is a pressure disturbance that originates from a vibrating object and then spreads via the molecules of an elastic medium. Sound waves, which are delivered by the stapes footplate to the perilymph, travel throughout the fluid of the inner ear, including up the scala vestibuli, to the apex of the cochlea (Fig. 20-6). The vestibular membrane is thin, so the sound vibrations from the scala vestibuli are readily transmitted into the scala media. Therefore, as far as sound conduction is concerned, the scala media and scala vestibuli function as a single chamber.

As the pressure wave descends through the endolymph of the scala media, it sets the entire basilar membrane vibrating. The basilar membrane, which becomes progressively larger from its base to its distal apex, resonates at higher frequencies near the base and at lower frequencies toward its apex as the fluid pressure wave travels up the cochlear spiral. This provides the major basis for recognition of sound, known as pitch.

On top of the basilar membrane and extending along its entire length is an elaborate arrangement of columnar epithelium called the *spiral organ of Corti* (Fig. 20-5). Continuous rows of hair cells separated into inner and outer rows can be found in the columnar arrangement of the spiral organ. The cells have hairlike cilia that protrude through openings and support the reticular membrane into the endolymph of the cochlear duct. A gelatinous mass, the tectorial membrane, extends from the medial side of the duct to enclose the cilia of the outer hair cells. The hair cells in the organ of Corti are programmed to respond to distortion of the cochlear duct induced by compression waves moving through the perilymph, which move up and down in the surrounding scala vestibuli and scala tympani. If enough hair cells are destroyed in a particular segment of the cochlea, hearing loss of particular tones can occur.

Neural Pathways

Information flows from the hair cells in the organ of Corti to neurons that have their cell bodies in the cochlear ganglion and follows a spiral course in the bony

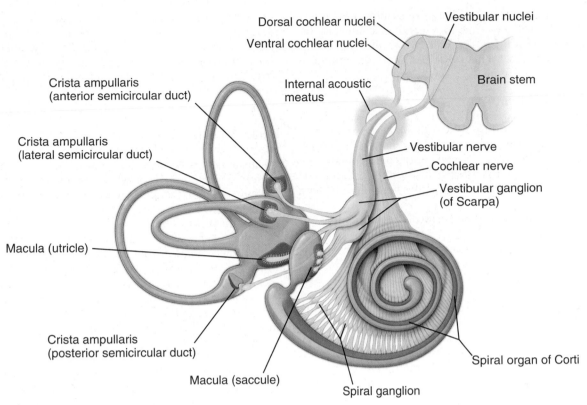

FIGURE 20-6. Spiral organ of Corti has been removed from the cochlear duct and greatly enlarged to show the inner and outer hair cells, the basilar membrane, and the cochlear nerve fibers. (From Pawlina W., Ross M. H. (2016). *Histology: A text and atlas with correlated cell and molecular biology* (7th ed., Figure 25.24, p. 954). Philadelphia, PA: Wolters Kluwer.)

modiolus of the cochlear spiral. Afferent fibers from the spiral ganglion (*i.e.*, vestibulocochlear or auditory nerve [CN VIII]) travel to the cochlear nuclei in the caudal pons. Consequently, impulses from either ear are transmitted through the auditory pathways to both sides of the brain stem.

From the inferior colliculus (located in the midbrain), the auditory pathway passes to the medial geniculate nucleus of the thalamus, where all the fibers synapse. From the medial geniculate nuclei, the auditory tract spreads through the auditory radiation to the primary auditory cortex (area 41), located mainly in the superior temporal gyrus and insula. This area and its corresponding higher-order thalamic nuclei are required for high-acuity loudness discrimination and precise discrimination of pitch. The auditory association cortex (areas 42 and 22) borders the primary cortex on the superior temporal gyrus. This area and its associated higher-order thalamic nuclei are necessary for auditory gnosis, or the meaningfulness of sound, to occur. Experience and the precise analysis of momentary auditory information are integrated during this process.

Tinnitus

Tinnitus (from the Latin word *tinniere*, meaning "to ring") is the perception of abnormal ear or head noises that are not produced by an external stimulus.[8] Although it is often described as "ringing of the ears," tinnitus may also assume a hissing, roaring, buzzing, or humming sound. Tinnitus may be constant or intermittent and unilateral or bilateral. Tinnitus affects 10% to 15% of the population; however, it is primarily associated with the elderly or those who work in loud areas.[8]

For clinical purposes, tinnitus is subdivided into objective and subjective tinnitus.[8] *Objective tinnitus* refers to those rare cases in which the sound is detected or potentially detectable by another observer. Typical causes of objective tinnitus include vascular abnormalities or neuromuscular disorders. In some vascular disorders, for example, sounds generated by turbulent blood flow (*e.g.*, arterial **bruits** or venous hums) are conducted to the auditory system. Vascular disorders typically produce a pulsatile form of tinnitus.

Subjective tinnitus refers to noise perception when there is no noise stimulation of the cochlea. A number of causes and conditions have been associated with subjective tinnitus. Intermittent periods of mild, high-pitched tinnitus lasting for several minutes are common in people who have normal hearing.

Etiology

Impacted cerumen is a benign cause of tinnitus, which resolves after the earwax is removed. Conditions associated with more persistent tinnitus include noise-induced hearing loss, presbycusis (sensorineural hearing loss that occurs with aging), hypertension, atherosclerosis, head injury, and cochlear or labyrinthine infection or inflammation.

The physiologic cause of subjective tinnitus is largely unknown. It is likely due to several mechanisms, including abnormal firing of auditory receptors, cochlear dysfunction, auditory nerve damage, or alterations in processing of the signal.

Diagnosis and Treatment

Because tinnitus is a symptom, the diagnosis relies heavily on the person's ability to describe the symptoms that have been impacting the person's hearing and other aspects of life. A history of medication or stimulant use and dietary factors that may cause tinnitus should be obtained. Tinnitus often accompanies hearing disorders, and tests of auditory function are usually done. Causes of objective tinnitus, such as serious vascular abnormalities, should be ruled out.

Treatment measures include elimination of drugs or other substances that are suspected of causing tinnitus, such as caffeine, some cheeses, red wine, and foods containing monosodium glutamate. The use of an externally produced sound (i.e., noise generators or tinnitus-masking devices) may be used to mask or inhibit the tinnitus. Medications (including antihistamines, anticonvulsant drugs, calcium channel blockers, benzodiazepines, and antidepressants) have been used for tinnitus alleviation, but most are not effective, and many produce undesirable side effects. For persistent tinnitus, psychological interventions may be needed to help the person deal with the stress and distraction associated with the condition. Tinnitus retraining therapy, which includes directive counseling and extended use of low-noise generators to facilitate auditory adaptation to the tinnitus, has met with considerable success. Surgical intervention (i.e., cochlear nerve section, vascular decompression) is a last resort for people in whom all other interventions have failed and in whom the disorder is disabling.

Disorders of the Central Auditory Pathways

The auditory pathways in the brain involve communication between the two sides of the brain at many levels. As a result, strokes, tumors, abscesses, and other focal abnormalities seldom produce more than a mild reduction in auditory acuity on the side opposite the lesion. For intelligibility of auditory language, lateral dominance becomes important. On the dominant side, usually the left side, the more medial and dorsal portion of the auditory association cortex is of crucial importance. This area is called the *Wernicke area*. People with damage to this area of the brain can speak intelligibly and read normally but are unable to understand the meaning of major aspects of audible speech. This condition is called auditory receptive aphasia.

Tumors or other irritative foci that affect the way sounds are perceived in the primary auditory cortex can produce roaring or clicking sounds, which can manifest as auditory hallucinations. Focal seizures that originate in or near the auditory cortex often are immediately preceded by a prodrome (i.e., an aura) and then the perception of ringing or other sounds. Damage to the auditory association cortex, especially if bilateral, results in an inability to recognize or remember sounds (i.e., auditory agnosia). If the damage is in the dominant hemisphere, speech recognition can be affected (i.e., sensory or receptive aphasia).

Hearing Loss

Hearing is a specialized sense that provides the ability to perceive vibration of sound waves. Functions of the ear include receiving sound waves, distinguishing their frequency, translating this information into nerve impulses, and transmitting these impulses to the central nervous system (CNS). The compression waves that produce sound have frequency and intensity. *Frequency* indicates the number of waves per unit time (reported in cycles per second or hertz). The human ear is most sensitive to waves in the frequency range of 1000 to 3000 Hz. Most people cannot hear compression waves that have a frequency higher than 20,000 Hz. Waves of higher frequency are called *ultrasonic waves*, meaning that they are above the audible range. In the audible frequency range, the subjective experience correlated with sonic frequency is the pitch of a sound. Waves below 20 to 30 Hz are experienced as a rattle or drumbeat rather than a tone.

Wave intensity is represented by amplitude or units of sound pressure. Generally, the intensity (in power units or ergs per square centimeter) of a sound is expressed as the ratio of intensities between the sound and a reference value. A 10-fold increase in sound pressure is called a *bel*, after Alexander Graham Bell. Because this representation is too crude to be of use, the decibel (dB), or 1/10 of a bel, is used.

Nearly 36 million Americans (17%) have hearing loss. Hearing loss in general is classified as:

- Mild (the most quiet sounds heard by people with their better ear are 26 to 40 dB)
- Moderate (the most quiet sounds heard by people with their better ear are 41 to 55 dB)
- Moderately severe (the most quiet sounds heard by people with their better ear are 56 to 70 dB)
- Severe (the most quiet sounds heard by people with their better ear are 71 to 90 dB)
- Profound (the most quiet sounds heard by people with their better ear are 91 dB or greater in adults and 70 dB or greater in children)[8]

The term "hard of hearing" is sometimes used for people who have difficulty hearing and is defined as hearing loss greater than 20 to 25 dB in adults and greater than 15 dB in children.

There are many causes of hearing loss or deafness. Age and suddenness of onset provide important clues as to the cause of hearing loss. Most hearing loss fits into the categories of conductive, sensorineural, or mixed deficiencies.[8] Hearing loss may be hereditary or acquired, sudden or progressive, unilateral or bilateral, partial or complete, and reversible or irreversible. Chart 20-1 summarizes common causes of conductive and sensorineural hearing loss.

CHART 20-1

COMMON CAUSES OF CONDUCTIVE AND SENSORINEURAL HEARING LOSS

Conductive Hearing Loss

- External ear conditions
  - Impacted earwax or foreign body
  - Otitis externa
- Middle ear conditions
  - Trauma
  - Otitis media (acute and with effusion)
  - Otosclerosis
  - Tumors

Sensorineural Hearing Loss

- Trauma
  - Head injury
  - Noise
- CNS infections (*e.g.*, meningitis)
- Degenerative conditions
  - Presbycusis
- Vascular
  - Atherosclerosis
  - Sudden deafness
- Ototoxic drugs (*e.g.*, aminoglycosides, salicylates, loop diuretics)
- Tumors
  - Vestibular schwannoma (acoustic neuroma)
  - Meningioma
  - Metastatic tumors
- Idiopathic
  - Ménière disease

Mixed Conductive and Sensorineural Hearing Loss

- Middle ear conditions
  - Barotrauma
  - Cholesteatoma
  - Otosclerosis
- Temporal bone fracture

KEY POINTS

Hearing Loss

- Hearing is a sensory function that incorporates the sound-transmitting properties of the external ear canal, the eardrum that separates the external and middle ear, the bony ossicles of the middle ear, the sensory receptors of the cochlea in the inner ear, the neural pathways of the vestibulocochlear or auditory nerve, and the primary auditory and auditory association cortices.

- Hearing loss can be caused by conductive disorders; this means that auditory stimuli are not transmitted properly through the structures of the ear to the sensory receptors in the inner ear. Hearing loss can also be caused by sensorineural disorders that affect the inner ear, auditory nerve, or auditory pathways. Hearing loss can also be a combination of conductive and sensorineural disorders (mixed hearing loss).

Conductive Hearing Loss

Conductive hearing loss occurs when auditory stimuli are not adequately transmitted through the auditory canal, tympanic membrane, middle ear, or ossicle chain to the inner ear.[9] Temporary hearing loss can occur as the result of impacted cerumen in the outer ear or fluid in the middle ear. Foreign bodies, including pieces of cotton and insects, may impair hearing. More permanent causes of hearing loss are thickening or damage of the tympanic membrane or involvement of the bony structures (ossicles and oval window) of the middle ear because of otosclerosis or Paget disease.

Sensorineural Hearing Loss

Sensorineural, or perceptive, hearing loss occurs with disorders that affect the inner ear, auditory nerve, or auditory pathways of the brain.[9] With this type of deafness, sound waves are conducted to the inner ear, but abnormalities of the cochlear apparatus or auditory nerve decrease or distort the transfer of information to the brain. Tinnitus often accompanies cochlear nerve irritation. Abnormal function resulting from damage or malformation of the central auditory pathways and circuitry is included in this category.

Etiology

Sensorineural hearing loss is usually irreversible and occurs most commonly in the higher frequencies. Sensorineural hearing loss may have a genetic cause or may result from intrauterine infections such as maternal rubella or developmental malformations of the inner ear. Genetic hearing loss may result from mutation in a single gene (monogenetic) or from a combination of mutations in different genes and environmental factors (multifactorial). Hearing loss may begin before development of speech (prelingual) or after speech development (postlingual). Most prelingual forms are present at birth. Hereditary forms of hearing loss also can be classified as being part of a syndrome in which other abnormalities are present or, as nonsyndromic, in which deafness is the only abnormality.

Sensorineural hearing loss also can result from trauma to the inner ear, tumors that encroach on the inner ear or sensory neurons, vascular disorders with hemorrhage, or thrombosis of vessels that supply the inner ear. Other causes of sensorineural deafness are infections and drugs. Sudden sensorineural hearing loss represents an abrupt loss of hearing that occurs instantaneously or on awakening. It is most commonly caused by viral infections, circulatory disorders, or rupture of the labyrinth membrane that can occur during tympanotomy.

Environmentally induced deafness can occur through direct exposure to an excessively intense sound, as in the workplace or at a concert. This is a particular problem in older adults who were working in noisy environments before the mid-1960s, when there were no laws mandating the use of devices for protective hearing. Sustained or repeated exposure to noise pollution at sound intensities greater than 100 to 120 dB can cause corresponding mechanical damage to the organ of Corti. If the damage is severe, permanent sensorineural deafness to the corresponding sound frequencies occurs. Wearing earplugs or ear protection is important under many industrial conditions and for musicians and music listeners exposed to high sound amplification.

A number of infections can cause hearing loss. Deafness or some degree of hearing impairment is the most common serious complication of bacterial meningitis in infants and children. The mechanism causing hearing impairment seems to be a suppurative labyrinthitis or neuritis resulting in the loss of hair cells and damage to the auditory nerve. Untreated suppurative OM also can extend into the inner ear and cause sensorineural hearing loss through the same mechanisms.

Among the neoplasms that impair hearing are *acoustic neuromas*, which are benign Schwann cell tumors affecting CN VIII. These tumors usually are unilateral and cause hearing loss by compressing the cochlear nerve or interfering with blood supply to the nerve and cochlea. Other neoplasms that can affect hearing include meningiomas and metastatic brain tumors. The temporal bone is a common site of metastases in people with cancer.

Drugs that damage inner ear structures are labeled *ototoxic*. Vestibular symptoms of ototoxicity include light-headedness and dizziness. If toxicity is severe, cochlear symptoms consisting of tinnitus or hearing loss occur. This type of hearing loss is sensorineural; it can occur in one or both ears and may be temporary or permanent. Several classes of drugs have been identified as having ototoxic potential, including aminoglycosides, antimalarials, some chemotherapeutic drugs, loop diuretics (*e.g.*, *furosemide [Lasix]*), and salicylates (*e.g.*, aspirin).[8] The symptoms of drug-induced hearing loss may be transient, as is often the case with salicylates and diuretics, or they may be permanent. The risk of ototoxicity depends on the total dose of the drug and its concentration in the bloodstream. This risk is increased in people with impaired kidney function because they are unable to excrete medications effectively, as well as those who have previously received another potentially ototoxic drug.

Diagnosis and Treatment

Diagnosis

Diagnosis of hearing loss is aided by obtaining a comprehensive history of associated otologic factors such as otalgia, otorrhea, tinnitus, and self-described hearing difficulties. Additionally, a thorough physical examination is needed to assess for otorrhea, impacted cerumen, or injury to the tympanic membrane. Hearing tests, including conventional audiometry and high-frequency audiometry, are most frequently used to diagnose ototoxicity.[8] A history of occupational and noise exposure is important, as is the use of medications with ototoxic potential. Testing for hearing loss includes a number of methods, including a person's reported ability to hear an observer's voice, use of a tuning fork to test air and bone conduction, audioscopes, and auditory brain stem evoked responses (ABRs).

Tuning forks are used to differentiate conductive and sensorineural hearing loss. A 512-Hz or higher-frequency tuning fork is used because frequencies below this level elicit a vibratory response.[9] The Weber test evaluates conductive hearing loss by lateralization of sound. The test is done by placing the lightly vibrating tuning fork on the forehead or top of the head. In people with conductive losses, the sound is louder on the side with the hearing loss, but in persons with sensorineural loss, the sound radiates to the side with the better hearing.[9] The Rinne test compares air and bone conduction.[9] The test is done by alternately placing the tuning fork on the mastoid bone and in front of the ear canal. In conductive losses, bone conduction exceeds air conduction. In sensorineural losses, the opposite occurs.[9]

An audioscope is a rechargeable battery–powered, handheld instrument that combines a pure-tone screening audiometer and otoscope into a single unit. It produces pure sounds at 500, 1000, 2000, and 4000 Hz, at loudness levels of 20, 25, and 40 dB. If a person cannot hear pure tones at 1000 to 2000 Hz (usual speech frequencies), referral for a full audiogram is indicated. The audiogram is an important method of analyzing a person's hearing and is generally considered the gold standard for diagnosis of hearing loss. It is done by an audiologist and requires highly specialized sound production and control equipment. Pure tones of controlled intensity are delivered, usually to one ear at a time, and the minimum intensity needed for hearing to be experienced is plotted as a function of frequency.

The ABR is a noninvasive method that permits functional evaluation of certain parts of the central auditory pathways. Electroencephalographic electrodes and high-gain amplifiers produce a record of the electrical wave activity elicited during repeated tests of either or both ears. ABR recording involves subjecting the ear to loud clicks and using a computer to pick up nerve impulses as they are processed in the midbrain. With this method, certain early waves that come from discrete portions of the pons and midbrain auditory pathways can be correlated with specific sensorineural abnormalities. Also, magnetic resonance imaging (MRI) and computed tomography are used to identify tumors in the brain.

Treatment

Hearing loss can have many consequences. Social isolation and depressive disorders are common in hearing-impaired elderly. Safety issues, both in and out of the home, may become significant.

Treatment of hearing loss can range from simple removal of impacted cerumen in the external auditory canal to surgical procedures such as those used to reconstruct the tympanic membrane. For other people, hearing aids and cochlear implants are an option. Although many assistive devices are available to people with hearing loss, understanding on the part of family and friends is perhaps the most important. It is important that those speaking to people with hearing impairment face the person and articulate so that lipreading cues can be used.

Hearing aids remain the mainstay of treatment for many people with conductive and sensorineural hearing loss. Other aids for the hearing impaired include alert and signal devices, assistive listening devices from telephone companies, and dogs trained to respond to various sounds.

Cochlear implants for profound hearing loss have been very effective, and over 200,000 people worldwide have received one.[8] These prostheses are inserted into the scala tympani of the cochlea and work by providing direct stimulation to the auditory nerve, bypassing the area that is absent or nonfunctional in a deaf cochlea. For the implant to work, the auditory nerve must be functional. Although early implants used a single electrode, current implants use multielectrode placement, enhancing speech perception. Most people who become deaf after learning speech derive substantial benefit when cochlear implants are used in conjunction with lipreading. Some are able to understand some speech without lipreading and some are able to communicate by telephone.

Hearing Loss in Infants and Children

Even slight or unilateral hearing loss can negatively impact the young child's language development. Although estimates vary depending on the group surveyed and testing methods used, 1 to 3 babies out of 1000 will be born with a permanent hearing loss. When considering less severe or transient conductive hearing loss that is commonly associated with middle ear disease in young children, the numbers are even greater.

The cause of hearing impairment in children may be conductive or sensorineural. Most conductive hearing loss is caused by middle ear infections. Causes of sensorineural hearing impairment include genetic, infectious, traumatic, and ototoxic factors. Genetic causes are probably responsible for as much as 50% of sensorineural hearing loss in children. Hearing loss affects 1 to 3 of 1000 newborns; this number increases if the newborn is in an intensive care setting.[10] Congenital cytomegalovirus is the most common cause of sensorineural hearing loss in newborns.[11]

Postnatal causes of sensorineural hearing loss include beta-hemolytic streptococcal sepsis in the newborn and bacterial meningitis. *Streptococcus pneumoniae* is the most common cause of bacterial meningitis that results in sensorineural hearing loss after the neonatal period. This cause may become less frequent with the routine administration of the conjugate pneumococcal vaccine. Other causes of sensorineural hearing loss are toxins and trauma. Early in pregnancy, the embryo is particularly sensitive to toxic substances, including ototoxic drugs such as the aminoglycosides and loop diuretics. Trauma, particularly head trauma, may cause sensorineural hearing loss.

The American Academy of Pediatrics (AAP) and the Joint Commission on Infant Hearing (JCIH) published a position paper calling for universal screening of all infants by physiologic measurements before 1 month of age, with proper intervention no later than 6 months of age.[12] Because many children become hearing impaired after the neonatal period and are not identified by neonatal screening programs, the AAP and JCIH recommend that all infants with risk factors for delayed onset of progressive hearing loss receive ongoing audiologic and medical monitoring and at appropriate intervals thereafter.[12] Once hearing loss has been identified, a full developmental and speech and language evaluation is needed.

Hearing Loss in Older Adults

The term *presbycusis* is used to describe degenerative hearing loss that occurs with advancing age.[13] Approximately 45% of the population aged 65 years and older is hearing impaired.[13] Because of its high prevalence, presbycusis is a common social and health problem.

The hearing loss associated with presbycusis is typically gradual, bilateral, and characterized by high-frequency hearing loss.[13] It is further characterized by reduced hearing sensitivity and speech understanding in noisy environments, slowed central processing of acoustic information, and impaired localization of sound sources. The disorder first reduces the ability to understand speech and, later, the ability to detect, identify, and localize sounds. The most common complaint of people with presbycusis is not that they cannot hear but rather that they cannot understand with clarity what is being said.[13] High-frequency warning sounds, such as beepers, turn signals, and escaping steam, are not heard and localized, with potentially dangerous results. Because the age at which problems occur varies widely, it seems likely that the disorder results from a mixture of acquired auditory stresses, trauma, and otologic diseases in addition to the aging process.

Given the high prevalence of presbycusis in people of retirement age and the adverse effects of hearing loss on well-being, screening for hearing loss should be performed at annual health care visits. The single question "do you have a hearing problem?" is usually an effective method of screening. Screening audiometry is a practical and cost-effective method for detecting significant hearing loss. The majority of hearing loss in older adults is sensorineural. In mild to severe hearing loss, the most effective treatment is hearing amplification with hearing aids, lipreading, and assistive listening devices (*e.g.*, hearing aids with the telephone, captioning on televised programs, flashing alarms). Cochlear implants are indicated at any age for people with bilateral hearing losses not materially helped by hearing aids.

SUMMARY CONCEPTS

Hearing is a specialized sense whose external stimulus is the vibration of sound waves. Our ears receive sound waves, distinguish their frequencies, translate this information into nerve impulses, and transmit them to the CNS. Anatomically, the auditory system consists of the outer ear, middle ear, and inner ear, the auditory pathways, and the auditory cortex. The middle ear is a tiny, air-filled cavity in the temporal bone. A connection exists between the middle ear and the nasopharynx. This connection, called the *eustachian tube*, allows equalization of pressure between the middle ear and the atmosphere. The inner ear contains the receptors for hearing.

Disorders of the auditory system include infections of the external and middle ear, otosclerosis, and conduction and sensorineural deafness. OE is an inflammatory process of the external ear. OM is an inflammation of the middle ear without reference to etiology or pathogenesis. AOM, which refers to an acute middle ear infection, is one of the most common illnesses in children. It usually follows an upper respiratory tract infection, has an abrupt onset, and is characterized by otalgia, fever, and hearing loss. OME refers to the presence of fluid in the inner ear without signs and symptoms of acute ear infection. The effusion that accompanies OM can persist for weeks or months, interfering with hearing and impairing speech development. It is important to differentiate OME from AOM to avoid unnecessary antimicrobial use. Otosclerosis is a familial disorder of the otic capsule. It causes bone resorption followed by excessive replacement with sclerotic bone. The disorder eventually causes immobilization of the stapes and conduction deafness.

Deafness, or hearing loss, can develop as the result of a number of auditory disorders. It can be conductive, sensorineural, or mixed. Conduction deafness occurs when transmission of sound waves from the external ear to the inner ear is impaired. Sensorineural deafness can involve cochlear structures of the inner ear or the neural pathways that transmit auditory stimuli. Sensorineural hearing loss can result from genetic or congenital disorders, trauma, infections, vascular disorders, tumors, or ototoxic drugs. Hearing loss in infants and young children impairs language and speech development. In the elderly, hearing loss is a common condition resulting in significant loss of social well-being. Treatment of hearing loss includes the use of hearing aids and, in some cases of profound deafness, implantation of cochlear prosthesis.

Disorders of Vestibular Function

The Vestibular System and Vestibular Reflexes

By about 24 weeks of gestational age, the vestibular system has reached adult form and size.[14] Located in the inner ear, the vestibular system is primarily responsible for balance. The vestibular system includes the vestibular apparatus, and CNS connections contribute to the reflex activity needed for detecting and maintaining postural orientation and perception of motion. Beyond maintaining posture and balance, the vestibular system also integrates visual input from the eyes and proprioceptive input from the peripheral nerves through the spinal cord.[15]

Disorders of the vestibular system are characterized by vertigo, nystagmus, tinnitus, nausea and vomiting, and autonomic nervous system manifestations. Despite the discomfort of these symptoms, few cases are life-threatening conditions.[15] There are many types of vestibular disorders (Table 20-1). These disorders can be a major cause for the sensation of dizziness, vision changes, or unsteadiness.

Peripheral Vestibular Apparatus

The peripheral vestibular apparatus is contained in the bony labyrinth of the inner ear. It has two chambers: outer bony labyrinth and outer bony labyrinth. The *outer bony labyrinth* is filled with perilymph fluid and the *inner membranous labyrinth* is filled with endolymph fluid. The membranous labyrinth has three semicircular canals and two otolithic organs (the utricle and saccule). Each ear contains these five structures, which supply sensory information to coordinate eye and head movement.[16]

TABLE 20-1 Common Disorders Affecting the Vestibular System

Type of Disorder	Pathology
Acoustic neuroma	A noncancerous growth or tumor on the vestibulocochlear nerve
Benign paroxysmal positional vertigo	Disorder of otoliths
Ménière disease	Dislodgement of otoliths that participate in the receptor function of the vestibular system
Motion sickness	Repeated stimulation of the vestibular system such as during car, air, and boat travel
Labyrinthitis	Acute viral or bacterial infection of the vestibular pathways
Vestibular migraine	Dizziness or vertigo occurs with or without headache; related to the neurotransmitter serotonin

The semicircular canals are located perpendicular to each other and detect rotational movement, whereas the utricle and saccule detect linear movement. The smaller saccule extends into the cochlea through the ductus reuniens, and the utricle lies between the cochlea and semicircular ducts (Fig. 20-7). Small patches of hair cells are located in a membranous **ampulla** of the three semicircular ducts and the maculae of the saccule and utricle.[5]

The cavities of the three semicircular canals—the lateral, anterior, and posterior canals—are oriented in one of three planes of space. The lateral (horizontal) canals are in the same plane, whereas the anterior (superior) canal of one side is parallel with the posterior (inferior) canal on the other side, and the two function as a pair. Located in each semicircular canal is a corresponding semicircular duct, which communicates with the utricle. Each of these ducts has an enlarged swelling at one end called an ampulla. The ampulla contains a ridge that is covered by a sensory epithelium with hair cells that are raised into a crest, called the *crista ampullaris* (Fig. 20-6). These hair cells are innervated by the primary afferents of the vestibular nerve, which is a subdivision of the eighth CN. The hair cells of the crista ampullaris extend into a flexible gelatinous mass called the *cupula*, which essentially closes off fluid flow through the semicircular ducts (Fig. 20-7). When the head begins to move, gravity produces a change in the endolymph, which causes the hair cells to bend, generating impulses carried by the vestibular branch of the eighth CN. Because all the hair cells in each semicircular canal share a common orientation, angular acceleration in one direction increases afferent nerve activity, whereas acceleration in the opposite direction diminishes nerve activity. Impulses from the semicircular ducts are particularly important in

reflex movement of the eyes and keep images steady on the retina when the head moves. Vestibular nystagmus is a complex phenomenon that occurs during and immediately after rotational motion.[17] As you rotate your head, your eyes slowly drift in the opposite direction and then jump rapidly back toward the direction of rotation to establish a new fixation point.

Both the saccule and utricle have an equilibrium receptor, called a macula, that relates to changes in head position. Each macula is a small, flat epithelial patch with supporting cells and sensory hair cells. The sides and bases synapse with sensory endings of the vestibular nerve (Fig. 20-8). Each group of hair cells has multiple small cilia called *stereocilia*, plus one large cilium, the *kinocilium*. The kinocilium is located at one side of the cell, and the stereocilia become progressively shorter toward the other side of the cell. Tiny short hairs connect the tip of each stereocilium to the next longer stereocilium and finally to the kinocilium. Movement of the head in one direction causes movement of the adjoined stereocilia and kinocilium and depolarization or activation of the receptor. Movement of the head in the other direction causes hyperpolarization or inactivation of the receptor.

The hair cells in both the utricular and saccular maculae are embedded in a flattened gelatinous mass, the *otolithic membrane*, which is studded with tiny stones (calcium carbonate crystals) called *otoliths*. Although they are small, the density of the otoliths increases the membrane's weight and its resistance to change in motion. When the head is tilted, the gelatinous mass shifts its position because of the pull of the gravitational field, bending the stereocilia of the macular hair cells. The otoliths are sensitive to static or changing head movements,

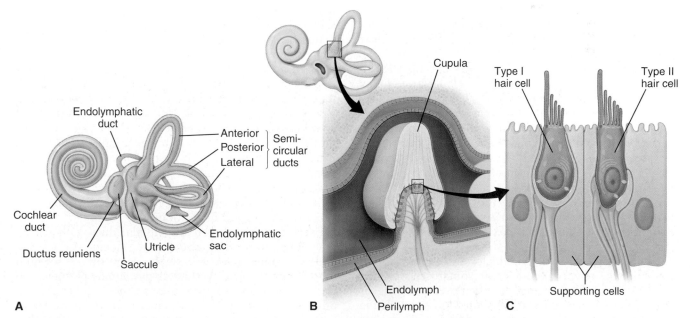

FIGURE 20-7. (**A**) The osseous and membranous labyrinth of the left ear showing the utricle and saccule with their maculae and three semicircular canals and their ampullae. (**B**) Location of the crista ampullaris and its connection to the vestibular branch of CN VIII. (**C**) The location of the cupula and movement of hair cells of the crista ampullaris with head movement. (From Pawlina W., Ross M. H. (2016). *Histology: A text and atlas with correlated cell and molecular biology* (7th ed., Figures 25.8C (p. 942), 25.12B and C (p. 946)). Philadelphia, PA: Wolters Kluwer.)

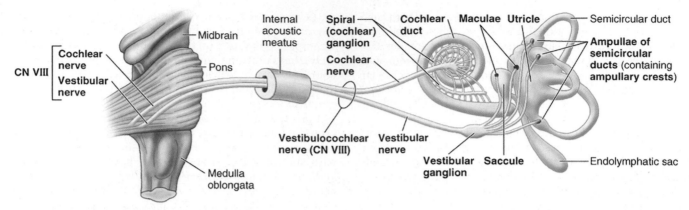

FIGURE 20-8. Vestibulocochlear nerve (CN VIII). (From Moore K. L., Anne M. R., Dalley A. F. (2014). *Essential clinical anatomy* (5th ed., Figure 7.78, p. 573). Philadelphia, PA: Lippincott Williams & Wilkins.)

depending on the direction that the cilia are bending. In a condition called *benign paroxysmal positional vertigo* (BPPV), changes in head position cause a sensation of whirling or spinning. With this condition, the otoliths become dislodged from their gelatinous base and drift into the semicircular canals, causing vertigo.

Neural Pathways

The response to body imbalance, such as stumbling, must be fast and reflexive. The vestibular system has extensive links with neural pathways controlling vision, hearing, and autonomic nervous system function. Information from the vestibular system goes directly to reflex centers in the brain stem rather than to the cerebral cortex. Ganglion cells associated with afferent nerve fibers relay sensory information to the peripheral vestibular apparatus. The central axons of these ganglion cells become the superior and inferior vestibular nerves, which become part of the vestibulocochlear nerve (CN VIII).

Impulses from the vestibular nerves initially pass to one of two destinations: the vestibular nuclear complex in the brain stem or the cerebellum. The vestibular nuclei receive input from visual and somatic receptors that report head position in space. These nuclei send impulses to the brain stem centers that control the extrinsic eye movements (CN III, IV, and VI) and reflex movements of the neck, limb, and trunk muscles (through the vestibulospinal tracts). The vestibulo-ocular reflexes (VORs) keep the eyes still as the head moves and the vestibulospinal reflexes enable the musculoskeletal system to make the quick adjustments needed to maintain or regain balance.

Neurons of the vestibular nuclei also project to the thalamus, the temporal cortex, the somatosensory area of the parietal cortex, and the chemoreceptor trigger zone. The thalamic and cortical projections provide the basis for the subjective experiences of position in space and of rotation. Connections with the chemoreceptor trigger zone stimulate the vomiting center in the brain. This is thought to account for the nausea and vomiting that accompany vestibular disorders.

Nystagmus

Nystagmus can be either physiologic or pathologic. Physiologically, nystagmus refers to the involuntary rhythmic and oscillatory eye movements caused by altered input from the vestibular nuclei during head movement.[18] The VOR produces slow compensatory conjugate eye rotations that occur in the opposite direction of head movement and stabilize fixation of both eyes on an object. This reflex can be demonstrated by holding a pencil vertically in front of the eyes and moving it from side to side through a 10-degree arc at a rate of approximately five times per second. At this rate of motion, the pencil appears blurred because a different and more complex reflex cannot compensate quickly enough. However, if the pencil is maintained in a stable position and the head is moved back and forth at the same rate, the image of the pencil is clearly defined. The eye movements are the same in both cases. The reason that the pencil image remains clear in the second situation is because the VOR keeps the image of the pencil on the retinal fovea. When compensatory VOR carries the conjugate eye rotations to their physical limit, a very rapid conjugate movement moves the eyes in the direction of head movement to a new fixation point, followed by a slow VOR as the head continues to rotate past the new fixation point. This pattern of slow–fast–slow movements is called *nystagmus*. Clinically, the direction of nystagmus is named for the fast phase of nystagmus.

Nystagmus can be classified according to the direction of eye movement: horizontal, vertical, rotary (torsional), or mixed. If head rotation is continued, friction between endolymph and semicircular duct walls results in endolymph rotating at the same velocity as the head, and nystagmus adapts to a stable eye posture. If rotation is suddenly stopped, vestibular nystagmus reappears in the direction precisely opposite to the angular accelerating nystagmus, because the inertia of the endolymph is again bending hair cells of a now stationary ampulla.

Pathologic nystagmus occurs without head movement or visual stimuli.[18] It seems to appear more readily and more severely with fatigue and to some extent can be influenced by psychological factors. Nystagmus because of a CNS pathologic process, in contrast to vestibular end organ or vestibulocochlear nerve sources, seldom is accompanied by vertigo. If present, the vertigo is mild. Nystagmus eye movements can be tested by caloric stimulation or rotation.

Vertigo

Disorders of vestibular function are characterized by a condition called vertigo, in which an illusion of motion occurs. Persons with vertigo frequently describe a sensation of spinning, "to-and-fro" motion, or falling.

 Concept Mastery Alert

> With vertigo, the person may be stationary and the environment in motion (*i.e.*, objective vertigo) or the person may be in motion and the environment stationary (*i.e.*, subjective vertigo).

Vertigo is different than light-headedness, faintness, or syncope. It is considered more of a spinning of oneself or the surroundings. Presyncope, which is characterized by a feeling of light-headedness or "blacking out," is commonly caused by postural hypotension or a global impairment of cerebral circulation that limits blood flow.[19] An inability to maintain normal gait may be described as dizziness despite the absence of objective vertigo. The unstable gait may be caused by disorders of sensory input (*e.g.*, proprioception), peripheral neuropathy, gait problems, or disorders other than vestibular function and usually is corrected by touching a stationary object such as a wall or table.

Vertigo or dizziness can result from central or peripheral vestibular disorders. The majority of cases result from a peripheral vestibular source rather than a central source.[20] Vertigo because of peripheral vestibular disorders tends to be severe in intensity and episodic or brief in duration. In contrast, vertigo because of central vestibular causes tends to be mild and constant and chronic in duration.

Objective vertigo is the sensation of the person being stationary and the environment in motion. Subjective vertigo is a sensation of a person who may be in motion and the environment stationary.

Motion Sickness

Motion sickness is a form of normal physiologic vertigo. It is caused by repeated rhythmic stimulation of the vestibular system, such as that encountered in car, air, or boat travel. Vertigo, malaise, nausea, and vomiting are the principal symptoms. Autonomic signs, including lowered blood pressure, tachycardia, and excessive sweating, may occur. Hyperventilation, which commonly accompanies motion sickness, produces changes in blood volume and pooling of blood in the lower extremities, leading to postural hypotension and sometimes to **syncope**. Some persons experience a variant of motion sickness, complaining of sensing the rocking motion of the boat after returning to ground. This usually resolves after the vestibular system becomes accustomed to the stationary influence of being back on land.

Motion sickness can usually be suppressed by supplying visual signals that more closely match the motion signals being supplied to the vestibular system. Anti-motion sickness drugs also may be used to reduce or relieve the symptoms. These drugs work by suppressing the activity of the vestibular system.

Disorders of Peripheral Vestibular Function

Disease or damage to the vestibular system can result in dysfunction of this system. Disorders of peripheral vestibular function occur when otolith debris enters the semicircular canals, causing gravitational sensitivity, as in BPPV, or is unbalanced by unilateral involvement of one of the vestibular organs, as in Ménière disease.[21] The inner ear is vulnerable to injury caused by fracture of the petrous portion of the temporal bones; by infection of nearby structures, including the middle ear and meninges; and by blood-borne toxins and infections. Damage to the vestibular system can occur as an adverse effect of certain drugs or from allergic reactions to foods. The aminoglycosides (*e.g.*, streptomycin, gentamicin) have a specific toxic affinity for the vestibular portion of the inner ear. Alcohol can cause transient episodes of vertigo. The cause of peripheral vertigo remains unknown in approximately half of the cases.

Severe irritation or damage of the vestibular end organs or nerves results in severe balance disorders reflected by instability of posture, ataxia, and falling accompanied by vertigo. With irritation, falling is away from the affected side. With destruction, it is toward the affected side. Adaptation to asymmetric stimulation occurs within a few days, after which the signs and symptoms diminish and eventually are lost. After recovery, there usually is a slightly reduced acuity for tilt, and the person walks with a somewhat broadened base to improve postural stability. The neurologic basis for this adaptation to unilateral loss of vestibular input is not understood. After adaptation to the loss of vestibular input from one side, the loss of function of the opposite vestibular apparatus produces signs and symptoms identical to those resulting from unilateral rather than bilateral loss. Within weeks, adaptation is again sufficient for movement and even for driving a car. Such a person relies heavily on visual and proprioceptive input from muscle and joint sensors and has severe orientation difficulty in the dark, particularly when moving over uneven areas.

Benign Paroxysmal Positional Vertigo

BPPV is the most common cause of pathologic vertigo and usually develops after the fourth decade of life. It is characterized by brief periods of vertigo, usually lasting less than 1 minute, that are precipitated by a change in head position. The most prominent symptom of BPPV is vertigo that occurs in bed when the person rolls into a lateral position.[21] It also commonly occurs when the person is getting in and out of bed, bending over and straightening up, or extending the head to look up. It can also be triggered by amusement rides that feature turns and twists.

BPPV is thought to result from damage to the delicate sensory organs of the inner ear, the semicircular ducts, and the otoliths. BPPV is a common recurrence with people who have Ménière disease or have experienced head trauma.[21] People experiencing BPPV have a movement of the otoliths from the utricle into the endolymph of the semicircular canal, which continue to move even when the head is stationary.[20] Movement of the otoliths or free-floating debris causes this portion of the vestibular system to become more sensitive such that any movement of the head in the plane parallel to the posterior duct may cause vertigo and nystagmus. There is usually a several second delay between head movement and onset of vertigo, representing the time it takes to generate the exaggerated endolymph activity. Symptoms usually subside with continued movement, probably because the movement causes the debris to be redistributed throughout the endolymph system and away from the posterior semicircular canal.

Diagnosis is based on tests that involve the use of a change in head position to elicit vertigo and nystagmus.[22] BPPV often is successfully treated with drug therapy to control vertigo-induced nausea. Nondrug therapies using the rolling over maneuver and canalith repositioning are successful for many people.[20] Canalith repositioning involves a series of maneuvers in which the head is moved to different positions in an effort to reposition the free-floating debris in the endolymph of the semicircular canals.

Acute Vestibular Neuronitis

Acute vestibular neuronitis, or labyrinthitis, represents an inflammation of the vestibular nerve and is characterized by an acute onset generally within a couple of hours. Manifestations include vertigo, nausea, and vomiting lasting several days and not associated with auditory or other neurologic presentations. Generally these symptoms resolve in about 10 to 14 days. A large percentage of people report an upper respiratory tract illness 1 to 2 weeks before onset of symptoms, suggesting a viral origin. The condition also can occur in people with herpes zoster oticus. In some people, attacks of acute vestibulopathy recur over months or years. There is no way to determine whether a person who experiences a first attack will have repeated attacks.

Ménière Disease

Ménière disease is a disorder of the inner ear because of distention of the endolymphatic compartment of the inner ear. The classic triad of symptoms includes hearing loss, vertigo, and tinnitus.[23] The primary lesion appears to be in the endolymphatic sac, which is thought to be responsible for endolymph filtration and excretion. A number of pathogenetic mechanisms have been postulated, including an increased production of endolymph, decreased production of perilymph accompanied by a compensatory increase in volume of the endolymphatic sac, and decreased absorption of endolymph caused by malfunction of the endolymphatic sac or blockage of endolymphatic pathways.

Etiology

The cause of Ménière disease is unknown, but it is known that this syndrome is of peripheral origin with vertigo. A number of conditions—such as trauma, infection, specific drugs (certain antibiotics), and toxins—have been identified as possible etiologies of Ménière disease. The most common form of the disease is classified as idiopathic and is thought to be caused by a single viral injury to the fluid transport system of the inner ear.[23]

Clinical Manifestations

Ménière disease is characterized by fluctuating episodes of tinnitus, feelings of ear fullness, and violent rotary vertigo that often render the person unable to sit or walk. There is a need to lie quietly with the head fixed in a comfortable position, avoiding all head movements that aggravate the vertigo. Symptoms referable to the autonomic nervous system, including pallor, sweating, nausea, and vomiting, usually are present. The more severe the attack, the more prominent are the autonomic manifestations. A fluctuating hearing loss occurs, which returns to normal after the episode subsides. Initially, the symptoms tend to be unilateral, resulting in rotary nystagmus caused by an imbalance in vestibular control of eye movements. Because initial involvement usually is unilateral and because the sense of hearing is bilateral, many people with the disorder are not aware of the full extent of their hearing loss. However, as the disease progresses, the person will experience worsening of hearing. The episodes of vertigo diminish and then disappear, although the person may be unsteady, especially in the dark.

Diagnosis and Treatment

Methods used in the diagnosis of Ménière disease include audiograms, vestibular testing by electronystagmography (ENG), and petrous pyramid radiographs. The administration of hyperosmolar substances, such as glycerin and urea, often produces acute temporary hearing improvement in persons with Ménière disease. This method sometimes is used as a diagnostic measure of endolymphatic hydrops. The diuretic furosemide also may be used for this purpose.

The management of Ménière disease focuses on attempts to reduce the distention of the endolymphatic space and can be medical or surgical. Pharmacologic management consists of suppressant drugs (e.g., prochlorperazine, promethazine, diazepam), which act centrally to decrease the activity of the vestibular system. Diuretics are used to reduce endolymph fluid volume. A low-sodium diet is recommended in addition to these medications. The steroid hormone, prednisone, may be used to maintain satisfactory hearing and resolve dizziness.

Surgical methods include the creation of an endolymphatic shunt in which excess endolymph from the inner ear is diverted into the subarachnoid space or the mastoid (endolymphatic sac surgery) and vestibular nerve section or chemical ablation.[24] Advances in vestibular nerve section have facilitated the monitoring of CN VII and CN VIII potentials.

Disorders of Central Vestibular Function

Abnormal nystagmus and vertigo can occur as a result of CNS lesions involving the cerebellum and lower brain stem. Central causes of vertigo include brain stem ischemia, tumors, and multiple sclerosis. When brain stem ischemia is the cause of vertigo, it is usually associated with other brain stem signs such as diplopia, ataxia, dysarthria, or facial weakness. Compression of the vestibular nuclei by cerebellar tumors invading the fourth ventricle results in progressively severe signs and symptoms. In addition to abnormal nystagmus and vertigo, vomiting and a broad-based and dystaxic gait become progressively more evident.

Centrally derived nystagmus usually has equal excursion in both directions (*i.e.*, pendular). In contrast to peripherally generated nystagmus, CNS-derived nystagmus is relatively constant rather than episodic. It can occur in any direction (rather than primarily in the horizontal or torsional [rotatory] dimensions), often changes direction through time, and cannot be suppressed by visual fixation. Repeated induction of nystagmus results in rapid diminution or "fatigue" of the reflex with peripheral abnormalities, but fatigue is not characteristic of central lesions. Abnormal nystagmus can make reading and other tasks that require precise eye positional control difficult.

Diagnosis and Treatment of Vestibular Disorders

Diagnostic Tests

Diagnosis of vestibular disorders is based on a description of the symptoms, a history of trauma or exposure to agents that are destructive to vestibular structures, and physical examination. Physical and neurologic examinations—including gait assessment, oculomotor assessment, and positional testing—are used to help make the diagnosis. Other tests performed when vestibular dysfunction is suspected are discussed next.

Romberg Test

The Romberg test is one of the oldest sensory tests used to demonstrate disorders of static vestibular function. The person being tested is requested to stand with feet together and arms extended forward so that the degree of sway and arm stability can be observed. The person then is asked to close his or her eyes. When visual clues are removed, postural stability is based on proprioceptive sensation from the joints, muscles, and tendons and from static vestibular reception. Deficiency in vestibular static input is indicated by greatly increased sway

and a tendency for the arms to drift toward the side of deficiency.

If vestibular input is severely deficient, the subject falls toward the deficient side. Care must be taken because defects of proprioceptive projection to the forebrain also result in some arm drift and postural instability toward the deficient side. Only if two-point discrimination and vibratory sensation from the lower and upper limbs are bilaterally normal, can the deficiency be attributed to the vestibular system.

Electronystagmography and Videonystagmography

ENG is an examination that records eye movements in response to vestibular, visual, cervical (vertigo triggered by somatosensory input from head and neck movements), rotational, and positional stimulation. Electrodes are placed lateral to the outer canthus of each eye and above and below each eye. A ground electrode is placed on the forehead. With ENG, the velocity, frequency, and amplitude of spontaneous or induced nystagmus and the changes in these measurements brought by a loss of fixation, with the eyes open or closed, can be quantified. The advantages of ENG are that it is easily administered, is noninvasive, does not interfere with vision, and does not require head restraint.

The videonystagmography, which has replaced the ENG in clinical practice, uses infrared goggles to record and measure eye movements on camera. The test captures ocular mobility using different eye maneuvers, eye tracking, head positioning, and caloric stimulation. Caloric testing has historically used water irrigation, but air has become the medium of choice. This test involves stimulating the inner ear, one ear at a time, with warm air followed by cold air and comparing measured responses.[23]

Other Tests

The rotational chair test rotates a person in the dark to stimulate nystagmus, and horizontal movements can be measured. A head MRI with contrast should also be considered when assessing vestibular dysfunction.[22]

In peripheral lesions, nystagmus is usually horizontal and with a rotary component; the fast beat usually beats away from the disease side. Several types of maneuvers can be used to provoke vertigo and observe for nystagmus. Usually, the examiner has the person sitting upright on an examining table with the head turned toward the examiner, with the person's eyes focused on the examiner's finger. The person is then properly supported and lowered rapidly to the supine position with the head extending over the upper end of the examining table and placed about 30 degrees lower than the body. The person is observed for nystagmus for about 30 seconds while in that position. The test can be performed with the head turned to either side or with the person looking straight ahead.

Vertigo arising from central lesions tends to develop gradually, and nystagmus is not always present, can occur in any direction, and can be dissociated in the two eyes. ENG is often useful in documenting the characteristics of the nystagmus. Further evaluation of central vertigo usually requires MRI.

Treatment

Pharmacologic Methods

Depending on the cause, vertigo may be treated pharmacologically. Medications used for symptomatic relief include antihistamines, anticholinergic agents, antiemetics, and benzodiazepines. Antihistamines and anticholinergic drugs suppress vestibular symptoms. Benzodiazepines and antiemetics can be sedating and are reserved for severe symptoms not responsive to other medications.[23] Although the antihistamines have long been used in treating vertigo, little is known about their mechanism of action.

Vestibular Rehabilitation Exercises

Vestibular rehabilitation has been shown to be helpful as a treatment for peripheral vestibular disorders. Physical therapists are usually involved in developing a program, including habituation exercises, balance retraining exercises, and a general conditioning program for people to use at home.[24]

SUMMARY CONCEPTS

The vestibular system plays an essential role in the equilibrium sense, which is closely integrated with the visual and proprioceptive (position) senses. Receptors in the semicircular canals, utricle, and saccule of the vestibular system, located in the inner ear, respond to changes in linear and angular acceleration of the head. The vestibular nerve fibers travel in CN VIII to the vestibular nuclei at the junction of the medulla and pons; some fibers pass through the nuclei to the cerebellum. Cerebellar connections are necessary for temporally smooth, coordinated movements during ongoing head movements, tilt, and angular acceleration. The vestibular nuclei also connect with nuclei of the oculomotor (CN III), trochlear (CN IV), and abducens (CN VI) nerves that control eye movement. *Nystagmus* is a term used to describe vestibular-controlled eye movements that occur in response to angular and rotational movements of the head. The vestibulospinal tract, which provides for the control of muscle tone in the axial muscles, including those of the back, provides the support for maintaining balance. Neurons of the vestibular nuclei also project to the thalamus, to the temporal cortex, and to the somatosensory area of the parietal cortex. The thalamic and cortical projections provide the basis for the subjective experiences of position in space and of rotation and vertigo.

Vertigo, an illusory sensation of motion of either oneself or one's surroundings, tinnitus, and hearing loss are common manifestations of vestibular dysfunction, as are autonomic manifestations such as perspiration, nausea, and vomiting. Common disorders of the vestibular system include motion sickness, BPPV, and Ménière disease.

BPPV is a condition believed to be caused by free-floating particles in the posterior semicircular canal. It presents as a sudden onset of dizziness or vertigo that is provoked by certain changes in head position. Ménière disease, which is caused by an overaccumulation of endolymph, is characterized by severe, disabling episodes of tinnitus, feelings of ear fullness, and violent rotary vertigo. The diagnosis of vestibular disorders is based on a description of the symptoms, a history of trauma or exposure to agents destructive to vestibular structures, and tests of eye movements (*i.e.*, nystagmus) and muscle control of balance and equilibrium. Among the methods used in treatment of the vertigo that accompanies vestibular disorders are habituation exercises and antivertigo drugs. These drugs act by diminishing the excitability of neurons in the vestibular nucleus.

Review Exercises

1. A mother notices that her 13-month-old child is fussy and tugging at his ear and he refuses to eat his breakfast. When she takes his temperature, it is 37.8°C (100°F). Although the child attends daycare, the mother has kept him home and made an appointment with the child's health care provider. In the provider's office, his temperature is 37.9°C (100.2°F), he is somewhat irritable, and he has a clear nasal drainage. His left tympanic membrane shows normal landmarks and mobility on pneumatic otoscopy. His right tympanic membrane is erythematous, and there is decreased mobility on pneumatic otoscopy.

   A. What risk factors are present that predispose this child to the development of AOM?
   B. Are his signs and symptoms typical of OM in a child of this age?
   C. What are the most likely pathogens? What treatment would be indicated?
   D. Later in the week, the mother notices that the child does not seem to hear as well as he did before developing the infection. Is this a common occurrence, and should the mother be concerned about transient hearing loss in a child of this age?

2. A granddaughter is worried that her grandfather is "losing his hearing." Lately, he has been staying away from social gatherings that he always enjoyed, saying everybody mumbles. He is defiant in maintaining that

there is nothing wrong with his hearing. However, he does complain that his ears have been ringing a lot lately.

A. What are common manifestations of hearing loss in older adults?

B. What type of evaluation would be appropriate for determining if this man has a hearing loss and the extent of his hearing loss?

C. What are some things that the granddaughter might do so that her grandfather could hear her better when she is talking to him?

3. A 70-year-old man complains that he gets this terrible feeling "like the room is moving around" and becomes nauseated when he rolls over in bed or bends over suddenly. It usually goes away once he has been up for a while. He has been told that his symptoms are consistent with BPPV.

A. What is the pathophysiology associated with this man's vertigo?

B. Why do the symptoms subside once he has been up for a while?

C. What methods are available for treatment of the disorder?

REFERENCES

1. Lemone P., Burke K. M., Bauldoff G., et al. (2015). *Medical-surgical nursing: Clinical reasoning in patient care* (6th ed.). Boston, MA: Pearson Education.
2. Schwartz S. R., Magit A. M., Rosenfeld R. M., et al. (2017). Clinical practice guideline (update): Earwax (cerumen impaction). *Sage Journals*. doi:10.1177/0194599816671491.
3. Waitzman A. A. (2017). Otitis externa. [Online]. Available: https://emedicine.medscape.com/article/994550-overview#a1. Accessed November 9, 2017.
4. Rosenfeld R. M., Schwartz S. P., Cannon C. R., et al. (2014). Clinical practice guideline: Acute otitis externa. *Otolaryngology—Head and Neck Surgery* 150(1 Suppl), S1–S24.
5. Scanlon V. C., Sanders T. (2015). *Essentials of anatomy and physiology* (7th ed.). Philadelphia, PA: F.A. Davis.
6. Porter R. S., Kaplan J. L. (2016). *Merck manual: Professional version*. Whitehouse Station, NJ: Merck Sharp & Dohme Corporation.
7. Burns C. E., Dunn A. M., Brady M. A., et al. (2017). *Pediatric primary care* (6th ed.). St. Louis, MO: Saunders Elsevier.
8. Pensak M. L., Choo D. I. (2015). *Clinical otology* (4th ed.). New York, NY: Thieme Medical Publishers, Inc.
9. Bickley L. S. (2017). *Bates' guide to physical examination and history taking* (12th ed.). Philadelphia, PA: Wolters Kluwer.
10. Simpson K. R., Creehan P. A. (2014). *Perinatal nursing* (4th ed.). Philadelphia, PA: Wolters Kluwer.
11. Youngkin E. Q., Davis M. S., Schadewald D. M., et al. (2013). *Women's health: A primary care clinical guide* (4th ed.). Upper Saddle River, NJ: Pearson Education Inc.
12. American Academy of Pediatrics. (2017). *Pediatric clinical practice guidelines & policies: A compendium of evidence-based research for pediatric practice* (17th ed.). Elk Grove Village, IL: American Academy of Pediatrics.
13. Cook R. L., Nelson K. C. (2018). Presbycusis. In *The 5-minute clinical consult* (26th ed.). Philadelphia, PA: Wolters Kluwer.
14. Hill M. (2017). Hearing development: Embryology of the ear. In Tharpe A. M., Seewald R. (Eds.), *Comprehensive handbook of pediatric audiology*. Kenilworth, NJ: Plural Publishing, Inc.
15. Kaplan J. L., Porter R. S. (2016). *Merck manual professional version*. Whitehouse Station, NJ: Merck Sharp & Dohme Corp., a subsidiary of Merck & Co., Inc.
16. Cacace A. T., Kleine E., Holt A. G., et al. (2016). *Scientific foundations of audiology: Perspectives from physics, biology, modeling, and medicine*. San Diego, CA: Plural Publishing, Inc.
17. Lambert S. R., Lyons C. J. (2017). *Taylor and Hoyt's pediatric ophthalmology and strabismus* (5th ed.). Edinburgh, Scotland: Elsevier.
18. Bowling B. (2016). *Kanski's clinical ophthalmology* (8th ed.). Edinburgh, Scotland: Elsevier.
19. Goldman L., Schafer A. (2016). *Goldman-Cecil medicine* (25th ed.). Philadelphia, PA: Elsevier.
20. Adams J. (2013). *Emergency medicine: Clinical essentials* (2nd ed.). Philadelphia, PA: Elsevier/Saunders.
21. Netter F. H., Jones H. R., Srinivasan J., et al. (2013). *Netter's neurology* (2nd ed.). Philadelphia, PA: Elsevier/Saunders.
22. Louis E. D., Mayer S. A., Rowland L. P. (2016). *Merritt's neurology* (13th ed.). Philadelphia, PA: Wolters Kluwer.
23. Samuels M. A. (2017). *Scientific American neurology*. Hamilton, ON: Decker Intellectual Properties, Inc.
24. O'Sullivan S. B., Schmitz T. J., Fulk G. D. (2014). *Physical rehabilitation* (6th ed.). Philadelphia, PA: F.A. Davis Company.

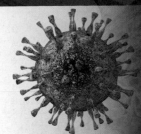
C H A P T E R 21

Blood Cells and the Hematopoietic System

Learning Objectives

After completing this chapter, the learner will be able to meet the following objectives:

1. Describe the composition and functions of plasma.
2. Understand the function and life span of blood cells.
3. Trace the process of hematopoiesis from stem cell to mature blood cell.
4. Describe the components of a complete blood count with differential.
5. Describe the various diagnostic tests used in determining laboratory values for red blood cells, white blood cells, and thrombocytes.

Blood is a specialized connective tissue that consists of blood cells (erythrocytes, leukocytes, and thrombocytes) suspended in an extracellular fluid, known as *plasma*. Blood accounts for about 7% to 8% of total body weight.[1] The total volume of blood in the average adult is about 5 to 6 L, and it circulates throughout the body within the confines of the circulatory system. Because blood circulates throughout the body, it is an ideal vehicle for transport of materials to and from the many cells of the body.

Composition of Blood and Formation of Blood Cells

Blood components are easily identified in the laboratory. When a blood specimen is spun in a centrifuge, it separates into distinct layers (Fig. 21-1).

The bottom layer (approximately 42% to 47% of the whole blood volume) contains the erythrocytes or red blood cells (RBCs). The intermediate layer (approximately 1%) containing the leukocytes, or white blood cells (WBCs), is white or gray. This layer is called the buffy coat.[2] Above the WBCs is a thin layer of thrombocytes that is not discernible to the naked eye. The translucent, yellowish fluid that forms above the RBCs, WBCs, and thrombocytes is the plasma, which comprises approximately 55% of the total blood volume.

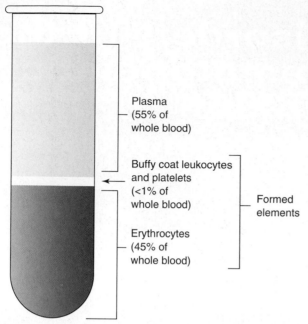

FIGURE 21-1. Layering of blood components in an anticoagulated and centrifuged blood sample.

KEY POINTS

Composition of the Blood

■ The most abundant type of blood cells, the RBC, functions in oxygen and carbon dioxide transport.

■ WBCs serve various roles in immunity and inflammation.

■ Thrombocytes are small cell fragments that are involved in blood clotting.

Plasma

By weight, plasma is 90% to 91% water, 6.5% to 8% proteins, and 2% other small molecular substances. Plasma serves a number of vital functions. It operates as a transport vehicle for nutrients, chemical messengers, metabolites, and other materials.[3] For example, plasma transports blood urea nitrogen, a waste product of metabolism, to the kidneys for excretion. Plasma also participates in electrolyte and acid–base balance, and it contains the plasma proteins that contribute to the osmotic regulation of body fluids. In addition, because water has a high capacity to hold heat, plasma can absorb and distribute much of the heat that is generated in the body.

Plasma Proteins

The plasma proteins are the most abundant solutes in plasma. It is the presence of these proteins that distinguishes the composition of plasma from that of interstitial fluid. The major types of plasma proteins are albumin, globulins, and fibrinogen. Most plasma proteins are produced by the liver, which secretes them into the blood. Albumin is the most abundant plasma protein, making up approximately 54% of all plasma proteins. It is too large to pass through the pores in the capillary wall; therefore, it remains in the circulation, where it contributes to the plasma osmotic pressure and maintenance of blood volume (see Chapter 14). Albumin also serves as a carrier for certain substances and acts as a blood buffer.

The globulins comprise approximately 38% of all plasma proteins. There are three types of globulins— the *alpha globulins* that transport bilirubin and steroids, the *beta globulins* that transport iron and copper, and the *gamma globulins* that constitute the antibodies of the immune system.

Fibrinogen makes up approximately 7% of the plasma proteins. Fibrinogen is a soluble protein that polymerizes to form the insoluble protein fibrin during blood clotting. The presence of fibrinogen and clotting factors differentiates plasma from serum. When these are removed from plasma, as occurs when a blood specimen is allowed to clot, the liquid that remains is the serum.[2]

A variety of proteins comprise the remaining 1% of the plasma proteins. These include hormones, enzymes, complement, and carriers for lipids.

Blood Cells

The formed elements in the blood—the RBCs, WBCs, and thrombocytes—originate in the bone marrow.[2] Figure 21-2 illustrates a blood smear. Although they are called blood cells, only the WBCs are true cells. RBCs have no nuclei or organelles, and thrombocytes are just cell fragments.

Most blood cells do not divide. Therefore, division of cells in the bone marrow must continually renew them. See Table A-2 in Appendix A for normal values of blood cells.

Erythrocytes

The erythrocytes, or RBCs, are the most numerous of the formed elements. They are small, biconcave disks[4] with a large surface area that, combined with their high elasticity, allow them to easily bend into virtually any shape needed in order to move through the small capillaries of the circulatory system.[4]

The primary function of RBCs is to carry oxygen to the body's tissues. This is accomplished by the oxygen-carrying protein, *hemoglobin*, which is contained within each RBC.[1] It is the hemoglobin that imparts the red color to these cells. In addition to transport of oxygen, RBCs contribute to carbon dioxide transport for excretion and to regulate acid–base balance.[1]

The life span of an RBC is approximately 120 days. In order to maintain sufficient numbers of RBCs, the bone marrow continually releases new RBCs as old or damaged RBCs are removed from the circulation.

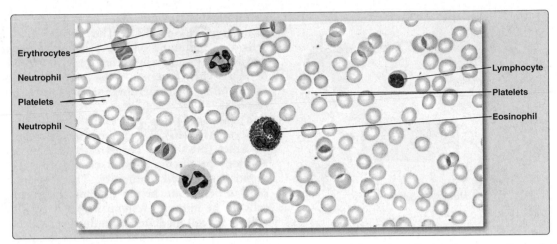

FIGURE 21-2. Human blood smear showing erythrocytes, neutrophils, eosinophils, lymphocytes, and platelets. (From Leeper-Woodford S. A., Adkinson L. R. (2016). *Lippincott illustrated reviews: Integrated systems* (Fig. 4.46). Philadelphia, PA: Wolters Kluwer.)

Leukocytes

The leukocytes, or WBCs, are 10 to 12 μm in diameter and thus are much larger than RBCs.[2] However, they constitute only 1% of the total blood volume. They originate in the bone marrow and circulate throughout the lymphoid tissues of the body.

WBCs are crucial to our defense against disease in the following ways:

- They are responsible for the immune response that protects against disease-causing microorganisms.
- They identify and destroy cancer cells.
- They participate in the inflammatory response and wound healing.

WBCs are commonly classified into two groups based on the presence or absence of specific cytoplasmic granules that can take up certain stains (Fig. 21-3). WBCs visibly containing these granules are classified as *granulocytes*. WBCs that lack these specific granules are classified as *agranulocytes*.[2]

Granulocytes

Granulocytes are spherical with distinctive nuclei that vary in shape. All are phagocytes, which have the ability to engulf microbes and other substances. The granules within the granulocyte's cytoplasm contain chemicals and enzymes that break down the engulfed microbes.[5]

Granulocytes are divided into three types—neutrophils, eosinophils, and basophils—according to the staining properties of their specific granules.[2]

Neutrophils. The neutrophils constitute 55% to 65% of the total WBCs.[2] Because these WBCs have nuclei that are divided into three to five lobes, they are often called *polymorphonuclear leukocytes*.[2]

The neutrophils are primarily responsible for maintaining normal host defenses against invading bacteria and fungi, cell debris, and a variety of foreign substances (see Chapter 13). Therefore, they increase in

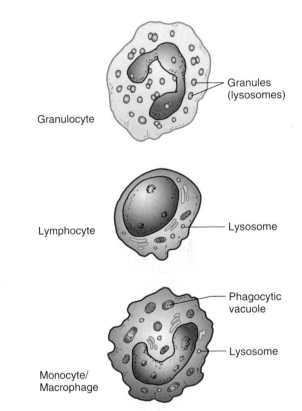

FIGURE 21-3. White blood cells.

number during bacterial and systemic fungal infections and other instances that call them into action. Neutrophils have a short life span that varies from 5 hours[6] to approximately 4 to 5 days.[1] The bone marrow releases large numbers of neutrophils in response to an acute systemic bacterial infection. Immature neutrophils, called *band cells*, are often released as part of this response. As the stores of mature neutrophils are depleted, band cells make up an increasing component of circulating WBCs. Figure 21-4 illustrates the development stages of the neutrophil.

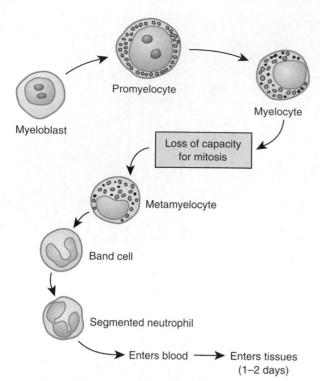

Myeloblast

Promyelocyte

Myelocyte

Loss of capacity for mitosis

Metamyelocyte

Band cell

Segmented neutrophil

Enters blood → Enters tissues (1–2 days)

FIGURE 21-4. Developmental stages of the neutrophil, which begins its development in the bone marrow as a myeloblast.

Eosinophils. Eosinophils are similar in size to neutrophils, but they contain bilobed (two-lobed) nuclei.[2] Eosinophils reside primarily in the tissues rather than within the circulation.[7] In the blood, they constitute 1% to 3% of the total WBCs.

Eosinophils have important host defense roles in allergic reactions, parasitic infections, and chronic immune responses associated with conditions such as asthma.[6] Therefore, eosinophils increase in number in response to allergic responses, worm infestations, and asthma.[2] In response to allergies, eosinophils release enzymes such as histaminase to inactivate histamine and other inflammatory substances, thereby decreasing the severity of inflammatory reactions.[2]

Basophils. The basophils, also of similar size to neutrophils, are the least numerous of the WBCs, accounting for only 0.3% to 0.5% of the total WBCs. These granules contain heparin, an anticoagulant; histamine, a vasodilator; and other mediators of inflammation such as bradykinin and leukotrienes.[2] Like the mast cells and the eosinophils, the basophils are involved in allergic and hypersensitivity reactions.[1]

Agranulocytes

Agranulocytes, also known as *mononuclear leukocytes*, are distinguished from granulocytes by their finer granules and their single-lobed nucleus. The granulocytes are divided into two types—lymphocytes and monocytes.

Lymphocytes. Lymphocytes account for 20% to 30% of the total blood WBCs.[2] They are the main functional cells of the immune system. They move between blood and lymph tissue, where they may be stored for hours or years. Their function in the lymph nodes or spleen is to defend against microorganisms through the immune response.

There are three types of lymphocytes—B lymphocytes (*B cells*), T lymphocytes (*T cells*), and natural killer (NK) cells. The *B cells* differentiate to form antibody-producing plasma cells and are involved in humoral-mediated immunity. The *T lymphocytes (T cells)* differentiate in the thymus. They activate other cells of the immune system (helper T cells) and are involved in cell-mediated immunity (cytotoxic T cells). *NK cells* participate in innate or natural immunity and their function is to destroy foreign cells. The breakdown of lymphocytes includes 80% T cells, 10% B cells, and 10% NK cells.[8] Major histocompatibility antigens, also known as human leukocyte antigens, are expressed on lymphocytes and are responsible for multiple aspects of the human immunologic response.[8]

Monocytes and Macrophages. Monocytes are the largest WBCs in size and constitute approximately 3% to 8% of the total leukocyte count. They are distinguished by a large amount of cytoplasm and a dark-stained nucleus in the shape of a kidney. These cells survive for months to years in the tissues; however, the life span of the circulating monocyte is approximately 1 to 3 days.[1]

Monocytes are produced in the bone marrow. After leaving the vascular system and entering the tissues, they transform into macrophages. The specific activity of macrophages depends on their location. The macrophages are known as *histiocytes* in loose connective tissue, *microglial cells* in the brain, and *Kupffer cells* in the liver. Other macrophages function in the alveoli, lymph nodes, and other tissues.[3]

Together, monocytes and macrophages comprise the mononuclear phagocyte system,[3] which is also known as the reticuloendothelial system.[5] Their primary role is host defense. They can engulf larger and greater quantities of foreign material than the neutrophils. Under the right conditions, they can convert into antigen-presenting cells (APCs). APCs are involved in the immune response by activating lymphocytes and by presenting antigen to T cells. Monocytes and macrophages also play an important role in chronic inflammation.

Thrombocytes

Thrombocytes, or platelets, are circulating cell fragments of the large megakaryocytes that are derived from the myeloid stem cell. They contribute to formation of the platelet plug to help control bleeding after injury to a vessel wall (Fig. 21-5). Their cytoplasmic granules release mediators required for the blood coagulation process. Thrombocytes have a membrane but no nucleus, cannot replicate, and, if not used, last approximately 10 days in the circulation before the phagocytic cells of the spleen remove them.[2]

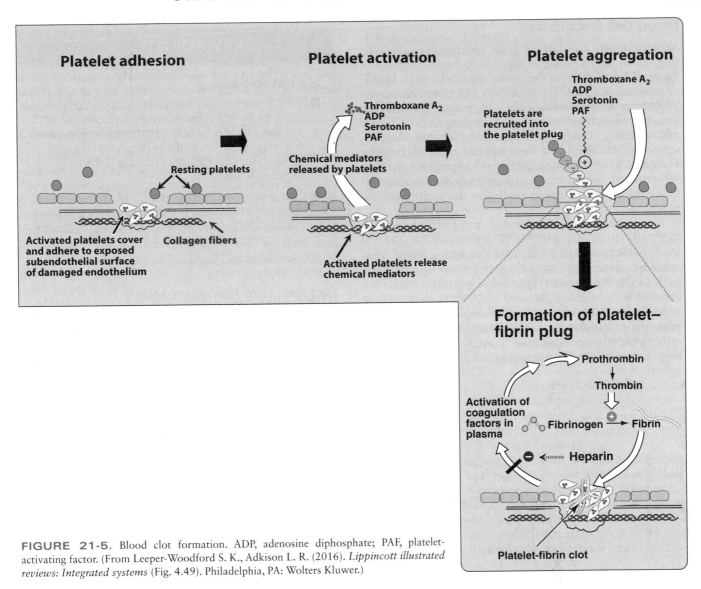

FIGURE 21-5. Blood clot formation. ADP, adenosine diphosphate; PAF, platelet-activating factor. (From Leeper-Woodford S. K., Adkison L. R. (2016). *Lippincott illustrated reviews: Integrated systems* (Fig. 4.49). Philadelphia, PA: Wolters Kluwer.)

Formation of Blood Cells (Hematopoiesis)

Hematopoiesis (from the Greek *haima*, "blood," and *poiesis*, "making") is the production of blood cells. It begins in the yolk sac during the second week of embryonic development[2] and then transitions to the liver and spleen around the second month of gestation. At approximately 7 months of gestation, this function is gradually taken over by the bone marrow.[4] The bone marrow continues to serve as the primary site of blood cell production throughout life. In children, this occurs primarily in the distal long bones. In adults, hematopoiesis is largely restricted to the flat bones of the axial skeleton.[4]

Medullary and Extramedullary Hematopoiesis

Medullary hematopoiesis refers to blood cell production that occurs within the bone marrow. The blood-forming population of bone marrow is made up of three types of cells—self-renewing stem cells, differentiated progenitor (parent) cells, and functional mature blood cells. During active skeletal growth, red (rich in RBCs) marrow in long bones is gradually replaced by yellow (fat cells) marrow. This occurs with the transition from long bone hematopoiesis to axial skeletal hematopoiesis. In adults, red marrow is largely restricted to the flat bones of the pelvis, ribs, and sternum. However, when the demand for red cell replacement increases, as in hemolytic anemia, there can be resubstitution of red marrow for yellow marrow.

Extramedullary hematopoiesis is blood cell production that occurs in places other than within the bone marrow. Although the liver and spleen cease hematopoiesis during fetal development, they retain hematopoietic ability. If the bone marrow becomes incapable of producing sufficient numbers of blood cells, as occurs during some pathologic conditions, the liver and spleen will resume hematopoiesis.[3]

determination of the erythroid to myeloid cell count (*i.e.*, normal ratio is 1:3), differential cell count, search for abnormal cells, evaluation of iron stores in reticulum cells, and special stains and immunochemical studies.[9]

Bone marrow biopsy is done with a special biopsy needle inserted into the posterior iliac crest.[9] Biopsy removes an actual sample of bone marrow tissue and allows study of the architecture of the tissue. It is used to determine the marrow-to-fat ratio and the presence of fibrosis, plasma cells, granulomas, and cancer cells. The major hazard of these procedures is the slight risk of hemorrhage. This risk is increased in people with a reduced platelet count or any type of bleeding tendency.

SUMMARY CONCEPTS

Diagnostic tests of the blood include CBC, ESR, and bone marrow aspiration and biopsy. The CBC is used to describe the number and characteristics of the RBCs, WBCs, and thrombocytes. The ESR is used to detect inflammation. Bone marrow aspiration is removal of the fluid portion of marrow from within the bone marrow cavity. Bone marrow aspirate analysis focuses on cellular morphology and determination of a differential cell count. A bone marrow biopsy removes a sample of solid bone marrow, which permits study of the marrow's overall cellularity and detection of focal lesions and the extent of the marrow by pathologic processes.

Review Exercises

1. A 14-year-old boy is admitted to the emergency department with severe abdominal pain and a tentative diagnosis of appendicitis. His WBC count shows an elevated number of WBCs with an increased percentage of "band cells."

   A. Explain the significance of this finding.

2. Many of the primary immunodeficiency disorders, in which there is a defect in the development of immune cells of T- or B-cell origin, can be cured with allogeneic stem cell transplantation from an unaffected donor.

   A. Explain why stem cells are used rather than mature lymphocytes. You might want to refer to Figure 21-6.
   B. Describe how the stem cells would go about the process of repopulating the bone marrow.

REFERENCES

1. Hall J. E. (2015). *Guyton and Hall textbook of medical physiology* (13th ed., pp. 445–464, 483–495). Philadelphia, PA: Elsevier Saunders.
2. Pawlina W. (2016). *Histology: A text and atlas with correlated cell and molecular biology* (7th ed., pp. 270–312). Philadelphia, PA: Wolters Kluwer.
3. McKenzie S. (2014). *Clinical laboratory hematology* (3rd ed., pp. 2–5, 26–34). Boston, MA: Pearson.
4. Ciesla B. (2012). *Hematology in practice* (2nd ed., pp. 32–58). Philadelphia, PA: F. A. Davis.
5. Hutson P. R. (2017). Hematology: Red and white blood cell tests. In Lee M. (Ed.), *Basic skills in interpreting laboratory data* (6th ed.). Bethesda, MD: American Society of Health-System Pharmacists.
6. Aster J. C., Bunn H. F. (2017). *Pathophysiology of blood disorders* (2nd ed.). New York, NY: McGraw-Hill.
7. Weller P. F., Klion A. D. (2017). Approach to the patient with unexplained eosinophilia. In Mahoney D. H., Bochner B. S. (Eds.), *UpToDate*. Waltham, MA: UpToDate Inc. Available: http://www.uptodate.com. Accessed May 4, 2019.
8. Warren J. S., Strayer D. S. (2015). Immunopathology. In Rubin R., Strayer D. (Eds.), *Rubin's pathology: Clinicopathologic foundations of medicine* (7th ed., pp. 131–168). Philadelphia, PA: Lippincott Williams & Wilkins.
9. Fischbach F., Dunning M. (2009). *A manual of laboratory and diagnostic tests* (8th ed.). Philadelphia, PA: Lippincott Williams & Wilkins.

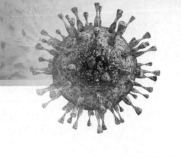

C H A P T E R **22**

Disorders of Hemostasis

Learning Objectives

**After completing this chapter, the learner
will be able to meet the following objectives:**

1. Describe the three stages of hemostasis.
2. Describe the purpose of blood coagulation.
3. Explain the functions of clot retraction and clot
   dissolution.
4. Compare normal and abnormal clotting.

5. Describe the causes and effects of increased
   platelet function.
6. State two conditions that contribute to increased
   clotting activity.
7. Differentiate between the mechanisms of
   drug-induced thrombocytopenia and idiopathic
   thrombocytopenia.
8. Describe the manifestations of thrombocytopenia.
9. State three common defects of coagulation factors
   and their etiologies.
10. Differentiate between the mechanisms of bleeding
    in hemophilia A and von Willebrand disease.
11. Describe the effect of vascular disorders on
    hemostasis.
12. Explain the physiologic basis of acute
    disseminated intravascular coagulation.

Hemostasis refers to the stoppage of blood flow. The normal process of hemostasis is regulated by a complex array of activators and inhibitors that maintain blood fluidity and prevent blood from leaving the vascular compartment. Hemostasis is normal when it seals a blood vessel to prevent blood loss and hemorrhage. It is abnormal when it causes inappropriate blood clotting or when clotting is insufficient to stop the flow of blood from the vascular compartment. Disorders of hemostasis fall into two main categories—the inappropriate formation of clots within the vascular system (thrombosis) and the failure of blood to clot in response to an appropriate stimulus (bleeding).

 ## Mechanisms of Hemostasis

Hemostasis is divided into three stages:

1. Vascular constriction
2. Formation of the platelet plug
3. Blood coagulation[1]

During the process of hemostasis, hair-like fibrin strands glue the aggregated platelets together to form the structural basis of the blood clot. In the presence of fibrin, plasma becomes gel-like and traps red blood cells and other formed elements in the blood. Hemostasis is complete when fibrous tissue grows into the clot and seals the hole in the vessel.

Vascular Constriction

Vessel spasm constricts the vessel and reduces blood flow. It is a transient event that usually lasts minutes or hours.[2] Vessel spasm is initiated by endothelial injury and caused by local and humoral mechanisms. Neural reflexes and thromboxane A_2 (TXA$_2$), a prostaglandin released from platelets and other mediators such as serotonin, contribute to vasoconstriction.[2] The most powerful vasoconstrictor is endothelin 1.[1] Prostacyclin, another prostaglandin released from the vessel endothelium, produces vasodilation and inhibits platelet aggregation in the surrounding uninjured endothelium.[2]

Formation of the Platelet Plug

Small breaks in the vessel wall are often sealed with a platelet plug rather than a blood clot. Platelets, or *thrombocytes*, arise from *megakaryocytes*.[1] The platelet has a half-life of approximately 8 to 12 days, and then, it is broken down and eliminated by macrophages.[1] The normal serum concentration is about 150,000 to 400,000 platelets per microliter (μL) of blood.[3] Platelet production is controlled by a protein called *thrombopoietin* that causes proliferation and maturation of megakaryocytes.[1] The sources of thrombopoietin include the liver, kidney, smooth muscle, and bone marrow.

Platelets are anuclear cell fragments but have many characteristics of cells. Platelets are spherically shaped, with an asymmetrical plasma membrane that is covered with a coat of glycoproteins, glycosaminoglycans, and coagulation proteins (Fig. 22-1). One of the important glycoproteins is GPIIb/IIIa, which binds fibrinogen and bridges platelets to one another.[1] The platelet shape is maintained by microtubules and actin and myosin filaments that support the cell membrane. Platelets have mitochondria and enzyme systems that are capable of producing adenosine triphosphate (ATP) and adenosine diphosphate (ADP). They also have the enzymes needed for synthesis of the prostaglandin, TXA$_2$, required for their function in hemostasis.

Platelets contain two specific types of granules (α- and δ-granules) that release mediators for hemostasis.[2] The α-granules express the P-selectin, an adhesive protein, on their surface and contain fibrinogen, von Willebrand factor (vWF), fibronectin, factors V and VIII, platelet factor 4 (a heparin-binding chemokine), platelet-derived growth factor (PDGF), transforming growth factor-alpha (TGF-α), and thrombospondin.[3] The release of growth factors results in the proliferation and growth of vascular endothelial cells, smooth muscle cells, and fibroblasts and is important in vessel repair. The δ-granules, or dense granules, contain ADP and ATP, ionized calcium, histamine, serotonin, and epinephrine, which contribute to vasoconstriction.[3]

Platelet plug formation involves activation, adhesion, and aggregation of platelets. Platelets are attracted to a damaged vessel wall, become activated, and change from smooth disks to spiny spheres, exposing glycoprotein receptors on their surfaces. Platelet adhesion requires a protein molecule called *von Willebrand factor*, which leaks into the injured tissue from the plasma.[1] This factor

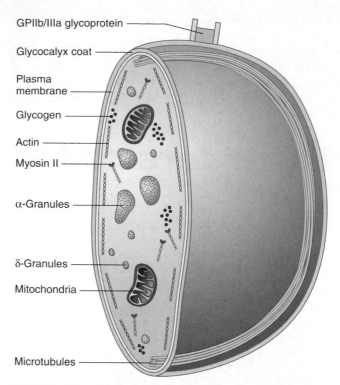

FIGURE 22-1. Platelet structure.

GPIIb/IIIa glycoprotein
Glycocalyx coat
Plasma membrane
Glycogen
Actin
Myosin II
α-Granules
δ-Granules
Mitochondria
Microtubules

is produced by the endothelial cells of blood vessels and circulates in the blood as a carrier protein for coagulation factor VIII. Adhesion to the vessel subendothelial layer occurs when the platelet receptor binds to vWF at the injury site, linking the platelet to exposed collagen fibers.[3]

Platelet aggregation occurs soon after adhesion. The secretion of the contents of the platelet granules and the release of the dense body contents are particularly important for platelet aggregation because calcium is required for the coagulation component of hemostasis and ADP is a mediator of platelet aggregation. ADP release also facilitates the release of ADP from other platelets, leading to amplification of the aggregation process. Besides ADP, platelets secrete the prostaglandin TXA$_2$, which is an important stimulus for platelet aggregation. The combined actions of ADP and TXA$_2$ lead to the expansion of the enlarging platelet aggregate, which becomes the primary hemostatic plug. Stabilization of the platelet plug occurs as the coagulation pathway is activated on the platelet surface, and fibrinogen is converted to fibrin. This creates a fibrin meshwork that cements the platelets and other blood components together.[1] P-selectin is also part of the platelet aggregation process because it binds leukocytes, which, with platelet substances such as PDGF, participate in healing of the vessel wall.[2]

The platelet membrane plays an important role in platelet adhesion and the coagulation process. The coat of glycoproteins on its surface controls interactions with the vessel endothelium. Platelets normally avoid adherence to the endothelium but interact with injured areas of the vessel wall and the deeper exposed collagen.[1] Glycoprotein (GPIIb/IIIa) receptors on the platelet membrane bind fibrinogen and link platelets together. Defective platelet plug formation causes bleeding in people who are deficient in platelets or vWF. In addition to sealing vascular breaks, platelets play an almost continuous role in maintaining normal vascular integrity. They may supply growth factors for endothelial and arterial smooth muscle cells.[1] Most platelet defects result in bleeding, which is usually superficial and localized.[4]

Platelet inhibitors are important pharmacologic agents that work at different points in the adhesion–activation–aggregation progression.[5] Cyclooxygenase-1 (COX-1) inhibitors (such as aspirin) prevent clot formation in people who are at risk for myocardial infarction, stroke, or peripheral artery disease. Low-dose aspirin therapy inhibits prostaglandin synthesis, including TXA_2. Thienopyridines (clopidogrel and ticlopidine) achieve their antiplatelet effects by inhibiting the ADP pathway in platelets. Unlike aspirin, these drugs have an effect on prostaglandin synthesis.[5]

KEY POINTS

Hemostasis

- Hemostasis is the orderly, stepwise process for stopping bleeding that involves vasospasm, formation of a platelet plug, and the development of a fibrin clot.
- The blood clotting process requires the presence of platelets produced in the bone marrow, vWF generated by the vessel endothelium, and clotting factors synthesized in the liver, using vitamin K.

Blood Coagulation

The coagulation cascade is part of the hemostatic process. It is a stepwise process, resulting in the conversion of the soluble plasma protein, fibrinogen, into fibrin. The insoluble fibrin strands create a meshwork that cements platelets and other blood components together to form the clot.

Many substances that promote clotting (procoagulation factors) or inhibit it (anticoagulation factors) control the coagulation process. Each of the procoagulation or coagulation factors, identified by Roman numerals, performs a specific step in the coagulation process. The activation of one procoagulation factor or proenzyme is designed to activate the next factor in the sequence (cascade effect). Because most of the inactive procoagulation factors are present in the blood at all times, the multistep process ensures that a massive episode of intravascular clotting does not occur. It also means that abnormalities of the clotting process occur when one or more of the factors are deficient or when conditions lead to inappropriate activation of any of the steps.

Most of the coagulation factors are proteins synthesized in the liver. Vitamin K is necessary for the synthesis of factors II, VII, IX, and X; prothrombin; and protein C. If there is a deficiency of vitamin K or liver failure so that not enough prothrombin is created, a bleeding tendency will develop.[1] Calcium (factor IV) is required in all but the first two steps of the clotting process.[1] The body usually has sufficient amounts of calcium for these reactions. Inactivation of the calcium ion prevents blood from clotting when it is removed from the body. The addition of citrate to blood stored for transfusion purposes prevents clotting by chelating ionic calcium. Ethylenediaminetetraacetic acid, another chelator, is often added to blood samples used for analysis in the clinical laboratory.

The coagulation process results from the activation of what have traditionally been designated the *intrinsic* and the *extrinsic* pathways, both of which form prothrombin activator[1,3,4] (Fig. 22-2). The intrinsic pathway, which is a relatively slow process (can cause clotting in 1 to 6 minutes), begins in the circulation with the activation of factor XII.[1] The extrinsic pathway, which is a much faster process (can cause clotting in 15 seconds), begins with trauma to the blood vessel or surrounding tissues and the release of tissue factor or tissue thromboplastin, an adhesive lipoprotein, from the subendothelial cells.[1,3] It is composed of phospholipids from the membranes along with a lipoprotein complex that acts as a proteolytic enzyme.[1] The terminal steps in both pathways are the same—the activation of factor X and the conversion of prothrombin to thrombin. Thrombin then acts as an enzyme to convert fibrinogen to fibrin, the material that stabilizes a clot. Both pathways are needed for normal hemostasis, and many interrelations exist between them. Each system is activated when blood passes out of the vascular system. The intrinsic system is activated as blood comes in contact with collagen in the injured vessel wall. The extrinsic system is activated when blood is exposed to tissue extracts. However, bleeding that occurs because of defects in the extrinsic system is usually not as severe as that resulting from defects in the intrinsic pathway.[1,3]

Blood coagulation is regulated by several natural anticoagulants. Antithrombin III inactivates coagulation factors and neutralizes thrombin, the last enzyme in the pathway for the conversion of fibrinogen to fibrin. When antithrombin III is complexed with naturally occurring heparin, its action is accelerated to inactivate thrombin, factor Xa, and other coagulation factors. This complex activation provides protection against uncontrolled thrombus formation on the endothelial surface.[1,5]

Protein C, a plasma protein, acts as an anticoagulant by inactivating factors V and VIII. Protein C or PC antigen (factor V Leiden) is produced in the liver and prevents thrombosis. Protein C deficiency is 35% to 58% congenital but can also be acquired if one has severe liver failure, vitamin K deficiency, or malignancy.[6] This disorder is an inherited defect in factor V and causes increased risk for clotting. It is able to be measured by a protein C resistance test, and the normal range should be between 0.60 and 1.25 of normal PC antigen.[6] Women with factor V Leiden combined with the prothrombotic influence of pregnancy are at high risk for adverse pregnancy outcomes, such as venous thromboembolism (VTE) disorders, preeclampsia, fetal loss, and placental abruption.[7]

Protein S, another plasma protein, accelerates the action of protein C. A deficiency of either protein C or protein S puts one at risk for thrombosis. A protein S test is performed to determine whether the deficiency is inherited or acquired because often people with autoimmune disorders are at risk for protein S deficiency.[4] The normal range for females is 0.50 to 1.20 of normal activity, and for males, the range is 0.60 to 1.30.[8]

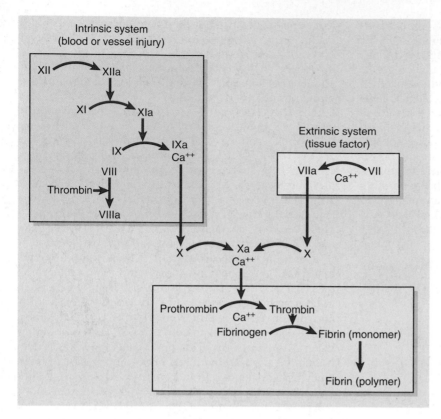

FIGURE 22-2. The intrinsic and extrinsic coagulation pathways. The terminal steps in both pathways are the same. Calcium, factors X and V, and platelet phospholipids combine to form prothrombin activator, which then converts prothrombin to thrombin. This interaction causes conversion of fibrinogen into the fibrin strands that create the insoluble blood clot.

Anticoagulant drugs, such as warfarin and heparin, are used to prevent thromboembolic disorder. Warfarin acts by decreasing prothrombin and other procoagulation factors. It alters vitamin K in a manner that reduces its ability to participate in synthesis of the vitamin K–dependent coagulation factors in the liver. Heparin is naturally formed and released in small amounts by mast cells in connective tissue surrounding capillaries. Heparin binds to antithrombin III, causing a conformational change that increases the ability of antithrombin III to inactivate thrombin, factor Xa, and other clotting factors. By promoting the inactivation of clotting factors, heparin ultimately suppresses the formation of fibrin.[9]

Clot Retraction

Clot retraction normally occurs within 20 to 60 minutes after a clot has formed, contributing to hemostasis by squeezing serum from the clot and joining the edges of the broken vessel.[1] Platelets, through the action of their actin and myosin filaments, also contribute to clot retraction and hemostasis. Clot retraction requires large numbers of platelets, and failure of clot retraction is indicative of a low platelet count.

Clot Dissolution

The dissolution of a blood clot begins shortly after its formation. This allows blood flow to be reestablished and permanent tissue repair to take place. The process by which a blood clot dissolves is called *fibrinolysis*. As with clot formation, clot dissolution requires a sequence of steps controlled by activators and inhibitors. Plasminogen, the proenzyme for the fibrinolytic process, normally is present in the blood in its inactive form. It is converted into its active form, plasmin, by plasminogen activators formed in the vascular endothelium, liver, and kidneys. The plasmin formed from plasminogen digests the fibrin strands of the clot and certain clotting factors, such as fibrinogen, factor V, factor VIII, prothrombin, and factor XII. Circulating plasmin is rapidly inactivated by α_2-plasmin inhibitor, which limits the fibrinolytic process to the local clot and prevents it from occurring in the entire circulation.[10]

Two naturally occurring plasminogen activators are tissue-type plasminogen activator and urokinase-type plasminogen activator. The liver, plasma, and vascular endothelium are the major sources of physiologic activators. These activators are released in response to a number of stimuli, including vasoactive drugs, venous occlusion, elevated body temperature, and exercise. The activators are unstable and rapidly inactivated by inhibitors synthesized by the endothelium and the liver. For this reason, chronic liver disease may cause altered fibrinolytic activity. A major inhibitor, plasminogen activator inhibitor-1, in high concentrations has been associated with deep vein thrombosis, coronary artery disease, and myocardial infarction.[1] Several tissue plasminogen activators (t-PAs) (alteplase, reteplase, and tenecteplase), produced by recombinant DNA technology, are available for use in the treatment of acute myocardial infarction, acute ischemic stroke, and pulmonary embolism.

UNDERSTANDING → Hemostasis

Hemostasis, which refers to the stoppage of blood flow, is divided into three stages:

1. Vessel vasoconstriction
2. Formation of the platelet plug
3. Development of a blood clot as a result of the coagulation process

Clot retraction and clot dissolution are also significant to hemostasis. The process involves the interaction of substrates, enzymes, protein cofactors, and calcium ions that circulate in the blood or are released from platelets and cells in the vessel wall.

① Vessel Vasoconstriction. Injury to a blood vessel causes vascular smooth muscle in the vessel wall to contract. This instantaneously reduces the flow of blood from the vessel rupture. Both local nervous reflexes and local humoral factors such as TXA_2, which is released from platelets, contribute to the vasoconstriction.

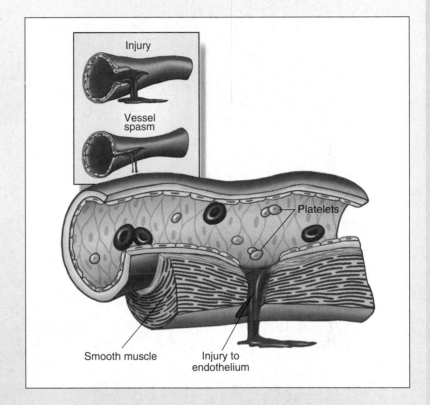

② Formation of the Platelet Plug. Seconds after vessel injury, vWF, released from the endothelium, binds to platelet receptors, causing adhesion of the platelets to the exposed collagen fibers (**inset**). As the platelets adhere to the collagen fibers on the damaged vessel wall, they become activated and release ADP and TXA_2. The ADP and TXA_2 attract additional platelets, leading to platelet aggregation.

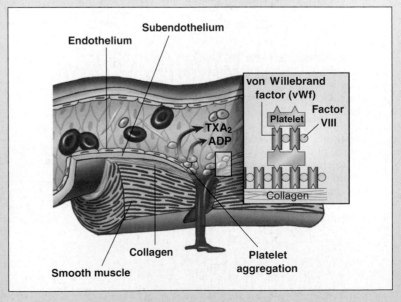

UNDERSTANDING ➡ Hemostasis (*continued*)

3

Blood Coagulation. The coagulation cascade was described earlier. Additionally, the two following processes occur that allow for dissolution of the newly formed clot.

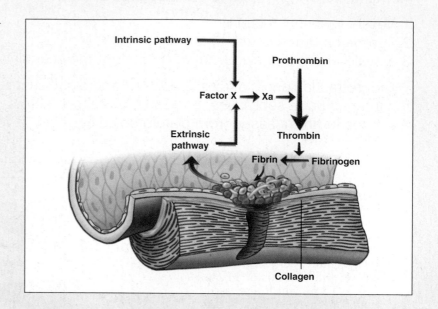

4

Clot Retraction. Within a few minutes after a clot is formed, the actin and myosin in the platelets that are trapped in the clot begin to contract in a manner similar to that in muscles. As a result, the fibrin strands of the clot are pulled toward the platelets, thereby squeezing serum (plasma without fibrinogen) from the clot and causing it to shrink.

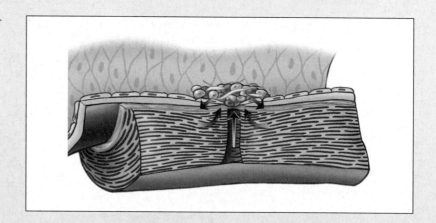

5

Clot Dissolution or Lysis. Clot dissolution begins shortly after a clot is formed. It begins with activation of plasminogen, an inactive precursor of the proteolytic enzyme, plasmin. When a clot is formed, large amounts of plasminogen are trapped in the clot. The slow release of a very powerful activator called t-PA from injured tissues and vascular endothelium converts plasminogen to plasmin, which digests the fibrin strands, causing the clot to dissolve.

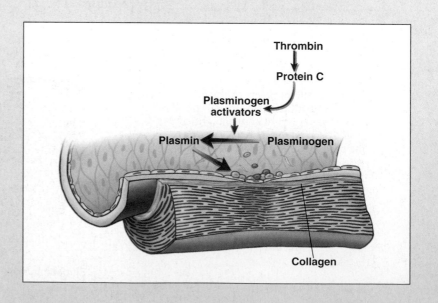

SUMMARY CONCEPTS

Hemostasis is designed to maintain the integrity of the vascular compartment. The process is divided into three phases—vessel vasoconstriction, which constricts the size of the vessel and reduces blood flow; platelet adherence and formation of the platelet plug; and formation of the fibrin clot, which cements the platelet plug together. Clot retraction, which pulls the edges of the injured vessel together, and clot dissolution, which involves the action of plasmin to dissolve the clot and allow blood flow to be reestablished and tissue healing to take place, are also important processes of hemostasis. Blood coagulation requires the stepwise activation of coagulation factors, carefully controlled by activators and inhibitors.

Hypercoagulability States

Hypercoagulability represents an exaggerated form of hemostasis that predisposes to thrombosis and blood vessel occlusion. There are two general forms of hypercoagulability states—conditions that create increased platelet function and conditions that cause accelerated activity of the coagulation system. Chart 22-1 summarizes conditions commonly associated with hypercoagulability states. Arterial thrombi are usually caused by turbulence and composed largely of platelet aggregates. On the other hand, venous thrombi are usually caused by stasis of flow and composed largely of platelet aggregates and fibrin complexes resulting from activation of the coagulation cascade.

CHART 22-1

CONDITIONS ASSOCIATED WITH HYPERCOAGULABILITY STATES

Increased Platelet Function

Atherosclerosis

Diabetes mellitus

Smoking

Elevated blood lipid and cholesterol levels

Increased platelet levels

Accelerated Activity of the Clotting System

Pregnancy and the puerperium

Use of oral contraceptives

Postsurgical state

Immobility

Congestive heart failure

Malignant diseases

Hypercoagulability Associated with Increased Platelet Function

Hypercoagulability because of increased platelet function results in platelet adhesion, formation of platelet clots, and disruption of blood flow. The causes of increased platelet function are disturbances in flow, endothelial damage, and increased sensitivity of platelets to factors that cause adhesiveness and aggregation. Atherosclerotic plaques disturb blood flow, causing endothelial damage and promoting platelet adherence. Platelets that adhere to the vessel wall release growth factors, which cause proliferation of smooth muscle and thereby contribute to the development of atherosclerosis. Smoking, elevated levels of blood lipids and cholesterol, hemodynamic stress, and diabetes mellitus predispose to vessel damage, platelet adherence, and eventual thrombosis.

Thrombocytosis

The term *thrombocytosis* is used to describe elevations in the platelet count above 1,000,000/μL. Thrombocytosis can occur as a reactive process (secondary thrombocytosis) or as an essential process (primary thrombocytosis).[11,12]

Etiology and Pathogenesis

Thrombopoietin is the key hormone in the regulation of megakaryocyte differentiation and platelet formation, although various cytokines (*e.g.*, interleukin-6 and interleukin-11) may also play a role.[2] Megakaryocytes and their platelet progeny have receptors for thrombopoietin. Thrombopoietin is carried in the plasma attached to receptors on the surface of circulating platelets and in an unbound form that is free to promote megakaryocyte proliferation. Platelet production is normally controlled in a negative feedback mechanism by the platelet count.[2]

The most common cause of secondary thrombocytosis is a disease state that stimulates thrombopoietin production. The result is increased megakaryocyte proliferation and platelet production. However, the platelet count seldom exceeds 1,000,000/μL. The common underlying causes of secondary thrombocytosis include tissue damage due to surgery, infection, cancer, and chronic inflammatory conditions such as rheumatoid arthritis and Crohn disease.[12] Usually, the only clinically apparent signs are those of the underlying disease. Thrombocytosis may also occur in other myeloproliferative disorders, such as polycythemia vera and myelogenous leukemia.

Primary or essential thrombocytosis represents a myeloproliferative (bone marrow) disorder of the hematopoietic stem cells.[11] Although thrombopoietin levels are often normal in essential thrombocytosis, abnormalities in the thrombopoietin receptor and platelet binding cause higher-than-expected levels of free thrombopoietin. This leads to increased megakaryocyte proliferation and platelet production. Dysfunction of the platelets produced contributes to the major clinical features of bleeding and thrombosis.

Clinical Manifestations and Treatment

The common clinical manifestations of essential thrombocytosis are thrombosis and hemorrhage. Thrombotic events include deep vein thrombosis and pulmonary embolism and portal and hepatic vein thrombosis. Some people experience erythromelalgia, a painful throbbing and burning of the fingers caused by occlusion of the arterioles by platelet aggregates. Typically, the disorder is characterized by long asymptomatic periods punctuated by occasional thrombotic episodes and hemorrhagic crises, both of which occur in people with very high platelet counts. Treatment includes the use of platelet-lowering drugs in high-risk cases.[12] Aspirin may be a highly effective adjunctive therapy in people with recurrent thrombotic complications.

> ## KEY POINTS
>
> ### Hypercoagulability States
> - Arterial thrombi are associated with conditions that produce turbulent blood flow and platelet adherence.
> - Venous thrombi are associated with conditions that cause stasis of blood flow with increased concentrations of coagulation factors.

Hypercoagulability Associated with Increased Clotting Activity

Thrombus formation because of activation of the coagulation system can result from primary (genetic) or secondary (acquired) disorders affecting the coagulation components of the blood clotting process (*i.e.*, an increase in procoagulation factors or a decrease in anticoagulation factors).

Inherited Disorders

A common hereditary thrombophilia, factor V Leiden, causes activated protein C resistance.[13] Activated protein C resistance accounts for approximately 20% of initial episodes of thrombosis, 50% of familial thrombosis, and 60% of thrombotic events in those with normal levels of protein C, protein S, antithrombin, and antiphospholipid antibodies.[13]

Hypercoagulability is associated with increased risk of VTE. High morbidity and mortality are associated with VTE.[14,15] VTE, which includes pulmonary embolism and deep vein thrombosis, can be divided into genetic and acquired. The incidence of genetic VTE is relatively low.[16]

Acquired Disorders

Among the acquired or secondary factors that lead to increased coagulation and thrombosis are venous stasis because of prolonged bed rest and immobility, myocardial infarction, cancer, hyperestrogenic states, smoking, obesity, and oral contraceptives.[17] People with a malignancy develop VTE more often than those without a malignancy. Approximately 20% to 25% of those presenting with primary VTE will be found to have an occult malignancy.[16]

Stasis of blood flow causes accumulation of activated clotting factors and platelets and prevents their interactions with inhibitors. Slow and disturbed flow is a common cause of venous thrombosis in the immobilized or post-surgical person. Inflammation is believed to contribute to stasis. Heart failure also contributes to venous congestion and thrombosis. Hyperviscosity syndromes (polycythemia) and deformed red blood cells in sickle cell disease increase the resistance to flow and cause small-vessel stasis.

The incidence of stroke, thromboemboli, and myocardial infarction is greater in women who use oral contraceptives, particularly those older than 35 years and those who are heavy smokers. Clotting factors are also increased during normal pregnancy. These changes, along with limited activity during the puerperium (immediate postpartum period), predispose to venous thrombosis.

Hypercoagulability is also common in cancer and sepsis. Many tumor cells are thought to release tissue factor molecules, which, along with the increased immobility and sepsis seen in people with malignant disease, contribute to thrombosis in these people.

As a result of these varied avenues for VTE to develop, prophylaxis has become a quality indicator of health care. The American College of Chest Physicians has developed and published standards for prevention of VTE, which include low-molecular-weight heparin, unfractionated heparin, and compression stockings and/or intermittent pneumatic stockings. These guidelines are to be implemented based on assessing the person's risk factors and current condition using the Caprini risk score. This score stratifies person into four risk categories. Interventions are then selected to prevent VTE.[15]

Antiphospholipid Syndrome

Another cause of increased venous and arterial thrombosis is the *antiphospholipid syndrome*. This condition is associated with autoantibodies (primarily immunoglobulin G) directed against protein-binding phospholipids, which results in increased coagulation activity.[16] The common features of antiphospholipid syndrome are venous and arterial thrombi, recurrent fetal loss, and thrombocytopenia. The disorder can be a primary condition occurring in isolation with signs of hypercoagulability or a secondary condition sometimes associated with systemic lupus erythematosus.[4]

Etiology and Pathogenesis
The mechanisms for this syndrome are unknown.

In addition to the action of the antibodies, it seems likely that other factors play a role in determining whether a person develops clinical manifestations of the disorder. Although speculative, these factors may include vascular trauma or the presence of infection that leads to cytokine production and endothelial cell activation.[4]

Clinical Manifestations
People with the disorder present with a variety of clinical manifestations, typically those characterized by recurrent venous and arterial thrombi. Cardiac valvular vegetations associated with adherence of thrombi and thrombocytopenia because of excessive platelet consumption may also occur. Venous thrombosis, especially in the deep leg veins, occurs in up to 50% of people with the syndrome, half of whom develop pulmonary emboli. Arterial thrombosis

involves the brain in up to 50% of cases, causing transient ischemic attacks or strokes.[16] Other sites for arterial thrombosis are the coronary arteries of the heart and the retinal, renal, and peripheral arteries. Women with the disorder commonly have a history of recurrent pregnancy losses because of ischemia and thrombosis of the placental vessels. These women also have increased risk of giving birth to a premature infant owing to pregnancy-associated hypertension and uteroplacental insufficiency.

In most people with antiphospholipid syndrome, the thrombotic events occur as a single episode at one anatomic site. In some people, recurrences may occur months or years later and mimic the initial event. Occasionally, someone may present with multiple vascular occlusions involving many organ systems. This rapid onset condition is termed *catastrophic antiphospholipid syndrome* and is associated with a high mortality rate.[18]

Treatment

Treatment of the syndrome focuses on removal or reduction in factors that predispose to thrombosis, including advice to stop smoking and counseling against use of estrogen-containing oral contraceptives by women. The acute thrombotic event is treated with anticoagulants (heparin and warfarin) and immune suppression in refractory cases. Aspirin and anticoagulant drugs, as well as newer, non–vitamin K anticoagulants, may be used to prevent future thrombosis.[18]

 SUMMARY CONCEPTS

Hypercoagulability causes excessive clotting and contributes to thrombus formation. It results from conditions that foster an increase in platelet numbers or function or accelerated activity of the coagulation system. Thrombocytosis, an elevation in the platelet count, can occur as a reactive process (secondary thrombocytosis) or an essential process (primary thrombocytosis). Increased platelet function usually results from disorders such as atherosclerosis that damage the vascular endothelium and disturb blood flow or from conditions such as smoking that increase sensitivity of platelets to factors that promote adhesiveness and aggregation.

Factors that cause accelerated activity of the coagulation system include blood flow stasis, resulting in an accumulation of coagulation factors, and alterations in the components of the coagulation system (*i.e.*, an increase in procoagulation factors or a decrease in anticoagulation factors). The antiphospholipid syndrome, an acquired venous and arterial clotting disorder, manifests as a primary disorder or can be a secondary disorder associated with systemic lupus erythematosus. It is associated with antiphospholipid antibodies, which promote thrombosis that can affect many organs.

Bleeding Disorders

Bleeding disorders or impairment of blood coagulation can result from defects in any of the factors that contribute to hemostasis. Bleeding can occur as a result of disorders associated with platelet number or function, coagulation factors, and blood vessel integrity.

Bleeding Associated with Platelet Disorders

Bleeding as a result of platelet disorders reflects a decrease in platelet number because of decreased production, increased destruction, or impaired function of platelets. Spontaneous bleeding from platelet disorders most often involves small vessels of the mucous membranes and skin. Common sites of bleeding are the mucous membranes of the nose, mouth, gastrointestinal tract, and uterine cavity. Cutaneous bleeding is seen as pinpoint hemorrhages (petechiae) and purple areas of bruising (purpura) in dependent areas where the capillary pressure is higher (Fig. 22-3). Petechiae are seen almost exclusively in conditions of platelet deficiency and not platelet dysfunction. Bleeding of the intracranial vessels is a rare danger with severe platelet depletion.

Thrombocytopenia

A reduction in platelet number, also referred to as *thrombocytopenia*, is an important cause of generalized bleeding. Thrombocytopenia usually refers to a decrease in the number of circulating platelets to a level less than 150,000/μL.[6] The greater the decrease in the platelet count, the greater the risk of bleeding. Thrombocytopenia can result from a decrease in platelet production, increased sequestration of platelets in the spleen, or decreased platelet survival.

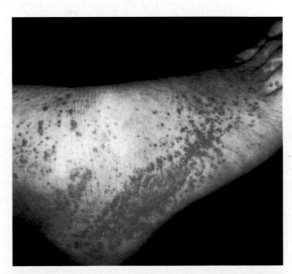

FIGURE 22-3. Clinically mild cutaneous vasculitis with palpable purpura and petechiae. (From Hall J. C., Hall B. J. (2017). *Sauer's manual of skin diseases* (11th ed., p. 176). Philadelphia, PA: Lippincott Williams & Wilkins.)

Decreased platelet production because of loss of bone marrow function occurs in aplastic anemia. Replacement of the bone marrow by malignant cells, such as that occurring in leukemia, also results in decreased production of platelets. Radiation therapy and drugs such as those used in the treatment of cancer may depress bone marrow function and reduce platelet production. Infection with human immunodeficiency virus (HIV) or cytomegalovirus may suppress the production of megakaryocytes, the platelet precursors.

Production of platelets may be normal, but excessive pooling of platelets in the spleen may occur. Although the spleen normally sequesters 30% to 40% of the platelets before release into the circulation, the proportion can be as great as 90% when the spleen is enlarged in splenomegaly.[1] When necessary, hypersplenic thrombocytopenia may be treated with splenectomy.

Reduced platelet survival is caused by a variety of immune and nonimmune mechanisms. Platelet destruction may be caused by antiplatelet antibodies. The antibodies may be directed against platelet self-antigens or against antigens on the platelets from blood transfusions or pregnancy. The antibodies target the platelet membrane glycoproteins GPIIb/IIIa and GPIb/IX. Nonimmune destruction of platelets results from mechanical injury because of prosthetic heart valves or malignant hypertension, which results in small-vessel narrowing. In acute disseminated intravascular coagulation (DIC) or thrombotic thrombocytopenic purpura (TTP), excessive platelet consumption leads to a deficiency.[4]

Drug-Induced Thrombocytopenia

Some drugs, such as aspirin, atorvastatin, and some antibiotics, may cause drug-induced immune thrombocytopenia (DITP).[6] These drugs induce an antigen–antibody response and formation of immune complexes that cause platelet destruction by complement-mediated lysis. In people with drug-associated thrombocytopenia, there is a rapid fall in the platelet count within 2 to 3 days of resuming a drug or 7 days or more (i.e., the time needed to mount an immune response) after starting a drug for the first time. The platelet count rises rapidly after the drug is discontinued.

Heparin-Induced Thrombocytopenia

Heparin-induced thrombocytopenia (HIT) is associated with the anticoagulant drug heparin. Ten percent of people treated with heparin develop a mild, transient thrombocytopenia within 2 to 5 days of starting the drug.[6] However, approximately 1% to 5% of people treated with heparin experience life-threatening thromboembolic events 1 to 2 weeks after the start of therapy.[4] HIT is caused by an immune reaction directed against a complex of heparin and platelet factor 4, a normal component of platelet granules that binds tightly to heparin. The binding of antibody to platelet factor 4 produces immune complexes that activate the remaining platelets, leading to thrombosis. In addition, prothrombotic platelet particles and induction of tissue factor continue to promote coagulation.[6]

The treatment of HIT requires the immediate discontinuation of heparin therapy and the use of alternative anticoagulants to prevent thrombosis recurrence. The newer low-molecular-weight heparin has been shown to be effective in reducing the incidence of heparin-induced complications compared with the older, high molecular weight form of the drug.

Immune Thrombocytopenic Purpura

Immune thrombocytopenic purpura (ITP) results in platelet antibody formation and excess destruction of platelets. Primary ITP is an autoimmune disease in which platelets are directly destroyed or their formation inhibited by the immune system. Primary ITP occurs in both genders and affects children and adults, though the incidence is highest in females aged 30 to 59 and in persons older than 60 years.[19] Primary ITP is classified as "newly diagnosed" (from diagnosis until 3 months), "persistent" (from diagnosis until 3 to 12 months), or "chronic" (from diagnosis until >12 months).[19] Immune thrombocytopenia purpura is also referred to as idiopathic or having unknown cause.

Autoimmune disorders and chronic infections such as *Helicobacter pylori*, hepatitis C virus, and HIV contribute to secondary forms of ITP. When these related diseases are present, expected hemorrhagic symptoms may be absent.[19]

Etiology and Pathogenesis. The thrombocytopenia that occurs in ITP is thought to result from multiple mechanisms, including antiplatelet antibodies against glycoproteins (GPIIb/IIIa and GPIb/IX) in the platelet membrane. The platelets, which are made more susceptible to phagocytosis because of the antibody, are destroyed in the spleen. Plasma levels of thrombopoietin, the major factor that stimulates growth and development of megakaryocytes, are not elevated in people with ITP.[20] Evidence suggests that ITP is caused by T-cell dysfunction, specifically CD4 and T regulatory cells, which trigger the autoimmune response and proceed to thrombocytopenia.[20]

Clinical Manifestations. Manifestations of ITP include a history of bruising, bleeding from gums, epistaxis (i.e., nosebleed), melena, and abnormal menstrual bleeding in those with moderately reduced platelet counts. Because the spleen is the site of platelet destruction, splenic enlargement may occur. The condition may be discovered incidentally or as a result of signs of bleeding, often into the skin (i.e., purpura and petechiae) or oral mucosa.

Diagnosis and Treatment. Diagnosis of ITP is usually based on severe thrombocytopenia (platelet counts <20,000 to 30,000/µL) and exclusion of other causes. Tests for the platelet-bound antibodies are available but lack specificity (e.g., they react with platelet antibodies from other sources). The secondary form of ITP sometimes mimics the idiopathic form of the disorder; therefore, the diagnosis is made only after excluding other known causes of thrombocytopenia.

The decision to treat ITP is based on the platelet count and the degree of bleeding. Many people with ITP do well without treatment. Corticosteroids are usually used as initial therapy. Other effective initial treatments include intravenous immunoglobulin. However, this treatment is expensive, and the beneficial effect lasts only 1 to 2 weeks.

Thrombotic Thrombocytopenic Purpura

TTP is a combination of thrombocytopenia, hemolytic anemia, renal failure, fever, and neurologic abnormalities. It is a rare disorder that likely results from introduction of platelet-aggregating substances into the circulation.[4]

Etiology and Pathogenesis. TTP is caused by a deficiency of ADAMTS13, which is responsible for severing large vWF multimers. The unchecked platelet aggregation results in microvascular occlusions, leading to end-organ failure. Approximately 1% of all TTP is hereditary, whereas the remaining 99% is acquired. The following are known to decrease ADAMTS13 activity: hemolytic uremic syndrome, cancer, infections, pregnancy, several drugs, and autoimmune diseases affecting connective tissues.[21]

The onset of TTP is abrupt, and the outcome may be fatal. Widespread vascular occlusions result from thrombi in the arterioles and capillaries of many organs, including the heart, brain, and kidneys. Erythrocytes become fragmented as they circulate through the partly occluded vessels, causing hemolytic anemia and jaundice.

Clinical Manifestations and Treatment. The clinical manifestations include purpura, petechiae, vaginal bleeding, and neurologic symptoms ranging from headache to seizures and altered consciousness. Emergency treatment for TTP includes *plasmapheresis*, a procedure that involves removal of plasma from withdrawn blood and replacement with fresh-frozen plasma. Plasma infusion provides the deficient enzyme. With plasmapheresis and plasma infusion treatment, there is a complete recovery in 80% of cases.[21]

Impaired Platelet Function

Impaired platelet function (also called *thrombocytopathia*) may result from inherited disorders of adhesion (*e.g.*, von Willebrand disease) or acquired defects resulting from drugs, disease, or surgery. Defective platelet function is also common in uremia, presumably because of unexcreted waste products. Chart 22-2 lists drugs that impair platelet function.

Concept Mastery Alert

The action of aspirin is irreversible acetylation of platelet COX activity. In contrast, ITP results in platelet antibody formation and excess destruction of platelets and can result from use of heparin or quinidine.

CHART 22-2

DRUGS THAT MAY PREDISPOSE TO BLEEDING*

Interference with Platelet Production or Function

Acetazolamide

Antimetabolite and anticancer drugs

Antibiotics such as penicillin and the cephalosporins

Aspirin and salicylates

Carbamazepine

Clofibrate

Colchicine

Dipyridamole

Thiazide diuretics

Gold salts

Heparin

NSAIDs

Quinine derivatives (quinidine and hydroxychloroquine)

Sulfonamides

Interference with Coagulation Factors

Amiodarone

Anabolic steroids

Warfarin

Heparin

Decrease in Vitamin K Levels

Antibiotics

Clofibrate

*This list is not intended to be inclusive.

KEY POINTS

Bleeding Disorders

■ Disorders of platelet plug formation include a decrease in platelet numbers because of inadequate platelet production (bone marrow dysfunction), excess platelet destruction (thrombocytopenia), abnormal platelet function (thrombocytopathia), or defects in vWF.

■ Impairment of the coagulation stage of hemostasis is caused by a deficiency in one or more of the clotting factors.

■ Disorders of blood vessel integrity result from structurally weak vessels or vessel damage because of inflammation and immune mechanisms.

Bleeding Associated with Coagulation Factor Deficiencies

Blood coagulation defects can result from deficiencies or impaired function of one or more of the clotting factors, including vWF. Deficiencies can arise because of inherited disease or defective synthesis or increased consumption of the clotting factors. Bleeding resulting from clotting factor deficiencies typically occurs after injury or trauma. Large bruises, hematomas, and prolonged bleeding into the gastrointestinal or urinary tracts or joints are common.

Inherited Disorders

Von Willebrand disease and hemophilia (A and B) are two of the most common inherited disorders of bleeding. Von Willebrand disease is considered the most frequent inherited coagulopathy and affects approximately 1% to 2% of the population.[4] Hemophilia A (factor VIII deficiency) affects 1 in 5000 male live births. Hemophilia B (factor IX deficiency) occurs in approximately 1 in 20,000 people, accounting for 15% of people with hemophilia.[4] It is genetically and clinically similar to hemophilia A. Von Willebrand disease and hemophilia A are caused by defects involving the factor VIII–vWF complex. vWF, which is synthesized by the endothelium and megakaryocytes, is required for platelet adhesion to the subendothelial matrix of the blood vessel. It also serves as the carrier for factor VIII and is important for the stability of factor VIII in the circulation by preventing its proteolysis. Factor VIII coagulant protein, the functional portion, is produced by the liver and endothelial cells. Thus, factor VIII and vWF, synthesized separately, come together and circulate in the plasma as a unit that serves to promote clotting and adhesion of platelets to the vessel wall.[4]

Von Willebrand Disease

Von Willebrand disease is a relatively common hereditary bleeding disorder characterized by a deficiency or defect in vWF. As many as 20 variants of von Willebrand disease have been described.[4] These variants can be grouped into two categories—types 1 and 3, which are associated with reduced levels of vWF, and type 2, which is characterized by defects in vWF.

Classification. Type 1, an *autosomal dominant disorder*, accounts for approximately 70% of cases and is relatively mild. Type 2, also an autosomal dominant disorder, accounts for about 25% of cases and is associated with mild-to-moderate bleeding. Type 3, which is a relatively rare *autosomal recessive disorder*, is associated with extremely low levels of functional vWF and correspondingly severe clinical manifestations.[4] People with von Willebrand disease have a compound defect involving platelet function and the coagulation pathway.

Clinical Manifestations. Clinical manifestations include spontaneous bleeding from the nose, mouth, and gastrointestinal tract; excessive menstrual flow; and a prolonged bleeding time in the presence of a normal platelet count. Most cases (*i.e.*, types 1 and 2) are mild and require no treatment, and many people with the disorder are diagnosed when surgery or dental extraction results in prolonged bleeding. In severe cases (*i.e.*, type 3), life-threatening gastrointestinal bleeding and joint hemorrhage may be similar to that seen in hemophilia.[4] The bleeding associated with von Willebrand disease is usually mild, and no treatment is routinely administered other than avoidance of aspirin.

Hemophilia A

Hemophilia A is an X-linked recessive disorder that primarily affects males. Although it is a hereditary disorder, there is no family history of the disorder in approximately 30% of newly diagnosed cases, suggesting that it has arisen as a new mutation in the factor VIII gene.[4] Approximately 90% of people with hemophilia produce insufficient quantities of the factor, and 10% produce a defective form. The percentage of normal factor VIII activity in the circulation depends on the genetic defect and determines the severity of hemophilia (*i.e.*, 6% to 30% in mild hemophilia, 2% to 5% in moderate hemophilia, and 1% or less in severe forms of hemophilia). In mild or moderate forms of the disease, bleeding usually does not occur unless there is a local lesion or trauma, such as surgery or a dental procedure. The mild disorder may not be detected in childhood. In severe hemophilia, bleeding usually occurs in childhood (*e.g.*, it may be noticed at the time of circumcision) and is spontaneous and severe, often occurring several times a month.

Clinical Manifestations. Characteristically, bleeding occurs in soft tissues, the gastrointestinal tract, and the hip, knee, elbow, and ankle joints. Spontaneous joint bleeding usually begins when a child begins to walk. Often, a target joint is prone to repeated bleeding. The bleeding causes inflammation of the synovium, with acute pain and swelling. Without proper treatment, chronic bleeding and inflammation cause joint fibrosis and contractures, resulting in major disability.

Treatment. The prevention of trauma is important in people with hemophilia. Aspirin and other nonsteroidal anti-inflammatory drugs (NSAIDs) that affect platelet function should be avoided. Factor VIII replacement therapy administered at home has reduced the typical musculoskeletal damage. It is initiated when bleeding occurs or as prophylaxis with repeated bleeding episodes. The recombinant products and continuous infusion pumps may allow prevention rather than therapy for hemorrhage. The development of inhibitory antibodies to recombinant factor VIII is still a major complication of treatment.

The cloning of the factor VIII gene and progress in gene delivery systems have led to the hope that hemophilia A may be cured by gene replacement therapy. Carrier detection and prenatal diagnosis can now be done by analysis of direct gene mutation or DNA linkage studies. Prenatal amniocentesis or chorionic villus sampling is used to predict complications and determine therapy.

Acquired Disorders

Coagulation factors V, VII, IX, X, XI, and XII; prothrombin; and fibrinogen are synthesized in the liver. In liver disease, synthesis of these clotting factors is reduced, and bleeding may result. Of the coagulation factors synthesized in the liver, factors II, VII, IX, and X and prothrombin require the presence of vitamin K for normal activity. In vitamin K deficiency, the liver produces the clotting factor but in an inactive form. Vitamin K is a fat-soluble vitamin that is continuously being synthesized by intestinal bacteria. This means that a deficiency in vitamin K is not likely to occur unless intestinal synthesis is interrupted or absorption of the vitamin is impaired. Vitamin K deficiency can occur in the newborn infant before the establishment of the intestinal flora. It can also occur as a result of treatment with broad-spectrum antibiotics that destroy intestinal flora. Because vitamin K is a fat soluble, its absorption requires bile salts. Vitamin K deficiency may result from impaired fat absorption caused by liver or gallbladder disease.

Bleeding Associated with Vascular Disorders

Bleeding resulting from vascular disorders is sometimes referred to as *nonthrombocytopenic purpura*. These disorders may occur because of structurally weak vessel walls or because of damage to vessels by inflammation or immune responses. Most often, they are characterized by easy bruising and the spontaneous appearance of petechiae and purpura of the skin and mucous membranes. In people with bleeding disorders caused by vascular defects, the platelet count and results of other tests for coagulation factors are normal.

Among the vascular disorders that cause bleeding are hemorrhagic telangiectasia, an uncommon autosomal dominant disorder characterized by thin-walled, dilated capillaries and arterioles; vitamin C deficiency (*i.e.,* scurvy), resulting in poor collagen synthesis and failure of the endothelial cells to be cemented together properly, which causes a fragile vascular wall; Cushing disease, causing protein wasting and loss of vessel tissue support because of excess cortisol; and senile purpura (*i.e.,* bruising in elderly persons), caused by impaired collagen synthesis in the aging process. Vascular defects also occur in the course of DIC or as a result of microthrombi and corticosteroid therapy.

Disseminated Intravascular Coagulation

DIC is a paradox in the hemostatic sequence and is characterized by widespread coagulation and bleeding in the vascular compartment. It is not a primary disease but occurs as a complication of a wide variety of conditions. DIC begins with massive activation of the coagulation sequence as a result of unregulated generation of thrombin, resulting in systemic formation of fibrin. In addition, levels of all the major anticoagulants are reduced (Fig. 22-4). The microthrombi that result cause vessel occlusion and tissue ischemia. Multiple organ failure may ensue. Clot formation consumes all available coagulation proteins and platelets, and severe hemorrhage results. Plasmin breaks down fibrin into fibrin degradation products that act as anticoagulants. It has been suggested that some of these natural anticoagulants may play a role in the bleeding that occurs with DIC.

Etiology and Pathogenesis

The disorder can be initiated by activation of the intrinsic or extrinsic pathway or both. Activation through the extrinsic pathway occurs with liberation of tissue factors and is associated with obstetric complications, trauma, bacterial sepsis, and cancers.

The intrinsic pathway may be activated through extensive endothelial damage, with activation of factor XII. Endothelial damage may be caused by viruses, infections, immune mechanisms, stasis of blood, or temperature extremes. Impaired anticoagulation pathways are also associated with reduced levels of antithrombin and the protein C anticoagulant system in DIC. There is evidence that the underlying cause of DIC is infection or inflammation and the cytokines (tumor necrosis factor, interleukin-1, and others) liberated in the process are the pivotal mediators.[22,23] These cytokines not only mediate inflammation but also can increase the expression of tissue factor on endothelial cells and simultaneously decrease the expression of thrombomodulin. Thrombomodulin, a glycoprotein that is present on the cell membrane of endothelial cells, binds thrombin and acts as an additional regulatory mechanism in coagulation. Common clinical conditions that may cause DIC include obstetric disorders, accounting for 50% of cases, massive trauma, shock, sepsis, and malignant disease.[22,23] Chart 22-3 summarizes the conditions associated with DIC.

The factors involved in the conditions that cause DIC are often interrelated. In obstetric complications, tissue factors released from necrotic placental or fetal tissue or amniotic fluid may be the trigger of DIC. The hypoxia, shock, and acidosis that may coexist also contribute by causing endothelial injury. Gram-negative bacterial infections result in the release of endotoxins, which activate both the extrinsic pathway by release of tissue factor and the intrinsic pathway through endothelial damage. Endotoxins also inhibit the activity of protein C.[22,23]

Clinical Manifestations

Although coagulation and formation of microemboli characterize DIC, its acute manifestations are usually more directly related to the bleeding problems

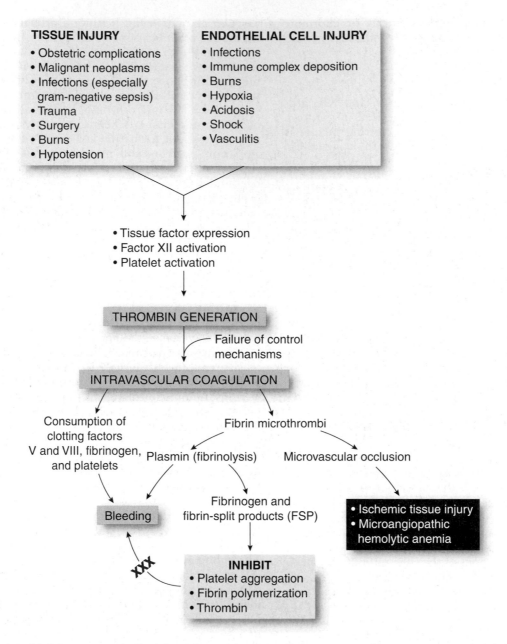

FIGURE 22-4. Pathophysiology of DIC. The DIC syndrome is triggered by tissue injury, endothelial cell injury, or a combination of both of these processes. Owing to the failure of the normal mechanisms controlling hemostasis, intravascular coagulation occurs. DIC, disseminated intravascular coagulation. (From Valdez R., Zutter M., Florea A. D., et al. (2015). Hematopathology. In Rubin R., Strayer D. (Eds.), *Rubin's pathology: Clinicopathologic foundations of medicine* (7th ed., p. 1113). Philadelphia, PA: Lippincott Williams & Wilkins.)

that occur. The bleeding may be present as petechiae, purpura, oozing from puncture sites, or severe hemorrhage.

Uncontrolled postpartum bleeding may indicate DIC. Microemboli may obstruct blood vessels and cause tissue hypoxia and necrotic damage to organ structures, such as the kidneys, heart, lungs, and brain. As a result, common clinical signs may be due to renal, circulatory, or respiratory failure, acute bleeding ulcers, or convulsions and coma. A form of hemolytic anemia may develop as red cells are damaged passing through vessels partially blocked by thrombus.[22,23]

Treatment

The treatment of DIC is directed toward managing the primary disease, replacing clotting components, and preventing further activation of clotting mechanisms. Transfusions of fresh-frozen plasma, platelets, or fibrinogen-containing cryoprecipitate may correct the clotting factor deficiency.

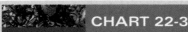

CHART 22-3

CONDITIONS THAT HAVE BEEN ASSOCIATED WITH DIC

Obstetric Conditions

Abruptio placentae

Dead fetus syndrome

Preeclampsia and eclampsia

Amniotic fluid embolism

Cancers

Metastatic cancer

Leukemia

Infections

Acute bacterial infections (*e.g.*, meningococcal meningitis)

Acute viral infections

Rickettsial infections (*e.g.*, Rocky Mountain spotted fever)

Parasitic infections (*e.g.*, malaria)

Shock

Septic shock

Severe hypovolemic shock

Trauma or Surgery

Burns

Massive trauma

Surgery involving extracorporeal circulation

Snake bite

Heat stroke

Hematologic Conditions

Blood transfusion reactions

SUMMARY CONCEPTS

Bleeding disorders or impairment of blood coagulation can result from defects in any of the factors that contribute to hemostasis: platelets, coagulation factors, or vascular integrity. The number of circulating platelets can be decreased (*i.e.*, thrombocytopenia) because of reduced bone marrow production, excess pooling in the spleen, or immune destruction. Impaired platelet function (*i.e.*, thrombocytopathia) is caused by inherited disorders (von Willebrand disease) or results from drugs or disease. Impairment of blood coagulation can result from deficiencies of one or more of the known clotting factors. Deficiencies can arise because of acquired disorders (*i.e.*, liver disease or vitamin K deficiency) or inherited diseases (*i.e.*, hemophilia A or von Willebrand disease). Bleeding may also occur from structurally weak vessels that result from impaired synthesis of vessel wall components (*i.e.*, vitamin C deficiency, excessive cortisol levels as in Cushing disease, or the aging process) or from damage by genetic mechanisms (*i.e.*, hemorrhagic telangiectasia) or the presence of microthrombi.

DIC is characterized by widespread coagulation and bleeding in the vascular compartment. It begins with massive activation of the coagulation cascade and generation of microthrombi that cause vessel occlusion and tissue ischemia. Clot formation consumes all available coagulation proteins and platelets, and severe hemorrhage results.

Review Exercises

1. A 55-year-old man has begun taking one 81-mg aspirin tablet daily on the recommendation of his physician. The physician had told him that this would help to prevent heart attack and stroke.

   A. What is the desired action of aspirin in terms of heart attack and stroke prevention?

2. A 29-year-old new mother, who delivered her infant 3 days ago, is admitted to the hospital with chest pain and is diagnosed as having venous thrombosis with pulmonary emboli.

   A. What factors would contribute to this woman's risk of developing thromboemboli?

3. The new mother is admitted to the intensive care unit and started on low-molecular-weight heparin and warfarin. She is told that she will be discharged in a day or 2 and will remain on the heparin for 5 days and the warfarin for at least 3 months.

   A. Anticoagulation with heparin and warfarin is not a definitive treatment for clot removal in pulmonary embolism but a form of secondary prevention. Explain.

REFERENCES

1. Hall J. E. (2016). *Guyton and Hall textbook of medical physiology* (13th ed., pp. 483–494). Philadelphia, PA: Elsevier.
2. Smith S. A., Travers R. J., Morrissey J. H. (2015). How it all starts: Initiation of the clotting cascade. *Critical Reviews in Biochemistry and Molecular Biology* 50(4), 326–336. doi:10.3109/10409238.2015.1050550.
3. Xu X. R., Zhang D., Oswald B. E., et al. (2016). Platelets are versatile cells: New discoveries in hemostasis, thrombosis,

immune responses, tumor metastasis and beyond. *Critical Reviews in Clinical Laboratory Sciences* 53(6), 409–430. doi:10.1080/10408363.2016.1200008.

4. Aster J. C., Bunn H. F. (2017). *Pathophysiology of blood disorders* (2nd ed., pp. 156–213). New York, NY: McGraw Hill Education.

5. Shifrin M. M., Widmar S. B. (2016). Platelet inhibitors. *Nursing Clinics of North America* 51, 29–43.

6. Pengo V., Banzato A., Bison E., et al. (2016). Efficacy and safety rivaroxaban vs. warfarin in high-risk patients with antiphospholipid syndrome: Rationale and design of the Trial on Rivaroxaban in AntiPhospholipid Syndrome (TRAPS) Trial. *Lupus* 25, 301–306.

7. Franchi F., Biguzzi E., Martinelli I., et al. (2013). Normal reference ranges of antithrombin, protein C and protein S: Effect of sex, age, and hormonal status. *Thrombosis Research* 132, e152–e157. doi:10.1016/j.thromres.2013.07.003.

8. Minuk L., Lazo-Langner A., Kovacs J., et al. (2010). Levels of protein C and protein S tested in the acute phase of a venous thrombolic event are not falsely elevated. *Thrombosis Journal* 8, 10. doi:10.1186/1477-9560-8-10.

9. Loffredo L., Perri L., Violi F. (2015). Impact of new oral anticoagulants on gastrointestinal bleeding in atrial fibrillation: A meta-analysis of interventional trials. *Digestive and Liver Disease* 47, 429–431.

10. Randi A. M., Laffan M. A. (2016). Von Willebrand factor and angiogenesis: Basic and applied issues. *Journal of Thrombosis and Haemostasis* 15, 13–20.

11. Chapin J. C., Hajjar K. A. (2015). Fibrinolysis and the control of blood coagulation. *Blood Reviews* 29, 17–24.

12. Nelson N. D., Marcogliese A., Bergstrom K., et al. (2016). Thrombopoietin measurement as a key component in the evaluation of pediatric thrombocytosis. *Pediatric Blood Cancer* 63, 1484–1487.

13. Sharma D., Singh G. (2017). Thrombocytosis in gynecological cancers. *Journal of Cancer Research and Therapeutics* 13(2), 193–197.

14. Cott M. V., Khor B., Zehnder J. L. (2016). Factor V Leiden. *American Journal of Hematology* 91, 46–49.

15. Wen S., Duan Q., Yang F., et al. (2017). Early diagnosis of venous thromboembolism as a clinical primary symptom of occult cancer: Core proteins of a venous thrombus (review). *Oncology Letters* 14, 491–496.

16. Tinholt M., Sandset P. M., Iversen N. (2016). Polymorphism of the coagulation system and risk of cancer. *Thrombosis Research* 140, S1, S49–S54.

17. Pollak A. W., McDane R. D. (2014). Succinct review of the new VTE prevention and management guidelines. *Mayo Clinic Proceedings* 89(3), 394–408.

18. Rosendaal F. R. (2016). Causes of venous thrombosis. *Thrombosis Journal* 14(Suppl 1), 24. doi:10.1186/s12959-016-0108-y.

19. Ali N., Auerbach H. E. (2017). New-onset acute thrombocytopenia in hospitalized patients: Pathophysiology and diagnostic approach. *Journal of Community Hospital Internal Medicine Perspectives* 7, 157–167.

20. Bădulescu O., Bădescu M., Ciocoiu M., et al. (2017). Immune thrombocytopenic purpura: Correlations between thrombocytopenia severity and its clinical symptoms. *Archives of the Balkan Medical Union* 52(1), 9–14.

21. Perer M., Garrido T. (2017). Advances in the pathophysiology of primary immune thrombocytopenia. *Hematology* 22, 42–53.

22. Kessler C. S., Khan B. A., Lai-Miller K. (2012). Thrombotic thrombocytopenic purpura: A hematological emergency. *Journal of Emergency Medicine* 43, 538–544.

23. Singh B. (2014). *Disseminated intravascular coagulation (DIC): Clinical manifestations, diagnosis, and treatment options*. New York, NY: Nova Science Publishers.

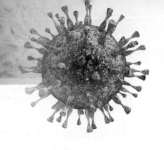

C H A P T E R **23**

Disorders of Red Blood Cells

Learning Objectives

After completing this chapter, the learner will be able to meet the following objectives:

1. Discuss the function of iron in the formation of hemoglobin.
2. Describe the formation, transport, and elimination of bilirubin.
3. Describe red blood cell count, percentage of reticulocytes, hemoglobin, hematocrit, mean corpuscular volume, and mean corpuscular hemoglobin concentration as it relates to the diagnosis of anemia.
4. Differentiate red cell antigens from antibodies in people with type A, B, AB, or O blood.
5. Explain the determination of the Rh factor.
6. List the signs and symptoms of a blood transfusion reaction.
7. Describe the manifestations of anemia and their mechanisms.
8. Compare characteristics of the red blood cells in acute blood loss, hereditary spherocytosis, sickle cell disease, iron deficiency anemia, and aplastic anemia.
9. Compare the causes and manifestations of polycythemia vera and secondary polycythemia.
10. Describe the function of hemoglobin F in the neonate, and describe the red blood cell changes that occur during the early neonatal period.
11. Cite the factors that predispose to hyperbilirubinemia in the infant.
12. Describe the pathogenesis of hemolytic disease of the newborn.
13. Compare conjugated and unconjugated bilirubin in terms of production of encephalopathy in the neonate.
14. State the changes in the red blood cells that occur with aging.

Although the lungs provide the means for gas exchange between the external and internal environments, it is the hemoglobin in the red blood cells that transports oxygen to the tissues. The red blood cells also function as carriers of carbon dioxide and participate in acid–base balance. This chapter focuses on the red blood cell, blood types and transfusion therapy, anemia, polycythemia, and age-related changes in the red blood cells.

The Red Blood Cell

The erythrocytes are 500 to 1000 times more numerous than other blood cells and are the most common type of blood cell.[1] The mature erythrocyte (also called a red blood cell or red cell) is a non-nucleated, biconcave disk (Fig. 23-1A). This unique shape contributes in two ways to the oxygen transport function of the erythrocyte. The biconcave shape provides a larger surface area for oxygen diffusion than would a spherical cell of the same volume, and the thinness of the cell membrane enables oxygen to diffuse rapidly between the exterior and the innermost regions of the cell (Fig. 23-1).

Another structural feature that facilitates the transport function of the red blood cell is the flexibility of its membrane. It can squeeze through capillaries easily and, therefore, has the ability to reach peripheral body tissue.[2] A complex network of fibrous proteins, especially one called *spectrin*, maintains the biconcave shape and flexibility of the red cell membrane (Fig. 23-2). Spectrin forms an attachment with another protein, called *ankyrin*, which resides on the inner surface of the membrane and is anchored to an integral protein that spans the membrane. This unique arrangement of proteins imparts elasticity and stability to the membrane and allows it to deform easily.[3]

The primary function of the red blood cell, facilitated by the hemoglobin molecule, is to transport oxygen to the tissues. Because oxygen is poorly soluble in plasma, about 95% to 98% is carried bound to hemoglobin. The hemoglobin molecule is composed of two pairs of structurally different alpha and beta polypeptide chains (see Fig. 23-1B). Each of the four polypeptide chains consists of a globin (protein) portion and a heme unit.[1] Thus, each molecule of hemoglobin can carry four molecules of oxygen. Hemoglobin is a natural pigment. Because of its iron content, it appears red when oxygen is attached and has a bluish cast when deoxygenated.[2] The production of each type of globin chain is controlled by individual structural genes with five different gene loci. Mutations, which can occur anywhere in these five loci, have resulted in over 550 types of abnormal hemoglobin molecules.[4]

The two major types of normal hemoglobin are adult hemoglobin (HbA) and fetal hemoglobin (HbF). HbA consists of a pair of alpha chains and a pair of beta chains. HbF is the predominant hemoglobin in the fetus from the third through the ninth month of gestation. It has a pair of gamma chains substituted for the alpha chains. Because of this chain substitution, HbF has a higher affinity for oxygen than HbA.[4] This affinity facilitates the transfer of oxygen across the placenta from the HbA in the mother's blood to the HbF in the fetus's blood. HbF is generally replaced within 6 months of birth with HbA.

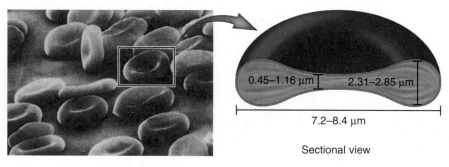

0.45–1.16 μm   2.31–2.85 μm

7.2–8.4 μm

Sectional view

A   Red blood cells

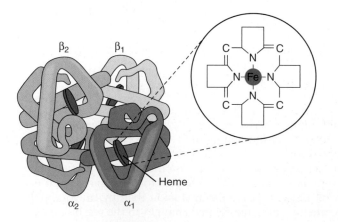

β_2 β_1

Heme

α_2 α_1

B   Hemoglobin

FIGURE 23-1. Physical characteristics of red blood cells. (**A**) RBCs are biconcave disks without nuclei. (**B**) Hemoglobin molecule showing the four iron (Fe)-containing heme subunits and their structure. (From Pawlina W. (2016). *Histology: A text and atlas: With correlated cell and molecular biology* (pp. 273, 276). Philadelphia, PA: Wolters Kluwer.)

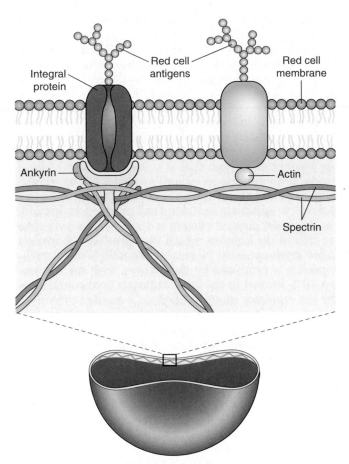

FIGURE 23-2. Cross-sectional side view of the biconcave structure of the red blood cell and diagram showing the cytoskeleton and flexible network of spectrin proteins that attach to the ankyrin protein, a transmembrane protein that resides on the inner surface of the membrane and is anchored to an integral protein that spans the membrane.

KEY POINTS

Red Blood Cells

■ The function of red blood cells, facilitated by the iron-containing hemoglobin molecule, is to transport oxygen from the lungs to the tissues.

■ The red blood cell, which has a life span of approximately 120 days, is broken down in the spleen; the degradation products such as iron and amino acids are recycled.

Hemoglobin Synthesis

The rate at which hemoglobin is synthesized depends on the availability of iron for heme synthesis. A lack of iron results in relatively small amounts of hemoglobin in the red blood cells. The amount of iron in the body is approximately 2 g in women and up to 6 g in men.[2] Body iron is found in several compartments. Most iron

(approximately 80%) is complexed to heme in hemoglobin, with small amounts found in the **myoglobin** of muscle, the **cytochromes**, and the iron-containing enzymes. The remaining 20% is stored in the bone marrow, liver, spleen, and other organs. Normally, some iron is sequestered in the intestinal epithelial cells and is lost in the feces as these cells slough off.

When red blood cells age and are destroyed in the spleen, the iron from their hemoglobin is released into the circulation and returned to the bone marrow for incorporation into new red blood cells. This recycled iron from old erythrocytes is the primary source of iron used in the production of new erythrocytes.[5]

Dietary iron also helps to maintain body stores. Iron, principally derived from meat, is absorbed in the small intestine, especially the duodenum (Fig. 23-3). When body stores of iron are diminished or erythropoiesis is stimulated, absorption is increased. (Conversely, in iron overload, excretion of iron is accelerated.) The iron that is absorbed enters the circulation, where it immediately combines with a beta globulin, *apotransferrin*, to form *transferrin*, which is then transported in the plasma.[1] From the plasma, iron can be deposited in tissues such as the liver, where it is stored as *ferritin*, a protein–iron complex, which can easily return to the circulation. Serum ferritin levels, which can be measured in the

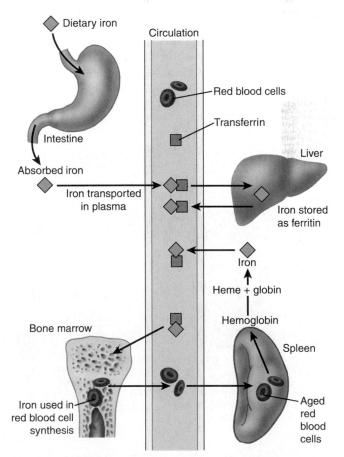

FIGURE 23-3. Diagrammatic representation of the iron cycle, including its absorption from the gastrointestinal tract, transport in the circulation, storage in the liver, recycling from aged red cells destroyed in the spleen, and use in the bone marrow synthesis of red blood cells.

laboratory, provide an index of body iron stores. Clinically, decreased ferritin levels usually indicate the need for prescription of iron supplements, such as ferrous sulfate. Transferrin can also deliver iron to the developing red cell in the bone marrow by binding to membrane receptors. This iron is taken up by the developing red cell, where it is used in heme synthesis.[5]

Red Cell Production

Erythropoiesis refers to the production of red blood cells. After birth, red cells are produced in the red bone marrow. Until 5 years of age, almost all bones produce red cells to meet the growth needs of a child, after which bone marrow activity in long bones gradually declines. In adults, red cell production takes place mainly in the membranous bones of the vertebrae, sternum, ribs, and pelvis.[3] With this reduction in activity, the red bone marrow is replaced with fatty yellow bone marrow.

The red blood cells are derived from precursor cells called *erythroblasts*, which are formed continuously from the *pluripotent stem cells* in the bone marrow (Fig. 23-4). The red cell precursors move through a series of divisions, each producing a smaller cell as they continue to develop into mature red blood cells. Hemoglobin synthesis begins at the early erythroblast stage and continues until the cell becomes a mature erythrocyte. During its transformation from normoblast to reticulocyte, the red blood cell accumulates hemoglobin as the nucleus condenses and is finally lost. The period from stem cell to emergence of the reticulocyte in the circulation normally takes approximately 1 week. Maturation of reticulocyte to erythrocyte takes approximately 24 to 48 hours. During this process, the red

cell loses its mitochondria and ribosomes, along with its ability to produce hemoglobin and engage in oxidative metabolism. Most maturing red cells enter the blood as reticulocytes. Approximately 1% of the body's total complement of red blood cells is generated from the bone marrow each day, and the reticulocyte count, therefore, serves as an index of the erythropoietic activity of the bone marrow.[2]

Erythropoiesis is governed for the most part by tissue oxygen needs. Any condition that causes a decrease in the amount of oxygen that is transported in the blood produces an increase in red cell production. The oxygen content of the blood does not act directly on the bone marrow to stimulate red blood cell production. Instead, the decreased oxygen content is sensed by the peritubular cells in the kidneys, which then produce a hormone called *erythropoietin*. Normally, about 90% of all erythropoietin is produced by the kidneys, with the remaining 10% formed in the liver. Although erythropoietin is the key regulator of erythropoiesis, a number of growth factors, including granulocyte colony–stimulating factor (G-CSF), granulocyte–macrophage (GM)-CSF, and insulin-like growth factor 1 (IGF-1), are involved in the early stages of erythropoiesis.[2] Erythropoietin acts primarily in later stages of erythropoiesis to induce the erythrocyte colony–forming units to proliferate and mature through the normoblast stage into reticulocytes and mature erythrocytes. In the absence of erythropoietin, as in kidney failure, hypoxia has little or no effect on red blood cell production.[2]

Because red blood cells are released into the blood as reticulocytes, the percentage of these cells is higher when there is a marked increase in red blood cell production. In some severe forms of anemia, the reticulocytes (normally about 1%) may account for as much as 30% of

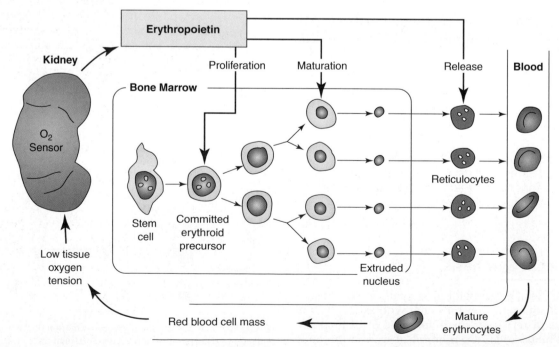

FIGURE 23-4. Red blood cell development involves the proliferation and differentiation of committed bone marrow cells through the erythroblast and normoblast stages to reticulocytes, which are released into the bloodstream and finally become erythrocytes.

the total red cell count. In some situations, red cell production is so accelerated that numerous erythroblasts appear in the blood.[2]

Red Cell Destruction

Mature red blood cells have a life span of approximately 4 months, or 120 days. As the red blood cell ages, a number of changes occur—metabolic activity in the cell decreases, enzyme activity declines, and adenosine triphosphate (ATP) decreases. Membrane lipids become reduced and the cell membrane becomes more fragile, causing the red cell to self-destruct as it passes through narrow places in the circulation and in the small trabecular spaces in the spleen.[2] The rate of red cell destruction (1% per day) normally is equal to the rate of red cell production, but in conditions such as hemolytic anemia, the cell's life span may be shorter.

The destruction of red blood cells is facilitated by a group of large phagocytic cells found in the spleen, liver, bone marrow, and lymph nodes. These phagocytic cells recognize old and defective red cells and then ingest and destroy them in a series of enzymatic reactions. During these reactions, the amino acids from the globulin chains and iron from the heme units are salvaged and reused (Fig. 23-5). The bulk of the heme unit is converted to bilirubin, the pigment of bile, which is insoluble in plasma and attaches to plasma proteins for transport. Bilirubin is removed from the blood by the liver and conjugated with glucuronide to render it water soluble so that it can be excreted in the bile. Excess elimination of bilirubin in the bile because of increased red cell destruction can lead to the development of bilirubin gallstones. The plasma-insoluble form of bilirubin is referred to as *unconjugated bilirubin* and the water-soluble form as *conjugated bilirubin*. Serum levels of conjugated and unconjugated bilirubin can be measured in the laboratory and are reported as direct and indirect, respectively. If red cell destruction and consequent bilirubin production are excessive, unconjugated bilirubin accumulates in the blood. This results in a yellow discoloration of the skin, called *jaundice*.[2]

When red blood cell destruction takes place in the circulation, as in hemolytic anemia, the hemoglobin remains in the plasma. The plasma contains a hemoglobin-binding protein called *haptoglobin*.[4] Other plasma proteins, such as albumin, can also bind hemoglobin. With extensive intravascular destruction of red blood cells, hemoglobin levels may exceed the hemoglobin-binding capacity of haptoglobin and other plasma proteins. When this happens, free hemoglobin appears in the blood (*i.e.*, hemoglobinemia) and is excreted in the urine (*i.e.*, hemoglobinuria).[4]

Red Cell Metabolism and Hemoglobin Oxidation

The red blood cell, which lacks mitochondria, relies on glucose and the glycolytic pathway for its metabolic needs. The enzyme-mediated anaerobic metabolism of glucose generates the ATP needed for normal membrane function and ion transport. The depletion of glucose or the functional deficiency of one of the glycolytic enzymes leads to the premature death of the red blood cell. An offshoot of the glycolytic pathway is the production of 2,3-diphosphoglycerate (2,3-DPG), which binds to the hemoglobin molecule and reduces the affinity of hemoglobin for oxygen. This facilitates the release of oxygen at the tissue level. An increase in the concentration of 2,3-DPG occurs in conditions of chronic hypoxia such as chronic lung disease, anemia, and residence at high altitudes.[1]

Certain chemicals (*e.g.*, nitrates and sulfates) and drugs that oxidize hemoglobin to an inactive form interrupt the oxidation of hemoglobin (the combination of hemoglobin with oxygen). The nitrite ion reacts with hemoglobin to produce methemoglobin, which has a low affinity for oxygen. Large doses of nitrites can result in high levels of methemoglobin, causing pseudocyanosis and tissue hypoxia.

A hereditary deficiency of glucose-6-phosphate dehydrogenase (G6PD) predisposes to oxidative denaturation of hemoglobin, with resultant red cell injury and lysis. Deficiency of G6PD is an anemia that is most frequently seen in African American men. Hemolysis usually occurs as the result of oxidative stress generated by either an infection or exposure to certain drugs or foods.

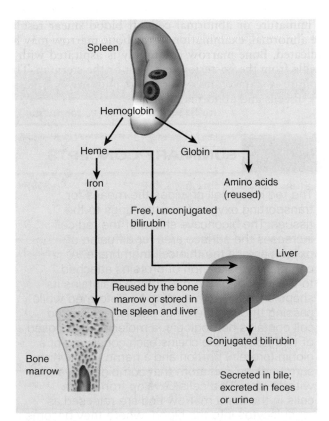

FIGURE 23-5. Destruction of red blood cells and fate of hemoglobin.

TABLE 23-2 Blood and Blood Components Commonly Used in Transfusion Therapy (continued)

Component	Composition	Indications and Considerations
Lymphocytes	Lymphocytes (number varies)	Stimulate graft-versus-.host disease effect
Cryoprecipitate	Fibrinogen ≥150 mg/bag, AHF (VIII:C) 80–110 units/bag, von Willebrand factor; fibronectin	von Willebrand disease Hypofibrinogenemia Hemophilia A
AHF	Factor VIII	Hemophilia A
Factor IX concentrate	Factor IX	Hemophilia B (Christmas disease)
Factor IX complex	Factors II, VII, IX, X	Hereditary factor VII, IX, and X deficiency; hemophilia A with factor VII inhibitors
Albumin	Albumin 5%, 25%	Hypoproteinemia; burns; volume expansion by 5% to ↑ blood volume; 25% leads to ↓ hematocrit
IV gamma globulin	Immunoglobulin G antibodies	Hypogammaglobulinemia (in CLL, recurrent infections); ITP; primary immunodeficiency states
Antithrombin III concentrate (AT III)	AT III (trace amounts of other plasma proteins)	AT III deficiency with or at risk for thrombosis

The composition of each type of blood component is described as well as the most common indications for using a given blood component. RBCs, platelets, and fresh-frozen plasma are the most commonly used blood products. When transfusing these blood products, it is important to realize that the individual product is always "contaminated" with very small amounts of other blood products (e.g., WBCs mixed in a unit of platelets). This contamination can cause some difficulties, particularly isosensitization, in certain people.
↑, increased; ↓, decreased; AHF, antihemophilic factor; CLL, chronic lymphocytic leukemia; ITP, idiopathic thrombocytopenic purpura; IV, intravenous; PRBCs, packed red blood cells; RBCs, red blood cells; WBCs, white blood cells.
Reprinted from Hinkle J. L., Cheever K. H. (2018). Brunner & Suddarth's textbook of medical-surgical nursing (14th ed., Table 32-4, p. 915). Philadelphia, PA: Wolters Kluwer; adapted from American Red Cross. (2015). Blood components. [Online]. Available: www.redcrossblood.org/learn-about-blood/blood components. Accessed September 14, 2015; Dzieczkowski J. S., Anderson K. C. (2015). Transfusion biology and therapy. In Kasper D., Fauci A., Hauser S., et al. (Eds.), Harrison's principles of internal medicine (19th ed.). Available: accessmedicine.mhmedical.com.laneproxy.stanford.edu/content.aspx?bookid=1130&Sectionid=79732248. Accessed May 25, 2016.

ABO Blood Groups

ABO compatibility is essential for effective transfusion therapy and requires knowledge of ABO antigens and antibodies. There are four major ABO blood groups determined by the presence or absence of two red cell antigens (A and B). People who have neither A nor B antigens are classified as having type O blood. Those with A antigens are classified as having type A blood; those with B antigens as having type B blood; and those with A and B antigens as having type AB blood (Table 23-3). The ABO blood groups are genetically determined. The type O gene is apparently functionless in production of a red cell antigen. Each of the other genes is expressed by the presence of a strong antigen on the surface of the red cell. Six genotypes, or gene combinations, result in four phenotypes, or blood type expressions. In the United States, types O and A are the most common.

ABO antibodies predictably develop in the serum of people whose red cells lack the corresponding antigen. Persons with type A antigens on their red cells develop type B antibodies; persons with type B antigens develop type A antibodies in their serum; people with type O blood develop type A and type B antibodies; and people with type AB blood develop neither A nor B antibodies. The ABO antibodies are usually not present at birth but begin to develop at 3 to 6 months of age and reach maximum levels between the ages of 5 and 10 years.[7]

TABLE 23-3 ABO Blood Group System

Genotype	Red Cell Antigens	Blood Type	Serum Antibodies
OO	None	O	AB
AO	A	A	B
AA	A	A	B
BO	B	B	A
BB	B	B	A
AB	AB	AB	None

Rh Types

The D antigen of the Rh system is also important in transfusion compatibility and is routinely tested. The Rh type is coded by three gene pairs—C, c; D, d; and E, e. Each allele, with the exception of d, codes for a specific antigen. The D antigen is the most immunogenic. People who express the D antigen are designated Rh-positive, and those who do not express the D antigen are Rh-negative. Unlike serum antibodies for the ABO blood types, which develop spontaneously after birth, Rh antibodies develop after exposure to one or more of the Rh antigens, usually through pregnancy or transfusions, and persist for many years.[2] Because it takes several weeks to produce antibodies, a reaction may be delayed and is usually mild. If subsequent transfusions of Rh-positive blood are given to a person who has become sensitized, the person may have a severe, immediate reaction.

Blood Transfusion Reactions

The seriousness of blood transfusion reactions prompts the need for extreme caution when blood is administered. Because most transfusion reactions result from administrative errors or misidentification, care should be taken to identify correctly the recipient and the transfusion source. The recipient's vital signs should be monitored before and during the transfusion, and careful observation for signs of transfusion reaction is imperative.

The Centers for Disease Control and Prevention (CDC) has identified 11 types of transfusion reactions.[9] The reactions and classification criteria are provided in Table 23-4. The most common or concerning reactions are addressed in the discussion that follows.

Acute Hemolytic Transfusion Reactions

Acute hemolytic transfusion reaction (AHTR) occurs when there is destruction of donor red cells by reaction with antibody in the recipient's serum.[7] It can be life-threatening, but fortunately, it is rare: It occurs in 1 of 76,000 transfusions. The majority of these (1 of 40,000 transfusions) is caused by ABO incompatibility. Typical signs and symptoms may occur following as little as 10 mL of blood transfusion.[7]

Hemoglobin that is released from the hemolyzed donor cells is filtered in the glomeruli of the kidneys. Because of the adverse effects of the filtered hemoglobin on renal tubular flow, two possible complications of an AHTR are oliguria and renal failure.[10] In addition to other testing, a urine specimen should be examined for the presence of hemoglobin, urobilinogen, and red blood cells.

TABLE 23-4 Classification of Blood Transfusion Reactions

Blood Transfusion Reaction	Case Definition*
Allergic reaction	**Definitive:** Two or more of the following occurring during or within 4 hours of cessation of transfusion: ■ Conjunctival edema ■ Edema of the lips, tongue, and uvula ■ Erythema and edema of the periorbital area ■ Generalized flushing ■ Hypotension ■ Localized angioedema ■ Maculopapular rash ■ Pruritus (itching) ■ Respiratory distress; bronchospasm ■ Urticaria (hives) **Probable:** *Any* one of the following occurring during or within 4 hours of cessation of transfusion: ■ Conjunctival edema ■ Edema of the lips, tongue, and uvula ■ Erythema and edema of the periorbital area ■ Localized angioedema ■ Maculopapular rash ■ Pruritus (itching) ■ Urticaria (hives)[8, p.12]
Acute hemolytic transfusion reaction	**Definitive:** Occurs during or within 24 hours of cessation of transfusion with new onset of *any* of the following signs/symptoms: ■ Back/flank pain ■ Chills/rigors ■ Disseminated intravascular coagulation ■ Epistaxis ■ Fever ■ Hematuria (gross visual hemolysis) ■ Hypotension ■ Oliguria/anuria ■ Pain and/or oozing at IV site ■ Renal failure

(*continued*)

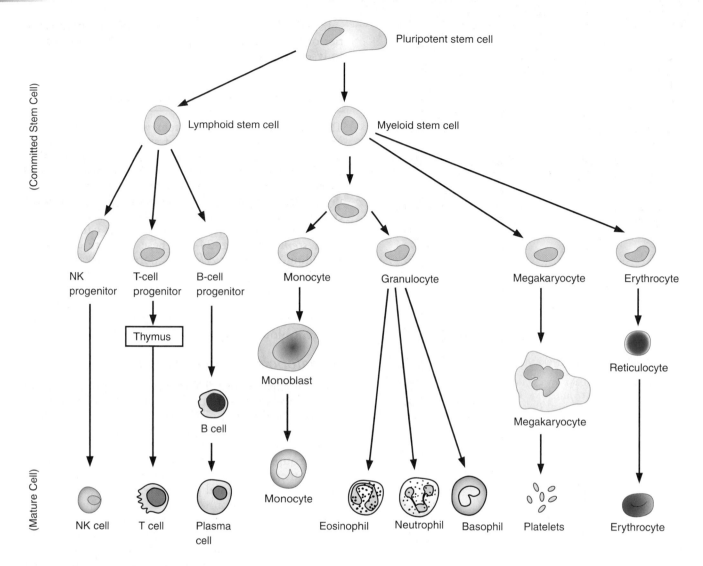

FIGURE 24-2. Major developmental stages of blood cells. NK, natural killer cell. (From Porth C. M. (2015). *Essentials of pathophysiology* (4th ed., Fig. 11-1, p. 242). Philadelphia, PA: Lippincott Williams & Wilkins.)

metamyelocyte stage, the nuclei distort and become arc-like, producing the band developmental stage. Maturation from metamyelocyte to mature neutrophil involves progressive condensation of nuclear chromatin, increasing nuclear lobulation, and the appearance of secondary (specific) granules. Eosinophils and basophils undergo similar developmental stages but develop different secondary granules. Like granulocytes, monocytes develop from the granulocyte–monocyte progenitor cell and progress through a monoblast and promonocyte stage. By contrast, lymphocytes derive from lymphoid stem cells and progress through the lymphoblast and prolymphocyte stages. The prolymphocytes leave the bone marrow and travel to the lymphoid tissues, where further differentiation into T and B lymphocytes occurs. The names of the various leukocyte developmental stages are often used in describing blood cell changes that occur in hematopoietic disorders.

KEY POINTS

Hematopoiesis

■ The white blood cells are formed from hematopoietic stem cells that differentiate into committed progenitor cells, which, in turn, develop into the myelocytic and lymphocytic lineages needed for the formation of the different types of white blood cell.

■ The life span of white blood cells is relatively short, so constant renewal is necessary to maintain normal blood levels. Any conditions that decrease the availability of stem cells or hematopoietic growth factors cause a decrease in white blood cells.

Lymphoid Tissues

The body's lymphatic system consists of the lymphatic vessels, lymphoid tissue and lymph nodes, thymus, and spleen (Fig. 24-3). Although both precursor B and T lymphocytes begin their development in the bone marrow, they migrate to peripheral lymphoid structures to complete the differentiation process. B lymphocytes leave the bone marrow, differentiate into plasma cells, and then move to the lymph nodes, where they continue to proliferate and produce antibodies. T lymphocytes leave the bone marrow as precursor T lymphocytes travel to the thymus, where they differentiate into CD4+ helper T cells and CD8+ cytotoxic T cells, after which many of them move to lymph nodes, where they undergo further proliferation.

Lymph nodes consist of organized collections of lymphoid tissue located along the lymphatic vessels.[3] Typically grayish white and ovoid or bean shaped, they range in size from 1 mm to about 1 to 2 cm in diameter. A fibrous capsule and radiating trabeculae provide a supporting structure, and a delicate reticular network contributes to internal support (Fig. 24-4). The parenchyma of the lymph

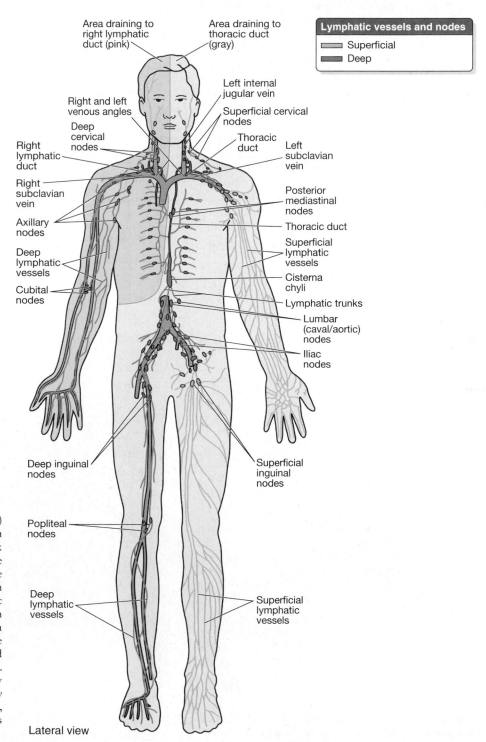

FIGURE 24-3. Lymphatic system. (**A**) The right lymphatic duct drains lymph from the right side of the head and neck and the right upper limbs (*shaded*). The thoracic duct drains the remainder of the body. Deep lymphatic vessels are shown on the right, and superficial lymphatic vessels are shown on the left. (**B**) Lymph flow from extracellular spaces through a lymph node. Small black arrows indicate the flow of interstitial fluid out of blood capillaries into the lymphatic capillaries. (From Moore K. L., Agur A. M., Dalley A. F. (2015). *Essential clinical anatomy* (5th ed., Fig. 1-18, p. 26). Philadelphia, PA: Wolters Kluwer/Lippincott Williams & Wilkins.)

Area draining to right lymphatic duct (pink)

Area draining to thoracic duct (gray)

Lymphatic vessels and nodes
Superficial
Deep

Right and left venous angles

Deep cervical nodes

Right lymphatic duct

Right subclavian vein

Axillary nodes

Deep lymphatic vessels

Cubital nodes

Left internal jugular vein

Superficial cervical nodes

Thoracic duct

Left subclavian vein

Posterior mediastinal nodes

Thoracic duct

Superficial lymphatic vessels

Cisterna chyli

Lymphatic trunks

Lumbar (caval/aortic) nodes

Iliac nodes

Deep inguinal nodes

Superficial inguinal nodes

Popliteal nodes

Deep lymphatic vessels

Superficial lymphatic vessels

Lateral view

node is divided into an outer or a superficial cortex and an inner medulla. The superficial cortex contains well-defined B-cell and T-cell domains. The B-cell–dependent cortex consists of two types of follicles: immunologically inactive follicles, called *primary follicles*, and active follicles that contain germinal centers, called *secondary follicles*. Germinal centers contain large lymphocytes (centroblasts) and small lymphocytes with cleaved nuclei (centrocytes). The mantle zone is the small layer of B cells surrounding the germinal centers. The portion of the cortex between the medullary and superficial cortex is called the *paracortex*. This region contains most of the T cells in the lymph nodes.

Although some lymphocytes enter the lymph nodes through the afferent lymphatic channels, most enter through the wall of postcapillary venules located in the deep cortex. These vessels, which are lined with specialized endothelial cells that possess receptors for antigen-primed lymphocytes, signal lymphocytes to leave the circulation and migrate through the lymph nodes. Both B and T cells leave the bloodstream through these channels.[1,4,5] Most lymphocytes leave the lymph node by entering the lymphatic sinuses, from which they enter the efferent lymphatic vessel.

The alimentary canal, respiratory passages, and genitourinary systems are guarded by accumulations of lymphoid tissue that are not enclosed in a capsule. This form of lymphoid tissue is called *diffuse lymphoid tissue* or *mucosa-associated lymphoid tissue* (MALT) because of its association with mucous membranes (Fig. 24-5).[3]

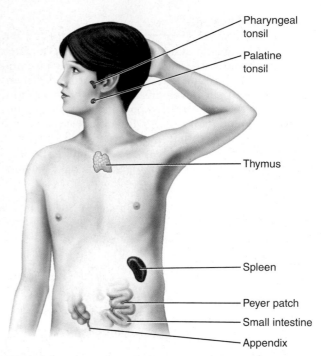

FIGURE 24-5. Mucosa-associated lymphoid tissue. This type of lymphoid tissue protects the body's entry points. (From McConnell T. H., Hull K. L. (2011). *Human form human function: Essentials of anatomy & physiology* (p. 473, Fig. 12-8). Philadelphia, PA: Wolters Kluwer/Lippincott Williams & Wilkins.)

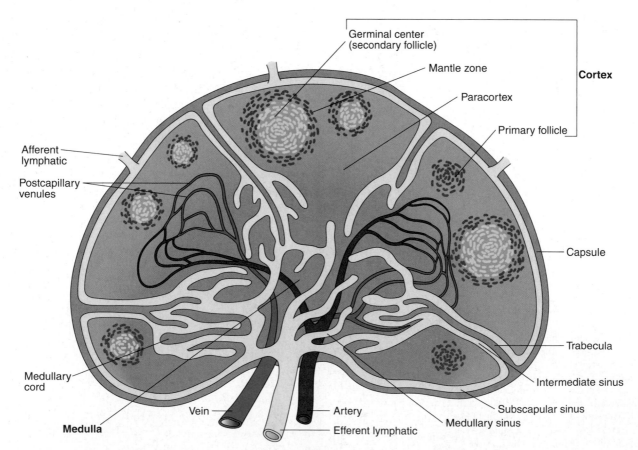

FIGURE 24-4. Structures of normal lymph node. (From Rubin R., Strayer D. E. (Eds.). (2015). *Rubin's pathology: Clinicopathologic foundations of medicine* (7th ed., Fig. 26-46, p. 1131). Philadelphia, PA: Lippincott Williams & Wilkins.)

Lymphocytes are found in the subepithelium of these tissues. Lymphomas can arise from MALT as well as lymph node tissue.

SUMMARY CONCEPTS

Leukocyte or white blood cell development begins with the myeloid and lymphoid stem cells in the bone marrow. The granulocyte and monocyte cell lines derive from the myeloid stem cells, and lymphocytes from the lymphoid stem cells. The immature precursor cells for each of the cell lines are called *blast cells*. The blast cells progress through subsequent maturational stages before becoming mature granulocytes, monocytes, or lymphocytes. The names of these developmental stages are often used in describing blood cell changes that occur in hematopoietic disorders.

The lymphatic system consists of a network of lymphatic vessels, nodes, and tissues where B and T lymphocytes complete their differentiation. Lymph nodes, which are the site where many lymphomas originate, exhibit an outer or a superficial cortex and an inner medulla.[4] The cortex contains well-defined B-cell and T-cell domains. The B-cell–dependent cortex consists of two types of follicles: immunologically inactive follicles, called *primary follicles*, and active follicles that contain germinal centers, called *secondary follicles*. Most of the T cells are contained in the paracortex, the area between the medullary and superficial cortex.

Non-neoplastic Disorders of White Blood Cells

The number of leukocytes, or white blood cells, in the peripheral circulation normally ranges from 5000 to 10,000 cells/μL (also expressed as 5 to 10 × 10³ cells/μL, or 5000 to 10,000 cells/mm³ of blood).[1]

Neutropenia (Agranulocytosis)

The term *leukopenia* describes a decrease in the absolute number of leukocytes in the blood. Although leukopenia may affect any of the specific types of white blood cells, it most often affects the neutrophil. Neutrophils constitute the majority of blood leukocytes and play a critical role in host–defense mechanisms against infection. They migrate to sites of infection and engulf, digest, and destroy microorganisms. Thus, a decrease in the number of neutrophils (neutropenia) places a person at risk for infection. The risk for and severity of neutropenia-associated infection are directly proportional to

the absolute neutrophil count (ANC) and duration of the neutropenia.[3] The ANC is determined with the following formula[5]:

$$\frac{segs + bands \times WBC}{100} = ANC$$

The normal ANC is 1000/μL, and if the ANC is less than 500 cells/mm³, the person is generally put on neutropenic precautions in the hospital to protect him or her from the environment.[6]

Neutropenia refers specifically to an abnormally low number of neutrophils and is commonly defined as a circulating neutrophil count of less than 1000/μL. *Agranulocytosis* denotes a virtual absence of neutrophils.

Neutropenia can result from decreased neutrophil production, accelerated utilization or destruction, or a shift from the blood to the tissue compartments. It can be present at birth (congenital) or arise from a number of factors that occur later in life and do not have a hereditary component (acquired).

Congenital Neutropenia

Inherited disorders of proliferation and maturation of myeloid stem cell lines are relatively rare and have a high degree of variability in severity and symptomatology. Approximately one half are caused by neutrophil elastase (*ELANE*) mutations.[7]

Congenital neutropenias can be divided into two subtypes: congenital (permanent) severe neutropenia and cyclic neutropenia, which has variable expression. Severe congenital neutropenia is usually diagnosed in infants under 6 months of age, and counts are usually less than 2 g/L.[7] Severe bacterial and/or fungal infections are associated with its discovery. The risk of severe infection is inversely related to the neutrophil count—that is, the lower the neutrophil count, the higher the risk of infection.

Cyclic (intermittent) neutropenia is often discovered in children under 2 years of age and is usually associated with acute stomatologic disorders. Cyclic neutropenia occurs with periodic oscillations between normal and abnormal neutrophils. In some instances, the bone marrow may function normally for a period of time. As a result, the risk of severe life-threatening infections exists, but frequency is reduced. The cycles may become less noticeable in older adults and then the disorder begins to resemble chronic neutropenia.

Severe congenital neutropenia, or *Kostmann syndrome*, is characterized by an arrest in myeloid maturation at the promyelocyte stage of development, which can be inherited as either an autosomal dominant or autosomal recessive trait.[8] The autosomal dominant disease is usually associated with mutations in the neutrophil elastase gene, which, in turn, leads to apoptosis of bone marrow myeloid cells. The autosomal recessive severe congenital neutropenia or Kostmann syndrome is caused by mutations in the *HAX-1* gene, which causes a loss of mitochondrial potential. The disorder is characterized by severe bacterial infections. Approximately 20% of people with the disorder develop acute myelogenous leukemia (AML).[8]

Acquired Neutropenia

Acquired neutropenia encompasses a broad spectrum of causative processes and includes primary and secondary autoimmune neutropenia, infection-related neutropenia, and drug-induced neutropenia (Chart 24-1). A number of bone marrow disorders, hematopoietic malignancies, and radiation therapy may induce neutropenia.

 CHART 24-1

PRINCIPAL CAUSES OF NEUTROPENIA

Congenital
- Alloimmune neonatal neutropenia (transfer of maternal antibodies)
- Cyclic neutropenia
- Kostmann syndrome (severe congenital neutropenia)

Acquired

Autoimmune
- Primary (rare, usually occurs in children and runs a benign course)
- Secondary
  - Systemic lupus erythematous
  - Felty syndrome in people with rheumatoid arthritis
- Infection related
- Many types of infections agents, but most commonly viruses
- Mechanisms include increased consumption of neutrophils, production of autoantibodies, direct infiltration of hematopoietic cells, and bone marrow suppression

Drug related
- Immune-mediated reactions in which drugs act as haptens (*e.g.*, penicillin, propylthiouracil, aminopyrine)
- Accelerated apoptosis (clozapine [antipsychotic agent])
- Cancer chemotherapeutic drugs (bone marrow depression)

Radiation therapy to bone marrow

Hematologic malignancies

Autoimmune Neutropenia

Autoimmune neutropenia results from antibodies directed against neutrophil cell membrane antigens or bone marrow progenitors. The autoimmune forms of neutropenia may be classified as primary (*i.e.*, those not associated with other detectable pathologic processes) or secondary (*i.e.*, those associated with another disease condition).[9]

Primary autoimmune neutropenia is a rare disorder of early childhood, during which a moderate-to-severe neutropenia is observed. The condition is usually benign, with mild-to-moderate infections for children. The disorder is rare in adults.

Secondary immune-associated neutropenia is often associated with systemic autoimmune disorders, mainly rheumatoid arthritis (RA), Felty syndrome (a variant of RA), and systemic lupus erythematosus (SLE).[9] Felty syndrome is a triad of splenomegaly, recurrent pulmonary infections, and neutropenia.

Several antibody-mediated mechanisms are believed to be responsible for the neutropenia seen in people with SLE. These include the development of antineutrophil antibodies, along with increased neutrophil apoptosis and decreased neutrophil production by the bone marrow.

Infection-Related Neutropenia

Many different types of infectious diseases, including viral, bacterial, rickettsial, and parasitic, may cause neutropenia, the most common being viral. Infections may produce neutropenia in multiple ways, such as decreased neutrophil production, loss of neutrophils by toxins, or problems resulting in neutrophil sequestration in the spleen. Neutropenia is also a common manifestation of acquired immunodeficiency syndrome, in which a virus-induced suppression of marrow cell proliferation is often aggravated by infectious consumption of neutrophils and by antiviral drugs.[4]

Drug-Related Neutropenia

Drug-induced neutropenia is attributed to a number of drugs, especially those used in the treatment of cancer.[10,11] Patient-related factors are age, disease burden, nutritional and hydration status, and prior history of anemia or neutropenia. Older adults are at higher risk than younger people because of age-related cellular changes in neutrophils.[12]

The term *idiosyncratic* is used to describe drug reactions that are different from the effect obtained in most people and that cannot be explained in terms of allergy. Idiosyncratic drug reactions occur as an immune-mediated or direct damage to myeloid precursors and cell lineage.[10] The reaction is reversible on discontinuation of the drug.

Febrile neutropenia (FN) is often related to chemotherapy-induced neutropenia and is associated with significant mortality and morbidity.[11] FN—defined as oral temperature greater than 38.3°C and an ANC less than $0.5 \times 10^9/L$[12]—is a key factor limiting the dose of many cytotoxic drugs.[11] Most cases are associated with bacterial infections, but FN may develop as a result of fungal or viral infections.[12]

Neutrophils provide the first line of defense against organisms that inhabit the skin and gastrointestinal tract. Thus, early signs of infection due to neutropenia, particularly those associated with a mild-to-moderate decrease in neutrophils, include mild skin lesions, stomatitis, pharyngitis, and diarrhea. Signs and symptoms of more severe neutropenia include malaise, chills, and fever, followed in sequence by marked weakness and fatigability. Untreated infections can be rapidly fatal, particularly if the ANC drops below 250/µL. With severe neutropenia, the usual signs of infection may not be present because of a lack of a sufficient number of neutrophils to produce an inflammatory response.

Infectious Mononucleosis

Infectious mononucleosis is a self-limiting lymphoproliferative disorder commonly caused by the Epstein–Barr virus (EBV), which belongs the herpesvirus family (Fig. 24-6).[13] Cytomegalovirus accounts for fewer cases of infectious mononucleosis. EBV occurs most often in adolescents and young adults.[13] Once an individual is infected, the virus will remain present in the B lymphocytes for a lifetime.[13]

Clinical Course

The onset of infectious mononucleosis is usually insidious. The incubation period lasts 4 to 6 weeks.[14] A prodromal period, which lasts for several days, follows and is characterized by malaise, anorexia, and chills. The prodromal period precedes the onset of fever, pharyngitis, and lymphadenopathy. Occasionally, the disorder comes on abruptly with a high fever. The lymph nodes are typically enlarged throughout the body, particularly in the cervical, axillary, and groin areas. Palatal petechiae may be present in those with sore throat and lymphadenopathy.[15]

A generalized maculopapular rash has been reported in 3% to 15% of people. The rash often follows treatment with β-lactam antibiotics.[16]

Complications

Splenomegaly occurs in approximately 50% to 60% of cases.[14] The spleen may be enlarged two to three times its normal size, and rupture of the spleen occurs in less than 0.5% of cases.[15] Hepatitis may also occur. These are thought to be immune-mediated. Other potential complications include myocarditis, upper airway obstruction, encephalitis, and hemolytic anemia.[15] Those who have X-linked lymphoproliferative syndrome have a higher risk of complications and are more likely to die from the infection.[15]

Blood testing includes the monospot and serologic testing. The monospot tests for heterophile antibodies, which are considered the hallmark of an EBV infection.[14] The development of the heterophile antibodies take time to develop, resulting in false-negatives early in the disease. An increase in IgM and IgG antibodies early in the disease are indicative of an EBV infection.

Most people with infectious mononucleosis recover without incident. The acute phase of the illness usually lasts for 2 to 3 weeks, after which recovery occurs rapidly. Some degree of debility and lethargy may persist for 2 to 3 months. Treatment is primarily symptomatic and supportive.

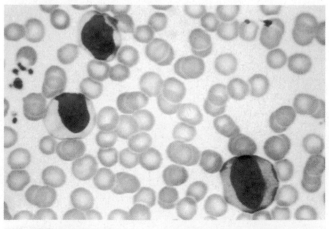

FIGURE 24-6. Infectious mononucleosis. An absolute lymphocytosis caused by a heterogeneous population of small and larger lymphoid cells, including atypical lymphocytes, is characteristic of the Epstein–Barr virus–driven disorder. (From Rubin R., Strayer D. E. (Eds.). (2015). *Rubin's pathology: Clinicopathologic foundations of medicine* (7th ed., Fig. 26-50, p. 1134). Philadelphia, PA: Lippincott Williams & Wilkins.)

 SUMMARY CONCEPTS

Neutropenia, which represents a marked reduction in the absolute number of neutrophils, is one of the major disorders of the white blood cells. It can occur as either a congenital or an acquired disorder. Congenital neutropenia consists primarily of cyclic neutropenia, which is characterized by cyclic (18- to 24-day) oscillations of peripheral neutrophils, and severe congenital neutropenia or Kostmann syndrome, which is associated with severe bacterial infections. The acquired neutropenias encompass a wide spectrum of causative processes, including immunologically mediated bone marrow suppression or neutrophil injury and destruction; infection-mediated mechanisms, including increased peripheral utilization; and drug-mediated mechanisms, particularly those related to the use of cancer chemotherapeutic agents. Neutropenia may also be caused by a number of bone marrow conditions, hematopoietic malignancies, and radiation therapy. Because the neutrophil is essential to host defenses against bacterial and fungal infections, severe and often life-threatening infections are common in people with neutropenia.

Infectious mononucleosis is a self-limited lymphoproliferative disorder caused by the B-lymphotropic EBV, a member of the herpesvirus family. The highest incidence of infectious mononucleosis is found in adolescents and young adults and is seen more frequently in the upper socioeconomic classes of developed countries. The virus is usually transmitted in the saliva. The disease is characterized by fever, generalized lymphadenopathy, sore throat, and the appearance in the blood of atypical lymphocytes and several antibodies, including the well-known heterophil antibodies that are used in the diagnosis of infectious mononucleosis. Most people with infectious mononucleosis recover without incident. Treatment is largely symptomatic and supportive.

Neoplastic Disorders of Lymphoid and Hematopoietic Origin

The neoplastic disorders of lymphoid origin represent the most important of the white blood cell disorders. The neoplasia of lymphoid origin can arise from both B and T cells as well as tumors representing various stages of lymphocyte development.[17,18] The major categories include non-Hodgkin lymphomas (NHLs), Hodgkin lymphoma (HL), lymphoid leukemias, and plasma cell dyscrasias. The clinical features of these neoplasms are largely determined by their cell of origin, the progenitor cell from which they originated, and the molecular events involved in their transformation into a malignant neoplasm. Because blood cells circulate throughout the body, these neoplasms are often disseminated from the onset.

Malignant Lymphomas

The lymphomas are a diverse group of solid tumors composed of neoplastic lymphoid cells that vary with respect to molecular features, genetics, clinical presentation, and treatment. NHL accounted 74,680 new cases and 19,910 deaths in the United States in 2018.[19]

Approximately 5% of cancers in children under 14 years of age are NHLs, including Burkitt lymphoma. HL accounts for 3%, occurring most often during adolescence.[19]

Non-Hodgkin Lymphomas

NHLs represent a clinically diverse group of B-cell, T-cell, or NK-cell origin. They represent about 4% of all new cases of cancer diagnosed in the United States.[19] The incidence of the disease has increased since the 1970s, and subtypes vary widely worldwide.[20] These variations are believed to occur because of environmental, genetic, and other unidentified factors.[20,21]

NHLs arise from the lymphocytes, and the site of their origination varies according to their common lymphoid progenitor.[22] Alterations in the developmental process of these cells can lead to any of the subtypes of lymphoid neoplasm with varying characteristics.[22] The exact cause of the alterations is unknown; however, pathogens such as EBV, human T-lymphotropic virus 1, and *Helicobacter pylori* have been linked to specific subtypes.[18]

Characterization of NHLs include cellular morphology, immunophenotype, clinical symptoms, and level of aggression.[18–20,22,23] Differential diagnosis is important in treatment planning, as is disease staging, disease location, and the person's general health and history, including any previous treatments for cancers.[18,23] Staging is accomplished using the Ann Arbor system.

Mature B-Cell Lymphomas

B-cell lymphomas are the most common NHL subtype and originate either from the germinal center B or activated B cells that have exited the germinal centers.[18,20] More commonly diagnosed B-cell subtypes include follicular lymphoma, immunoblastic large cell lymphoma, and mantle cell lymphoma.[24]

Follicular lymphomas are derived from germinal center B cells and consist of a mixture of centroblasts and centrocytes (Fig. 24-7). Follicular lymphoma tumors resemble primary lymphoid follicles, secrete cytokines, induce T-cell exhaustion and apoptosis, and interact with resident T helper cells to promote their survival and proliferation.[25] Follicular lymphomas are usually indolent, and prognosis for long-term survival is good.[26] However, there is an increased risk for second cancers for those over 65 years, males, and those treated with radiation.[26] The lymphoma predominantly affects lymph nodes. Other sites of involvement include the spleen, bone marrow, peripheral blood, head and neck region, gastrointestinal tract, and skin. Over time, approximately one of three follicular lymphomas transforms into a fast-growing diffuse large B-cell lymphoma.[17]

Diffuse large B-cell lymphomas are a heterogeneous group of aggressive germinal or post–germinal center neoplasms. The disease occurs in all age groups but is most prevalent between the ages of 60 and 70 years. The cause of diffuse large B-cell lymphoma is unknown, but may involve EBV or HIV infections. It is a rapidly

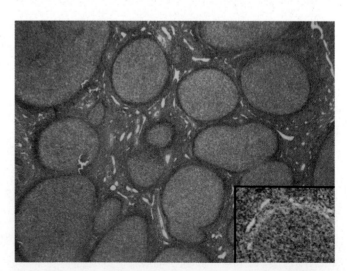

FIGURE 24-7. Follicular lymphoma. The normal lymph node architecture is replaced by malignant lymphoid follicles in a back-to-back pattern. The *inset* illustrates malignant lymphoid follicle germinal centers. (From Rubin R., Strayer D. E. (Eds.). (2015). *Rubin's pathology: Clinicopathologic foundations of medicine* (7th ed., Fig. 26-58, p. 1144). Philadelphia, PA: Lippincott Williams & Wilkins.)

evolving, multifocal, nodal, and extranodal tumor. Manifestations are typically seen at the time of presentation. As a group, diffuse large B-cell lymphomas are rapidly fatal if untreated.

Burkitt lymphoma, one of the most aggressive and rapidly growing tumors of the NHLs, is a disorder of germinal center B cells.[17] It is endemic in regions of Africa, where both EBV and malarial infection are common.[21] Virtually, 100% of people with African Burkitt lymphoma have evidence of previous EBV infection (Fig. 24-8).

Mantle cell lymphomas constitute less than 10% of NHLs and have their origin in the naive B cell. After the precursor stage, B cells undergo Ig gene rearrangements and develop into surface IgM- and IgD-positive naive B cells. These cells give rise to mantle cell lymphoma. Mantle cell lymphomas do not occur in children, but affect older people (median age, 60 years). They have a rapid rate of progression, and half of people do not tend to survive 3 years.

Marginal zone lymphoma (MZL) refers to related forms of NHL that affect B cells, including MALT, nodal MZL, and splenic MZL. MALT involves late-stage memory B cells that reside in the marginal zone or outermost compartment of the lymph node follicle. MALT lymphomas tend to remain localized for prolonged periods and to follow an indolent course. MALT develops in epithelial tissues of the gastrointestinal and respiratory tracts and remains localized. Prolonged inflammation promotes continued mutations. These additional mutations allow the tumor to become antigen independent and metastasize.[27]

Clinical Manifestations

The manifestations of NHL depend on lymphoma type (*i.e.*, indolent or aggressive) and the stage of the disease. People with indolent or slow-growing lymphomas usually present with painless lymphadenopathy, which may be isolated or widespread. Involved lymph nodes may be present in the retroperitoneum, mesentery, and pelvis. The indolent lymphomas are usually disseminated at the time of diagnosis, and bone marrow involvement is frequent. With or without treatment, the natural course of the disease may fluctuate 5 to 10 years or more. Many low-grade lymphomas eventually transform into more aggressive forms of lymphoma/leukemia.

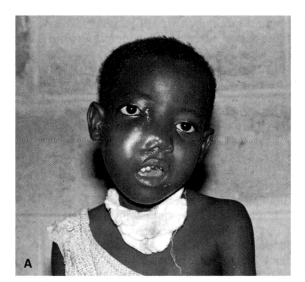
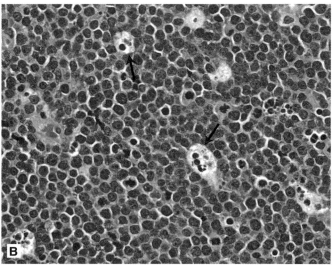
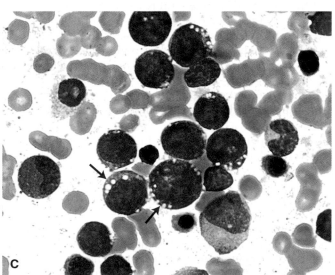

FIGURE 24-8. Burkitt lymphoma. (**A**) A tumor of the jaw distorts the child's face. (**B**) Lymph node is effaced by neoplastic lymphocytes with macrophages (see *arrows*), and (**C**) bone marrow aspiration illustrates typical cytologic features of Burkitt lymphoma (*arrows* indicate lipid vacuoles and basophilic cytoplasm). (From Rubin R., Strayer D. E. (Eds.). (2015). *Rubin's pathology: Clinicopathologic foundations of medicine* (7th ed., Fig. 26-64, p. 1149). Philadelphia, PA: Lippincott Williams & Wilkins.)

UNDERSTANDING ➡ The Hemodynamics of Blood Flow

1

Pressure, Resistance, and Flow. The flow (F) of fluid through a tube is directly related to a pressure difference $(P_1 - P_2)$ between the two ends of the tube and inversely proportional to the resistance (R) encountered.

The resistance to flow, peripheral resistance units (PRUs), is determined by blood viscosity, vessel radius, and if vessels are aligned in series or in parallel. In vessels aligned in series, resistance becomes additive (*e.g.*, 2 + 2 + 2 = 6 PRU). In vessels aligned in parallel, blood can travel through several parallel channels, and resistance becomes the reciprocal of the total resistance (*i.e.*, 1/R). There is no loss of pressure, and total resistance (*e.g.*, 1/2 + 1/2 + 1/2 = 3/2 PRU) is less than the resistance of any of the channels (*i.e.*, 2) taken separately.

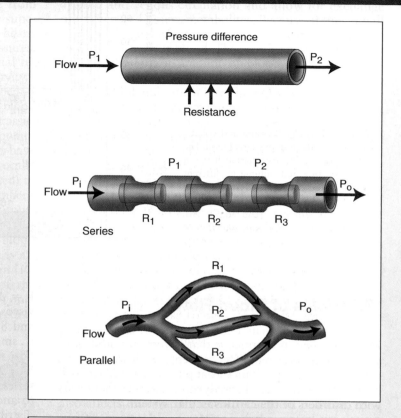

2

Vessel Radius. In addition to pressure and resistance, the rate of blood flow through a vessel is affected by the fourth power of its radius.

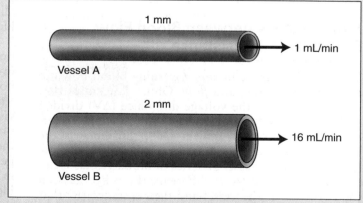

3

Cross-sectional Area and Velocity of Flow. The velocity of blood is affected by the cross-sectional area of a blood vessel. As cross-sectional area increases (sections 1 and 3), blood must flow laterally as well as forward to fill the increased area. As a result, mean forward velocity decreases. When the cross-sectional area is decreased (section 2), the lateral flow decreases and mean forward velocity is increased.

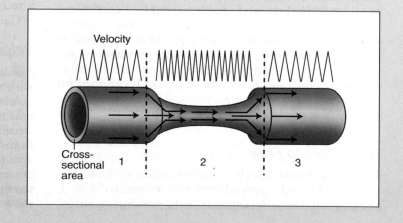

4

Laminar and Turbulent Flow.
Blood flow is laminar, a layered flow in which a thin layer of plasma adheres to the vessel wall and layers of blood cells and platelets shear against this motionless layer. Each layer moves at a slightly faster velocity, with the greatest velocity in the central part of the bloodstream.

Turbulent blood flow is when blood elements develop vortices that push blood cells and platelets against the vessel wall. More pressure is required to move blood through a vessel or valve when flow is turbulent rather than laminar. Turbulence can result from increased velocity of flow, decreased vessel diameter, or low blood viscosity. Turbulence is usually accompanied by vibrations of the fluid and surrounding structures, which may be detected as murmurs or bruits.

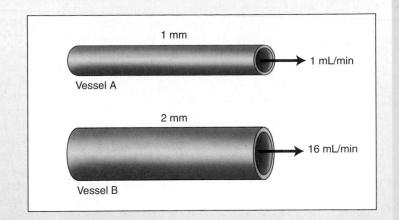

The linear velocity of blood flow in the circulatory system varies from 30 to 35 cm/second in the aorta to 0.2 to 0.3 mm/second in the capillaries. This is because although each individual capillary is small, the total cross-sectional area of all systemic capillaries exceeds the cross-sectional area of other parts of the circulation. The slower movement of blood allows time for exchange of nutrients, gases, and metabolites between tissues and blood.

Laminar versus Turbulent Flow

Ideally, blood flow is *laminar*, which means that blood components are arranged so that plasma is adjacent to the endothelial surface of the blood vessel, and the blood elements, including the platelets, are in the center of the bloodstream. The molecules that touch the side of the vessel wall move slower because of adherence to the wall.[1] This arrangement allows blood layers to slide smoothly over one another, and the middle layers have the most rapid rate of flow.

In turbulent flow, laminar stream is disrupted. Because energy is wasted in propelling blood radially and axially, more energy (pressure) is required to drive turbulent flow than laminar flow. Turbulent flow can be caused by high velocity of flow, change in diameter, obstruction, and low blood viscosity. Tendency for turbulence increases in proportion to velocity of flow.

Low blood viscosity allows for faster blood flow and accounts for transient heart murmurs in people who are severely anemic (decreased hematocrit). Vibrations of blood and surrounding structures often accompany turbulence and may be heard with a stethoscope (*e.g.*, heart murmur results from turbulent flow through a diseased heart valve that may be too narrow, stiff, or floppy).

Wall Tension, Radius, and Pressure

Wall tension is the force in the vessel wall that opposes distending pressure inside the vessel. The *law of Laplace* is expressed by $P = T/r$ (T is wall tension, P is intraluminal pressure, r is vessel radius).[3] Accordingly, P expands the vessel until it is balanced by T. The smaller the radius, the greater the pressure needed to balance the wall tension. The law of Laplace can also be used to express the effect of radius on wall tension ($T = P \times r$). The principle holds true for an arterial aneurysm, in which T and risk of rupture increase as the aneurysm (r) grows.

The law of Laplace can also include wall thickness ($T = P \times r$/wall thickness). T is inversely related to wall thickness: a thicker vessel wall results in lower tension. In hypertension, arterial vessel walls hypertrophy develops and becomes thicker, reducing the tension and minimizing wall stress.

The law of Laplace can be applied to the pressure required to maintain patency of small vessels. Provided that wall thickness is constant, it takes more pressure to overcome wall tension and keep a vessel open as its radius decreases. The *critical closing pressure* is the point at which blood vessels collapse. In circulatory shock, there is a decrease in blood volume and vessel radii and a drop in blood pressure. Many small blood vessels collapse as blood pressure drops. Collapse of peripheral veins makes it difficult to insert venous lines needed for fluid and blood replacement.

Distention and Compliance

Compliance is the quantity of blood that can be stored in a portion of circulation for each mm Hg rise in pressure. Compliance is the increase in volume divided by increase in pressure, or the ability of a vessel to distend and increase volume with increasing pressure. Veins are the most distensible vessels and can increase volume with only slight changes in pressure. Thus, veins store large quantities of blood that can be returned to circulation when needed. Vein compliance is 24 times that of its corresponding artery because it is 8× as distensible and has 3× the volume.

 SUMMARY CONCEPTS

The rate of blood flow is directly related to the pressure difference between the two ends of the vessel and the vessel radius and inversely related to vessel length and blood viscosity. As the cross-sectional area decreases, the velocity is increased and vice versa. Laminar blood flow is a flow in which there is layering of blood components in the center of the bloodstream, which reduces friction. Turbulent flow is disordered flow, in which the blood moves crosswise and lengthwise in blood vessels. The law of Laplace states that the pressure needed to overcome wall tension becomes greater as the radius decreases. Wall thickness also affects wall tension. It increases as the wall becomes thinner and decreases as the wall becomes thicker. Compliance of blood vessels refers to the total quantity of blood that can be stored in a given part of the circulatory system for each mm Hg rise in pressure.

The Systemic Circulation and Control of Blood Flow

Blood vessels are dynamic structures that constrict and relax to adjust blood pressure and flow to meet the varying needs of the many different tissue types and organ systems. Structures such as the heart, brain, liver, and kidneys require a large and continuous flow, whereas in other tissues, such as the skin and skeletal muscle, the need for blood flow varies with the level of function.

Blood Vessels

All blood vessels, except the capillaries, have walls composed of three *tunicae* (Fig. 25-12). The outermost layer, the *tunica externa* or *tunica adventitia*, is composed primarily of loosely woven collagen fibers that protect the blood vessel and anchor it to surrounding structures. The middle layer, the *tunica media*, is largely a smooth muscle layer that constricts to regulate the diameter of the vessel. Larger arteries have an external elastic lamina that separates the tunica media from the externa. The innermost layer, the *tunica intima*, consists of a single layer of flattened endothelial cells with minimal underlying subendothelial connective tissue. The endothelial layer provides a smooth inner surface that prevents platelet adherence and blood clotting.

Layers of different vessels vary with function. Walls of arterioles, which control blood pressure, have large amounts of smooth muscle. Veins are thin-walled, distensible, and collapsible vessels. Capillaries are single-cell–thick vessels designed for the exchange of gases, nutrients, and waste.

Vascular Smooth Muscle

Vascular smooth muscle cells form the predominant cellular layer in the tunica media and produce constriction or dilation of blood vessels. Smooth muscle contracts slowly and generates high forces for long periods with

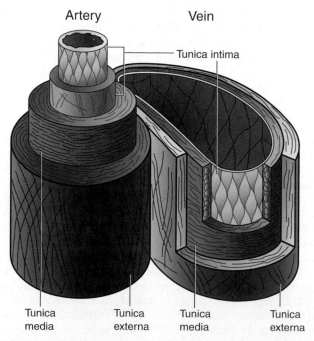

FIGURE 25-12. Medium-sized artery and vein showing the relative thicknesses of the three layers.

low energy requirements, which is important in structures, such as blood vessels, that must constantly maintain their tone.

Compared with skeletal and cardiac muscles, smooth muscle has less sarcoplasmic reticula for storing intracellular calcium and fewer fast sodium channels. Depolarization of smooth muscle relies largely on extracellular calcium, which enters through calcium channels in the muscle membrane. Sympathetic nervous system control of vascular smooth muscle tone occurs through receptor-activated opening and closing of calcium channels. In general, α-adrenergic receptors are excitatory and cause channels to open, producing vasoconstriction. β-Adrenergic receptors are inhibitory and cause channels to close, producing vasodilation. Calcium channel–blocking drugs cause vasodilation by blocking calcium entry through the calcium channels.

Smooth muscle contraction and relaxation also occur in response to local tissue factors such as lack of O_2, increased H^+ concentrations, and excess CO_2. Nitric oxide (NO) acts locally to produce smooth muscle relaxation and regulate blood flow…

KEY POINTS

The Vascular System and Control of Blood Flow

■ The vascular system, which consists of the arterial system (a high-pressure system delivering blood to tissues), the venous system (a low-pressure system that collects blood from the capillaries), and the capillaries, functions in the delivery of oxygen and nutrients and in the removal of wastes from the tissues.

■ Local control of blood flow is regulated by mechanisms that match blood flow to the metabolic needs of the tissue. Over the short term, tissues autoregulate flow through the synthesis of vasodilators and vasoconstrictors derived from the tissue, smooth muscle, or endothelial cells; over the long term, blood flow is regulated by creation of collateral circulation.

Arterial System

The arterial system consists of the large- and medium-sized arteries and the arterioles. Arteries are thick-walled vessels with large amounts of elastic fibers. The elasticity allows them to stretch during systole and to recoil during diastole. The arterioles, which are predominantly smooth muscle, serve as resistance vessels for the circulatory system. They act as control valves through which blood is released as it moves into the capillaries. The activity of sympathetic fibers that innervate these vessels causes them to constrict or to relax as needed to maintain blood pressure.

Arterial Pressure Pulsations

Delivery of blood to body tissues depends on pressure pulsations generated by the intermittent ejection of blood from the left ventricle into the distensible aorta and large arteries. The arterial pressure pulse is the energy transmitted from molecule to molecule along the length of the vessel (Fig. 25-13). In the aorta, this pressure pulse is transmitted at 4 to 6 m/second, 20 times faster than the flow of blood. Therefore, pressure pulse has no direct relation to blood flow and could occur if there was no flow. Pressure pulses are felt when taking a pulse and produce Korotkoff sounds heard during blood pressure measurement. Maximum deflection of the pressure pulsation coincides with systolic blood pressure, and the minimum point of deflection coincides with diastolic pressure. Pulse pressure is the difference between the systolic and diastolic pressure, and the magnitude of pulse pressure reflects the volume of blood ejected from the left ventricle per beat.

The pressure values and pressure wave change as it moves through the peripheral arteries, such that systolic pressure and pulse pressure in the large arteries are greater than those in the aorta (see Fig. 25-13). This increase in pulse pressure is because, immediately after ejection from the left ventricle, the pressure wave travels at a higher velocity than the blood itself, augmenting the downhill pressure. Furthermore, pressure points are reflected backward at branch points, which also augment pressure at those sites. With peripheral arterial disease, there is a delay in the transmission of the reflected wave and pulse decreases rather than increases in amplitude.

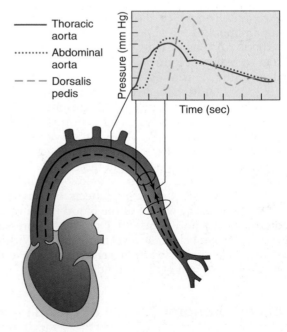

FIGURE 25-13. Amplification of the arterial pressure wave as it moves forward in the peripheral arteries. This amplification occurs as a forward-moving pressure wave merges with a backward-moving reflected pressure wave. **(Inset)** The amplitude of the pressure pulse increases in the thoracic aorta, abdominal aorta, and dorsalis pedis.

After its initial amplification, pressure pulse becomes smaller as it moves through arteries and arterioles, until it disappears almost entirely in the capillaries. The damping of pressure pulse is caused by the vessel's resistance and ability to distend. The increased resistance of small vessels impedes the transmission of the pressure waves, and their ability to distend is enough that any small change in flow does not cause a pressure change. Although pressure pulses are not usually transmitted to the capillaries, it may occur, for example, when injury results in a throbbing sensation. In this case, extreme dilation of small vessels in the injured area produces reduced dampening of the pressure pulse. Capillary pulsations also occur in conditions that cause exaggeration of aortic pressure pulses, such as aortic **regurgitation** or patent ductus arteriosus.

Venous System

The venous system is a low-pressure system. Venules collect blood from the capillaries, and veins transport blood to the right heart. Therefore, the pressure in the right atrium is the *central venous pressure*. Right atrial pressure is regulated by the ability of the right ventricle to pump blood into the lungs and the tendency of blood to flow from peripheral veins into the atrium. Normal right atrial pressure is 0 mm Hg (equal to atmospheric pressure). It can increase to 20 to 30 mm Hg in conditions such as right heart failure and transfusion of blood at a rate that greatly increases total blood volume and causes excess blood to attempt to flow into the heart.

Veins and venules are thin-walled, distensible, collapsible vessels. Veins are capable of enlarging and storing large quantities of blood. Although thin walled, veins are muscular, which allows them to accommodate varying amounts of blood. Veins are innervated by the sympathetic nervous system. When blood is lost, veins constrict to maintain intravascular volume.

Valves in the veins of extremities prevent retrograde flow (Fig. 25-14). With the help of skeletal muscles that surround and compress leg veins, blood is moved to the heart through one-way valves. This action is known as the *venous* or *muscle pump*. There are no valves in abdominal or thoracic veins, so pressure changes in these cavities cause venous blood flow in these veins.

Because the venous system is a low-pressure system, blood flow must oppose the effects of gravity. In a standing person, the weight of the blood in the vascular column causes an increase of 1 mm Hg in pressure for every 13.6 mm below the level of the heart. Without valves and skeletal muscle action, venous pressure in the feet would be +90 mm Hg in a standing adult.

Local and Humoral Control of Blood Flow

Tissue blood flow is regulated acutely in relation to tissue needs and longer term through development of collateral circulation. Neural mechanisms regulate the CO and blood pressure needed to support these local mechanisms.

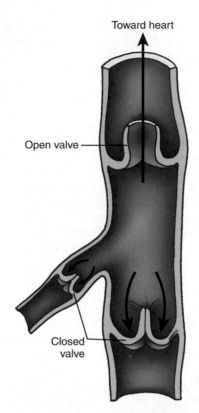

FIGURE 25-14. Portion of a femoral vein opened, to show the valves. The direction of flow is upward. Backward flow closes the valve.

Short-Term Autoregulation

Local control of blood flow is governed by the nutritional needs of the tissue, and blood flow to the heart, brain, and kidneys remains relatively constant despite blood pressure variations. The ability to maintain constant changes in perfusion pressure is *autoregulation* and is mediated by changes in vessel tone resulting from changes in flow or by local tissue factors, such as lack of oxygen or accumulation of metabolites. Changes in systemic arterial pressure (*e.g.*, hypotension in circulatory shock) lead to autoregulation in organs to ensure blood flow and oxygen delivery.

Reactive Hyperemia

An increase in local blood flow following a brief period of ischemia is *reactive hyperemia*. An increase in blood flow with increased activity, such as exercise, is *functional hyperemia*. When the blood supply to an area has been occluded and then restored, local blood flow increases within seconds to restore metabolic equilibrium. The transient redness seen after leaning on a hard surface is an example of reactive hyperemia. Local control mechanisms rely on continuous flow from the main arteries, so hyperemia cannot occur when arteries supplying the capillaries are narrowed. For example, if a major coronary artery becomes occluded, opening channels supplied by that vessel cannot restore blood flow.

Endothelial Control of Vascular Function

An important function of endothelial cells lining arterioles and small arteries is synthesis and release of factors that control vessel dilation. Intact endothelium produces

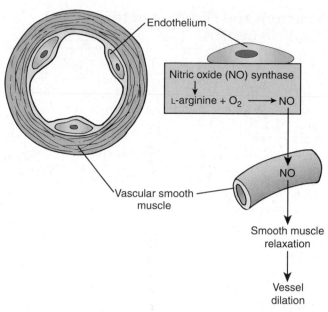

FIGURE 25-15. Function of nitric oxide in smooth muscle relaxation.

NO, which relaxes vascular smooth muscle. Normal endothelium maintains a continuous release of NO, which is formed from L-arginine and oxygen through via NO *synthase* (Fig. 25-15). NO production can be stimulated by a variety of endothelial *agonists*, including acetylcholine, bradykinin, histamine, and thrombin. *Shear stress* on the endothelium (from increased blood flow or blood pressure) also stimulates NO production and vessel relaxation. NO inhibits platelet aggregation and secretion of platelet contents, many of which cause vasoconstriction. NO is released into the vessel lumen (to inactivate platelets) and away from the lumen (to relax smooth muscle) and protects against both thrombosis and vasoconstriction. Nitroglycerin is used in the treatment of angina by causing release of NO in vascular smooth muscle of the target tissues.

Endothelium also produces a number of vasoconstrictor substances, including *angiotensin II*, vasoconstrictor prostaglandins, and *endothelin-1*. Endothelin-1 is present in all endothelial cells and requires very small amounts to cause vasoconstriction. After a blood vessel is damaged, local endothelin is released to vasoconstrict the vessel and prevent extensive bleeding.[2]

Long-Term Regulation of Blood Flow

Long-term regulation allows a more complete control of blood flow. *Angiogenesis* is the process of changing the amount of vascularity over a prolonged period. If tissue metabolism is increased for a long period of time, vascularity increases and vice versa. This regeneration is better in younger compared to older tissue. In addition, *vascular endothelial growth factor, fibroblast growth factor, and angiotensin* have been isolated in tissues that have insufficient blood supply. These growth factors cause new vessels to spring new growth. Blood vessels can also disappear due to other substances, such as *angiostatin* and *endostatin*.

Oxygen also plays a role in long-term blood flow regulation.[2,3] If the atmospheric oxygen is low, vascularity increases to compensate. This is seen in animals that live in higher altitude where oxygen levels are low.

Collateral circulation is also a mechanism for long-term regulation of local blood flow. In the heart and other vital structures, anastomotic channels exist between some smaller arteries that permit perfusion of an area by more than one artery. If one artery is occluded, anastomotic channels increase in size, allowing blood from a patent artery to perfuse the area. People with extensive obstruction of a coronary blood vessel may rely on collateral circulation to meet the oxygen needs of the myocardial tissue. As with other long-term compensatory mechanisms, the recruitment of collateral circulation is most efficient when obstruction to flow is gradual.

Humoral Control of Vascular Function

Humoral control of blood flow involves the effect of vasodilator and vasoconstrictor substances. Some are formed by glands and transported throughout the circulation. Others are formed in local tissues and aid in the local control of blood flow. Humoral factors include norepinephrine and epinephrine, angiotensin II, histamine, serotonin, bradykinin, and the prostaglandins.

Norepinephrine and Epinephrine

Norepinephrine is a powerful vasoconstrictor hormone. Epinephrine is less so and, in some tissues (*e.g.*, skeletal muscle), causes mild vasodilation. Stimulation of the sympathetic nervous system during stress or exercise causes local constriction of veins and arterioles because of the release of norepinephrine from sympathetic nerve endings. Sympathetic stimulation also causes the adrenal medullae to secrete norepinephrine and epinephrine into the blood. These then circulate in the blood, causing direct sympathetic stimulation of blood vessels in all parts of the body.

Angiotensin II

Angiotensin II is another powerful vasoconstrictor. Angiotensin II is produced as a part of the renin–angiotensin–aldosterone system and normally acts on arterioles to increase PVR, thereby increasing the arterial blood pressure.

Histamine

Histamine has a powerful vasodilator effect on arterioles and increases capillary permeability, allowing leakage of fluid and plasma proteins into tissues. Histamine is largely from mast cells in injured tissues and basophils in the blood. In certain tissues, the activity of mast cells is mediated by the sympathetic nervous system, which, when withdrawn, allows mast cells to release histamine.

Serotonin

Serotonin is liberated from aggregating platelets during the clotting process. It causes vasoconstriction and plays a major role in control of bleeding.

Bradykinin

The kinins (*i.e.*, kallidins and bradykinin) are liberated from the globulin kininogen. Bradykinin causes intense dilation of arterioles, increased capillary permeability, and constriction of venules.

Prostaglandins

Prostaglandins are synthesized from *arachidonic acid* in the cell membrane, which is released with tissue injury. There are several prostaglandins (*e.g.*, E_2, F_2, D_2), which are subgrouped according to their solubility. Those in the E group are vasodilators, and those in the F group are vasoconstrictors. The corticosteroid hormones produce an anti-inflammatory response by blocking the release of arachidonic acid, preventing prostaglandin synthesis.

SUMMARY CONCEPTS

The walls of all blood vessels, except the capillaries, are composed of three layers—tunica externa, tunica media, and tunica intima—which vary with vessel function. Arteries are thick-walled vessels with large amounts of elastic fibers. The walls of the arterioles, which control blood pressure, have large amounts of smooth muscle. Veins are thin-walled, distensible, and collapsible vessels. Venous flow returns blood to the heart. It is a low-pressure system and relies on valves and muscle pumps to offset the effects of gravity.

The delivery of blood to the tissues of the body depends on pressure pulses generated by the intermittent ejection of blood from the left ventricle into the distensible aorta and large arteries of the arterial system. The arteries' ability to distend and their resistance to flow reduce pressure pulsations so that constant blood flow occurs by the time blood reaches the capillaries.

Mechanisms to control local blood flow ensure adequate delivery of blood to the capillaries in the microcirculation, where exchange of cellular nutrients and wastes occurs. Local control is governed largely by tissue needs and is regulated by local factors such as lack of oxygen and accumulation of metabolites. Reactive hyperemia is a local increase in blood flow that occurs after temporary occlusion of blood flow. It is a compensatory mechanism that decreases oxygen debt of deprived tissues. Long-term regulation of blood flow includes angiogenesis, vascular endothelial growth factor, fibroblast growth factor, and angiotensin, which increase tissue vascularity, where angiostatin and endostatin dissolve blood vessels. Collateral circulation improves local blood flow.[2,3] NO and humoral factors contribute to regulation of blood flow.

The Microcirculation and Lymphatic System

Microcirculation is the functions of the smallest blood vessels, the capillaries, and lymphatic vessels, which transport nutrients to tissues and remove wastes from cells.

Structure and Function of the Microcirculation

The structures of the microcirculation include the arterioles, capillaries, and venules. Blood enters the microcirculation through an arteriole, passes through metarterioles and capillaries, and leaves through a venule (Fig. 25-16). Small cuffs of smooth muscle, precapillary sphincters, are positioned at the arterial end of the capillary. The smooth muscle tone of the arterioles, venules, and precapillary sphincters control blood flow through the capillary bed. Depending on venous pressure, blood flows through capillary channels when precapillary sphincters are open.

Capillary Structure and Function

Capillaries are microscopic vessels that connect arterial and venous segments. There are about 10 billion capillaries in a person, with a total surface area of 500 to 700 m.² Capillary walls are composed of a single layer of endothelial cells and their basement membrane (Fig. 25-17). Endothelial cells form a tube just large enough to allow passage of red blood cells, one at a time.

Water-filled junctions (*capillary pores*) join capillary endothelial cells and provide a path for passage of substances. Pore size varies with capillary function. In the brain, endothelial cells are joined by tight junctions to form the blood–brain barrier, which prevents substances that would alter neural excitability from leaving the capillary. In organs that process blood contents, such as the liver, capillaries have large pores so that substances can pass easily. Glomerular capillaries in the kidney have small openings (*fenestrations*) that pass through the middle of the endothelial cells. This allows large amounts of small molecular and ionic substances to filter through the glomeruli without having to pass through the clefts between the endothelial cells.

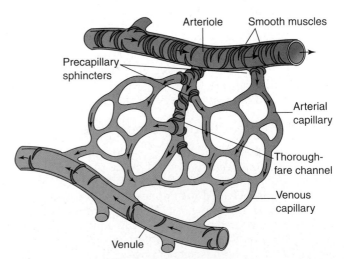

FIGURE 25-16. Capillary bed. Precapillary sphincters control the flow of blood through the capillary network. Thoroughfare channels (*i.e.*, arteriovenous shunts) allow blood to move directly from the arteriole into the venule without moving through nutrient channels of the capillary.

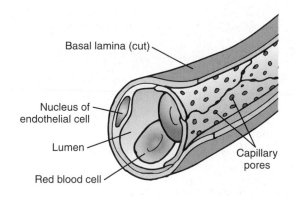

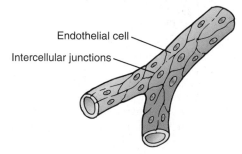

FIGURE 25-17. Endothelial cells and intercellular junctions in a section of the capillary.

Because of their thin walls and close proximity to cells of metabolically active tissues, the capillaries are well suited for the exchange of gases and metabolites between cells and the bloodstream. This exchange occurs through spaces between tissue cells called the *interstitium*, which is supported by *collagen* and *elastin* fibers and filled with *proteoglycan* (sugar–protein) molecules that combine with water to form a tissue gel. The tissue gel traps the interstitial fluid and provides for distribution of the fluid, even to those cells that are most distant from the capillary.

Exchange of gases and fluids across the capillary wall occurs by simple diffusion. Lipid-soluble substances, such as oxygen and carbon dioxide, readily exchange across the endothelial cells by diffusion. Water flows through endothelial cell membranes via *aquaporins*. Water and water-soluble substances, such as electrolytes, glucose, and amino acids, diffuse between endothelial cells in capillary pores. Pinocytosis moves white blood cells and large protein molecules.

Control of Blood Flow in the Microcirculation

Nutrient flow is blood flow through capillary channels designed for exchange of nutrients and metabolites. In some areas, blood flow bypasses the capillary bed, moving through an *arteriovenous shunt*, which directly connects an arteriole and a venule. This type of blood flow is called *non-nutrient flow* because it does not allow for nutrient exchange. Non-nutrient channels are common in the skin and are important for heat exchange and temperature regulation.

Capillary–Interstitial Fluid Exchange

The hydrostatic and osmotic pressures of the capillary and interstitial fluids and the permeability of the capillary wall largely control the direction and magnitude of fluid movement across the capillary wall. *Filtration* is net fluid movement out of the capillary into the interstitial spaces. Absorption is net movement from the interstitium into the capillary (Fig. 25-18).

Capillary hydrostatic pressure is the fluid pressure that pushes water and its dissolved substances through capillary pores into the interstitium. Osmotic pressure caused by plasma proteins pulls fluid from interstitial spaces back into the capillary (*colloidal osmotic pressure*). Capillary permeability controls movement of water and substances into the interstitial spaces. The lymphatic system removes excess fluid, osmotically active proteins and large particles from the interstitial spaces and returns them to circulation.

Hydrostatic Forces

Capillary hydrostatic pressure is the principal force in capillary filtration. Both the arterial and venous pressures determine hydrostatic pressure within the capillaries. An increase in small artery and arterial pressure elevates capillary hydrostatic pressure. A change in venous pressure has a greater effect on capillary hydrostatic pressure than the same change in arterial pressure. About 80% of increased venous pressure, such as that due to venous thrombosis or congestive heart failure, is transmitted back to the capillary. Gravity also affects capillary hydrostatic pressure: when a person stands, hydrostatic pressure is greater in the legs and lower in the head.

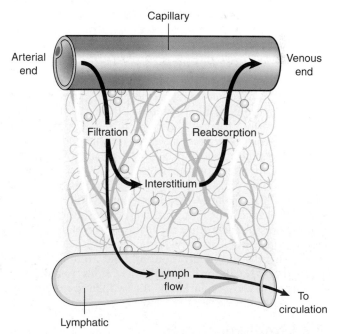

FIGURE 25-18. Capillary filtration and lymph flow. Fluid is filtered out of the capillary and into the interstitium at the arterial end of the capillary. Most of the fluid is reabsorbed at the venous end of the capillary, with the rest of the fluid entering the terminal lymphatics for return to the circulation.

Interstitial hydrostatic pressure is the pressure exerted by interstitial fluids outside the capillary. A positive interstitial fluid pressure opposes capillary filtration, and a negative interstitial fluid pressure increases the movement of fluid out of the capillary into the interstitium. In the normal nonedematous state, the interstitial hydrostatic pressure is close to zero or slightly negative (−1 to −4 mm Hg) and has little effect on capillary filtration or outward movement of fluid.

Osmotic Forces

The key factor that restrains fluid loss from the capillaries is colloidal osmotic pressure (28 mm Hg) generated by plasma proteins. Because the capillary membrane is almost impermeable to plasma proteins, these particles exert an osmotic force that pulls fluid into the capillary and offsets the pushing of capillary filtration pressure. Plasma proteins include albumin, globulins, and fibrinogen. Albumin is the smallest and most abundant and accounts for 70% of the total osmotic pressure. It is the number of the particles in solution that controls osmotic pressure.

Although the size of the capillary pores prevents most proteins from leaving the capillary, small amounts escape into interstitial spaces and exert an osmotic force that pulls fluid from the capillary into the interstitium. This is increased in conditions such as inflammation in which an increase in capillary permeability allows plasma proteins to escape into the interstitium. The lymphatic system is responsible for removing proteins from the interstitium. In the absence of a functioning lymphatic system, interstitial colloidal osmotic pressure increases, causing fluid to accumulate. Normally, a few white blood cells, plasma proteins, and other large molecules enter the interstitial spaces. These are too large to reenter the capillary and rely on the loosely structured wall of the lymphatic vessels for return to the vascular compartment.

Balance of Hydrostatic and Osmotic Forces

Movement of fluid between the capillary bed and interstitial spaces is continuous. Equilibrium exists as long as equal amounts of fluid enter and leave the interstitial spaces ("Starling forces" illustrated in Fig. 25-19). In the diagram, hydrostatic pressure at the arterial end is higher than at the venous end.[5,6] The pushing force of capillary hydrostatic pressure on the arterial end of the capillary and the pulling effects of the interstitial colloidal osmotic pressure allow net outward movement of fluid. The capillary colloidal osmotic pressure and opposing interstitial osmotic pressure determine the reabsorption of fluid at the venous end of the capillary. A slight imbalance in forces causes slightly more filtration of fluid into interstitial spaces than absorption back into the capillary. This fluid is returned to the circulation by the lymphatic system.

The Lymphatic System

The lymphatic system is an accessory route through which fluid can flow into the blood from interstitial spaces.[3] This system serves almost all body tissues,

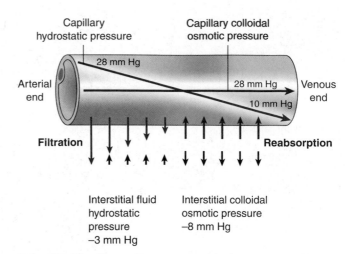

FIGURE 25-19. Capillary–interstitial fluid exchange equilibrium. Normally, the forces (capillary hydrostatic pressure, interstitial colloidal osmotic pressure, and the opposing interstitial fluid pressure) that control the outward movement of fluid from the capillary (filtration) are almost balanced by the forces (capillary colloidal osmotic pressure and interstitial colloidal osmotic pressure) that pull fluid back into the capillary (reabsorption).

except the cartilage, bone, epithelial tissue, and tissues of the central nervous system (CNS). Most of these tissues have prelymphatic channels that eventually flow into areas supplied by the lymphatics. Lymph contains plasma proteins and other osmotically active particles that rely on the lymphatics for movement back into the circulatory system. The lymphatic system is also

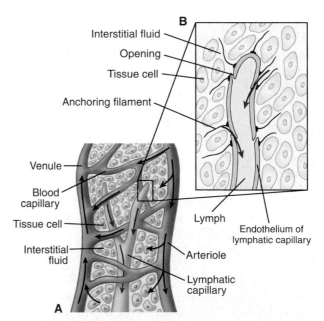

FIGURE 25-20. (A) Location of the lymphatic capillary. Fluid from the arterial side of the capillary bed moves into the interstitial spaces and is reabsorbed in the venous side of the capillary bed. (B) Details of the lymphatic capillary with its anchoring filaments and overlapping edges that serve as valves and can be pushed open, allowing the inflow of interstitial fluid and its suspended particles.

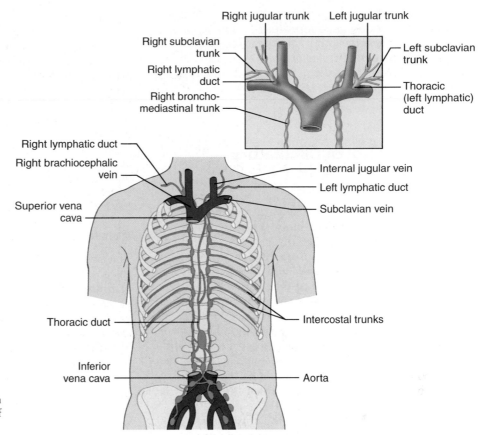

FIGURE 25-21. Lymphatic system showing the thoracic duct and position of the left and right lymphatic ducts (**inset**).

the main route for absorption of nutrients, particularly fats, from the gastrointestinal tract. The lymphatic system also filters the fluid at lymph nodes and removes foreign particles such as bacteria. When lymph flow is obstructed, *lymphedema* occurs. Involvement of lymphatic structures by malignant tumors and removal of lymph nodes with surgery are common causes of lymphedema.

The lymphatic system is made up of vessels similar to those of the circulatory system. These vessels travel along with an arteriole or a venule or with its companion artery and vein. Terminal lymphatic vessels are made up of a single layer of connective tissue with an endothelial lining and resemble blood capillaries. Lymphatic vessels lack tight junctions and are loosely anchored to surrounding tissues by fine filaments (Fig. 25-20). The loose junctions permit entry of large particles, and filaments hold the vessels open under conditions of edema when the pressure of the surrounding tissues would otherwise cause them to collapse. The lymph capillaries drain into larger lymph vessels that empty into the right and left thoracic ducts (Fig. 25-21). The thoracic ducts empty into the circulation at the junctions of the subclavian and internal jugular veins. The total amount of lymph normally transported is 2 to 3 L/day.[2]

Although the divisions are not as distinct as in the circulatory system, larger lymph vessels show evidence of intimal, medial, and adventitial layers similar to blood vessels. The intima of these channels contains elastic tissue and an endothelial layer, and the larger collecting lymph channels contain smooth muscle in their medial layer. Contraction of this smooth muscle assists in propelling lymph toward the thorax. External compression of lymph channels by pulsating blood vessels in the vicinity and active and passive movements of body parts aid in forward propulsion of lymph. The interstitial fluid pressure and activity of lymph pumps determine the rate of flow (approximately 120 mL/hour) through the lymphatic system via all of the lymph channels.

SUMMARY CONCEPTS

Exchange of fluids between the vascular compartment and the interstitial spaces occurs at the capillary level. Capillary hydrostatic pressure pushes fluids out of the capillaries, and colloidal osmotic pressure exerted by the plasma proteins pulls fluids back into the capillaries. Albumin, which is the smallest and most abundant plasma protein, provides the major osmotic force for return of fluid to the vascular compartment. Normally, slightly more fluid leaves the capillary bed than can be reabsorbed. This excess fluid is returned to circulation via lymphatic channels.

Neural Control of Circulatory Function

The neural control centers for integration and modulation of cardiac function and blood pressure are in the medulla oblongata. There are three distinct groups of medullary cardiovascular neurons that provide sympathetic innervation of the heart and blood vessels and parasympathetic innervation of the heart. The first two, the *vasomotor center*, control sympathetic-mediated acceleration of HR and blood vessel tone. The third, the *cardioinhibitory* center, controls parasympathetic-mediated slowing of HR. These centers receive information from many areas of the nervous system. Arterial baroreceptors and chemoreceptors provide the medullary cardiovascular center with continuous information regarding changes in blood pressure.

Autonomic Nervous System Regulation

Circulatory system neural control occurs primarily through *sympathetic* and *parasympathetic* divisions of the autonomic nervous system (ANS). The ANS modulates cardiac (*i.e.*, HR and cardiac contractility) and vascular (*i.e.*, PVR) functions.

Autonomic Regulation of Cardiac Function

Parasympathetic innervation of the heart is achieved by the *vagus nerve*. Parasympathetic outflow to the heart originates from the vagal nucleus in the medulla. Axons of these neurons pass to the heart in the cardiac branches of the vagus nerve. The effect of vagal stimulation on heart function is largely limited to HR: increased vagal activity slows the pulse through the release of acetylcholine. Sympathetic outflow to the heart and blood vessels arises from neurons in the reticular formation of the brain stem. Axons of these neurons exit the thoracic segments of the spinal cord to synapse with the postganglionic neurons that innervate the heart. Cardiac sympathetic fibers are widely distributed to SA and AV nodes and the myocardium. Increased sympathetic activity produces increased HR and velocity and force of cardiac contraction.

Autonomic Regulation of Vascular Function

The sympathetic nervous system is the final common pathway for controlling the smooth muscle tone of blood vessels. Most sympathetic preganglionic fibers that control vessel function originate in the vasomotor center of the brain stem, travel down the spinal cord, and exit in the thoracic and lumbar segments. Sympathetic neurons maintain blood vessels in a state of tonic activity so that blood vessels are partially constricted even under resting conditions. Constriction and relaxation are accomplished by altering this basal input. Increasing sympathetic activity causes constriction of some vessels, such as those of the skin, gastrointestinal tract, and kidneys. Blood vessels in skeletal muscle are supplied by both vasoconstrictor and vasodilator fibers. Activation of sympathetic vasodilator fibers causes vessel relaxation and provides muscles with increased blood flow during exercise. Although the parasympathetic nervous system contributes to the regulation of heart function, it has little or no control over blood vessels.

Autonomic Neurotransmitters

The actions of the ANS are mediated by chemical neurotransmitters. *Acetylcholine* is the postganglionic neurotransmitter for parasympathetic neurons, and *norepinephrine* is the main neurotransmitter for postganglionic sympathetic neurons. Sympathetic neurons also respond to epinephrine, which is released into the bloodstream by the adrenal medulla. The neurotransmitter *dopamine* can also act as a neurotransmitter for some sympathetic neurons.

Central Nervous System Responses

The CNS, which plays an essential role in regulating vasomotor tone and blood pressure, has a mechanism for controlling blood flow to the brain centers that control circulatory function. When interruption of blood flow to the brain causes ischemia of the vasomotor center, these vasomotor neurons become strongly excited. This causes massive vasoconstriction to raise blood pressure to levels as high as the heart can pump against. This is called the *CNS ischemic response* and can raise blood pressure to levels as high as 270 mm Hg for as long as 10 minutes.[1] It does not become activated until blood pressure has fallen to at least 60 mm Hg, and it is most effective in the range of 15 to 20 mm Hg. If the cerebral circulation is not reestablished within 3 to 10 minutes, the neurons of the vasomotor center cease to function. As a result, the tonic impulses to the blood vessels stop and the blood pressure falls precipitously.

The *Cushing reaction* is a CNS response resulting from increase in intracranial pressure.[1,3] When intracranial pressure rises to levels that equal intra-arterial pressure, blood vessels to the vasomotor center become compressed, initiating the CNS ischemic response. This reflex produces a rise in arterial pressure to levels above intracranial pressure to reestablish blood flow to the vasomotor center. Should intracranial pressure rise to the point that blood supply to the vasomotor center becomes inadequate, vasoconstrictor tone is lost, and the blood pressure begins to fall. The elevation in blood pressure associated with the Cushing reflex is usually of short duration and helps protect the vital centers of the brain from nutrition loss if the CNS fluid rises high enough to compress the cerebral arteries.[3] The brain and other cerebral structures are located within the rigid confines of the skull, with no room for expansion. Therefore, any increase in intracranial pressure tends to compress the blood vessels that supply the brain.

 SUMMARY CONCEPTS

Neural control centers for the regulation of cardiac function and blood pressure are located in the reticular formation of the lower pons and medulla of the brain stem, where the integration and modulation of ANS responses occur. These brain stem centers receive information from many areas of the nervous system, including the hypothalamus. The parasympathetic and sympathetic nervous systems innervate the heart. The parasympathetic nervous system functions in regulating HR through the vagus nerve, with increased vagal activity slowing the HR. The sympathetic nervous system has an excitatory influence on HR and contractility and serves as the final common pathway for controlling the smooth muscle tone of the blood vessels.

Review Exercises

1. In people with atherosclerosis of the coronary arteries, symptoms of myocardial ischemia do not usually occur until the vessel has been 75% occluded.

   A. Use the Poiseuille law to explain.

2. Once an arterial aneurysm has begun to form, it continues to enlarge as the result of the increased tension in its wall.

   A. Explain the continued increase in size using the law of Laplace.
   B. Using information related to cross-sectional area and velocity of flow, explain why there is stasis of blood flow with the tendency to form clots in aneurysms with a large cross-sectional area.

3. Use events in the cardiac cycle depicted in Figure 25-10 to explain:

   A. The effect of hypertension on the isovolumetric contraction period.
   B. The effect of an increase in HR on the time spent in diastole.
   C. The effect of an increase in the isovolumetric relaxation period on the diastolic filling of the ventricle.

4. Use the Frank-Starling ventricular function curve depicted in Figure 25-11 to explain the changes in CO that occur with changes in respiratory effort.

   A. What happens to CO during increased inspiratory effort in which a marked decrease in intrathoracic pressure produces an increase in venous return to the right heart?
   B. What happens to CO during increased expiratory effort in which a marked increase in intrathoracic pressure produces a decrease in venous return to the right heart?
   C. Given these changes in CO that occur during increased respiratory effort, what would you propose as one of the functions of the Frank-Starling curve?

REFERENCES

1. St. John S., Cerkvenic J., Borlaug B., et al. (2015). Effects of cardiac resynchronization therapy on cardiac remodeling and contractile function: Results from resynchronization reverses remodeling in systolic left ventricular dysfunction (REVERSE). *Journal of the American Heart Association* 4(9), 1–9.
2. Mohrman D., Heller L. (2010). *Cardiovascular physiology* (7th ed.). New York: McGraw-Hill.
3. Guyton A., Hall J. E. (2011). *Textbook of medical physiology* (12th ed., pp. 157–189, 191–211). Philadelphia, PA: Saunders.
4. Freeman W., Kobayashi Y. (2016). Invasive assessment of the coronary microcirculation. *JACC: Cardiovascular Interventions* 25(9), 802–804.
5. Yolmaz-Erol A., Atasever B., Mathura K., et al. (2007). Cardiac resynchronization improves microcirculation. *Journal of Cardiac Failure* 13(2), 95–99.
6. Brunner L. S., Suddarth D. S., Smeltzer S. O., et al. (2018). *Brunner and Suddarth's textbook of medical-surgical nursing* (14th ed., p. 678). Philadelphia, PA: Lippincott.

Disorders of Blood Flow and Blood Pressure Regulation

Learning Objectives

After completing this chapter, the learner will be able to meet the following objectives:

1. Describe the functions of the endothelial cells and define the term *endothelial dysfunction*.
2. Describe the function of vascular smooth muscle and its role in vascular repair.
3. Define the terms *systolic blood pressure, diastolic blood pressure, pulse pressure,* and *mean arterial blood pressure*.

4. Explain how cardiac output and peripheral vascular resistance interact in determining systolic and diastolic blood pressure.
5. Describe possible mechanisms involved in the development of atherosclerosis.
6. Describe the pathology associated with the vasculitides and relate it to disease conditions associated with vasculitis.
7. Distinguish between the pathology and manifestations of aortic aneurysms and dissection of the aorta.
8. Describe venous return of blood from the lower extremities, including the function of the muscle pumps and the effects of gravity, and relate this to the development of varicose veins.
9. Characterize the pathology of venous insufficiency and relate this to the development of stasis dermatitis and venous ulcers.
10. List the four most common causes of lower leg ulcer.
11. Define hypertension and identify the blood pressure limits that are used clinically to identify the presence of hypertension.
12. Describe how hypertension contributes to target-organ damage. Identify the organs most commonly affected by target-organ damage and discuss the pathophysiologic changes.
13. Describe the four types of hypertension that can occur during pregnancy.
14. Define the term *orthostatic hypotension*.
15. Describe the cardiovascular, neurohumoral, and muscular responses that serve to maintain blood pressure when moving from the supine to standing position.
16. Explain how fluid deficit, medications, aging, disorders of the autonomic nervous system, and bed rest contribute to the development of orthostatic hypotension.

Blood flow requires a system of patent blood vessels and adequate perfusion pressure. Structural disorders of arteries and arterioles decrease blood flow to the tissues, causing impaired delivery of oxygen and nutrients and accumulation of waste. Venous structural disorders interfere with blood outflow from capillary beds, trapping fluid, and cellular waste products in the tissues.

Blood pressure is highly variable and must be carefully regulated. Assuring constant blood flow to vital organs such as the heart, brain, and kidneys is essential to life. While a critical decrease in blood flow (hypotension) can produce an immediate threat to life, continuous elevation (hypertension) contributes to premature death and disability because of damage to blood vessels.

Blood Vessel Structure and Function

The walls of all blood vessels, except the capillaries, are composed of a *tunica externa*, *tunica media*, and *tunica intima* (Fig 26-1). Thin capillaries consist of a single layer of endothelial cells surrounded intermittently by *pericytes*. Pericytes share some characteristics with

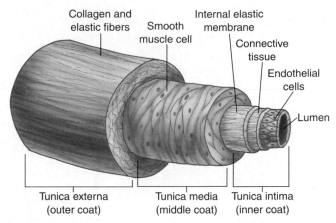

FIGURE 26-1. Diagram of a typical artery showing the tunica externa, tunica media, and tunica intima.

smooth muscle cells (SMCs).[1] Figure 26-2 illustrates the comparative microanatomy of veins, arteries, and capillaries. Table 26-1 describes the structure and function of the blood vessels.

Endothelium

The *endothelium* is 60,000 miles of specialized squamous epithelial cells that form a continuous, semipermeable lining for the vascular system.[2] It is essential for homeostatic functions such as transfer across the vascular wall, platelet adhesion, blood clotting, modulation of blood flow and vascular resistance, metabolism of hormones, regulation of immune and inflammatory reactions, and elaboration of factors that influence cell growth (particularly vascular SMCs).[3]

Endothelial cells respond to various stimuli by structural and functional alterations, described as *endothelial dysfunction*. This can be caused by factors such as inflammation, hemodynamic stress, certain lipid molecules, and hypoxia. Dysfunctional endothelial cells secrete a variety of biologically active products. They also influence the reactivity of underlying SMCs through production of both relaxing factors (*e.g.*, NO) and contracting factors (*e.g.*, endothelins).[1,2]

Vascular Smooth Muscle Cells

Vascular SMCs in the tunica media constrict and dilate blood vessels in response to hormonal and neural stimulation (particularly in response to the sympathetic branch of the autonomic nervous system [ANS]). Norepinephrine diffuses into the tunica media. Action potentials are then propagated along SMCs through gap junctions, causing contraction of the muscle layer and reducing lumen radius, which increases the resistance to flow through the vessel.[2]

Vascular SMCs also synthesize biologic molecules such as collagen, elastin, growth factors, and cytokines. When injured, SMCs migrate into the tunica intima and proliferate.[1] SMCs are important in normal vascular repair and

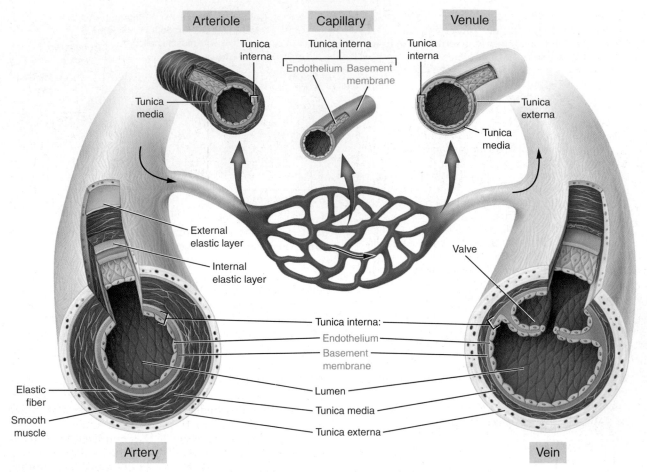

FIGURE 26-2. Blood vessels—microanatomy of the artery, vein, and capillary beds. (From McConnell T. H., Hull K. L. (2011). *Human form, human function: Essentials of anatomy & physiology* (Figure 11-12, p. 433). Philadelphia, PA: Wolters Kluwer/Lippincott Williams & Wilkins.)

TABLE 26-1. Structure and Function of the Blood Vessels

Vessel	Structure	Function
Artery	Three-layered wall with thick tunica media, which gives it the properties of contractility and elasticity	Transport of blood away from the heart, maintenance of blood pressure
Arteriole	Three-layered wall, with much thinner layers and smaller lumen than in arteries	Transport of blood away from the heart, help control blood pressure by regulation of peripheral resistance through vasoconstriction and vasodilation
Capillary	Microscopic size with single-layered wall of endothelium	Thin walls permit the exchange of materials between the blood and interstitial fluid
Venule	Three-layered wall with very thin layers, which gradually enlarge as they near the heart	Transport of blood from capillary beds toward the heart
Vein	Three-layered wall, with thinner tunica media and larger lumen than in arteries. Include internal valves to aid in the unidirectional flow of blood toward the heart	Transport of blood from venules toward the heart

From Wingerd B. (2014). The human body: Concepts of anatomy and physiology. Philadelphia, PA: Lippincott Williams & Wilkins.

in pathologic processes such as atherosclerosis. Growth promoters (*i.e.*, platelet-derived growth factor and thrombin) and inhibitors (*i.e.*, nitric oxide) stimulate the migratory and proliferative activities of vascular SMCs.[3,4]

SUMMARY CONCEPTS

With the exception of capillaries, blood vessels walls are composed of three layers. Capillaries are composed a single layer of endothelial cells. Vascular endothelial cells control the transfer of molecules across capillary walls and are actively involved in modulating the processes of platelet adhesion and coagulation and in regulating blood flow and vascular resistance. Endothelial cells also play a role in regulating immune and inflammatory reactions and elaborating factors that are important in both normal vascular repair and pathologic processes. *Endothelial dysfunction* is potentially reversible changes in function that occurs in response to environmental stimuli.

Regulation of Systemic Arterial Blood Pressure

Blood pressure rises during systole (as the left ventricle contracts) and falls as the heart relaxes during diastole. The arterial pressure tracing (Fig. 26-3) illustrates pressure

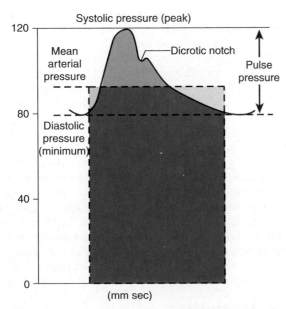

FIGURE 26-3. Intra-arterial pressure tracing made from the brachial artery. Pulse pressure is the difference between systolic and diastolic pressure. The darker area represents the mean arterial pressure, which can be calculated using the formula: mean arterial pressure = diastolic pressure + pulse pressure/3.

changes within the large arteries of systemic circulation. A rapid upstroke in pulse occurs during left ventricular contraction, followed by a slower rise to the peak blood pressure. Seventy percent of blood that leaves the left ventricle is ejected during the first third of systole, accounting for the rapid rise in pressure. The end of systole is marked by a brief downward deflection and the *dicrotic notch*: the point at which ventricular pressure falls below aortic pressure and triggers sudden closure of the aortic valve. This leads to a small rise in intra-aortic pressure resulting from continued contraction of the aorta and other large vessels against the closed aortic valve. As ventricles relax and blood flows into the peripheral vessels during diastole, the arterial pressure falls rapidly at first, then declines more slowly as the driving force decreases.[3]

The pressure at the height of the pressure pulse (*systolic pressure*) ideally is less than 120 mm Hg in adults, with the lowest pressure (*diastolic pressure*) less than 80 mm Hg (Fig. 26-3). The difference between pressures (40 mm Hg in healthy adults) is the *pulse pressure*. Two major factors affect the magnitude of pulse pressure—volume of blood ejected from the left ventricle during a beat (*stroke volume or SV*) and the degree of distensibility within the arterial tree (reflecting the ability of arterial vasculature to accept ejected blood). Arterial distensibility is determined by the (1) elastic properties of the aorta and large arteries and (2) degree of resistance to flow into smaller vessels. *Mean arterial pressure (MAP)*, which is 90 to 100 mm Hg in adults, is the average pressure in the arterial system during ventricular contraction and relaxation. MAP is an indicator of tissue perfusion and is 60% of diastolic pressure and 40% of systolic pressure.[3]

The components of *cardiac output* (CO) are SV and *heart rate* (HR): CO = SV × HR. MAP can be expressed as: MAP = CO × PVR. *Peripheral vascular resistance* (PVR) reflects changes in arteriole radius and viscosity of the blood. Arterioles are referred to as *resistance vessels*: they constrict or relax to control resistance to outflow of blood into the capillaries. The body maintains blood pressure by (a) adjusting CO to compensate for changes in PVR and (b) adjusting PVR to compensate for CO changes.[3]

Mechanisms of Blood Pressure Regulation

Although some tissues can autoregulate blood flow, it is necessary for arterial pressure to remain relatively constant to ensure adequate tissue perfusion[3] (see Fig. 26-4).

Acute Regulation

Acute regulation of blood pressure (seconds to minutes) is necessary to correct temporary imbalances and during life-threatening situations. Acute blood pressure control relies mainly on neural and humoral mechanisms, with neural mechanisms producing the most rapid response.[3]

Neural Mechanisms

The neural control centers for blood pressure regulation are in the reticular formation of the medulla and

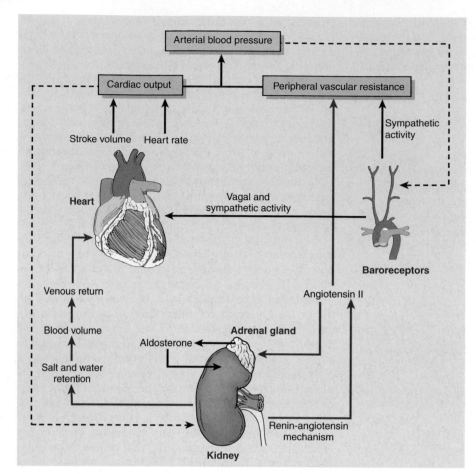

FIGURE 26-4. Mechanisms of blood pressure regulation. The *solid lines* represent the mechanisms for renal and baroreceptor control of blood pressure through changes in CO and PVR. The *dashed lines* represent the stimulus for regulation of blood pressure by the baroreceptors and the kidneys. CO, cardiac output; PVR, peripheral vascular resistance.

lower third of the pons, where integration and modulation of ANS responses occur. This area contains vasomotor and cardiac control centers. This cardiovascular center transmits parasympathetic impulses to the heart through the vagus nerve and sympathetic impulses to the heart and blood vessels through the spinal cord and peripheral sympathetic nerves. Vagal stimulation slows HR, sympathetic stimulation increases HR and cardiac contractility. Blood vessels are selectively innervated by the sympathetic nervous system (SNS). Increased sympathetic activity constricts the small arteries and arterioles, thereby increasing PVR.[3]

ANS control of blood pressure is mediated through intrinsic and extrinsic reflexes, and higher neural control centers. The *intrinsic reflexes*, including *baroreceptor* and *chemoreceptor reflexes*, are controlled within the circulatory system and are essential for rapid and short-term blood pressure regulation. Sensors for *extrinsic reflexes* are outside the circulation and include responses associated with factors such as pain and cold. The neural pathways are more diffuse, and their responses are less consistent than with intrinsic reflexes. Many responses are channeled through the hypothalamus, which plays an essential role in control of SNS responses.[3]

Baroreceptors or *pressoreceptors* are pressure-sensitive receptors in the walls of blood vessels and the heart. The carotid and aortic baroreceptors are in areas between the heart and the brain (Fig. 26-5). They respond to

changes in vessel wall stretch via impulses to the cardiovascular centers in the brain stem to alter HR, strength of cardiac contraction, and vascular smooth muscle tone. For example, the fall in blood pressure that occurs upon moving to a standing position produces a decrease in the stretch of baroreceptors. This triggers an increase in HR and a sympathetically induced vasoconstriction that produces an increase in PVR.[3]

Arterial chemoreceptors are chemosensitive cells that monitor blood levels of oxygen, carbon dioxide, and hydrogen ions and are in the carotid and aortic bodies (Fig. 26-5). Chemoreceptors are in close contact with arterial blood, and although their main function is to regulate ventilation, they also communicate with brain stem cardiovascular centers for widespread vasoconstriction. When arterial blood pressure drops, chemoreceptors are stimulated because of diminished oxygen and buildup of carbon dioxide and hydrogen ions.[3] In chronic lung disease, systemic and pulmonary hypertension may develop in response to hypoxemia. People with sleep apnea may also experience increased blood pressure due to hypoxemia during apneic periods.[1,4-6]

Humoral Mechanisms
Humoral mechanisms that contribute to blood pressure regulation include the *renin–angiotensin–aldosterone system*, *vasopressin*, and *epinephrine/norepinephrine*. These substances acutely regulate blood pressure by

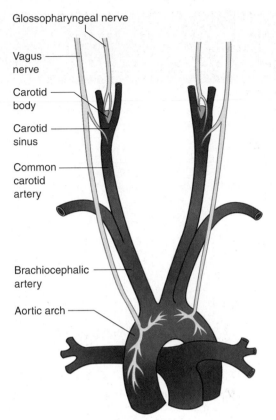

FIGURE 26-5. Location and innervation of the aortic arch and carotid sinus baroreceptors and carotid body chemoreceptors.

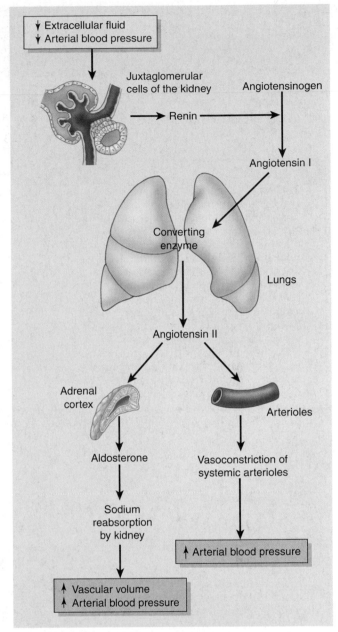

FIGURE 26-6. Control of blood pressure by the renin–angiotensin–aldosterone system. Renin enzymatically converts the plasma protein angiotensinogen to angiotensin I; angiotensin-converting enzyme in the lung converts angiotensin I to angiotensin II; and angiotensin II produces vasoconstriction and increases salt and water retention through direct action on the kidney and through increased aldosterone secretion by the adrenal cortex.

altering vascular tone. Norepinephrine/epinephrine modifies blood pressure by increasing HR and cardiac contractility.[3]

Renin is an enzyme that is synthesized, stored, and released by kidney **juxtaglomerular** cells. Renin release occurs with increased SNS activity or decreased blood pressure, extracellular fluid volume, or extracellular sodium concentration. Most renin leaves the kidney. In the bloodstream, it converts an inactive circulating plasma protein, *angiotensinogen*, to angiotensin I (Fig. 26-6). Angiotensin I is converted to angiotensin II while blood is flowing through the lungs, catalyzed by *angiotensin-converting enzyme* produced in the endothelium of lung blood vessels. While angiotensin II has a half-life of several minutes, renin persists for 30 minutes to 1 hour, leading to production of additional angiotensin II during this time.[3]

Angiotensin II functions in short- and long-term blood pressure regulation. It is a vasoconstrictor of arterioles and, to a lesser extent, veins. Arteriole constriction increases PVR, contributing to short-term regulation of blood pressure. Angiotensin II reduces sodium excretion by increasing sodium reabsorption by kidney proximal tubules. Angiotensin II stimulates adrenal gland aldosterone secretion, which contributes to long-term regulation of blood pressure by increasing kidney salt and water retention.[3]

Vasopressin (or antidiuretic hormone, ADH) is released from the posterior pituitary gland in response to decreased blood volume or blood pressure, or increased osmolality of body fluid. It has a direct vasoconstrictor effect, particularly on vessels of splanchnic circulation that supply abdominal viscera, but long-term increases cannot maintain increased blood pressure.[3]

The catecholamines epinephrine and, to a lesser extent, norepinephrine are released from the adrenal gland into the bloodstream when the SNS is activated. Catecholamines increase blood pressure by inducing vasoconstriction and increasing HR and cardiac contractility.[3]

UNDERSTANDING ➡ Determinants of Blood Pressure

Arterial blood pressure moves blood through the arterial system. It is determined by factors including blood volume, elasticity of blood vessels, CO, and PVR.

1

Arterial Blood Pressure. The highest arterial pressure is systolic pressure (coinciding with ventricular contraction), and the lowest is diastolic pressure (coinciding with relaxation). Arterioles regulate blood distribution to capillary beds. Because arteries are compliant and arterioles provide high resistance to flow, the arterial system converts pulsatile flow into a steady, nonpulsating flow through the capillaries. As blood exits capillary beds, the low-pressure venous system collects blood and returns it to the heart, maintaining the diastolic filling pressure needed for adequate CO.

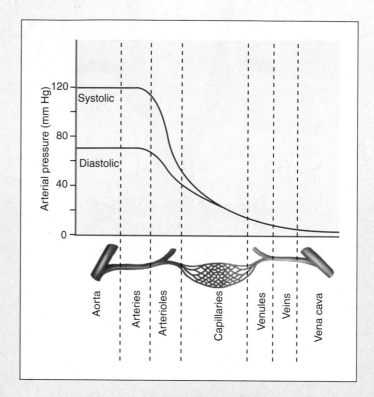

2

Systolic Pressure. Systolic blood pressure reflects the (a) volume of blood (SV) ejected from the ventricles with each beat; (b) rate and force of blood ejection; and (c) elasticity, or compliance, of the aorta and large arteries. Blood ejected during systole does not move directly through circulation. Instead, a substantial fraction of SV is stored in large arteries. Because these vessels walls are elastic, they can stretch to accommodate a large volume without a significant change in pressure. Systolic pressure often increases with age as the aorta and large arteries lose elasticity.

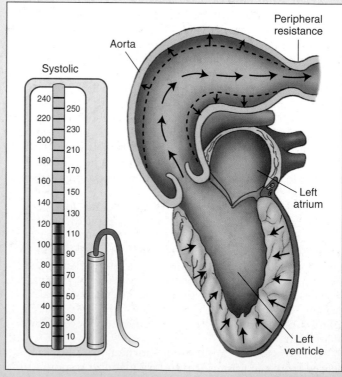

3 **Diastolic Pressure.** Diastolic blood pressure reflects the (a) closure of the aortic valve, (b) energy stored in the elastic fibers of the large arteries during systole, and (c) resistance to flow through arterioles into the capillaries. Aortic valve closure at the onset of diastole and recoil of elastic fibers in the aorta and large arteries drive the blood forward. These effects convert the pulsatile systolic flow in the ascending aorta into a continuous, nonpulsating flow in the peripheral arteries and arterioles.

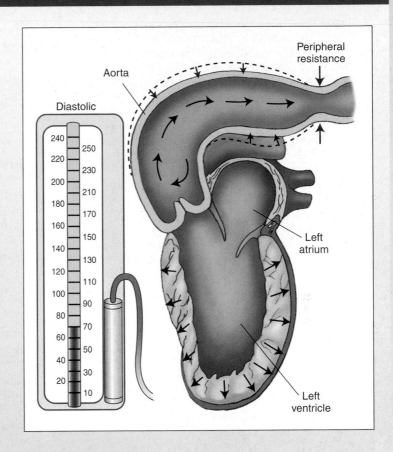

Long-Term Regulation

Neural and hormonal mechanisms involved in the short-term regulation of blood pressure are unable to maintain effectiveness over time. Instead, long-term regulation of blood pressure is largely vested in the kidneys and their role in the regulation of extracellular fluid volume.[3]

Extracellular fluid volume and arterial blood pressure are regulated near an equilibrium point.[3] Arterial pressure rises when increased water and salt intake increase extracellular fluid. This increases the rate of kidney water (*pressure diuresis*) and salt (*pressure natriuresis*) excretion. Arterial pressure can be increased by (a) shifting elimination of salt and water to a higher pressure level and (b) changing the fluid level at which diuresis and natriuresis occur. Long-term blood pressure regulation by the kidneys can be influenced by excess sympathetic nerve activity or release of vasoconstrictor substances. Similarly, changes in neural and humoral control can shift diuresis–natriuresis to a higher fluid or pressure level, increasing arterial pressure.[3]

Increased fluid volume can elevate blood pressure through (a) a direct effect on the preload component of CO and (b) an indirect effect on PVR through mechanisms that autoregulate blood flow. Autoregulatory mechanisms distribute blood flow to body tissues according to metabolic needs. When blood flow is excessive, local vessels constrict, and when flow is deficient, local vessels dilate (autoregulation of blood flow). With increased extracellular fluid volume and a resultant increase in CO, all tissues are exposed to the same increase in flow. This results in a generalized constriction of arterioles and an increase in the PVR (and blood pressure).[3]

Circadian Variations in Blood Pressure

Acute and chronic mechanisms regulate blood pressure around a set point. This set point varies in a circadian pattern: nocturnal blood pressure declines 10% to 20%. Decreased nocturnal dipping of blood pressure is a useful predictor of adverse cardiovascular events and has been noted in people with repetitively shortened sleep periods.[7]

SUMMARY CONCEPTS

Alternating contraction and relaxation of ventricular muscle produce a pressure pulse that moves blood through the circulatory system. Elastic walls of the aorta stretch during systole and relax during diastole to maintain diastolic pressure. *Systolic blood pressure* denotes the highest point of the pressure pulse and *diastolic blood pressure* the lowest point. *Pulse pressure* is the difference between systolic and diastolic pressure. *MAP* is the average blood pressure in systemic circulation. Systolic pressure is determined by characteristics of *SV*, and diastolic pressure is determined by *PVR*, reflecting the condition of arteries and arterioles and their abilities to accept the runoff of blood from the aorta.

The acute mechanisms are responsible for regulating blood pressure on a minute-by-minute or hour-by-hour basis during activities such as physical exercise and changes in body position. It relies mainly on neural and humoral mechanisms. Long-term mechanisms are largely vested in the kidney and the regulation of extracellular fluid volume.

Disorders of Systemic Arterial Blood Flow

Large, elastic arteries function mainly in transport of blood. Medium-sized arteries are composed of circular and spirally arranged SMCs. Distribution of blood flow is controlled by contraction and relaxation of the vessel smooth muscle. Small arteries and arterioles regulate capillary blood flow. Each of these types of arteries can be affected by different disease processes.[1,3,4]

The effect of impaired blood flow on the body depends on the structures involved and the extent of altered flow. *Ischemia* is the reduction in arterial flow to a level that is insufficient to meet the oxygen demands of the tissues. *Infarction* refers to an area of ischemic necrosis in an organ produced by occlusion of its arterial blood supply or venous drainage.

KEY POINTS

Disorders of Systemic Arterial Blood Flow

■ Atherosclerosis is a progressive disease characterized by formation of fibrofatty plaques in the intima of large- and medium-sized vessels. Major risk factors are hypercholesterolemia and inflammation.

■ Vasculitis is an inflammation of the blood vessel wall, resulting in tissue injury and necrosis. Arteries, capillaries, and veins may be affected. The inflammatory process may be initiated by direct injury, infectious agents, or immune processes.

■ Aneurysms are an abnormal localized dilatation of an artery because of a weakness in the vessel wall. As it increases in size, the tension in the vessel wall increases, and it may rupture. The increased size of the vessel may also exert pressure on adjacent structures.

Dyslipidemia

Dyslipidemia is a condition of imbalance of the lipid components (triglycerides, phospholipids, and cholesterol) of the blood. Triglycerides are used in energy metabolism and are combinations of three fatty acids and a single glycerol molecule. Phospholipids contain a phosphate group and are important structural constituents of lipoproteins, blood-clotting components, the myelin sheath, and cell membranes. Cholesterol has a steroid nucleus synthesized from fatty acids, and its chemical and physical activities are similar to that of other lipid substances.[3]

Classification of Lipoproteins

Cholesterol and triglyceride combine with water-soluble proteins called *apoproteins* in order to travel through the plasma, forming a transport molecule called a *lipoprotein* (Fig. 26-7). Lipoproteins transport cholesterol and triglycerides to various tissues for energy utilization, lipid deposition, steroid hormone production, and bile acid formation.[3]

Lipoproteins are classified into five types according to their densities: chylomicrons, very-low-density lipoprotein (VLDL), intermediate-density lipoprotein (IDL), low-density lipoprotein (LDL), and high-density lipoprotein (HDL). VLDL carries large amounts of triglycerides, which have a lower density than cholesterol, and lesser amounts of cholesterol. LDL is the main carrier of cholesterol, whereas HDL is actually 50% protein (Fig. 26-7).[3]

Various classes and subtypes of apoproteins have been identified.[8,9,10] Apolipoprotein (apoprotein B) combines with lipids, and its involvement in lipid metabolism and role as the primary protein of VLDL and LDL contributes to plaque formation and atherosclerosis.

The small intestine and liver are the sites of lipoprotein synthesis. Chylomicrons are the largest lipoprotein molecules and are synthesized in the wall of the small intestine. They are involved in transport of dietary triglycerides and cholesterol absorbed from the gastrointestinal tract. Chylomicrons transfer triglycerides to adipose and skeletal muscle cells. Cholesterol remains in remnant chylomicron particles after triglycerides are removed. Residual cholesterol is taken up by the liver, which synthesizes it for development of VLDL and/or excretes it in the bile.[3]

The liver synthesizes and releases VLDL and HDL. VLDLs provide the primary pathway for transport of

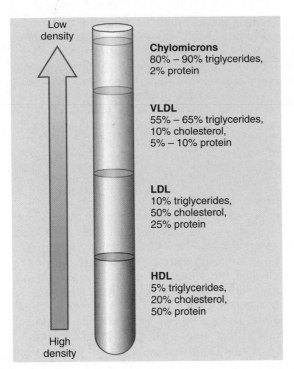

FIGURE 26-7. Lipoproteins are named based on their protein content, which is measured in density. Because fats are less dense than proteins, as the proportion of triglycerides decreases, the density increases. HLD, high-density lipoprotein; LDL, low-density lipoprotein; VLDL, very-low-density lipoprotein.

endogenous triglycerides produced in the liver and are the body's main source of energy during prolonged fasting.[1] Like chylomicrons, VLDLs carry triglycerides to fat and muscle cells, where triglycerides are removed. Resulting IDL fragments travel to the liver where they are recycled to reform VLDL, or are converted to LDL in the vascular compartment. IDLs are the main source of LDL[3] (Fig. 26-8).

LDL is the primary transport molecule for cholesterol. Seventy percent of LDL is removed from circulation through the LDL receptor–mediated pathway, and the remainder is removed by the scavenger pathway.[1] Seventy five percent of LDL receptors are located on hepatocytes. LDL receptor–mediated removal involves binding of LDL to cell surface receptors, followed by *endocytosis.* The endocytic vesicles fuse with lysosomes and the LDL molecule is enzymatically degraded, releasing free cholesterol into the cellular cytoplasm. Nonhepatic tissues also use the LDL receptor–mediated pathway to obtain cholesterol for membrane and hormone synthesis. These tissues can control cholesterol intake by adding or removing LDL receptors.[1,3,4]

The scavenger pathway of LDL removal involves ingestion by phagocytic monocytes and macrophages, which have receptors that bind oxidized or chemically modified LDL. The amount of LDL removed is related to plasma cholesterol level. When LDL receptors are decreased or when levels exceed receptor availability, LDL removed by

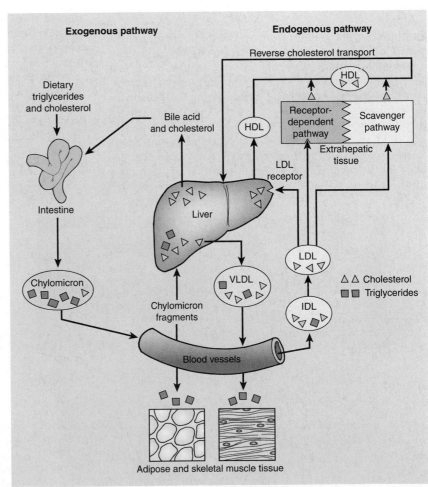

FIGURE 26-8. Schematic representation of the exogenous and endogenous pathways for triglyceride and cholesterol transport. HLD, high-density lipoprotein; LDL, low-density lipoprotein; VLDL, very-low-density lipoprotein.

scavenger cells increases. Uptake of LDL by macrophages in the arterial wall can lead to atherosclerosis.[1,3,4]

HDL facilitates reverse transport of cholesterol (carrying cholesterol from peripheral tissues back to the liver, where it is secreted into the bile).[5] Exercise, moderate alcohol consumption, and certain lipid medications increase HDL levels, whereas smoking, the metabolic syndrome, and excess alcohol consumption are associated with decreased levels of HDL.[1,4,11]

Etiology and Pathogenesis of Dyslipidemia

Serum cholesterol levels may be elevated because of increases in any lipoprotein, and classification of dyslipidemia can be based on the lipoprotein type involved. Factors that can raise blood lipid levels include nutrition, genetics, medications, comorbid conditions, and metabolic diseases.[4]

Primary dyslipidemia is abnormalities in lipid and cholesterol levels developing independent of other health problems or behaviors, and secondary dyslipidemia is associated with other health problems and behaviors. Dyslipidemia is characterized by increased triglycerides, increased total blood cholesterol, increased LDL cholesterol, and decreased HDL cholesterol.[12]

Primary Dyslipidemia

Primary dyslipidemia may have a genetic basis. There may be a defective synthesis of apoproteins, a lack of receptors for lipids, defective lipid receptors, or genetically determined defects in the handling of cholesterol by cells.[4]

Familial Hypercholesterolemia. The LDL receptor is deficient or defective in *familial hypercholesterolemia*, an autosomal dominant disorder that causes a mutation in a gene that codes for an LDL receptor.[4] Because most circulating cholesterol is removed through receptor-dependent mechanisms, cholesterol levels are elevated in people with this disorder. The heterozygous form occurs in 1 in 500 adults in the United States. The recessive homozygous form is more rare, with an incidence of 1 case per million.[4] In the heterozygous form, blood LDL levels have a mean value of 350 mg/dL. Although they commonly have elevated cholesterol levels from birth, they do not develop symptoms until adult life, when they often develop *xanthomas* (cholesterol deposits) along the tendons (Fig. 26-9) and atherosclerosis. People with the homozygous form may experience LDL blood levels up to1,000 mg/dL. They typically develop tendon xanthomas and atherosclerotic vascular lesions during childhood and are at higher risk for death from myocardial ischemic disease during the young adult years. Thus, it is important for people with the homozygous form to receive early pharmacologic treatment to lower blood levels of LDL.[4]

Secondary Dyslipidemia

The causes of secondary dyslipidemia include dietary factors, obesity, and the metabolic changes associated with type 2 diabetes mellitus. Recommendations are to adopt a diet high in fruits, vegetables, whole grains, dairy products, chicken, fish, legumes, and nuts. Intake of sweets and red meat should be minimized. These recommendations are consistent with the DASH diet (*D*ietary *A*pproaches to *S*top *H*ypertension) or a Mediterranean approach.[13]

Dyslipidemia associated with obesity typically consists of elevated triglycerides, elevated LDL cholesterol, and decreased HDL cholesterol and appears to be related to the chemical activity of adipose tissue. The combination of adipokine secretion and macrophage activity leads to a chronic low-grade state of systemic inflammation in some people with obesity. Elevated free fatty acids and systemic inflammation together may disrupt glucose homeostatic mechanisms, contributing to the development of insulin resistance. Insulin resistance results in use of nonglucose energy sources, leading to further increases blood lipid levels.[14]

Type 2 diabetes mellitus is characterized by the development of a state of insulin resistance along with a collection of metabolic alterations, including dyslipidemia, called the *metabolic syndrome*. The metabolic syndrome is defined as the presence of three or more of the following:

- Elevated fasting blood glucose (or current treatment for diabetes)

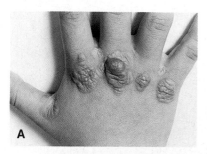
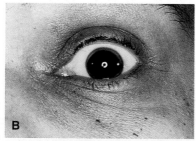
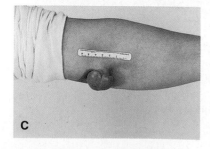
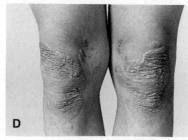

FIGURE 26-9. Xanthomas in the skin and tendons (**A, C, D**). Arcus lipoides represents the deposition of lipids in the peripheral cornea (**B**). (From Strayer D., Rubin R., Saffitz J. E., et al. (Eds.). (2015). *Rubin's pathology: Clinicopathologic foundations of medicine* (7th ed., Figure 26-24, p. 600). Philadelphia, PA: Wolters Kluwer.)

- Elevated blood pressure (or current treatment for hypertension)
- Elevated waist circumference (country-specific norms) and increased abdominal fat deposits
- Dyslipidemia reflected by increased blood triglycerides and/or decreased HDL cholesterol in the blood (or receiving current treatment for dyslipidemia).[15]

Other systemic disorders that can elevate lipids include hypothyroidism, nephrotic syndrome, and obstructive liver disease.[1,4] Medications such as beta-blockers, estrogens, and protease inhibitors (used in the treatment of HIV infection) can also increase lipid levels.[16]

Atherosclerosis

Atherosclerosis is the hardening of the arteries characterized by the formation of fibrofatty lesions in the intimal lining of large- and medium-sized arteries (Fig. 26-10).

Etiology and Risk Factors

The major risk factor for atherosclerosis is hypercholesterolemia and elevations in LDL cholesterol levels. Hypercholesterolemia is one of several risk factors for atherosclerosis that can be modified by dietary and lifestyle changes and medications. Additional risk factors include increasing age, family history of heart disease, and male sex. Genetically determined alterations in lipoprotein and cholesterol metabolism have also been identified.[4] Males are at higher risk for development of atherosclerotic coronary vascular disease than premenopausal females. After menopause, the incidence of atherosclerosis-related diseases in women increases, and the frequency of myocardial infarction in men and women tends to equalize.[1,3,4]

Cigarette smoking, obesity and visceral fat, hypertension, and diabetes mellitus are also risk factors for atherosclerosis. Toxins that enter the bloodstream with cigarette smoking can damage endothelial tissue. Prolonged smoking of one pack or more per day doubles damage to the endothelium. Stopping smoking reduces risk of endothelial damage significantly.[1]

The presence of either hypertension or diabetes mellitus increases the risk for atherosclerosis by twofold. When hypertension and diabetes mellitus exist together, the risk increases eightfold. In the presence of hypertension, diabetes, and hyperlipidemia, the risk increases 20-fold.[3]

Other factors associated with an increased risk for atherosclerosis include physical inactivity, stressful life patterns, blood levels of C-reactive protein (CRP), and serum homocysteine levels.[4] CRP is an acute-phase reactant protein of the inflammatory process and has been noted within some atherosclerotic plaques, further implicating inflammation in plaque formation. Blood levels of CRP serve as a clinical marker of risk for atherosclerotic vascular disease (see Chapter 9).[4] The high-sensitivity CRP test can detect smaller quantities of CRP, making it useful as a screening test for cardiovascular risk in apparently healthy people.[17]

Homocysteine is derived from the metabolism of dietary methionine, an amino acid abundant in animal protein. Metabolism of homocysteine requires adequate folate, vitamin B_6, vitamin B_{12}, and riboflavin.

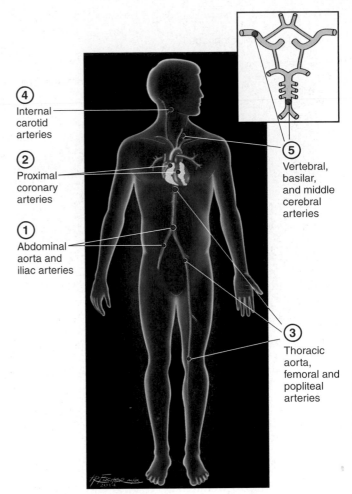

FIGURE 26-10. Sites of severe atherosclerosis in order of frequency. (From Strayer D., Rubin R., Saffitz J. E., et al. (Eds.). (2015). *Rubin's pathology: Clinicopathologic foundations of medicine* (6th ed., Figure 16-17, p. 594). Philadelphia, PA: Wolters Kluwer.)

Homocysteine inhibits elements of the anticoagulant cascade and is associated with endothelial damage.[1,4] A rare autosomal recessive disorder, homocystinuria, is caused by a defect in the production of an enzyme to metabolize homocysteine, resulting in high serum levels of homocysteine. People with homocystinuria are at risk for early development of severe atherosclerosis because of high blood levels of homocysteine.[4,18]

Pathogenesis

The three types of lesions associated with atherosclerosis are fatty streak, fibrous atheromatous plaque, and complicated lesion (Fig. 26-11). The latter two are responsible for the clinically significant manifestations of the disease.

Fatty streaks are thin, flat, yellow intimal discolorations that become thicker and slightly elevated as they grow in length. Histologically, they consist of macrophages and SMCs that have become distended with lipid to form foam cells. Fatty streaks are present in children.[1,2] This occurs regardless of geographic setting, sex, or race. They increase in number until about 20 years of age and then remain static or regress. Endothelium damage is an early marker for atherosclerosis, and, once damaged, circulating monocytes and lipids begin to adhere to the area.

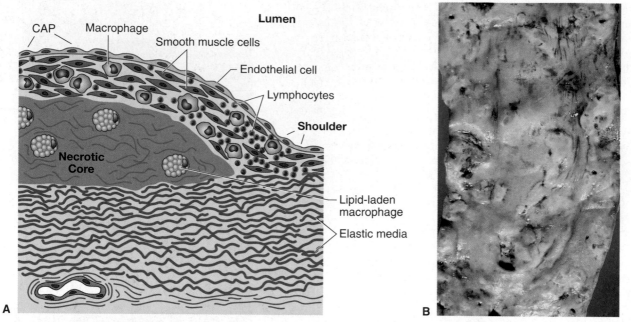

FIGURE 26-11. Fibrofatty plaque of atherosclerosis. **(A)** In this fully developed fibrous plaque, the core contains lipid-filled macrophages and necrotic smooth muscle cell (SMC) debris. The "fibrous" cap is composed largely of SMCs, which produce collagen, small amounts of elastin, and glycosaminoglycans. Also shown are infiltrating macrophages and lymphocytes. Note that the endothelium over the surface of the fibrous cap frequently appears intact. **(B)** The aorta shows discrete raised, tan plaques. Focal plaque ulcerations are also evident. (From Rubin R., Strayer D. S., Saffitz J. E., et al. (Eds.). (2015). *Rubin's pathology: Clinicopathologic foundations of medicine* (7th ed., Fig. 16-12A and D, p. 589). Philadelphia, PA: Wolters Kluwer.)

This *fibrous atheromatous plaque* is characterized by a gray to pearly white appearance because macrophages ingest and oxidize accumulated lipoproteins. Over time, the fatty streaks grow and proliferate into the smooth muscle, encroaching on the lumen of the artery. The macrophages cause inflammation, which may occlude the vessel or predispose to thrombus formation, causing a reduction of blood flow.[3] Because flow is inversely related to the fourth power of the vessel radius, reduction in blood flow becomes greater as the disease progresses.[3]

More advanced complicated lesions contain hemorrhage, ulceration, and scar tissue deposits. Thrombosis is the most important complication of atherosclerosis. The thrombus may cause occlusion of small vessels in the heart and brain. Aneurysms may develop in arteries weakened by extensive plaque formation.[4]

Although risk factors associated with atherosclerosis have been identified, many unanswered questions remain regarding the development of atherosclerosis. One hypothesis of plaque formation suggests that injury to the endothelial vessel layer is the initiating factor in the development of atherosclerosis.[1,4] That atherosclerotic lesions tend to form where vessels branch or where there is turbulent flow suggests that hemodynamic factors also play a role.

Hyperlipidemia may also play a role in the pathogenesis of atherosclerotic lesions, with special concern related to increased blood levels of LDL because of its higher cholesterol content.[4]

Activated macrophages release free radicals that oxidize LDL. Oxidized LDL is toxic, causing endothelial loss and exposure of the subendothelial tissue to blood components. This leads to platelet adhesion, platelet aggregation, and fibrin deposition.[1,4] Activated macrophages also ingest oxidized LDL to become foam cells, which are present in all stages of atherosclerotic plaque formation. Lipids released from necrotic foam cells accumulate to form the lipid core of unstable plaques. Histologically, a large central lipid core, inflammatory infiltrate, and a thin fibrous cap characterize unstable atherosclerotic plaques[1,4] (see Fig. 26-12.) These "vulnerable plaques" are at risk of rupture, which often occurs at the shoulder of the plaque where the fibrous cap is thinnest and the mechanical stresses highest.[1,4]

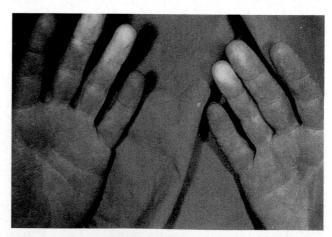

FIGURE 26-12. Raynaud phenomenon. The tips of the fingers show marked pallor. (From Rubin R., Strayer D. S., Saffitz J. E., et al. (Eds.). (2015). *Rubin's pathology: Clinicopathologic foundations of medicine* (7th ed., Figure 16-29, p. 604). Philadelphia, PA: Wolters Kluwer.)

UNDERSTANDING → The Development of Atherosclerosis

Atherosclerosis is characterized by the development of atheromatous lesions within the intimal lining of the large- and medium-sized arteries that protrude into and can eventually obstruct blood flow. The development of atherosclerotic lesions is a progressive process involving (a) endothelial cell injury, (b) migration of inflammatory cells, (c) SMC proliferation and lipid deposition, and (d) gradual development of the atheromatous plaque with a lipid core.

1

Endothelial Cell Injury. The vascular endothelium consists of a single layer of cells with cell-to-cell attachments that protects subendothelial layers from interacting with blood components. Smoking, elevated LDL levels, immune mechanisms, and mechanical stress associated with hypertension share the potential for causing endothelial injury with adhesion of monocytes and platelets.

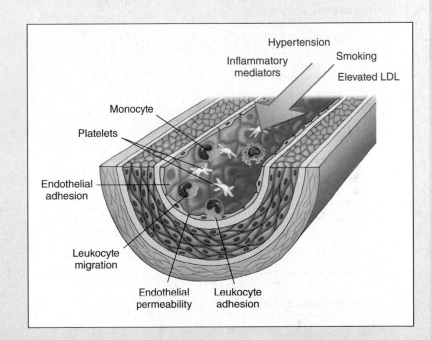

2

Migration of Inflammatory Cells. Early in the development of atherosclerotic lesions, endothelial cells express selective adhesion molecules that bind monocytes and other inflammatory cells that initiate the atherosclerotic lesions. After monocytes adhere to the endothelium, they migrate between the endothelial cells to localize in the intima of the vascular wall. Monocytes then transform into macrophages, which engulf lipoproteins, particularly LDL. Activated macrophages become *foam cells* when they release toxic oxygen species that oxidize the engulfed LDL.

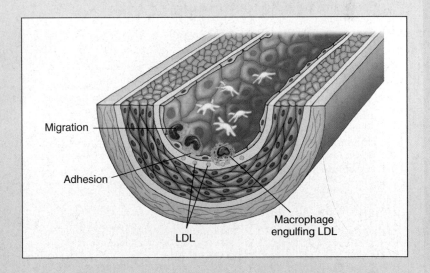

(continued)

UNDERSTANDING ➔ The Development of Atherosclerosis (*continued*)

3

Lipid Accumulation and Smooth Muscle Cell Proliferation. The recruitment of monocytes and their transformation into foam cells is protective because it removes excess lipids from circulation. However, accumulation of foam cells in the vessel wall eventually leads to lesion progression. Macrophages produce growth factors that contribute to migration and proliferation of SMCs and elaboration of extracellular matrix (ECM) in the vascular wall. Ultimately, foam cell macrophages die, depositing necrotic cellular debris and lipids within the vascular wall.

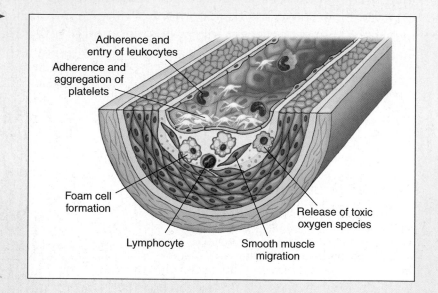

Adherence and entry of leukocytes

Adherence and aggregation of platelets

Foam cell formation

Lymphocyte

Release of toxic oxygen species

Smooth muscle migration

4

Plaque Structure. Atherosclerotic plaques consist of SMCs, macrophages, and other leukocytes; ECM, including collagen and elastic fibers; and intracellular and extracellular lipids. Typically, the superficial fibrous cap is composed of SMCs and dense ECM. Beneath and to the side of the fibrous cap is the "shoulder" consisting of macrophages, SMCs, and lymphocytes. Below the cap is a central core of lipid-laden foam cells and fatty debris. Rupture, ulceration, or erosion of a vulnerable fibrous cap may lead to hemorrhage into the plaque or thrombotic occlusion of the vessel lumen.

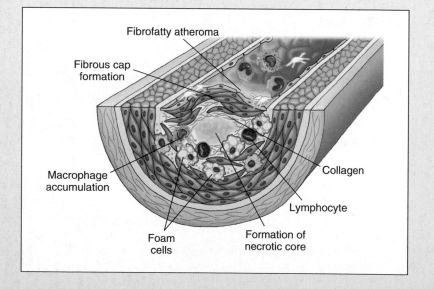

Fibrofatty atheroma

Fibrous cap formation

Macrophage accumulation

Foam cells

Formation of necrotic core

Collagen

Lymphocyte

Clinical Manifestations

Clinical manifestations of atherosclerosis typically do not become evident for 20 years or longer. Clinical manifestations depend on the vessels involved and the extent of vessel obstruction.[4]

Atherosclerotic plaques (lesions) produce their effects through narrowing of the vessel and production of ischemia, sudden vessel obstruction because of plaque hemorrhage or rupture, thrombosis and formation of emboli resulting from damage to the vessel endothelium, or aneurysm formation because of weakening of the vessel wall.[1,4]

In larger vessels, important complications are thrombus formation and weakening of the vessel wall. In medium-sized arteries, ischemia and infarction because of vessel occlusion are more common. Although atherosclerosis can affect any organ or tissue, the arteries supplying the heart, brain, kidneys, lower extremities, and small intestine are most frequently involved.[4]

Vasculitis

The vasculitides are a group of vascular disorders that cause inflammatory injury and necrosis of the blood vessel wall (*i.e.*, vasculitis). The vasculitides, which are a common pathway for tissue and organ involvement in many different disease conditions, involve the endothelial cells and SMCs of the vessel wall.[2] Because they may affect veins and capillaries, *vasculitis*, *angiitis*, and *arteritis* are often used interchangeably. Clinical manifestations often include fever, myalgia, arthralgia, and malaise. Vasculitis may result from direct injury to the vessel, infectious agents, or immune processes, or they may be secondary to other disease states such as systemic lupus erythematosus. Physical agents such as cold, irradiation, mechanical injury, immune mechanisms, and toxins may secondarily cause vessel damage, often leading to necrosis of the vessels. Small vessel vasculitides are sometimes associated with *antineutrophil cytoplasmic antibodies* (ANCAs). ANCAs are antibodies directed against certain proteins in the cytoplasm of neutrophils that may cause endothelial damage.[1] Serum ANCA titers, which can correlate with disease activity, may serve as a useful quantitative diagnostic marker for these disorders.

The vasculitides are classified based on etiology, pathologic findings, and prognosis. One system divides the conditions into (a) small vessel, (b) medium-sized vessel, and (c) large vessel vasculitides[1,4] (Table 26-2). The small vessel vasculitides are involved in a number of different diseases, most of which are mediated by type III immune complex hypersensitivity reaction. They commonly involve the skin and are a complication of an underlying disease and exposure to environmental agents. ANCA-positive small vessel vasculitis includes microscopic polyangiitis, Wegener granulomatosis, and the Churg–Strauss syndrome.[19]

Medium-sized vessel vasculitides produce necrotizing damage to medium-sized muscular arteries of major organ systems. This group includes polyarteritis nodosa, Kawasaki disease, and thromboangiitis obliterans. Large vessel vasculitides involve large elastic arteries. They include giant cell arteritis, polymyalgia rheumatica, and Takayasu arteritis.

TABLE 26-2. Classification of the Vasculitides

Group	Examples	Characteristics
Small vessel vasculitis	Microscopic polyangiitis	Necrotizing vasculitis with few or no immune deposits affecting medium and small blood vessels, including capillaries, venules, and arterioles; necrotizing glomerulonephritis and involvement of the pulmonary capillaries are common
	Wegener granulomatosis	Granulomatous inflammation involving the respiratory tract and necrotizing vasculitis affecting capillaries, venules, arterioles, and arteries; necrotizing glomerulonephritis is common
Medium-sized vessel vasculitis	Polyarteritis nodosa	Necrotizing inflammation of medium-sized or small arteries without vasculitis in arteries, capillaries, or venules; usually associated with underlying disease or environmental agents
	Kawasaki disease	Involves large, medium-sized, and small arteries (frequently the coronaries) and is associated with mucocutaneous lymph node syndrome; usually occurs in small children
	Thromboangiitis obliterans	Segmental, thrombosing, acute and chronic inflammation of the medium-sized and small arteries, principally the tibial and radial arteries but sometimes extending to the veins and nerves of the extremities; occurs almost exclusively in men who are heavy smokers
Large vessel vasculitis	Giant cell (temporal) arteritis	Granulomatous inflammation of the aorta and its major branches with predilection for extracranial vessels of the carotid artery; infiltration of vessel wall with giant cells and mononuclear cells; usually occurs in people older than 50 years of age and is often associated with polymyalgia rheumatic
	Takayasu arteritis	Granulomatous inflammation of the aorta and its branches; usually occurs in people younger than 50 years of age

Giant Cell Temporal Arteritis

Temporal arteritis (*i.e.*, giant cell arteritis), the most common of the vasculitides, is a focal inflammatory condition of medium-sized and large arteries. It predominantly affects arteries originating from the aortic arch. It progresses to the entire artery wall with focal necrosis and granulomatous inflammation involving multinucleated giant cells. It is more common in older adults, with a 2:1 female-to-male ratio. The cause is unknown.[1] The disorder is often insidious in onset and may be heralded by the sudden onset of headache, tenderness over the artery, swelling and redness of the overlying skin, blurred vision or diplopia, and facial pain. Almost half of affected people have systemic involvement in the form of polymyalgia rheumatica. Up to 10% of people with giant cell arteritis go on to develop aortic aneurysm (especially thoracic).

Arterial Disease of the Extremities

Peripheral vascular disorders are disorders of circulation in the extremities. These are similar to disorders affecting coronary and cerebral arteries—they produce ischemia, pain, impaired function, and, in some cases, infarction and tissue necrosis.

Acute Arterial Occlusion

Acute arterial occlusion is a sudden event that interrupts arterial flow to the affected tissues or organ. Most acute arterial occlusions are the result of an embolus or a thrombus. Less commonly, trauma or arterial spasm caused by arterial cannulation can also cause acute arterial occlusion.

Etiology and Pathogenesis

An embolus is a freely moving particle, such as a blood clot, that breaks loose and travels in the larger vessels of the circulation until lodging in a smaller vessel and occluding blood flow. Most emboli arise in the heart and are caused by conditions that cause blood clots to develop on a heart chamber wall or valve surface. Emboli are usually a complication of heart disease: ischemic heart disease, atrial fibrillation, or rheumatic heart disease. Prosthetic heart valves can be a source of emboli. Other types of emboli are fat emboli that originate from the bone marrow of fractured bones, air emboli from the lung, and amniotic fluid emboli that develop during childbirth.

A thrombus is a blood clot on the wall of a vessel that continues to grow until obstructing blood flow. Thrombi often arise from erosion or rupture of the fibrous cap of an arteriosclerotic plaque.

Clinical Manifestations

The symptoms of acute arterial occlusion depend on the artery involved and the adequacy of collateral circulation. Emboli often lodge in bifurcations of major arteries, including the aorta and iliac, femoral, and popliteal arteries.[4] Presentation is often described by the seven "Ps": pistol shot (acute onset), pallor, polar (cold), pulselessness, pain, paresthesia, and paralysis.

Occlusion in an extremity causes sudden onset of acute pain with numbness, tingling, weakness, pallor, and coldness. There is often a line between the oxygenated tissue above and the ischemic tissue below the obstruction. Pulses are absent below the level of the occlusion. This is followed rapidly by cyanosis, mottling, and loss of sensory, reflex, and motor function. Tissue death occurs unless blood flow is restored.[1,4]

Diagnosis and Treatment

Diagnosis of acute arterial occlusion uses visual assessment, palpation of pulses, and methods to assess blood flow. Treatment is aimed at restoring blood flow. An embolectomy, surgical removal of the embolus, is the optimal therapy when a large artery is occluded.[1,4]

Thrombolytic therapy (*i.e.*, streptokinase or tissue plasminogen activator) may dissolve the clot. Anticoagulant therapy (*i.e.*, heparin) is usually given to prevent extension of the embolus and to prevent progression of the original thrombus. Cold should be avoided, and the extremity should be protected from injury caused by hard surfaces and overlying bedclothes.[1,4,16]

Atherosclerotic Occlusive Disease (Peripheral Artery Disease)

Atherosclerosis is an important cause of peripheral artery disease (PAD) and is common in the lower extremities (*i.e.*, superficial femoral and popliteal arteries). When lesions develop in the lower leg and foot, the tibial, common peroneal, or pedal vessels are most commonly affected. The disease is seen commonly with advanced age.[1,4]

Etiology

Risk factors are similar to those for atherosclerosis. Cigarette smoking contributes to the progress of atherosclerosis of the lower extremities and development of symptoms of ischemia. People with diabetes mellitus develop more extensive and rapidly progressive vascular disease.[1,4]

Clinical Manifestations

The symptoms of vessel occlusion are gradual. Usually, there is a 50% narrowing of the vessel before symptoms of ischemia arise. The primary symptom of chronic obstructive arterial disease is *intermittent claudication* (pain with walking).[1,4] People often complain of calf pain (the gastrocnemius has the highest oxygen consumption of all leg muscles required for walking). Some may complain of a vague aching feeling or numbness. Other activities such as swimming and bicycling use other muscle groups and may not incite the same degree of discomfort.[1,4]

Other signs of ischemia include atrophic changes and thinning of skin and subcutaneous tissues of the lower leg and reduced size of leg muscles. The foot may be cool, and popliteal and pedal pulses weak or absent. Limb color blanches with leg elevation because of the effects of gravity on perfusion pressure and becomes deep red when the leg is in the dependent position because of an autoregulatory increase in blood flow and a gravitational increase in perfusion pressure.[1,4]

When blood flow no longer meets the minimal needs of muscle and nerves, ischemic pain at rest, ulceration, and gangrene develop. As necrosis develops, there is often severe pain in the region of breakdown, which is worse at night with limb elevation and is improved with standing.[1,4]

Diagnosis

Diagnostic methods include inspection of the limbs for signs of chronic low-grade ischemia, such as subcutaneous atrophy, brittle toenails, hair loss, pallor, coolness, or dependent rubor. Palpation or Doppler ultrasound of the femoral, popliteal, posterior tibial, and dorsalis pedis pulses allows for an estimation of the level and degree of obstruction. Blood pressures may be taken at various levels on the leg to determine the level of obstruction. Ultrasound imaging, magnetic resonance imaging (MRI) arteriography, spiral computed tomography (CT) arteriography, and invasive contrast angiography may also be used as diagnostic methods.[1,4]

Treatment

The goals of treatment for PAD are to (1) decrease considerable cardiovascular risk and (2) reduce symptoms. A person with PAD should be evaluated for coexisting coronary and cerebrovascular atherosclerosis. Other cardiovascular risk factors, including smoking, hypertension, high lipid levels, and diabetes, should also be addressed. Useful medications include antiplatelet agents to minimize thrombosis and statins to lower cholesterol. Tissues affected by atherosclerosis are easily injured and slow to heal. Treatment includes measures to protect the affected tissues and preserve functional capacity. Walking (slowly) to the point of claudication may be encouraged to increase collateral circulation. Percutaneous or surgical vascular intervention is typically reserved for disabling claudication or limb-threatening ischemia.[1,4,16]

Thromboangiitis Obliterans

Thromboangiitis obliterans, or Buerger disease, is an inflammatory (*i.e.*, vasculitis) arterial disorder that causes thrombus formation. It affects medium-sized arteries, usually the plantar and digital vessels in the foot and lower leg. Arteries in the arm and hand may also be affected. It is characterized by segmental, thrombosing, and acute and chronic inflammation. Although primarily an arterial disorder, the inflammatory process may extend to adjacent veins and nerves. It is often seen in people less than 35 years of age who are heavy cigarette smokers.[1,4]

Etiology and Pathogenesis

The pathogenesis of Buerger disease remains speculative. However, cigarette smoking and, in some instances, tobacco chewing seem to be involved.[1] Genetic influences are suggested.

Clinical Manifestations

Pain is the predominant symptom and is usually related to distal arterial ischemia. During the early stages, there is intermittent claudication in the arch of the foot and digits. In severe cases, pain is present at rest. Impaired circulation increases sensitivity to cold. Peripheral pulses are diminished or absent, and there are changes in extremity color. In moderately advanced cases, the extremity becomes cyanotic when in a dependent position, and digits may turn reddish blue even when in a nondependent position. With lack of blood flow, the skin assumes a thin, shiny look and hair growth and skin nutrition suffer. Chronic ischemia causes thick, malformed nails. Tissues eventually ulcerate, and gangrenous changes arise that may necessitate amputation.[1,4]

Diagnosis and Treatment

Diagnostic methods are similar to those for atherosclerotic disease of the lower extremities. As part of the treatment program, nicotine and tobacco use must be eliminated. Other treatment measures are of secondary importance and focus on methods for producing vasodilation and preventing tissue injury.[1,4]

Raynaud Disease and Phenomenon

Raynaud disease or phenomenon is a functional disorder caused by intense vasospasm of the arteries and arterioles in the fingers and, less often, toes. It affects 3% to 5% of the population and is more common in females than males. The primary type, *Raynaud disease*, occurs without demonstrable cause, and the secondary type, *Raynaud phenomenon*, is associated with other disease states or known causes of vasospasm.[1,4]

Etiology and Pathogenesis

Vasospasm is an excessive vasoconstrictor response to stimuli that normally produce moderate vasoconstriction. Cutaneous vessels of the fingers and toes are innervated only by sympathetic vasoconstrictor fibers, and vasodilation occurs by withdrawal of sympathetic stimulation. Cooling specific body parts such as the head, neck, and trunk produces a sympathetic-mediated reduction in digital blood flow, as does emotional stress.[1,4]

Raynaud disease is precipitated by exposure to cold or strong emotions and is usually limited to the fingers. It seldom causes tissue necrosis. The cause of vasospasm in primary Raynaud disease is unknown. Raynaud phenomenon is associated with previous vessel injury, such as frostbite, occupational trauma associated with the use of heavy vibrating tools or exposure to alternating hot and cold temperatures, neurologic disorders, and chronic arterial occlusive disorders. It is a first symptom of collagen diseases, such as scleroderma and systemic lupus erythematosus.[1,4]

Clinical Manifestations

In Raynaud disease and phenomenon, ischemia due to vasospasm causes changes in skin color that progress from pallor to cyanosis, a sensation of cold, and changes in sensory perception, such as numbness and tingling. Color changes are usually first noticed in the tips of the fingers, moving into one or more of the distal phalanges (Fig. 26-12). After the ischemic episode, there is hyperemia with intense redness, throbbing, and paresthesias, followed by a return to normal color. Although all fingers are usually affected symmetrically, occasionally only one or two digits are involved, or only a portion of the digit is affected.[1,4]

In severe, progressive cases usually associated with Raynaud phenomenon, the nails may become brittle, and the skin over the tips of affected fingers may thicken. Nutritional impairment of these structures may cause arthritis. Ulceration and superficial gangrene of fingers may occur.[1,4]

Diagnosis and Treatment

Initial diagnosis is based on history of vasospastic attacks supported by other findings. Treatment aims to eliminate factors that cause vasospasm and protect digits from trauma during an ischemic episode. Smoking abstinence, cold protection, and emotional stress control are priorities.[1,4]

Aneurysms

An *aneurysm* is an abnormal localized dilation of a blood vessel. Aneurysms can occur in the arteries and veins, but they are most common in the aorta. Aneurysms can assume several forms and may be classified according to their cause, location, and anatomic features (Fig. 26-13).

A *true aneurysm* is bounded by a complete vessel wall, and the blood remains within the vascular compartment. *False aneurysm* is a localized *dissection* or tear in the inner wall of the artery with formation of an extravascular hematoma that causes vessel enlargement. Only the outer layers of the vessel wall or supporting tissues bound false aneurysms.[1,4]

A *berry aneurysm* (Fig. 26-14A) is a true aneurysm that consists of a small, spherical dilation of the vessel at a bifurcation.[1,4] It is usually found in the circle of Willis. A *fusiform aneurysm* (Fig. 26-14C) is a true aneurysm that involves the entire circumference of the vessel with gradual and progressive vessel dilation. These vary in diameter and length and may involve ascending and transverse portions of the thoracic aorta or may extend over large segments of the abdominal aorta. A *saccular aneurysm* is a true aneurysm that extends over part of the circumference of the vessel (appears saclike).[4] A *dissecting aneurysm* (Fig. 26-14B) is a false aneurysm resulting from a tear in the intimal layer of the vessel that allows blood to enter the vessel wall, dissecting its layers to create a blood-filled cavity. Dissection in the aorta is a life-threatening condition.

Weakness that leads to aneurysm formation may be due to congenital defects, trauma, infections, and atherosclerosis. Once initiated, the aneurysm grows larger as the tension in the vessel increases because the tension in the vessel wall equals pressure multiplied by radius.

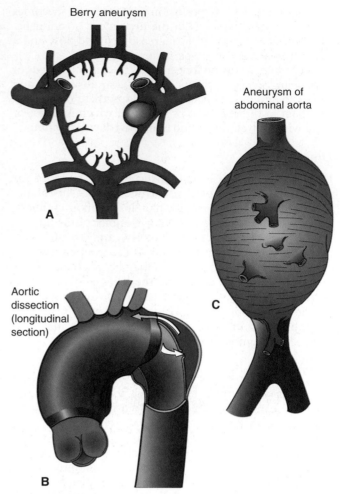

FIGURE 26-13. Three forms of aneurysms: (**A**) berry aneurysm in the circle of Willis, (**B**) aortic dissection, and (**C**) fusiform-type aneurysm of the abdominal aorta.

As an aneurysm increases in diameter, the tension in the wall of the vessel increases in proportion to its increased size. If untreated, the aneurysm may rupture. Even an unruptured aneurysm can cause damage by exerting pressure on adjacent structures and interrupting blood flow.

Aortic Aneurysms

Aortic aneurysms may involve any part of the aorta. Multiple aneurysms may be present (Fig. 26-14).

Etiology

The two common causes of aortic aneurysms are atherosclerosis and degeneration of the vessel media. Half of the people with aortic aneurysms have hypertension. Aortic aneurysms develop more frequently in males after the age of 50 years who smoke cigarettes.[4]

Clinical Manifestations

An aneurysm may be asymptomatic, with the first evidence being vessel rupture. Aneurysms of thoracic aorta are less common than abdominal aorta and may present

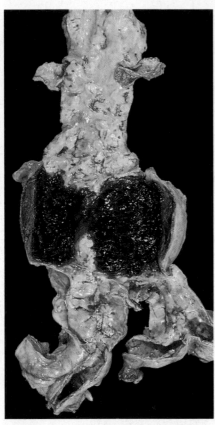

FIGURE 26-14. Atherosclerotic aneurysm of the abdominal aorta. The aneurysm has been opened longitudinally to reveal a large thrombus in the lumen. The aorta and common iliac arteries display complicated lesions of atherosclerosis. (From Rubin R., Strayer D. S., Saffitz J. E., et al. (Eds.). (2015). *Rubin's pathology: Clinicopathologic foundations of medicine* (7th ed., Figure 16-38, p. 611). Philadelphia, PA: Wolters Kluwer.)

with substernal, back, and neck pain. There may be dyspnea, stridor, or brassy cough caused by pressure on the trachea. Hoarseness may result from pressure on the recurrent laryngeal nerve, and there may be difficulty swallowing because of pressure on the esophagus. The aneurysm may compress the superior vena cava, causing distention of neck veins and edema of the face and neck.[1,4]

Abdominal aortic aneurysms are commonly found below the level of the renal artery and involve bifurcation of the aorta and proximal end of the common iliac arteries.[1,4] The infrarenal aorta is 2 cm in diameter; an aneurysm is an aortic diameter greater than 3 cm. They can involve any part of the vessel circumference (saccular) or extend to the entire circumference (fusiform). Most abdominal aneurysms are asymptomatic. Because an aneurysm is of arterial origin, a pulsating mass may provide the first evidence of the disorder. Typically, aneurysms larger than 4 cm are palpable. Calcification, which frequently exists on the wall of the aneurysm, may be detected during abdominal radiologic examination. Pain may be present and varies from mild mid-abdominal or lumbar discomfort to severe abdominal and back pain. As the aneurysm expands, it may compress lumbar nerve roots, causing lower back pain

that radiates to the posterior aspects of the legs. The aneurysm may extend to and impinge on the renal, iliac, or mesenteric arteries or to the vertebral arteries that supply the spinal cord. An abdominal aneurysm may also cause erosion of vertebrae. Stasis of blood favors thrombus formation along the wall of the vessel (Fig. 26-14), and peripheral emboli may develop, causing symptomatic arterial insufficiency.[1,4]

With thoracic and abdominal aneurysms, the most dreaded complication is rupture. Likelihood of rupture correlates with aneurysm size: risk of rupture rises from less than 2% for small abdominal aneurysms to 5% to 10% per year for aneurysms larger than 5 cm in diameter.[4]

Diagnosis and Treatment

Diagnostic methods include use of ultrasonography, echocardiography, CT scans, and MRI. Surgical repair frequently is the treatment of choice.[1,4]

Aortic Dissection

Aortic dissection (dissecting aneurysm) is an acute, life-threatening condition. It involves hemorrhage into the vessel wall with longitudinal tearing to form a blood-filled channel (Fig. 26-15). Aortic dissection often occurs without evidence of previous vessel dilation. Over 95% of cases show a transverse tear in the intima and internal media. The dissection can originate anywhere along the length of the aorta.[4] The most common site is the ascending aorta, and the second most common site is the thoracic aorta, just distal to the origin of the subclavian artery.

Etiology and Pathogenesis

Aortic dissection is caused by conditions that weaken or degenerate the elastic and smooth muscle layers of the aorta. It is most common in the 40- to 60-year-old age group and more prevalent in males than females.[1] Two risk factors predispose to aortic dissection—hypertension and degeneration of the medial layer of the vessel wall. Aortic dissection is also associated with connective tissue diseases, such as Marfan syndrome. It may also occur during pregnancy because of changes in the aorta. Other factors are congenital defects of the aortic valve (*i.e.*, bicuspid or unicuspid valve structures) and aortic coarctation. Aortic dissection is a potential complication of cardiac surgery or catheterization. Surgically related dissection may occur at the points where the aorta has been incised or cross-clamped.

Aortic dissections are commonly classified by the level of dissection. The more common (and potentially more serious in terms of complications) proximal lesions involving the ascending aorta only or both the ascending and the descending aorta, are designated *type A*. Those not involving the ascending aorta and usually beginning distal to the subclavian artery are designated *type B*.[1] Aortic dissections are also classified according to time of onset as acute or chronic, with acute dissections occurring within 14 days of the onset of symptoms.[20]

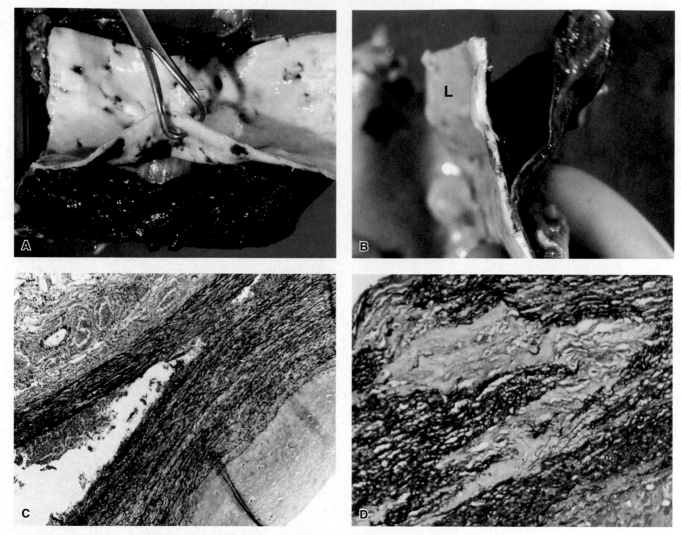

FIGURE 26-15. Dissecting aortic aneurysm. **(A)** Thoracic aorta with metal clamps revealing the dissection and hematoma in the wall with old blood clot. **(B)** The thoracic aorta has been opened longitudinally and reveals clotted blood dissecting the media of the vessel. **(C)** Atherosclerotic aorta with dissection along the outer third of the media (elastic stain). **(D)** A section of the aortic wall stained with aldehyde fuchsin showing pools of metachromatic material characteristic of the degenerative process known as cystic medial necrosis. L, lumen. (From Strayer D., Rubin R., Saffitz J. E., et al. (Eds.). (2015). *Rubin's pathology: Clinicopathologic foundations of medicine* (7th ed., Figure 16-39, p. 613). Philadelphia, PA: Wolters Kluwer.)

Clinical Manifestations

A major symptom of a dissecting aneurysm is the abrupt presence of excruciating pain, described as tearing or ripping. Pain associated with dissection of the ascending aorta is frequently located in the anterior chest, and pain associated with dissection of the descending aorta is often located in the back. In the early stages, blood pressure is typically moderately or markedly elevated. Later, the blood pressure and the pulse rate become unobtainable in one or both arms as the dissection disrupts arterial flow to the arms. Syncope, hemiplegia, or paralysis of the lower extremities may occur because of occlusion of blood vessels that supply the brain or spinal cord. Heart failure may develop when the aortic valve is involved.[1,4]

Diagnosis and Treatment

Diagnosis of aortic dissection is based on history and physical examination supported by vascular imaging, CT, and MRI. The treatment may be medical or surgical depending on the type and whether it is acute or chronic. Because aortic dissection is a life-threatening emergency, people with a probable diagnosis are stabilized medically before the diagnosis is confirmed. Two factors that propagate dissection are high blood pressure and steepness of the pulse wave, which will continue to cause extension of the dissection. Medical treatment focuses on control of hypertension and drugs that lessen the force of systolic blood ejection from the heart. Surgical treatment consists of resection of the involved segment and replacement with a prosthetic graft. The mortality rate of untreated dissecting aneurysm is high.[1,4]

SUMMARY CONCEPTS

Lesions of the arterial system exert their effects through ischemia or impaired blood flow. There are two types of arterial disorders: diseases such as atherosclerosis, vasculitis, and peripheral arterial diseases that obstruct flow and disorders such as aneurysms that weaken the vessel wall.

Cholesterol relies on lipoproteins for transport in the blood. LDLs, which are atherogenic, carry cholesterol to peripheral tissues. HDLs, which are protective, remove cholesterol from the tissues and carry it back to the liver for disposal. LDL receptors play a major role in removing cholesterol from the blood; people with reduced numbers of receptors are at higher risk for development of atherosclerosis.

Atherosclerosis affects large- and medium-sized arteries. It has an insidious onset, and its lesions are usually far advanced before symptoms appear. Although the mechanisms of atherosclerosis are uncertain, risk factors include heredity, sex, and age, and factors such as smoking, high blood pressure, high serum cholesterol levels, diabetes, obesity, and inflammation.

The vasculitides are a group of vascular disorders characterized by vasculitis or inflammation and necrosis of the blood vessels. They can be caused by injury to the vessel, infectious agents, or immune processes or can occur secondary to other disease states such as systemic lupus erythematosus.

Occlusive disorders interrupt arterial flow of blood and interfere with delivery of oxygen and nutrients to the tissues. Occlusion of flow can result from a thrombus, emboli, vessel compression, vasospasm, or structural changes in the vessel. Peripheral arterial diseases affect blood vessels outside the heart and thorax. They include Raynaud disease or phenomenon and thromboangiitis obliterans (Buerger disease).

Aneurysms are localized areas of vessel dilation caused by weakness of the arterial wall. A berry aneurysm, often found in the circle of Willis, consists of a small, spherical vessel dilation. Fusiform and saccular aneurysms, often found in the thoracic and abdominal aorta, are characterized by gradual and progressive enlargement of the aorta. They can involve part of the vessel circumference (saccular) or extend to involve the entire circumference of the vessel (fusiform). A dissecting aneurysm is an acute, life-threatening condition. It involves hemorrhage into the vessel wall with longitudinal tearing (dissection) of the vessel wall to form a blood-filled channel. The most serious consequence of aneurysms is rupture.

Disorders of Systemic Venous Circulation

Veins are low-pressure, thin-walled vessels that rely on the action of skeletal muscle pumps and changes in abdominal and intrathoracic pressure to return blood to the heart. The venous system in the legs consists of the superficial veins (*i.e.*, saphenous vein and its tributaries) and the deep venous channels. Perforating, or communicating, veins connect these two systems. Blood from the skin and subcutaneous tissues in the leg collects in superficial veins and is then transported across the communicating veins into the deeper venous channels for return to the heart.[3]

The venous system has valves that prevent retrograde flow of blood. Valves are almost always at junctions where communicating veins merge with larger deep veins and where two veins meet. The number of venous valves differs per person, as does their structural competence. This may explain the familial predisposition to development of varicose veins.[1,3,4]

When a person walks, leg muscles increase flow in the deep venous channels and return venous blood to the heart (Fig. 26-16). This function of the leg muscles is referred to as the *skeletal muscle pump*.[4] During muscle contraction, valves in the communicating channels close to prevent backward flow of blood into the superficial system, as blood in the deep veins is moved forward by the action of the contracting muscles. During muscle relaxation, the communicating valves open, allowing blood from the superficial veins to move into the deep veins.

Although its structure enables the venous system to serve as a storage area for blood, it also renders the system susceptible to problems related to stasis and venous insufficiency.

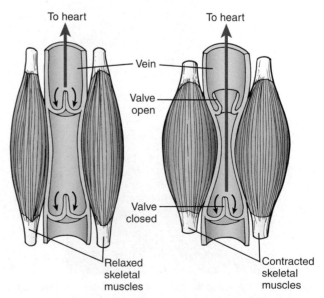

FIGURE 26-16. The skeletal muscle pumps and their function in promoting blood flow in the deep and superficial calf vessels of the leg.

Varicose Veins

Varicose, or dilated, tortuous veins of the lower extremities are common and often lead to secondary problems of venous insufficiency (Fig. 26-17). *Primary varicose veins* originate in the superficial saphenous veins, and *secondary varicose* veins result from impaired flow in the deep venous channels. In all, 80% to 90% of venous blood from the lower extremities is transported through the deep channels. Secondary varicose veins develop when flow in deep channels is impaired or blocked. The most common cause of secondary varicose veins is deep vein thrombosis (DVT). Other causes include congenital or acquired arteriovenous (AV) fistulas, congenital venous malformations, and pressure on the abdominal veins as result of pregnancy or a tumor.[1,3,4]

The prevalence of varicose veins is 50% in people over 50 years of age. It is more common in females between 30 and 50 years of age, especially if there is a familial predisposition.[4] There is also a higher incidence in people with obesity, because of increased intra-abdominal pressure, and among people who stand for the majority of their day (*e.g.*, nurses).

Etiology and Pathogenesis

Prolonged standing increases venous pressure and causes dilation and stretching of the vessel wall. When a person is in the erect position, the full weight of the venous columns of blood is transmitted to the leg veins. The effects of gravity are compounded in people who stand for long periods without using their leg muscles to assist in pumping blood back to the heart.[1,3,4]

Because there are no valves in the inferior vena cava or common iliac veins, blood in the abdominal veins must be supported by valves located in the external iliac or femoral veins. When intra-abdominal pressure increases, as it does during pregnancy and obesity, or when the valves in these two veins are absent or defective, the stress on the saphenofemoral junction is increased. The high incidence of varicose veins with pregnancy also suggests a hormonal effect on venous smooth muscle, contributing to venous dilation and valvular incompetence. Lifting also increases intra-abdominal pressure and decreases flow of blood through abdominal veins. Occupations that require repeated heavy lifting predispose to development of varicose veins.[1,3,4]

Prolonged exposure to increased pressure causes venous valves to become incompetent, so they no longer close properly. Reflux of blood causes further venous enlargement, pulling the valve leaflet apart and causing more valvular incompetence in sections of adjacent distal veins. Another consideration in the development of varicose veins is that superficial veins have only subcutaneous fat and superficial fascia for support, but the deep venous channels are supported by the muscle, bone, and connective tissue. Obesity reduces the support provided by the superficial fascia and tissues, increasing the risk for development of varicose veins.[1,3,4]

Clinical Manifestations

The signs and symptoms associated with primary varicose veins vary. In many cases, aching in the lower extremities and edema, especially after long periods of standing, may occur. The edema usually subsides at night when legs are elevated. When the communicating veins are incompetent, symptoms are more common.[21]

Diagnosis and Treatment

Diagnosis can often be made after a thorough history and physical examination, especially inspection of extremities involved. The Doppler ultrasonic flow probe

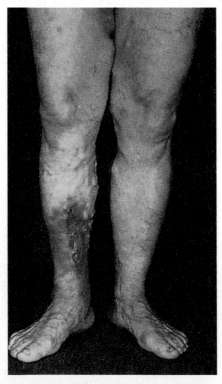

FIGURE 26-17. Varicose veins of the legs. Severe varicosities of the superficial leg veins have led to stasis dermatitis and secondary ulcerations. (From Strayer D., Rubin R., Saffitz J. E., et al. (Eds.). (2015). *Rubin's pathology: Clinicopathologic foundations of medicine* (7th ed., Figure 16-41, p. 614). Philadelphia, PA: Wolters Kluwer.)

can assess flow in large vessels. Angiographic studies using a radiopaque contrast can assess venous function.[21]

After the venous channels have been repeatedly stretched and the valves rendered incompetent, little can be done to restore normal venous tone and function. Measures to prevent development and progression of varicose veins include weight loss and measures to avoid activities, such as continued standing, that produce prolonged elevation of venous pressure. Treatment measures focus on improving venous flow and preventing tissue injury. Elastic support stockings compress superficial veins and prevent distention. Prescription stockings measured to fit afford the most precise control and should be applied before the standing, when the leg veins are empty.[21]

Sclerotherapy is used in the treatment of small residual varicosities and involves injection of a sclerosing agent into the collapsed superficial veins to produce fibrosis of the vessel lumen. Surgical treatment removes the varicosities and the incompetent perforating veins; however, this is limited to people with patent deep venous channels.[21]

Chronic Venous Insufficiency

The term *venous insufficiency* refers to the pathophysiologic condition of persistent venous hypertension on the structure and function of the venous system of the lower extremities.

Etiology and Pathogenesis

The causation includes factors such as increased venous hydrostatic pressure (as with prolonged standing), incompetent valves in the veins, deep vein obstructions (as with DVT), decreased skeletal muscle pump function, inflammatory processes, and endothelial dysfunction.[1,4,22]

With venous insufficiency, effective unidirectional flow and emptying of the deep veins cannot occur. If muscle pumps are ineffective, blood may be driven retrogradely. Secondary failure of communicating and superficial veins subjects subcutaneous tissues to high pressures.[1,4,22]

Clinical Manifestations

Venous insufficiency leads to tissue congestion, edema, and eventual impairment of tissue nutrition. Edema is exacerbated by long periods of standing. Necrosis of subcutaneous fat deposits can occur, followed by skin atrophy. Brown pigmentation of the skin is caused by hemosiderin deposits resulting from the breakdown of red blood cells. Secondary lymphatic insufficiency may occur, with progressive sclerosis of lymph channels because of increased demand for clearance of interstitial fluid. People with long-standing venous insufficiency may also experience stiffening of the ankle joint and loss of muscle mass and strength.[1,4,22]

In advanced venous insufficiency, impaired tissue nutrition causes stasis dermatitis and stasis or venous ulcers (Fig. 26-17). Stasis dermatitis is characterized by thin, shiny, bluish brown, irregularly pigmented desquamative skin that lacks the support of underlying subcutaneous tissues. Minor injury leads to relatively painless ulcerations that are difficult to heal. The lower part of the leg is prone to development of stasis dermatitis and venous ulcers. Most lesions are located medially over the ankle and lower leg, with the highest frequency above the medial malleolus. Venous insufficiency is the most common cause of lower leg ulcers.[1,4,22] Treatment includes compression therapy with dressings and inelastic or elastic bandages.

Venous Thrombosis

Venous thrombosis (*thrombophlebitis*) is the presence of thrombus and the accompanying inflammatory response in the vein wall. Thrombi can develop in superficial or deep veins.[5] Superficial venous thrombosis (SVT) can occur on any superficial vein. In some cases, SVT leads to complications such as reoccurrence of SVT, DVT, and pulmonary embolus.[23] DVT most commonly occurs in the lower extremities and is a serious disorder characterized by pulmonary embolism, recurrent episodes of DVT, and development of chronic venous insufficiency. Most postoperative thrombi arise in the soleal sinuses or the large veins draining the gastrocnemius muscles.[4] Isolated calf thrombi are often asymptomatic. If untreated, they may extend to larger, more proximal veins, with an increased risk of pulmonary emboli.[4]

Etiology and Pathogenesis

Venous thrombosis is associated with stasis of blood, increased blood coagulability, and vessel wall injury.[4] Bed rest and immobilization are associated with decreased blood flow and stasis, venous pooling in the lower extremities, and increased risk of DVT. People immobilized by a hip fracture, joint replacement, or spinal cord injury are particularly vulnerable to DVT. The risk of DVT is increased with impaired cardiac function. This may account for the high incidence in people with acute myocardial infarction and congestive heart failure. Older adults are more susceptible, likely because disorders that produce venous stasis occur more frequently in older adults. Long airplane travel poses a particular threat in people predisposed to DVT because of prolonged sitting and increased blood viscosity because of dehydration.[1]

Hypercoagulability is a state of increased clot formation that increases the likelihood of DVT. Hypercoagulable states can be caused by inherited or acquired deficiencies in certain plasma proteins that normally inhibit thrombus formation. Inherited disorders of factor V Leiden and prothrombin can also produce a hypercoagulable state. Oral contraceptives and hormone replacement therapy increase coagulability and predispose to venous thrombosis, a risk that is further increased with smoking cigarettes. Certain cancers are associated with increased clotting tendencies, although the reason for this is largely unknown. When body fluid is lost due to injury or disease, resulting hemoconcentration concentrates clotting factors. Other important risk factors include the antiphospholipid syndrome and myeloproliferative disorders.[1,4]

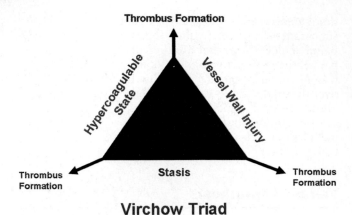

Virchow Triad

FIGURE 26-18. The Virchow triad of thrombus formation. (From Zierler, R. E., Dawson, D. L. (2016). *Strandness's duplex scanning in vascular disorders*. Philadelphia, PA: Wolters Kluwer.)

Vessel injury can result from trauma and surgery, may occur secondary to infection or inflammation of the vessel wall, and result from vascular injury caused by venous catheters. Risk factors for venous thrombosis include bed rest, immobility, spinal cord injury, acute myocardial infarction, congestive heart failure, shock, and venous obstruction. The Virchow triad illustrates three key factors leading to thrombus formation (Fig. 26–18).

Clinical Manifestations

Many people with venous thrombosis are asymptomatic. Lack of signs is likely due to the vein not being totally occluded or the presence of collateral circulation. Common signs and symptoms are related to the inflammatory process, including pain, swelling, and deep muscle tenderness. Fever, general malaise, and an elevated white blood cell count and erythrocyte sedimentation rate are accompanying indications of inflammation. There may be tenderness and pain along the vein. Swelling may vary from minimal to maximal.[1,4]

The site of thrombus formation determines the location of physical findings. The most common site is in the venous sinuses in the soleus muscle and posterior tibial and peroneal veins. Swelling in these cases involves the foot and ankle, although it may be slight or absent. Calf pain and tenderness are common. Femoral vein thrombosis produces pain and tenderness in the distal thigh and popliteal area. Thrombi in iliofemoral veins produce the most profound manifestations, with swelling, pain, and tenderness of the entire extremity.[1,4]

Diagnosis and Treatment

Diagnostic tests include venography, ultrasonography, and plasma D-dimer assessment. When possible, venous thrombosis should be prevented in preference to being treated. Early ambulation after childbirth and surgery decreases the risk of thrombus formation. Exercising the legs and wearing support stockings improve venous flow. Further precautions include avoiding body positions that favor venous pooling. Properly fitted antiembolism stockings should be used routinely in people at risk for

DVT. A sequential pneumatic compression device is used for immobile people at risk for DVT. This consists of a plastic sleeve that encircles the legs and provides alternating periods of compression on the lower extremity. These devices enhance venous emptying to augment flow and reduce stasis. Prophylactic anticoagulation drug therapy is often used in people who are at high risk for development of venous thrombi.[1,4,24]

Treatment is aimed at preventing formation of additional thrombi, preventing extension and embolization of existing thrombi, and minimizing venous valve damage. Leg elevation can help prevent stasis of blood flow. Heat applied to the leg can relieve venospasm and aid in resolving the inflammatory process. Bed rest is maintained until local tenderness and swelling subside, followed by gradual ambulation with elastic support and avoidance of prolonged periods of standing or sitting, which should be continued after the resolution of the DVT.[1,4,24]

Anticoagulation drug therapy (*i.e.*, heparin and warfarin) is used to prevent further thrombus formation. Treatment is initiated with an injectable form of a heparin-based anticoagulant. The patient is transitioned to either an oral anticoagulant or subcutaneous injections for outpatient management. Thrombolytic therapy may be used in an attempt to dissolve the clot.[1,4,24]

Percutaneous insertion of intracaval filters may be done in people at high risk for development of pulmonary emboli. This procedure prevents large clots from moving through the vessel. However, an increase in thrombosis occurs at the site of the filter itself in the absence of anticoagulation. Additional risks include the potential for filter breakage or migration.[1,4,24]

SUMMARY CONCEPTS

The storage function of the venous system renders it susceptible to venous insufficiency, stasis, and thrombus formation. Varicose veins occur with prolonged distention and stretching of the superficial veins owing to venous insufficiency. Varicosities can arise because of defects in the superficial veins (*i.e.*, primary varicose veins) or because of impaired blood flow in the deep venous channels (*i.e.*, secondary varicose veins). Venous insufficiency reflects chronic venous stasis resulting from valvular incompetence. It is associated with stasis dermatitis and stasis or venous ulcers. Venous thrombosis is the presence of thrombus in a vein and the accompanying inflammatory response in the vessel wall. It is associated with vessel injury, stasis of venous flow, and hypercoagulability states. Thrombi can develop in superficial or deep veins. Thrombus formation in deep veins is a precursor to venous insufficiency and embolus formation.

Disorders of Blood Pressure Regulation

Blood pressure must be closely regulated to ensure adequate perfusion of body tissues and to prevent damage to blood vessels. If blood pressure is too low, tissues do not receive sufficient flow to ensure delivery of nutrients and removal of waste products. High pressures can easily damage the delicate endothelial tissue, increasing the likelihood of atherosclerotic vascular disease and vascular rupture. High blood pressure can also seriously damage the perfused organs.

 ## Hypertension

Hypertension is a sustained elevation of blood pressure within the arterial circuit. It is a primary risk factor for cardiovascular disease and a leading cause of morbidity and mortality worldwide.[25] Populations with special considerations regarding to the diagnosis and management of hypertension are pregnant women, children and adolescents, and older adults.

Etiology and Pathogenesis

Hypertension is broadly classified based on etiology as either primary (essential) hypertension or secondary hypertension. Primary hypertension refers to the clinical presence of hypertension without evidence of a specific causative clinical condition.

Nonmodifiable Risk Factors for Primary Hypertension

Risk factors for primary hypertension include nonmodifiable factors such as age, gender, race, family history, and genetics.

Age. Primary hypertension is more common in adults than in children. Historically, hypertension in children was more likely to be secondary hypertension, often due to congenital cardiac disorders or renal disease. The incidence of primary hypertension in children and adolescents is rising, corresponding to the increase in obesity and type 2 diabetes mellitus in children.[4,26] The likelihood of hypertension increases with increasing age, as does the likelihood of hypertension-associated cardiovascular morbidities. Elevations of blood pressure increase the risk for cardiovascular disorders, including ischemic heart disease, heart failure, ischemic stroke, peripheral arterial disease, aortic aneurysm, and renal vascular disease.[25] Rising blood pressures with aging are related to a stiffening of arterial walls, which particularly affects systolic pressure. The ability of the kidneys to excrete sodium also decreases with age, with sodium retention contributing to hypertension.[27]

Gender and Race. In the United States, hypertension is more prevalent and more severe in African Americans. African American populations tend to develop hypertension at an earlier age than other populations.[28] Adverse events attributable to hypertension were more likely to occur in females than males and in black people than in white people.[29] The general prevalence of hypertension is higher in males than females across age.[30]

Family History and Genetics. Hypertension is seen most frequently among people with a family history of high blood pressure. The genetic contribution to hypertension may approach 50%. Although many genetic loci are associated to hypertension, they do not account for a large proportion of the incidence. The environment interacts with genetics, as evidenced by many disorders that do not have a commonly identified genetic locus yet recur within families.[31]

Modifiable Risk Factors for Primary Hypertension

Modifiable risk factors for primary hypertension include diet, levels of blood lipids, tobacco and alcohol consumption, fitness and activity level, overweight/obesity, and blood glucose control. Pathophysiologic pathways that may be common contributing factors among these lifestyle factors include disruptions in the renin–angiotensin–aldosterone system, alterations of natriuretic peptide mechanisms, SNS activation, and alteration of endothelial cell function.[25]

Dietary Factors. A physiologic trait for salt sensitivity with respect to blood pressure regulation appears to be normally distributed throughout the human population. To maintain adequate renal salt elimination, the pressure natriuresis system adapts: blood pressure rises to maintain adequate renal salt elimination.[32] Current recommendation for people with hypertension is to restrict dietary sodium intake.[13] Dietary intake of fats and cholesterol also contributes to hypertension, partially because of the contribution of dietary fat intake to the development of dyslipidemia.

Dyslipidemia. Dyslipidemia contributes to an increased risk for hypertension. Atherosclerotic plaques within arteries increase resistance to blood flow, contributing to a rise in arterial blood pressure to overcome increased resistance. Increased risk for hypertension is associated when blood lipids have higher levels of cholesterol, triglycerides, and LDLs; low levels of HDLs are also associated with higher risk for hypertension.[25]

Tobacco. Cigarette smoking has long been associated with the development of hypertension; however, causal connections have not yet been clearly identified. This pathogenetic connection between tobacco and hypertension may also be extended to other forms of tobacco use.[33]

 Concept Mastery Alert

Smoking is an independent risk factor for the development of coronary artery disease and should be avoided, but it has not been identified as a direct cause of hypertension.

Alcohol Consumption. Alcohol consumption has a direct relational effect with hypertension, with higher levels of alcohol associated with development of hypertension. Excess alcohol consumption may account for as much as 10% of the population occurrence of hypertension, with alcohol-related hypertension more prevalent in males than females. In contrast, evidence indicates that modest levels of alcohol intake are associated with a protective effect against heart disease.[25]

Fitness Level. Research evidence indicates that higher levels of fitness and exercise are associated with lower blood pressures and more favorable blood lipid levels. Overall, cardiovascular risk is decreased with higher levels of fitness and regular exercise.[13]

Obesity. Excessive body weight is commonly associated with hypertension. Weight reduction of as little as 4.5 kg (10 lb) can decrease blood pressure in people who are overweight with hypertension. The pattern of fat distribution may be a more critical indicator of hypertension risk than weight or body mass index. Waist-to-hip ratio is used to differentiate central obesity (with fat cells located in the abdomen and viscera) from peripheral obesity (with fat cell deposits in the buttocks and legs). There may be a link between hypertension and increased waist-to-hip ratio (*i.e.*, central obesity). Abdominal or visceral fat seems to cause more insulin resistance, glucose intolerance, dyslipidemia, hypertension, and chronic kidney disease than subcutaneous fat. Leptin, an adipocyte-derived hormone, may link adiposity and increased cardiovascular sympathetic activity. Besides its effect on appetite and metabolism, leptin acts on the hypothalamus to increase blood pressure through activation of the SNS. High levels of circulating free fatty acids in people with obesity also participate in activation of the SNS.[4,14,33]

Insulin Resistance and Metabolic Abnormalities. Hypertension is one of the components of the metabolic syndrome and insulin resistance associated with type 2 diabetes mellitus.[15]

Obstructive Sleep Apnea. Obstructive sleep apnea has been directly connected to hypertension, thought to be in part because disrupted sleep interferes with the normal circadian nocturnal "dipping" of blood pressure. Repetitive interruptions of sleep and decreased duration or quality of sleep are associated with less nocturnal "dipping" of blood pressure.[7,34]

Secondary Hypertension

Secondary hypertension is elevation in blood pressure because of another disease condition. Unlike primary hypertension, many conditions causing secondary hypertension can be corrected by surgery or specific medical treatment. Secondary hypertension is seen in people younger than 30 and older than 50 years of age. Cocaine, amphetamines, and other illicit drugs can cause significant hypertension, as can sympathomimetic agents (decongestants and anorectics), erythropoietin, and licorice. Common causes of secondary hypertension are kidney disease, disorders of adrenal cortical hormones, pheochromocytoma, coarctation of the aorta, and use of oral contraceptive agents.[25,35-38]

Renal Hypertension. The largest cause of secondary hypertension is renal disease. Decreased urine formation, retention of salt and water, and hypertension are common complications of acute kidney disorders. Hypertension also occurs with chronic pyelonephritis, polycystic kidney disease, diabetic nephropathy, and end-stage renal disease. In older adults, the sudden onset of secondary hypertension is often associated with atherosclerotic disease of renal blood vessels.[1,3,4]

Renovascular hypertension is caused by reduced renal blood flow and activation of the renin–angiotensin–aldosterone mechanism. It is the most common cause of secondary hypertension, accounting for 1% to 2% of all hypertension cases.[36] Reduced renal blood flow causes the affected kidney to release excess renin, increasing circulating levels of angiotensin II, which acts as a vasoconstrictor to increase PVR and as a stimulus for increased aldosterone levels and sodium retention by the kidney. When the renal artery of one kidney is involved, the unaffected kidney is subjected to the effects of the elevated blood pressure.[1,3,4]

Two major types of renovascular disease are atherosclerosis of the proximal renal artery and fibromuscular dysplasia, a noninflammatory vascular disease that affects the renal arteries and branch vessels. Atherosclerotic stenosis of the renal artery is seen often in older adults, particularly with comorbidities for atherosclerosis. Fibromuscular dysplasia is common in females and in younger age groups, particularly 30- to 50-year age range. Pathogenic mechanisms are uncertain; however, the incidence increases with environmental factors such as smoking.[36]

Disorders of Adrenocortical Hormones. Increased levels of adrenocortical hormones can also give rise to hypertension because of hormonally induced renal retention of salt and water. Primary hyperaldosteronism (excess production of aldosterone because of adrenocortical hyperplasia or adenoma) and excess levels of glucocorticoid (Cushing disease or syndrome) tend to raise the blood pressure.[38]

Pheochromocytoma. A pheochromocytoma is a tumor of chromaffin tissue, which contains sympathetic nerve cells that release catecholamine. The tumor is most commonly located in the adrenal medulla. Although rare, the presence of a pheochromocytoma can cause serious hypertensive crises.[37]

Coarctation of the Aorta. Coarctation of the aorta is a congenital condition in which there is a narrowing in the area of the arch of the aorta. Narrowing increases resistance to blood flow, causing the left ventricle to increase pressure to overcome resistance. Because the subclavian arteries arise above the location of the narrowing, the result is hypertension in the upper extremities and normal or low blood pressures in the lower extremities. Coarctation can be surgically repaired.[39]

Oral Contraceptive Drugs. The use of oral contraceptives is a common cause of secondary hypertension. The cause is largely unknown, although it has been suggested that the probable cause is volume expansion because both estrogens and synthetic progesterones cause sodium retention. Fortunately, the hypertension associated with oral contraceptives usually disappears after the drug has been discontinued, although it may take as long as 3 months.[4,16]

Clinical Manifestations of Hypertension

Primary hypertension is typically an asymptomatic disorder. When symptoms do occur, they are often related to long-term effects of hypertension on *target-organ* systems, such as the kidneys, heart, eyes, and blood vessels. *Target-organ damage* varies markedly among people with similar levels of hypertension. People with secondary hypertension are also at risk for these target-organ effects; however, those people may also demonstrate clinical manifestations related to the primary disease process that is causing the secondary hypertension (Chart 26-1).

Target-Organ Damage
Increased perfusion pressure can damage target organs, and increased intravascular pressure can damage vascular endothelial cells, which increases the risk for the development of atherosclerotic vascular disease (which further impairs organ perfusion). Target-organ damage particularly affects organs that are highly vascular or dependent on adequate blood supply for appropriate

---

CHART 26-1

CONSEQUENCES OF TARGET-ORGAN DAMAGE IN HYPERTENSION

- Heart
  - Angina (due to myocardial ischemia)
  - Myocardial infarction
  - Heart failure
- Brain
  - Stroke or transient ischemic attack
- Chronic kidney disease or kidney failure
- Peripheral artery disease
- Retinopathy
- Sexual dysfunction

Source: American Heart Association (2018). Health Threats from High Blood Pressure. Downloaded from: http://www.heart.org/HEARTORG/Conditions/HighBloodPressure/LearnHowHBPHarmsYourHealth/Health-Threats-From-High-Blood-Pressure_UCM_002051_Article.jsp.

---

function. Therefore, hypertension is a leading cause of ischemic heart and brain disease, end-stage renal disease, and visual impairment or blindness caused by retinopathy.[4,25]

Hypertension is a major risk factor for atherosclerosis because it promotes plaque formation and rupture. It predisposes to coronary heart disease, heart failure, stroke, and PAD. The risk for coronary artery disease and stroke depends on other risk factors, such as obesity, smoking, dyslipidemia, and genetic predisposition.[1,4]

Elevated blood pressure increases the workload of the left ventricle by increasing the pressure against which the heart must pump as it ejects blood into the systemic circulation. Over time, the left ventricular wall remodels and hypertrophies to compensate for the increased pressure work. This is a major risk factor for coronary heart disease, cardiac dysrhythmias, sudden death, and congestive heart failure because it cannot pump efficiently.[1,4]

Chronic hypertension leads to nephrosclerosis, a common cause of chronic kidney disease. One way hypertension causes damage to the kidneys is through glomerular hypoperfusion, which causes glomerulosclerosis and tubulointerstitial fibrosis. Other ways include endothelial dysfunction resulting from high glomerular pressures. Hypertensive kidney disease is more common in African American populations. Hypertension also plays an important role in accelerating the course of other types of kidney disease, particularly diabetic nephropathy.[1,4]

Dementia and cognitive impairment occur more commonly in people with hypertension. Hypertension, particularly systolic hypertension, is a major risk factor for ischemic stroke and intracerebral hemorrhage.[1,4] Narrowing and sclerosis of small penetrating arteries in the subcortical regions of the brain are common findings on autopsy in people with chronic hypertension.[1,4] These changes contribute to hypoperfusion, loss of autoregulation of blood flow, and impairment of the blood–brain barrier, ultimately leading to subcortical white matter demyelination. Effective antihypertensive therapy reduces the risk of significant white matter changes. However, once established, white matter changes do not appear to be reversible.[1,4]

Hypertensive retinopathy affects the retina through a series of microvascular changes.[1,4] The eye will initially have increased vasomotor tone, which causes generalized arteriolar narrowing. As hypertension persists, arteriosclerotic changes include media wall hyperplasia, intimal thickening, and hyaline degeneration. These long-term changes can cause more severe AV nicking and may cause blindness (Fig. 26-19). Acute increases in blood pressure can lead to hemorrhages, microaneurysms, and hard exudates. Eyes need to be evaluated regularly in person with hypertension to prevent extensive damage.[1,4]

Hypertensive Emergency
Rarely, people with hypertension develop an accelerated and potentially fatal form hypertension called a *hypertensive emergency*, characterized by sudden elevations

Drug-Induced Hypotension

Antihypertensive drugs and psychotropic drugs are common causes of chronic orthostatic hypotension. If the hypotension causes lightheadedness or syncope, dosage is usually reduced or a different drug substituted.[16]

Disorders of the Autonomic Nervous System

Sympathetic stimulation increases HR and cardiac contractility and causes constriction of peripheral veins and arterioles. Orthostatic hypotension caused by altered ANS function is common in peripheral neuropathies associated with diabetes mellitus, after injury or disease of the spinal cord, or disruption of sympathetic outflow from the brain stem.[1,3,4]

Diagnosis and Treatment

Orthostatic hypotension can be assessed with the auscultatory method. A second person should be available when blood pressure is measured to prevent injury should the person become faint. A thorough physical examination and history should be taken for information about symptoms, dizziness and history of syncope and falls; medical conditions, such as diabetes mellitus; medications; and symptoms of ANS dysfunction, such as erectile or bladder dysfunction. Blood pressure and HR should be measured in both arms while in the supine, sitting, and standing positions. Noninvasive, 24-hour ambulatory blood pressure monitoring may determine blood pressure responses to stimuli of daily life, such as food ingestion and exertion.[44-47]

Treatment is directed toward alleviating the cause, coping with symptoms and preventing falls and injuries. Measures designed to help people prevent symptomatic orthostatic drops in blood pressure include gradual ambulation to allow the circulatory system to adjust; avoidance of situations that encourage excessive vasodilation; and avoidance of excess diuresis, diaphoresis, or loss of body fluids. Tight-fitting elastic support hose or an abdominal support garment may help prevent pooling of blood in the lower extremities and abdomen.[44-47]

 SUMMARY CONCEPTS

Hypertension is one of the most common cardiovascular disorders. It may occur as a primary disorder or as a symptom of some other disease. Incidence of primary hypertension increases with age, is seen more frequently among African Americans, and may be associated with a family history of high blood pressure, metabolic syndrome, obesity, and increased sodium intake. Causes of secondary hypertension include kidney disease and adrenal cortical disorders, which increase sodium and water retention; pheochromocytomas, which increase catecholamine levels; and coarctation of the aorta, which produces an increase in blood flow and systolic blood pressure in the arms and a decrease in blood flow and systolic pressure in the legs. Uncontrolled hypertension increases the risk of heart disease, renal complications, retinopathy, and stroke.

Hypertension occurring during pregnancy includes preeclampsia–eclampsia, chronic hypertension, chronic hypertension with superimposed preeclampsia, and gestational hypertension. Preeclampsia–eclampsia is a life-threatening complication that is thought to be related to the placenta and widespread endothelial dysfunction. Gestational hypertension is a new onset finding of increased blood pressure after 20 weeks' gestation, without signs of preeclampsia.

Hypertension in children and adolescents is increasing, partly as a result of increased childhood obesity and lifestyle factors such as inactivity and increased intake of high-calorie and high-salt foods. Hypertension is a common pathophysiologic condition in older adults.

Orthostatic hypotension is an abnormal decrease in systolic and diastolic blood pressures that occur on assumption of the upright position, causing dizziness and syncope. Among the factors that contribute to its occurrence are decreased fluid volume, medications, aging, defective function of the ANS, and immobility. Diagnosis relies on blood pressure measurements in the supine and upright positions, and a history of symptomatology, medication use, and disease conditions that contribute to a postural drop in blood pressure. Treatment includes correcting the reversible causes and compensating for the disorder and prevent falls and injuries.

Review Exercises

1. A 55-year-old male executive presents at the clinic for his regular checkup. He was diagnosed with hypertension 5 years ago and has been taking a diuretic and a β-adrenergic blocker to control his blood pressure. His blood pressure is currently being maintained at about 135/70 mm Hg. His total cholesterol level is 180 mg/dL, and his HDL cholesterol is 30 mg/dL. He is otherwise well. He is a nonsmoker. He has recently read in the media about "inflammation" and the heart and expresses concern about his risk of CHD.
   A. Identify risk factors for atherosclerosis present in this history.
   B. Explain the role of HDL in the prevention of atherosclerosis.

2. A 62-year-old man presents at the emergency department of his local hospital with

complaints of excruciating, "ripping" pain in his upper back. He has a history of poorly controlled hypertension. His radial pulse and blood pressure, which, on admission, were 92 and 140/80 mm Hg, respectively, become unobtainable in both arms. A transesophageal echocardiogram reveals a dissection of the descending aorta. Aggressive blood pressure control is initiated with the goal of reducing the systolic pressure and pulsatile blood flow (pulse pressure).

A. Explain how aortic dissection differs from a thoracic aorta aneurysm.
B. Explain the role of poorly controlled hypertension as an etiologic factor in dissecting aneurysms.
C. Why did his radial pulse and blood pressure become unobtainable?
D. Explain the need for aggressive control of aortic pressure and pulsatile blood flow.

3. A 34-year-old, otherwise healthy woman complains of episodes lasting several hours in which her fingers become pale and numb. This is followed by a period during which the fingers become red, throbbing, and painful. She lives in the Northeast and notices it more in the fall and winter months.

A. What do you think is causing this woman's problem?
B. She relates that the episodes often occur when her fingers become cold or when she becomes upset. Explain the possible underlying mechanisms.
C. What types of measures could be used to treat this woman?

4. A 47-year-old African American man who is an executive in a law firm has his blood pressure taken at a screening program and is told that his pressure is 142/90 mm Hg. His father and older brother have hypertension, and his paternal grandparents had a history of stroke and myocardial infarction. He enjoys salty foods and routinely uses a saltshaker to add salt to meals his wife prepares, drinks about four beers while watching television in the evening, and gained 15 lb in the past year. Although his family has encouraged him to engage in physical activities with them, he states he is either too busy or too tired.

A. According to the 2017 ACC/AHA guidelines, into what category does the patient's blood pressure fall? What are his risk factors for hypertension?
B. Explain how an increased salt intake might contribute to his increase in blood pressure.

C. What lifestyle changes would you suggest to the patient? Explain the rationale for your suggestions.

5. A 36-year-old woman enters the clinic complaining of headache and not feeling well. Her blood pressure is 175/90 mm Hg. Her renal test results are abnormal, and follow-up tests confirm that she has a stricture of the left renal artery.

A. Would this woman's hypertension be classified as primary or secondary?
B. Explain the physiologic mechanisms underlying her blood pressure elevation.

6. A 75-year-old woman residing in an extended care facility has multiple health problems, including diabetes, hypertension, and heart failure. Lately, she has been feeling dizzy when she stands up, and she has almost fallen on several occasions. Her family is concerned and wants to know why this is happening and what they can do to prevent her from falling and breaking her hip.

A. How would you go about assessing this woman for orthostatic hypotension?
B. What are some causes of orthostatic hypotension in elderly people?
C. How might this woman's medical conditions and their treatment contribute to her orthostatic hypotension?

REFERENCES

1. Kumar V., Abbas A. K., Aster J. C. (2015). *Robbins & Cotran pathologic basis of disease* (9th ed.). Philadelphia, PA: Elsevier Saunders.
2. Ross M., Pawlina W. (2015). *Histology: A text and atlas* (7th ed.). Philadelphia, PA: Lippincott Williams & Wilkins.
3. Hall J. E. (2015). *Guyton and Hall textbook of medical physiology* (13th ed.). Philadelphia, PA: Elsevier.
4. Rubin R., Strayer D. S., Saffitz J. E., et al. (Eds.) (2015). *Rubin's pathology: Clinicopathologic foundations of medicine* (7th ed.). Philadelphia, PA: Wolters Kluwer.
5. Hopps E., Caimi G. (2015). Obstructive sleep apnea syndrome: Links between pathophysiology and cardiovascular complications. *Clinical and Investigative Medicine* 38(6), E362–E370.
6. Wang L., Li N., Yao X., et al. (2017). Detection of secondary causes and coexisting diseases in hypertensive patients: OSA and PA are the common causes associated with hypertension. *BioMed Research International* 2017, 8. doi:10.1155/2017/8295010.
7. Yang H., Haack M., Gautam S., et al. (2017). Repetitive exposure to shortened sleep leads to blunted sleep-associated blood pressure dipping. *Journal of Hypertension* 35(6), 1187–1194.
8. Missala I., Kassner U., Steinhagen-Thiessen E. (2012). A systematic literature review of the association of lipoprotein(a) and autoimmune diseases and atherosclerosis. *International Journal of Rheumatology* 2012, 10. doi:10.1155/2012/480784.

9. Schmitz G., Orso E. (2015). Lipoprotein(a) hyperlipidemia as cardiovascular risk factor: Pathophysiological aspects. *Clinical Research in Cardiology Supplement* 10, 21–25.

10. Tsimikas S. (2016). The re-emergence of lipoprotein(a) in a broader clinical arena. *Progress in Cardiovascular Diseases* 59(2), 135–144.

11. Wakabayashi I. (2016). A U-shaped relationship between alcohol consumption and cardiometabolic index in middle-aged men. *Lipids in Health and Disease* 15(50), 1–7. doi:10.1186/s12944-016-0217-4.

12. Kennedy M. J., Jellerson K. D., Snow M. Z., et al. (2013). Challenges in the pharmacologic management of obesity in children and adolescents. *Pediatric Drugs* 15, 335–342. doi:10.1007/s40272-013-0028-2.

13. Eckel R. H., Jakicic J. M., Ard J. D., et al. (2013). AHA/ACC guideline on lifestyle management to reduce cardiovascular risk: A report of the American College of Cardiology American/Heart Association Task Force on Practice Guidelines. *Circulation* 2013;129(25 Suppl 2):S76–S99.

14. Heymsfield S. B., Wadden T. A. (2017). Mechanisms, pathophysiology, and management of obesity. *New England Journal of Medicine* 376, 254–266. doi:10.1056/NEJMra1514009.

15. McCracken E., Monaghan M., Sreenivasan S. (2018). Pathophysiology of the metabolic syndrome. *Clinics in Dermatology* 36, 14–20. doi:10.1016/j.clindermatol.2017.09.004.

16. Lehne R. A. (2016). *Pharmacology for nursing care* (9th ed.). St. Louis, MO: Elsevier.

17. American Association of Clinical Chemistry Lab Tests Online. (2018). High-sensitivity C-reactive protein. Available: https://labtestsonline.org/tests/high-sensitivity-c-reactive-protein-hs-crp. Accessed February 6, 2019.

18. Goff D. C. Jr, Lloyd-Jones D. M., Bennett G., et al. (2013). 2013 ACC/AHA guideline on the assessment of cardiovascular: A report of the American College of Cardiology/American Heart Association Task Force on Practice Guidelines. *Circulation* 29(25 Suppl 2), S49–S73. doi:10.1161/01.cir.0000437741.48606.98.

19. Jennette J. C. (2013). Overview of the 2012 revised international Chapel Hill Consensus Conference nomenclature of vasculotides. *Clinical and Experimental Nephrology* 17(5), 603–606.

20. Steuer J., Bjorck M., Mayer D., et al. (2013). Distinction between acute and chronic type B aortic dissection: Is there a sub-acute phase? *European Journal of Vascular and Endovascular Surgery* 45(6), 627–631.

21. Chen J. C. (2017). Current therapy for primary varicose veins. *British Columbia Medical Journal* 59(8), 418–423.

22. Mazuchova J., Pec M., Halasova E., et al. (2016). News in pathogenesis of chronic venous insufficiency. *Acta Medica Martiniana* 16(2), 5–8. doi:10.1515/acm-2016-0006.

23. Nasr H., Scriven J. M. (2015). Superficial thrombophlebitis (superficial venous thrombosis). *The British Medical Journal* 350, h2039. doi:10.1136/bmj.h2039.

24. Douketis J. D. (2016). Deep venous thrombosis (DVT). Merck Manual Professional Edition. Available: http://www.merckmanuals.com/professional/cardiovascular-disorders/peripheral-venous-disorders/deep-venous-thrombosis-dvt. Accessed May 14, 2019.

25. Whelton P. K., Carey R. M., Aronow W. S., et al. (2017). ACC/AHA/AAPA/ABC/ACPM/AGS/APhA/ASH/ASPC/NMA/PCNA guideline for the prevention, detection, evaluation, and management of high blood pressure in adults: A report of the American College of Cardiology/American Heart Association Task Force on Clinical Practice Guidelines. *Hypertension* 71(6), 1269–1324.

26. Flynn J. T., Kaelber D. C., Baker-Smith C. M., et al. (2017). Clinical practice guidelines for screening and management of high blood pressure in children and adolescents. *Pediatrics* 140(3), e20171904.

27. Garfinkle M. A. (2017). Salt and essential hypertension: Pathophysiology and implications for treatment. *Journal of the American Society of Hypertension* 11(6), 385–391. doi:10.1016/j.jash.2017.04.006.

28. American Heart Association. (2016). High blood pressure and African Americans. Available: http://www.heart.org/HEARTORG/Conditions/HighBloodPressure/UnderstandSymptomsRisks/High-Blood-Pressure-and-African-Americans_UCM_301832_Article.jsp. Accessed May 14, 2019.

29. Willey J. Z., Moon Y. P., Kahn E., et al. (2014). Population attributable risks of hypertension and diabetes for cardiovascular disease and stroke in the northern Manhattan study. *Journal of the American Heart Association* 3, e001106. doi:10.1161/JAHA.114.001106.

30. Everett B., Zajacova A. (2015). Gender differences in hypertension and hypertension awareness among young adults. *Biodemography and Social Biology* 61(1), 1–17. doi:10.1080/19485565.2014.929488.

31. Han L., Liu Y., Duan S., et al. (2016). DNA methylation and hypertension: Emerging evidence and challenges. *Briefings in Functional Genomics* 15(6), 460–469. doi:10.1093/bfgp/elw014.

32. Elijovich F., Weinberger M. H., Anderson C. A. M.; on behalf of the American Heart Association Professional and Public Education Committee of the Council on Hypertension; Council on Functional Genomics and Translational Biology; and Stroke Council. (2016). Salt sensitivity of blood pressure: A scientific statement from the American Heart Association. *Hypertension* 68, e7–e46. doi:10.1161/HYP.0000000000000047.

33. McEvoy J. W., Blaha M. J., DeFilippis A. P., et al. (2015). Cigarette smoking and cardiovascular events: Role of inflammation and subclinical atherosclerosis. *Arteriosclerosis, Thrombosis, and Vascular Biology* 35(3), 700–709.

34. Ahmad M., Makati D., Akbar S. (2017). Review of and updates on hypertension in obstructive sleep apnea. *International Journal of Hypertension* 2017 , 13. doi:10.1155/2017/1848375.

35. Foster C. A., Church K. S., Poddar M. (2017). Licorice-induced hypertension: A case of pseudohyperaldosteronism due to jelly bean ingestion. *Postgraduate Medicine* 129(3), 329–331.

36. Samadian F., Dalli N., Jamalian A. (2017). New insights into pathophysiology, diagnosis, and treatment of renovascular hypertension. *Iranian Journal of Kidney Diseases* 11(2), 79–89.

37. Lenders J. W. M., Duo Q. Y., Eisenhofer G., et al. (2014). Pheochromocytoma and paraganglioma: An endocrine society clinical practice guideline. *Journal of Clinical Endocrinology and Metabolism* 99(6), 1915–1942.

38. Funder J. W., Carey R. M., Mantero F., et al. (2016). The management of primary aldosteronism: Case detection, diagnosis, and treatment: An endocrine society clinical practice guideline. *Journal of Clinical Endocrinology and Metabolism* 101(5), 1889–1916.

39. American Heart Association. (2017). Coarctation of the aorta. Available: http://www.heart.org/HEARTORG/Conditions/CongenitalHeartDefects/AboutCongenitalHeartDefects/Coarctation-of-the-Aorta-CoA_UCM_307022_Article.jsp. Accessed May 14, 2019.

40. Golshani C., Lieberman R. M., Fischer R. M., et al. (2017). Hypertensive crisis with massive retinal and choroidal infarction. *American Journal of Ophthalmology Case Reports* 6, 58–60.

41. American Heart Association. (2017). Hypertensive crisis: When you should call 9-1-1 for blood pressure. Available: http://www.heart.org/HEARTORG/Conditions/HighBlood Pressure/GettheFactsAboutHighBloodPressure/Hypertensive-Crisis-When-You-Should-Call-9-1-1-for-High-Blood-Pressure_UCM_301782_Article.jsp

42. American College of Obstetricians and Gynecologists Task Force on Hypertension in Pregnancy. (2013). Hypertension in Pregnancy. Available: https://www.acog.org/Resources-And-Publications/Task-Force-and-Work-Group-Reports/Hypertension-in-Pregnancy

43. Jena M., Mishra S., Jena S., et al. (2016). Pregnancy induced hypertension & pre-eclampsia: Pathophysiology & recent management trends: A review. *International Journal of Pharmaceutical Research and Allied Sciences* 5(3), 326–334.

44. Freeman R., Wieling W., Axelrod F. B., et al. (2011). Consensus statement on the definition 47(4), orthostatic hypotension, neutrally mediated syncope and the postural tachycardia syndrome. *Autonomic Neuroscience: Basic and Clinical* 161, 46–48. doi:10.1016/j.autneu. 2011.02.004.

45. Chisolm P. Anpalahan M. (2017). Orthostatic hypotension: Pathophysiology, assessment, treatment and the paradox of supine hypotension. *Internal Medicine Journal* 47(4), 370–379. doi:10.1111/imj.13171.

46. Wieling W., vanDijk N., Thijs R. D., et al. (2014). Physical countermeasures to increase orthostatic tolerance. *Journal of Internal Medicine* 277(1), 69–82. doi:10.1111/joim.12249.

47. Shaw B. H., Claydon V. E. (2014). The relationship between orthostatic hypotension and falling in older adults. *Clinical Autonomic Research* 24, 3–13. doi:10.1007/s10286-013-0219-5.

Disorders of Cardiac Function, and Heart Failure and Circulatory Shock

Learning Objectives

After completing this chapter, the learner will be able to meet the following objectives:

1. Characterize the function of the pericardium.
2. Compare the clinical manifestations of acute pericarditis and chronic pericarditis.
3. Describe the physiologic impact of pleural effusion on cardiac function and relate it to cardiac tamponade.
4. Describe blood flow in the coronary circulation and relate it to the determinants of myocardial oxygen supply and demand.
5. Define the term *acute coronary syndrome* (ACS) and distinguish among chronic stable angina, unstable angina (UA), non–ST-segment elevation myocardial infarction (NSTEMI), and ST-segment elevation myocardial infarction (STEMI) in terms of pathology, symptomatology, electrocardiographic changes, and serum cardiac markers.
6. Define the treatment goal for ACS.
7. Define *cardiomyopathy* as it relates to mechanical and electrical myocardium functions.
8. Differentiate among the pathophysiologic changes that occur with hypertrophic cardiomyopathy (HCM), arrhythmogenic right ventricular cardiomyopathy (ARVC), dilated cardiomyopathies, and myocarditis.
9. Describe the treatment strategies of both primary and secondary cardiomyopathy.
10. Distinguish between the roles of infectious organisms in infective endocarditis (IE) and rheumatic fever (RF).
11. Describe the relation between the infective vegetations associated with IE and the extracardiac manifestations of the disease.
12. Describe the long-term effects of RF and outline primary and secondary prevention strategies for RF and rheumatic heart disease.
13. State the function of the heart valves and relate alterations in hemodynamic function of the heart that occur with valvular disease.
14. Compare the effects of stenotic and regurgitant mitral and aortic valvular heart disease on cardiovascular function.
15. Explain how the Frank-Starling mechanism, sympathetic nervous system, renin–angiotensin–aldosterone mechanism, natriuretic peptides (NPs), endothelins, and myocardial hypertrophy and remodeling function as adaptive and maladaptive mechanisms in heart failure.
16. Differentiate high-output versus low-output heart failure, systolic versus diastolic heart failure, and right-sided versus left-sided heart failure in terms of causes, impact on cardiac function, and major manifestations.
17. Differentiate chronic heart failure from acute heart failure syndromes (AHFS) and methods of diagnosis, assessment, and management.
18. Describe the flow of blood in the fetal circulation, state the function of the foramen ovale and ductus arteriosus, and describe the changes in circulatory function that occur at birth.

19. Describe the anatomic defects and altered patterns of blood flow in children with atrial septal defects, ventricular septal defects, endocardial cushion defects, pulmonary stenosis, tetralogy of Fallot, patent ductus arteriosus, transposition of the great vessels, coarctation of the aorta, and single-ventricle anatomy.
20. Describe the manifestations related to the acute, subacute, and convalescent phases of Kawasaki disease.
21. Describe the causes of heart failure in infants and children.
22. Explain how aging affects cardiac function and predisposes to ventricular dysfunction.
23. Identify how signs and symptoms of heart failure may differ in younger and older adults.
24. Compare the causes, pathophysiology, and chief characteristics of cardiogenic, hypovolemic, obstructive, and distributive shock.
25. Describe the complications of shock as they relate to the lungs, kidneys, gastrointestinal tract, and blood clotting.
26. State the rationale for treatment measures to correct and reverse shock.

This chapter focuses on common heart problems that affect persons in all age groups. The "Disorders of Cardiac Function" part of this chapter includes disorders of the pericardium, coronary artery disease (CAD), cardiomyopathies, infectious and immunologic disorders of the heart, and valvular heart disease. The "Heart Failure and Circulatory Shock" part includes heart disease (in infants and children), heart failure (in children, adults, and older adults), and circulatory shock. Although cardiovascular disease (CVD) and heart failure are often thought to be the same, CVD typically refers to conditions with narrow or blocked vessels, whereas heart failure refers to failure of the heart as a pump.

DISORDERS OF CARDIAC FUNCTION

CVD is the leading cause of death in both males and females in the United States. Low- and middle-income countries are seeing an accelerated increase in CVD, surpassing infectious diseases.[1]

Disorders of the Pericardium

The pericardium, or the *pericardial sac*, is a double-layered serous membrane that isolates the heart from other thoracic structures, maintains its position in the thorax, prevents it from overfilling, and serves as a barrier to infection. It consists of two layers: a thin inner layer, called the *visceral pericardium*, that adheres to the epicardium; and an outer fibrous layer, called the *parietal pericardium*, that is attached to the great vessels that enter and leave the heart, sternum, and diaphragm. These two layers are separated by a potential space, the *pericardial cavity*, which contains about 50 mL of serous fluid. This fluid acts as a lubricant that prevents frictional forces from developing as the heart contracts and relaxes. There is little blood supply to the pericardium but it is well innervated, and inflammation can cause severe pain.[2]

The pericardium is subject to many of the same pathologic processes that affect other structures of the body. Pericardial disorders are frequently associated with or result from another disease in the heart or the surrounding structures.

Acute Pericarditis

Pericarditis is an inflammatory process of the pericardium. *Acute pericarditis*, pericardial inflammation of less than 2 weeks, may occur as an isolated disease or the result of systemic disease. Viral infections (*e.g.*, with coxsackieviruses and echoviruses) are the most common cause of pericarditis. Other causes include bacterial or mycobacterial infections, connective tissue diseases (*e.g.*, systemic lupus erythematosus, rheumatoid arthritis), uremia, postcardiac surgery, neoplastic invasion of the pericardium, radiation, trauma, drug toxicity, and contiguous inflammatory processes of the myocardium or lung.[2,3]

Acute pericarditis is often associated with increased capillary permeability. The capillaries that supply the serous pericardium become permeable, allowing plasma proteins to leave capillaries and enter the pericardial space. Acute pericarditis is associated with a fibrin-containing exudate (Fig. 27-1), which heals or progresses to scar tissue and forms adhesions between the layers of serous pericardium. Inflammation may involve superficial myocardium and adjacent pleura.

Clinical Manifestations

The manifestations of acute pericarditis include a triad of chest pain, pericardial friction rub, and electrocardiographic (ECG) changes. Nearly all people with acute pericarditis have chest pain, which is usually abrupt in onset and sharp, occurring in the precordial area, and may radiate to the neck, back, abdomen, or side. The pain is typically worse with deep breathing, coughing, swallowing, and positional changes because of changes in venous return and cardiac filling. The person often finds relief by sitting up and leaning forward. It is important to differentiate the chest pain from pericarditis from acute myocardial infarction (MI) or pulmonary embolism (PE).

Diagnosis

Diagnosis is based on clinical manifestations, ECG, chest radiography, and echocardiography. A pericardial friction rub results from the rubbing and friction between inflamed pericardial surfaces. It is typically described as having three components: atrial systole,

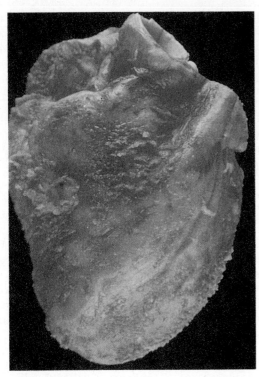

FIGURE 27-1. Fibrinous pericarditis. The heart of a person who died of untreated uremia displays a shaggy, fibrinous exudate covering the visceral pericardium. (From Strayer D. E., Rubin R. (Eds.) (2015). *Rubin's pathology: Clinicopathologic foundations of medicine* (7th ed., Fig. 17-52, p. 675). Philadelphia, PA: Lippincott Williams & Wilkins.)

ventricular systole, and rapid filling of the ventricle. Because it results from the rubbing of inflamed pericardial surfaces, large effusions are unlikely to produce a friction rub. Except in uremic pericarditis, ECG changes in pericarditis evolve through four progressive stages: diffuse ST-segment elevations and PR-segment depression, normalization of the ST and PR segments, widespread T-wave inversions, and normalization of T waves. Laboratory markers of systemic inflammation may also be present, including an elevated white blood cell count, elevated erythrocyte sedimentation rate (ESR), and increased C-reactive protein (CRP).[3]

Treatment

Acute idiopathic pericarditis is frequently self-limiting. Symptoms are usually successfully treated with nonsteroidal anti-inflammatory drugs (NSAIDs).[2,3] Colchicine can be added to the treatment regimen in people who have a slow response to NSAIDs. When infection is present, antibiotics specific for the causative agent are usually prescribed. Corticosteroids may be used for the treatment of person with connective tissue disease or severely symptomatic pericarditis that is not responsive to NSAIDs and colchicine. Corticosteroids should be avoided owing to side effects, recurrences, and hospitalizations.

Relapsing pericarditis can occur in up to 30% of people with acute pericarditis who respond to treatment.[2] A minority develop recurrent bouts of pericardial pain, which can be chronic and debilitating. The process is commonly associated with autoimmune disorders, but may also occur following viral pericarditis. Treatment includes anti-inflammatory medications such as NSAIDs initially and then colchicine. If reoccurrence continues, colchicine prophylaxis is warranted. If colchicine is not tolerated, then low-dose corticosteroids can be initiated.[2]

Pericardial Effusion and Cardiac Tamponade

Pericardial effusion is the accumulation of fluid in the pericardial cavity, usually as a result of an inflammatory or infectious process. It may also develop as the result of neoplasms, cardiac surgery, trauma, cardiac rupture due to MI, and dissecting aortic aneurysm. The pressure–volume relationship between the normal pericardial and cardiac volumes can be dramatically affected once critical levels of effusion are present. As right heart filling pressures are lower than the left, increases in pressure are usually reflected in right-sided heart failure.

Pathogenesis

The amount of fluid, the rapidity with which it accumulates, and the elasticity of the pericardium determine the effect the effusion on cardiac function. Even a large effusion that develops slowly may cause no symptoms if the pericardium can stretch and avoid compressing the heart. But a sudden accumulation of 200 mL may raise intracardiac pressure to levels that seriously limit the venous return to the heart.[3] Symptoms of cardiac compression may occur with smaller amounts of fluid if the pericardium is thickened by scar tissue or neoplastic infiltrations.

Pericardial effusion can lead to *cardiac tamponade*, the compression of the heart caused by the accumulation of fluid, pus, or blood in the pericardial sac. This life-threatening condition can be caused by infections, neoplasms, and bleeding.[2,3] It results in increased intracardiac pressure, limitation of ventricular diastolic filling, and reductions in stroke volume (SV) and cardiac output (CO). The severity of disorder depends on the amount of fluid and the rate at which it accumulates.

Significant accumulation of fluid in the pericardium results in increased adrenergic stimulation, which leads to tachycardia and increased cardiac contractility. There is elevation of central venous pressure (CVP), jugular venous distention, a fall in systolic blood pressure, narrowed pulse pressure, muffled heart sounds, and signs of circulatory shock.

Diagnosis

Pulsus paradoxus is an exaggeration in the systemic arterial pulse volume with respiration.[2,3] Normally, the decrease in intrathoracic pressure during inspiration accelerates venous flow, increasing right heart filling. Because the interventricular septum will bulge into the left heart, there is a decrease in left ventricular (LV) filling, SV, and systolic blood pressure. In cardiac **tamponade**, LV is compressed by the interventricular septum and the pericardium (Fig. 27-2), which decreases LV filling

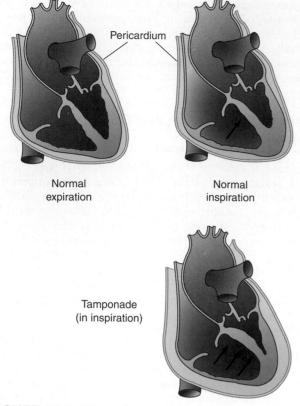

Normal
expiration

Normal
inspiration

Tamponade
(in inspiration)

FIGURE 27-2. Effects of respiration and cardiac tamponade on ventricular filling and cardiac output. During inspiration, venous flow into the right heart increases, causing the interventricular septum to bulge into the left ventricle (LV). This produces a decrease in LV volume, with a subsequent decrease in stroke volume output. In cardiac tamponade, the fluid in the pericardial sac produces further compression of the LV, causing an exaggeration of the normal inspiratory decrease in stroke volume and systolic blood pressure.

and LV SV. With pulsus paradoxus, the arterial pulse is weakened or absent during inspiration and is stronger during expiration.

The echocardiogram is a widely used method of evaluating pericardial effusion. The ECG often reveals non-specific T-wave changes and low QRS voltage.

Treatment

Treatment depends on the progression to cardiac tamponade. In small pericardial effusions or mild cardiac tamponade, NSAIDs, colchicine, or corticosteroids may minimize fluid accumulation. Pericardiocentesis (removal of fluid from the pericardial sac), with the aid of ECG, is the treatment of choice. Closed pericardiocentesis, performed with a needle inserted through the chest wall, may be an emergency measure in severe cardiac tamponade. Open pericardiocentesis may be used for recurrent or loculated effusions. Aspiration and laboratory evaluation of the pericardial fluid may be used to identify the causative agent.

Constrictive Pericarditis

In constrictive pericarditis, fibrous, calcified scar tissue develops between the visceral and parietal layers of the serous pericardium. The scar tissue contracts and interferes with diastolic filling, and CO and cardiac reserve become fixed. The equalization of end-diastolic pressures in all four cardiac chambers is the pathophysiologic hallmark of constrictive pericarditis.[4]

Effusive–constrictive pericarditis is a combination of effusion–tamponade and constriction. It is detected when hemodynamic measurements fail to stabilize after pericardiocentesis. The most common cause is idiopathic. People with the disorder usually require pericardiectomy.[2,4]

Etiology and Clinical Manifestations

Long-standing inflammation from mediastinal radiation, cardiac surgery, or infection is usually the cause. Ascites is a prominent early finding, along with pedal edema, dyspnea on exertion, and fatigue. The Kussmaul sign is an inspiratory distention of the jugular veins caused by the inability of the right atrium to accommodate increased venous with inspiration. Exercise intolerance, muscle wasting, and weight loss develop in end-stage constrictive pericarditis.

Diagnosis

Doppler echocardiogram, cardiac catheterization, computed tomography (CT), and magnetic resonance imaging (MRI) can distinguish constrictive pericarditis from restrictive cardiomyopathy. In chronic constrictive pericarditis, surgical removal or resection of the pericardium is often the treatment of choice.[2]

SUMMARY CONCEPTS

The pericardium is a two-layered membranous sac that isolates the heart from other thoracic structures, maintains its position, and prevents it from overfilling. Disorders include acute and chronic pericarditis, pericardial effusion and cardiac tamponade, and constrictive and effusive–constrictive pericarditis. A major threat of pericardial disease is compression of heart chambers.

Acute pericarditis is characterized by chest pain, ECG changes, and pericardial friction rub. Recurrent pericarditis is associated with autoimmune disorders. Pericardial effusion can increase intracardiac pressure, compress the heart, and interfere with venous return. The amount of exudate, the rapidity of accumulation, and elasticity of the pericardium determine the effect on cardiac function. Cardiac tamponade is a life-threatening compression of the heart resulting from excess fluid in the pericardial sac. In constrictive pericarditis, scar tissue develops between the visceral and parietal layers. In time, the scar tissue contracts and interferes with cardiac filling.

Coronary Artery Disease

CAD is caused by impaired coronary blood flow. In most cases, CAD is caused by atherosclerosis. CAD can cause myocardial ischemia and angina, MI or heart attack, cardiac arrhythmias, conduction defects, heart failure, and sudden death. Over 790,000 Americans have new or recurrent MIs each year.[5]

Major risk factors include cigarette smoking, elevated blood pressure, elevated serum total and low-density lipoprotein cholesterol, low serum high-density lipoprotein cholesterol, diabetes, age, abdominal obesity, and physical inactivity.[6] Diabetes and metabolic syndrome increase risk and morbidity.[6]

 ## Coronary Circulation

The Coronary Arteries

The two main coronary arteries arise from the coronary sinus just above the aortic valve (Fig. 27-3). The *left main coronary artery* divides into the left anterior descending and circumflex branches. The *left anterior descending artery* passes through the groove between the ventricles, giving off diagonal branches that supply the LV and perforating branches that supply the anterior portion of the interventricular septum and the anterior papillary muscle of the LV. The *circumflex branch* of the left coronary artery moves in the groove that separates the atrium and ventricle, giving off branches that supply the left lateral LV wall. The *right coronary artery* lies in the right atrioventricular (AV) groove, and its branches supply most of the right ventricle and the posterior LV.

The right coronary artery forms the *posterior descending artery*, which supplies the posterior heart, interventricular septum, sinoatrial (SA) and AV nodes, and posterior papillary muscle. The coronary artery that supplies the posterior third of the septum (either the right coronary artery or the left circumflex) is *dominant*. In a right dominant circulation, present in four fifths of people, the left circumflex perfuses the lateral LV wall, and the right coronary artery supplies the right ventricular free wall and the posterior third of the septum.

Large epicardial coronary arteries lie on the surface of the heart, with smaller arteries branching and penetrating the myocardium before merging with a plexus of subendocardial vessels. There are anastomotic channels that join the small arteries. With gradual occlusion of larger vessels, smaller collateral vessels increase in size. One reasons CAD does not produce symptoms until it is advanced is that collateral channels develop as atherosclerotic changes are occurring.

Blood flow in the coronary arteries is controlled by physical, neural, and metabolic factors. Perfusion of coronary arteries is dependent on aortic blood pressure, which is generated by the heart. Myocardial blood flow is largely regulated by the metabolic activity of the myocardium and autoregulatory mechanisms that control vessel dilation. The contracting heart compresses its intramyocardial and subendocardial blood vessels during systole. The autonomic nervous system exerts its effects via changes in heart rate (HR), cardiac contractility, and blood pressure.

Coronary blood flow is regulated by the need of the cardiac muscle for oxygen. During rest, blood flows through the coronary arteries at about 225 mL/minute. Coronary arteries can increase their flow up to four- to fivefold during periods of increased activity.

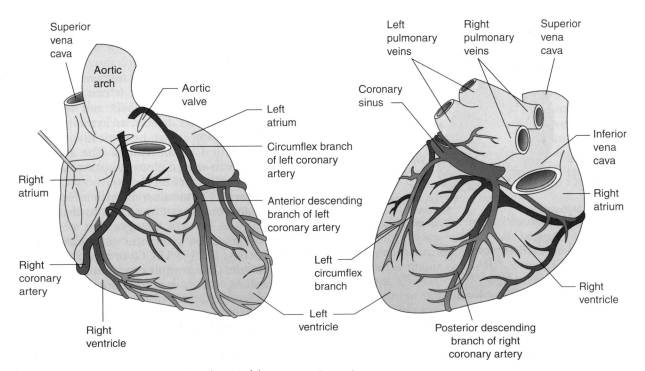

FIGURE 27-3. Coronary arteries and some of the coronary sinus veins.

Diagnosis

Diagnosis of angina is based on a detailed pain history, the presence of risk factors, invasive and noninvasive studies, and laboratory data. Noncoronary causes of chest pain, such as esophageal reflux or musculoskeletal disorders, are ruled out.

Noninvasive testing includes ECG, echocardiography, exercise stress testing, nuclear imaging studies, CT, and, possibly, cardiac MRI. Resting ECG is often normal, and exercise testing is often used. Ischemia that is asymptomatic at rest is detected by precipitation of typical chest pain or ST-segment changes on the ECG. Cardiac catheterization and coronary arteriography are needed for definitive diagnosis.[13,17] Serum biochemical markers for MI are normal in chronic stable angina. Metabolic abnormalities are frequently detected, such as hypercholesterolemia and other dyslipidemias, carbohydrate intolerance, and insulin resistance.

Treatment

The treatment goals for stable angina are directed toward symptom reduction and prevention of MI through nonpharmacologic strategies, pharmacologic therapy, and coronary interventions. PCI relieves symptoms for people with chronic stable angina but does not extend life span. CABG is indicated in people with double- or triple-vessel disease.[21]

Nonpharmacologic methods are aimed at symptom control and lifestyle modifications to reduce risk factors for coronary disease. They include smoking cessation, stress reduction, a regular exercise program, limiting dietary intake of cholesterol and saturated fats, weight reduction if obesity is present, and avoidance of cold that produces vasoconstriction. Pharmacologic agents used in chronic stable angina include aspirin or clopidogrel, beta-blockers in people without contraindications or calcium antagonists when beta-blockers are contraindicated, and ACE inhibitors in people who also have diabetes or LV systolic dysfunction. In people with established CAD, the use of lipid-lowering agents or statins is recommended.

Nitrates, both short acting and long acting, are vasodilators used in the treatment of chronic stable angina and in silent myocardial ischemia.[23] Nitrates decrease venous return to the heart with a resultant decrease in intraventricular volume. Arterial pressure also decreases. Decreased intraventricular pressure and volume are associated with decreased wall tension and myocardial oxygen requirement. Beta-blocking drugs are useful in management of angina associated with effort. The benefits of beta-blocking agents are primarily because of their hemodynamic effects that decrease myocardial oxygen requirements at rest and during exercise. Calcium channel–blocking drugs block activated and inactivated L-type calcium channels in cardiac and smooth muscle. The therapeutic effects result from coronary and peripheral artery dilation and from decreased myocardial metabolism associated with the decrease in myocardial contractility. Person with variant angina usually respond to treatment with calcium antagonists.

SUMMARY CONCEPTS

CAD is a disorder of impaired coronary blood flow, usually caused by atherosclerosis. Myocardial ischemia occurs when there is a disparity between myocardial oxygen supply and demand and can present as chronic ischemic heart disease or ACS. Diagnostic methods for CAD include ECG, exercise stress testing, nuclear imaging studies, CT, MRI, and angiographic studies in the cardiac catheterization laboratory.

The ACS, which includes UA/NSTEMI and STEMI, results from multiple pathophysiologic processes, including unstable atherosclerotic plaques, platelet aggregation, and thrombus formation. UA is an accelerated form of angina in which the pain occurs more frequently, is more severe, and lasts longer than in chronic stable angina. Myocardial infarction refers to the ischemic death of myocardial tissue associated with obstructed blood flow in the coronary arteries because of plaque disruption and occlusion of blood flow. NSTEMI and STEMI differ in terms of extent of myocardial damage. The complications of STEMI include potentially fatal arrhythmias, heart failure and cardiogenic shock, pericarditis, thromboemboli, rupture of cardiac structures, and ventricular aneurysms. Diagnostic methods include the use of ECG monitoring and serum biomarkers. Treatment goals focus on reestablishment of myocardial blood flow through rapid reperfusion of the occluded coronary artery, prevention of clot extension through use of aspirin and other antiplatelet and antithrombotic agents, alleviation of pain, administration of oxygen, and the use of vasodilators (nitroglycerin) and β-adrenergic blocking agents to reduce the work demands on the heart.

Chronic ischemic heart diseases include chronic stable angina, silent myocardial ischemia, variant (vasospastic) angina, chest pain with normal angiography, and ischemic cardiomyopathy. Chronic stable angina is associated with a fixed atherosclerotic obstruction and pain that is precipitated by increased work demands on the heart and relieved by rest. Variant angina can result from spasms of the coronary arteries or other dysfunctions. Silent myocardial ischemia and ischemic cardiomyopathy occur without CAD symptoms.

Cardiomyopathies

Cardiomyopathies are "a heterogeneous group of diseases of the myocardium associated with mechanical and/or electrical dysfunction that usually (but not invariably) exhibit inappropriate ventricular hypertrophy or dilatation and are due to a variety of causes that frequently are genetic. Cardiomyopathies either are confined to the heart or are part of generalized systemic disorders, often leading to cardiovascular death or progressive heart failure–related disability."[24]

Primary cardiomyopathies are heart disorders that confined to the myocardium, whereas *secondary cardiomyopathies* are myocardial changes that occur with a variety of systemic (multiorgan) disorders. Cardiomyopathies are usually associated with disorders related to mechanical (*e.g.*, heart failure) or electrical (*e.g.*, life-threatening arrhythmias) mechanisms.

Primary Cardiomyopathies

Primary cardiomyopathies are genetic, mixed, or acquired, based on their etiology.[24] Genetic cardiomyopathies include hypertrophic cardiomyopathy (HCM), arrhythmogenic right ventricular cardiomyopathy (ARVC), LV noncompaction cardiomyopathy, inherited conduction system disorders, and ion channelopathies. Mixed cardiomyopathies, which include dilated cardiomyopathy (DCM), are of both genetic and nongenetic origin. Acquired cardiomyopathies include those that have their origin in the inflammatory process (*e.g.*, myocarditis), stress ("Takotsubo" pericarditis), or pregnancy (peripartum cardiomyopathy). *Idiopathic cardiomyopathy* is when the cause is unknown.

Genetic Cardiomyopathies

Hypertrophic Cardiomyopathy

HCM is unexplained LV hypertrophy with disproportionate thickening of the interventricular septum, abnormal diastolic filling, cardiac arrhythmias, and, in some cases, intermittent LV outflow obstruction[25] (Fig. 27-14). It is one of the most common types of cardiomyopathy, occurring in 1 in 500 persons.[25] HCM is the most common cause of SCD in young athletes. The propensity to sudden death seems to be genetic, and implantable cardioverter–defibrillators (ICDs) are lifesaving.[25] Complications include atrial fibrillation, stroke, and heart failure.

HCM is an autosomal dominant heart disease caused by mutations in the genes encoding proteins of the cardiac sarcomere contractile proteins. Histologically, HCM appears as myocyte hypertrophy with myofibril disarray and increased cardiac fibrosis.[25] Although HCM is inherited, it may present anywhere from early childhood to late adulthood. The basic physiologic abnormalities in HCM are reduced LV chamber size, poor compliance with reduced SV that results from impaired

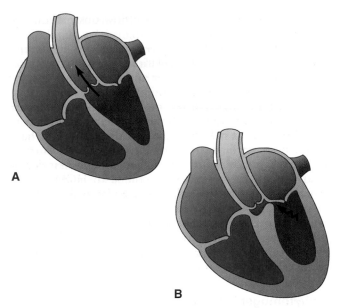

FIGURE 27-14. Vertical section of the heart showing (**A**) a normal heart and (**B**) a heart with HCM in which disproportionate thickening of interventricular septum causes intermittent left ventricular outflow obstruction. HCM, hypertrophic cardiomyopathy.

diastolic filling, mitral regurgitation, and, in about 25% of cases, dynamic obstruction of LV outflow.[25] Clinical manifestations are usually asymptomatic but may include dyspnea, chest pain during exertion, exercise intolerance, syncope, and arrhythmias. Owing to massive hypertrophy, high LV chamber pressure, and potentially abnormal **intramural** arteries, focal myocardial ischemia often develops even in the absence of CAD; thus, anginal pain is common. HCM is frequently associated with the development of LV outflow obstruction during rest or exertion that is caused by systolic anterior motion of the mitral valve and contact of the mitral valve with the ventricular septum. Clinical manifestations are variable and may progress to end-stage heart failure with LV remodeling and systolic dysfunction.

Diagnosis is frequently established with 2-D echocardiography, demonstrating nondilated LV hypertrophy, in the absence of other cardiac or systemic diseases. ECG is abnormal in 95% of the cases showing LV hypertrophy. Continuous ambulatory monitoring is useful to detect arrhythmias. MRI can also be helpful in determining the site and extent of hypertrophy. Genetic testing, through bidirectional DNA sequence analysis, provides accurate diagnosis and precise identification of gene mutations, if the gene involved is one that can be identified via testing.[25]

Medical management is focused on people with obstructive HCM who are symptomatic. The first-line approach to relief of symptoms is pharmacologic therapy designed to block the effects of catecholamines that exacerbate outflow obstruction and to slow HR to enhance diastolic filling. β-Adrenergic blockers are generally the initial choice for person with symptomatic HCM. The calcium channel blocker verapamil can also be used. It can exacerbate LV outflow obstruction and have been proposed. Some females exhibit inflammatory cells in biopsies taken during the symptomatic phase of the disorder, suggesting a disordered immune response. It presents as shortness of breath at rest and/or exertional, palpitations, edema, and orthopnea.

Diagnosis can be challenging because symptoms that can occur in late pregnancy are similar to early signs of heart failure. The criteria for peripartum cardiomyopathy are (1) heart failure in the last month of pregnancy or within 5 months after delivery; (2) no identifiable cause of heart failure; (3) no identifiable cause of heart failure before the last month of pregnancy; and (4) evidence of systolic dysfunction.[32] Management includes standard therapy for heart failure.

Teratogenic effects and excretion of drugs during breastfeeding should be considered. Therapy aims to reduce fluid and salt intake, reduce preload and afterload, increase contractility, and prevent complications such as mortality. Prognosis depends on resolution of heart failure. Half of females with peripartum cardiomyopathy spontaneously recover normal cardiac function; the other half have persistent LV dysfunction or progress to overt heart failure and early death.[32]

Stress or Takotsubo ("Broken Heart Syndrome") Cardiomyopathy

Stress or takotsubo cardiomyopathy is as a transient, reversible LV dysfunction in response to profound psychological or emotional stress. It occurs primarily in middle-aged females who present with acute STEMI but have no evidence of CAD. There is impaired contractility characterized by apical ballooning of the LV with hypercontractility of the basal LV.[33]

The mechanism for myocardial stunning is unclear. When catecholamine levels return to normal, the interventricular gradient resolves and LV function recovers.[33] Treatment is the same as that for heart failure, including short-term use of anticoagulants; most people demonstrate rapid improvement and an excellent prognosis.

Secondary Cardiomyopathies

Secondary cardiomyopathy is a heart muscle disease in the presence of a multisystem disorder (Chart 27-1). There are numerous conditions reported to involve the myocardium. Some of these disorders produce accumulation of abnormal substances between myocytes (extracellular), whereas others produce accumulation of abnormal substances within myocytes (intracellular).

Almost 100 distinct myocardial diseases can result in the clinical features of DCM. Alcoholic cardiomyopathy is the most common identifiable cause of DCM in the United States and Europe. Doxorubicin and other anthracycline drugs, used in the treatment of cancer, are potent agents whose use is limited by cumulative dose-dependent cardiac toxicity. Another chemotherapeutic agent with cardiotoxic potential is cyclophosphamide. The principal insult with cyclophosphamide appears to be vascular, leading to myocardial hemorrhage.

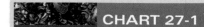

CHART 27-1

CONDITIONS ASSOCIATED WITH SECONDARY CARDIOMYOPATHIES*

Autoimmune Disorders
Systemic lupus erythematosus
Rheumatoid arthritis
Scleroderma
Polyarteritis nodosa

Endocrine Disorders
Acromegaly
Diabetes mellitus
Hypothyroidism and hyperthyroidism
Hyperparathyroidism

Familial Storage Diseases
Glycogen storage disease
Mucopolysaccharidoses
Hemochromatosis

Infiltrative Disorders
Amyloidosis
Sarcoidosis
Radiation-induced fibrosis

Neuromuscular/Neurologic Disorders
Friedreich ataxia
Muscular dystrophy
Neurofibromatosis

Nutritional Deficiencies
Thiamine (beriberi)
Protein (**kwashiorkor**)

Toxins
Alcohol and its metabolites
Arsenic
Cancer chemotherapeutic agents (anthracyclines [doxorubicin, daunorubicin], cyclophosphamide)
Catecholamines
Hydrocarbons

* Not intended to be inclusive.

SUMMARY CONCEPTS

The cardiomyopathies involve both mechanical and electrical etiologies of myocardial dysfunction. They are currently identified as either primary or secondary cardiomyopathies, based on genetic or other organ system involvement. Symptoms related to most cardiomyopathies, whether primary or secondary, are those associated with heart failure and SCD. Treatments are related to symptom management and prevention of lethal arrhythmias.

The primary cardiomyopathies include genetic, mixed, or acquired types. The genetic cardiomyopathies include HCM, ARVC, left ventricular noncompaction cardiomyopathy, inherited conduction system disorders, and ion channelopathies. The mixed cardiomyopathies, which include DCM, are of both genetic and acquired origin. Acquired cardiomyopathies include those that have their origin in the inflammatory process (*e.g.,* myocarditis), stress (takotsubo), or pregnancy (peripartum cardiomyopathy). In many cases, the cause is unknown, in which case the cardiomyopathy is referred to as *idiopathic*.

The secondary cardiomyopathies are heart diseases in which myocardial involvement occurs as part of a generalized systemic (multiorgan) disorder. They include cardiomyopathies associated with drugs, diabetes mellitus, muscular dystrophy, autoimmune disorders, and cancer treatment agents (radiation and chemotherapeutic drugs).

Infectious and Immunologic Disorders

Infective Endocarditis

Infective endocarditis (IE) is a serious and potentially life-threatening infection of the inner heart surface, characterized by invasion of the heart valves and mural endocardium by a microbial agent, leading to the formation of bulky, friable vegetations and destruction of underlying cardiac tissues.[34]

Common causes are mitral valve prolapse, congenital heart disease, prosthetic heart valves, and implantable devices such as pacemakers and defibrillators.[34,35] Host factors such as neutropenia, immunodeficiency, malignancy, therapeutic immunosuppression, diabetes, and alcohol or IV drug use are predisposing factors. Infections of these intracardiac, arterial, and venous devices are nosocomially acquired in medical centers in the developed world.[34]

IE is classified into acute or subacute–chronic forms, depending on the onset, etiology, and severity of the disease. Usually, onset of acute cases is rapid and involves people with normal cardiac valves who are either healthy with a history of IV drug use or are debilitated. Subacute–chronic cases evolve over months, usually in people with valve abnormalities. Increases in drug-resistant strains of microorganisms and in immunocompromised persons have made classification of acute and subacute–chronic cases more difficult.[35]

Etiology and Pathogenesis

Staphylococcal infections are the leading cause of IE, with streptococci and enterococci as the other common causes. Other causative agents include the HACEK group (*Haemophilus* species, *Actinobacillus actinomycetemcomitans*, *Cardiobacterium hominis*, *Eikenella corrodens*, and *Kingella kingae*), gram-negative bacilli, and fungi.[35] Causative agents differ in major high-risk groups: *Staphylococcus aureus* is the major offender in IV drug abusers, whereas prosthetic heart valve IE is caused by coagulase-negative staphylococci (*e.g.,* *Staphylococcus epidermidis*). *S. epidermidis* has been associated with implantable devices and health care–associated infections.[35] The major factor leading IE is seeding of the blood with microbes. The portal of entry may be an obvious infection, a dental or surgical procedure, injection of a contaminated substance directly into the blood, or an occult source in the oral cavity or gut. Endothelial injury, bacteremia, and altered hemodynamics can incite the formation of a fibrin–platelet thrombus along the endothelial lining. The thrombus is susceptible to bacterial seeding from transient bacteremia, causing continued monocyte activation and cytokine and tissue factor production. This results in progressive enlargement of infected valvular vegetations.

In both forms of IE, friable, bulky, and potentially destructive vegetative lesions form on the heart valves (Fig. 27-16). Aortic and mitral valves are common sites of infection, although the right heart may be involved particularly in IV drug abusers. These lesions are a collection of infectious organisms and cellular debris enmeshed in the fibrin strands of clotted blood. The lesions may be singular or multiple, may grow up to several centimeters, and are usually found loosely attached to free edges of the valve surface.[35] Infectious loci are a source of persistent bacteremia. As lesions grow, they cause valve destruction, leading to valvular regurgitation, ring abscesses with heart block, pericarditis, aneurysm, and valve perforation.

Intracardiac vegetative lesions have local and distant systemic effects.[35] Loose organization of these lesions permits the organisms and fragments of the lesions to form emboli and travel in the bloodstream, causing cerebral, systemic, or pulmonary emboli. Fragments may lodge in small vessels, causing small hemorrhages, abscesses, and infarction. Bacteremia can initiate immune responses responsible for skin manifestations, polyarthritis, and other immune disorders.

Clinical Manifestations

The incubation period for onset of symptoms is 2 weeks or less in over 80% of people. If the infection is *Candida* related, the incubation period can be up to 5 months. Initial symptoms can include fever and signs of systemic infection, change in the character of an existing heart murmur, and evidence of embolic distribution of the

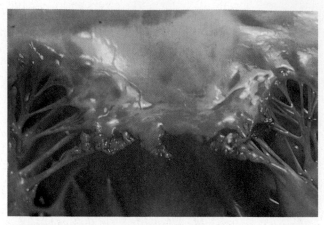

FIGURE 27-16. Bacterial endocarditis. The mitral valve shows destructive vegetations, which have eroded through the free margin of the valve leaflet. (From Strayer D. E., Rubin R. (Eds.) (2015). *Rubin's pathology: Clinicopathologic foundations of medicine* (7th ed., Fig. 17-34, p. 657). Philadelphia, PA: Lippincott Williams & Wilkins.)

vegetative lesions.[35] In the acute form, the fever is usually spiking and accompanied by chills. In the subacute form, the fever is usually low grade, of gradual onset, and accompanied by other systemic signs of inflammation, such as spleen enlargement, anorexia, malaise, and lethargy. Small petechial hemorrhages frequently result when emboli lodge in the small vessels of the skin, nail beds, and mucous membranes. Splinter hemorrhages under the nails of the fingers and toes are common.[35] Cough, dyspnea, arthralgia or arthritis, diarrhea, and abdominal or flank pain may occur as the result of systemic emboli. Congestive heart failure can develop from valve destruction, coronary artery embolism, or myocarditis. Renal insufficiency can also develop from destruction or antimicrobial toxicities.

Diagnosis

IE poses major challenges in diagnosis and treatment. Diagnosis includes the use of clinical, laboratory, and echocardiographic features.[35] The modified Duke criteria are classified into major criteria (positive blood culture for IE, evidence of endocardial involvement) and minor criteria (predisposition to IE, predisposing heart condition, or IV drug use; temperature over 38°C; vascular phenomenon, *i.e.*, evidence of arterial emboli; immunologic phenomenon such as glomerulonephritis; microbiologic evidence that does not meet major criteria). Cases are "definite" if they fulfill two major criteria, one major and two minor criteria, or five minor criteria. Cases are "possible" if they fulfill one major and one minor criterion, or three minor criteria. Diagnosis is rejected if an alternative diagnosis is made, the infection resolves with antibiotic treatment for 4 days or less, or there is no histologic evidence of infection.[34]

The blood culture is the most definitive diagnostic procedure. Three sets of blood cultures from three separate sites should be obtained within 24 hours. The indiscriminate use of antibiotics has made identifying the causative organism difficult. The modified Duke criteria

recommend inclusion of *S. aureus*, *Viridans streptococci*, *Streptococcus bovis*, and HACEK groups as a major criterion. A single positive blood culture for *Coxiella burnetii* and an anti–phase I immunoglobulin G antibody titer greater than 1:800 are also considered major criteria. Negative blood cultures can delay diagnosis and treatment and have a profound effect on outcome.[35] This can occur because of prior antibiotic administration or because the causative organisms are not readily cultured.

Echocardiography is the primary technique for detection of vegetations and cardiac complications resulting from IE. The American College of Cardiology/American Heart Association (ACC/AHA) recommends echocardiography in all people who are suspected of having IE. Echocardiographic evidence of endocardial involvement is now the major criterion in the modified Duke criteria. Transthoracic echocardiography is recommended in low initial risk or low clinical suspicion, and transesophageal echocardiography be used in moderate-to-high clinical suspicion. High-suspicion individuals include prosthetic valves, prior IE, complex congenital disease, heart failure, or new-onset heart murmur.[34]

Treatment

Treatment focuses on identifying and eliminating the causative microorganism, minimizing the residual cardiac effects, and treating the pathologic effect of emboli. The choice of antimicrobial therapy depends on the organism cultured and whether it occurs in a native or prosthetic valve. *S. aureus* is primarily the result of nosocomial infections from intravascular catheters, surgical wounds, and indwelling prosthetic devices.[34,35] In addition to antibiotic therapy, surgery may be needed for unresolved infection, severe heart failure, and significant emboli.

The majority of IE is cured with medical or surgical treatment. People who have had IE should be educated about its symptoms and informed of the possibility of recurrence. Prophylaxis with antibiotics is recommended only for people with previous IE, congenital heart disease (such as unrepaired cyanotic coronary heart disease repaired with prosthetic material or with residual defects), prosthetic cardiac valve, and cardiac transplantation with cardiac valvulopathy.[34,35]

Rheumatic Heart Disease

Rheumatic fever (RF) and rheumatic heart disease (RHD) are complications of the immune-mediated response to group A (beta-hemolytic) streptococcal (GAS) throat infection.[36] RF can develop into chronic valvular disorders that produce permanent cardiac dysfunction and may eventually cause fatal heart failure. RF and RHD are major health problems in countries with inadequate health care, poor nutrition, and crowded living conditions.[36,37]

Pathogenesis

The pathogenesis of RF still remains unclear. The time frame for development of symptoms and the presence of antibodies to GAS suggests an immunologic origin.[36,37] Although a small percentage of person with untreated GAS pharyngitis develop RF, the incidence of recurrence with a subsequent untreated infection is great.

Clinical Manifestations

RF can manifest as an acute, recurrent, or chronic disorder. The *acute stage* of RF includes a history of an initiating streptococcal infection and subsequent involvement of the connective tissue elements of the heart, blood vessels, joints, and subcutaneous tissues. Common to all is the *Aschoff body*,[36,37] a localized area of tissue necrosis surrounded by immune cells. The *recurrent phase* usually involves extension of the cardiac effects of the disease. The *chronic phase* of RF is permanent deformity of the heart valves and is a common cause of mitral valve stenosis. Chronic RHD usually does not appear until at least 10 years after the initial attack.

Most people with RF have a history of sore throat, headache, fever (101°F to 104°F), abdominal pain, nausea, vomiting, swollen glands (usually at the angle of the jaw), and other symptoms of streptococcal infection. Other clinical manifestations associated with an acute episode of RF are related to the acute inflammatory process and the structures involved. The course of the disease is characterized by findings including migratory polyarthritis of large joints, carditis, erythema marginatum, subcutaneous nodules, and Sydenham chorea.[36,37] Laboratory markers of acute inflammation include an elevated white blood cell count, ESR, and CRP. These elevated levels of acute-phase reactants provide evidence of an acute inflammatory response.

Polyarthritis

Polyarthritis is the most common and the first manifestation of RF in 75% of cases. The arthritis, which may range from arthralgia to disabling arthritis, often involves the larger joints. It is almost always migratory, affecting one joint and moving to another. Untreated, the arthritis lasts approximately 4 weeks. A striking feature of rheumatic arthritis is the dramatic response (usually within 48 hours) to salicylates. Arthritis usually heals completely leaving no functional residua.

Carditis

Acute rheumatic carditis can affect the endocardium, myocardium, or pericardium. Involvement of the endocardium and valvular structures produces the permanent and disabling effects of RF. Carditis mostly manifests itself as mitral regurgitation and less commonly aortic regurgitation, though all four valves can be involved. During the acute inflammatory stage of the disease, the valvular structures become red and swollen, and small vegetative lesions develop on the valve leaflets. The acute inflammatory changes gradually proceed to development of fibrous scar tissue, which tends to contract deforming the valve leaflets and shortening the chordae tendineae. In some cases, the edges or commissures of the valve leaflets fuse together during healing.

Clinical features of endocarditis/valvulitis without a history of RHD include apical holosystolic murmur of mitral regurgitation or a basal early diastolic murmur of aortic regurgitation. Features in someone with an RHD history include a change in the character of murmurs or a new murmur.

Subcutaneous nodules, Erythema marginatum, and Sydenham chorea

Subcutaneous nodules are hard, painless, and freely movable and usually occur over the extensor muscles of the wrist, elbow, ankle, and knee joints, ranging in size from 0.5 to 2 cm. Subcutaneous nodules occur most often in association with moderate-to-severe carditis.

Erythema marginatum lesions are maplike, macular areas most commonly seen on the trunk or inner aspects of the upper arm and thigh. They occur early in a rheumatic attack and may occur with subcutaneous nodules and carditis. They disappear during the course of the disease.

Sydenham chorea is the major central nervous system manifestation of RF. It is seen most frequently in young females and rarely occurs after 20 years of age. There is typically an onset of irritability and other behavior problems. The child is often fidgety, cries easily, begins to walk clumsily, and drops things. Choreiform movements are spontaneous, rapid, purposeless jerking movements that interfere with voluntary activities. Facial grimaces are common, and speech may be affected. The chorea is self-limited, but recurrences are not uncommon. A streptococcal infection can be detected only in about two thirds of cases, making differential diagnosis difficult.

Diagnosis

There are no laboratory tests that can establish a diagnosis of RF. The Jones criteria divide the clinical features of RF into major and minor categories, based on prevalence and specificity. The presence of two major signs (*i.e.*, carditis, polyarthritis, chorea, erythema marginatum, and subcutaneous nodules) or one major and two minor signs (*i.e.*, arthralgia, fever, and elevated ESR, CRP, or leukocyte count), accompanied by evidence of a preceding GAS infection, indicates a high probability of RF.

The use of echocardiography has enhanced the understanding of acute and chronic RHD. It is useful in assessing the severity of valvular stenosis and regurgitation, chamber size and function, and the presence and size of pleural effusions. Doppler ultrasonography may identify cardiac lesions in person who do not show typical signs of cardiac involvement during an attack of RF but is not considered either a Jones criterion.

Treatment and Prevention

Streptococcal infections must be promptly diagnosed and treated to prevent RF. However, it takes 24 to 48 hours to produce a result in throat cultures. Development of rapid tests for direct detection of GAS antigens has provided a partial solution for this problem. Both throat culture and the rapid antigen tests are highly specific for GAS infection but are limited in sensitivity. A negative antigen test result should be confirmed with a throat culture when a streptococcal infection is suspected.[36] The presence of GAS in the upper respiratory tract can indicate either a carrier or infectious state, the latter of which can be defined by a rising antibody response. Serologic examinations for streptococcal antibodies are measured for retrospective confirmation of recent streptococcal infections in person thought to have acute RF.

Treatment of acute RF aims to control the acute inflammatory response and prevent cardiac complications and recurrence. Penicillin, or erythromycin in penicillin-allergic people, is the treatment of choice for GAS infection.[36] Salicylates and corticosteroids can be used to suppress the inflammatory response but should not be given until diagnosis is confirmed. Surgery is indicated for chronic rheumatic valve disease and is determined by the severity of the symptom or the evidence that cardiac function is significantly impaired. Procedures include closed mitral commissurotomy, valve repair, and valve replacement.

The person who has had an attack of RF is at high risk for recurrence after subsequent GAS throat infections. Secondary prophylaxis is achieved with penicillin, and the duration depends on if residual valvular disease is present or absent. Compliance with a plan for prophylactic administration of penicillin requires that the person understand the morbidity associated with such recurrent infections. People are also urged to promptly report streptococcal infections for adequate treatment and to their dentists for adequate protection during dental procedures.

SUMMARY CONCEPTS

IE involves the invasion of the endocardium by pathogens that produce vegetative lesions on the endocardial surface. The loose organization of these lesions permits the organisms and fragments of the lesions to be disseminated throughout the systemic circulation. Although several organisms can cause the condition, staphylococci have now become the leading cause of IE. Treatment of IE focuses on identifying and eliminating the causative microorganism, minimizing the residual cardiac effects, and treating the pathologic effect of emboli.

RF, which is associated with an antecedent GAS throat infection, is an important cause of heart disease. Its most serious and disabling effects result from involvement of the heart valves. Because there is no single laboratory test result, sign, or symptom that is pathognomonic for acute RF, the Jones criteria are used to establish the diagnosis during the acute stage of the disease. Primary and secondary prevention strategies focus on appropriate antibiotic therapy.

Valvular Heart Disease

Hemodynamic Derangements

The function of the heart valves is to promote unidirectional flow of blood through the chambers of the heart. Dysfunction of the heart valves can result from a number of disorders, including congenital defects, trauma, ischemic damage, degenerative changes, and inflammation. The most commonly affected valves are the mitral and aortic valves. Disorders of the pulmonary and tricuspid valves are not as common because of the low pressure in the right side of the heart.

The heart valves consist of thin leaflets of tough, flexible, endothelium-covered fibrous tissue firmly attached at the base to the fibrous valve rings. Capillaries and smooth muscle are present at the base of the leaflet, but do not extend up into the valve. The leaflets of the heart valves may be injured or become the site of an inflammatory process that can deform their line of closure. Healing of the valve leaflets is often associated with increased collagen content and scarring, causing the leaflets to shorten and become stiffer. The edges of the healing valve leaflets can fuse together so that the valve does not open or close properly.

Two types of mechanical disruptions occur with valvular heart disease: narrowing of the valve opening so it does not open properly and distortion of the valve so it does not close properly (Fig. 27-17). *Stenosis* refers to a narrowing of the valve orifice and failure of the valve leaflets to open normally. Blood flow through a normal valve can increase by five to seven times the resting volume; consequently, valvular stenosis must be severe before it causes problems. Significant narrowing of the valve orifice increases the resistance to blood flow through the valve, converting the normally smooth laminar flow to a less efficient turbulent flow.

This increases the volume and work of the chamber emptying through the narrowed valve. Symptoms are usually noticed first during situations of increased flow, such as exercise. An incompetent or regurgitant valve permits backward flow to occur when the valve should be closed—flowing back into the LV during diastole

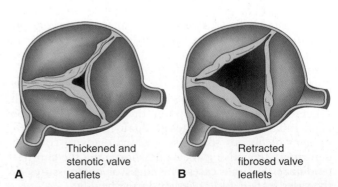

FIGURE 27-17. Disease of the aortic valve as viewed from the aorta. (**A**) Stenosis of the valve opening. (**B**) An incompetent or regurgitant valve that is unable to close completely.

Within the figure:
A — Thickened and stenotic valve leaflets
B — Retracted fibrosed valve leaflets

when the aortic valve is affected and back into the left atrium during systole when the mitral valve is diseased.

The effects of valvular heart disease on cardiac function are related to alterations in blood flow and increased work demands on the heart. Many valvular heart defects are defined by heart murmurs resulting from turbulent blood flow through a diseased valve (Fig. 27-18).

Echocardiography allows visualization in valvular motion and closing patterns as well as blood flow. Pulsed Doppler ultrasonography provides a semiquantitative or qualitative estimation of the severity of transvalvular gradients, right ventricular systolic pressure, and valvular regurgitation. Color flow Doppler provides a visual pattern of flow velocities over the anatomic 2-D or 3-D echocardiographic image, demonstrating turbulence from stenotic/regurgitant valves.

Transesophageal echocardiography with Doppler ultrasonography is used for echocardiographic data when surface sound transmission is poor. It provides clearer images and allows better visualization of the AV valves and prosthetic heart valves.

Mitral Valve Disorders

The edges or cusps of AV valves are thinner than semilunar valves and are anchored to papillary muscles by the chordae tendineae. During much of systole, the mitral valve is subjected to the high pressure generated by the LV, and the chordae tendineae prevent the eversion of the valve leaflets into the left atrium.

Mitral Valve Stenosis

Mitral valve stenosis is the incomplete opening of the mitral valve during diastole, causing left atrial distention and impaired LV filling. It is most commonly the result of RF.[26,38] Less frequently, the defect is congenital and manifests during infancy or early childhood or in older adults related to annular calcification. Mitral valve stenosis is a continuous, progressive, lifelong disorder consisting of a slow, stable course early and progressive acceleration in later years.

Pathogenesis

Mitral valve stenosis is characterized by fibrous replacement of valvular tissue, and stiffness and fusion of the valve apparatus (Fig. 27-18). Mitral cusps fuse at the edges and involvement of chordae tendineae pulls valvular structures deeply into the ventricles. As resistance to flow through the valve increases, the left atrium dilates and left atrial pressure rises.[38] Increased left atrial pressure is transmitted to the pulmonary venous system, causing pulmonary congestion.

The rate of flow across the valve depends on the size of the valve orifice, the driving pressure, and the time available for flow during diastole. The normal mitral valve area is 4 to 5 cm². Symptoms develop as the gradient across the valve becomes worse. As the condition progresses, symptoms of decreased CO occur with extreme exertion or situations that cause tachycardia and reduced diastolic filling time. In the late stages, pulmonary vascular resistance increases with the development of pulmonary hypertension;

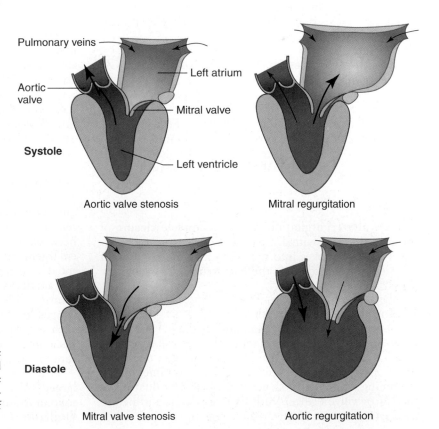

FIGURE 27-18. Alterations in hemodynamic function that accompany aortic valve stenosis, mitral valve regurgitation, mitral valve stenosis, and aortic valve regurgitation. The *thin arrows* indicate direction of normal flow and *thick arrows* the direction of abnormal flow.

Pulmonary veins

Aortic valve

Left atrium

Mitral valve

Systole

Left ventricle

Aortic valve stenosis

Mitral regurgitation

Diastole

Mitral valve stenosis

Aortic regurgitation

this increases the pressure against which the right heart must pump and leads to right-sided heart failure.

Clinical Manifestations

The signs of mitral valve stenosis depend on the severity of the obstruction and are related to the elevation in left atrial pressure and pulmonary congestion, decreased CO owing to impaired LV filling, and left atrial enlargement with development of atrial arrhythmias and mural thrombi. The symptoms are those of heart failure development, including pulmonary congestion, nocturnal paroxysmal dyspnea, and orthopnea. Palpitations, chest pain, weakness, and fatigue are common.

Premature atrial beats, paroxysmal atrial tachycardia, and atrial fibrillation may occur as a result of distention of the left atrium. Fibrosis of the internodal and interatrial tracts, along with damage to the SA node, may occur from the rheumatic process itself. Atrial fibrillation develops in 30% to 40% of people with symptomatic mitral stenosis.[38] Together, the fibrillation and distention predispose to mural thrombus formation. The risk of arterial embolization, particularly stroke, is significantly increased in people with atrial fibrillation.

Diagnosis

The murmur of mitral valve stenosis is heard during diastole when blood is flowing through the constricted valve orifice; it is characteristically a low-pitched, rumbling murmur, best heard at the apex of the heart. Two-dimensional and Doppler echocardiograms are used to diagnose mitral stenosis. They confirm diagnosis of mitral stenosis, evaluate mitral valve morphology and hemodynamics, measure pulmonary artery pressures, and assist in identifying the most appropriate treatment.

Treatment

Medical treatment aims to relieve signs of decreased CO and pulmonary congestion. Loop diuretics are initiated to relieve some congestion. In atrial fibrillation, the goals are to control ventricular rate and prevent systemic embolization with anticoagulation therapy. Surgical interventions, including balloon valvotomy, commissurotomy, and valve repair or replacement, may be used to treat degenerative and functional mitral valve disease.[38,39]

Mitral Valve Regurgitation

Mitral valve regurgitation is the incomplete closure of the mitral valve, with LV SV divided between the forward SV that moves into the aorta and the regurgitant SV that moves back into the left atrium during systole (Fig. 27-19).

Etiology and Pathogenesis

RHD is associated with a rigid and thickened valve that does not open or close completely. Mitral regurgitation can result from rupture of the chordae tendineae or papillary muscles, papillary muscle dysfunction, or stretching of the valve structures caused by dilation of the LV or valve orifice. Mitral valve prolapse is a common cause of mitral valve regurgitation.

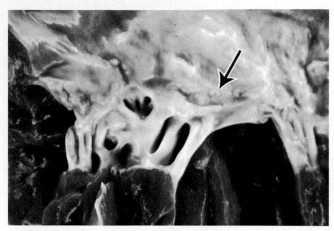

FIGURE 27-19. Chronic rheumatic valvulitis. A view of the mitral valve from the left atrium showing rigid, thickened, and fused leaflets with a narrow orifice, creating the characteristic "fish-mouth" (*arrow*) appearance of rheumatic mitral stenosis. (From Strayer D. E., Rubin R. (Eds.) (2015). *Rubin's pathology: Clinicopathologic foundations of medicine* (7th ed., Fig. 17-30, p. 654). Philadelphia, PA: Lippincott Williams & Wilkins.)

Acute mitral valve regurgitation may occur abruptly, such as with papillary muscle dysfunction after MI, valve perforation in IE, or ruptured chordae tendineae in mitral valve prolapse. In acute severe mitral regurgitation, acute volume overload increases LV preload, allowing a modest increase in LV SV. The forward SV is reduced, and the regurgitant SV leads to a rapid rise in left atrial pressure and pulmonary edema and decrease in CO. Acute mitral valve regurgitation is almost always symptomatic.

The hemodynamic changes associated with chronic mitral valve regurgitation occur more slowly, allowing for recruitment of compensatory mechanisms. An increase in LVED volume permits an increase in total SV, with restoration of forward flow into the aorta. Augmented preload and reduced or normal afterload facilitate LV ejection. Simultaneously, gradual increase in left atrial size allows for accommodation of the regurgitant volume at a lower filling pressure.

Clinical Manifestations

The increased volume work associated with mitral regurgitation is relatively well tolerated, and people may remain asymptomatic for years, developing symptoms between 6 and 10 years after diagnosis. The degree of LV enlargement reflects the severity of regurgitation.[40] As the disorder progresses, LV function becomes impaired, the aortic SV decreases, and the left atrial pressure increases, with the subsequent development of pulmonary congestion. Typical symptoms are those of LV failure such as dyspnea on exertion, paroxysmal nocturnal dyspnea, and orthopnea. Surgery should be performed before the onset of these symptoms.

Features of mitral valve regurgitation are an enlarged LV, a hyperdynamic LV impulse, and a pansystolic murmur. Mitral regurgitation predisposes to atrial fibrillation.

Diagnosis and Treatment

The 2-D Doppler echocardiogram is useful to evaluate LV and atrial size, measure the ejection fraction, and assess severity of regurgitation. Preload reduction can be beneficial and may be treated with ACE inhibitors and biventricular pacing. Surgeries include mitral valve repair and replacement with or without removal of the mitral apparatus. Surgery is recommended in severe mitral regurgitation or where mitral valve regurgitation is possibly underestimated. Mitral valve repair avoids the use of anticoagulation needed with artificial valves.[39,40]

Mitral Valve Prolapse

Mitral valve prolapse occurs in 1% to 2.5% of the general population. The disorder is seen more frequently in females than males and may have a familial basis. Familial mitral valve prolapse is an autosomal trait. Although the exact cause of the disorder is usually unknown, it is associated with Marfan syndrome, osteogenesis imperfecta, and other connective tissue disorders and with cardiac, hematologic, neuroendocrine, metabolic, and psychological disorders.

Pathogenesis

Pathologic findings in people with mitral valve prolapse include a myxedematous (mucinous) degeneration of mitral valve leaflets that causes them to become enlarged and floppy so that they prolapse or balloon back into the left atrium during systole (Fig. 27-20).

Secondary fibrotic changes reflect the stresses and injury that the ballooning movements impose on the valve. Certain forms of mitral valve prolapse may arise from disorders of the myocardium that place undue stress on the mitral valve because of abnormal movement of the ventricular wall or papillary muscle. Mitral valve prolapse may or may not cause mitral regurgitation.

Clinical Manifestations and Diagnosis

Most people with mitral valve prolapse are asymptomatic, and the disorder is discovered during a routine physical examination. A minority have chest pain mimicking angina, dyspnea, fatigue, anxiety, palpitations, and lightheadedness. Chest pain is often prolonged, ill defined, and not associated with exercise or exertion. The pain has been attributed to ischemia resulting from traction of prolapsing valve leaflets. Anxiety, palpitations, and arrhythmias may result from abnormal autonomic nervous system function. The disorder is characterized by a spectrum of auscultatory findings, ranging from a silent form to one or more midsystolic clicks followed by a late systolic or holosystolic murmur. Clicks are caused by the sudden tensing of the mitral valve apparatus as the leaflets prolapse. The 2-D and Doppler echocardiographies are valuable noninvasive studies used to diagnose mitral valve prolapse.

Treatment

Treatment focuses on relief of symptoms and prevention of complications.[39] People with palpitations and mild tachyarrhythmias or increased adrenergic symptoms and those with chest discomfort, anxiety, and fatigue often respond to β-adrenergic blocking drugs. Cessation of

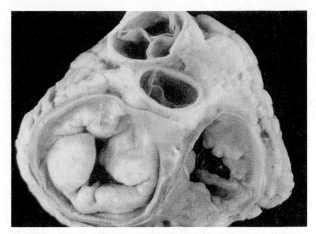

FIGURE 27-20. Mitral valve prolapse. A view of the mitral valve from the left atrium showing redundant and deformed leaflets that billow into the left atrial cavity. (From Strayer D. E., Rubin R. (Eds.) (2015). *Rubin's pathology: Clinicopathologic foundations of medicine* (7th ed., Fig. 17-38A, p. 659). Philadelphia, PA: Lippincott Williams & Wilkins.)

stimulants, such as caffeine, alcohol, and cigarettes, may be sufficient to control symptoms. Transient ischemic attacks occur more frequently in person with mitral valve prolapse. Therefore, in people with documented events who are in sinus rhythm with no atrial thrombi, daily aspirin therapy is recommended. Most people with mitral valve prolapse are encouraged to participate in regular exercise and lead a normal life. People who develop severe valve dysfunction may require valve surgery.

Aortic Valve Disorders

The aortic valve (*aortic semilunar valve*) has three cusps and no chordae tendineae (Fig. 27-17). The cusps are thicker than those of the mitral valve. The middle layer is thickened near the middle, where the leaflets meet, ensuring a tight seal. Between the thickened tissue and their free margins, the leaflets are thinner and flimsy.

The orifices for the two main coronary arteries are located behind the valve and at right angles to the direction of blood flow. The lateral pressure in the aorta propels blood into the coronary arteries. During the ejection phase of the cardiac cycle, the lateral pressure is diminished by conversion of potential energy to kinetic energy as blood moves forward into the aorta. This process is grossly exaggerated in aortic valve stenosis because of the high-flow velocities.

Aortic Valve Stenosis

Aortic valve stenosis is characterized by increased resistance to ejection of blood from LV into the aorta (Fig. 27-18). Congenital malformations may result in unicuspid, bicuspid, or misshaped valve leaflets. Acquired aortic stenosis is usually caused by calcification associated with normal "wear and tear" of a previously normal aortic valve or congenitally bicuspid valves.[41] The incidence of acquired aortic valve stenosis is 2% to 4% in adults older than 65 years.[41]

Pathogenesis

The progression of calcific aortic stenosis is usually slow. Valve changes range from mild thickening without obstruction to severe calcification with impaired leaflet motion and obstructed LV outflow.[41] Processes in the development of calcific aortic valve disease have been shown to be similar to those in CAD. Both conditions are more common in males, older persons, and person with hypercholesterolemia derived in part from an active inflammatory process.[41] Early lesions of aortic sclerosis show focal subendothelial plaquelike lesions. Aortic sclerosis is distinguished from aortic stenosis by the degree of valve impairment. In aortic sclerosis, the valve leaflets are abnormally thickened, but the obstruction to outflow is minimal, whereas in aortic stenosis, the functional area of the valve has decreased enough to cause measurable obstruction to outflow. Calcification of the aortic valve progresses from the base of the cusps to the leaflets. This reduces leaflet motion and effective valve area but without commissural fusion. As calcification progresses, leaflets become more rigid, there is worsening obstruction to LV outflow, and fusion of the commissures leads to aortic stenosis.

Because aortic stenosis develops gradually, the LV has time to adapt. With increased systolic pressure from obstruction, LV wall becomes thicker (hypertrophies), but a chamber volume is maintained. This increased wall thickness can maintain a normal ejection fraction. Little hemodynamic disturbance occurs as the valve area is reduced by half its area, but an additional reduction to one fourth of its normal size produces severe obstruction to flow and a progressive pressure overload on LV. Increased work of the heart begins to exceed the coronary blood flow reserve, causing both systolic and diastolic dysfunction and signs of heart failure.[39,41]

Diagnosis

Aortic stenosis is usually first diagnosed with auscultation of a loud systolic ejection murmur or a single or paradoxically split second heart sound. Eventually, the classic symptoms of angina, syncope, and heart failure develop, although more subtle signs of a decrease in exercise tolerance or exertional dyspnea should be monitored. Angina occurs in two thirds of people with advanced aortic stenosis. Dyspnea, marked fatigability, peripheral cyanosis, and other signs of low-output heart failure are not usually prominent until late in the course of the disease. Syncope (fainting) is most commonly caused by the reduced cerebral circulation that occurs during exertion when the arterial pressure declines consequent to vasodilation in the presence of a fixed CO.

Echocardiography can evaluate the severity of calcified aortic lesions, LV size and function, degree of ventricular hypertrophy, and presence of associated valve disorders and plays a major part in decision-making for aortic valve replacement. Evaluation is recommended yearly in people with severe aortic stenosis, every 1 to 2 years with moderate stenosis, and every 3 to 5 years with mild stenosis.

Treatment

There is no effective medical therapy for severe aortic stenosis, although aggressive risk factor modification is indicated.[39,41] In children with congenital aortic stenosis, the valve leaflets are merely fused, and balloon valvotomy may provide substantial benefit; valve replacement is the most effective treatment. Medical interventions are prescribed to relieve symptoms of heart failure for those people who are ineligible for surgical intervention. For people with symptomatic aortic stenosis, valve replacement almost always improves symptoms.

Aortic Valve Regurgitation

Aortic valve regurgitation (aortic regurgitation) is the result of an incompetent aortic valve that allows blood to flow back to the LV during diastole (Fig. 27-18). The LV must increase its SV to include blood entering from the lungs and leaking back through the regurgitant valve.

Etiology and Pathogenesis

This defect may result from conditions that cause scarring of valve leaflets or from enlargement of the valve orifice to the extent that the valve leaflets no longer meet. Causes include RF, idiopathic dilation of the aorta, congenital abnormalities, IE, and Marfan syndrome. Other causes include hypertension, trauma, and failure of a prosthetic valve.

Acute aortic regurgitation is characterized by a sudden, large regurgitant volume to an LV of normal size that has not had time to adapt. It is commonly caused by IE, trauma, or aortic dissection. Although the heart responds with Frank-Starling mechanisms and an increased HR, these compensatory mechanisms fail to maintain CO. As a result, there is severe elevation in LVED pressure, which is transmitted to the left atrium and pulmonary veins, culminating in pulmonary edema. A decrease in CO leads to sympathetic stimulation and a resultant increase in HR and peripheral vascular resistance that worsens regurgitation. Death from pulmonary edema, ventricular arrhythmias, or circulatory collapse is common in severe acute aortic regurgitation.

Chronic aortic regurgitation, which usually has a gradual onset, represents combined LV volume and pressure overload. As the valve deformity increases, regurgitant flow into the LV increases, diastolic blood pressure falls, and the LV progressively enlarges. Increase in LV volume results in the ejection of a large SV that is usually adequate to maintain the forward CO until late in the course of the disease. Most persons remain asymptomatic during this compensated phase, which may last for decades. The only sign may be a soft systolic aortic murmur.

Clinical Manifestations and Diagnosis

As the disease progresses, signs of LV failure begin to appear. These include exertional dyspnea, orthopnea, and paroxysmal nocturnal dyspnea. Failure of aortic valve closure during diastole causes an abnormal drop in diastolic pressure. Because coronary blood flow is greatest during diastole, this produces a decrease in coronary perfusion. Although angina is rare, it may occur when HR and diastolic pressure fall to low levels. People with severe aortic regurgitation often complain of an uncomfortable awareness of heartbeat when lying down, and chest discomfort caused by pounding of the heart against the chest wall. Tachycardia, occurring with emotional stress or exertion, may produce palpitations, head pounding, and premature ventricular contractions.

The major physical findings relate to the widening of arterial pulse pressure. Korotkoff sounds may persist to zero, even though intra-arterial pressure rarely falls below 30 mm Hg.[39,41] Large SV and wide pulse pressure may result in prominent carotid pulsations in the neck (Corrigan's pulse), head bobbing (de Musset's sign), systolic pulsations in the fingernail bed on gentle pressure (Quincke's pulse), throbbing peripheral pulses, and LV impulse that causes the chest to move with each beat. The hyperkinetic pulse of more severe aortic regurgitation (*water-hammer pulse*) is characterized by distention and quick collapse of the artery. Turbulence of flow across the aortic valve produces a holodiastolic decrescendo murmur heard best at the left sternal border. In severe cases, a mid-diastolic rumble at the apex can be heard (*Austin Flint* murmur).

Treatment

Treatment is aortic valve replacement. Surgery is recommended when people are symptomatic, regardless of LV function. In asymptomatic people, valve replacement remains controversial. However, in people with LV systolic dysfunction or with severe LV dilation, valve replacement is also recommended, even if asymptomatic.[39,41]

The goal of medical therapy is to improve forward SV and reduce regurgitant volume, usually through the use of afterload reducers. The first-line agent that is recommended in people with asymptomatic severe aortic regurgitation, especially in people with hypertension, is ACE inhibitors. Surgery remains the primary therapy for symptomatic severe aortic regurgitation.[41]

SUMMARY CONCEPTS

Dysfunction of the heart valves can result from a number of disorders, including congenital defects, trauma, ischemic heart disease, degenerative changes, and inflammation. Rheumatic endocarditis is a common cause. Valvular heart disease produces its effects through disturbances of blood flow. A stenotic valvular defect is one that causes a decrease in blood flow through a valve, resulting in impaired emptying and increased work demands on the heart chamber that empties blood across the diseased valve. A regurgitant valvular defect permits the blood flow to continue when the valve is closed. Valvular heart disorders produce blood flow turbulence and often are detected through cardiac auscultation.

HEART FAILURE AND CIRCULATORY SHOCK

Adequate perfusion of body tissues depends on the pumping ability of the heart. Heart failure and circulatory shock reflect failure of the circulatory system. Both conditions exhibit common compensatory mechanisms, even though they differ in terms of pathogenesis and causes.

Heart Failure in Adults

Heart failure is a complex syndrome resulting from any functional or structural disorder of the heart that results in or increases the risk of developing manifestations of low CO and/or pulmonary or systemic congestion.[42] Heart failure can occur in any age group but primarily affects older adults. Although morbidity and mortality rates from other CVDs have decreased over the past several decades, the incidence of heart failure is increasing at an alarming rate.

The syndrome of heart failure can be produced by any heart condition that reduces the pumping ability of the heart. The most common causes of heart failure are CAD, hypertension, DCM, and valvular heart disease.[42] Because many of the processes leading to heart failure are long-standing and progress gradually, heart failure can often be prevented or its progression slowed by early detection and intervention. The ACC/AHA guidelines have incorporated a classification system of heart failure that includes four stages: Stage A—High risk for developing heart failure, but no identified structural abnormalities and no signs of heart failure; Stage B—The presence of structural heart disease, but no history of signs and symptoms of heart failure; Stage C—Current or prior symptoms of heart failure with structural heart disease; and Stage D—Advanced structural heart disease and symptoms of heart failure at rest on maximum medical therapy.[42,43]

This system recognizes established risk factors and structural abnormalities of the four stages of heart failure. People normally progress from one stage to another unless slowed by treatment.

Pathophysiology of Heart Failure

The heart has the capacity to adjust CO to meet the varying needs of the body. The ability to increase CO during increased activity is the *cardiac reserve*. During exercise, CO can increase up to five to six times resting level.[44] People with heart failure often use their cardiac reserve at rest, and mild activity may cause shortness of breath because of exceeding their cardiac reserve.

 Control of Cardiac Performance and Output

CO, the major determinant of cardiac performance, reflects how often the heart beats per minute (HR) and how much blood it pumps per beat (SV) and can be expressed as CO = HR × SV. HR is regulated by the sympathetic nervous system, which produces an increase in HR, and the parasympathetic nervous system, which slows it down, whereas the SV is a function of preload, afterload, and myocardial contractility.[7,44]

Preload and Afterload

The work the heart performs is mainly ejecting blood that has returned to the ventricles into the pulmonary or systemic circulation. It is determined largely by *preload* and *afterload*.

Preload reflects the volume or loading conditions of the ventricle at the end of diastole, just before the onset of systole. It is the volume of blood stretching the heart muscle at the end of diastole and is normally determined by the venous return to the heart. The maximum volume of blood filling the ventricle is present at the end of diastole (*end-diastolic volume*). This volume increases the length of the myocardial muscle fibers. Within limits, as end-diastolic volume or preload increases, the SV increases in accord with the Frank-Starling mechanism.

Afterload is the force that the heart muscle must generate to eject blood from the filled heart. The main components of afterload are the systemic (peripheral) vascular resistance and ventricular wall tension. When the systemic vascular resistance is elevated, as with arterial hypertension, an increased left intraventricular pressure must be generated to open the aortic valve and then move blood into the systemic circulation. This increased pressure equates to an increase in ventricular wall stress or tension. Excess afterload may impair ventricular ejection and increase wall tension.

Myocardial Contractility

Myocardial contractility (*inotropy*) is the ability of the contractile elements (actin and myosin filaments) of the heart muscle to interact and shorten against a load. Contractility increases CO independent of preload and afterload.

Interaction between actin and myosin filaments during cardiac muscle contraction and relaxation requires energy supplied by the breakdown of ATP and the presence of calcium ions (Ca++).

When an action potential passes over the cardiac muscle fiber, the impulse spreads to the interior of the muscle fiber along the transverse (T) tubules. T tubule action potentials act to release Ca++ from the sarcoplasmic reticulum (Fig. 27-21). Ca++ ions diffuse into the

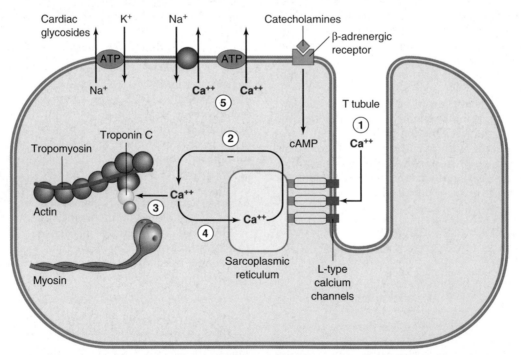

FIGURE 27-21. Schematic representation of the role of calcium ions (Ca++) in cardiac excitation–contraction coupling. The influx (site 1) of extracellular Ca++ through the L-type Ca++ channels in the transverse (T) tubules during excitation triggers (site 2) release of Ca++ by the sarcoplasmic reticulum. This Ca++ binds to TnC (site 3). The Ca++–troponin complex interacts with tropomyosin to unblock active sites on the actin and myosin filaments, allowing cross-bridge attachment and contraction of the myofibrils (systole). Relaxation (diastole) occurs as a result of calcium reuptake by the sarcoplasmic reticulum (site 4) and extrusion of intracellular Ca++ by the sodium Na+/Ca++ exchange transporter or, to a lesser extent, by the Ca++ ATPase pump (site 5). Mechanisms that raise systolic Ca++ increase the level of developed force (inotropy). Binding of catecholamines to β-adrenergic receptors increases Ca++ entry by phosphorylation of the Ca++ channels through a cAMP-dependent second messenger mechanism. The cardiac glycosides increase intracellular Ca++ by inhibiting the Na+/K+–ATPase pump. The elevated intracellular Na+ reverses the Na+/Ca++ exchange transporter (site 5), so less Ca++ is removed from the cell. cAMP, cyclic adenosine monophosphate. (Modified from Klabunde R. E. (2005). *Cardiovascular physiology concepts* (p. 46). Philadelphia, PA: Lippincott Williams & Wilkins.)

myofibrils to promote sliding of the actin and myosin filaments along one another to produce muscle shortening. A large quantity of extracellular Ca^{++} also diffuses into the sarcoplasm through voltage-dependent L-type Ca^{++} channels in T tubules at the time of the action potential. Opening of L-type Ca^{++} channels is facilitated by the second messenger cyclic adenosine monophosphate, the formation of which is coupled to β-adrenergic receptors. The catecholamines (norepinephrine and epinephrine) exert their inotropic effects by binding to these receptors. Dihydropyridine Ca^{++} channel–blocking drugs (*e.g.*, nifedipine) exert their effects by binding to one site of the L-type Ca^{++} channel, and diltiazem and verapamil bind to closely related receptors in another region. Blockade of the Ca^{++} channels in cardiac muscle results in a reduction in contractility throughout the heart and a decrease in sinus node pacemaker rate and in AV node conduction velocity.

Another mechanism that can modulate inotropy is the sodium ion $(Na^+)/Ca^{++}$ exchange pump and the ATPase-dependent Ca^{++} pump on the myocardial cell membrane (Fig. 27-21). These pumps transport Ca^{++} out of the cell, preventing the cell from becoming overloaded with Ca^{++}. If Ca^{++} extrusion is inhibited, rise in intracellular Ca^{++} can increase inotropy. Digitalis and related cardiac glycosides are inotropic agents that exert their effects by inhibiting the Na^+/potassium ion (K^+)–ATPase pump, which increases intracellular Na^+; this, in turn, leads to an increase in intracellular Ca^{++} through the Na^+/Ca^{++} exchange pump.

Systolic versus Diastolic Dysfunction

Classification separates the pathophysiology of heart failure into systolic and diastolic failure or dysfunction based on the ventricular ejection fraction.[45,46] *Ejection fraction* is the blood pumped out of the ventricles with each contraction, normally about 55% to 70%. In systolic ventricular dysfunction, myocardial contractility is impaired, leading to a decreased ejection fraction and CO. In diastolic ventricular dysfunction, ejection fraction is normal but diastolic ventricular relaxation is impaired, leading to a decrease in ventricular filling that ultimately causes a decrease in preload, SV, and CO. Many people with heart failure have combined elements of both systolic and diastolic ventricular dysfunction, and the division between the two may be somewhat artificial, particularly as it relates to manifestations and treatment.[46] Ventricular dysfunction is not synonymous with heart failure, but it can lead to heart failure. With both systolic and diastolic ventricular dysfunction, compensatory mechanisms are usually able to maintain adequate resting cardiac function until the later stages of heart failure.

Systolic Dysfunction

Systolic dysfunction is a decrease in myocardial contractility and an ejection fraction under 40%. In systolic heart failure, the ejection fraction declines with increasing degrees of myocardial dysfunction. In severe heart failure, the ejection fraction may drop under 10%. With decreased ejection fraction, there is an increase in end-diastolic volume (preload), ventricular dilation, and ventricular wall tension and a rise in ventricular end-diastolic pressure.[4] Increased volume, added to normal venous return, leads to an increase in ventricular preload. Although it serves as a compensatory mechanism, increased preload can also lead to accumulation of blood in the atria and the venous system (which empties into the atria), causing pulmonary or peripheral edema.

Systolic dysfunction commonly results from conditions that impair the contractile performance of the heart, produce a volume overload, or generate a pressure overload on the heart. The extent of systolic ventricular dysfunction can be estimated by measuring CO and ejection fraction and by assessment for manifestations of left-sided heart failure, particularly pulmonary congestion.

Diastolic Dysfunction

Although heart failure is commonly associated with impaired systolic function, in about 55% of cases, systolic function is preserved and heart failure occurs exclusively on the basis of LV diastolic dysfunction.[47,48] Although such hearts contract normally, relaxation is abnormal. Abnormal ventricle filling compromises CO, especially during exercise. For any ventricular volume, ventricular pressures are elevated, leading to signs of pulmonary and systemic venous congestion. The prevalence of diastolic failure increases with age and is higher in females than in males and in people with hypertension and atrial fibrillation.[47,48]

Conditions that cause diastolic dysfunction include those that impede expansion of the ventricle (*e.g.*, pericardial effusion, constrictive pericarditis), those that increase wall thickness and reduce chamber size, and those that delay diastolic relaxation.[47,48] Aging is often accompanied by a delay in relaxation during diastole such that diastolic filling begins while the ventricle is still resistant to stretching to accept an increase in volume. A similar delay occurs in myocardial ischemia because of a lack of energy to break the rigor between the actin and myosin filaments and to move Ca^{++} back into the sarcoplasmic reticulum.[47,48]

Diastolic function is influenced by HR, which determines the time available for ventricular filling. An increase in HR shortens diastolic filling time.[7] Thus, diastolic dysfunction can be aggravated by tachycardia or arrhythmia and improved by a reduction in HR.

With diastolic dysfunction, blood is unable to move freely into the LV, causing an increase in intraventricular pressure at any volume. Elevated pressures are transferred from the LV into the left atrium and pulmonary venous system, causing a decrease in lung compliance, increasing the work of breathing, and evoking dyspnea. CO is decreased because of a decrease in the volume (preload) available for adequate CO. Inadequate CO during exercise may lead to fatigue of the legs and accessory muscles of respiration.

Right versus Left Ventricular Dysfunction

Although heart failure is classified by the side of the heart primarily affected, long-term heart failure usually involves both sides (Fig. 27-22). The pathophysiologic

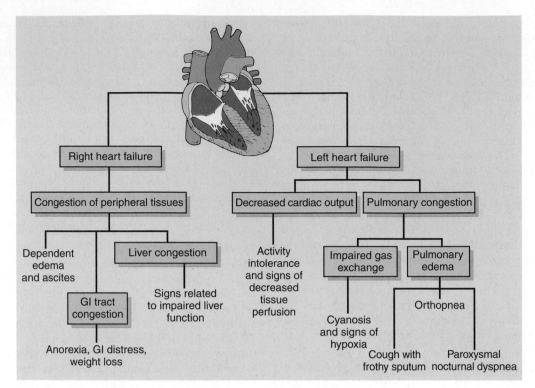

FIGURE 27-22. Manifestations of left- and right-sided heart failure. GI, gastrointestinal.

changes that occur in the myocardium are similar between the two sides.

Right Ventricular Dysfunction

When the right ventricle fails, there is reduced deoxygenated blood moving into the pulmonary circulation and a reduction in LV CO. If the right ventricle does not move the blood forward, there is congestion of blood into the systemic venous system. This increases right ventricular end-diastolic, right atrial, and systemic venous pressures. A major effect of right-sided heart failure is peripheral edema (Fig. 27-22). Because of the effects of gravity, when the person is upright, edema is seen in the lower extremities; when the person is supine, edema is seen in the area over the sacrum. The accumulation of edema fluid is evidenced by a gain in weight (1 pint [568 mL] of accumulated fluid results in a 1 lb [0.45 kg] weight gain). Weight gain of more than 2 lb (0.90 kg) in 24 hours or 5 lb (2.27 kg) in 1 week is a sign of worsening failure.[47]

Right-sided heart failure also produces congestion of the viscera. As venous distention progresses, blood backs up in the hepatic veins that drain into the inferior vena cava, and the liver becomes engorged. This may cause hepatomegaly and right upper quadrant pain. In severe and prolonged right-sided heart failure, liver function is impaired, and hepatic cells may die. Portal circulation congestion may also lead to spleen engorgement and development of ascites. GI tract congestion may interfere with digestion and absorption of nutrients, causing anorexia and abdominal discomfort. Jugular veins are normally not visible when standing or when sitting with the head at higher than 30 degrees. In severe right-sided

heart failure, the external jugular veins become distended and can be seen when sitting up or standing.

Causes include conditions that impede blood flow into the lungs or compromise the pumping of the right ventricle. LV failure is the most common cause of right ventricular failure. Sustained pulmonary hypertension is also a cause. Pulmonary hypertension occurs in people with chronic pulmonary disease, severe pneumonia, pulmonary embolus, or aortic or mitral stenosis. *Cor pulmonale* is when right-sided heart failure occurs due to chronic pulmonary disease.[47] Other causes include stenosis or regurgitation of tricuspid or pulmonic valves, right ventricular infarction, and cardiomyopathy. Right ventricular dysfunction with heart failure is also caused by congenital heart defects, such as tetralogy of Fallot and ventricular septal defect (VSD).

Left Ventricular Dysfunction

Left-sided heart failure impairs movement of blood from the low-pressure pulmonary circulation into the high-pressure arterial side of the systemic circulation. Impairment of left heart function decreases CO to the systemic circulation. Blood accumulates in LV, left atrium, and pulmonary circulation, which causes an elevation in pulmonary venous pressure (Fig. 27-22). When the pressure in the pulmonary capillaries (10 mm Hg) exceeds capillary osmotic pressure (25 mm Hg), there is a shift of intravascular fluid into the interstitium of the lung, resulting in pulmonary edema (Fig. 27-23). Pulmonary edema often occurs at night, after the person has been reclining and gravitational forces have been removed from the circulatory system. It is then that the edema fluid that had been sequestered in the lower extremities

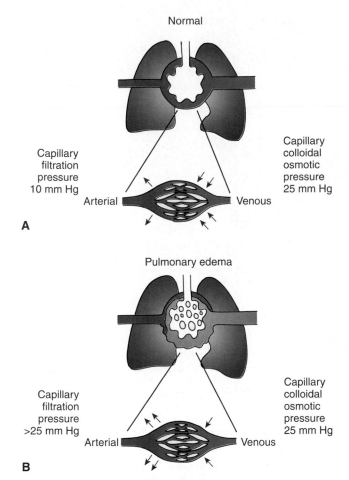

FIGURE 27-23. Mechanism of respiratory symptoms in left-sided heart failure. In the normal exchange of fluid in the pulmonary capillaries (**A**), the capillary filtration pressure that moves fluid out of the capillary into the lung is less than the capillary colloidal osmotic pressure that pulls fluid back into the capillary. Development of pulmonary edema (**B**) occurs when the capillary filtration pressure exceeds the capillary colloidal osmotic pressure that pulls fluid back into the capillary.

during the day is returned to the vascular compartment and redistributed to the pulmonary circulation.

Common causes of LV dysfunction are hypertension and acute MI. LV heart failure and pulmonary congestion can develop rapidly with acute MI. Even if the infarcted area is small, there may be surrounding areas of ischemic tissue that can cause large regions of LV wall hypokinesis or akinesis and rapid onset of pulmonary congestion and edema. Stenosis or regurgitation of the valves also creates left-sided backflow, resulting in pulmonary congestion. As pulmonary pressure rises, it may progress to produce right-sided heart failure.

High-Output versus Low-Output Failure

High-output failure is an uncommon type of heart failure caused by an excessive need for CO. Hear function may be supranormal but inadequate because of excessive metabolic needs. Causes include severe anemia, conditions that cause arteriovenous shunting, and Paget disease.

Low-output failure is caused by disorders that impair the pumping ability of the heart, such as ischemic heart disease and cardiomyopathy. Low-output failure is characterized by clinical evidence of systemic vasoconstriction with cold, pale, and often cyanotic extremities.[47,48] In advanced forms, marked reductions in SV are evidenced by pulse pressure narrowing. In high-output failure, extremities are warm and flushed, and pulse pressure is widened or normal.

Compensatory Mechanisms

In heart failure, cardiac reserve is maintained through compensatory responses (Fig. 27-24).

The first of these adaptations occurs over minutes to hours of myocardial dysfunction and may be adequate to maintain overall pumping performance. Myocardial hypertrophy and remodeling occur over months to years and are important in the long-term adaptation to hemodynamic overload. In the failing heart, early decreases in cardiac function may go unnoticed because these compensatory mechanisms maintain the CO. However, these mechanisms contribute not only to the adaptation of the failing heart but also to the pathophysiology of heart failure.[48]

Frank-Starling Mechanism

Increased diastolic filling increases myocardial fiber stretching and more optimal lining up of the myosin heads with the troponin-binding sites, increasing the force of the next contraction. The Frank-Starling mechanism matches the outputs of the two ventricles. An increase in contractility, or inotropy, will increase CO at any end-diastolic volume, causing the curve to move up and to the left. A decrease in inotropy will move the curve down and to the right (Fig. 27-25). In heart failure, inotropy is decreased compared with normal. Thus, the SV will not be as high as with normal inotropy, regardless of the increase in preload.

In heart failure, decreased CO and renal blood flow lead to increased sodium and water retention, an increase in vascular volume and venous return to the heart, and an increase in ventricular end-diastolic volume. Within limits, as preload and ventricular end-diastolic volume increase, there is an increase in CO. Although this may preserve resting CO, resulting chronic elevation of LVED pressure is transmitted to the atria and the pulmonary circulation, causing pulmonary congestion.

An increase in muscle stretch also increases ventricular wall tension and myocardial oxygen consumption. This can produce ischemia and contribute to further impairment of inotropy. In this situation, increased worsens heart failure. The use of diuretics helps reduce vascular volume and ventricular filling, thereby unloading the heart and reducing ventricular wall tension.

Sympathetic Nervous System Activity

Stimulation of the sympathetic nervous system plays an important role in the compensatory response to decreased CO and SV. Cardiac sympathetic tone and catecholamine levels are elevated during the late stages

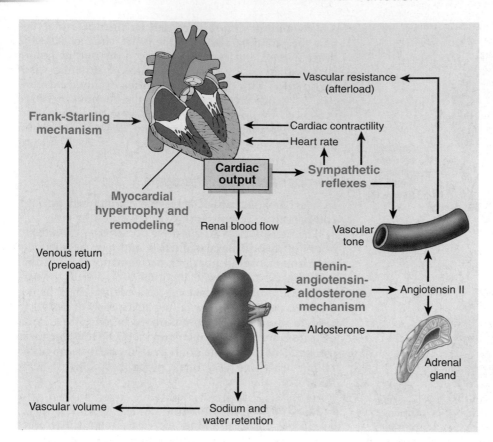

FIGURE 27-24. Compensatory mechanisms in heart failure. The Frank-Starling mechanism, sympathetic reflexes, renin–angiotensin–aldosterone mechanism, and myocardial hypertrophy function in maintaining cardiac output for the failing heart.

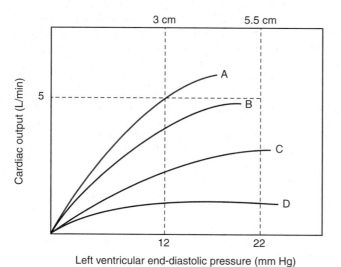

FIGURE 27-25. Left ventricular function curves. *Curve A:* Normal function curve, with a normal cardiac output and optimal left ventricular end-diastolic (LVED) filling pressure. *Curve B:* Compensated heart failure with normal cardiac output at higher LVED pressures. *Curve C:* Decompensated heart failure with a decrease in cardiac output and elevated LVED, with eventual elevation of pulmonary capillary pressure and development of pulmonary congestion. *Curve D:* Cardiogenic shock, with an extreme decrease in cardiac output and marked increase in LVED pressures.

of most heart failure. By direct stimulation of HR and cardiac contractility, regulation of vascular tone, and enhancement of renal sodium and water retention, the sympathetic nervous system initially helps maintain perfusion of the body organs. In more severe heart failure, blood is diverted to the critical cerebral and coronary circulations.

An increase in sympathetic activity by stimulation of β-adrenergic receptors leads to tachycardia, vasoconstriction, and cardiac arrhythmias. Acutely, tachycardia increases the workload of the heart, increasing oxygen demand; and cardiac ischemia and cardiomyopathy both worsen heart failure. By promoting arrhythmias, catecholamines released with sympathetic nervous system stimulation may contribute to the high rate of sudden death seen with heart failure.

Renin–Angiotensin–Aldosterone Mechanism

One of the most important effects of lowered CO in heart failure is reduction in renal blood flow and glomerular filtration rate, which leads to sodium and water retention. With decreased renal blood flow, there is a progressive increase in renin secretion by the kidneys and increases in circulating levels of angiotensin II. The increased concentration of angiotensin II contributes directly to a generalized and excessive vasoconstriction, and facilitates norepinephrine release and inhibits reuptake of norepinephrine by the sympathetic nervous system.

Angiotensin II provides a powerful stimulus for aldosterone production. Aldosterone increases tubular reabsorption of sodium and water. Because aldosterone is metabolized in the liver, its levels are further increased when heart failure causes liver congestion. Angiotensin II also increases antidiuretic hormone (ADH), a vasoconstrictor and an inhibitor of water excretion. In heart failure, progressive accumulation of fluid leads to ventricular dilation and increased wall tension. The increased oxygen demand eventually outweighs the compensatory Frank-Starling mechanism, reducing inotropy and progressing heart failure.

Angiotensin II and aldosterone are also involved in regulating the inflammatory and reparative processes that follow tissue injury. They stimulate inflammatory cytokine production, attract inflammatory cells, activate macrophages at sites of injury and repair, and stimulate growth of fibroblasts and synthesis of collagen fibers. Fibroblast and collagen deposition results in ventricular hypertrophy and myocardial wall fibrosis, which decreases compliance, causing heart remodeling and progression of both systolic and diastolic ventricular dysfunction.[48]

Natriuretic Peptides

The heart muscle produces and secretes a family of related peptide hormones (natriuretic peptides or NPs) that have potent diuretic, natriuretic, and vascular smooth muscle effects and interact with other neurohumoral mechanisms that affect cardiovascular function. The NPs commonly associated with heart failure are atrial natriuretic peptide (ANP) and brain natriuretic peptide (BNP).

ANP is released from atrial cells in response to atrial stretch, pressure, or fluid overload. BNP is secreted by ventricles in response to increased ventricular pressure or fluid overload. ANP and BNP promote rapid, transient natriuresis and diuresis via increased glomerular filtration rate and inhibited tubular sodium and water reabsorption.

NPs inhibit the sympathetic nervous system, the renin–angiotensin–aldosterone system, endothelin inflammatory cytokines, and vasopressin. Suppression of the sympathetic nervous system causes venous and arterial dilation and reduction in venous return to the heart and cardiac filling pressures and a decrease in afterload. Inhibition of angiotensin II and vasopressin by NPs reduces renal fluid retention. In addition, NPs directly affect the central nervous system and the brain, inhibiting secretion of vasopressin and the function of the salt appetite and thirst center.

Circulating levels of both ANP and BNP are reportedly elevated in people with heart failure. BNP and NT-proBNP levels can be detected in the blood, and concentrations are correlated with the extent of ventricular dysfunction. Medications used to treat heart failure often reduce BNP concentrations. Therefore, many people with chronic stable heart failure have BNP levels in the normal diagnostic range. However, digoxin and beta-blockers appear to increase BNP levels.

Endothelins

The endothelins, released from endothelial cells, are potent vasoconstrictor peptides. Endothelins induce vascular smooth muscle cell proliferation and cardiac myocyte hypertrophy; increase release of ANP, aldosterone, and catecholamines; and exert antinatriuretic effects on the kidneys. Production of endothelin 1 (ET-1) is regulated by factors that are significant for cardiovascular function

and have implications for heart failure. Plasma ET-1 levels correlate with pulmonary vascular resistance. Type A endothelin receptor is associated with smooth muscle constriction and hypertrophy, and type B endothelin receptor is associated with vasodilation. Because ET-1 can act on the heart to cause hypertrophy and sodium and water retention, an endothelin receptor antagonist can be used in people with pulmonary arterial hypertension due to severe heart failure.

Inflammatory Mediators

Elevated CRP levels have been associated with adverse consequences in people with heart failure and may be predictive of development of heart failure in high-risk groups. Of particular interest are interactions between CRP and mediators, such as angiotensin II and norepinephrine.

Myocardial Hypertrophy and Remodeling

The development of myocardial hypertrophy is one of the principal mechanisms of compensation for increased workload.[47,48] Inappropriate hypertrophy and remodeling can result in changes in structure and function that often lead to further pump dysfunction and hemodynamic overload.

The myocardium is composed of myocytes and nonmyocytes. Myocyte growth is limited by an increment in cell size, as opposed to an increase in cell number. Nonmyocytes include cardiac macrophages, fibroblasts, vascular smooth muscle, and endothelial cells. These cells are present in the interstitial space and provide support for the myocytes. Nonmyocytes determine many of the inappropriate changes that occur during myocardial hypertrophy: uncontrolled cardiac fibroblast growth is associated with increased synthesis of collagen fibers, myocardial fibrosis, and ventricular wall stiffness. Fibrosis and remodeling may lead to electrical conduction abnormalities in which the heart contracts in an uncoordinated manner, known as *cardiac dyssynchrony*, causing reduced systolic heart function.[46]

Cardiac muscle cells respond to stimuli from stress on the ventricular wall by initiating several different processes that lead to hypertrophy. These include stimuli that produce *symmetric hypertrophy* with a proportionate increase in muscle length and width, as occurs in athletes; *concentric hypertrophy* with an increase in wall thickness, as occurs in hypertension; and *eccentric hypertrophy* with a disproportionate increase in muscle length, as in DCM (Fig. 27-26).

When the primary stimulus for hypertrophy is *pressure overload*, the increase in wall stress leads to replication of myofibrils, thickening individual myocytes, and concentric hypertrophy. Concentric hypertrophy may preserve systolic function for a time, but eventually the work performed by the ventricle exceeds the vascular reserve, predisposing to ischemia. When the primary stimulus is *ventricular volume overload*, increase in wall stress leads to replication of myofibrils in series, elongation of myocytes, and eccentric hypertrophy. Eccentric hypertrophy leads to decreased ventricular wall thickness and increased diastolic volume and wall tension.

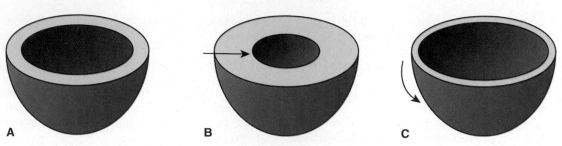

FIGURE 27-26. Different types of myocardial hypertrophy. (A) Normal symmetric hypertrophy with proportionate increases in myocardial wall thickness and length. (B) Concentric hypertrophy with a disproportionate increase in wall thickness. (C) Eccentric hypertrophy with a disproportionate decrease in wall thickness and ventricular dilation.

Acute Heart Failure Syndromes

Acute heart failure syndromes (AHFS) are "defined as gradual or rapid changes in heart failure signs and symptoms resulting in a need for urgent therapy."[49] Symptoms are primarily due to severe pulmonary edema because of elevated LV filling pressures, with or without a low CO.[49] AHFS are commonly seen in emergency departments, and chronic heart failure is the most common cause of the syndrome.

AHFS are thought to encompass three different types of conditions: worsening of chronic systolic or diastolic dysfunction that appears to respond to treatment (80%); new-onset acute heart failure that occurs secondary to a precipitating event; worsening of end-stage/advanced heart failure that is refractory to treatment.[49,50]

The degree of physiologic response is more pronounced in the new-onset AHFS and subtler in AHFS caused by chronic heart failure because of compensatory pathophysiology. Because of the compensatory mechanisms in chronic heart failure, they tolerate higher pulmonary vascular pressures. Chronic changes in neurohormonal regulation lead to stronger activation of the angiotensin–aldosterone system with a resultant volume overload, and venous congestion becomes more prominent in both the systemic and pulmonary circulations.

Clinical Manifestations of Heart Failure

The manifestations of heart failure depend on the extent and type of cardiac dysfunction present and rapidity of development. A person with previously stable compensated heart failure may develop signs of heart failure when the condition advances to a critical point. Overt heart failure may be precipitated by conditions such as infection, emotional stress, uncontrolled hypertension, or fluid overload.[49] Many people with serious underlying heart disease may be relatively asymptomatic as long as they carefully adhere to their treatment regimen. A dietary excess of sodium is a frequent cause of sudden cardiac decompensation.

The manifestations of heart failure reflect the physiologic effects of impaired pumping ability of the heart, decreased renal blood flow, and activation of sympathetic compensatory mechanisms. The severity and progression of symptoms depend on the extent and type of dysfunction present. Signs and symptoms include shortness of breath and other respiratory manifestations; fatigue and limited exercise tolerance; fluid retention and edema; cachexia and malnutrition; and cyanosis. People with severe heart failure may exhibit diaphoresis and tachycardia.

Respiratory Manifestations

Shortness of breath caused by congestion of pulmonary circulation is a major symptom of left-sided heart failure. Perceived shortness of breath is *dyspnea* and, when related to increased activity, is *exertional dyspnea*. *Orthopnea* is shortness of breath occurring when supine. Gravitational forces cause fluid to sequester in lower legs and feet when standing or sitting. When the person assumes the recumbent position, fluid from the legs and dependent parts of the body is mobilized and redistributed to an already distended pulmonary circulation. *Paroxysmal nocturnal dyspnea* is a sudden attack of dyspnea during sleep. The person awakens feeling extreme suffocation that resolves when sitting. The experience may be interpreted as awakening from a bad dream.

A subtle symptom of heart failure is a chronic dry, nonproductive cough that becomes worse when the person is lying down. Bronchospasm caused by congestion of the bronchial mucosa may result in wheezing and difficulty in breathing (*cardiac asthma*).[49]

Cheyne-Stokes Respiration
Cheyne-Stokes respiration is a pattern of periodic breathing characterized by gradual increase in depth (and sometimes rate) of breathing to a maximum, followed by a decrease resulting in apnea. It is an independent risk factor for worsening of heart failure. During sleep, Cheyne-Stokes breathing causes recurrent awakening and reduces slow-wave and range of motion sleep. Nocturnal oxygen may improve sleep, exercise tolerance, and cognitive function.

Acute Pulmonary Edema
Acute pulmonary edema is a life-threatening condition in which capillary fluid moves into the alveoli.[49,51] The accumulated fluid causes lung stiffness, makes lung expansion more difficult, and impairs the gas exchange

function. The hemoglobin leaves the pulmonary circulation without being fully oxygenated, resulting in shortness of breath and cyanosis.

A person with severe pulmonary edema is usually seen sitting and gasping for air. Pulse is rapid, skin is moist and cool, and lips and nail beds are cyanotic. As the pulmonary edema worsens and oxygen to the brain drops, confusion and stupor appear. Dyspnea and air hunger accompany a productive cough with frothy and often blood-tinged sputum—the effect of air mixing with the serum albumin and red blood cells that have moved into the alveoli. The movement of air through the alveolar fluid produces fine crepitant sounds called *crackles*, which can be heard with chest auscultation. As fluid moves into larger airways, crackles become louder and coarser.

Fatigue, Weakness, and Mental Confusion

Fatigue and weakness often accompany diminished LV output. Cardiac fatigue is usually not present in the morning but appears and progresses as activity increases during the day.

In acute or severe left-sided heart failure, CO may fall to levels that are insufficient for providing the brain with adequate oxygen, thus causing confusion and disturbed behavior. Confusion, impairment of memory, anxiety, restlessness, and insomnia are common in elderly person with advanced heart failure, particularly in those with cerebral atherosclerosis. These symptoms may confuse diagnosis of heart failure because of their myriad of other causes associated with aging.

Fluid Retention and Edema

Many of the manifestations of heart failure result from increased capillary pressures that develop in peripheral circulation with right-sided heart failure and in the pulmonary circulation with left-sided heart failure. Increased capillary pressure reflects vascular system overfilling because of increased sodium and water retention and venous congestion (*backward* failure).[49,51]

Nocturia is a nightly increase in urine output that occurs relatively early in the course of heart failure. It occurs because of increased CO, renal blood flow, and glomerular filtration rate that follow the increased blood return to the heart when the person is supine. *Oliguria*, a decrease in urine output, is a late sign related to a severely reduced CO and resultant renal failure.

Transudation of fluid into the pleural cavity (hydrothorax) or the peritoneal cavity (ascites) may occur with advanced heart failure. Because pleural veins drain into the systemic and pulmonary venous beds, hydrothorax is common in hypertension involving both venous systems.[49] Pleural effusion occurs as excess fluid in the lung interstitial spaces crosses the visceral pleura, which overwhelms the pulmonary lymphatic system. Ascites occurs with increased pressure in the hepatic veins and veins draining the peritoneum. It usually reflects right ventricular failure and long-standing elevation of systemic venous pressure in chronic heart failure.[49,50]

Cachexia and Malnutrition

Cardiac cachexia is a condition of malnutrition and tissue wasting that occurs in people with end-stage heart failure. Factors contributing to its development may include fatigue and depression that interfere with food intake, congestion of the liver and GI structures that impairs digestion and absorption and produces feelings of fullness, and circulating toxins and mediators released from poorly perfused tissues that impair appetite and contribute to tissue wasting.

Cyanosis

Cyanosis is the bluish discoloration of the skin and mucous membranes caused by excess desaturated hemoglobin in the blood. Cyanosis may be central, caused by arterial desaturation resulting from impaired pulmonary gas exchange, or peripheral, caused by venous desaturation resulting from extensive extraction of oxygen at the capillary level. Central cyanosis is caused by conditions that impair oxygenation of the arterial blood, such as pulmonary edema, left heart failure, or right-to-left cardiac shunting. Peripheral cyanosis is caused by conditions such as low-output heart failure that result in delivery of poorly oxygenated blood to the peripheral tissues or by conditions such as peripheral vasoconstriction that cause excessive removal of oxygen from the blood. Central cyanosis is best monitored in the lips and mucous membranes because these areas are not subject to conditions, such as a cold environment, that cause peripheral cyanosis. People with right-sided or left-sided heart failure may develop cyanosis around the lips and in the peripheral parts of the extremities.

Arrhythmias and Sudden Cardiac Death

Atrial fibrillation is the most common arrhythmia. Clinical manifestations are related to loss of atrial contraction, tachycardia, irregular HR, and a drop in blood pressure.[49-51] People with heart failure are at increased risk for sudden cardiac arrest, death that occurs within 1 hour of symptom onset.[49-51] In people with ventricular dysfunction, sudden death is caused most commonly by ventricular tachycardia or ventricular fibrillation.

Diagnosis and Treatment

Diagnosis

Diagnostic methods are directed toward establishing the cause of the disorder and determining the extent of dysfunction. Because heart failure represents the failure of the heart as a pump and can occur in the course of a number of heart diseases or other systemic disorders, the diagnosis of heart failure is often based on signs and symptoms related to the failing heart itself, such as shortness of breath and fatigue. The functional classification of the New York Heart Association is a guide to classifying the extent of dysfunction[49]: Class I—People who have known heart disease without symptoms during ordinary activity; Class II—People with heart disease who have slight limitations, but not extreme fatigue, palpitations, dyspnea, or angina pain during regular activity; Class III—People with heart disease who are comfortable at rest, but ordinary activity does result in fatigue, palpitations, dyspnea, and angina pain; and Class IV—People who have marked progressive cardiac disease and are not comfortable at rest or minimal activity.

Methods used in the diagnosis of heart failure include risk factor assessment, history and physical examination, laboratory studies, ECG, chest radiography, and echocardiography. History should include information related to dyspnea, cough, nocturia, generalized fatigue, and other signs and symptoms of heart failure. Physical examination includes assessment of HR, heart sounds, blood pressure, jugular veins for venous congestion, lungs for signs of pulmonary congestion, and lower extremities for edema. Laboratory tests diagnose anemia and electrolyte imbalances and detect signs of chronic liver congestion. Measurements of BNP and NT-proBNP can be useful if the diagnosis of heart failure is uncertain and as risk stratification.

Invasive hemodynamic monitoring may be used for assessment in acute, life-threatening episodes of heart failure. These methods include CVP, pulmonary artery pressure monitoring, thermodilution measurements of CO, and intra-arterial measurements of blood pressure. CVP reflects the amount of blood returning to the heart, which decreases in hypovolemia and increases in right-sided heart failure. The changes that occur in CVP over time are usually more significant than the absolute numeric values obtained during a single reading.

Ventricular volume pressures are obtained by means of a flow-directed, balloon-tipped pulmonary artery catheter (Fig. 27-27). The catheter monitors pulmonary capillary pressures (*PCWP*), which is in direct communication with pressures from the left heart. PCWP assess the pumping ability of the left heart.

Intra-arterial blood pressure monitoring allows for continuous monitoring of blood pressure. It is used in people with acute heart failure when aggressive IV medication therapy or a mechanical assist device is required. The system displays the contour of the pressure waveform and the systolic, diastolic, and mean arterial pressures, along with the HR and rhythm.

Treatment

Treatment goals are determined by rapidity of onset and severity of the heart failure. People with AHFS require urgent therapy directed at stabilizing and correcting the cause. For people with chronic heart failure, the goals of treatment are directed toward relieving the symptoms, improving the quality of life, and reducing or eliminating risk factors with a long-term goal of slowing, halting, or reversing the cardiac dysfunction.[49-52]

Treatment measures for both acute and chronic heart failure include nonpharmacologic and pharmacologic approaches. Mechanical support devices, including the intra-aortic balloon pump (for acute failure) and the ventricular assist device (VAD), sustain life in severe heart failure. Heart transplantation is the treatment of choice for many with end-stage heart failure.

Nonpharmacologic Methods

Exercise intolerance is typical in people with chronic heart failure.[50] Consequently, exercise training is important to maximize muscle conditioning. Sodium and fluid restriction and weight management are important and should be individualized. Counseling and ongoing evaluation programs help people with heart failure to manage and cope with their treatment regimen.

Pharmacologic Treatment

Once heart failure is moderate to severe, adding pharmacologic management is important to prevent and treat acute heart failure and manage chronic heart failure. This includes diuretics, ACE inhibitors or angiotensin II receptor blockers, β-adrenergic blockers, and digoxin.[49-52] The choice of agents is based on symptomatology of the person.

Thiazide and loop *diuretics* are frequently prescribed and promote the excretion of fluid and help to sustain CO and tissue perfusion by reducing preload and allowing the heart to operate at a more optimal part of the Frank-Starling curve.[49-52] In emergencies, such as acute pulmonary edema, loop diuretics such as furosemide can be administered IV. When given as a **bolus** infusion, IV furosemide acts within minutes to increase venous capacitance so that right ventricular output and pulmonary capillary pressures are decreased.

ACE inhibitors, which prevent the conversion of angiotensin I to angiotensin II, are used in the treatment of chronic heart failure. The renin–angiotensin–aldosterone system is activated early in heart failure and increases angiotensin II, which causes vasoconstriction, unregulated ventricular remodeling, and increased aldosterone production with a subsequent increase in

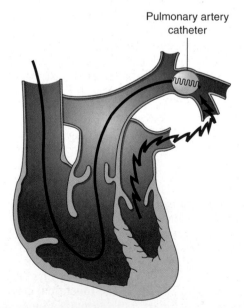

Pulmonary artery catheter

FIGURE 27-27. Balloon-tipped pulmonary artery catheter positioned in a small pulmonary vessel. The PCWP, which reflects the left ventricular diastolic pressure, is measured with the balloon inflated. PCWP, pulmonary capillary wedge pressure.

sodium and water retention by the kidneys. ACE inhibitors limit these harmful complications. *Angiotensin II receptor blockers* have similar but more limited beneficial effects. They have the advantage of not causing a cough. *Aldosterone receptor antagonists* may be used in combination with other agents for people with moderately severe to severe heart failure.

β-*Adrenergic receptor blocking drugs* decrease LV dysfunction associated with activation of the sympathetic nervous system. The mechanism remains unclear, but it is likely that chronic elevations of catecholamines and sympathetic nervous system activity cause progressive myocardial damage, leading to a worsening of LV function and a poorer prognosis.[51,52]

The various forms of *digitalis* are called *cardiac glycosides*, which improve cardiac function by increasing the force and strength of ventricular contractions. By decreasing SA node activity and conduction through the AV node, they also slow HR and increase diastolic filling time. Digitalis promotes urine output by improving CO and renal blood flow.

Vasodilator drugs can be effective in symptom management. Agents such as isosorbide dinitrate and hydralazine may be added to other standard medications for people with chronic heart failure. Vasodilators such as nitroglycerin, nitroprusside, and nesiritide (B-type NP) are used in AHFS to improve left heart performance by decreasing the preload (through vasodilation) or reducing the afterload (through arteriolar dilation) or both.[51,52]

Oxygen Therapy

Oxygen therapy increases the oxygen content of the blood and is most often used in acute episodes of heart failure. Continuous positive airway pressure (CPAP) is recommended to reduce the need for endotracheal intubation in people with AHFS. CPAP increases intrathoracic pressure, which may decrease venous return and LV preload, thereby improving the cardiac ejection fraction and stabilizing the hemodynamic status in severe heart failure. Bilevel positive airway pressure is like CPAP, but also delivers higher pressures during inspiration.[52]

Cardiac Resynchronization and Implantable Cardioverter–Defibrillators

Some people with heart failure have abnormal intraventricular conduction that results in dyssynchronous and ineffective contractions. Cardiac resynchronization therapy places pacing leads into the right ventricle and LV to resynchronizing the contraction of the two ventricles. Cardiac resynchronization has been shown to improve ventricular function and blood pressure, improve quality of life, and reduce the risk of death.[53]

People with heart failure are at significant risk of SCD from ventricular fibrillation or ventricular tachycardia. Implantation of a cardioverter–defibrillator is indicated in selected people with heart failure to prevent SCD.[53] It has the capacity to pace the heart and deliver electrical shocks to terminate lethal arrhythmias when needed.

Mechanical Support and Heart Transplantation

Refractory heart failure reflects deterioration in cardiac function that is unresponsive to interventions. With improved methods of treatment, more people are reaching a point where a cure is unachievable and death is imminent without mechanical support or heart transplantation.

VAD are mechanical pumps that decrease the workload of the myocardium while maintaining CO and systemic arterial pressure. This allows the ventricle to rest and recover. They may be used in people who fail or have difficulty being weaned from cardiopulmonary bypass after cardiac surgery, those who develop cardiogenic shock after MI, those with end-stage cardiomyopathy, and those who are awaiting cardiac transplantation. Earlier and more aggressive use of VADs as a bridge to transplantation and destination therapy increases survival.[54] VADs that allow the person to be mobile and managed at home are sometimes used for long-term or permanent support for treatment of end-stage heart failure. VADs can be used to support the function of the LV or right ventricle or both.[54]

Heart transplantation is the preferred treatment for people with end-stage cardiac failure and otherwise good life expectancy.[54] Despite the overall success of heart transplantation, donor availability remains a key problem, and only about 5000 procedures are completed each year, with thousands being denied transplantation each year.

Other novel surgical therapies that are being explored include LV remodeling, a surgical procedure designed to restore the size and shape of the ventricle. It is thought to be a viable surgical alternative to cardiac transplantation for people with severe LV dysfunction.[54]

SUMMARY CONCEPTS

Heart failure occurs when the heart fails to pump sufficient blood to meet the metabolic needs of body tissues. The physiology of heart failure reflects the interplay between a decrease in cardiac output that accompanies impaired function of the failing heart and the compensatory mechanisms that preserve the cardiac reserve. Compensatory mechanisms include the Frank-Starling mechanism, sympathetic nervous system activation, the renin–angiotensin–aldosterone mechanism, NPs, the endothelins, and myocardial hypertrophy and remodeling. In the failing heart, early decreases in cardiac function may go unnoticed because these compensatory mechanisms maintain the cardiac output. In severe and prolonged heart failure, the compensatory mechanisms no longer are effective and instead contribute to the progression of heart failure.

Heart failure may be described in terms of systolic versus diastolic dysfunction and right ventricular versus left ventricular dysfunction. With systolic dysfunction, there is impaired ejection of blood from the heart during systole; with diastolic dysfunction, there is impaired filling of the heart during diastole. Right ventricular dysfunction is characterized by congestion in the peripheral circulation and left ventricular dysfunction by congestion in the pulmonary circulation. Heart failure can present as a chronic condition characterized by decreased cardiac function or as an AHFS. The AHFS represents a gradual or rapid change in heart failure signs and symptoms, indicating need for urgent therapy. These symptoms are primarily the result of pulmonary congestion because of elevated left ventricular filling pressures with or without a low cardiac output.

The manifestations of heart failure include edema, nocturia, fatigue and impaired exercise tolerance, cyanosis, signs of increased sympathetic nervous system activity, and impaired gastrointestinal function and malnutrition. In right-sided heart failure, there is dependent edema of the lower parts of the body, engorgement of the liver, and ascites. In left-sided heart failure, pulmonary congestion with shortness of breath and chronic, nonproductive cough are common.

The diagnostic methods in heart failure are directed toward establishing the cause and extent of the disorder. Treatment is directed toward correcting the cause whenever possible, improving cardiac function, maintaining the fluid volume within a compensatory range, and developing an activity pattern consistent with individual limitations in cardiac reserve. Among the medications used in the treatment of heart failure are diuretics, ACE inhibitors and angiotensin receptor blocking agents, β-adrenergic receptor blockers, digoxin, and vasodilators. Mechanical support devices, including the VADs, sustain life in people with severe heart failure. Heart transplantation remains the treatment of choice for many people with end-stage heart failure.

Heart Disease in Infants and Children

Approximately 1 in 115 to 125 infants born has a congenital heart defect, making this the most common form of structural birth defect.[1] Advances in diagnostic methods and surgical treatment have greatly increased the long-term survival and outcomes for children born with congenital heart defects. Surgical correction of most defects is now possible, often within the first weeks of life, and the majority of affected children are expected to survive into adulthood.

Although thousands of infants born each year will have a congenital heart disease, other children will develop an acquired heart disease, including Kawasaki disease.

Embryonic Development of the Heart

The heart is the first functioning organ in the embryo: its pulsatile movements begin in the third week after conception. Early development of the heart is essential to the rapidly growing embryo in order to circulate nutrients and remove waste products. Most of the development of the heart and blood vessels occurs between the third and eighth weeks of embryonic life.[55]

The developing heart begins as two endothelial tubes that fuse into a single tubular structure.[55] Early structures develop as the heart elongates and forms dilations and constrictions. A single atrium and ventricle along with the bulbus cordis develop, followed by formation of the truncus arteriosus and sinus venosus (Fig. 27-28). Early pulsatile movements begin in the sinus venosus and move blood out of the heart via the bulbus cordis, truncus arteriosus, and aortic arches.

A differential growth rate in the early cardiac structures and fixation at the venous and arterial ends causes the tubular heart to bend over on itself. As the heart bends, the atrium and the sinus venosus come to lie behind the bulbus cordis, truncus arteriosus, and ventricle. This looping results in the heart's alignment in the left side of the chest with the atrium located behind the

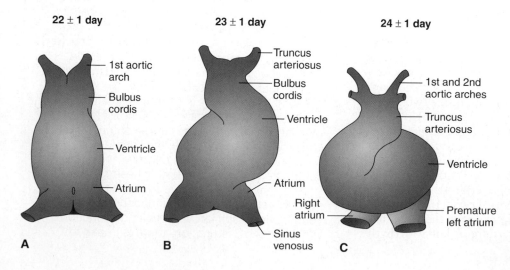

22 ± 1 day

1st aortic arch
Bulbus cordis
Ventricle
Atrium

A

23 ± 1 day

Truncus arteriosus
Bulbus cordis
Ventricle
Atrium
Right atrium
Sinus venosus

B

24 ± 1 day

1st and 2nd aortic arches
Truncus arteriosus
Ventricle
Premature left atrium

C

FIGURE 27-28. Ventral view of the developing heart. **(A)** Fusion of the heart tubes to form a single tube; it is at this stage that the heart begins to beat. **(B)** Cardiac looping, in which the heart begins to bend ventrally and to the right, bringing the primitive ventricle leftward and in continuity with the sinus venosus (future left and right atria), with the future right ventricle being shifted rightward and in continuity with the bulbus cordis (future aorta and pulmonary artery), and **(C)** folding is complete.

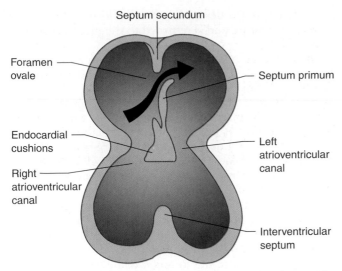

FIGURE 27-29. Development of the endocardial cushions, right and left AV canals, interventricular septum, and septum primum and septum secundum of the foramen ovale. Note that blood from the right atrium flows through the foramen ovale to the left atrium. AV, atrioventricular.

ventricle. Malrotation can cause various malpositions, such as dextroposition of the heart.

Partitioning of the AV canal, atrium, and ventricle begins in the fourth week and is complete by the fifth week. Septation begins as tissue bundles (*endocardial cushions*) form in the midportion of the dorsal and ventral walls of the heart in the region of the AV canal and begin to grow inward. As the endocardial cushions enlarge, they meet and fuse to form separate right and left AV canals (Fig. 27-29). The mitral and tricuspid valves develop in these canals. The endocardial cushions also contribute to formation of parts of the atrial and ventricular septa. Defects in endocardial cushion formation can result in atrial septal defects and VSD, complete AV canal defects, and anomalies of the mitral and tricuspid valves.

Compartmentalization of ventricles begins with the growth of the interventricular septum from the floor of the ventricle moving upward to the endocardial cushions. Fusion of the endocardial cushions with the interventricular septum is completed by the end of the seventh week.

Partitioning of the atrial septum begins with the formation of a thin, crescent-shaped membrane (*septum primum*) that emerges from the anterosuperior portion of the heart and grows toward the endocardial cushions, leaving an opening called the *foramen primum* between its lower edge and the endocardial cushions. A second membrane, called *septum secundum*, also begins to grow from the upper wall of the atrium on the right side of the septum primum. As this membrane grows toward the endocardial cushions, it gradually overlaps an opening in the upper part of the septum primum, forming an oval opening with a flap-type valve called the *foramen ovale* (Fig. 27-22). The upper part of the septum primum gradually disappears, with the remaining part becoming the valve of the foramen ovale. The foramen ovale forms a communicating channel between the two upper chambers of the heart. This opening typically closes shortly after birth and allows blood from the umbilical vein to pass directly into the left heart, bypassing the lungs.

Finally, blood pumped from the right side of the heart, which is to be diverted into the pulmonary circulation, must be separated from the blood pumped from the left side of the heart, which is to be pumped to the systemic circulation. This is accomplished by developmental changes in the outflow channels of the tubular heart, the *bulbus cordis* and *truncus arteriosus*, which undergo spiral twisting and vertical partitioning (Fig. 27-30). As these vessels spiral and divide, the aorta takes up position posterior to and to the right of the pulmonary artery. Impaired spiraling during this stage can lead to defects such as *transposition of the great vessels*.

In the process of forming a separate pulmonary trunk and aorta, a vessel called the *ductus arteriosus* develops. This vessel, which connects the pulmonary artery and the aorta, allows blood entering the pulmonary trunk to be shunted into the aorta as a means of bypassing the lungs. Like the foramen ovale, the ductus arteriosus usually closes shortly after birth.[55]

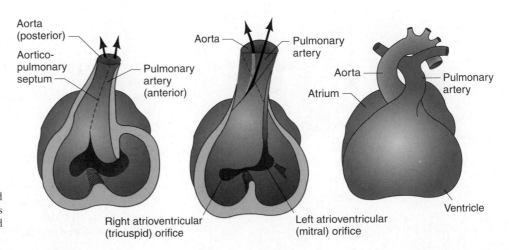

FIGURE 27-30. Separation and twisting of the truncus arteriosus to form the pulmonary artery and aorta.

Fetal and Perinatal Circulation

Blood flow in the fetal circulation occurs in parallel rather than in series, with the right ventricle delivering most of its output to the placenta for oxygen uptake and the LV pumping blood to the heart, brain, and primarily upper body of the fetus.[56] Before birth, oxygenation of blood occurs through the placenta, and after birth, it occurs through the lungs. The fetus is maintained in a low-oxygen state. To compensate, fetal CO is higher than at any other time in life, and fetal hemoglobin has a higher affinity for oxygen.[56] Pulmonary vessels are markedly constricted because of the fluid-filled lungs and heightened hypoxic stimulus for vasoconstriction that is present in the fetus. As a result, blood flow through the lungs is less than at any other time in life.

In the fetus, blood enters the circulation through the umbilical vein and returns to the placenta through the two umbilical arteries (Fig. 27-31). The *ductus venosus* allows the majority of the blood from the umbilical vein to bypass the hepatic circulation and pass directly into the inferior vena cava. From the inferior vena cava, blood flows into the right atrium, where 40% of the blood volume moves through the foramen ovale into the left atrium. It then passes into the LV and is ejected into the ascending aorta to perfuse the head and upper extremities. Thus, the best-oxygenated blood perfuses the brain. Simultaneously, venous blood from the head and upper extremities returns to the right side of the heart through the superior vena cava, moves into the right ventricle, and is ejected into the pulmonary artery. Because of the high pulmonary vascular resistance, 90% of blood ejected gets diverted through the ductus

arteriosus into the descending aorta. This blood perfuses lower extremities and is returned to the placenta by umbilical arteries.

At birth, the infant takes its first breath and switches from placental to pulmonary oxygenation of the blood. Within minutes of birth, pulmonary blood flow increases from 35 to 160 to 200 mL/kg/minute.[56] The pressure in the pulmonary circulation and the right side of the heart falls as fetal lung fluid is replaced by air and as lung expansion decreases the pressure transmitted to the pulmonary blood vessels. With lung inflation, the alveolar oxygen tension increases, causing reversal of the hypoxemia-induced pulmonary vasoconstriction of the fetal circulation. Removal of the low-resistance placental circulation produces an increase in systemic vascular resistance and a resultant increase in LV pressure. The decrease in right atrial pressure and increase in left atrial pressure close the foramen ovale. Reversal of the fetal hypoxemic state also produces constriction of ductal smooth muscle, contributing to closure of the ductus arteriosus by 72 hours after birth. After the initial precipitous fall in pulmonary vascular resistance, a more gradual decrease in pulmonary vascular resistance is related to regression of the medial smooth muscle layer in the pulmonary arteries. During the first 2 to 9 weeks of life, gradual thinning of the smooth muscle layer further decreases pulmonary vascular resistance. By the time a healthy infant is several weeks old, pulmonary vascular resistance falls to adult levels.

Several factors, including alveolar hypoxia, prematurity, lung disease, and congenital heart defects, may affect postnatal pulmonary vascular development. Alveolar hypoxia is one of the most potent stimuli of pulmonary vasoconstriction and pulmonary hypertension in the neonate. During this period, the pulmonary arteries remain highly reactive and can constrict in response to hypoxia, acidosis, hyperinflation of the alveoli, and hypothermia. Thus, hypoxia during the first days of life may delay or prevent the normal decrease in pulmonary vascular resistance.

Much of the development of the smooth muscle layer in the pulmonary arterioles occurs during late gestation; as a result, infants born prematurely have less medial smooth muscle. These infants follow the same pattern of smooth muscle regression, but because less muscle exists, the muscle layer may regress in a shorter time. The pulmonary vascular smooth muscle in premature infants may also be less responsive to hypoxia. For these reasons, a premature infant may demonstrate a larger decrease in pulmonary vascular resistance and a resultant shunting of blood from the aorta through the ductus arteriosus to the pulmonary artery within hours of birth.

Congenital Heart Defects

Most congenital heart defects are multifactorial in origin, resulting from an interaction between a genetic predisposition toward development of a heart defect and environmental influences.

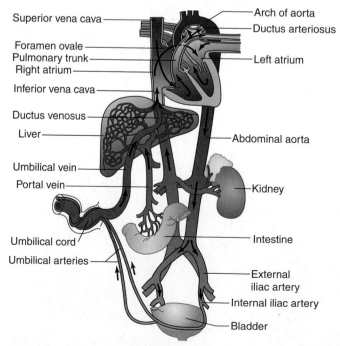

Superior vena cava
Arch of aorta
Ductus arteriosus
Foramen ovale
Pulmonary trunk
Right atrium
Left atrium
Inferior vena cava
Ductus venosus
Liver
Abdominal aorta
Umbilical vein
Portal vein
Kidney
Umbilical cord
Intestine
Umbilical arteries
External iliac artery
Internal iliac artery
Bladder

FIGURE 27-31. Fetal circulation.

Some heart defects, such as aortic stenosis, atrial septal defect of the secundum type, pulmonary valve stenosis, tetralogy of Fallot, and certain VSDs, have a stronger familial predisposition than others.

Chromosomal abnormalities are associated with congenital heart defects, and as much as 30% of children with congenital heart disease have an associated chromosomal abnormality. Heart disease is found in nearly 100% of children with trisomy 18, 50% of those with trisomy 21, and 35% of those with Turner syndrome. Williams syndrome (7q11.23 microdeletion) is associated with supravalvar aortic and pulmonary stenosis.

As much as 30% of congenital cardiac defects may be attributable to identifiable and potentially modifiable risk factors, including teratogenic influences, and adverse maternal conditions such as febrile illnesses, systemic lupus erythematosus, diabetes mellitus, maternal alcohol ingestion, and treatment with anticonvulsant medications, retinoids, lithium, and other prescription or nonprescription drugs. Proper prenatal care, especially periconceptive multivitamin intake with folic acid, may reduce the risk of cardiac disease in the fetus.

Pathophysiology

Congenital heart defects produce their effects mainly through abnormal shunting of blood, production of cyanosis, and disruption of pulmonary blood flow.

Abnormal Shunting of Blood

Shunting of blood is the diversion of blood flow from the arterial to the venous system (left-to-right shunt) or from the venous to the arterial system (right-to-left shunt). Shunting of blood in congenital heart defects is determined by the presence, position, and size of an abnormal opening between the right and left circulations and degree of resistance to flow through the opening.

Because of the high pulmonary vascular resistance in the neonate, atrial septal defects and VSDs usually do not produce significant shunt or symptoms during the first weeks of life.

As the pulmonary vascular smooth muscle regresses in the neonate, the resistance in the pulmonary circulation falls below that of the systemic circulation; in uncomplicated atrial septal defects or VSDs, blood shunts from the left side of the heart to the right. In more complicated VSDs, increased resistance to outflow may affect the pattern of shunting. For example, defects that increase resistance to aortic outflow (*e.g.*, aortic valve stenosis, coarctation of the aorta, hypoplastic left heart syndrome) increase left-to-right shunting, and defects that obstruct pulmonary outflow (*e.g.*, pulmonary valve stenosis, tetralogy of Fallot) increase right-to-left shunting.[57] Crying, defecating, or the stress of feeding may increase pulmonary vascular resistance and cause an increase in right-to-left shunting and cyanosis in infants with septal defects.

Cyanotic versus Acyanotic Disorders

Congenital heart diseases are divided into acyanotic and cyanotic. Defects that result in a left-to-right shunt are usually acyanotic because shunted systemic circulation blood mixing with pulmonary circulation blood is not enough to significantly change the levels of oxygen saturation.

Defects that produce shunting of blood from the right to the left side of the heart or result in obstruction of pulmonary blood flow are categorized as cyanotic disorders.[57] Cyanosis, most notable in the nail beds and mucous membranes, develops when sufficient deoxygenated blood from the right side of the heart mixes with oxygenated blood in the left side of the heart. Abnormal color becomes obvious when the oxygen saturation falls below 80% in the capillaries.

A right-to-left shunt results in deoxygenated blood moving from the right side of the heart to the left side and then being ejected into the systemic circulation. With a left-to-right shunt, oxygenated blood intended for ejection into the systemic circulation is recirculated through the right side of the heart and back through the lungs. This increased volume distends the right side of the heart and pulmonary circulation and increases the workload placed on the right ventricle. A child with a defect that causes left-to-right shunting usually has an enlarged right side of the heart and pulmonary blood vessels. Patent ductus arteriosus, atrial septal defects and VSDs, endocardial cushion defects, pulmonary valve stenosis, and coarctation of the aorta are considered defects with little or no cyanosis; tetralogy of Fallot, transposition of the great vessels, and single-ventricle anatomy are considered defects with cyanosis.

Disruption of Pulmonary Blood Flow

Defects that reduce pulmonary blood flow typically cause symptoms of fatigue, dyspnea, and failure to thrive. Arterioles in the pulmonary circulation are normally thin-walled vessels that can accommodate various volumes ejected from the right heart. Thinning of pulmonary vessels occurs during the first weeks after birth, during which pulmonary vascular resistance decreases. In a term infant who has a congenital heart defect that produces markedly increased pulmonary blood flow, the increased flow stimulates pulmonary vasoconstriction and delays or reduces the normal involutional thinning of the small pulmonary arterioles. In most cases during early infancy, pulmonary vascular resistance is only slightly elevated, and the major contribution to pulmonary hypertension is the increased blood flow. However, in some infants with a large right-to-left shunt, the pulmonary vascular resistance never decreases.

Congenital heart defects that persistently increase pulmonary blood flow or pulmonary vascular resistance have the potential of causing pulmonary hypertension and producing irreversible pathologic changes in the pulmonary vasculature. When shunting of systemic blood flow into the pulmonary circulation threatens permanent injury to the pulmonary vessels, a surgical procedure should be done to reduce the flow temporarily or permanently. Pulmonary artery banding consists of placing a constrictive band around the main pulmonary artery, thereby increasing resistance to outflow from the right ventricle. This is a temporary measure to alleviate symptoms and protect the pulmonary vasculature in anticipation of later surgical repair of the defect.

Manifestations and Treatment

Infants can be evaluated shortly after birth to confirm diagnosis and develop a treatment plan. Reliable diagnostic images of the fetal heart can be obtained as early as 12 weeks of gestation. Disorders that can be diagnosed with certainty by fetal echocardiography include AV septal defects, hypoplastic left heart syndrome, aortic valve stenosis, HCM, pulmonic valve stenosis, and transposition of the great arteries. Disorders that result in an abnormal four-chamber view, an image typically obtained during prenatal ultrasonography, are likely to be detected.[58]

In the postnatal period, congenital heart defects may present with numerous signs and symptoms. Some defects, such as patent ductus arteriosus and small VSDs, close spontaneously. In other, less severe defects, there may be no obvious signs and symptoms, and the disorder may be discovered during a routine health examination. Cyanosis, pulmonary congestion, cardiac failure, and decreased peripheral perfusion are the chief concerns in children with more severe defects. Such defects often cause problems immediately after birth or early in infancy. The child may exhibit cyanosis, respiratory difficulty, and fatigability and is likely to have difficulty with feeding and failure to thrive. A generalized cyanosis that persists longer than 3 hours after birth suggests congenital heart disease.[59]

An oxygen challenge (100% oxygen for 10 minutes) can help determine whether congenital heart disease is present in a cyanotic newborn. An arterial blood sample is taken during this time. If the partial pressure of oxygen (PO_2) is greater than 250 mm Hg, cyanotic heart disease can be ruled out; if the PO_2 is 160 to 250 mm Hg, heart disease is unlikely; failure of the PO_2 to rise to these levels is strongly suggestive of cyanotic heart disease.[57] Because infant cyanosis may appear as duskiness, it is important to assess the color of the mucous membranes, fingernails, toenails, tongue, and lips. Pulmonary congestion in the infant causes an increase in respiratory rate, orthopnea, grunting, wheezing, coughing, and crackles. The infant whose peripheral perfusion is markedly decreased may be in a shock-like state.

Heart failure manifests itself as tachypnea or dyspnea at rest or on exertion. For the infant, this most commonly occurs during feeding. Recurrent respiratory infections and excessive sweating may also be reported. Also, syncope or near syncope can occur. Growth failure results from unresolved heart failure.[59] The treatment plan usually includes supportive therapy (digoxin, diuretics, and feeding supplementation) designed to help the infant compensate for the limitations in cardiac reserve and to prevent complications. Surgical intervention is often required for severe defects. It may be done in the early weeks of life or, conditions permitting, delayed until the child is older. Children with structural congenital heart disease and those who have had corrective surgery may have a higher-than-expected risk for development of IE. Prophylactic antibiotic therapy before dental procedures or other periods of increased risk for bacteremia is suggested for children with unrepaired cyanotic heart disease, prior IE, prosthetic cardiac valves, prosthetic material used for cardiac valve repair, and cardiac transplant with valve regurgitation.[60,61]

Types of Defects

Congenital heart defects can affect almost any cardiac structure or central blood vessels. The particular defect reflects the embryo's stage of development at the time it occurred. Multiple defects can be present, and for some congenital heart disorders, there may be several defects.

The development of the heart is simultaneous and sequential; a heart defect may reflect the multiple developmental events that were occurring simultaneously or sequentially. Most infants who have a congenital heart defect usually do not have a major problem during infancy. Only about one third of infants who are born with anomalies have a disease state that is critical. Over 40 types of defects have been identified, the most common being VSDs, which are responsible for 28% to 42% of all congenital heart disorders.[59]

Patent Ductus Arteriosus

The ductus arteriosus diverts blood from the right side of the heart and away from the lungs to the systemic circulation during fetal life (Fig. 27-32G). With spontaneous respiration after birth, muscular constriction of the ductal tissue typically closes this vessel. The initiating step of ductal closure in the healthy infant is believed to be the sharp increase in arterial oxygen saturation and subsequent fall in pulmonary vascular resistance after birth. After constriction, the lumen of the ductus becomes permanently sealed with fibrous tissue within 2 to 3 weeks.

For 90% of full-term infants, the ductus is functionally closed by 48 hours of age.[62] Full-term infants with abnormalities of circulation or ventilation and premature infants are those most likely to exhibit persistent patency of the ductus arteriosus. Arterial oxygenation, circulating prostaglandins, genetic predetermination, and other unknown factors interact to determine the mechanism of ductal closure.[62] Circulating prostaglandin levels are directly related to gestational age, and the incidence of patent ductus arteriosus in infants with birth weights less than 1000 g may be as high as 50%.[62]

Persistent patency of the ductus arteriosus is a duct that remains open beyond 3 months in the full-term infant. The size of the persistent ductus and the difference between the systemic and pulmonary vascular resistance determine its clinical manifestations. Blood typically shunts across the ductus from the higher pressure left side to the lower pressure right. A murmur is typically detected within days or weeks of birth. The murmur is loudest at the second left intercostal space, is continuous through systole and diastole, and has a characteristic "machinery" sound.[59,62] A widened pulse pressure is common because of the continuous runoff of aortic blood into the pulmonary artery. Diagnostic methods include chest radiography and echocardiography. There are increased pulmonary markings on chest radiography and enlargement of the left heart from the increased pulmonary venous return if it is a larger shunt. Chest x-rays are normal in small shunts.[59] Echocardiography

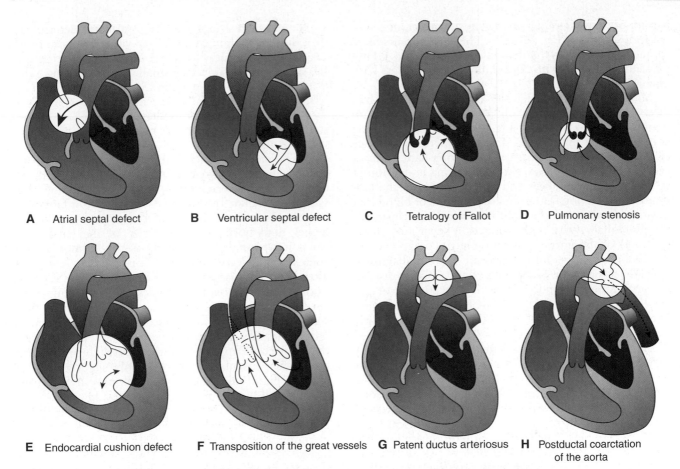

A Atrial septal defect **B** Ventricular septal defect **C** Tetralogy of Fallot **D** Pulmonary stenosis

E Endocardial cushion defect **F** Transposition of the great vessels **G** Patent ductus arteriosus **H** Postductal coarctation of the aorta

FIGURE 27-32. Congenital heart defects. **(A)** Atrial septal defect. Blood is shunted from left to right. **(B)** Ventricular septal defect. Blood is usually shunted from left to right. **(C)** Tetralogy of Fallot. This involves a ventricular septal defect, dextroposition of the aorta, right ventricular outflow obstruction, and right ventricular hypertrophy. Blood is shunted from right to left. **(D)** Pulmonary stenosis, with decreased pulmonary blood flow and right ventricular hypertrophy. **(E)** Endocardial cushion defects. Blood flows between the chambers of the heart. **(F)** Transposition of the great vessels. The pulmonary artery is attached to the left side of the heart and the aorta to the right side. **(G)** Patent ductus arteriosus. The high-pressure blood of the aorta is shunted back to the pulmonary artery. **(H)** Postductal coarctation of the aorta.

determines the presence, size, direction (*i.e.*, left to right or right to left), and physical consequences of the shunt.

An untreated patent ductus can result in important long-term complications, which may include congestive heart failure, IE, pulmonary vascular disease, aneurysm formation, thromboembolism, and calcification.[59] The potential risk of complications and the extremely low procedural morbidity and mortality justify closure of a patent ductus even when the shunt is small. In the premature infant, a patent ductus can produce respiratory distress and impede weaning from mechanical ventilation. Indomethacin, an inhibitor of prostaglandin synthesis and an NSAID, has proven effective in the treatment of patent ductus in premature infants.[59] NSAIDs result in the functional closure of patent ductus in about 80% of people.

If medical management fails, surgical intervention is recommended. In the full-term infant or older child, closure can be achieved with surgical ligation or device occlusion. Surgery typically involves a small left thoracotomy or thoracoscopic approach for vessel ligation. Implantable devices allow ductus closure to be done in

the catheterization laboratory on an outpatient basis. The anatomy of the ductus and size of the person are key determinants for this technique.

Deliberate maintenance of ductal patency can be a lifesaving therapy in complex forms of congenital heart disease with ductal-dependent pulmonary or systemic blood flow or those with obligatory mixing of the arterial and venous circulations (*i.e.*, transposition of the great arteries). Infusion of prostaglandin E_1 is effective in maintaining ductal patency or reopening the ductus in newborns and is routinely administered to newborns with suspected congenital heart defects, until they can be transported to a specialized center where a diagnosis can be confirmed.[59]

Atrial Septal Defects

Any persistent opening that allows shunting of blood across the atrial septum is an atrial septal defect. The may be single or multiple and vary from a small, asymptomatic opening to a large, symptomatic opening. The typology is determined by its position and may include a secundum atrial defect (the most common form), an ostium primum defect, a sinus venosus defect, or a patent foramen ovale (Fig. 27-32A). The defect occurs more frequently in females than in males at a 2:1 ratio.[59] Fifty percent of children with congenital heart disorders have an atrial septal defect.

Many atrial septal defects are asymptomatic and discovered incidentally during a routine physical examination at a few years of age.[62] Intracardiac shunting is usually from left to right and may increase with age as the right ventricle becomes more compliant. In most cases, there is a moderate shunt, resulting in dilation of the right heart chambers and overperfusion of the pulmonary circulation. The increased volume of blood that must be ejected from the right heart prolongs closure of the pulmonary valve and produces a separation (fixed splitting) of the aortic and pulmonary components of the second heart sound. Children with undiagnosed atrial defects are at risk for pulmonary vascular disease, although this is a rare occurrence before 20 years of age. Rarely, infants with a large shunt may develop congestive heart failure and failure to thrive, prompting early closure of the defect.[59,62]

Atrial septal defects over 8 years of age are unlikely to undergo spontaneous closure. Smaller defects may be observed for spontaneous closure in the young child. However, surgical or transcatheter closure is recommended in children with persistent defects to reduce the long-term risk of pulmonary vascular disease and atrial arrhythmias.[62] Both transcatheter device and surgical closures are effective and of low risk. Transcatheter device closure is particularly effective for small to medium-sized secundum septal defects and patent foramen ovale. Sinus venosus defects, which are frequently associated with partial anomalous pulmonary venous return and ostium primum defects, require surgical closure. Surgery requires the use of cardiopulmonary bypass and mild hypothermia. Most defects are effectively closed using the person's native septal tissue or a pericardial or synthetic patch. There is a very low incidence of residual sequelae or need for reintervention if closure occurred during the first two decades of life.

Ventricular Septal Defects

A VSD is an opening in the ventricular septum that results from an incomplete separation of the ventricles during early fetal development (Fig. 27-32B). These defects may be single or multiple and may occur in any position along the ventricular septum. VSDs are the most common form of congenital heart defect, accounting for 28% to 42% of congenital heart disorders.[63]

The ventricular septum originates from the interventricular groove of the folded tubular heart that gives rise to the muscular part of the septum and the endocardial cushions that extend to form the membranous portion of the septum. The upper membranous portion of the septum is the last area to close, typically by the seventh week of gestation, and it is where most defects occur. Depending on the size of the opening and pulmonary vascular resistance, the symptoms of a VSD may range from asymptomatic murmur to congestive heart failure.[59]

The physical size of the VSD is a major determinant of left-to-right shunt. Pulmonary vascular resistance in relation to systemic vascular resistance also determines the shunt's magnitude. In a small communicating defect (<0.5 cm^2), higher pressure in LV drives the shunt to the left, and the size of the defect limits the magnitude of the shunt. Most children with such defects are asymptomatic and have a low risk of developing pulmonary vascular disease.

In a larger, nonrestrictive shunt (usually >1 cm^2), right ventricular and LV pressure is equalized, and the degree of shunting is determined by the ratio of pulmonary to systemic vascular resistance. After birth in infants with large VSDs, pulmonary vascular resistance may remain higher than normal, and the size of the left-to-right shunt may initially be limited. As the pulmonary vascular resistance continues to fall in the first few weeks after birth because of normal involution of the media of the small pulmonary arterioles, the magnitude of the left-to-right shunt increases. Eventually, a large left-to-right shunt develops, and clinical symptoms (e.g., tachypnea; diaphoresis, especially with feeding; and failure to thrive) become apparent. In most cases during infancy, pulmonary vascular pressure is only slightly elevated, and the major contributor to pulmonary hypertension is an increase in pulmonary blood flow. In some infants with a large septal defect, pulmonary arteriolar thickness never decreases. With continued exposure to high pulmonary blood flow, pulmonary vascular obstructive disease develops. In untreated people, the pulmonary vascular resistance can eventually exceed the systemic resistance. In this case, a reversal of shunt flow occurs, and the child demonstrates progressive cyanosis as deoxygenated blood moves from the right to the left side of the heart. These symptoms, coupled with irreversible changes in the pulmonary vasculature, represent an end-stage form of congenital heart disease called *Eisenmenger complex*. People who develop this have a life expectancy of about 43 years, and the cause of death is progressive heart failure.[59]

Treatment depends on the size of the defect, accompanying hemodynamic derangements, and symptomatology. Children with small or medium-sized defects may be followed without intervention if they remain free from signs of congestive heart failure or pulmonary hypertension.[62] Two-dimensional echocardiography is usually adequate to diagnose the size and position of a defect and to estimate pulmonary pressures. Cardiac catheterization is usually reserved for cases where it is necessary to confirm degree and reversibility of pulmonary vascular resistance.

Congestive heart failure is treated medically. Symptomatic infants may require feeding supplements or tube feeding to promote growth and development. In the symptomatic infant in whom complete repair cannot be achieved, a palliative procedure may be performed to reduce symptoms. Pulmonary artery banding can reduce pulmonary blood flow until complete repair can be accomplished. Surgical closure of the defect is completed by placement of a synthetic or autologous patch effectively to close the shunt across the ventricular septum.

These procedures are typically done electively in the infant or young child and are associated with low morbidity and mortality rates. Transcatheter device closure of VSDs is another option for defect closure with improved complication risk in the recent years.

Endocardial Cushion Defects

The AV canal connects the atria to the ventricles during early cardiac development. The endocardial cushions surround this canal and contribute tissue to the lower part of the atrial septum, the upper part of the ventricular septum, the septal leaflet of the tricuspid valve, and the anterior leaflet of the mitral valve.[63] Any flaw in the development of these tissues results in an endocardial cushion defect. Approximately 3% of all congenital heart defects are endocardial cushion defects. Endocardial cushion defects have a strong association with trisomy 21 and are seen in as much as 50% of children with this genetic disorder.[63]

Endocardial cushion defects may be described as *partial* or *complete*. The anatomy of the AV valve determines its classification. In partial AV canal defects, the two AV valve rings are complete and separate. The most common type of partial AV canal defect is an ostium primum defect, often associated with a cleft in the mitral valve. In a complete canal defect, there is a common AV valve orifice along with defects in both the atrial and ventricular septal tissue (Fig. 27-32E). Other cardiac defects may be associated with endocardial cushion defects and most commonly include cardiac malposition defects and tetralogy of Fallot.[64,65]

Physiologically, endocardial cushion defects result in abnormalities similar to those described for atrial septal defects or VSDs. The direction and magnitude of a shunt in a child with an endocardial cushion defect are determined by the combination of defects and the child's pulmonary and systemic vascular resistances. The hemodynamic effects of an isolated ostium primum defect are those of the previously described atrial septal defect. These children are largely asymptomatic during childhood. With a complete AV canal defect, pulmonary blood flow is increased after pulmonary vascular resistance falls because of left-to-right shunting across both the ventricular and atrial septal defects. Children with complete defects often have effort intolerance, easy fatigability, failure to thrive, recurrent infections, and other signs of congestive heart failure, particularly when the shunt is large. Pulmonary hypertension and increased pulmonary vascular resistance result if the lesion is left untreated.

The timing of treatment for endocardial cushion defects is determined by the severity of the defect and symptoms. With an ostium primum defect, surgical repair is usually planned on an elective basis before the child reaches school age. The defect in the atrial septum is closed with a patch, and mitral valvuloplasty is performed if the valve is regurgitant. Corrective surgery is required for all complete AV canal defects. This is typically performed early in the infant's life and requires patching of both the atrial septal defects and VSDs and separation of the AV valve apparatus to create competent mitral and tricuspid valves. Infants with severe symptoms may require a palliative procedure, where the main pulmonary artery is banded to reduce pulmonary blood flow. This typically improves the infant's ability to grow and develop until a complete repair can be performed. Total surgical repair of complete AV canal defects can be accomplished with low operative risk. Reoperation may be required in 11.7% of children.

Pulmonary Stenosis

Obstruction of blood flow from the right ventricle to the pulmonary circulation is *pulmonary stenosis*. Obstruction can be an isolated valvular lesion, within the right ventricular chamber, in pulmonary arteries, or as a combination of stenoses in multiple areas. It is relatively common, accounting for 10% of congenital cardiac disease, and is often associated with other defects.[62]

Pulmonary valvular defects, the most common type of obstruction, usually produce some impairment of pulmonary blood flow and increase the workload imposed on the right side of the heart (Fig. 27-32D). Most children with pulmonary valve stenosis have mild stenosis that does not increase in severity. They are largely asymptomatic and diagnosed by the presence of a systolic murmur. Moderate or greater stenosis has been shown to progress over time, particularly before 12 years of age. Critical pulmonary stenosis in the neonate is evidenced by cyanosis caused by right-to-left atrial-level shunting and right ventricular hypertension. These infants require prostaglandin E_1 to maintain circulation to the lungs through the ductus arteriosus.[33]

Pulmonary valvotomy is the treatment for all valvular defects with pressure gradients from right ventricle to pulmonary circulation greater than 30 mm Hg. Transcatheter balloon valvuloplasty is quite successful. Stenosis in the peripheral pulmonary arteries can also be effectively treated with balloon angioplasty.[62] Stents are used for children with pulmonary artery stenosis to keep the vessels open. This is used when balloon dilation has failed.[59]

Tetralogy of Fallot

Tetralogy of Fallot is the most common cyanotic congenital heart defect.[59] As the name implies, tetralogy of Fallot consists of four associated defects: (1) a VSD involving the membranous septum and the anterior portion of the muscular septum; (2) dextroposition or shifting to the right of the aorta so that it overrides the right ventricle and is in communication with the septal defect; (3) obstruction or narrowing of the pulmonary outflow channel, including pulmonary valve stenosis, a decrease in the size of the pulmonary trunk, or both; and (4) hypertrophy of the right ventricle because of the increased work required to pump blood through the obstructed pulmonary channels[65] (Fig. 27-32C). Variations of the defect can be a right aortic arch and a persistent left superior vena cava. When this is seen, it is called *pentalogy of Fallot*.[59]

Cyanosis is caused by a right-to-left shunt across the VSD. The degree of cyanosis is determined by the restriction of blood flow into the pulmonary bed. Right ventricular outflow obstruction causes deoxygenated blood from the right ventricle to shunt across the VSD and be ejected into the systemic circulation. The degree of obstruction may be dynamic and can increase during periods of stress, causing hypercyanotic attacks. These spells typically occur in the morning during crying, feeding, or defecating, which increase the infant's oxygen requirements. Crying and defecation may further increase pulmonary vascular resistance, thereby increasing right-to-left shunting and decreasing pulmonary blood flow. The infant becomes acutely cyanotic, hyperpneic, irritable, and diaphoretic. Later in the spell, the infant becomes limp and may lose consciousness. Placing the infant in the knee–chest position increases systemic vascular resistance, thus decreasing right-to-left shunting and increasing pulmonary blood flow. During a hypercyanotic spell, toddlers and older children may spontaneously assume the squatting position, which functions like the knee–chest position to relieve the spell. Turbulent flow across the narrow right ventricular outflow track produces a characteristic harsh systolic ejection murmur. Auscultation during a hypercyanotic spell reveals a diminished or absent murmur as a result of the dramatic reduction in pulmonary blood flow.[65]

Surgical correction is required for all children with tetralogy of Fallot. Iron deficiency anemia should be addressed in order to prevent stroke prior to surgery. Dehydration is monitored closely to prevent thrombotic complications, propranolol can be administered to prevent hypoxic spells, and sodium bicarbonate and α-adrenergic agonists are administered if acidosis is present.

When extreme cyanosis is present in a small infant or when there is associated marked hypoplasia of the pulmonary arteries, a palliative procedure to facilitate pulmonary blood flow may be necessary. This is accomplished by a prosthetic shunt between a systemic artery and the pulmonary artery. Balloon dilation of the pulmonary valve may also afford palliation in some infants. Total correction is then carried out later in infancy or early childhood. Complete repair includes patch closure of the VSD and relief of any right ventricular outflow tract obstruction. Repair is associated with a mortality rate under 3%; however, people need long-term follow-up to monitor for residual lesions, right ventricular dilation or dysfunction, and arrhythmias.[65] They also need to be monitored because they continue to be at risk for IE.

Transposition of the Great Arteries

In complete transposition of the great arteries, the aorta arises from the right ventricle and the pulmonary artery from the LV (Fig. 27-32F). It occurs in 1 per 4000 live births.

Cyanosis is the most common presenting symptom resulting from an anomaly that allows the systemic venous return to be circulated through the right heart and ejected into the aorta and the pulmonary venous return to be recirculated to the lungs through the LV and main pulmonary artery.[59] In infants born with this

defect, survival depends on communication between the right and left sides of the heart in the form of a patent ductus arteriosus or septal defect. VSDs are present in 50% of infants, of which 10% have a small VSD, with transposition of the great arteries at birth and may allow effective mixing of blood. Prostaglandin E$_1$ should be administered when this lesion is suspected in an effort to maintain the patency of the ductus arteriosus. Balloon atrial septostomy may be done to increase the blood flow between the two sides of the heart. In this procedure, a balloon-tipped catheter is inserted into the heart through the vena cava and then passed through the foramen ovale into the left atrium. The balloon is then inflated and pulled back through the foramen ovale, enlarging the opening as it goes.

Corrective surgery is essential for long-term survival. An arterial switch procedure has survival rates greater than 90%.[59] This procedure, which corrects the relation of the systemic and pulmonary blood flows, is preferably performed in the first 2 to 3 weeks of life, before the postnatal reduction in pulmonary vascular resistance occurs. The coronary arteries are moved to the left-sided great artery, and any VSDs are closed during the same operation. Complications of the arterial switch procedure may include coronary insufficiency, supravalvar pulmonary stenosis, neoaortic regurgitation, and rhythm abnormalities.[64]

Coarctation of the Aorta

Coarctation of the aorta is a localized narrowing of the aorta, proximal to (preductal), distal to (postductal), or opposite the entry of the ductus arteriosus (juxtaductal; see Fig. 27-32H). In all, 98% of coarctations are juxtaductal. The anomaly occurs more often in males than in females, as much as 3:1. It is frequently associated with other congenital cardiac lesions, most commonly bicuspid aortic valve (46%), and occurs in approximately 10% of people with Turner syndrome.[59,62]

The classic sign of coarctation of the aorta is a disparity in pulsations and blood pressures in the arms and legs. The femoral, popliteal, and dorsalis pedis pulsations are weak or delayed compared with the bounding pulses of the arms and carotid vessels. Normally, the systolic blood pressure in the legs obtained by the cuff method is 10 to 20 mm Hg higher than that in the arms. In coarctation, the pressure in the legs is lower and may be difficult to obtain. People with coarctation are often identified during a diagnostic workup for hypertension. Most with moderate coarctation remain otherwise asymptomatic owing to collateral vessels that form around the area of narrowing. Left untreated, however, coarctation will result in LV hypertension and hypertrophy and significant systemic hypertension. Infants with severe coarctation demonstrate early symptoms of heart failure and may present in critical condition upon ductal closure. Reopening of the duct with prostaglandin E$_1$, if possible, and emergent surgery are needed.[62]

Children with coarctation causing a blood pressure gradient between the arms and the legs of 20 mm Hg or greater should be treated ideally by 2 years of age to reduce the likelihood of persistent hypertension.[62]

Surgical typically involves resection of the narrowed segment of the aorta and end-to-end anastomosis of healthy tissue. This can be accomplished without cardiopulmonary bypass, with a mortality rate near zero. Balloon angioplasty with or without stent placement has also been used.[59,62] Common complications after repair are persistent hypertension and recoarctation. Operative mortality rates increase if an associated defect is present.

Functional Single-Ventricle Anatomy

Several forms of complex congenital heart disease result in only one functional ventricle. There may be a single right or a single LV or a ventricle of indeterminate morphology. Hypoplastic left heart syndrome is the most common form of single right ventricular anatomy. Tricuspid valve atresia is the most common cause of a single LV. Several other forms of double-inlet ventricle have been described; however, all forms of this disease result in similar pathologic effects and follow a common pathway of intervention.[59]

All forms of single-ventricle anatomy result in a common mixing chamber of pulmonary and systemic venous return and cause varying degrees of cyanosis. The single ventricle must supply both the pulmonary and systemic circulations.[59] The amount of blood flow to each circulation is determined by the resistance in each system. As pulmonary vascular resistance falls, flow to the pulmonary circulation will be preferential, and systemic circulation will be compromised. In some defects, such as hypoplastic left heart syndrome, systemic flow depends on a patent ductus arteriosus. Neonates with this lesion typically present with extreme cyanosis and symptoms of heart failure as the ductus begins to close.[62]

The goal of surgical palliation is to redirect systemic venous return directly to the pulmonary arteries and allow the single ventricle to deliver oxygenated blood to the systemic circulation. This is accomplished in a series of two- to three-staged surgical procedures during the first years of life. Cardiac transplantation is also used as an intervention for the most complex forms of single-ventricle congenital heart disease (Fig. 27-33).

Survival rates for children with complex forms of single-ventricle heart disease have improved markedly, but ventricular dysfunction, arrhythmias, and thromboses plague this population. Defining the optimal medical and surgical management strategies for these people remains an active area of research in pediatric cardiology and cardiac surgery.[59]

Adults with Congenital Heart Disease

Successful treatment of congenital heart disease in the pediatric population has resulted in a growing number of adult survivors with a variety of repaired, unrepaired, and palliated congenital cardiac lesions. An epidemiologic study on the prevalence and age distribution of congenital heart disease identified a prevalence of 6 in 1000 adults.[59,66]

Most congenital heart defects must be considered chronic conditions requiring long-term surveillance and care.[66] Chronic physiologic concerns include

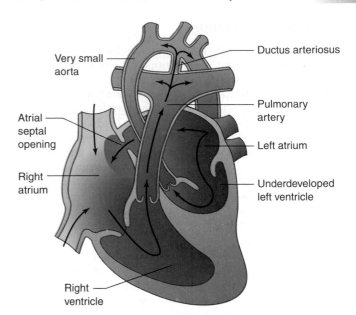

FIGURE 27-33. Functional single-ventricle anatomy with an underdeveloped left ventricular (LV) and small ascending aorta. Because of the markedly decreased LV compliance, most of the pulmonary venous blood returning to the left atrium shunts left to right at the atrial level. Pulmonary arterial blood flows into the pulmonary arteries as well as right to left across a patent ductus arteriosus into the aorta.

arrhythmias, hemodynamic problems, complications of prolonged cyanosis, endocarditis, residual lesions, and the need for reoperation. The underlying defect can also have implications for other aspects of health, such as exercise tolerance, noncardiac surgery, and pregnancy. Several important psychosocial issues also require consideration, including neurocognitive achievement, employment, insurability, family planning, treatment adherence, and understanding of the underlying condition and risks.

Kawasaki Disease

Kawasaki disease (*mucocutaneous lymph node syndrome*) is an acute febrile disease of young children. The disease affects the skin, brain, eyes, joints, liver, lymph nodes, and heart. It is the most common cause of acquired heart disease in young children, with 15% to 25% of cases resulting in coronary artery aneurysms or ectasias that may lead to MI, sudden death, or chronic coronary insufficiency.[37,67] Over 80% of people with the disease are 4 years or younger, with a male-to-female ratio of 1.5:1. Although it is most common in Japan, the disease affects children of many races, occurs worldwide, and is increasing in frequency.

Pathogenesis

The disease is characterized by a vasculitis that begins in the small vessels and progresses to involve some of the larger arteries, such as the coronaries. The exact etiology and pathogenesis of the disease remain unknown, but it is thought to be of immunologic origin.

Sympathetic stimulation produces peripheral vaso-constriction and diaphoresis. Decreased renal blood flow often results in a decrease in urine output despite adequate fluid intake.

When right ventricular function is impaired, systemic venous congestion develops. Hepatomegaly caused by liver congestion is often one of the first signs of systemic venous congestion in infants and children. However, dependent edema or ascites is rarely seen, unless the CVP is extremely high. Jugular venous distention is difficult to detect in infants. A third heart sound, or gallop rhythm, is common in infants and children with heart failure. It results from rapid filling of a noncompliant ventricle. However, it is difficult to distinguish at high HRs.

Most commonly, children develop interstitial pulmonary edema rather than alveolar pulmonary edema. This reduces lung compliance and increases the work of breathing, causing tachypnea and increased respiratory effort. Older children display use of accessory muscles. Head bobbing and nasal flaring may be observed in infants. Signs of respiratory distress are often the first indication of heart failure in infants and young children. Pulmonary congestion may be mistaken for bronchiolitis or lower respiratory tract infection. An infant or young child with respiratory distress may grunt with expiration (exhaling against a closed glottis), which is an instinctive effort to increase end-expiratory pressures and prevent collapse of small airways and the development of atelectasis. Respiratory crackles are uncommon in infants and suggest a respiratory tract infection. Wheezes may be heard if there is a large left-to-right shunt.

Infants with heart failure often show increased tachypnea, fatigue, and diaphoresis during feeding.[68] Weight gain is slow owing to high energy requirements and low calorie intake. Diaphoresis occurs particularly over the head and neck. They may have repeated lower respiratory tract infections. Peripheral perfusion is usually poor, with cool extremities; tachycardia is common; and the respiratory rate is increased.[68]

Diagnosis and Treatment

Diagnosis of heart failure in infants and children is based on symptomatology, chest radiographic films, ECG findings, and echocardiographic techniques to assess cardiac structures and ventricular function, arterial blood gases to determine intracardiac shunting and ventilation–perfusion inequalities, and other studies to determine anemia and electrolyte imbalances.

Treatment of heart failure in infants and children includes measures aimed at improving cardiac function and eliminating excess intravascular fluid. Oxygen delivery must be supported and oxygen demands controlled or minimized. Whenever possible, the cause of the disorder is corrected. With congenital anomalies that are amenable to surgery, medical treatment is often needed for a time before surgery and is usually continued in the immediate postoperative period. For some children, only medical management can be provided.

Medical management of heart failure in infants and children is similar to that in the adult, although it is

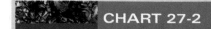

CHART 27-2

CAUSES OF HEART FAILURE IN CHILDREN

Newborn Period
Congenital heart defects
Severe left ventricular outflow disorders
Hypoplastic left heart
Critical aortic stenosis or coarctation of the aorta
Large arteriovenous shunts
Ventricular septal defects
Patent ductus arteriosus
Transposition of the great vessels
Heart muscle dysfunction (secondary)
Asphyxia
Sepsis
Hypoglycemia
Hematologic disorders (*e.g.,* anemia)

Infants 1 to 6 Months
Congenital heart disease
Large arteriovenous shunts (ventricular septal defect)
Heart muscle dysfunction
Myocarditis
Cardiomyopathy
Pulmonary abnormalities
Bronchopulmonary dysplasia
Persistent pulmonary hypertension

Toddlers, Children, and Adolescents
Acquired heart disease
Cardiomyopathy
Viral myocarditis
Rheumatic fever
Endocarditis
Systemic disease
Sepsis
Kawasaki disease
Renal disease
Sickle cell disease
Congenital heart defects
Nonsurgically treated disorders
Surgically treated disorders

tailored to the special developmental needs of the child. Inotropic agents such as digitalis are often used to increase cardiac contractility. Diuretics may be given to reduce preload, and vasodilating medications used to manipulate the afterload. Medication doses must be controlled for weight and conditions such as reduced renal function. Daily weighing and accurate measurement of intake and output are imperative during acute episodes of failure. Most children feel better in the semi-upright position. An infant seat is useful for infants with chronic heart failure. Activity restrictions are usually designed to allow children to be as active as possible within the limitations of their heart disease. Small, frequent feedings are usually more successful than larger, less frequent feedings. Severely ill infants may need to be tube-fed.

The treatment of heart failure in children should be designed to allow optimal physical and psychosocial development. It requires the full involvement of the parents, who are often the primary care providers. Therefore, parent education and support are essential.

Heart Failure in Older Adults

Heart failure is largely a disease of aging. It is one of the most common causes of disability in older adults and is the most frequent hospital admission and discharge diagnosis for older adults (those older than 65 years) in the United States and Canada.[69] Among the factors contributing to the increased numbers of older adults with heart failure are improved therapies for ischemic and hypertensive heart disease.[70] Advances in treatment of other diseases have also contributed indirectly to the rising prevalence of heart failure in the older population.

Coronary heart disease, hypertension, arrhythmias, and valvular heart disease (particularly aortic stenosis and mitral regurgitation) are common causes of heart failure in older adults.[71] In contrast to the etiology in middle-aged people with heart failure, factors other than systolic failure contribute to heart failure in older adults. Preserved LV function may be seen in 40% to 80% of older adults with heart failure. Aging is associated with impaired LV filling caused by changes in myocardial relaxation and compliance. These alterations lead to a shift in the LV pressure–volume relationship, such that small increases in LV volume lead to greater increases in LV diastolic pressure. This increase in diastolic pressure further compromises LV filling and leads to increases in left atrial, pulmonary venous, and pulmonary capillary pressures and thus predisposes to pulmonary congestion and heart failure.[70,71] Although diastolic heart failure accounts for less than 10% of heart failure cases in people younger than 60 years, it accounts for greater than 50% of cases after age 75 years.[70,71]

There are a number of changes associated with aging that contribute to the development of heart failure in older adults.[70,71] First, reduced responsiveness to β-adrenergic stimulation limits the heart's capacity to maximally increase HR and contractility. A second major effect of aging is increased vascular stiffness, which leads to a progressive increase in systolic blood pressure with advancing age, contributing to LV hypertrophy and altered diastolic filling. Third, in addition to increased vascular stiffness, the heart itself becomes stiffer and less compliant with age. The changes in diastolic stiffness

result in important alterations in diastolic filling and atrial function. A reduction in ventricular filling not only affects CO, but produces an elevation in diastolic pressure that is transmitted back to the left atrium, where it stretches the muscle wall and predisposes to atrial ectopic beats and atrial fibrillation. The fourth major effect is altered myocardial metabolism in mitochondria. Although older mitochondria may be able to generate sufficient ATP to meet the normal energy needs, they may not be able to respond under stress.

Clinical Manifestations

The manifestations of heart failure in older adults are often masked by other disease conditions.[52] Nocturia and nocturnal incontinence are early symptoms but may be caused by other conditions such as prostatic hypertrophy. Lower extremity edema may reflect venous insufficiency. Impaired perfusion of the GI tract is a common cause of anorexia and profound loss of lean body mass. Loss of lean body mass may be masked by edema. Exertional dyspnea, orthopnea, and impaired exercise tolerance are cardinal symptoms of heart failure in both younger and older adults with heart failure. However, with increasing age, which is often accompanied by a more sedentary lifestyle, exertional dyspnea becomes less prominent. Instead of dyspnea, the prominent sign may be restlessness (Chart 27-3).

Physical signs of heart failure, such as elevated jugular venous pressure, hepatic congestion, S_3 gallop, and pulmonary crackles, occur less commonly in older adults, in part because of the increased incidence of diastolic failure, in which signs of right-sided heart failure are late manifestations and a third heart sound is typically absent.[70]

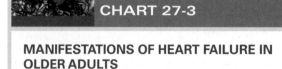

CHART 27-3

MANIFESTATIONS OF HEART FAILURE IN OLDER ADULTS

Symptoms

Nocturia or nocturnal incontinence

Fatigue

Cognitive impairment (*e.g.*, problem-solving, decision-making)

Depression

Restlessness/acute delirium

Sleep disturbance

History of falls

Loss of appetite

Signs

Dependent edema (ankle edema when sitting up and sacral edema when supine)

Pulmonary crackles (usually late sign)

Instead, behavioral changes and altered cognition such as short-term memory loss and impaired problem-solving are more common. Depression is common in older adults with heart failure and shares the symptoms of sleep disturbances, cognitive changes, and fatigue.[52]

During the managed symptom state, they are relatively symptom free while adhering to their treatment regimen. Acute symptom exacerbation, often requiring emergency medical treatment, can be precipitated by minor conditions such as poor adherence to sodium restriction, infection, or stress. Failure to promptly seek medical care is a common cause of progressive acceleration of symptoms.

Diagnosis and Treatment

The diagnosis of heart failure in older adults is based on the history, physical examination, chest radiograph, and ECG findings.[17,70,71] The presenting symptoms are often difficult to evaluate. Symptoms of dyspnea on exertion are often interpreted as a sign of "getting older" or attributed to deconditioning from other diseases. Ankle edema is not unusual because of decreased skin turgor and the tendency of older adults to be more sedentary.

Treatment of heart failure in older adults involves medication dose adaptations to reduce age-related adverse and toxic events.[52] ACE inhibitors may preserve cognitive and functional capacities.[52] Activities may be restricted to a level that is commensurate with the cardiac reserve. Bed rest causes rapid deconditioning of skeletal muscles and increases the risk of complications such as orthostatic hypotension and thromboemboli. Instead, carefully prescribed exercise programs can help maintain activity tolerance. Sodium restriction is usually indicated. Because older adults have the highest hospital readmission rates, education is important, and it is imperative to involve the family members and caregivers in management and treatment. It is also important to have a multidisciplinary approach with frequent contact because they will have other comorbid conditions and can deteriorate rapidly.

SUMMARY CONCEPTS

The mechanisms of heart failure in children and older adults are similar to those in adults. However, the causes and manifestations may differ because of age. In children, heart failure is seen most commonly during infancy and immediately after heart surgery. It can be caused by congenital and acquired heart defects and is characterized by fatigue, effort intolerance, cough, anorexia, abdominal pain, and impaired growth. Treatment of heart failure in children includes correction of the underlying cause whenever possible. For congenital anomalies that are amenable to surgery, medical treatment often is needed for a time before surgery and usually is continued in the immediate postoperative period. For many children, only medical management can be provided.

In older adults, age-related changes in cardiovascular function contribute to heart failure but are not in themselves sufficient to cause heart failure.[70] The clinical manifestations of heart failure often are different and superimposed on other disease conditions. Therefore, heart failure often is more difficult to diagnose in older adults than in younger people. Because older adults are more susceptible to adverse and toxic medication reactions, medication doses need to be adapted and more closely monitored.

Circulatory Failure (Shock)

Circulatory shock is an acute failure of the circulatory system to supply the peripheral tissues and organs of the body with an adequate blood supply, resulting in cellular hypoxia.[72] Most often, hypotension and hypoperfusion are present, but shock may occur in the presence of normal vital signs. Shock is a syndrome that can occur in the course of many life-threatening traumatic conditions or disease states. It can be caused by an alteration in cardiac function (cardiogenic shock), a decrease in blood volume (hypovolemic shock), excessive vasodilation with maldistribution of blood flow (distributive shock), or obstruction of blood flow through the circulatory system (obstructive shock) (Chart 27-4; Fig. 27-35).

Pathophysiology of Circulatory Shock

Circulatory failure results in hypoperfusion of organs and tissues, resulting in insufficient supply of oxygen and nutrients for cellular function. There are compensatory physiologic responses that eventually decompensate into various shock states if the condition is not properly treated in a timely manner. The most immediate of the compensatory mechanisms are the sympathetic and renin systems, which are designed to maintain CO and blood pressure.

The two types of adrenergic receptors for the sympathetic nervous system are α and β. The β-receptors are further subdivided into β_1 and β_2 receptors. Stimulation of the α-receptors causes vasoconstriction, stimulation of β_1-receptors causes an increase in HR and force of myocardial contraction, and of β_2-receptors vasodilation of the skeletal muscle beds and relaxation of the bronchioles. In shock, there is an increase in sympathetic outflow that results in increased epinephrine and norepinephrine release and activation of both α- and β-receptors. Thus, increases in HR and vasoconstriction

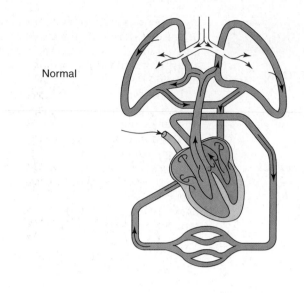

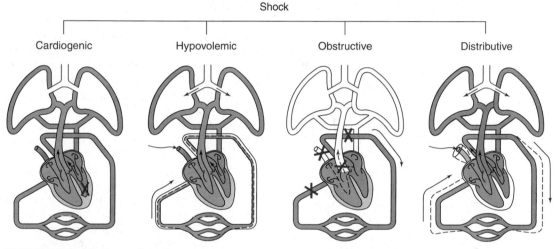

FIGURE 27-35. Types of shock.

occur in most types of shock. There is also an increase in renin release, leading to an increase in angiotensin II, which augments vasoconstriction and leads to an aldosterone-mediated increase in sodium and water retention by the kidneys. There is also local release of vasoconstrictors, which contribute to arterial and venous vasoconstriction.

The compensatory mechanisms that the body recruits are not effective over the long term and become detrimental when the shock state is prolonged. The intense vasoconstriction causes a decrease in tissue perfusion and insufficient supply of oxygen. Cellular metabolism is impaired, vasoactive inflammatory mediators such as histamine are released, production of oxygen free radicals is increased, and excessive lactic acid and hydrogen ions result in intracellular acidity.[73] Each of these factors promotes cellular dysfunction or death. Whether the shock is irreversible or the person will survive is determined largely at the cellular level.

Shock ultimately exerts its effect at the cellular level, with failure of the circulation to supply the cell with the oxygen and nutrients needed for production of ATP. The cell uses anaerobic and aerobic pathways to convert

nutrients to energy. The anaerobic glycolytic pathway converts glucose to ATP and pyruvate. The aerobic pathway moves converts pyruvate from the glycolytic pathway into ATP, carbon dioxide, and water. When oxygen is lacking, pyruvate does not enter the citric acid cycle; instead, it is converted to lactic acid. The anaerobic pathway is relatively inefficient and produces significantly less ATP than the aerobic pathway.

In severe shock, cellular metabolic processes are essentially anaerobic because of the decreased availability of oxygen. Excess lactic acid accumulates in both the cellular and the extracellular compartments, and limited amounts of ATP are produced. Without sufficient energy production, normal cell function cannot be maintained. The sodium–potassium membrane pump is impaired, resulting in excess sodium inside the cells and potassium loss from cells. The increase in intracellular sodium results in cellular edema and increased cell membrane permeability. Mitochondrial activity becomes severely depressed and lysosomal membranes may rupture, resulting in the release of enzymes that cause further intracellular destruction. This is followed by cell death and the release of intracellular contents into the extracellular

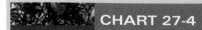

CHART 27-4

CLASSIFICATION OF CIRCULATORY SHOCK

Cardiogenic

Myocardial damage (myocardial infarction, contusion)

Sustained arrhythmias

Acute valve damage, ventricular septal defect

Cardiac surgery

Hypovolemic

Loss of whole blood

Loss of plasma

Loss of extracellular fluid

Obstructive

Inability of the heart to fill properly (cardiac tamponade)

Obstruction to outflow from the heart (pulmonary embolus, cardiac myxoma, pneumothorax, or dissecting aneurysm)

Distributive

Loss of sympathetic vasomotor tone (neurogenic shock)

Presence of vasodilating substances in the blood (anaphylactic shock)

Presence of inflammatory mediators (septic shock)

space. The destruction of the cell membrane activates the arachidonic acid cascade, release of inflammatory mediators, and production of oxygen free radicals that extend cellular damage.

The extent of the microvascular injury and organ dysfunction is primarily determined by the extent of the shock state and whether it is prolonged. Interventions are targeted at both prevention and early intervention, when possible.

Cardiogenic Shock

Cardiogenic shock occurs when the heart fails to pump blood sufficiently to meet the body's demands (Fig. 27-35). It is defined as decreased CO, hypotension, hypoperfusion, and indications of tissue hypoxia, despite adequate intravascular volume.[74,75] Cardiogenic shock may occur suddenly from a number of causes, including MI, myocardial contusion, sustained arrhythmias, and cardiac surgery. Cardiogenic shock may also ensue as an end-stage condition of CAD or cardiomyopathy.

Pathophysiology

The most common cause of cardiogenic shock is MI. Most people who die of cardiogenic shock have had extensive damage to the contracting muscle of the LV because of a recent infarct or a combination of recent and old infarctions.[76] Cardiogenic shock can occur with other types of shock because of inadequate coronary blood flow.

People with cardiogenic shock have a decrease in SV and CO, which results in insufficient perfusion to meet cellular demands. The poor CO is a result of decreased myocardial contractility, increased afterload, and excessive preload.[74,75] Mediators and neurotransmitters, including norepinephrine, produce an increase in systemic vascular resistance, which increases afterload and contributes to the deterioration of cardiac function. Preload, or the filling pressure of the heart, is increased as blood returning to the heart is added to blood that previously was not pumped forward, resulting in an increase in LV end-systolic volume. Activation of the renin–angiotensin–aldosterone mechanism worsens both preload and afterload by producing an aldosterone-mediated increase in fluid retention and an angiotensin II–mediated increase in vasoconstriction. The increased resistance (*i.e.*, afterload) to ejection of blood from the LV, in combination with a decrease in myocardial contractility, results in an increase in end-systolic ventricular volume and preload, which further impairs the heart's ability to pump effectively.

Eventually, coronary artery perfusion is impaired because of increased preload and afterload, and cardiac function decreases because of poor myocardial oxygen supply. There is an increase in intracardiac pressures because of volume overload and ventricular wall tension in both diastole and systole. Excessive pressures decrease coronary artery perfusion during diastole, and increased wall tension decreases coronary artery perfusion during systole. If treatment is unsuccessful, cardiogenic shock may result in a systemic inflammatory response, evidenced by increased white blood cell count and temperature, and release of inflammatory markers such as CRP.[74,75]

Clinical Manifestations

Symptoms of cardiogenic shock include hypoperfusion with hypotension, although a preshock state of hypoperfusion may occur with a normal blood pressure. The lips, nail beds, and skin may become cyanotic because of stagnation of blood flow and increased extraction of oxygen from the hemoglobin as it passes through the capillary bed. Mean arterial and systolic blood pressures decrease because of poor SV, and there is a narrow pulse pressure and near-normal diastolic blood pressure because of arterial vasoconstriction.[76] Urine output decreases because of lower renal perfusion pressures and increased release of aldosterone. Elevated preload is reflected in a rise in CVP and PCWP. Neurologic changes, such as alterations in cognition or consciousness, may occur because of low CO and poor cerebral perfusion.

Treatment

Treatment of cardiogenic shock requires striking a balance between improving CO, reducing the workload and oxygen needs of the myocardium, and increasing coronary perfusion. Fluid volume must be tightly regulated to maintain the filling pressure and optimize SV in people who are fluid overloaded. Pulmonary edema and arrhythmias should be monitored, corrected, or prevented to increase SV and decrease the oxygen demands of the heart. Coronary artery perfusion is increased by promoting coronary artery vasodilation, increasing blood pressure, decreasing ventricular wall tension, and decreasing intracardiac pressures.

Pharmacologic treatment includes the use of vasodilators such as nitroprusside and nitroglycerin.[74,75] At lower doses, the main effects of nitroglycerin are on the venous vascular beds and coronary arteries. At high doses, it also dilates the arterial beds. The systolic arterial pressure is maintained by an increase in ventricular SV, which is ejected against the lowered systemic vascular resistance. The improvement in heart function increases SV and enables blood to be redistributed from the pulmonary vascular bed to the systemic circulation.

Positive inotropic agents are used to improve cardiac contractility. Dobutamine and milrinone are effective medications and result in increased contractility and arterial vasodilation. The increase in SV results in a decrease in end-systolic volume and a reduction in preload. With a decrease in preload pressures, coronary artery perfusion is improved during diastole. Thus, SV and myocardial oxygen supply are improved with a minimal increase in myocardial oxygen demand. Catecholamines increase cardiac contractility but must be used with extreme caution because they also result in arterial constriction and increased HRs, which worsen the imbalance between myocardial oxygen supply and demand.

The intra-aortic balloon pump (*counterpulsation*) enhances coronary and systemic perfusion yet decreases afterload and myocardial oxygen demands.[73] The device, which pumps in synchrony with the heart, is a 10-inch-long balloon inserted through a catheter into the descending aorta (Fig. 27-36). The balloon inflates during ventricular diastole and deflates just before ventricular systole. Diastolic inflation creates a pressure wave in the ascending aorta that increases coronary artery blood flow and a less intense wave in the lower aorta that enhances organ perfusion. The abrupt balloon deflation at the onset of systole results in a displacement of blood volume that lowers the resistance to ejection of blood from the LV. Thus, pumping efficiency and myocardial oxygen supply are increased, and myocardial oxygen consumption is decreased.

When cardiogenic shock is caused by MI, several interventions can be used. Fibrinolytic therapy, PCI, or CABG may prevent or treat shock.[76] Reperfusion of the coronary arteries is expected to improve myocardial function.

Hypovolemic Shock

Hypovolemic shock is diminished blood volume causing inadequate filling of the vascular compartment[72,74,75] (Fig. 27-35). It occurs with an acute loss of 15% to 20% of circulating blood volume. The decrease may be caused by an external loss of whole blood (hemorrhage),

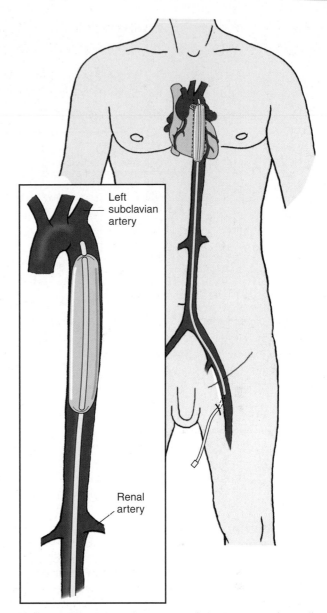

FIGURE 27-36. Proper position of the balloon catheter illustrating percutaneous insertion. (From Morton P. G., Fontaine D. K. (2018). *Critical care nursing: A holistic approach* (11th ed., Fig. 18-18, p. 293). Philadelphia, PA: JB Lippincott.)

plasma (severe burns), or extracellular fluid (severe dehydration loss of GI fluids). Hypovolemic shock can also result from internal hemorrhage or third-space losses, when extracellular fluid shifts from the vascular compartment to the interstitial compartment.

Pathophysiology

Figure 27-37 shows the effect of removing blood from the circulatory system during approximately 30 minutes.[72] Overall, 10% of total blood volume can be removed without changing CO or arterial pressure. As increasing amounts of blood (10% to 25%) are removed, SV falls, but arterial pressure is maintained because of sympathetic-mediated increases in HR and vasoconstriction. Vasoconstriction results in increased diastolic pressure and narrow pulse pressure. Blood pressure

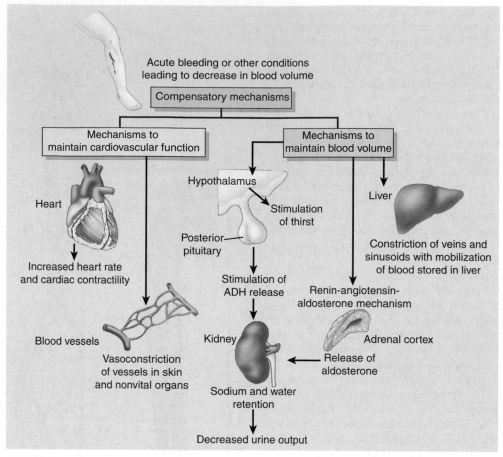

FIGURE 27-37. Compensatory mechanisms used to maintain circulatory function and blood volume in hypovolemic shock. ADH, antidiuretic hormone.

is the product of CO and systemic vascular resistance (blood pressure = cardiac output × systemic vascular resistance). An increase in systemic vascular resistance maintains mean arterial pressure for a short time despite decreased CO. CO and tissue perfusion decrease before signs of hypotension appear. CO and arterial pressure fall to zero when approximately 30% to 40% of the total blood volume has been removed.[72,74,75]

Compensatory Mechanisms

The most immediate of the compensatory mechanisms are the sympathetic-mediated responses designed to maintain CO and blood pressure (Fig. 27-37). Within seconds after the onset of hemorrhage or the loss of blood volume, tachycardia, increased cardiac contractility, vasoconstriction, and other signs of sympathetic and adrenal medullary activity appear. The sympathetic vasoconstrictor response also mobilizes blood stored in the venous side of the circulation. There is considerable capacity for blood storage in the large veins of the abdomen, and approximately 350 mL of blood that can be mobilized in shock is stored in the liver.[72] Sympathetic stimulation does not initially cause constriction of the cerebral and coronary vessels, and blood flow to the heart and brain is maintained at essentially normal levels as long as the mean arterial pressure remains above 70 mm Hg.[72]

Compensatory mechanisms designed to restore blood volume include absorption of fluid from the interstitial spaces, conservation of sodium and water by the kidneys, and thirst. Extracellular fluid is distributed between interstitial spaces and vascular compartment. When there is a loss of vascular volume, capillary pressures decrease, and water is drawn into the vascular compartment from the interstitial spaces. The maintenance of vascular volume is further enhanced by renal mechanisms that conserve fluid. A decrease in renal blood flow and glomerular filtration rate results in activation of the renin–angiotensin–aldosterone mechanism, which produces an increase in sodium reabsorption by the kidneys. The decrease in blood volume also stimulates centers in the hypothalamus that regulate ADH release and thirst. ADH (*vasopressin*) constricts peripheral arteries and veins and greatly increases water retention by the kidneys. A decrease of 10% to 15% in blood volume serves as a strong stimulus for thirst.[72,74,75]

During the early stages of hypovolemic shock, vasoconstriction decreases the size of the vascular compartment and increases systemic vascular resistance. As hypovolemic shock progresses, vasoconstriction of the blood vessels that supply the skin, skeletal muscles, kidneys, and abdominal organs becomes more severe, with a further decrease in blood flow and conversion to anaerobic metabolism resulting in cellular injury.

Clinical Manifestations

The signs and symptoms of hypovolemic shock depend on its severity and are closely related to low peripheral blood flow and excessive sympathetic stimulation. They include thirst, increased HR, cool and clammy skin, decreased arterial blood pressure, decreased urine output, and changes in mentation. Laboratory tests of hemoglobin and hematocrit provide information regarding the severity of blood loss or hemoconcentration because of dehydration. Serum lactate and arterial pH provide information about the severity of acidosis because of anaerobic metabolism. Metabolic acidosis revealed by arterial blood gas measurement is the gold-standard diagnostic test.[74,75] Acute, fatal hemorrhagic shock is characterized by metabolic acidosis, coagulopathy, and hypothermia, followed by circulatory failure.[74,75]

An increase in HR is an early sign of hypovolemic shock, as the body tries to maintain CO despite the decrease in SV. As shock progresses, the pulse becomes weak and thready, indicating vasoconstriction and reduced filling of the vascular compartment. Thirst is an early symptom in hypovolemic shock.

Arterial blood pressure is decreased in moderate-to-severe shock, but compensatory mechanisms tend to preserve blood pressure until shock is relatively far advanced. Normal arterial pressure also does not ensure adequate perfusion and oxygenation of vital organs at the cellular level.

As shock progresses, the respirations become rapid and deep, to compensate for the increased production of acid and decreased availability of oxygen. Decreased intravascular volume results in decreased venous return to the heart and a decreased CVP. When shock becomes severe, the peripheral veins may collapse. Sympathetic stimulation leads to intense vasoconstriction of the skin vessels, which results in cool and mottled skin. In hemorrhagic shock, the loss of red blood cells results in pallor of the skin and mucous membranes.

Urine output decreases very quickly in hypovolemic shock. Compensatory mechanisms decrease renal blood flow as a means of diverting blood flow to the heart and brain. Oliguria of 20 mL/hour or less indicates inadequate renal perfusion. Continuous measurement of urine output is essential for assessing the circulatory and volume status of the person in shock.

Restlessness, agitation, and apprehension are common in early shock because of increased sympathetic outflow and increased levels of epinephrine. As the shock progresses and blood flow to the brain decreases, restlessness is replaced by altered arousal and mentation. Loss of consciousness and coma may occur if the person does not receive or respond to treatment.

Treatment

The duration and amount of fluid loss are directly related to mortality. Therefore, the treatment of hypovolemic shock is directed toward correcting or controlling the underlying cause and improving tissue perfusion. Ongoing loss of blood must be corrected. Oxygen is administered to increase oxygen delivery to the tissues.

Medications are usually administered IV. Frequent measurements of HR and cardiac rhythm, blood pressure, and urine output are used to assess the severity of circulatory compromise and to monitor treatment.

The goal of treatment is to restore vascular volume.[74,75] This can be accomplished through IV administration of fluids and blood. The crystalloids (e.g., isotonic saline and Ringer lactate) are readily available and effective, at least temporarily. Plasma volume expanders (e.g., pentastarch and colloidal albumin) have high molecular weight, do not necessitate blood typing, and remain in the vascular space for longer periods than crystalloids. Blood or blood products are administered based on hematocrit and hemodynamic findings. Fluids and blood are best administered based on volume indicators, such as CVP and urine output.

Vasoactive medications constrict or dilate blood vessels. As a general rule, vasoconstrictor agents are not used as a primary form of therapy in hypovolemic shock and may be detrimental. They are given only when volume deficits have been corrected yet hypotension persists.

Distributive Shock

Distributive or vasodilatory shock is characterized by loss of blood vessel tone, enlargement of the vascular compartment, and displacement of the vascular volume away from the heart and central circulation.[74,75,77] In distributive shock, the capacity of the vascular compartment expands to the extent that a normal volume of blood does not fill the circulatory system (Fig. 27-35). Therefore, this type of shock is also referred to as *normovolemic shock*. Two main causes result in loss of vascular tone: a decrease in the sympathetic control of vasomotor tone and the release of excessive vasodilator substances. It can also occur as a complication of vessel damage resulting from prolonged and severe hypotension due to hemorrhage (*irreversible* or *late-phase hemorrhagic shock*).[77] There are three shock states that share the basic circulatory pattern of distributive shock: neurogenic shock, anaphylactic shock, and septic shock.[74,75]

Neurogenic Shock

Neurogenic shock is caused by decreased sympathetic control of blood vessel tone resulting from a defect in the vasomotor center in the brain stem or the sympathetic outflow to the blood vessels.[72] *Spinal shock* describes the neurogenic shock that occurs in people with spinal cord injury. Output from the vasomotor center can be interrupted by brain injury, the depressant action of drugs, general anesthesia, hypoxia, or lack of glucose (e.g., insulin reaction). Fainting as a result of emotional causes is a transient form of impaired sympathetic outflow. Many general anesthetic agents can cause a neurogenic shock–like reaction, especially during induction, because of interference with sympathetic nervous system function. Spinal anesthesia or spinal cord injury above the midthoracic region can interrupt the transmission of outflow from the vasomotor center. In contrast to other shock states, owing to the loss of blood volume or impaired cardiac function, the HR in neurogenic shock is often slower than normal, and the skin is dry and warm. This type of distributive shock is rare and usually transitory.

Anaphylactic Shock

Anaphylaxis is a clinical syndrome that represents the most severe systemic allergic reaction.[8] Anaphylactic shock results from an immunologically mediated reaction in which vasodilator substances such as histamine are released into the blood. These substances cause vasodilation of arterioles and venules along with a marked increase in capillary permeability. The vascular response in anaphylaxis is often accompanied by life-threatening laryngeal edema and bronchospasm, circulatory collapse, contraction of GI and uterine smooth muscle, and urticaria (hives) or angioedema.

Etiology

Among the most frequent causes of anaphylactic shock are reactions to medications, such as penicillin; foods, such as nuts and shellfish; and insect venoms. The most common cause is stings from insects of the order Hymenoptera (*i.e.*, bees, wasps, and fire ants). Latex allergy causes life-threatening anaphylaxis in a growing segment of the population. Health care workers and others who are exposed to latex are developing latex sensitivities that range from mild urticaria, contact dermatitis, and mild respiratory distress to anaphylactic shock.[74,75,78] The onset and severity of anaphylaxis depend on the sensitivity of the person and the rate and quantity of antigen exposure.

Clinical Manifestations

Signs and symptoms associated with impending anaphylactic shock include abdominal cramps, apprehension, warm or burning sensation of the skin, itching, urticaria (*i.e.*, hives), coughing, choking, wheezing, chest tightness, and difficulty in breathing.

After blood begins to pool peripherally, there is a precipitous drop in blood pressure, and the pulse becomes so weak that it is difficult to detect. Life-threatening airway obstruction may be caused by laryngeal angioedema or bronchial spasm. Anaphylactic shock may develop suddenly; death can occur within minutes unless appropriate medical intervention is promptly instituted.

Treatment

Treatment includes immediate discontinuation of the inciting agent or institution of measures to decrease its absorption (*e.g.*, application of ice to the site of an insect bite), close monitoring of cardiovascular and respiratory function, and maintenance of respiratory gas exchange, CO, and tissue perfusion. Epinephrine is given in an anaphylactic reaction because it constricts blood vessels and relaxes the smooth muscle in the bronchioles, thus restoring cardiac and respiratory function.[78,79] Other treatment measures include the administration of oxygen, antihistamine drugs, and corticosteroids. The person should be placed in a supine

position. This is important because venous return can be severely compromised in the sitting position. This, in turn, produces a pulseless mechanical contraction of the heart and predisposes to arrhythmias. In several cases, death has occurred immediately after assuming the sitting position.[78,79]

Prevention

The prevention of anaphylactic shock is preferable to treatment. Once sensitized to an antigen, the risk of repeated anaphylactic reactions with subsequent exposure is high. All health care providers should question people regarding previous drug reactions and inform people as to the name of the medication they are to receive before it is administered or prescribed. People with known hypersensitivities should wear MedicAlert jewelry and carry an identification card to alert medical personnel if they become unable to relate this information. People who are at risk for anaphylaxis should be provided with emergency medications (*e.g.*, epinephrine autoinjector) and instructed in procedures to follow in case they are inadvertently exposed.[78,79]

Sepsis and Septic Shock

Septic shock, which is the most common type of vasodilatory shock, is associated with severe infection and the systemic response to infection (Fig. 27-38).[80,81] *Sepsis* is currently defined as suspected or proven infection, plus a systemic inflammatory response syndrome (*e.g.*, fever, tachycardia, tachypnea, elevated white blood cell count, altered mental state, and hyperglycemia in the absence of diabetes).[80,81] *Septic shock* is defined as severe sepsis with hypotension, despite fluid resuscitation, with a high risk for mortality.[80]

It is estimated that sepsis occurs in 1.5 million people each year in the United States, and about 250,000 die.[82] The growing incidence has been attributed to enhanced awareness of the diagnosis, increased number of resistant organisms, growing number of immunocompromised and older adults, and greater use of invasive procedures. With early intervention and advances in treatment methods, the mortality rate has decreased.[80-82]

Pathophysiology

The pathogenesis of sepsis involves a complex process of cellular activation, resulting in the release of pro-inflammatory mediators such as cytokines, recruitment of neutrophils and monocytes, involvement of neuroendocrine reflexes, and activation of complement, coagulation, and fibrinolytic systems. Initiation of the response begins with activation of the innate immune system by pattern recognition receptors (*e.g.*, Toll-like receptors [TLRs]) that interact with specific molecules present on microorganisms. Binding of TLRs to epitopes on microorganisms stimulates transcription and release of a number of pro-inflammatory and anti-inflammatory mediators. Two of these mediators, tumor necrosis factor α (TNF-α) and interleukin-1, are involved in leukocyte adhesion, local inflammation, neutrophil activation, suppression of erythropoiesis, generation of fever, tachycardia, lactic acidosis,

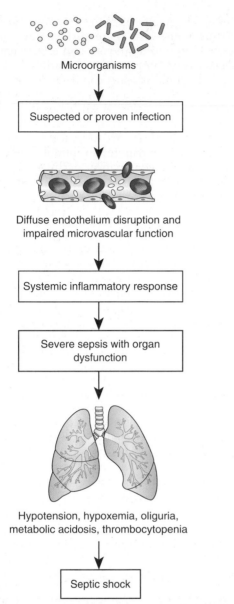

Microorganisms

↓

Suspected or proven infection

↓

Diffuse endothelium disruption and impaired microvascular function

↓

Systemic inflammatory response

↓

Severe sepsis with organ dysfunction

↓

Hypotension, hypoxemia, oliguria, metabolic acidosis, thrombocytopenia

↓

Septic shock

FIGURE 27-38. Pathogenic mechanisms leading to infection to septic shock.

ventilation–perfusion abnormalities, and other signs of sepsis as discussed earlier. Activated neutrophils also injure the endothelium by releasing mediators that increase vascular permeability. Activated endothelial cells release nitric oxide, a potent vasodilator that acts as a key mediator of septic shock.

Another important aspect of sepsis is an alteration of the procoagulation–anticoagulation balance with an increase in procoagulation factors and a decrease in anticoagulation factors. Lipopolysaccharide on the surface of microorganisms stimulates endothelial cells lining the blood vessels to increase their production of tissue factor, thus activating coagulation. Fibrinogen is then converted to fibrin, leading to the formation of microvascular thrombi that further amplify tissue injury. In addition, sepsis lowers levels of protein C, protein S, antithrombin III, and tissue factor pathway inhibitor, substances that modulate and inhibit coagulation.

Lipopolysaccharide and TNF-α also decrease the synthesis of thrombomodulin and endothelial protein C receptor, impairing activation of protein C, and they increase the synthesis of plasminogen activator inhibitor-1, impairing fibrinolysis.[80,82]

Clinical Manifestations

Sepsis and septic shock typically manifest with hypotension and warm, flushed skin. Whereas other forms of shock (*i.e.*, cardiogenic, hypovolemic, and obstructive) are characterized by a compensatory increase in systemic vascular resistance, septic shock often presents with a decrease in systemic vascular resistance. There is hypovolemia due to arterial and venous dilation, plus leakage of plasma into the interstitial spaces. Abrupt changes in cognition or behavior are caused by reduced cerebral blood flow and may be early indications of septic shock. Regardless of the underlying cause, fever and increased leukocytes are present. An elevated serum lactate or metabolic acidosis indicates anaerobic metabolism due to tissue hypoxia or cellular dysfunction and altered cellular metabolism.[80,81] Tissue hypoxia produces continued production and activation of inflammatory mediators, resulting in further increases in vascular permeability, impaired vascular regulation, and altered hemostasis.

Treatment

The treatment focuses on control of the causative agent and support of the circulation. Early use of antibiotics is essential, followed by antibiotic therapy specific to the infectious agent.[80,81] Airway management to treat hypoxemia along with early administration of fluids (aggressive administration to include crystalloids) within the first 3 hours and empiric broad-spectrum antibiotics are priority treatments for sepsis. Mechanical ventilation may be needed to reduce the workload of breathing, especially if encephalopathy is present. Central venous access is recommended because of infusion of IV fluids, medications, and frequent blood draws. Complete blood counts with differential, coagulation studies including D-dimer levels, serum lactate, and liver function tests are diagnostic and indicate the severity. Blood cultures from at least two different sites are obtained prior to antibiotic therapy.[81]

Obstructive Shock

Obstructive shock describes circulatory shock that results from mechanical obstruction of the flow of blood through the central circulation (great veins, heart, or lungs; Fig. 27-35). It may be caused by a number of conditions, including dissecting aortic aneurysm, cardiac tamponade, pneumothorax, atrial myxoma, and **evisceration** of abdominal contents into the thoracic cavity because of a ruptured hemidiaphragm. The most frequent cause of obstructive shock is PE.

The primary physiologic result of obstructive shock is elevated right heart pressure because of impaired right ventricular function. Pressures are increased despite impaired venous return to the heart. Signs of right-sided heart failure occur, including elevation of CVP and jugular venous distention. Treatment focuses on correcting the cause of the disorder, frequently with surgical interventions such as pulmonary embolectomy, pericardiocentesis (*i.e.*, removal of fluid from the pericardial sac) for cardiac tamponade, or the insertion of a chest tube for correction of a tension pneumothorax or hemothorax. In severe or massive pulmonary embolus, fibrinolytic drugs may be used to break down the clots causing the obstruction.

Complications of Shock

Many body systems are destroyed by shock. Five major complications of severe shock are pulmonary injury, acute renal failure, GI ulceration, disseminated intravascular coagulation (DIC), and multiple organ dysfunction syndrome (MODS). These complications of shock are serious and often fatal.

Acute Lung Injury/Acute Respiratory Distress Syndrome

Acute lung injury/acute respiratory distress syndrome (ALI/ARDS) is a potentially lethal form of pulmonary injury that may be either the cause or result of shock. ARDS is a more severe aspect of ALI and is differentiated primarily for early intervention, prevention, and research purposes.

ALI/ARDS is marked by the rapid onset of profound dyspnea that usually occurs 12 to 48 hours after the initiating event. The respiratory rate and effort of breathing increase. Arterial blood gas analysis establishes the presence of profound hypoxemia that is refractory to supplemental oxygen. The hypoxemia results from impaired matching of ventilation and perfusion and from the greatly reduced diffusion of blood gases across the thickened alveolar membranes.

The Berlin definition of ARDS requires that the following criteria be present:

- Respiratory symptoms are present within 1 week of known clinical insult or new/worsening symptoms during the week.
- Chest x-ray or CT shows bilateral opacities found with pulmonary edema not caused by pleural effusion, atelectasis, or pulmonary nodules.
- Cardiac failure or hypervolemia must not be the only cause for respiratory failure.
- Impairment of oxygenation must be present; severity of the hypoxemia determines the severity of the ARDS.[83]

Interventions for ALI/ARDS focus on increasing the oxygen concentration in the inspired air and supporting ventilation mechanically to optimize gas exchange while avoiding oxygen toxicity and preventing further lung injury. Although the delivery of high levels of oxygen using high-pressure mechanical ventilatory support and positive end-expiratory pressure may correct the hypoxemia, the mortality rate, which was previously greater than 50%, has declined.[84] The use of sedation and analgesic agents increases tolerance to mechanical ventilation while also decreasing energy consumption. Evidence surrounding the use and effectiveness of muscle relaxants to improve oxygenation lacks scientific proof. Nutritional support can decrease catabolic losses and improve the immune response. Nosocomial pneumonia is a complication of ARDS leading to prolonged mechanical ventilation and increased rate of mortality. Even with prophylactic treatment, the risk of DVT and PE is high and contributes to immobility, trauma, and activation of the coagulation pathway. To prevent GI complications such as risk for GI bleed, prophylaxis against stress ulcers is recommended.[84]

Acute Renal Failure

The renal tubules are particularly vulnerable to ischemia, and acute renal failure is an important factor in mortality due to severe shock. Most cases of acute renal failure are caused by impaired renal perfusion or direct injury to the kidneys. The degree of renal damage is related to the severity and duration of shock. The normal kidney is able to tolerate severe ischemia for 15 to 20 minutes. The renal dysfunction most frequently seen after severe shock is acute tubular necrosis. Acute tubular necrosis is usually reversible, although return to normal renal function may require weeks or months. Continuous monitoring of urinary output during shock provides a means for assessing renal blood flow. Frequent monitoring of serum creatinine and blood urea nitrogen levels also provides valuable information regarding renal status.

Mediators implicated in septic shock are powerful vasoconstrictors capable of activating the sympathetic nervous system and causing intravascular clotting. They trigger all the separate physiologic mechanisms that contribute to the onset of acute renal failure.

Gastrointestinal Complications

The most important risk factors for GI complications are shock and administration of drugs used to treat shock. Splanchnic perfusion and intolerance to enteral nutrition may lead to hypoperfusion of the gut. The GI tract is particularly vulnerable to ischemia because of the changes in distribution of blood flow to its mucosal surface. In shock, there is widespread constriction of blood vessels that supply the GI tract, causing a redistribution of blood flow and a severe decrease in mucosal perfusion. People may experience loss of appetite, nausea, or vomiting. Superficial mucosal lesions of the stomach and duodenum can develop within hours of severe trauma, sepsis, or burns. Bowel obstruction or bleeding may occur after the decrease in perfusion in shock. Hemorrhage usually has its onset within 2 to 10 days after the original insult and often begins without warning. Poor perfusion in the GI tract has been credited with allowing intestinal bacteria to enter the bloodstream, thereby contributing to the development of sepsis and shock.[74,75] Shock can result in intestinal and gastric mucosa tissue damage because of decreased supply of ATP during shock states. When ischemia is present, the GI tract is at risk for reperfusion injury, where oxygen supply that is restored produces free radicals, leading to tissue damage. The glycoprotein mucous layer that forms a protective physical barrier in the gut is decreased during shock states.

Histamine type 2 receptor antagonists, proton pump inhibitors, or sucralfate may be given prophylactically to prevent GI ulcerations caused by shock. Nasogastric tubes, when attached to intermittent suction, also help diminish the accumulation of hydrogen ions in the stomach. Enteral nutrition may also reduce the risk of GI bleed. IV proton pump inhibitors are used to treat severe upper GI bleeding.[74,85]

Disseminated Intravascular Coagulation

DIC is characterized by widespread activation of the coagulation system with resultant formation of fibrin clots and thrombotic occlusion of small- and medium-sized vessels. The systemic formation of fibrin results from increased generation of thrombin, the simultaneous suppression of physiologic anticoagulation mechanisms, and the delayed removal of fibrin as a consequence of impaired fibrinolysis. Clinically overt DIC is reported to occur in as much as 1% of hospitalized people and in 30% to 50% of people with sepsis.[85] As with other systemic inflammatory responses, the derangement of coagulation and fibrinolysis is thought to be mediated by inflammatory mediators and cytokines.

The contribution of DIC to morbidity and mortality in sepsis depends on the underlying clinical condition and the intensity of the coagulation disorder. Depletion of the platelets and coagulation factors increases the risk of bleeding. Deposition of fibrin in the vasculature of organs contributes to ischemic damage and organ failure. It remains uncertain whether DIC was a predictor of unfavorable outcome or merely a marker of the condition causing the DIC.

The management of sepsis-induced DIC focuses on treatment of the underlying disorder and measures to interrupt the coagulation process. Platelet and factor replacement to correct bleeding and heparin for people with excessive fibrin deposits is recommended.[86,87]

Multiple Organ Dysfunction Syndrome

MODS reflects the presence of altered organ function in a person who is acutely ill, such that homeostasis cannot be maintained without intervention. As the name implies, MODS commonly affects multiple organ systems, including the kidneys, lungs, liver, brain, and heart. MODS is a particularly life-threatening complication of shock, especially septic shock. It is the most frequent cause of death in the noncoronary intensive care unit. Mortality rates vary but range from 40% to 75% in people with MODS due to sepsis.[88] Mortality rates increase with an increased number of organs failing. A high mortality rate is associated with failure of the brain, liver, kidneys, and lungs. The pathogenesis of MODS is not clearly understood, and current management is, therefore, primarily supportive. Elevated levels of endotoxins consistent with septic shock are also found

in multiple organ dysfunction. Apoptosis is also delayed during sepsis, contributing to multiple organ failure. Major risk factors for the development of MODS are severe trauma, sepsis, prolonged periods of hypotension, hepatic dysfunction, infarcted bowel, advanced age, and alcohol abuse. Interventions for multiple organ failure are focused on support of the affected organs.[88,89]

SUMMARY CONCEPTS

Circulatory shock is an acute emergency in which body tissues are deprived of oxygen and cellular nutrients or are unable to use these materials in their metabolic processes. Circulatory shock may develop because the heart is unable to adequately pump blood through the circulatory system (cardiogenic shock), there is insufficient blood in the circulatory system (*i.e.*, hypovolemic shock), there is a maldistribution of blood due to abnormalities in the vascular resistance (*i.e.*, distributive shock), or blood flow or venous return is obstructed (*i.e.*, obstructive shock). Three types of shock share the basic circulatory pattern of distributive shock: neurogenic shock, anaphylactic shock, and septic shock. Septic shock, which is the most common of the three types, is associated with a severe, overwhelming inflammatory response and has a high mortality rate.

The manifestations of hypovolemic shock, which serves as a prototype for circulatory shock, are related to low peripheral blood flow and excessive sympathetic stimulation. The low peripheral blood flow produces thirst, changes in skin temperature, decreased blood pressure, increased heart rate, decreased venous pressure, decreased urine output, and changes in the sensorium. The intense vasoconstriction that serves to maintain blood flow to the heart and brain causes a decrease in tissue perfusion, impaired cellular metabolism, liberation of lactic acid, and, eventually, cell death. Whether the shock is irreversible or the person will survive is determined largely by changes that occur at the cellular level.

The complications of shock result from the deprivation of blood flow to vital organs or systems, such as the lungs, kidneys, gastrointestinal tract, and blood coagulation system. Shock can cause or be accompanied by ALI/ARDS, which is characterized by changes in the permeability of the alveolar–capillary membrane with development of interstitial edema and severe hypoxemia that does not respond to oxygen therapy. The renal tubules are particularly vulnerable to ischemia, and acute renal failure is an important complication of shock. Gastrointestinal ischemia may lead to gastrointestinal bleeding and increased vascular permeability to intestinal bacteria, which can cause further sepsis and shock. DIC is characterized by formation of small clots in the circulation. It is thought to be caused by inappropriate activation of the coagulation cascade because of toxins or other products released as a result of the shock state. Multiple organ failure, perhaps the most ominous complication of shock, rapidly depletes the body's ability to compensate and recover from a shock state.

Review Exercises

1. A 45-year-old man presents in the emergency department complaining of substernal chest pain that is also felt in his left shoulder. He is short of breath and nauseated. His blood pressure is 160/90 mm Hg, and his HR is 100 beats/minute. His ECG shows an ST-segment elevation in leads II, III, and aVF. He is given oxygen, aspirin, and nitroglycerin. Blood tests reveal elevated CK-MB and TnI.

   A. What is the probable cause of the man's symptoms?
   B. What is the significance of the ST-segment changes?
   C. What is the significance of elevated CK-MB and TnI?
   D. Relate the actions of aspirin, nitroglycerin, and oxygen to the treatment of this man's condition.

2. A 50-year-old woman presents with complaints of paroxysmal nocturnal dyspnea and orthopnea, palpitations, and fatigue. An echocardiogram demonstrates a thickened, immobile mitral valve with anterior and posterior leaflets moving together, slow early diastolic filling of the ventricle, and left atrial enlargement.

   A. What is the probable cause of this woman's symptoms?
   B. Explain the pathologic significance of the slow early diastolic filling, distended left atrium, and palpitations.
   C. Given the echocardiographic data, what type of cardiac murmur would you expect to find in this woman?
   D. Which circulation (systemic or pulmonary) would you expect to be affected as this woman's mitral valve disorder progresses?

3. A 75-year-old male with long-standing hypertension and angina due to coronary heart disease presents with ankle edema, nocturia, increased shortness of breath with activity, and

a chronic nonproductive cough. He has a past history of smoking two packs/day and drinking, but he says he now does not smoke and is now sober. His blood pressure is 170/80 and his HR is 100. ECG and chest radiography indicate the presence of LV hypertrophy.

   A. Relate the presence of uncontrolled hypertension and CAD to the development of heart failure in this man.
   B. Explain the significance of LV hypertrophy in terms of both a compensatory mechanism and a pathologic mechanism in the progression of heart failure.
   C. Explain the management and treatment for this diagnosis.

4. A 4-month-old male infant is brought into the pediatric clinic by his mother. She reports that she noted over the past several weeks that her baby's lips and mouth and his fingernails and toenails have become a bluish gray color. She also states that he seems to tire easily and that even nursing seems to wear him out. Lately, he has had several spells where he has suddenly turned blue, has had difficulty breathing, and has been very irritable. During one of these spells, he turned limp and seemed to have passed out for a short time. An echocardiogram reveals a thickening of the right ventricular wall with overriding of the aorta, a large subaortic VSD, and narrowing of the pulmonary outflow with stenosis of the pulmonary valve.

   A. What is this infant's probable diagnosis?
   B. Describe the shunting of blood that occurs with this disorder and its relationship to the development of cyanosis.
   C. The surgical creation of a shunt between the aorta and pulmonary artery may be performed as a palliative procedure for infants with marked hypoplasia of the pulmonary artery, with corrective surgery performed later in childhood. Explain how this procedure increases blood flow to the lungs.

5. A 21-year-old man is admitted to the emergency department with excessive blood loss after an automobile injury. He is alert and anxious, his skin is cool and moist, his HR is 135, and his blood pressure is 100/85. He is receiving IV fluids, which were started at the scene of the accident by an emergency medical technician. He has been typed and cross-matched for blood transfusions, and a urinary catheter has been inserted to monitor his urinary output. His urinary output has been less than 10 mL since admission, and his blood pressure has dropped to 85/70. Efforts to control his bleeding have been unsuccessful, and he is being prepared for emergency surgery.

A. Use information regarding the compensatory mechanisms in circulatory shock to explain this man's presenting symptoms, including urinary output.

B. The treatment of hypovolemic shock is usually directed at maintaining the circulatory volume through fluid resuscitation rather than maintaining the blood pressure through the use of vasoactive medications. Explain.

REFERENCES

1. Gaziano T. A., Prabhakaran D., Gaziano J. M. (2015). Global burden of cardiovascular disease. In Mann D. L., Zipes D. P., Libby P., et al. (Eds.), *Braunwald's heart disease: A textbook of cardiovascular medicine* (10th ed., pp. 1–20). Philadelphia, PA: Elsevier Saunders.

2. Roger V. L., Go A. S., Lloyd-Jones D., et al. (2012). Heart disease and stroke statistics—2012 update. A report from the American Heart Association Statistics Committee and Stroke Statistics Subcommittee. *Circulation* 125, e2–e220.

3. LeWinter M. M., Tischler M. D. (2015). Pericardial diseases. In Mann D. L., Zipes D. P., Libby P. (Eds.), *Braunwald's heart disease: A textbook of cardiovascular medicine* (10th ed., pp. 1636–1657). Philadelphia, PA: Elsevier Saunders.

4. O'Gara P. T., Kushner F. G., Ascheim D. D., et al. (2013). ACC/AHA guidelines for the management of patients with ST-elevation myocardial infarction. *Circulation* 110, e362–e425.

5. Guyton A. C., Hall J. E. (2016). *Textbook of medical physiology* (13th ed., pp. 259–270). Philadelphia, PA: Elsevier Saunders.

6. Center for Disease Control. (2017). Heart attack. Available: https://www.cdc.gov/heartdisease/heart_attack.htm. Accessed February 28, 2018.

7. Opie L. H., Bers D. M. (2015). Mechanisms of cardiac contraction and relaxation. In Mann D. L., Zipes D. P., Libby P., et al. (Eds.), *Braunwald's heart disease: A textbook of cardiovascular medicine* (10th ed., pp. 429–453). Philadelphia, PA: Elsevier Saunders.

8. Myers J. (2011). Exercise testing. In Woods S. L., Froelicher E. S., Motzer S. U., et al. (Eds.), *Cardiac nursing* (6th ed., pp. 420–435). Philadelphia, PA: Lippincott Williams & Wilkins.

9. Solomon S. D., Wu J., Gillam L. D. (2015). Echocardiography. In Mann D. L., Zipes D. P., Libby P., et al. (Eds.), *Braunwald's heart disease: A textbook of cardiovascular medicine* (10th ed., pp. 179–260). Philadelphia, PA: Elsevier Saunders.

10. Udelson J. E., Dilsizian V., Bonow R. O. (2015). Nuclear cardiology. In Mann D. L., Zipes D. P., Libby P., et al. (Eds.), *Braunwald's heart disease: A textbook of cardiovascular medicine* (10th ed., pp. 271–319). Philadelphia, PA: Elsevier Saunders.

11. Kwong R. Y. (2015). Cardiovascular magnetic resonance. In Mann D. L., Zipes D. P., Libby P., et al. (Eds.), *Braunwald's heart disease: A textbook of cardiovascular medicine* (10th ed., pp. 320–340). Philadelphia, PA: Elsevier Saunders.

12. Taylor A. J. (2015). Cardiac computed tomography. In Mann D. L., Zipes D. P., Libby P., et al. (Eds.), *Braunwald's heart disease: A textbook of cardiovascular medicine* (10th ed., pp. 341–363). Philadelphia, PA: Elsevier Saunders.

13. Davidson C. J., Bonow R. O. (2015). Cardiac catheterization. In Mann D. L., Zipes D. P., Libby P., et al. (Eds.), *Braunwald's heart disease: A textbook of cardiovascular medicine* (10th ed., pp. 364–391). Philadelphia, PA: Elsevier Saunders.

14. Falk E., Fuster V. (2017). Atherothrombosis: Disease burden, activity, and vulnerability. In Fuster V., Walsh R. A., Harrington R. A., et al. (Eds.), *Hurst's the heart* (14th ed., Chapter 32). New York, NY: McGraw-Hill.

15. Badimon J. J., Ibanez B., Fuster V., et al. (2017). Coronary thrombosis: Local and systemic factors. In Fuster V., Walsh R. A., Harrington R. A., et al. (Eds.), *Hurst's the heart* (14th ed., Chapter 33). New York, NY: McGraw-Hill.

16. Mirvis D. M., Goldberger A. L. (2015). Electrocardiography. In Mann D. L., Zipes D. P., Libby P., et al. (Eds.), *Braunwald's heart disease: A textbook of cardiovascular medicine* (10th ed., pp. 114–154). Philadelphia, PA: Elsevier Saunders.

17. Scirica B. M., Morrow D. A. (2015). ST-elevation myocardial infarction: Pathology, pathophysiology, and clinical features; and ST-elevation myocardial infarction: Management. In Bonow R. O., Mann D. L., Zipes D., et al. (Eds.), *Braunwald's heart disease: A textbook of cardiovascular medicine* (10th ed., pp. 1068–1094). Philadelphia, PA: Elsevier Saunders.

18. Giugliano R. P., Cannon C. P., Braunwald E. (2015). Non-ST elevation acute coronary syndromes. In Bonow R. O., Mann D. L., Zipes D. P., et al. (Eds.), *Braunwald's heart disease: A textbook of cardiovascular medicine* (10th ed., pp. 1155–1181). Philadelphia, PA: Elsevier Saunders.

19. Canty J. M., Duncker D. J. (2015). Coronary blood flow and myocardial ischemia. In Bonow R. O., Mann D. L., Zipes D. P., et al. (Eds.), *Braunwald's heart disease: A textbook of cardiovascular medicine* (10th ed., pp. 1029–1056). Philadelphia, PA: Elsevier Saunders.

20. Mauri L., Bhatt D. (2015). Percutaneous coronary interventions. In Mann D. L., Zipes D. P., Libby P., et al. (Eds.), *Braunwald's heart disease: A textbook of cardiovascular medicine* (10th ed., pp. 1245–1268). Philadelphia, PA: Elsevier Saunders.

21. Hills L. D., Smith P. K., Anderson J. L., et al. (2011). 2011 ACC/AHA Guideline for coronary artery bypass graft surgery. *Circulation* 124, e652–e735.

22. Thompson P. D. (2015). Exercise-based, comprehensive rehabilitation. In Mann D. L., Zipes D. P., Libby P., et al. (Eds.), *Braunwald's heart disease: A textbook of cardiovascular medicine* (10th ed., pp. 1015–1020). Philadelphia, PA: Elsevier Saunders.

23. Morrow D. A., Boden W. B. (2015). Stable ischemic heart disease. In Mann D. L., Zipes D. P., Libby P., et al. (Eds.), *Braunwald's heart disease: A textbook of cardiovascular medicine* (10th ed., pp. 1182–1244). Philadelphia, PA: Elsevier Saunders.

24. Maron B. J., Towbin J. A., Thiene G., et al. (2006). Contemporary definitions and classification of the cardiomyopathies. *Circulation* 113, 1807–1816.

25. Chowdhry S., Jacoby D., Moon J. C., et al. (2016). Update on hypertrophic cardiomyopathy and a guide to the guidelines. *Nature Reviews Cardiology* 13, 651–675.

26. Otto C. M., Bonow R. O. (2015). Valvular heart disease. In Mann D. L., Zipes D. P., Libby P., et al. (Eds.), *Braunwald's heart disease: A textbook of cardiovascular medicine* (10th ed., pp. 1446–1523). Philadelphia, PA: Elsevier Saunders.

27. Arbustini E., Favalli B., Narula N., et al. (2017). Genetic basis of cardiovascular disease. In Fuster V., Walsh R. A., Harrington R. A., et al. (Eds.) *Hurst's the heart* (14th ed., Chapter 9). New York, NY: McGraw-Hill.

28. Priori S., Napolitano C. (2017). Genetics of channelopathies and clinical implications. In Fuster V., Walsh R. A., Harrington R. A., et al. (Eds.), *Hurst's the heart* (14th ed., Chapter 80). New York, NY: McGraw-Hill.

29. Arbustini E., Serrio A., Favalli V., et al. (2017). Dilated cardiomyopathies. In Fuster V., Walsh R. A., Harrington R. A., et al. (Eds.), *Hurst's the heart* (14th ed., Chapter 58). New York, NY: McGraw-Hill.

30. Arbustini E., Agozzino M., Favalli V., et al. (2017). Myocarditis. In Fuster V., Walsh R. A., Harrington R. A., et al. (Eds.), *Hurst's the heart* (14th ed., Chapter 63). New York, NY: McGraw-Hill.

31. Maisch B., Pankuweit S. (2013). Standard and etiology-directed evidence-based therapies in myocarditis: State of the art and future perspectives. *Heart Failure Reviews* 18, 761–795.

32. Johnson-Coyle L., Jensen L., Sobey A. (2012). Peripartum cardiomyopathy: Review and practice guidelines. *American Journal of Critical Care* 21, 89–98.

33. Tarkin J. M., Khetyar M., Kaski J. C. (2008). Management of Takotsubo syndrome. *Cardiovascular Drugs and Therapy* 22, 71–77.

34. Baddour L. M., Freeman W. K., Suri R. M., et al. (2015). Cardiovascular infections. In Mann D. L., Zipes D. P., Libby P., et al. (Eds.), *Braunwald's heart disease: A textbook of cardiovascular medicine* (10th ed., pp. 1524–1550). Philadelphia, PA: Elsevier Saunders.

35. Badour L., Wilson W., Bayer A. (2015). Infective endocarditis: Diagnosis, antimicrobial therapy, and management of complications. *Circulation* 132, 1435–1486.

36. Mayosi B. M. (2015). Rheumatic fever. In Bonow R. O., Mann D. L., Zipes D. P., et al. (Eds.), *Braunwald's heart disease: A textbook of cardiovascular medicine* (10th ed., pp. 1834–1842). Philadelphia, PA: Elsevier Saunders.

37. Mason J. C. (2015). Rheumatic diseases and the cardiovascular system. In Bonow R. O., Mann D. L., Zipes D. P., et al. (Eds.), *Braunwald's heart disease: A textbook of cardiovascular medicine* (10th ed., pp. 1876–1892). Philadelphia, PA: Elsevier Saunders.

38. Bahl V. K., Math R. S., Carabello B. A. (2017). Mitral stenosis. In Fuster V., Walsh R. A., Harrington R. A., et al. (Eds.), *Hurst's the heart* (14th ed., Chapter 50). New York, NY: McGraw-Hill.

39. Nishimura R. A., Otto C. M., Bonow R. O., et al. (2014). ACC/AHA 2014 Guideline for the management of patients with valvular heart disease. *Circulation* 129, e521–e643.

40. Groarke J. D., Carabello B. A., O'Gara P. T. (2017). Ischemic mitral regurgitation. In Fuster V., Walsh R. A., Harrington R. A., et al. (Eds.), *Hurst's the heart* (14th ed., Chapter 49). New York, NY: McGraw-Hill.

41. Carabello B. A., Hahn R. T. (2017). Aortic valve disease. In Fuster V., Walsh R. A., Harrington R. A., et al. (Eds.), *Hurst's the heart* (14th ed., Chapter 47). New York, NY: McGraw-Hill.

42. Yancy C. W., Jessup M., Bozkurt B., et al. (2013). 2013 ACC/AHA 2013 Guidelines for the management of heart failure. *Circulation* 128, e240–e327.

43. Yancy C. W., Jessup M., Bozkurt B., et al. (2016). 2016 ACCF/AHA/HFSA Focused update on new pharmacological therapy for heart failure. *Circulation* 134, 1977–2016.

44. Guyton A. C., Hall J. E. (2016). *Textbook of medical physiology* (13th ed., pp. 245–258). Philadelphia, PA: Elsevier Saunders.

45. Januzzi J. L., Mann D. L. (2015). Clinical assessment of heart failure. In Bonow R. O., Mann D. L., Zipes D. P., et al. (Eds.), *Braunwald's heart disease: A textbook of cardiovascular medicine* (10th ed., pp. 473–483). Philadelphia, PA: Elsevier Saunders.

46. Mann D. (2015). Management of heart failure with reduced ejection fraction. In Bonow R. O., Mann D. L., Zipes D. P., et al. (Eds.), *Braunwald's heart disease: A textbook of cardiovascular medicine* (10th ed., pp. 512–546). Philadelphia, PA: Elsevier Saunders.

47. Hasenfuss G., Mann D. (2015). Pathophysiology of heart failure. In Bonow R. O., Mann D. L., Zipes D. P., et al. (Eds.) *Braunwald's heart disease: A textbook of cardiovascular medicine* (10th ed., pp. 454–472). Philadelphia, PA: Elsevier Saunders.

48. Gaggin H. K., Dec G. W. (2017). Pathophysiology of heart failure. In Fuster V., Walsh R. A., Harrington R. A., et al. (Eds.), *Hurst's the heart* (14th ed., Chapter 68). New York, NY: McGraw-Hill.

49. Felker G. M., Teerlink J. R. (2015). Diagnosis and management of acute heart failure. In Bonow R. O., Mann D. L., Zipes D. P., et al. (Eds.), *Braunwald's heart disease: A textbook of cardiovascular medicine* (10th ed., pp. 484–511). Philadelphia, PA: Elsevier Saunders.

50. Ahmad T., Butler J., Borlaug B. (2017). The diagnosis and management of chronic heart failure. In Fuster V., Walsh R. A., Harrington R. A., et al. (Eds.), *Hurst's the heart* (14th ed., Chapter 70). New York, NY: McGraw-Hill.

51. Bloom M. W., Cole R. T., Butler J. (2017). Evaluation and management of acute heart failure. In Fuster V., Walsh R. A., Harrington R. A., et al. (Eds.), *Hurst's the heart* (14th ed., Chapter 71). New York, NY: McGraw-Hill.

52. Yancy C. W., Jessup M. (2017). 2017 ACC/AHA/HFSA Focused update of the 2013 ACCF/AHA Guideline for the management of heart failure. *Circulation* 136, e137–e161.

53. Upadhyay G. A., Singh J. P. (2017). Pacemakers and defibrillators. In Fuster V., Walsh R. A., Harrington R. A., et al. (Eds.), *Hurst's the heart* (14th ed., Chapter 89). New York, NY: McGraw-Hill.

54. Jessup M., Acker M. A. (2015). Surgical management of heart failure. In Bonow R. O., Mann D. L., Zipes D. P., et al. (Eds.), *Braunwald's heart disease: A textbook of cardiovascular medicine* (10th ed., pp. 575–589). Philadelphia, PA: Elsevier Saunders.

55. Van Praagh R. (2006). Embryology. In Keane J. F., Lock J. E., Fyler D. C. (Eds.), *Nadas pediatric cardiology* (2nd ed., pp. 13–25). Philadelphia, PA: Elsevier Saunders.

56. Freed M. D. (2006). Fetal and transitional circulation. In Keane J. F., Lock J. E., Fyler D. C. (Eds.), *Nadas' pediatric cardiology* (2nd ed., pp. 75–79). Philadelphia, PA: Elsevier Saunders.

57. Nadas A. S., Fyler D. C. (2006). Hypoxemia. In Keane J. F., Lock J. E., Fyler D. C. (Eds.), *Nadas' pediatric cardiology* (2nd ed., pp. 97–101). Philadelphia, PA: Elsevier Saunders.

58. Webb G. D., Smallhorn J. F., Therrien J., et al. (2015). Congenital heart disease. In Mann D. L., Zipes D. P., et al. (Eds.), *Braunwald's heart disease: A textbook of cardiovascular medicine* (10th ed., pp. 1391–1445). Philadelphia, PA: Elsevier Saunders.

59. Lin J. P., Child J. S. (2017). Congenital heart disease in adolescents and adults. In Fuster V., Walsh R. A., Harrington R. A., et al. (Eds.), *Hurst's the heart* (14th ed., Chapter 56). New York, NY: McGraw-Hill.

60. Colan S. D. (2006). Cardiomyopathies. In Keane J. F., Lock J. E., Fyler D. C. (Eds.), *Nadas' pediatric cardiology* (2nd ed., pp. 415–445). Philadelphia, PA: Elsevier Saunders.

61. Nishimura R. A., Otto C. M., Bonow R. O., et al. (2017). 2017 ACC/AHA Focused update of the 2014 guideline for the management of patients with valvular heart disease. *Circulation* 135(25), e1159–e1195.

62. Keane J. F., Geva T., Fyler D. C. (2006). Atrial septal defect, ventricular septal defect, coarctation of the aorta, single ventricle, pulmonary stenosis. In Keane J. F., Lock J. E., Fyler D. C. (Eds.), *Nadas' pediatric cardiology* (2nd ed., pp. 527–558, 603–616, 627–644, 743–752). Philadelphia, PA: Elsevier Saunders.

63. Marx G. R., Fyler D. C. (2006). Endocardial cushion defects. In Keane J. F., Lock J. E., Fyler D. C. (Eds.), *Nadas' pediatric cardiology* (2nd ed., pp. 663–674). Philadelphia, PA: Elsevier Saunders.

64. Fulton D. R., Fyler D. C. (2006). D-Transposition of the great arteries. In Keane J. F., Lock J. E., Fyler D. C. (Eds.), *Nadas' pediatric cardiology* (2nd ed., pp. 645–662). Philadelphia, PA: Elsevier Saunders.

65. LoBreitbart R. E., Fyler D. C. (2006). Tetralogy of Fallot. In Keane J. F., Lock J. E., Fyler D. C. (Eds.), *Nadas' pediatric cardiology* (2nd ed., pp. 559–580). Philadelphia, PA: Elsevier Saunders.

66. Landzberg M. (2006). Adult congenital heart disease. In Keane J. F., Lock J. E., Fyler D. C. (Eds.), *Nadas' pediatric cardiology* (2nd ed., pp. 833–841). Philadelphia, PA: Elsevier Saunders.

67. Fulton D. R., Newburger J. W. (2006). Kawasaki disease. In Keane J. F., Lock J. E., Fyler D. C. (Eds.), *Nadas' pediatric cardiology* (2nd ed., pp. 401–413). Philadelphia, PA: Elsevier Saunders.

68. Bernstein D. (2016). Heart failure. In Kliegman R. M., Stanton B. F., St Geme J. W., et al. (Eds.), *Nelson textbook of pediatrics* (20th ed., pp. 2282–2288). Philadelphia, PA: Elsevier Saunders.

69. American Heart Association. (2017). Heart disease and stroke statistics: 2017 update at a glance. [Online]. Available: www.americanheart.org/downloadable/heart/.pdf. Accessed October 12, 2017.

70. Rich M. W. (2011). Heart failure in older adults. *Medical Clinics of North America 95*(3), 439–461.

71. Schwartz J. B., Zipes D. P. (2015). Cardiovascular disease in the elderly. In Bonow R. O., Mann D. L., Zipes D. P., et al. (Eds.), *Braunwald's heart disease: A textbook of cardiovascular medicine* (10th ed., pp. 1711–1743). Philadelphia, PA: Elsevier Saunders.

72. Guyton A. C., Hall J. E. (2016). *Textbook of medical physiology* (13th ed., pp. 169–291). Philadelphia, PA: Elsevier.

73. Bloom M. M., Cole R. T., Butler J. (2018). Evaluation and management of acute heart failure. In Fuster V., Harrington R. A., Narula J., et al. (Eds.), *Hurst's the heart* (14th ed.). New York, NY: McGraw-Hill. http://accessmedicine.mhmedical.com/content.aspx?bookid=2046&sectionid=176562062. Accessed May 22, 2018

74. Gaieski D. F., Mikkelsen M. (2018). Evaluation of and initial approach to the adult patient with undifferentiated hypotension and shock. In Finley G. (Ed.), *UpToDate*. Available: https://www.uptodate.com/contents/evaluation-of-and-initial-approach-to-the-adult-patient-with-undifferentiated-hypotension-and-shock. Accessed May 18, 2019.

75. Gaieski D. F., Mikkelsen M. E. (2018). Definition, classification, etiology, and pathophysiology of shock in adults. In Finlay G. (Ed.), *UpToDate*. Available: https://www.uptodate.com/contents/definition-classification-etiology-and-pathophysiology-of-shock-in-adults. Accessed May 18, 2019.

76. Hochman J. S., Reyentovich A. Prognosis and treatment of cardiogenic shock complicating acute myocardial infarction. In Saperia G. M. (Ed.), *UpToDate*. Available: https://www.uptodate.com/contents/prognosis-and-treatment-of-cardiogenic-shock-complicating-acute-myocardial-infarction. Accessed May 18, 2019.

77. Smith N., Jamil R. T., Silberman M. (2019). Distributive Shock. In *StatPearls* [Internet]. Available: https://www.ncbi.nlm.nih.gov/pubmed/29261964. Accessed June 25, 2019.

78. Kelso J. M. (2018). Anaphylaxis: Confirming the diagnosis and determining the cause(s). In Feldweg A. M. (Ed.), *UpToDate*. Available: https://www.uptodate.com/contents/anaphylaxis-confirming-the-diagnosis-and-determining-the-causes. Accessed May 18, 2019.

79. Campbell R. L., Kelso J. M. (2017). Anaphylaxis: Emergency treatment. In Feldweg A. M. (Ed.), *UpToDate*. Available: https://www.uptodate.com/contents/anaphylaxis-emergency-treatment. Accessed May 18, 2019.

80. Neviere R. (2018). Sepsis syndromes in adults: Epidemiology, definitions, clinical presentation, diagnosis, and prognosis. In Finlay G. (Ed.), *UpToDate*. Available: https://www.uptodate.com/contents/sepsis-syndromes-in-adults-epidemiology-definitions-clinical-presentation-diagnosis-and-prognosis. Accessed May 18, 2019.

81. Schmidt G. A., Mandel J. (2018). Evaluation and management of suspected sepsis and septic shock in Adults. In Finlay G. (Ed.), *UpToDate*. Available: https://www.uptodate.com/contents/evaluation-and-management-of-suspected-sepsis-and-septic-shock-in-adults. Accessed May 18, 2019.

82. Center for Disease Control and Prevention. (2017). Sepsis. Available: https://www.cdc.gov/sepsis/index.html. Accessed May 18, 2019.

83. Siegel M. D. (2017). Acute respiratory distress syndrome: Clinical features and diagnosis in adults. In Finlay G. (Ed.), *UpToDate*. Available: https://www.uptodate.com/contents/acute-respiratory-distress-syndrome-clinical-features-diagnosis-and-complications-in-adults. Accessed May 18, 2019.

84. Siegel M. D. (2018). Acute respiratory distress syndrome: Supportive care and oxygenation in adults. In Finlay G. (Ed.), *UpToDate*. Available: https://www.uptodate.com/contents/acute-respiratory-distress-syndrome-supportive-care-and-oxygenation-in-adults. Accessed May 18, 2019.

85. Weinhouse G. L. (2018). Stress ulcer prophylaxis in the intensive care unit. In Finlay G. (Ed.), *UpToDate*. Available: https://www.uptodate.com/contents/stress-ulcer-prophylaxis-in-the-intensive-care-unit. Accessed May 18, 2019.

86. Levi M. M. (2017). Disseminated intravascular coagulation clinical presentation. Available: https://emedicine.medscape.com/article/199627-clinical#b3. Accessed May 15, 2018.

87. Leung L. L. K. (2017). Clinical features, diagnosis, and treatment of disseminated intravascular coagulation in adults. In Timjauer J. S. (Ed.), *UpToDate*. Available: https://www.uptodate.com/contents/clinical-features-diagnosis-and-treatment-of-disseminated-intravascular-coagulation-in-adults. Accessed May 18, 2019.

88. La-Khafaji A. H. (2018). Multiple organ dysfunction syndrome in sepsis. Available: https://emedicine.medscape.com/article/169640-overview. Accessed May 15, 2018.

89. Neviere R. (2018). Pathophysiology of sepsis. In Finlay G. (Ed.), *UpToDate*. Available: https://www.uptodate.com/contents/pathophysiology-of-sepsis. Accessed May 18, 2019.

Disorders of Cardiac Conduction and Rhythm

Learning Objectives

After completing this chapter, the learner will be able to meet the following objectives:

1. Describe the cardiac conduction system, including the five phases of cardiac action potential.
2. Illustrate an electrocardiogram tracing labeling the electrical signals of the conduction system of the heart.
3. Characterize the effects of atrial arrhythmias including atrial flutter and atrial fibrillation on heart rhythm.
4. Describe the characteristics of first-, second-, and third-degree heart block; ventricular tachycardia; and ventricular fibrillation.

Heart muscle is unique in that it is capable of generating and rapidly conducting its own electrical impulses or action potentials. These action potentials result in excitation of muscle fibers throughout the myocardium. Impulse formation and conduction result in weak electrical currents that spread throughout the body. It is these impulses that are recorded on an electrocardiogram (ECG). Disorders of cardiac impulse generation and conduction range from benign arrhythmias to those causing serious disruption of heart function and sudden cardiac death.

Cardiac Conduction System

In certain areas of the heart, the myocardial cells have been modified to form the specialized cells of the conduction system. These specialized cells have the ability to self-excitation, which is the capability of initiating and conducting impulses.[1] It is the conduction system that maintains the pumping efficiency of the heart. Specialized pacemaker cells generate impulses at a faster rate than other types of heart tissue, and the conduction tissue transmits these impulses more rapidly than other cardiac cell types. Because of these properties, a normal conduction system controls the rhythm of the heart.

The specialized excitatory and conduction system of the heart consists of the sinoatrial (SA) node, in which the normal rhythmic impulse is generated; the internodal pathways between the atria and the ventricles; the atrioventricular (AV) node and bundle of His, which conduct the impulse from the atria to the ventricles; and the Purkinje fibers, which conduct the impulses through the entire tissue of the right and left ventricles (Fig. 28-1).

The heart essentially has two conduction systems: one that controls atrial activity and one that controls ventricular activity. The atrial conduction begins with the SA node, which has the fastest intrinsic rate of firing (60 to 100 beats/minute), normally serving as the

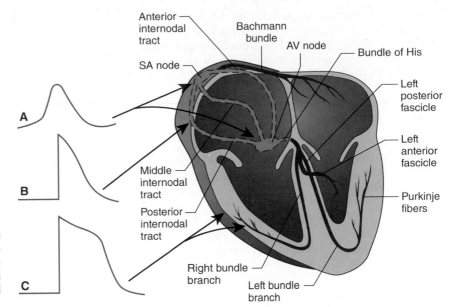

FIGURE 28-1. Conduction system of the heart and action potentials. (*A*) Action potential of sinoatrial (SA) and atrioventricular (AV) nodes; (*B*) atrial muscle action potential; and (*C*) action potential of ventricular muscle and Purkinje fibers.

pacemaker of the heart. It is a spindle-shaped strip of specialized muscle tissue, about 10 to 20 mm in length and 2 to 3 mm wide, located in the posterior wall of the right atrium just below the opening of the superior vena cava and less than 1 mm from the epicardial surface.[2] Impulses originating in the SA node travel through the atria to the AV node. Because of the anatomic location of the SA node, the progression of atrial depolarization occurs in an inferior, leftward, and somewhat posterior direction, and the right atrium is depolarized slightly before the left atrium.[1,3] There are three internodal pathways between the SA node and the AV node, including the anterior (Bachmann), middle (Wenckebach), and posterior (Thorel) internodal tracts. These three tracts anastomose with each other proximally to the AV node. This large muscle bundle originates along the anterior border of the SA node and travels posteriorly around the aorta to the left atrium.[1,4]

The AV junction connects the two conduction systems and provides for one-way conduction between the atria and the ventricles. The AV node is a compact, ovoid structure measuring approximately 1 mm × 3 mm × 5 mm and located on the posterior wall slightly beneath the right atrial endocardium, anterior to the opening of the coronary sinus, and immediately above the insertion of the septal leaflet of the tricuspid valve.[1,4] It is important to note that everywhere except for the AV node in a healthy heart, the atrial muscle is separated from the ventricular muscle in order to prevent cardiac impulses firing inappropriately.

The AV node is divided into three functional regions:

- The AN or transitional region, located between the atria and the rest of the node
- The N or middle region
- The NH region, in which nodal fibers merge with the bundle of His, which is the upper portion of the specialized conduction system[1,5]

In the AN portion of the node, atrial fibers connect with very small junctional fibers of the node itself. The velocity of conduction through the AN and N fibers is very slow (approximately one half that of normal cardiac muscle), which greatly delays transmission of the impulse.[1,4] A further delay occurs as the impulse travels through the N region into the NH region, which connects with the *bundle of His* (also called the *AV bundle*). This delay provides a mechanical advantage whereby the atria complete their ejection of blood before ventricular contraction begins. Its main function is to coordinate atrial and ventricular conduction. The atria and ventricles would beat independently of each other if the transmission of impulses through the AV node were blocked.

The *Purkinje system*, which initiates ventricular conduction, has large fibers that allow for rapid conduction. Once the impulse enters the Purkinje system, it spreads almost immediately to the whole ventricle (0.03 second).[1] This rapid rate of conduction throughout the Purkinje system is necessary for the swift and efficient ejection of blood from the heart. The fibers of the Purkinje system originate in the AV node and proceed to form the bundle of His, which extends through the fibrous tissue between the valves of the heart and into the ventricular system. Because of its proximity to the aortic valve and the mitral valve ring, the bundle of His is predisposed to inflammation and deposits of calcified debris that can interfere with impulse conduction.[1] The bundle of His penetrates into the ventricles and almost immediately divides into *right* and *left bundle branches* that straddle the interventricular septum. Branches from the anterior and posterior descending coronary arteries provide the blood supply for the His bundle, making this conduction site less susceptible to ischemic damage, unless the damage is extensive.[2] The bundle branches move through the subendocardial tissues toward the papillary muscles and then subdivide into the Purkinje fibers, which branch out and supply the outer walls of the ventricles. The main trunk of the left bundle branch extends for approximately 1 to 2 cm before fanning out as it enters the septal area and divides further into two segments: the *left posterior* and *anterior fascicles*. These Purkinje fibers transmit the impulse almost simultaneously to the right and left ventricular endothelium in a healthy conduction system.

The AV nodal fibers, when not stimulated, discharge at an intrinsic rate of 40 to 60 times/minute, and the Purkinje fibers discharge 15 to 40 times/minute. Although the AV node and Purkinje system have the ability to control the rhythm of the heart, they do not normally do so because the discharge rate of the SA node is considerably faster. Each time the SA node discharges, its impulses are conducted into the AV node and Purkinje fibers, causing them to fire. The AV node can assume the pacemaker function of the heart, should the SA node fail to discharge, and the Purkinje system can assume the pacemaker function of the ventricles, should the AV node fail to conduct impulses from the atria to the ventricles. Under these circumstances, the heart rate reflects the intrinsic firing rate of the prevailing structures.

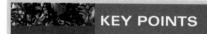

KEY POINTS

Cardiac Conduction System

■ Normally, impulses are generated in the SA node, which has the fastest rate of firing and travel through the AV node to the Purkinje system in the ventricles.

Action Potentials

An action potential represents the sequential change in electrical potential that occurs across a cell membrane when excitation occurs and causes the heart to conduct this electrical impulse across the atrium and ventricle. These potential or voltage differences, often referred to as *membrane potentials*, represent the flow of current associated with the passage of ions through ion channels in the cell membrane. The sodium (Na^+), potassium (K^+), and calcium (Ca^{++}) ions are the major charge carriers in cardiac muscle cells. Disorders of the ion channels, along with disruption in the flow of these current-carrying ions, are increasingly being linked to the generation of cardiac arrhythmias and conduction disorders.

Action potentials can be divided into three phases:

1. Resting or unexcited state
2. Depolarization
3. Repolarization

During the resting phase, cardiac cells exhibit a resting membrane potential that typically ranges from -60 to -90 mV. The negative sign before the voltage indicates that the inside of the membrane is negatively charged in relation to the outside (Fig. 28-2A). Although different

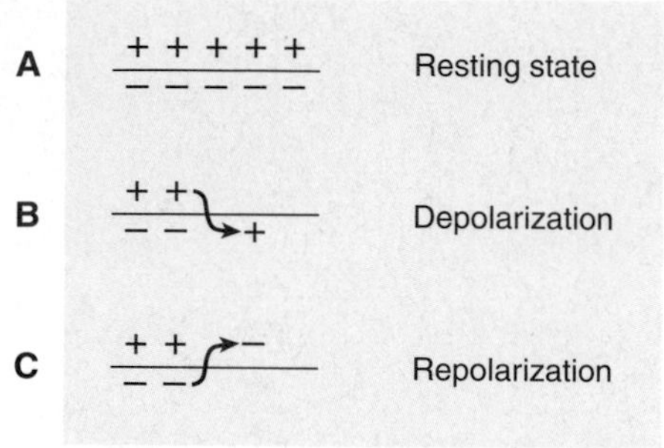

FIGURE 28-2. The flow of charge during impulse generation in excitable tissue. During the resting state (*A*), opposite charges are separated by the cell membrane. Depolarization (*B*) represents the flow of charge across the membrane, and repolarization (*C*) denotes the return of the membrane potential to its resting state.

kinds of ions are found both inside and outside the membrane, the membrane potential is determined largely by Na^+ and K^+ and the membrane permeability for these two ions. During the resting phase of the membrane potential, the membrane is selectively permeable to K^+ and nearly impermeable to Na^+. As a result, K^+ diffuses out of the cell along its concentration gradient, causing a relative loss of positive ions from inside the membrane. The result is an uneven distribution of charge with negativity on the inside and positivity on the outside.

Depolarization represents the period of time (measured in milliseconds [ms]) during which the polarity of the membrane potential is reversed. It occurs when the cell membrane suddenly becomes selectively permeable to a current-carrying ion such as Na^+, allowing it to move into a cell and change the membrane potential so it becomes positive on the inside and negative on the outside (Fig. 28-2B).

Repolarization involves reestablishment of the resting membrane potential. It has a somewhat slower process, involving the outward flow of electrical charges and the return of the membrane potential to its resting state.[6] During repolarization, membrane permeability for K^+ again increases, allowing the positively charged K^+ to move outward across the membrane. This outward movement removes positive charges from inside the cell; thus, the voltage across the membrane again becomes negative on the inside and positive on the outside (Fig. 28-2C). The adenosine triphosphatase (ATPase)-dependent sodium–potassium pump assists in repolarization by pumping positively charged Na^+ out across the cell membrane and returning K^+ to the inside of the membrane.[7]

Action Potential Phases

The action potentials in cardiac muscle are typically divided into five phases:

1. *Phase 0*—upstroke or rapid depolarization
2. *Phase 1*—rapid repolarization period
3. *Phase 2*—plateau
4. *Phase 3*—final, rapid repolarization period
5. *Phase 4*—diastolic depolarization (Fig. 28-3B)

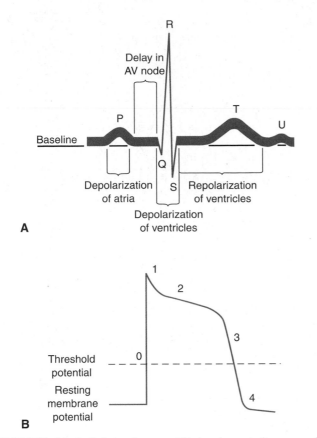

FIGURE 28-3. Relation between (**A**) the electrocardiogram and (**B**) phases of the ventricular action potential. AV, atrioventricular.

Cardiac muscle has three types of membrane ion channels that contribute to the voltage changes that occur during the different phases of the cardiac action potential. They are the fast Na^+ channels, slow calcium (Ca^{++}) channels, and K^+ channels.

During *phase 0*, in atrial and ventricular muscle and in the Purkinje system, the fast Na^+ channels in the cell membrane are stimulated to open, resulting in the rapid influx of Na^+. The point at which the Na^+ channels open is called the *depolarization threshold*. The exterior of the cell now is negatively charged in relation to the highly positive interior of the cell. This influx of Na^+ produces a rapid, positively directed change in the membrane potential, resulting in the electrical spike during phase 0 of the action potential.[2,6] The membrane potential shifts from a resting membrane potential of approximately −90 to +20 mV. The rapid depolarization that comprises phase 0 is responsible for the QRS complex on the ECG (Fig. 28-3A). Depolarization of a cardiac cell causes adjacent cells to depolarize and stimulating the Na^+ channels in nearby cells to open, resulting in a wave of depolarization across the heart, cell by cell.

Phase 1 occurs at the peak of the action potential as a result of inactivation of the fast Na^+ channels with an abrupt decrease in sodium permeability. The slight downward slope is thought to be caused by the influx of a small amount of negatively charged chloride ions and efflux of potassium.[2] The decrease in intracellular

positivity reduces the membrane potential to a level near 0 mV, from which the plateau, or phase 2, arises.

Phase 2 represents the plateau of the action potential. If K^+ permeability increased to its resting level at this time, as it does in nerve fibers or skeletal muscle, the cell would repolarize rapidly. Instead, K^+ permeability is low, allowing the membrane to remain depolarized throughout the phase 2 plateau. A simultaneous influx of Ca^{++} into the cell through the slow Ca^{++} channels produces the contractile process and contributes to the phase 2 plateau.[2,7] These unique features of the phase 2 plateau cause the action potential and contractility of cardiac muscle to last longer than that of skeletal muscle.[1] The phase 2 plateau coincides with the ST segment of the ECG.

Phase 3 reflects rapid repolarization and begins with the downslope of the action potential. During the phase 3 repolarization period, the slow Ca^{++} channels close and the influx of Ca^{++} and Na^+ ceases. There is a sharp rise in K^+ permeability moving K^+ out and reestablishment of the resting membrane potential (−90 mV). At the conclusion of phase 3, the membrane returns to the normal resting state. The T wave on the ECG corresponds with phase 3 of the action potential.

Phase 4 represents the resting membrane potential. During phase 4, the activity of the Na^+/K^+-ATPase pump contributes to maintaining the resting membrane potential by transporting Na^+ out of the cell and moving K^+ back in. Phase 4 corresponds to diastole.[2]

Fast and Slow Responses

There are two main types of action potentials in the heart—the fast response and the slow response. The *fast response* occurs in the normal myocardial cells of the atria, the ventricles, and the Purkinje fibers (Fig. 28-4A). It is characterized by the opening of voltage-dependent Na^+ channels called the *fast sodium channels*. The fast response cardiac cells do not normally initiate cardiac action potentials. The fast response cells have a constant resting potential, rapid depolarization, and then a longer period of sustained depolarization before repolarization. This allows impulse conduction to be rapid to adjacent cells. Myocardial fibers with a fast response are capable of conducting electrical activity at relatively rapid rates (0.5 to 5.0 m/second), thereby providing a high safety factor for conduction.[8]

The *slow response* occurs in the SA node, which is the natural pacemaker of the heart, and the conduction fibers of the AV node (Fig. 28-4B). The hallmark of these pacemaker cells is a spontaneous phase 4 depolarization. The membrane permeability of these cells allows a slow inward leak of current to occur through the slow channels during phase 4. This leak continues until the threshold for firing is reached, at which point the cell spontaneously depolarizes. Under normal conditions, the primary role of this slow response, sometimes referred to as the *calcium current*, in normal atrial and ventricular cells is to provide for the entrance of calcium for the excitation and resultant muscle contraction.

The rate of pacemaker cell discharge varies with the resting membrane potential and the slope of phase 4 depolarization (Fig. 28-3). Catecholamines

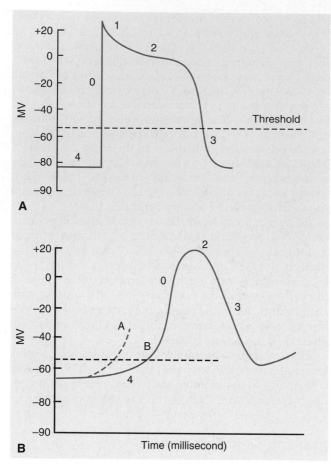

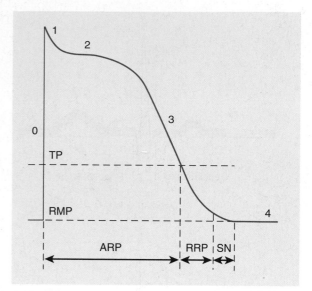

FIGURE 28-5. Diagram of an action potential of a ventricular muscle cell, showing the threshold potential (TP), resting membrane potential (RMP), absolute refractory period (ARP), relative refractory period (RRP), and supernormal (SN) period.

FIGURE 28-4. Changes in action potential recorded from a fast response in cardiac muscle cell (**A**) and from a slow response recorded in the sinoatrial and atrioventricular nodes (**B**). The phases of the action potential are identified by numbers: phase 4, resting membrane potential; phase 0, depolarization; phase 1, brief period of repolarization; phase 2, plateau; and phase 3, repolarization. The slow response is characterized by a slow, spontaneous rise in the phase 4 membrane potential to threshold levels; it has a lesser amplitude and shorter duration than the fast response. Increased automaticity (A) occurs when the rate of phase 4 depolarization is increased.

(*i.e.*, epinephrine and norepinephrine) increase heart rate by increasing the slope or rate of phase 4 depolarization. Acetylcholine, a parasympathetic mediator, slows the heart rate by decreasing the slope of phase 4.

The fast response of atrial and ventricular muscle can be converted to a slow pacemaker response under certain conditions. For example, such conversions may occur spontaneously in people with severe coronary artery disease and in areas of the heart where blood supply has been markedly compromised. Impulses generated by these cells can lead to ectopic beats and serious arrhythmias.

Absolute and Relative Refractory Periods

The pumping action of the heart requires alternating contraction and relaxation. There is a period in the action potential during which the membrane cannot be stimulated to depolarize under any condition to generate another action potential (Fig. 28-5). This period,

known as the *absolute or effective refractory period*, includes phases 0, 1, and 2 and part of phase 3. This acts as a safety margin for the heart in order to prevent any stimulation or generate any extra beats. During the *relative refractory period,* the cell is capable of responding to a greater-than-normal stimulus. The relative refractory period begins when the membrane potential in phase 3 reaches threshold level and ends just before the end of phase 3. After the relative refractory period is a short period called the *supernormal excitatory period,* during which a weak stimulus can evoke a response. The supernormal excitatory period extends from the terminal portion of phase 3 until the beginning of phase 4. It is during this period that cardiac arrhythmias develop.[8]

Electrocardiography

The ECG is a graphic recording of the electrical activity of the heart or a picture of the heart as it contracts. The electrical currents generated by the heart spread through the body to the skin, where they can be sensed by appropriately placed electrodes, amplified, and viewed on an oscilloscope or chart recorder.

The deflection points of an ECG are designated by the letters P, Q, R, S, and T. The P wave represents the SA node and atrial depolarization; the QRS complex (*i.e.,* beginning of the Q wave to the end of the S wave) depicts ventricular depolarization; and the T wave portrays ventricular repolarization. The isoelectric line between the P wave and the Q wave represents depolarization of the AV node, bundle branches, and Purkinje system. Atrial repolarization occurs during ventricular depolarization and is hidden in the QRS complex. Figure 28-6 depicts the electrical activity of the conduction system on an ECG tracing.

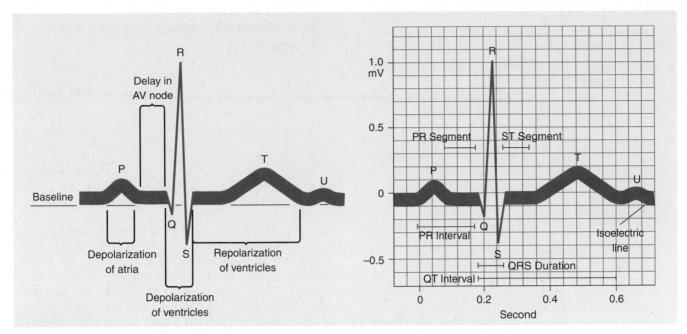

FIGURE 28-6. Diagram of the electrocardiogram (lead II) and representative depolarization and repolarization of the atria and ventricles. The P wave represents atrial depolarization, the QRS complex ventricular depolarization, and the T wave ventricular repolarization. Atrial repolarization occurs during ventricular depolarization and is hidden under the QRS complex. AV, atrioventricular.

The ECG records the potential difference in charge between two electrodes as the depolarization and repolarization waves move through the heart and are conducted to the skin surface. The shape of the recorder tracing is determined by the direction in which the impulse spreads through the heart muscle in relation to electrode placement. A depolarization wave that moves toward the recording electrode registers as a positive, or upward, deflection. Conversely, if the impulse moves away from the recording electrode, the deflection is downward, or negative. When there is no flow of charge between electrodes, the potential is zero, and a straight line is recorded at the baseline of the chart.

Conventionally, 12 leads (six limb leads and six chest leads) are recorded for a diagnostic ECG, each providing a unique view of the electrical forces of the heart from a different position on the body's surface. The six limb leads view the electrical forces as they pass through the heart on the frontal or vertical plane. The electrodes are attached to the four extremities or representative areas on the body near the shoulders and lower chest or abdomen. The six chest leads provide a view of the electrical forces as they pass through the heart on the horizontal plane. They are moved to different positions on the chest, including the right and left sternal borders and the left anterior surface (Fig. 28-7). The right lower extremity lead is used as a ground electrode.[8] When indicated, additional electrodes may be applied to other areas of the body, such as the back or right anterior chest to record from other areas of the heart. However, this is not done routinely.

Research has shown that ECG monitoring is more sensitive than a person's report of symptoms for identifying transient ongoing myocardial ischemia. ECG monitoring also provides for more accurate and timely detection of ischemic events that predict early complications.

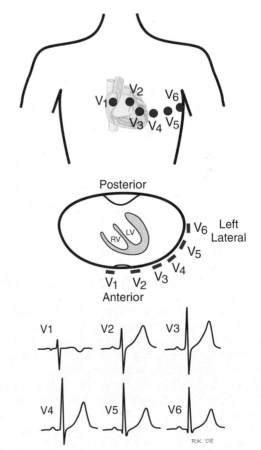

FIGURE 28-7. Placement of the six precordial chest leads and the normal appearance of the electrocardiogram recording for leads V_1–V_6. These electrodes record electrical activity in the horizontal plane, which is perpendicular to the frontal plane of the limb leads. (From Klabunde R. E. (2012). *Cardiovascular physiology concepts* (2nd ed., Fig. 2.20, p. 35). Philadelphia, PA: Wolters Kluwer.)

The American Heart Association recently published practice standards for ECG monitoring in hospital settings.[8] This rating system includes three categories:

■ Class I—cardiac monitoring is necessary in most, if not all, people in this group.
■ Class II—cardiac monitoring may be beneficial in some people, but it is not an essential component of care for these people.
■ Class III—cardiac monitoring is not indicated because the risk of a serious event for these people is so low that monitoring is not viewed as therapeutic.

SUMMARY CONCEPTS

The rhythmic contraction and relaxation of the heart rely on the specialized cells of the heart's conduction system. Specialized cells in the SA node have the fastest inherent rate of impulse generation known as *automaticity* and act as the pacemaker of the heart. Impulses from the SA node travel through the atria to the AV node and then to the AV bundle and the ventricular Purkinje system. The AV node provides the only connection between the atrial and ventricular conduction systems. The atria and the ventricles function independently of each other when AV node conduction is blocked.

Action potentials represent the sequential changes in electrical potentials that are associated with the movement of current-carrying ions through ion channels in the cell membrane. The action potentials of cardiac muscle are divided into five phases: phase 0 represents depolarization and is characterized by the rapid upstroke of the action potential; phase 1 is characterized by a brief period of repolarization; phase 2 consists of a plateau, which prolongs the duration of the action potential; phase 3 represents repolarization; and phase 4 is the resting membrane potential. After an action potential, there is a refractory period during which the membrane is resistant to a second stimulus. During the absolute refractory period, the membrane is insensitive to stimulation. This period is followed by the relative refractory period, during which a more intense stimulus is needed to initiate an action potential. The relative refractory period is followed by a supernormal excitatory period, during which a weak stimulus can evoke a response.

The ECG provides a means for monitoring the electrical activity of the heart. Conventionally, 12 leads (six limb leads and six chest leads) are recorded for a diagnostic ECG, each providing a unique view of the electrical forces of the heart from a different position on the body's surface. This procedure allows for advanced arrhythmia detection and early identification of ischemia- and infarction-related changes in people with acute coronary syndrome.

Disorders of Cardiac Rhythm and Conduction

There are two types of disorders of the cardiac conduction system: disorders of rhythm and disorders of impulse conduction. There are many causes of cardiac arrhythmias and conduction disorders, including congenital defects or degenerative changes in the conduction system, myocardial ischemia and myocardial infarction (MI), fluid and electrolyte imbalances, and the effects of pharmacologic agents. Arrhythmias are not necessarily pathologic; they can occur in both healthy and diseased hearts. Disturbances in cardiac rhythms exert their harmful effects by interfering with the heart's pumping ability. Excessively rapid heart rates (tachyarrhythmias) reduce the diastolic filling time, causing a subsequent decrease in the stroke volume output and in coronary perfusion while increasing the myocardial oxygen needs. Abnormally slow heart rates (bradyarrhythmias) may impair blood flow to vital organs such as the brain.

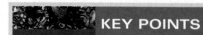

KEY POINTS

Physiologic Basis of Arrhythmia Generation

■ Cardiac arrhythmias represent disorders of cardiac rhythm related to alterations in automaticity, excitability, conductivity, or refractoriness of specialized cells in the conduction system of the heart.

Mechanisms of Arrhythmias and Conduction Disorders

The specialized cells in the conduction system manifest four inherent properties that contribute to the genesis of all cardiac rhythms, both normal and abnormal. They are automaticity, excitability, conductivity, and refractoriness. An alteration in any of these four properties may produce arrhythmias or conduction defects.

The ability of certain cells in the conduction system spontaneously to initiate an impulse or action potential is referred to as *automaticity*. The SA node has an inherent discharge rate of 60 to 100 times/minute. It normally acts as the pacemaker of the heart because it reaches the threshold for excitation before other parts of the conduction system have recovered sufficiently to be depolarized. If the SA node fires more slowly or SA node conduction is blocked, another site that is capable of automaticity takes over as pacemaker.[1,3] Other regions that are capable of automaticity include the atrial fibers that have plateau-type action potentials, the AV node, the bundle of His, and the bundle branch Purkinje fibers. These pacemakers have a slower rate of discharge than the SA node. The AV node has an inherent firing rate of 40 to 60 times/minute, and the Purkinje system fires at a rate of 15 to 40 times/minute. The SA node may be functioning properly, but because of additional precipitating factors, other cardiac cells can assume accelerated properties of automaticity and begin to initiate impulses. These additional factors might include injury, hypoxia, electrolyte disturbances, enlargement or hypertrophy of the atria or ventricles, and exposure to certain chemicals or drugs.

An *ectopic pacemaker* is an excitable focus outside the normally functioning SA node. A premature contraction occurs when an ectopic pacemaker initiates a beat. Premature contractions do not follow the normal conduction pathways, they are not coupled with normal mechanical events, and they often render the heart refractory or incapable of responding to the next normal impulse arising in the SA node. They occur without incident in person with healthy hearts in response to sympathetic nervous system stimulation or other stimulants, such as caffeine. In the diseased heart, premature contractions may lead to more serious arrhythmias.

Excitability describes the ability of a cell to respond to an impulse and generate an action potential. Myocardial cells that have been injured or replaced by scar tissue do not possess normal excitability.

Conductivity is the ability to conduct impulses, and *refractoriness* refers to the extent to which the cell is able to respond to an incoming stimulus. The refractory period of cardiac muscle is the interval in the repolarization period during which an excitable cell has not recovered sufficiently to be excited again. Disturbances in conductivity or refractoriness predispose to arrhythmias.

The phenomenon, known as *reentry*, is the cause of many *tachyarrhythmias*.[1,5] Under normal conditions, an electrical impulse is conducted through the heart in an orderly, sequential manner. The electrical impulse then dies out and does not reenter adjacent tissue because that tissue has already been depolarized and is refractory to immediate stimulation. For reentry to occur, there must be areas of slow conduction and a unidirectional conduction block (Fig. 28-8). Reentry requires a triggering stimulus, such as an extrasystole, to start the circuit.

Reentry may occur anywhere in the conduction system. The functional components of a reentry circuit can be large and include an entire specialized conduction system, or the circuit can be microscopic. Factors contributing to the development of a reentrant circuit include ischemia, infarction, and elevated serum potassium levels. There are several forms of reentry. The first is anatomic reentry. It involves an anatomic obstacle around which the circulating current must pass and results in an excitation wave that travels in a set pathway.[2] Arrhythmias that arise as a result of anatomic reentry are paroxysmal supraventricular tachycardias, as seen in Wolff–Parkinson–White syndrome, atrial fibrillation (AF), atrial flutter, AV nodal reentry, and some ventricular tachycardias. Functional reentry depends on the local differences in conduction velocity and refractoriness among neighboring fibers that allow an impulse to circulate repeatedly around an area.[2] The last type of reentry is spiral reentry. It is initiated by a current that does not proceed down a regular pathway; rather, it breaks away, then curls and rotates. These impulses become erratic and irregular in the atrium. This is what is seen in AF.

Types of Arrhythmias and Conduction Disorders

In a healthy heart driven by sinus node discharge, the rate ranges between 60 and 100 beats/minute. On the ECG, a P wave may be observed to precede every QRS complex. Normal sinus rhythm has been considered the "normal" rhythm of a healthy heart. In normal sinus rhythm, a P wave precedes each QRS complex, and the R-R intervals remain relatively constant over time (Fig. 28-9). A normal

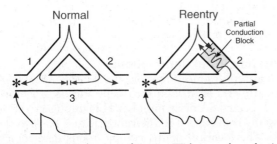

FIGURE 28-8. Mechanism of reentry. With normal conduction of action potentials, impulses traveling down branches *1* and *2* cancel out each other in branch *3*. Reentry can occur if branch *2* has impaired conduction and blocks orthograde impulses but slowly conducts retrograde impulses. If a retrograde impulse emerging from branch *2* reaches excitable tissue (after the effective refractory period, but before the next normal impulse), a premature action potential can be conducted down branch *1*. If this occurs with successive action potentials, tachycardia occurs. (From Klabunde R. E. (2012). *Cardiovascular physiology concepts* (2nd ed., Fig. 2.11, p. 24). Philadelphia, PA: Wolters Kluwer.)

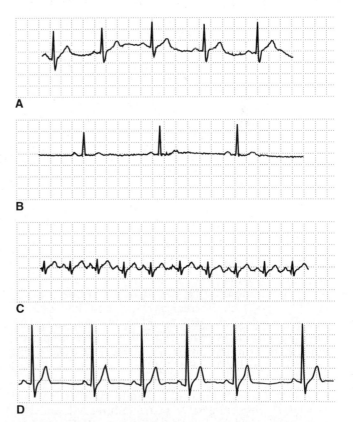

FIGURE 28-9. Electrocardiographic tracings of rhythms originating in the sinus node. (**A**) Normal sinus rhythm (60 to 100 beats/minute). (**B**) Sinus bradycardia (<60 beats/minute). (**C**) Sinus tachycardia (>100 beats/minute). (**D**) Respiratory sinus arrhythmia, characterized by gradual lengthening and shortening of R-R intervals.

P wave and PR interval (0.12 to 0.20 second) indicates that the impulse originated in the SA node rather than in another area of the conduction system that has a slower inherent rate.

Sinus Node Arrhythmias

Alterations in the function of the SA node lead to changes in rate or rhythm of the heartbeat.

For example, respiratory sinus arrhythmia is a cardiac rhythm characterized by gradual lengthening and shortening of R-R intervals (see Fig. 28-9). This variation in cardiac cycles is related to intrathoracic pressure changes that occur with respiration and resultant alterations in autonomic control of the SA node. Inspiration causes acceleration of the heart rate, and expiration causes slowing and does not require any treatment. Respiratory sinus arrhythmia accounts for most heart rate variability in healthy people. A decreased heart rate variability has been associated with altered health states, including MI, congestive heart failure, hypertension, stable angina, diabetes mellitus, and chronic obstructive pulmonary disease (COPD).[9]

Sinus Bradycardia

Sinus bradycardia describes a slow (<60 beats/minute) heart rate (see Fig. 28-9). In sinus bradycardia, a P wave precedes each QRS. Vagal stimulation as well as some medications decreases the firing rate of the SA node and conduction through the AV node to cause a decrease in heart rate. This rhythm may be normal in trained athletes, who maintain a large stroke volume, and during sleep. In most cases, sinus bradycardia is benign unless it is associated with hemodynamic decompensation, such as dizziness and fatigue.[10]

Sinus Pause or Arrest

Sinus arrest refers to failure of the SA node to discharge and results in an irregular pulse. The impulse fails to proceed through the AV node. An escape rhythm develops as another pacemaker takes over. Sinus arrest may result in prolonged periods of asystole and often predisposes to other arrhythmias. Causes of sinus arrest include disease of the SA node, digitalis toxicity, stroke, MI, acute myocarditis, excessive vagal tone, sleep apnea, quinidine, lidocaine, and hyperkalemia or hypokalemia.[10,11]

Sinus Tachycardia

Sinus tachycardia refers to a rapid heart rate (>100 beats/minute) that has its origin in the SA node (see Fig. 28-9). A normal P wave and PR interval should precede each QRS complex. The mechanism of sinus tachycardia is enhanced automaticity related to sympathetic stimulation or withdrawal of vagal tone. Sinus tachycardia is a normal response during fever, blood loss, anxiety, pain, and exercise, and in situations that incite sympathetic stimulation. It may be associated with congestive heart failure, MI, and hyperthyroidism. Pharmacologic agents, such as atropine, isoproterenol, epinephrine, and quinidine, can also cause sinus tachycardia.[11,12]

Sick Sinus Syndrome

Sick sinus syndrome (SSS) is a term that describes a number of forms of cardiac impulse formation and intra-atrial and AV conduction abnormalities.[11-14] The syndrome is most frequently the result of total or subtotal destruction of the SA node, areas of nodal–atrial discontinuity, inflammatory or degenerative changes of the nerves and ganglia surrounding the node, or pathologic changes in the atrial wall.[10] In addition, occlusion of the sinus node artery may be a significant contributing factor. SSS is most often idiopathic, but can be seen in people with coronary artery disease, fibrosis infective processes, certain drugs, and collagen vascular diseases.[12,13] In children, the syndrome is most commonly associated with congenital heart defects, particularly after corrective cardiac surgery.[14]

The most common manifestations of SSS are lightheadedness, dizziness, and syncope, and these symptoms are related to the bradyarrhythmias.[14] When person with SSS experiences palpitations, he or she is generally the result of tachyarrhythmias.

Treatment depends on the rhythm problem and frequently involves the implantation of a permanent pacemaker combined with drug therapy.[10,11]

KEY POINTS

Supraventricular and Ventricular Arrhythmias

- Supraventricular arrhythmias represent disorders of atrial rhythm or conduction above the ventricles.
- Ventricular arrhythmias represent disorders of ventricular rhythm or conduction and can be life-threatening.

Arrhythmias of Atrial Origin

Impulses from the SA node pass through the conductive pathways in the atria to the AV node. Arrhythmias of atrial origin include premature atrial contractions (PACs), multifocal and focal atrial tachycardia, atrial flutter, and AF (Fig. 28-10).

Premature Atrial Contractions

PACs are contractions that originate in the atrial conduction pathways or atrial muscle cells and occur before the next expected SA node impulse. This impulse to contract is usually transmitted to the ventricle and back to the SA node. The location of the ectopic focus determines the configuration of the P wave. The retrograde transmission to the SA node often interrupts the timing of the next sinus beat, such that a pause occurs between the two normally conducted beats. In healthy people, PACs may be the result of stress, alcohol, tobacco, or caffeine. They have also been associated with MI, digitalis toxicity, low serum potassium or magnesium levels, and hypoxia.

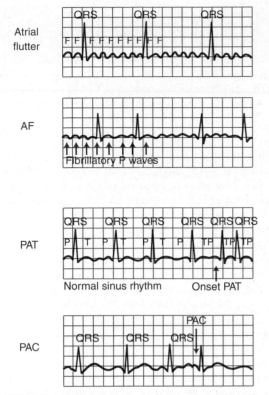

FIGURE 28-10. Electrocardiographic tracings of atrial arrhythmias. Atrial flutter (*first tracing*) is characterized by the atrial flutter (*F*) waves occurring at a rate of 240 to 450 beats/minute. The ventricular rate remains regular because of the conduction of every sixth atrial contraction. Atrial fibrillation (AF) (*second tracing*) has grossly disorganized atrial electrical activity that is irregular with respect to rate and rhythm. The ventricular response is irregular, and no distinct *P* waves are visible. The *third tracing* illustrates paroxysmal atrial tachycardia (PAT), preceded by a normal sinus rhythm. The *fourth tracing* illustrates premature atrial contractions (PACs).

Atrial Tachycardia

Atrial tachycardia can be from one source (focal) or several areas (multifocal). In multifocal atrial tachycardia, the P waves look different based on where they originate in the atrium and become irregular with rates greater than 100 beats/minute. Focal atrial tachycardia is regular, with rates around 100 to 250 beats/minute. Multifocal atrial tachycardia is usually seen in older adults with COPDs, hypoxia, and electrolyte disorders. Focal atrial tachycardia is usually associated with caffeine, alcohol intake, mitral valve disease, rheumatic heart disease, acute MI, COPD, hypokalemia, and digitalis toxicity. Multifocal atrial tachycardia is treated by addressing the underlying disease. Focal can be treated by identifying the underlying cause, the use of antiarrhythmics, or (if those fail) a radiofrequency (RF) catheter ablation of the ectopic focus causing the atrial tachycardia.[15]

Atrial Flutter

Atrial flutter is a rapid atrial ectopic tachycardia. There are two types of atrial flutter: typical and atypical flutter.[10,15] The most common, typical atrial flutter (sometimes called type I), is a result of a reentry rhythm in the right atrium, which can be entrained and interrupted

with atrial pacing techniques. The atrial rate in typical type I flutter can range from 240 to 340 beats/minute and reveals a defined sawtooth pattern in leads AVF, V_1, and V_5.[16] The ventricular response rate and regularity are variable and depend on the AV conduction sequence. The QRS complex may be normal or abnormal.

People who are at particularly high risk for development of atrial flutter include children, adolescents, and young adults who have undergone corrective surgery for complex congenital heart diseases.[15]

Atrial Fibrillation

AF is characterized as rapid disorganized atrial activation ranging from 400 to 600 beats/minute and uncoordinated contraction by the atria.[17] In most cases, multiple, small reentrant circuits are constantly arising in the atria characterized by a grossly disorganized irregular pattern of atrial activity without discernible P waves known as fibrillatory (f) waves. Fibrillation occurs when the atrial cells cannot repolarize in time for the next incoming stimulus. Because of the blocked random conduction through the AV node, QRS complexes appear in an irregular pattern and rate ranging from 80 to 180 beats/minute. Not all ventricular beats produce a palpable pulse. The difference between the apical rate and the palpable peripheral pulses is called the *pulse deficit*.

AF is classified into three categories—paroxysmal, persistent, and permanent.[17] Paroxysmal AF self-terminates and lasts no longer than 7 days, whereas persistent lasts greater than 7 days and usually requires intervention such as a cardioversion. AF is classified as permanent when attempts to terminate are failed and the person remains in AF.

AF can be seen in people without any apparent disease, or it may occur in people with coronary artery disease, mitral valve disease, ischemic heart disease, hypertension, MI, pericarditis, congestive heart failure, digitalis toxicity, and hyperthyroidism. Spontaneous conversion to sinus rhythm within 24 hours of AF is common.[17]

AF is the most common chronic arrhythmia, with an incidence and prevalence that increase with age. The prevalence is also greater in men than that in women.[17]

The symptoms of chronic AF vary from minimal to severe symptoms to ranging from palpitations to acute pulmonary edema. Fatigue and other nonspecific symptoms are common in the elderly. The condition predisposes people to thrombus formation in the atria, with subsequent risk of embolic stroke.

AF can be treated with antiarrhythmic medications to control rate or medically convert to sinus rhythm. Anticoagulant medications may be used to prevent embolic stroke depending on their risk for stroke.[18] Cardioversion may be considered in some persons, particularly when pulmonary edema or unstable cardiac status is present.

Paroxysmal Supraventricular Tachycardia

Paroxysmal supraventricular tachycardia refers to tachyarrhythmias that originate above the bifurcation of the bundle of His and have a sudden onset and termination. The heart rate may be 140 to 240 beats/minute and be perfectly regular despite exercise or change in position.

Most people remain asymptomatic except for an awareness of the rapid heartbeat, but some may experience shortness of breath, especially if the episodes are prolonged. The most common mechanism for paroxysmal supraventricular tachycardia is reentry.

Junctional Arrhythmias

The AV node can act as a pacemaker in the event the SA node fails to initiate an impulse. Junctional rhythms can be transient or permanent, and they usually have a rate of 40 to 60 beats/minute. Junctional fibers in the AV node or bundle of His can also serve as ectopic pacemakers, producing premature junctional complexes. Nonparoxysmal junctional tachycardia is of gradual onset and termination but may occur abruptly if the dominant pacemaker slows sufficiently. The rate associated with ranges from 70 to 130 beats/minute, but it may be faster.[2] The P waves may precede, be buried in, or follow the QRS complexes, depending on the site of the originating impulses. The clinical significance of nonparoxysmal junctional tachycardia is the same as for atrial tachycardias. Catheter ablation therapy has been used successfully to treat some people with recurrent or intractable junctional tachycardia. Nonparoxysmal junctional tachycardia is observed most frequently in people with underlying heart disease, such as inferior wall MI or myocarditis, or after open heart surgery. It may also be present in person with digitalis toxicity.

Disorders of Ventricular Conduction and Rhythm

The junctional fibers in the AV node join with the bundle of His, which divides to form the right and left bundle branches. The bundle branches continue to divide and form the Purkinje fibers, which supply the walls of the ventricles (see Fig. 28-1). As the cardiac impulse leaves the junctional fibers, it travels through the AV bundle. Next, the impulse moves down the right and left bundle branches that lie beneath the endocardium on either side of the septum. It then spreads out through the walls of the ventricles. Interruption of impulse conduction through the bundle branches is called *bundle-branch block*. These blocks usually do not cause alterations in the rhythm of the heartbeat. Instead, a bundle-branch block interrupts the normal progression of depolarization, causing the ventricles to depolarize one after the other because the impulses must travel through muscle tissue rather than through the specialized conduction tissue. This prolonged conduction causes the QRS complex to be wider than the normal 0.08 to 0.12 second. The left bundle branch bifurcates into the left anterior and posterior fascicles.

Long QT Syndrome and Torsade de Pointes

The *long QT syndrome* (LQTS) is characterized by a prolongation of the QT interval that may result in a characteristic type of polymorphic ventricular tachycardia called *torsade de pointes* and sudden cardiac death.[10,12] (Fig. 28-11). *Torsade de pointes* refers to the polarity of

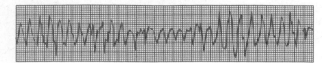

FIGURE 28-11. Torsade de pointes. (From Morton P. G., Fontaine D. K. (2018). *Critical care nursing: A holistic approach* (11th ed., Fig. 17-27B, p. 227). Philadelphia, PA: Wolters Kluwer.)

the QRS complex and is characterized by large, bizarre, polymorphic QRS complexes that vary in amplitude and direction, as well as in rotation of the complexes around the isoelectric line. The rate of tachycardia is 100 to 180, but it can be as fast as 200 to 300 per minute. The rhythm is highly unstable and may terminate in ventricular fibrillation or revert to sinus rhythm.

LQTSs have been classified into inherited and acquired forms. The hereditary forms of LQTS are caused by disorders of membrane ion channel proteins, with either potassium channel defects or sodium channel defects.[19,20] Acquired LQTS are lined to cocaine use, exposure to organophosphorus compounds, electrolyte imbalances, bradycardia, MI, subarachnoid hemorrhage, autonomic neuropathy, human immunodeficiency virus infection, and protein-sparing fasting.[20] Medications linked to LQTS include digitalis, antiarrhythmic agents, verapamil, haloperidol, and erythromycin.[21]

A QT_c greater than 440 ms in men and greater than 460 ms in women has been linked with episodes of sudden arrhythmia death syndromes.

Treatment of acquired forms of LQTS is directed primarily at identifying and withdrawing the offending agent.

Ventricular Arrhythmias

Arrhythmias that arise in the ventricles generally are considered more serious than those that arise in the atria because they afford the potential for interfering with the pumping action of the heart.

Premature Ventricular Contractions

A premature ventricular contraction (PVC) is caused by a ventricular ectopic pacemaker that renders the ventricle unable to repolarize and sufficiently respond to the next electrical impulse. This delay, commonly referred to as a *compensatory pause*, occurs while the ventricle waits to reestablish its previous rhythm (Fig. 28-12). Because the diastolic volume is usually insufficient for ejection of blood into the arterial system, a palpable pulse is absent or significantly diminished. In the absence of heart disease, PVCs are typically not clinically significant. The incidence of PVCs is greatest with ischemia, MI ventricular hypertrophy, infection, increased sympathetic nervous system activity, or increased heart rate.[22] PVCs can also be the result of electrolyte disturbances or medications.

A special pattern of PVC called *ventricular bigeminy* is a condition in which each normal beat is followed by or paired with a PVC. This pattern is often an indication of digitalis toxicity or heart disease. The occurrence of

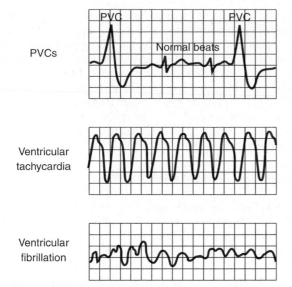

FIGURE 28-12. Electrocardiographic (ECG) tracings of ventricular arrhythmias. Premature ventricular contractions (PVCs) (*top tracing*) originate from an ectopic focus in the ventricles, causing a distortion of the QRS complex. Because the ventricle usually cannot repolarize sufficiently to respond to the next impulse that arises in the SA node, a PVC is frequently followed by a compensatory pause. Ventricular tachycardia (*middle tracing*) is characterized by a rapid ventricular rate of 70 to 250 beats/minute and the absence of P waves. In ventricular fibrillation (*bottom tracing*), there are no regular or effective ventricular contractions, and the ECG tracing is totally disorganized.

frequent PVCs in the diseased heart predisposes to the development of other, more serious arrhythmias, including ventricular tachycardia and ventricular fibrillation.

Ventricular Tachycardia
Ventricular tachycardia describes a cardiac rhythm originating distal to the bifurcation of the bundle of His or in the specialized conduction system in ventricular muscle or both.[2] It is characterized by a ventricular rate of 70 to 250 beats/minute, and the onset can be either sudden or insidious. Usually, ventricular tachycardia is exhibited electrocardiographically by wide, tall, bizarre-looking QRS complexes that persist longer than 0.12 second (see Fig. 28-12). QRS complexes can be uniform in appearance, *monomorphic*, or they can vary randomly (polymorphic).[12] Ventricular tachycardia can be sustained or stop spontaneously. This rhythm is dangerous because it eliminates atrial filling and can cause a reduction in diastolic filling time to the point at which cardiac output is severely diminished or nonexistent.

Ventricular Flutter and Fibrillation
These arrhythmias represent severe derangements of cardiac rhythm that terminate fatally within minutes unless corrective measures are taken promptly. The ECG pattern in ventricular flutter has a sine-wave appearance, with large oscillations occurring at a rate of 150 to 300 per minute.[10] In ventricular fibrillation, the ventricle quivers, but does not contract. The classic ECG pattern of ventricular fibrillation is that of gross disorganization without identifiable waveforms or intervals

(see Fig. 28-12). When the ventricles do not contract, there is no cardiac output and no palpable or audible pulses. Immediate defibrillation using a nonsynchronized, direct-current electrical shock is mandatory for ventricular fibrillation and for ventricular flutter that has caused loss of consciousness.[10]

Disorders of Atrioventricular Conduction

Conduction defects of the AV node are most commonly associated with fibrosis or scar tissue in fibers of the conduction system. Conduction defects may also result from medications, including digoxin, β-adrenergic–blocking agents, calcium channel–blocking agents, and class 1A antiarrhythmic agents.[23] Additional contributing factors include electrolyte imbalances, acute MI, idiopathic fibrosis of the conduction system, inflammatory disease, or cardiac surgery. Some other less common causes include infections, autoimmune, oncologic, and **iatrogenic** disorders.

Heart block refers to abnormalities of impulse conduction. It may be normal, physiologic (*e.g.*, vagal tone), or pathologic. It may occur from a conduction block in the atrium, AV nodal fibers, or in the AV bundle that is continuous with the Purkinje conduction system that supplies the ventricles. The PR interval on the ECG corresponds with the time it takes for the cardiac impulse to travel from the SA node to the ventricular pathways. Normally, the PR interval ranges from 0.12 to 0.20 second.

First-Degree Atrioventricular Block
First-degree AV block is characterized by a prolonged PR interval (>0.20 second; Fig. 28-13). The prolonged PR interval indicates delayed AV conduction, but all atrial

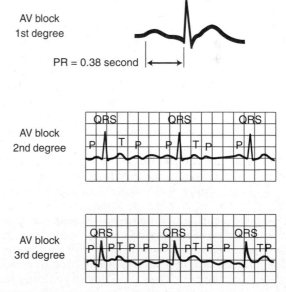

FIGURE 28-13. Electrocardiographic changes that occur with alterations in atrioventricular (AV) node conduction. The *top tracing* shows the prolongation of the PR interval, which is characteristic of first-degree AV block. The *middle tracing* illustrates Mobitz type II second-degree AV block, in which the conduction of one or more P waves is blocked. In third-degree AV block (*bottom tracing*), impulses conducted through the AV node are completely blocked, and the atria and ventricles develop their own rates of impulse generation.

impulses are conducted to the ventricles. This condition usually produces a regular atrial and ventricular rhythm. Clinically significant PR interval prolongation can result from conduction delays in the AV node itself or the His–Purkinje system or both.[18] First-degree block may be the result of disease in the AV node, such as ischemia or infarction, or of infections such as rheumatic fever or myocarditis.[20,23] Isolated first-degree heart block is usually not symptomatic, and temporary or permanent cardiac pacing is not indicated but should be monitored.

Second-Degree Atrioventricular Block

Second-degree AV block is characterized by intermittent failure of conduction of one or more impulses from the atria to the ventricles. The nonconducted P wave can appear intermittently or frequently, whereas the conducted P wave is related to recurring PR intervals.[18] Second-degree AV block has been divided into two types: type I (*i.e.*, Mobitz type I or Wenckebach phenomenon) and type II (*i.e.*, Mobitz type II). A *Mobitz type I* AV block is characterized by progressive lengthening of the PR interval until an impulse is blocked and the sequence begins again. It frequently occurs in person with inferior wall MI, particularly with concomitant right ventricular infarction. The condition is usually associated with an adequate ventricular rate and is rarely symptomatic. It is usually transient and does not require temporary pacing.[18] In the *Mobitz type II* AV block, an intermittent block of atrial impulses occurs, with a constant PR interval (see Fig. 28-13). It frequently accompanies anterior wall MI and can require temporary or permanent pacing. This condition is associated with a high mortality rate. In addition, Mobitz type II AV block is associated with other types of organic heart disease and often progresses to complete heart block.

Third-Degree Atrioventricular Block

Third-degree, or complete, AV block occurs when the conduction link between the atria and the ventricles is lost owing to interruption at the AV node (usually congenital), bundle of His, or Purkinje system (usually acquired), resulting in atrial and ventricular depolarization being controlled by separate pacemakers (see Fig. 28-13). The atrial pacemaker can be sinus or ectopic in origin. The ventricular pacemaker is usually located just below the region of the block. The atria usually continue to beat at a normal rate, and the ventricles develop their own rate, which is normally slow (30 to 40 beats/minute).

Complete heart block causes a decrease in cardiac output with possible periods of syncope (fainting), known as a *Stokes–Adams attack*.[18] Other symptoms include dizziness, fatigue, exercise intolerance, or episodes of acute heart failure.[1] Most people with complete heart block require a permanent cardiac pacemaker.

Inherited Types of Arrhythmias

For many years, people who had died suddenly were referred to as having *idiopathic ventricular fibrillation* when, in fact, ion channel abnormalities or channelopathies were the underlying cause.[24] Evidence now indicates that these cases are genetically determined abnormalities of proteins in the ion channels that control the electrical activity of the heart. Many genes have been associated with inherited arrhythmogenic channelopathies, and it is expected that more will be identified and linked to sudden death in people with apparently healthy hearts.[24,25] Among the inherited arrhythmogenic disorders are congenital LQTS, short QT syndrome (SQTS), Brugada syndrome, and catecholaminergic polymorphic ventricular tachycardia (CPVT).

Congenital Long QT Syndrome

Congenital LQTS is an inherited arrhythmogenic disease characterized by prolonged QT interval, abnormal T wave, and torsade de pointes. Hundreds of gene mutations have been identified on the three major and nine minor LQTS susceptible genes.[19] The severity of the clinical manifestations in LQTS varies, ranging from full-blown disease to no arrhythmias or syncopal episodes.

Depending on which gene is affected, long-term treatment with β-adrenergic receptor blockers, permanent pacing, or left cardiac sympathetic denervation is frequently effective.[25] Placement of an implantable cardioverter–defibrillator is recommended for people in whom recurrent syncope, sustained ventricular arrhythmias, or sudden cardiac arrest occurs despite drug treatment.

Short QT Syndrome

SQTS, an inherited channelopathy, was first described in 2000 and is associated with a QT interval less than 330 ms. It is an autosomal dominant disorder with some people having a family history of heart disease. Most people with this disorder are asymptomatic, and some have history of syncope. The treatment of choice remains an implantable cardioverter–defibrillator to prevent sudden cardiac death.[16,26]

Brugada Syndrome

First described in 1992, Brugada syndrome is an autosomal dominant disorder characterized by ST-segment elevation in precordial leads V_1 to V_3, right bundle-branch block, and susceptibility to ventricular tachycardia.[25] Symptoms associated with this ECG include syncope, palpitations, chest discomfort, cardiac arrest, and nocturnal agonal respiration. It has so far been associated with a single gene encoding for the cardiac sodium channel. The disorder typically manifests in adulthood with very incomplete penetrance, and a high percentage of mutation carriers are asymptomatic.[26] Even though the disorder is inherited as an autosomal trait, a male-to-female ratio of 8:1 is observed in clinical manifestations.[24]

Catecholaminergic Polymorphic Ventricular Tachycardia

CPVT is a disorder characterized by ventricular tachycardia, syncope, and sudden death occurring in familial or sporadic cases in the absence of cardiac disease or ECG abnormalities.

The ECG of people with CPVT is usually remarkably normal, and they do not have structural heart disease. Physical activity and acute emotions are the specific triggers for arrhythmias in people with CPVT. The complexity of the arrhythmias can range from isolated PVCs to ventricular tachycardia depending on workload. It is particularly important to perform genetic analyses to identify mutations. Antiadrenergic treatment with beta-blockers is the cornerstone of therapy for CPVT. The use of an implantable cardioverter–defibrillator may be necessary when exercise stress testing.

Diagnostic Methods

The diagnosis of cardiac rhythm and conduction disorders is usually made on the basis of the surface ECG, Holter ECG monitoring, or implantable loop ECG recording. Further clarification of conduction defects and cardiac arrhythmias can be obtained using exercise stress testing and electrophysiologic studies.

Surface Electrocardiogram

A resting surface ECG records the impulses originating in the heart as they are recorded at the body surface. These impulses are recorded for a limited time and during periods of inactivity. Although there are no complications related to the procedure, errors related to misdiagnosis may result in incorrect diagnosis and treatment.[5,6] The resting ECG is the first approach to the clinical diagnosis of disorders of cardiac rhythm and conduction, but it is limited to events that occur during the period the ECG is being monitored.

Holter Electrocardiogram Monitoring

Holter monitoring is one form of long-term monitoring during which a person wears a device that digitally records two or three ECG leads for up to 48 hours. During this time, the person keeps a diary of his or her activities or symptoms, which later are correlated with the ECG recording. Most recording devices also have an event marker button that can be pressed when the individual experiences symptoms, which assists the technician or physician in correlating the diary, symptoms, and ECG changes during analysis. Event recorders can either recognize abnormalities or allow the individual to activate the unit when symptomatic.[27]

Implantable Loop Electrocardiogram Recorder

If Holter and event monitors do not produce any diagnostic information and a person continues to have symptoms, a loop recorder can be implanted. This device is implanted under the skin in the left upper chest area. It continuously monitors the person's ECG and can be programmed to store patient-activated events when they are symptomatic. The loop recorder can be in place for as long as 3 years. It is useful for documenting arrhythmias, antiarrhythmic drug efficacy, episodes of myocardial ischemia, QT prolongation, pauses, and heart rate variability.

Exercise Stress Testing

The exercise stress test elicits the body's response to measured increases in acute exercise measuring changes in heart rate, blood pressure, respiration, and perceived level of exercise. It is useful in determining exercise-induced alterations in hemodynamic response and ECG ischemic-type ST-segment changes and can detect and classify disturbances in cardiac rhythm and conduction associated with exercise.[28] The stress echocardiogram includes an echocardiogram following the exercise stress test to determine whether there is lack of blood flow to a certain area of the heart.

Electrophysiologic Studies

Electrophysiologic testing is used for the diagnosis and management of complex arrhythmias. It involves the passage of two or more electrode catheters into the right side of the heart.[3] The electrode catheters are used to stimulate the heart and record intracardiac ECGs.

The primary indications for electrophysiologic testing are:

- To determine a person's potential for arrhythmia formation
- To evaluate recurrent syncope of cardiac origin, when ambulatory ECG has not provided the diagnosis
- To differentiate supraventricular from ventricular arrhythmias
- To locate arrhythmogenic foci for therapeutic interventions, such as catheter ablation procedures or antitachycardia devices[11]

Most electrophysiologic studies do not involve left-sided heart access, and therefore, the risk of MI, stroke, or systemic embolism is less than observed with coronary arteriography unless ablation therapy is indicated increasing the risk for venous thrombosis and pulmonary emboli.[29]

Treatment

The treatment of cardiac rhythm or conduction disorders is directed toward controlling the arrhythmia, correcting the cause, and preventing more serious or fatal arrhythmias. Correction may involve simply adjusting an electrolyte disturbance or withholding a medication such as digitalis. Preventing more serious arrhythmias often involves drug therapy, electrical stimulation, or surgical intervention.

Pharmacologic Treatment

Antiarrhythmic drugs act by modifying the disordered formation and conduction of impulses that induce cardiac muscle contraction. These drugs are classified into four major groups (class I through class IV) according to the drug's effect on the action potential of the cardiac cells.[11] Two other types of antiarrhythmic drugs, the cardiac glycosides and adenosine, are not included in this classification schema. The cardiac glycosides (i.e., digitalis drugs) slow the heart rate and are used in the management of arrhythmias, such as atrial tachycardia, atrial flutter, and AF. Adenosine, an endogenous nucleoside that is present in every cell, is used for emergency intravenous treatment of paroxysmal supraventricular tachycardia involving the AV node. It interrupts AV node conduction and slows SA node firing.[30,31]

Class I Drugs

Class I drugs act by blocking the fast sodium channels. These drugs affect impulse conduction, excitability, and automaticity to various degrees and, therefore, have been divided into three groups (IA, IB, and IC) based on the kinetics of their sodium channel effects. Class IA are used in supraventricular and ventricular tachycardias. Class IB are used to treat ventricular arrhythmias. Class IC are effecting for atrial and ventricular premature beats, ventricular tachycardias, atrial and ventricular fibrillation, and flutter.[30,31] Each class has a unique effect on phases of the action potential.

Class II Drugs

Class II drugs are β-adrenergic–blocking drugs that act by blunting the effect of sympathetic nervous system stimulation on the heart, thereby inhibiting calcium channel opening. These drugs decrease automaticity by depressing phase 4 of the action potential. They also decrease heart rate and cardiac contractility. These medications are effective for treatment of supraventricular arrhythmias and tachyarrhythmias by counteracting action on arrhythmogenesis of catecholamines.[24]

Class III Drugs

Class III drugs act by inhibiting the potassium current and repolarization, thereby extending the action potential and refractoriness. They have little inhibiting effect on depolarizing currents. These agents are used in the treatment of serious ventricular arrhythmias.

Class IV Drugs

Class IV drugs act by blocking the slow calcium channels, thereby depressing phase 4 and lengthening phases 1 and 2 of the action potential. By blocking the release of intracellular calcium ions, these agents reduce the force of myocardial contractility, thereby decreasing myocardial oxygen demand. These drugs are used to slow the SA node pacemaker and inhibit conduction in the AV node, slowing the ventricular response in atrial tachycardias, and to terminate reentrant paroxysmal supraventricular tachycardias when the AV node functions as a reentrant pathway.[24]

Electrical Interventions

The correction of conduction defects, bradycardias, and tachycardias can involve the use of a pacemaker, cardioversion, or defibrillation. Electrical interventions can be used in emergency and elective situations.

Cardiac Pacemaker

A cardiac pacemaker is an electronic device that delivers an electrical stimulus to the heart. It is used to initiate heartbeats in situations when the normal pacemaker of the heart is defective. These situations include certain types of AV heart block, symptomatic bradycardia in which the rate of cardiac contraction and consequent cardiac output are inadequate to perfuse vital tissues, as well as other cardiac arrhythmias. A pacemaker may be used as a temporary or permanent measure. Pacemaker leads can pace the atria, the ventricles, or the atria and ventricles sequentially, or overdrive pacing can be used.

Overdrive pacing may be used to try to treat recurrent ventricular tachycardia and reentrant atrial or ventricular tachyarrhythmias and to terminate atrial flutter.[22]

Synchronized Cardioversion and Defibrillation

Synchronized cardioversion and defibrillation are two reliable methods for treating ventricular tachycardia, and cardioversion is the definitive treatment for AF. The discharge of electrical energy that is synchronized with the R wave of the ECG is referred to as *synchronized cardioversion*, and unsynchronized discharge is known as *defibrillation*. The goal of both of these techniques is to provide an electrical pulse to the heart in such a way as to depolarize the heart completely during passage of the current. This electrical current interrupts the disorganized impulses, allowing the SA node to regain control of the heart.[32]

 Concept Mastery Alert

The electricity in nonsynchronized defibrillation depolarizes the entire heart, interrupting the chaotic rhythm and allowing the SA node to take control.

Automatic implantable cardioverter–defibrillators (AICDs) are being used successfully to treat people with life-threatening ventricular tachyarrhythmias by the use of intrathoracic electrical countershock.[32] The AICD can also be programmed to provide antitachycardia pacing, which will pace faster than the ventricular rate to try to terminate the arrhythmia. All AICDs respond to ventricular tachyarrhythmia at fast rates by delivering an electrical shock between intrathoracic electrodes within 10 to 20 seconds of its onset.[22]

Ablation and Surgical Interventions

Ablation therapy is used for treating recurrent, life-threatening supraventricular and ventricular tachyarrhythmias. Ablative therapy may be performed by catheter or surgical techniques. It involves localized destruction, isolation, or excision of cardiac tissue that is considered to be arrhythmogenic.[3,28]

RF ablation uses RF waves to destroy defective or aberrant electrical conduction pathways. RF ablation remains the most common method for ablating cardiac arrhythmias. An additional kind of energy that was developed was cryoenergy, or freezing. Cryoablation involves the direct application of an extremely cold probe to arrhythmogenic cardiac tissue.[23]

Coronary artery bypass surgery improves myocardial oxygenation by increasing blood supply to the myocardium. Ventriculotomy involves the removal of aneurysm tissue and the resuturing of the myocardial walls to eliminate the paradoxical ventricular movement and the foci of arrhythmias. In endocardial resection, endocardial tissue that has been identified as arrhythmogenic through the use of electrophysiologic testing or intraoperative mapping is surgically removed. Ventriculotomy and endocardial resection have been performed with cryoablation or laser ablation as an adjunctive therapy.[33]

SUMMARY CONCEPTS

Disorders of cardiac rhythm arise as the result of disturbances in impulse generation or conduction in the heart. Normal sinus rhythm and respiratory sinus arrhythmia are considered normal cardiac rhythms. Cardiac arrhythmias are not necessarily pathologic; they occur in healthy and diseased hearts. Sinus arrhythmias originate in the SA node and include sinus bradycardia, sinus tachycardia, sinus arrest, and SSS.

Atrial arrhythmias arise from alterations in impulse generation that occur in the conduction pathways or muscle of the atria. They include PACs, atrial flutter, and AF. Atrial arrhythmias often go unnoticed unless they are transmitted to the ventricles.

Arrhythmias that arise in the ventricles are commonly considered more serious than those that arise in the atria because they afford the potential for interfering with the pumping action of the heart. The LQTS represents a prolongation of the QT interval that may result in torsade de pointes and sudden cardiac death. A PVC is caused by a ventricular ectopic pacemaker. Ventricular tachycardia is characterized by a ventricular rate of 70 to 250 beats/minute. Ventricular fibrillation is a fatal arrhythmia unless it is successfully treated with defibrillation. Arrhythmogenic cardiomyopathies are inherited disorders of the ion channels that control the electrical activity of the heart. Among the inherited arrhythmogenic disorders are congenital LQTS, SQTS, Brugada syndrome, and CPVT.

Alterations in the conduction of impulses through the AV node lead to disturbances in the transmission of impulses from the atria to the ventricles. There can be a delay in transmission (*i.e.*, first-degree heart block), failure to conduct one or more impulses (*i.e.*, second-degree heart block), or complete failure to conduct impulses between the atria and the ventricles (*i.e.*, third-degree heart block). Conduction disorders of the bundle of His and Purkinje system, called *bundle-branch blocks*, cause a widening of and changes in the configuration of the QRS complex of the ECG.

The diagnosis of disorders of cardiac rhythm and conduction is typically accomplished using surface ECG recordings or electrophysiologic studies. Surface electrodes can be used to obtain a 12-lead ECG; signal-averaged electrocardiographic studies in which multiple samples of QRS waves are averaged to detect ventricular late action potentials; and Holter monitoring, which provides continuous ECG recordings for up to 48 hours, and loop recording, which provides continuous recording up to 3 years. Electrophysiologic studies use electrode catheters inserted into the right heart through a peripheral vein as a means of directly stimulating the heart while obtaining an intracardiac ECG recording.

Both medications and electrical devices are used in the treatment of arrhythmias and conduction disorders. Antiarrhythmic drugs act by modifying disordered formation and conduction of impulses that induce cardiac muscle contraction. They include drugs that act by blocking the fast sodium channels, β-adrenergic–blocking drugs that decrease sympathetic outflow to the heart, drugs that act by inhibiting the potassium current and repolarization, calcium channel–blocking agents, cardiac glycosides (*i.e.*, digitalis drugs), and adenosine, which is used for emergency intravenous treatment of paroxysmal supraventricular tachycardia involving the AV mode. Electrical devices include temporary and permanent cardiac pacemakers that are used to treat symptomatic bradycardias or to provide overdrive pacing procedures; defibrillators that are used to treat atrial and ventricular fibrillation; external or internally implanted cardioversion devices, which can be used to treat ventricular tachycardia; and RF ablation and cryoablation therapy, which are used to destroy specific irritable foci in the heart. Surgical procedures can be performed to excise irritable or dysfunctional tissue, to replace cardiac valves, or to provide better blood supply to the myocardial muscle wall.

Review Exercises

1. A 75-year-old woman with a history of congestive heart failure presents to the clinic complaining of feeling tired. Her heart rate is 121 beats/minute, and the rhythm is irregular.

   A. What type of arrhythmia do you think she might be having? What would it look like if you were to obtain an ECG?
   B. What causes this irregularity?
   C. Why do you think she is feeling tired?
   D. What are some of the concerns with this type of arrhythmia?

2. A 45-year-old man appears at the urgent care center with complaints of chest discomfort, shortness of breath, and generally not feeling well. You assess vital signs and find that his temperature is 99.2°F, blood pressure 180/90, pulse 90 and slightly irregular, and respiratory rate 26. You do an ECG, and the readings from the anterior leads indicate that he is experiencing an ischemic episode.

   A. You attach him to a cardiac monitor and see that his underlying rhythm is normal sinus rhythm, but he is having frequent premature contractions that are more than 0.10 second in duration. What type of premature contractions do you suspect?

B. What would you expect his pulse to feel like?

C. What do you think the etiology of this arrhythmia might be? How might it be treated?

REFERENCES

1. Guyton A. C., Hall J. E. (2016). *Textbook of medical physiology* (131th ed., pp. 109–123, 155–165, 1115–1127, 1157). Philadelphia, PA: Elsevier Saunders.
2. Rubart M., Zipes D. P. (2012). Genesis of cardiac arrhythmias: Electrophysiologic considerations. In Bonow R. O., Mann D. L., Zipes D. P., et al. (Eds.), *Braunwald's heart disease: A textbook of cardiovascular medicine* (9th ed., pp. 653–687). Philadelphia, PA: Elsevier Saunders.
3. Fogoros R. N. (2012). *Electrophysiologic testing* (5th ed., pp. 4–12, 210–256). Hoboken, NJ: Wiley-Blackwell.
4. Klabunde R. (2012). *Cardiovascular physiology concepts* (2nd ed., pp. 1–67). Philadelphia, PA: Lippincott Williams & Wilkins.
5. Rao B. N. V. R. (2017). *Clinical examination in cardiology* (2nd ed., p. 48). Philadelphia, PA: Elsevier Saunders.
6. Garcia T. (2015). Acquiring the 12 lead electrocardiogram doing it right every time. *Journal of Emergency Nursing* 41(6), 474–478.
7. Morton P. G., Fontaine D. K. (2018). Anatomy and physiology of the cardiovascular system. In *Critical care nursing: A holistic approach* (11th ed., pp. 173–183). Philadelphia, PA: Wolters Kluwer.
8. Drew B., Califf R., Funk M., et al. (2004). Practice standards for electrocardiographic monitoring in hospital settings. *Circulation* 110, 2721–2746.
9. Jones T., Goldberger Z. (2016). Errors in electrocardiography monitoring, computerized EGC, other sites of ECG recording. In Stroobandt R. X., Serge Barold S., Sinnaeve A. F. (Eds.), *ECG from basics to essentials: Step by step*. Chichester, UK: John Wiley & Sons, Ltd.
10. Olgin J. L., Zipes D. P. (2012). Specific arrhythmias: Diagnosis and treatment. In Bonow R. O., Mann D. L., Zipes D. P., et al. (Eds.), *Braunwald's heart disease: A textbook of cardiovascular medicine* (13th ed., pp. 771–823). Philadelphia, PA: Elsevier Saunders.
11. Bashore T. M., Granger C. B., Jackson K., et al. (2017). The heart. In Papadakis M. A., McPhee S. J., Rabow M. W. (Eds.), *Current medical diagnosis and treatment* (56th ed., pp. 322–438). New York: McGraw-Hill.
12. Morton P. G., Reck K., Headley J. M. (2018). Patient assessment: Cardiovascular system. In Morton P. G., Fontaine D. K. (Eds.), *Critical care nursing: A holistic approach* (11th ed., pp. 184–261). Philadelphia, PA: Wolters Kluwer.
13. Ewy G. (2014). Sick sinus syndrome. *Journal of the American College of Cardiology* 64(6), 539–540.
14. Semelka M., Gera J., Usman S.(2013). Sick sinus syndrome: A review. *American Academy of Family Physicians* 87(10), 691–696.
15. Page R. L., Joglar J. A., Caldwell M. A., et al. (2016). 2015 ACC/AHA/HRS guideline for the management of adult patients with supraventricular tachycardia. *Journal of the American College of Cardiology* 67(13), e27–e115. doi:10.1016/j.jacc.2015.08.856.
16. Mazzanti A., Kanthan A., Montefore N., et al. (2014). Novel insight into the natural history of short QT syndrome. *Journal of the American College of Cardiology* 63(13), 1300–1308.
17. Members W. C., January C. T., Wann L. S., et al. (2014). 2014 AHA/ACC/HRS guideline for the management of patients with atrial fibrillation: A report of the American College of Cardiology/American Heart Association Task Force on Practice Guidelines and the Heart Rhythm Society. *Circulation* 130(23), e199.
18. Curtis A. (2013). Practice implication of the atrial fibrillation guidelines. *American Journal of Cardiology* 111, 1660–1670.
19. Nakano Y., Shimizu W. (2015). Genetics of long QT syndrome. *Journal of Human Genetics* 61, 51–55.
20. Abrams D., MacRae C. (2014). Long QT syndrome. *Circulation* 129, 1524–1529.
21. Earl G., Hankins S. (2016). Drug-induced long QT syndrome. *Nursing Critical Care* 11(5), 5–10.
22. Knight B. P. (2017). Patient education: Implantable cardioverter-defibrillators (Beyond the Basics). *UpToDate* [Online]. Available: https://www.uptodate.com/contents/implantable-cardioverter-defibrillators-beyond-the-basics. Accessed May 16, 2019.
23. Garg J., Chaudhary R., Palaniswamy C., et al. (2016). Cryoballoon versus radiofrequency ablation for atrial fibrillation: A meta-analysis of 16 clinical trials. *Journal of Atrial Fibrillation* 9(3), 1429.
24. Steinberg J., Mittal S. (2017). *Electrophysiology: The basics* (2nd ed., pp. 301–322, 271–298). Philadelphia, PA: Wolters Kluwer.
25. Tester D. J., Ackerman M. J. (2012). Genetics of cardiac arrhythmias. In Bonow R. O., Mann D. L., Zipes D. P., et al. (Eds.), *Braunwald's heart disease: A textbook of cardiovascular medicine* (9th ed., pp. 81–90). Philadelphia, PA: Elsevier Saunders.
26. Khera S., Jacobson J. T. (2016). Short QT syndrome in current clinical practice. *Cardiology in Review* 24(4), 190–193.
27. Miller J. M., Zipes D. P. (2012). Diagnosis of cardiac arrhythmias. In Bonow R. O., Mann D. L., Zipes D. P., et al. (Eds.), *Braunwald's heart disease: A textbook of cardiovascular medicine* (9th ed., pp. 702–709). Philadelphia, PA: Elsevier Saunders.
28. Garner K. K., Pomeroy W., Arnold J. J. (2017). Exercise stress testing: Indications and common questions. *American Family Physician* 96(5), 293–299.
29. Synder M. L., Coombs V. J., Barquist K. C., et al. (2018). Patient management: Cardiovascular system. In Morton P. G., Fontaine D. K. (Eds.), *Critical care nursing: A holistic approach* (11th ed., pp. 261–336). Philadelphia, PA: Wolters Kluwer.
30. Kumar K., Zimetbaum P. J. (2013). Antiarrhythmic drugs 2013: State of the art. *Invasive Electrophysiology and Pacing* 14, 409–416.
31. Parker M., Sanoski C. (2016). Clinical Pearls in using antiarrhythmic drugs in the outpatient setting. *Journal of Pharmacy Practice* 29(1), 77–86.
32. Fisher J. D., Furman S., Kim S. G., et al. (1992). Antitachycardia pacing, cardioversion, and defibrillation: From the past to the future. In Alt E., Klein H., Griffin J. C. (Eds.), *The implantable cardioverter/defibrillator*. Berlin, Heidelberg: Springer.
33. Eliopoulos C. (2018). Circulation. In *Gerontological nursing* (9th ed., pp. 268–291). Philadelphia, PA: Wolters Kluwer.

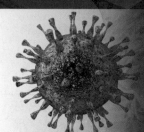
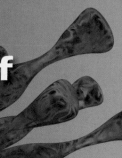

UNIT 9

Disorders of Respiratory Function

CHAPTER 29

Structure and Function of the Respiratory System

Structural Organization of the Respiratory System

Conducting Airways
Nasopharyngeal Airways
Larynx
Tracheobronchial Tree
Lungs and Respiratory Airways
Lobules
Alveoli
Pulmonary Vasculature and Lymphatic Supply
Pulmonary and Bronchial Circulations
Lymphatic Circulation
Innervation
Pleura

Exchange of Gases between the Atmosphere and the Lungs

Basic Properties of Gases
Ventilation and the Mechanics of Breathing
Respiratory Pressures
Chest Cage and Respiratory Muscles
Lung Compliance
Airway Airflow
Lung Volumes
Pulmonary Function Studies
Efficiency and the Work of Breathing

Exchange and Transport of Gases

Ventilation
Distribution of Ventilation
Dead Air Space
Perfusion
Distribution of Blood Flow

Hypoxia-Induced Vasoconstriction
Shunt
Mismatching of Ventilation and Perfusion
Diffusion
Oxygen and Carbon Dioxide Transport
Oxygen Transport
Carbon Dioxide Transport

Control of Breathing

Respiratory Center
Regulation of Breathing
Chemoreceptors
Lung Receptors
Cough Reflex
Dyspnea

Learning Objectives

After completing this chapter, the learner will be able to meet the following objectives:

1. State the difference between the conducting and the respiratory airways.
2. Trace the movement of air through the airways, beginning in the nose and oropharynx and moving into the respiratory tissues of the lung.
3. Differentiate the function of the bronchial and pulmonary circulations that supply the lungs.
4. Describe the basic properties of gases in relation to their partial pressures and their pressures in relation to volume and temperature.
5. Compare intrathoracic, intrapleural, and intra-alveolar pressures, in relation to how each of these pressures changes in relation to

atmospheric pressure during inspiration and expiration.

6. Define inspiratory reserve, expiratory reserve, vital capacity, residual lung volume, and $FEV_{1.0}$.
7. Differentiate between pulmonary and alveolar ventilation.
8. Explain why ventilation and perfusion must be matched.
9. Describe the difference between dead air space and shunt.
10. Explain the significance of a shift to the right and a shift to the left in the oxygen–hemoglobin dissociation curve.
11. Compare the neural control of the respiratory muscles, which control breathing, with that of cardiac muscle, which controls the pumping action of the heart.
12. Trace the integration of the cough reflex from stimulus to explosive expulsion of air that constitutes the cough.
13. List three types of conditions in which dyspnea occurs.

The primary function of the respiratory system, which consists of the airways and lungs, is gas exchange. Oxygen from the air is transferred to the blood, and carbon dioxide from the blood is eliminated into the atmosphere. In addition to gas exchange, the lungs serve as a host defense by providing a barrier between the external environment and the inside of the body. Finally, the lung is also a metabolic organ that synthesizes and metabolizes different compounds.

This chapter focuses on the structural organization of the respiratory system, exchange of gases between the atmosphere and the lungs, exchange of gases in the lungs and its transport in the blood, and control of breathing.

Structural Organization of the Respiratory System

The respiratory system consists of the air passages (two lungs) and the blood vessels that supply them. It also consists of the structures that provide a ventilator mechanism, that is, the rib cage and the respiratory muscles, which include the diaphragm—the principal respiratory muscle.

The lungs are soft, spongy, cone-shaped organs located side by side in the chest cavity (Fig. 29-1). They are separated from each other by the *mediastinum* (*i.e.,* the space between the lungs) and its contents—the heart, blood vessels, lymph nodes, nerve fibers, thymus gland, and esophagus. The upper part of the lung, which lies against the top of the thoracic cavity, is called the *apex*, and the lower part, which lies against the diaphragm, is called the *base*. The lungs are divided into lobes, three in the right lung and two in the left.

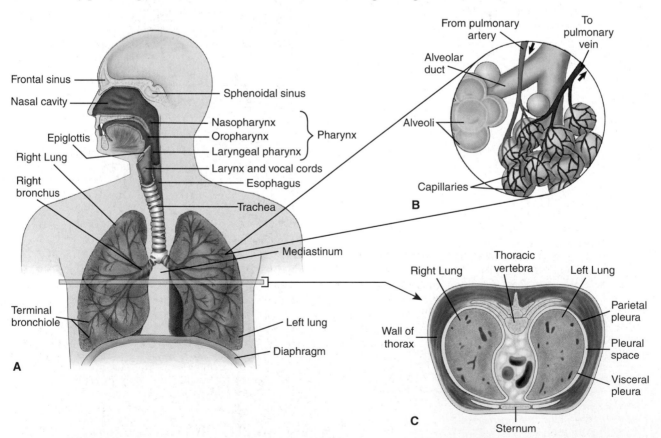

FIGURE 29-1. The respiratory system. (**A**) Upper respiratory structures and the structures of the thorax. (**B**) Alveoli. (**C**) A horizontal cross section of the lungs. (From Hinkle J. L., Cheever K. H. (2018). *Brunner & Suddarth's textbook of medical-surgical nursing* (14th ed., Fig. 20-3, p. 482). Philadelphia, PA: Wolters Kluwer.)

Functionally, the respiratory system can be divided into two parts: the *conducting airways*, through which air moves as it passes between the atmosphere and the lungs, and the *respiratory tissues* of the lungs, where gas exchange takes place.

KEY POINTS

Conducting and Respiratory Airways

- Respiration requires ventilation, or movement of gases into and out of the lungs; perfusion, or movement of blood through the lungs; and diffusion of gases between the lungs and the blood.

- Ventilation depends on the conducting airways, including the nasopharynx and oropharynx, larynx, and tracheobronchial tree, which move air into and out of the lungs but do not participate in gas exchange.

- Gas exchange takes place in the respiratory airways of the lungs, where gases diffuse across the alveolar–capillary membrane as they are exchanged between the air in the lungs and the blood that flows through the pulmonary capillaries.

Conducting Airways

The conducting airways consist of the nasal passages, mouth and pharynx, larynx, trachea, bronchi, and bronchioles (see Fig. 29-1). Besides functioning as a conduit for airflow, the conducting airways serve to "condition" the inspired air. The air we breathe is warmed, filtered, and moistened as it moves through these structures. Heat is transferred to the air from the blood flowing through the walls of the respiratory passages. The mucociliary blanket removes foreign materials, and water from the mucous membranes is used to moisten the air.

A combination of cartilage, elastic and collagen fibers, and smooth muscle provides the airways with the rigidity and flexibility needed to maintain airway patency and ensure an uninterrupted supply of air. Most of the conducting airways are lined with ciliated pseudostratified columnar epithelium, containing a mosaic of mucus-secreting glands, ciliated cells with hairlike projections, and serous glands that secrete a watery fluid containing antibacterial enzymes (Fig. 29-2). The epithelial layer gradually becomes thinner as it moves from the pseudostratified epithelium of the bronchi to cuboidal epithelium of the bronchioles and then to squamous epithelium of the alveoli.

The mucus produced by the epithelial cells in the conducting airways forms a layer, called the *mucociliary blanket*. This layer protects the respiratory system by entrapping dust, bacteria, and other foreign particles that enter the airways. The cilia, which are in constant motion, move the mucociliary blanket with its entrapped particles in an escalator-like manner toward the oropharynx. At this point, the mucociliary blanket is expectorated or swallowed. The function of cilia in clearing the lower airways is optimal at normal oxygen levels. Drying conditions, such as breathing heated but unhumidified indoor air during the winter months, also impair function. Cigarette smoking slows down or paralyzes the motility of the cilia. This slowing allows the residue from tobacco smoke, dust, and other particles to accumulate in the lungs, decreasing the efficiency of this pulmonary defense system. These changes are thought to contribute to the development of chronic bronchitis and emphysema.

Water contained in the mucous membranes of the upper airways and the tracheobronchial tree keeps the conducting airways moist. The capacity of the air to contain moisture without condensation increases as the temperature rises. Thus, the air in the alveoli, which is maintained at body temperature, usually contains

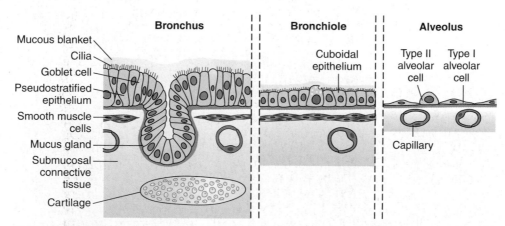

FIGURE 29-2. Airway wall structure: bronchus, bronchiole, and alveolus. The bronchial wall contains pseudostratified epithelium, smooth muscle cells, mucus glands, connective tissue, and cartilage. In smaller bronchioles, a simple epithelium is found, cartilage is absent, and the wall is thinner. The alveolar wall is designed for gas exchange rather than structural support. (From Porth C. M. (2015). *Essentials of pathophysiology* (4th ed., Fig. 21-6, p. 517). Philadelphia, PA: Lippincott Williams & Wilkins.)

considerably more moisture than does the atmosphere—temperature air that we breathe. The difference between the moisture contained in the air we breathe and that found in the alveoli is drawn from the moist surface of the mucous membranes that line the conducting airways. This is a source of insensible water loss. When a person has a fever, the water vapor in the lungs increases, causing more water to be lost from the respiratory mucosa. Also, fever is usually accompanied by an increase in respiratory rate so that more air needing to be moisturized passes through the airways. As a result, respiratory secretions thicken, preventing free movement of the cilia and impairing the protective function of the mucociliary defense system. This is particularly true in people whose fluid intake is inadequate and/or who have dehydration as a result of another pathologic cause.

Nasopharyngeal Airways

The nose is the preferred route for the entrance of air into the respiratory tract during normal breathing. As air passes through the nasal passages, it is filtered, warmed, and humidified. The outer nasal passages are lined with coarse hairs, which filter and trap dust and other large particles from the air. The upper portion of the nasal cavity is lined with a mucous membrane that contains a rich network of small blood vessels. This portion of the nasal cavity supplies warmth and moisture to the air we breathe.

The mouth serves as an alternative airway when the nasal passages are plugged or when there is a need for the exchange of large amounts of air. The oropharynx extends posteriorly from the soft palate to the epiglottis and is the only opening between the nose, mouth, and lungs. Both swallowed food on its way to the esophagus and air on its way to the larynx pass through it. Obstruction of the oropharynx leads to immediate cessation of ventilation. Neural control of the tongue and pharyngeal muscles may be impaired in coma and other neurologic disorders, allowing the tongue falls back into the pharynx and obstructs the airway, particularly if the person is lying on his or her back. Swelling of the pharyngeal structures caused by injury, infection, or severe allergic reaction or the presence of a foreign body also predisposes a person to airway obstruction.

Larynx

The larynx connects the oropharynx with the trachea. It is located between the upper airways and the lungs. The walls of the larynx are supported by firm cartilaginous structures that prevent collapse during inspiration. The functions of the larynx can be divided into two categories: those associated with speech and those associated with protecting the lungs from substances other than air.

The cavity of the larynx is divided into two pairs of shelflike folds stretching from front to back with an opening in the midline (Fig. 29-3). The upper pair of folds, called the *vestibular folds*, has a protective function. The lower pair of folds, called the *vocal folds*, produces the vibrations required for making vocal sounds. The vocal folds and the elongated opening between them are called the *glottis*. A complex set of muscles controls the opening and closing of the glottis. The *epiglottis*, which is located above the larynx, is a large, leaf-shaped piece of cartilage that is covered with epithelium. When

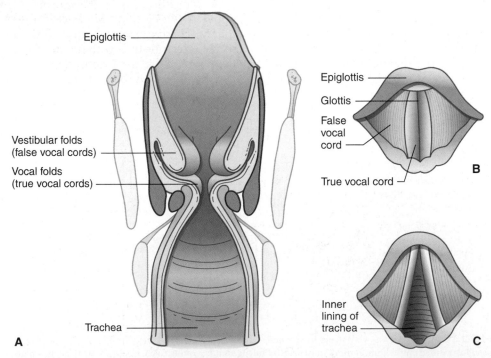

FIGURE 29-3. (A) Coronal section showing the position of the epiglottis, the vestibular folds (true vocal cords), vocal folds (false vocal cords), and glottis. (B) Vocal cords viewed from above with glottis closed and (C) with glottis open.

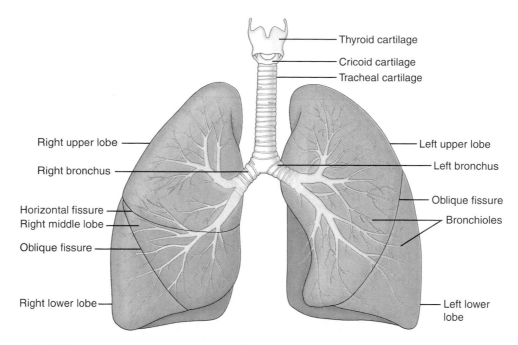

FIGURE 29-4. Anterior view of the lungs. The lungs consist of five lobes. The right lung has three lobes (upper, middle, and lower); the left has two lobes (upper and lower). The lobes are further subdivided into fissures. The bronchial tree, another lung structure, inflates with air to fill the lobes. (From Hinkle J. L., Cheever K. H. (2018). *Brunner & Suddarth's textbook of medical-surgical nursing* (14th ed., Fig. 20-4, p. 483). Philadelphia, PA: Wolters Kluwer.)

only air is flowing through the larynx, the inlet of the larynx is open and the free edges of the epiglottis point upward. During swallowing, the larynx is pulled superiorly and the free edges of the epiglottis move downward to cover the larynx, thus routing liquids and foods into the esophagus.

In addition to opening and closing the glottis for speech, the vocal folds of the larynx can perform a sphincter function, closing off the airways. When confronted with substances other than air, the laryngeal muscles contract and close off the airway. At the same time, the cough reflex is initiated as a means of removing a foreign substance from the airway. If the swallowing mechanism is partially or totally paralyzed, food and fluids can enter the airways instead of the esophagus when a person attempts to swallow. Substances entering the airways can cause a serious inflammatory condition called *aspiration pneumonia.*

Tracheobronchial Tree

The tracheobronchial tree, which consists of the trachea, bronchi, and bronchioles, can be viewed as a system of branching tubes flowing through the lobes of the lungs. There are approximately 23 levels of branching, beginning with the conducting airways and ending with the respiratory airways, where gas exchange takes place (see Fig. 29-4).

The trachea, or windpipe, is a continuous tube that connects the larynx and the major bronchi of the lungs. The walls of the trachea are supported by horseshoe- or C-shaped rings of hyaline cartilage, which prevent it from collapsing when the pressure in the thorax

becomes negative (Fig. 29-5). The open part of the C ring, which abuts the esophagus, is connected by smooth muscle. Because this portion of the trachea is not rigid, the esophagus can expand anteriorly as swallowed food passes through it.

The trachea extends from the larynx where it divides to form the right and left main or primary bronchi. The

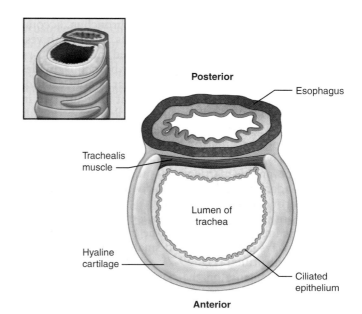

FIGURE 29-5. Cross section of the trachea illustrating its relationship to the esophagus, the position of the supporting hyaline cartilage rings in its wall, and the trachealis muscle connecting the free ends of the cartilage rings.

pneumonia. The characteristics of the gas and its molecular weight and solubility constitute the diffusion coefficient and determine how rapidly a gas diffuses through the respiratory membranes. For example, carbon dioxide diffuses 20 times more rapidly than oxygen because of its greater solubility in the respiratory membranes.

The diffusing capacity provides a measure of the rate of gas transfer in the lungs per partial pressure gradient. Because the initial alveolar–capillary difference for oxygen cannot be measured, carbon monoxide (CO) is used to determine the diffusing capacity.

Oxygen and Carbon Dioxide Transport

Although the lungs are responsible for the exchange of gases with the external environment, it is the blood that transports these gases between the lungs and body tissues. The blood carries oxygen and carbon dioxide in the physically dissolved state and in combination with hemoglobin. Carbon dioxide is also converted to bicarbonate and transported in that form.

Dissolved oxygen and carbon dioxide exert a partial pressure that is designated in the same manner as the partial pressures in the gas state. In the clinical setting, blood gas measurements are used to determine the partial pressure of oxygen (PO_2) and carbon dioxide (PCO_2) in the blood.

Concept Mastery Alert

Arterial blood is commonly used for measuring blood gases. Venous blood is not used because venous levels of oxygen and carbon dioxide reflect the metabolic demands of the tissues rather than the gas exchange function of the lungs.

Normally, the arterial blood gases (ABGs) are the same or nearly the same as the partial pressure (Pa) of the gases in the alveoli. For example, the arterial PO_2 is often written PaO_2. This text uses PO_2 and PCO_2 to designate both arterial and alveolar levels of the gases. See Table 29-3 for normal range of ABGs.

Oxygen Transport

Oxygen is transported in two forms:

- In chemical combination with hemoglobin
- In the dissolved state

TABLE 29-3 Arterial Blood Gas Ranges

Parameter	Range
1. pH = acid or base	7.35–7.45
2. PCO_2 = partial pressure of carbon dioxide	35–45 mm Hg
3. HCO_3^- = bicarbonate	22–26 mEq/L
4. PO_2 = partial pressure of oxygen	80–100 mm Hg

Hemoglobin carries about 98% to 99% of oxygen in the blood and is the main transporter of oxygen. The remaining 1% to 2% of the oxygen is carried in the dissolved state. Only the dissolved form of oxygen passes through the capillary wall, diffuses through the cell membrane, and makes itself available for use in cell metabolism. The oxygen content (measured in mL/100 mL) of the blood includes the oxygen carried by hemoglobin and is in the dissolved state.

Hemoglobin Transport

Hemoglobin is a highly efficient carrier of oxygen. Hemoglobin with bound oxygen is called *oxyhemoglobin*. When oxygen is removed, it is called *deoxygenated* or *reduced hemoglobin*. Each gram of hemoglobin carries approximately 1.34 mL of oxygen when it is fully saturated. This means that a person with a hemoglobin level of 14 g/100 mL carries 18.8 mL of oxygen per 100 mL of blood.

In the lungs, oxygen moves across the alveolar–capillary membrane, through the plasma, and into the red blood cell, where it forms a loose and reversible bond with the hemoglobin molecule. In normal lungs, this process is rapid. Therefore, even with a fast heart rate, the hemoglobin is almost completely saturated with oxygen during the short time it spends in the pulmonary capillaries. As the oxygen moves out of the capillaries in response to the needs of the tissues, the hemoglobin saturation drops. It is approximately 95% to 97% saturated as the blood leaves the left side of the heart. It then drops to approximately 75% saturation as the mixed venous blood returns to the right side of the heart.

Binding Affinity of Hemoglobin for Oxygen

The efficiency of the hemoglobin transport system depends on the ability of the hemoglobin molecule to bind oxygen in the lungs and release it as it is needed in the tissues. Oxygen that remains bound to hemoglobin cannot participate in tissue metabolism. The term *affinity* refers to hemoglobin's ability to bind oxygen. Hemoglobin binds oxygen more readily when its affinity is increased and releases it more readily when its affinity is decreased.

The hemoglobin molecule is composed of four polypeptide chains with an iron-containing heme group. Because oxygen binds to the iron atom, each hemoglobin molecule can bind four molecules of oxygen when it is fully saturated. Oxygen binds cooperatively with the heme groups on the hemoglobin molecule. After the first molecule of oxygen binds to hemoglobin, the molecule undergoes a change in shape. As a result, the second and third molecules bind more readily, and binding of the fourth molecule is even easier. In a like manner, the unloading of the first molecule of oxygen enhances the unloading of the next molecule and so on. Thus, the affinity of hemoglobin for oxygen changes with hemoglobin saturation.

Hemoglobin's affinity for oxygen is also influenced by pH, carbon dioxide concentration, and body temperature. It binds oxygen more readily under conditions of increased pH (alkalosis), decreased carbon dioxide concentration, and decreased body temperature, and it releases it more readily under conditions of decreased pH (acidosis), increased carbon dioxide concentration, and fever. For example, increased tissue metabolism generates carbon dioxide and metabolic acids and thereby decreases the affinity of hemoglobin for oxygen. Heat is also a by-product of tissue metabolism, explaining the effect of fever on oxygen binding.

Red blood cells contain a metabolic intermediate called *2,3-diphosphoglycerate (2,3-DPG)* that also affects the affinity of hemoglobin for oxygen. An increase in 2,3-DPG enhances unloading of oxygen from hemoglobin at the tissue level. Conditions that increase 2,3-DPG include exercise, hypoxia that occurs at high altitude, and chronic lung disease.[1]

The Oxygen Dissociation Curve

The relation between the oxygen carried in combination with hemoglobin and the PO_2 of the blood is described by the *oxygen–hemoglobin dissociation curve*, which is shown in Figure 29-21. The x-axis of the graph depicts the PO_2 or dissolved oxygen. It reflects the partial pressure of the oxygen in the lungs (*i.e.*, the PO_2 is approximately 100 mm Hg when room air is being breathed, but can rise to 200 mm Hg or higher when oxygen-enriched air is breathed). The left y-axis depicts hemoglobin saturation or the amount of oxygen that is carried by the hemoglobin. The right y-axis depicts oxygen content or total amount of the oxygen content being carried in the blood.

The S-shaped oxygen dissociation curve has a flat top portion representing binding of oxygen to hemoglobin in the lungs and a steep portion representing its release into the tissue capillaries (see Fig. 29-21A). The S shape of the curve reflects the effect that oxygen saturation has on the conformation of the hemoglobin molecule and its affinity for oxygen.

The steep portion of the dissociation curve—between 60 and 40 mm Hg—represents the removal of oxygen from the hemoglobin as it moves through the tissue capillaries. This portion of the curve reflects a considerable transfer of oxygen from hemoglobin to the tissues with only a small drop in PO_2. This ensures a gradient for oxygen to move into body cells.

Hemoglobin can be regarded as a buffer system that regulates the delivery of oxygen to the tissues. In order to function as a buffer system, the affinity of hemoglobin for oxygen must change with the metabolic needs of the tissues. This change is represented by a shift to the right or left in the dissociation curve (see Fig. 29-21B). A shift to the right indicates that the tissue PO_2 is greater for any given level of hemoglobin saturation and represents reduced affinity of the hemoglobin for oxygen at any given PO_2. It is usually caused by conditions that reflect increased tissue metabolism, such as fever or acidosis, or by an increase in PCO_2. High altitude and conditions such as pulmonary insufficiency, heart failure, and severe anemia also cause the oxygen dissociation curve to shift to the right. A shift to the left in the oxygen dissociation curve represents an increased affinity of hemoglobin for oxygen. It occurs in situations associated with a decrease in tissue metabolism, such as alkalosis, decreased body temperature, and decreased PCO_2 levels. The degree of shift can be determined by the P_{50}, or the partial pressure of oxygen that is needed to achieve a 50% saturation of hemoglobin. Returning to Figure 29-21B, the dissociation curve on the left has a P_{50} of approximately 20 mm Hg; the normal curve, a P_{50} of 26 mm Hg; and the curve on the right, a P_{50} of 39 mm Hg.

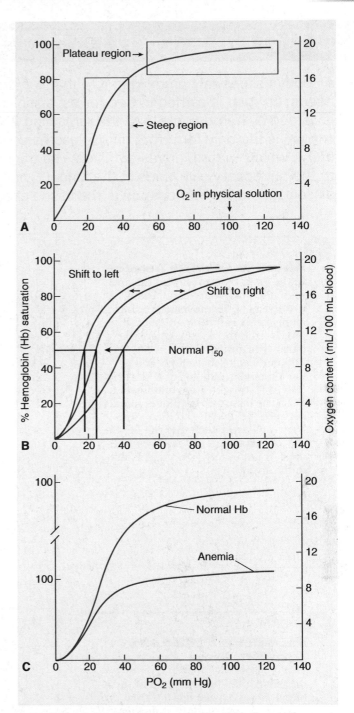

FIGURE 29-21. Oxygen–hemoglobin (Hb) dissociation curve. **(A)** Left-boxed area represents the steep portion of the curve where oxygen is released from Hb to the tissues, and the top-boxed area the plateau of the curve where oxygen is loaded onto Hb in the lung. **(B)** The effect of body temperature, arterial PCO_2, and pH on Hb affinity for oxygen as indicated by a shift in the curve and position of the P_{50}. A shift of the curve to the right because of an increase in temperature or PCO_2 or decreased pH favors release of oxygen to the tissues. A decrease in temperature or PCO_2 or increase in pH shifts the curve to the left and has the opposite effect. The P_{50} is the partial pressure of oxygen required to saturate 50% of Hb with oxygen. **(C)** Effect of anemia on the oxygen-carrying capacity of blood. The Hb can be completely saturated, but the oxygen content of the blood is reduced.

UNDERSTANDING → Oxygen Transport

All body tissues rely on oxygen (O_2) that is transported in the blood to meet their metabolic needs. Oxygen is carried in two forms: dissolved and bound to hemoglobin. About 98% of O_2 is carried by hemoglobin, and the remaining 2% is carried in the dissolved state. Dissolved oxygen is the only form that diffuses across cell membranes and produces a partial pressure (PO_2), which, in turn, drives diffusion. The transport of O_2 involves (1) transfer from the alveoli to the pulmonary capillaries in the lung, (2) hemoglobin binding and transport, and (3) the dissociation from hemoglobin in the tissue capillaries.

1 **Alveoli-to-Capillary Transfer.** In the lung, O_2 moves from the alveoli to the pulmonary capillaries as a dissolved gas. Its movement occurs along a concentration gradient. It moves from the alveoli, where the partial pressure of PO_2 is about 100 mm Hg, to the venous end of the pulmonary capillaries with their lesser O_2 concentration and lower PO_2. The dissolved O_2 moves rapidly between the alveoli and the pulmonary capillaries, such that the PO_2 at the arterial end of the capillary is almost, if not exactly, the same as that in the alveoli.

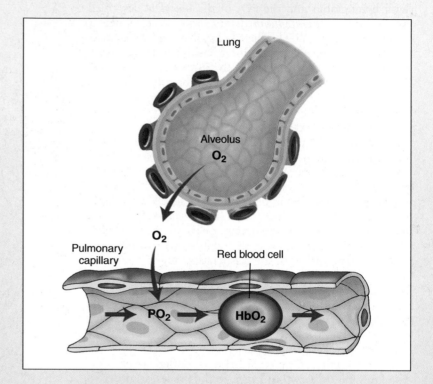

2 **Hemoglobin Binding and Transport.** Oxygen, which is relatively insoluble in plasma, relies on hemoglobin for transport in the blood. Once oxygen has diffused into the pulmonary capillary, it moves rapidly into the red blood cells and reversibly binds to hemoglobin to form HbO_2. The hemoglobin molecule contains four heme units, each capable of attaching an oxygen molecule. Hemoglobin is 100% saturated when all four units are occupied and is usually about 97% saturated in the systemic arterial blood. The capacity of the blood to carry O_2 is dependent both on hemoglobin levels and the ability of the lungs to oxygenate the hemoglobin.

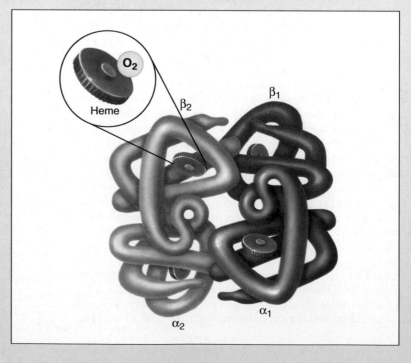

③ Oxygen Dissociation in the Tissues. The dissociation or release of O_2 from hemoglobin occurs in the tissue capillaries where the PO_2 is less than that of the arterial blood. As oxygen dissociates from hemoglobin, it dissolves in the plasma and then moves into the tissues where the PO_2 is less than that in the capillaries. The affinity of hemoglobin for O_2 is influenced by the carbon dioxide (PCO_2) content of the blood and its pH temperature and 2,3-DPG, a by-product of glycolysis in red blood cells. Under conditions of high metabolic demand, in which the PCO_2 is increased and the pH is decreased, the binding affinity of hemoglobin is decreased. During decreased metabolic demand, when the PCO_2 is decreased and the pH is increased, the affinity is increased.

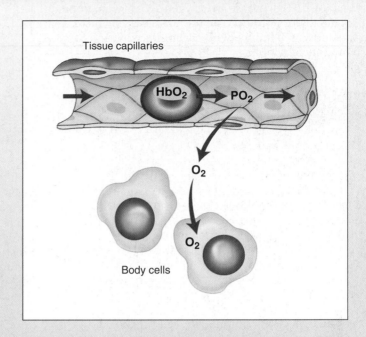

The oxygen content (measured in mL/dL blood) represents the total amount of oxygen carried in the blood, including the dissolved oxygen and that carried by the hemoglobin (see Fig. 29-21C). The amount of hemoglobin-bound oxygen is determined by the concentration of hemoglobin (in g/dL), the oxygen-binding capacity of hemoglobin (1.34 mL O_2/g hemoglobin), and the percentage saturation of the hemoglobin. The dissolved oxygen content is the product of the oxygen solubility (0.0003 mL O_2/dL) times the PO_2. Thus, an anemic person may have a normal PO_2 and hemoglobin saturation level but decreased oxygen content because of the lower amount of hemoglobin for binding oxygen.

Carbon Dioxide Transport

Carbon dioxide is transported in the blood in three forms:

- As dissolved carbon dioxide (10%)
- Attached to hemoglobin (30%)
- As bicarbonate (60%)

Acid–base balance is influenced by the amount of dissolved carbon dioxide and the bicarbonate level in the blood.

As carbon dioxide is formed during the metabolic process, it diffuses out of cells into the tissue spaces and then into the capillaries. The partial pressure of the gas and its solubility coefficient (0.03 mL/100 mL/1 mm Hg PCO_2) determine the amount of dissolved carbon dioxide that can be carried in plasma. Carbon dioxide is 20 times more soluble in plasma than is oxygen. Thus, the dissolved state plays a greater role in transport of carbon dioxide compared with oxygen.

Most of the carbon dioxide diffuses into the red blood cells, where it either forms carbonic acid or combines with hemoglobin. *Carbonic acid* (H_2CO_3) is formed when carbon dioxide combines with water. The process is catalyzed by an enzyme called *carbonic anhydrase*, which is present in large quantities in red blood cells. Carbonic anhydrase increases the rate of the reaction between carbon dioxide and water approximately 5000-fold. Carbonic acid readily ionizes to form bicarbonate (HCO_3^-) and hydrogen (H^+) ions. The hydrogen ion combines with the hemoglobin, which is a powerful acid–base buffer, and the bicarbonate ion diffuses into plasma in exchange for a chloride ion. This exchange is made possible by a special bicarbonate–chloride carrier protein in the red blood cell membrane. As a result of the bicarbonate–chloride shift, the chloride and water content of the red blood cell is greater in venous blood than in arterial blood.

In addition to the carbonic anhydrase–mediated reaction with water, carbon dioxide reacts directly with hemoglobin to form *carbaminohemoglobin*. The combination of carbon dioxide with hemoglobin is a reversible reaction that involves a loose bond. This allows transport of carbon dioxide from tissues to the lungs, where it is released into the alveoli for exchange with the external environment. The release of oxygen from hemoglobin in the tissues enhances the binding of carbon dioxide to hemoglobin. In the lungs, the combining of oxygen with hemoglobin displaces carbon dioxide. The binding of carbon dioxide to hemoglobin is determined by the acidic nature of hemoglobin. Binding with carbon dioxide causes the hemoglobin to become a stronger acid.

In the lungs, the highly acidic hemoglobin has a lesser tendency to form carbaminohemoglobin, and carbon dioxide is released from hemoglobin into the alveoli. In the tissues, the release of oxygen from hemoglobin causes hemoglobin to become less acid, thereby increasing its ability to combine with carbon dioxide and form carbaminohemoglobin.

SUMMARY CONCEPTS

The primary functions of the lungs are oxygenation of the blood and removal of carbon dioxide. Pulmonary gas exchange is conventionally divided into three processes: ventilation, or the flow of gases into the alveoli of the lungs; perfusion, or movement of blood through the adjacent pulmonary capillaries; and diffusion, or transfer of gases between the alveoli and the pulmonary capillaries.

Ventilation is the movement of air between the atmosphere and the lungs, and perfusion is the flow of blood into and out of the gas exchange portions of the lung. Pulmonary ventilation refers to the total exchange of gases between the atmosphere and the lungs, and alveolar ventilation to ventilation in the gas exchange portion of the lungs. The distribution of alveolar ventilation and pulmonary capillary blood flow varies with lung volume and body position. In the upright position and at high lung volumes, ventilation is greatest in the lower parts of the lungs. The upright position also produces a decrease in blood flow to the upper parts of the lung, resulting from the distance above the level of the heart and the low mean arterial pressure in the pulmonary circulation. The efficiency of gas exchange requires matching of ventilation and perfusion so that equal amounts of air and blood enter the respiratory portion of the lungs. Two conditions interfere with matching of ventilation and perfusion: dead air space, in which areas of the lungs are ventilated but not perfused, and shunt, in which areas of the lungs are perfused but not ventilated.

The diffusion of gases in the lungs is influenced by four factors: the surface area available for diffusion; the thickness of the alveolar–capillary membrane, through which the gases diffuse; the differences in the partial pressure of the gas on either side of the membrane; and the diffusion characteristics of the gas.

The blood transports oxygen to the cells and returns carbon dioxide to the lungs. Oxygen is transported in two forms: in chemical combination with hemoglobin and physically dissolved in plasma (PO_2). Hemoglobin is an efficient carrier of oxygen. Approximately 98% to 99% of oxygen is transported in this manner. The relationship between the oxygen carried in combination with hemoglobin and the oxygen–hemoglobin dissociation curve describes the PO_2 of the blood. Carbon dioxide is carried in three forms: attached to hemoglobin (30%), dissolved carbon dioxide (10%), and bicarbonate (60%).

Control of Breathing

Unlike the heart, which has inherent rhythmic properties and can beat independently of the nervous system, the muscles that control respiration require continuous input from the nervous system. Movement of the diaphragm, intercostal muscles, sternocleidomastoid, and other accessory muscles that control ventilation is integrated by neurons located in the pons and medulla. These neurons are collectively referred to as the *respiratory center* (Fig. 29-22).

Respiratory Center

The respiratory center consists of two dense, bilateral aggregates of respiratory neurons. These neurons are involved in initiating inspiration and expiration and incorporating afferent impulses into motor responses of the respiratory muscles. The first, or dorsal, group of neurons in the respiratory center is concerned primarily with inspiration. These neurons control the activity of the phrenic nerves that innervate the diaphragm and drive the second, or ventral, group of respiratory neurons. They are thought to integrate sensory input from the lungs and airways into the ventilatory response. The second group of neurons, which contains inspiratory and expiratory neurons, controls the spinal motor neurons of the intercostal and abdominal muscles.

The pacemaker properties of the respiratory center result from the cycling of the two groups of respiratory neurons: the *pneumotaxic center* in the upper pons and the *apneustic center* in the lower pons (see Fig. 29-22). These two groups of neurons contribute to the function of the respiratory center in the medulla. The apneustic center has an excitatory effect on inspiration, tending to prolong inspiration. The pneumotaxic center switches inspiration off, assisting in the control of respiratory rate and inspiratory volume. Brain injuries that damage the connection between the pneumotaxic and apneustic centers result in an irregular breathing pattern that consists of prolonged inspiratory gasps interrupted by expiratory efforts.

Axons from the neurons in the respiratory center cross in the midline and descend in the ventrolateral columns of the spinal cord. The tracts that control expiration and inspiration are spatially separated in the cord, as are the tracts that transmit specialized reflexes (*i.e.*, coughing and hiccupping) and voluntary

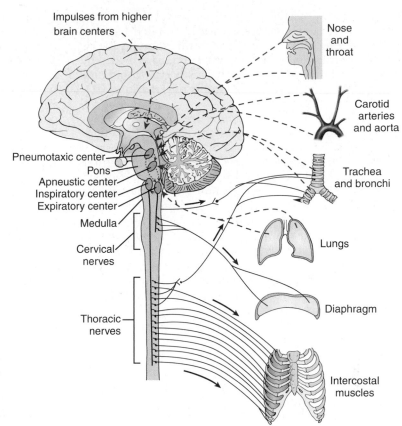

FIGURE 29-22. Schematic representation of activity in the respiratory center. Impulses traveling over afferent neurons (*dashed lines*) communicate with central neurons, which activate efferent neurons that supply the muscles of respiration. Respiratory movements can be altered by a variety of stimuli.

control of ventilation. Only at the level of the spinal cord are the respiratory impulses integrated to produce a reflex response.

Regulation of Breathing

The control of breathing has automatic and voluntary components. The automatic regulation of ventilation is controlled by input from two types of sensors or receptors: chemoreceptors and lung receptors. Chemoreceptors monitor blood levels of oxygen, carbon dioxide, and pH and adjust ventilation to meet the changing metabolic needs of the body. Lung receptors monitor breathing patterns and lung function.

Voluntary regulation of ventilation integrates breathing with voluntary acts such as speaking, blowing, and singing. These acts, which are initiated by the motor and premotor cortex, cause a temporary suspension of automatic breathing. The automatic and voluntary components of respiration are regulated by afferent impulses transmitted to the respiratory center from a number of sources. Afferent input from higher brain centers is evidenced by the fact that a person can consciously alter the depth and rate of respiration. Fever, pain, and emotion exert their influence through lower brain centers. Vagal afferents from sensory receptors in the lungs and airways are integrated in the dorsal area of the respiratory center.

Chemoreceptors

Tissue needs for oxygen and the removal of carbon dioxide are regulated by chemoreceptors that monitor blood levels of these gases. Input from these sensors is transmitted to the respiratory center, and ventilation is adjusted to maintain the ABGs within a normal range.

There are two types of chemoreceptors: central and peripheral. The most important chemoreceptors for sensing changes in the PCO_2 of the blood are the *central chemoreceptors*, which are located in chemosensitive regions near the respiratory center in the medulla. The central chemoreceptors are surrounded by brain extracellular fluid and respond to changes in its hydrogen ion (H^+) concentration. The composition of the extracellular fluid surrounding the chemoreceptors is governed by the cerebrospinal fluid (CSF), local blood flow, and tissue metabolism. Of these, the CSF is apparently the most important. The CSF is separated from the blood by the blood–brain barrier, which permits free diffusion of carbon dioxide but not bicarbonate (HCO_3^-) or H^+. The carbon dioxide combines rapidly with water to form carbonic acid (H_2CO_3), which dissociates into H^+ and HCO_3^-. When the PCO_2 rises, carbon dioxide from the blood diffuses into the CSF, liberating H^+, which then stimulates the chemoreceptors. The central chemoreceptors are extremely sensitive to short-term changes in PCO_2. An increase in PCO_2 levels produces an increase in ventilation that reaches its peak within a minute or so and then declines if the PCO_2 level remains elevated. Thus, people with chronically elevated levels of PCO_2 no longer have a response to this stimulus for increased ventilation but rely on the stimulus provided by a decrease in blood PO_2 levels. This occurs commonly with people who have COPD and is referred to as CO_2 narcosis.

The *peripheral chemoreceptors* are located in the carotid and aortic bodies, which are found at the bifurcation of the common carotid arteries and in the arch of the aorta, respectively (see Fig. 29-22). Although the peripheral chemoreceptors also monitor carbon dioxide, they play a much more important role in monitoring oxygen levels. These receptors exert little control over ventilation until the PO_2 has dropped below 60 mm Hg. Thus, hypoxia is the main stimulus for ventilation in people with chronically elevated levels of carbon dioxide. If these people are given oxygen therapy at a level sufficient to increase the PO_2 above that needed to stimulate the peripheral chemoreceptors, their ventilation may be seriously depressed.

Lung Receptors

Lung and chest wall receptors monitor the status of breathing in terms of airway resistance and lung expansion. There are three types of lung receptors: stretch, irritant, and juxtacapillary receptors.

Stretch receptors are located in the smooth muscle layers of the conducting airways. They respond to changes in pressure in the walls of the airways. When the lungs are inflated, these receptors inhibit inspiration and promote expiration. They are important in establishing breathing patterns and minimizing the work of breathing by adjusting respiratory rate and V_T to accommodate changes in lung compliance and airway resistance.

The *irritant receptors* are located between the airway epithelial cells. They are stimulated by noxious gases, cigarette smoke, inhaled dust, and cold air. Stimulation of the irritant receptors leads to airway constriction and a pattern of rapid, shallow breathing. This pattern of breathing probably protects respiratory tissues from the damaging effects of toxic inhalants. It is also thought that the mechanical stimulation of these receptors may ensure more uniform lung expansion by initiating periodic sighing and yawning. It is also possible that these receptors are involved in the bronchoconstriction response that occurs in some people with bronchial asthma.

The *juxtacapillary* or *J receptors* are located in the alveolar wall, close to the pulmonary capillaries. It is thought that these receptors sense lung congestion. These receptors may be responsible for the rapid, shallow breathing that occurs with pulmonary edema, pulmonary embolism, and pneumonia.[4]

Cough Reflex

Coughing is a neurally mediated reflex that protects the lungs from accumulation of secretions and from entry of irritating and destructive substances. It is one of the primary defense mechanisms of the respiratory tract. The cough reflex is initiated by receptors located in the tracheobronchial wall. These receptors are extremely sensitive to irritating substances and to the presence of excess secretions. Afferent impulses from these receptors are transmitted through the vagus to the medullary center, which integrates the cough response.

Coughing itself requires the rapid inspiration of a large volume of air (usually about 2.5 L), followed by rapid closure of the glottis and forceful contraction of the abdominal and expiratory muscles. As these muscles contract, intrathoracic pressures are elevated to levels of 100 mm Hg or more. The rapid opening of the glottis at this point leads to an explosive expulsion of air.

Many conditions can interfere with the cough reflex and its protective function. The reflex is impaired in people whose abdominal or respiratory muscles are weak. This problem can be caused by disease conditions that lead to muscle weakness or paralysis, by prolonged inactivity, or as an outcome of surgery involving these muscles. Bed rest interferes with expansion of the chest and limits the amount of air that can be taken into the lungs in preparation for coughing, making the cough weak and ineffective. Disease conditions that prevent effective closure of the glottis and laryngeal muscles interfere with production of the marked increase in intrathoracic pressure that is needed for effective coughing. The cough reflex is also impaired when there is depressed function of the medullary centers in the brain that integrate the cough reflex. Interruption of the central integration aspect of the cough reflex can arise as the result of disease of this part of the brain or the action of drugs that depress the cough center.

Dyspnea

Dyspnea is a subjective sensation or a person's perception of difficulty in breathing that includes the perception of labored breathing and the reaction to that sensation. The terms *dyspnea*, *breathlessness*, and *shortness of breath* are often used interchangeably. Dyspnea is observed in at least three major cardiopulmonary disease states:

- Primary lung diseases, such as pneumonia, asthma, and emphysema
- Heart disease that is characterized by pulmonary congestion
- Neuromuscular disorders, such as myasthenia gravis and muscular dystrophy, that affect the respiratory muscles

Although dyspnea is commonly associated with respiratory disease, it also occurs for some people only during exercise and is referred to as exercise-induced reactive airway disorder or exercise-induced asthma.

The cause of dyspnea is unknown. Four types of mechanisms have been proposed to explain the sensation. The first of the suggested mechanisms is stimulation of lung receptors. These receptors are stimulated by the contraction of bronchial smooth muscle, the stretch of the bronchial wall, pulmonary congestion, and conditions that decrease lung compliance. The second category of proposed mechanisms focuses on central nervous system mechanisms that transmit information to the cortex regarding respiratory muscle weakness or a discrepancy between the increased effort of breathing and inadequate respiratory muscle contraction. The third type of mechanism focuses on a reduction in ventilatory capacity or breathing reserve. A reduction in breathing reserve to less than 65% to 75% usually correlates with dyspnea. The fourth possible mechanism is stimulation of muscle and joint receptors in the respiratory musculature because of a discrepancy in the tension generated by these muscles and the V_T that results. These receptors, once stimulated, transmit signals that bring about an awareness of the breathing discrepancy. Like other subjective symptoms, such as fatigue and pain, dyspnea is difficult to quantify because it relies on a person's perception of the problem.

The most common method for measuring dyspnea is a retrospective self-perceived determination of the level of daily activity at which a person experiences dyspnea. The visual analog scale may be used to assess breathing difficulty that occurs with a given activity, such as walking a certain distance. The visual analog scale consists of a continuum line (often 10 cm in length) with descriptors such as "easy to breathe" on one end and "very difficult to breathe" on the other. The person being assessed selects a point on the scale that describes his or her perceived dyspnea.

The treatment of dyspnea depends on the cause. For example, people with impaired respiratory function may require oxygen therapy, and those with pulmonary edema may require measures to improve heart function. Methods to decrease anxiety, breathing retraining, and energy conservation measures may be used to decrease the subjective sensation of dyspnea.

SUMMARY CONCEPTS

The respiratory system requires continuous input from the nervous system. Movement of the diaphragm, intercostal muscles, and other respiratory muscles is controlled by neurons of the respiratory center located in the pons and medulla. The control of breathing has automatic and voluntary components. The automatic regulation of ventilation is controlled by two types of receptors: lung receptors, which protect respiratory structures, and chemoreceptors, which monitor the gas exchange function of the lungs by sensing changes in blood levels of carbon dioxide, oxygen, and pH. There are three types of lung receptors: stretch receptors, which monitor lung inflation; irritant receptors, which protect against the damaging effects of toxic inhalants; and J receptors, which are thought to sense lung congestion. There are two groups of chemoreceptors: central and peripheral. The central chemoreceptors are the most important in sensing changes in carbon dioxide levels, and the peripheral chemoreceptors function in sensing arterial blood oxygen levels.

Voluntary respiratory control is needed for integrating breathing and actions, such as speaking, blowing, and singing. These acts, which are initiated by the motor and premotor cortex, cause temporary suspension of automatic breathing. The cough reflex protects the lungs from the accumulation of secretions and from the entry of irritating and destructive substances; it is one of the primary defense mechanisms of the respiratory tract. Dyspnea is a subjective sensation of difficulty in breathing that is seen in cardiac, pulmonary, and neuromuscular disorders that affect the respiratory muscles.

Review Exercises

1. Calculate the *partial pressure* of oxygen (PO_2) in the alveoli at an atmospheric pressure at sea level (760 mm Hg); Denver, Colorado, at 5431 feet (621 mm Hg); and Berthoud Pass, Colorado, at 12,490 feet (477 mm Hg). Consider that the oxygen concentration is 21% and the water vapor pressure in the lungs is 47 mm Hg. Use the solubility coefficient for oxygen and the oxygen dissociation curve depicted in Figure 29-21 to answer the following questions:

   A. What is the hemoglobin saturation at a high altitude in which the barometric pressure is 500 mm Hg (consider oxygen to represent 21% of the total gases)?

   B. It is usually recommended that the hemoglobin saturation of people with chronic lung disease be maintained at about 89% to 90% when they are receiving supplemental low-flow oxygen. What would their PO_2 be at this level of hemoglobin saturation, and what is the rationale for keeping the PO_2 at this level?

   C. What is the oxygen content of a person with a hemoglobin level of 6 g/dL who is breathing room air?

   D. What is the oxygen content of a person with CO poisoning who is receiving 100% oxygen at 3 atmospheres' pressure in a hyperbaric chamber? Consider that most of the person's hemoglobin is saturated with CO.

REFERENCES

1. Boron W. F., Boulpaep E. L. (2017). *Medical physiology* (3rd ed.). Philadelphia, PA: WB Saunders.
2. Coleman W. B., Songalis T. (2018). *Molecular pathology: The molecular basis of human disease* (2nd ed.). San Diego, CA: Elsevier.
3. Andreoli T., Benjamin I., Griggs R., et al. (Eds.). (2016). *Andreoli and Carpenter's Cecil essentials of medicine* (9th ed.). St. Louis, MO: Elsevier.
4. West J. B. (2012). *Respiratory physiology: The essentials* (9th ed.). Philadelphia, PA: Lippincott Williams & Wilkins.

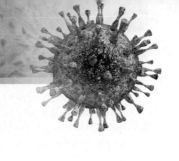

C H A P T E R **30**

Respiratory Tract Infections, Neoplasms, and Childhood Disorders

Learning Objectives

After completing this chapter, the learner will be able to meet the following objectives:

1. Compare community-acquired pneumonia, hospital-acquired pneumonia, and pneumonia in immunocompromised people in terms of pathogens, manifestations, and prognosis.
2. Describe the immunologic properties of the tubercle bacillus, and differentiate between primary tuberculosis and reactivated tuberculosis on the basis of their pathophysiology.
3. Compare small cell lung cancer and non–small cell lung cancer in terms of histopathology, prognosis, and treatment methods.
4. Describe three paraneoplastic manifestations of lung cancer.
5. Describe the role of surfactant in lung function in the neonate.
6. Describe the possible cause and manifestations of respiratory distress syndrome and broncho-pulmonary dysplasia.
7. List the signs of impending respiratory failure in small children.

Respiratory illnesses represent one of the more common reasons for visits to the physician, admission to the hospital, and forced inactivity among all age groups. The common cold, although not usually serious, is a frequent cause of missed work and school days. Pneumonia is the eighth leading cause of death in the United States, particularly among the elderly and those with compromised immune function.[1] In addition, it is the largest infectious cause of death among children in the world.[2] Tuberculosis (TB) remains one of the deadliest diseases in the world and affects one third of the world population.[3] A large number of people have multidrug-resistant TB, and many are immunocompromised. The most frequently seen fungal infections include histoplasmosis, coccidioidomycosis, and blastomycosis. Lung cancer remains the leading cause of cancer death worldwide.[1,4] Children with upper and lower airway infections represent a large number of visits to primary care providers. Premature infants, especially those who experience respiratory distress syndrome (RDS), are at high risk for chronic respiratory infections and other complications such as bronchopulmonary dysplasia (BPD).

Respiratory Tract Infections

The respiratory tract is susceptible to infectious processes caused by multiple types of microorganisms. Infections can involve the upper respiratory tract (*i.e.*, nose, oropharynx, and larynx), the lower respiratory tract (*i.e.*, lower airways and lungs), or the upper and lower airways. The signs and symptoms of respiratory tract infections depend on the function of the structure involved, the severity of the infectious process, and the person's age and general health status. This chapter focuses on the common cold, rhinosinusitis, influenza, pneumonia, TB, fungal infections of the lung, and acute respiratory infections in children.

Viruses are the most frequent cause of respiratory tract infections ranging from a self-limited cold to life-threatening pneumonia. Viral infections can damage bronchial epithelium, obstruct airways, and lead to secondary bacterial infections. Each viral species has its own pattern of respiratory tract involvement.[5] Viruses are able to move from the nasal cavity to the upper airways by binding to the intercellular adhesion molecule 1. People with compromised immunologic response are most susceptible to having a virus that causes serious gas exchange or ventilation problems.[6]

Other microorganisms, such as bacteria, mycobacteria, fungi, and opportunistic organisms, also produce infections of the lung. Many of these infections produce significant morbidity and mortality.

The Common Cold

The common cold, the most common respiratory tract infection, is a viral infection of the upper respiratory tract. Most adults have three to four episodes of the common cold per year, whereas the average school child may have up to 6 to 8 per year.[6]

Etiology and Pathogenesis

The common cold is now recognized to be associated with a number of viruses.[6] The rhinoviruses are the most common cause of colds. Other viral causes include parainfluenza viruses, respiratory syncytial virus (RSV), human metapneumovirus, coronaviruses, and adenoviruses. In children, a new virus, bocavirus, causes respiratory tract infections. The season of the year and the person's age, immunologic state, and prior exposure are important factors in identifying the type of virus causing the infection and the type of symptoms that occur. For example, outbreaks of the common cold because of rhinoviruses are most common in early fall and late spring. Common colds caused by RSV peak in the winter and spring months, and infections caused by adenoviruses and coronaviruses are more frequent during the winter and spring months. Infections resulting from the RSV and parainfluenza viruses are most common and severe in infants and children younger than 6 years. Infections occur less frequently and with milder symptoms with increasing age until after 65 years of age. Parainfluenza viruses often produce lower respiratory symptoms with first infections, but less severe upper respiratory symptoms with reinfections.

The "cold viruses" are spread rapidly from person to person. Children are the major reservoir of cold viruses, often acquiring a new virus from another child in school or day care. The fingers are the greatest source of spread, and the nasal mucosa and conjunctival surface of the eyes are the most common portals for entry of the virus. The illness lasts, on average, about 7 days with an incubation period of about 2 days.[7] Aerosol spread of colds through coughing and sneezing is much less important than the spread through direct mucous membrane contact by fingers picking up the virus from contaminated surfaces and carrying it to the nasal membranes and eyes.[7]

Clinical Manifestations

The condition usually begins with a feeling of dryness and stuffiness, affecting mainly the nasopharynx. This is followed by excessive production of nasal secretions and tearing of the eyes, which is often referred to as rhinitis. Usually, the secretions remain clear and watery. The mucous membranes of the upper respiratory tract become reddened and swollen. Often, there is postnasal dripping, which irritates the pharynx and larynx, causing sore throat and hoarseness. The affected person may experience headache and generalized malaise. In severe cases, there may be chills, fever, and exhaustion. Viral shedding may begin shortly before symptoms.[7]

Treatment

The common cold is an acute and self-limited illness in people who are otherwise healthy. Therefore, symptomatic treatment with rest and antipyretic drugs is usually all that is needed. Antibiotics are ineffective against viral infections and are not recommended. Antihistamines are popular over-the-counter drugs because of their action in drying nasal secretions but lack evidence to shorten the duration of the cold. Decongestant drugs constrict the blood vessels in the swollen nasal mucosa and reduce nasal swelling.[8]

Vitamin C intake has been found to be beneficial in shortening the duration of the cold if taken before the onset of the cold, but it has shown no true effect on incidence with the general population.[8]

Rhinosinusitis

Rhinosinusitis refers to inflammation involving the nasal sinuses.

The paranasal sinuses are air sacs that develop during embryogenesis developing into outpouchings from these furrows that become lined with ciliated respiratory epithelium and invade the surrounding facial bones to become the major sinuses. Each sinus remains in constant communication with the nasal cavity through narrow openings or *ostia*. The sinuses are named for the bone in which they are located—frontal, ethmoid, maxillary, and sphenoidal (Fig. 30-1A). The *frontal sinuses* open into the middle meatus of the nasal cavity. The *ethmoid sinuses* consist of 3 to 15 air cells on each side of the ethmoid, with each maintaining a separate path to the nasal chamber. The anterior ethmoid, frontal, and maxillary sinuses all drain into the nasal cavity through a narrow passage called the *ostiomeatal complex* (see Fig. 30-1B). Defects in the anterior ethmoid sinus can obstruct the ostiomeatal complex and cause secondary disease of the frontal or maxillary sinuses. The *maxillary sinuses* are located inferior to the bony orbit and superior to the hard palate, and their openings are located superiorly and medially in the sinus, a location that impedes drainage. The *sphenoidal sinuses* are located just anterior to the pituitary fossa behind the posterior ethmoid sinuses, with their openings draining into the sphenoethmoid recess at the top of the nasal cavity (see Fig. 30-1C).

An active mucociliary clearance mechanism helps move fluid and microorganisms out of the sinuses and into the nasal cavity. Mucociliary clearance, along with innate and adaptive immune mechanisms, helps to keep the sinuses sterile. The lower oxygen content in the sinuses facilitates the growth of organisms, impairs local defenses, and alters the function of immune cells.

Etiology and Pathogenesis

The most common causes of rhinosinusitis are conditions that obstruct the narrow ostia that drain the sinuses.[9] Most commonly, rhinosinusitis develops when a viral upper respiratory tract infection or allergic rhinitis, which causes mucosal swelling, obstructs the ostia and impairs the mucociliary clearance mechanism. Nasal polyps can also obstruct the sinus openings and facilitate sinus infection. Barotrauma caused by changes in barometric pressure may lead to impaired sinus ventilation and clearance of secretions. Swimming, diving, and abuse of nasal decongestants are other causes of sinus irritation and impaired drainage.

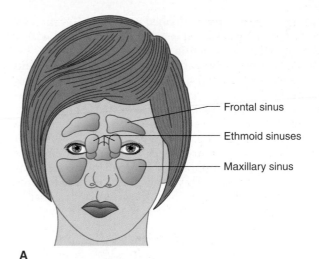

A

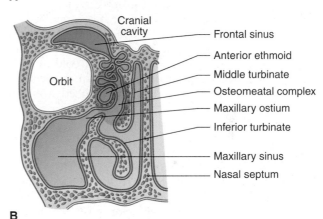

B

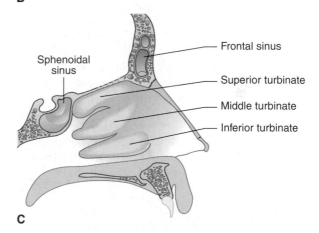

C

FIGURE 30-1. Paranasal sinuses. **(A)** Frontal view showing the frontal, ethmoid, and maxillary sinuses. **(B)** Cross section of nasal cavity (*anterior view*). The *shaded area* is the osteomeatal complex, which is the final common pathway for drainage of the anterior ethmoid, frontal, and maxillary sinuses. **(C)** Lateral wall, left nasal cavity showing the frontal sphenoidal sinuses and the superior, middle, and inferior turbinates.

Rhinosinusitis can be classified as acute or chronic.[9] Acute rhinosinusitis may be of viral, bacterial, or mixed viral–bacterial origin and may last up to 4 weeks.[9] Acute, community-acquired bacterial rhinosinusitis most commonly results from infection with *Haemophilus influenzae* or *Streptococcus pneumoniae* pathogens.

Chronic rhinosinusitis is defined as having duration of greater than 12 weeks and is generally associated with a bacterial or fungal infection.[9]

In chronic rhinosinusitis, anaerobic organisms tend to predominate, alone or in combination with aerobes such as the *Streptococcus* species or *Staphylococcus aureus*.[9] People with chronic rhinosinusitis and otitis media and effusion have been found to have accumulation of *Pseudomonas aeruginosa*, which forms biofilm in various ear, nose, and throat areas.[9] The presence of biofilms with chronic ear, nose, and throat infections lends support to signs and symptoms caused by the chronic inflammation related to chronic otitis, rhinosinusitis, and effusion.[9]

Clinical Manifestations

The symptoms of acute viral rhinosinusitis are often difficult to differentiate from those of the common cold and allergic rhinitis. They include facial pain, headache, purulent nasal discharge, decreased sense of smell, and fever. A history of a preceding common cold and the presence of purulent nasal drainage, pain on bending, unilateral maxillary pain, and pain in the teeth are common with involvement of the maxillary sinuses. The symptoms of acute viral rhinosinusitis usually resolve within 5 to 7 days without medical treatment.[6] Acute bacterial rhinosinusitis is suggested by symptoms that worsen after 5 to 7 days or persist beyond 10 days, or symptoms that are out of proportion to those usually associated with a viral upper respiratory tract infection.[9] People who are immunocompromised often present with fever of unknown origin, rhinorrhea, or facial edema. Often, other signs of inflammation such as purulent drainage are absent.

In people with chronic rhinosinusitis, symptoms may consist of sinus pressure with nasal congestion. The symptoms may persist for years with periods of greater severity than others.[9] The person may complain of a headache that is dull and constant. People with chronic rhinosinusitis may have superimposed bouts of acute rhinosinusitis. The epithelial changes that occur during acute rhinosinusitis are usually reversible, but the mucosal changes that occur with chronic rhinosinusitis are often irreversible.

Diagnosis and Treatment

The diagnosis of rhinosinusitis is usually based on symptom history and a physical examination that includes inspection of the nose and throat.[9] Headache due to sinusitis needs to be differentiated from other types of headache. Bending forward, coughing, or sneezing usually exaggerates sinusitis headache. Physical examination findings in acute bacterial sinusitis and viral sinusitis are often times difficult to differentiate with regard to diagnosis.[9] Sinus radiographs and computed tomography (CT) scans may be used.[9] Treatment of rhinosinusitis depends on the cause and includes appropriate use of antibiotics, mucolytic agents, and symptom relief measures. About two thirds of people with acute bacterial rhinosinusitis improve without antibiotic treatment. Most people with viral upper respiratory

infections improve within 7 days. Treatment of bacterial infections consists of repeated courses of antibiotics that are culture guided. Treatment may also consist of mechanical nasal irrigation and intranasal glucocorticoids.[9] Oral and topical decongestants may be used to promote adequate nasal drainage and congestion. Mucolytic agents may be used to thin secretions. Topical corticosteroids may be used to decrease inflammation in people with allergic rhinitis or rhinosinusitis. Nonpharmacologic measures include saline nasal sprays, nasal irrigation, and mist humidification.

Surgical intervention directed at correcting obstruction of the ostiomeatal openings includes obstructive nasal polyps and obstructive nasal deformities.

Complications

Because of the sinuses' proximity to the brain and orbital wall, sinusitis can lead to intracranial and orbital wall complications. Intracranial complications are seen most commonly with infection of the frontal and ethmoid sinuses because of their proximity to the dura and drainage of the veins from the frontal sinus into the dural sinus. Orbital complications can range from edema of the eyelids to orbital cellulitis and subperiosteal abscess formation. Facial swelling over the involved sinus, abnormal extraocular movements, protrusion of the eyeball, periorbital edema, or changes in mental status may indicate intracranial complications and require immediate medical attention.[10]

Influenza

Influenza is one of the most important causes of acute upper respiratory tract infection in humans. Rates of infection are highest among children and older adults, but rates of serious illness and death are highest among people aged 65 years or older.[11]

The viruses that cause influenza belong to the Orthomyxoviridae family, whose members are characterized by a segmented, single-stranded ribonucleic acid (RNA) genome.[12] There are three types of influenza viruses that cause epidemics in humans: types A, B, and C. Influenza A differs in its ability to infect multiple species, including avian and mammalian species. The influenza A virus is further divided into subtypes based on two surface glycoproteins: hemagglutinin (HA) and neuraminidase (NA).[12] HA is an attachment protein that allows the virus to enter epithelial cells in the respiratory tract, and NA facilitates viral replication from the cell.[12] Contagion results from the ability of the influenza A virus to develop new HA and NA subtypes against which the population is not protected. An antigenic shift, which involves a major genetic rearrangement in either antigen, may lead to epidemic or pandemic infection. Lesser changes, called *antigenic drift*, find the population partially protected by cross-reacting antibodies. Influenza B and C undergo less frequent antigenic shifts than influenza A, probably because few related viruses exist in mammalian or avian species.[12]

Influenza is more contagious than bacterial respiratory tract infections. Transmission occurs by inhalation of droplet nuclei rather than touching contaminated objects. Most infected people develop symptoms of the disease, increasing the likelihood of contagion through spread of infectious droplets. Young children are most likely to become infected and also to spread the infection. The incubation period for influenza is 1 to 4 days, with 2 days being the average. People become infectious starting 1 day before their symptoms begin and remain infectious through approximately 1 week after illness onset.[12] Viral shedding can continue for approximately 3 weeks.

Pathogenesis

The influenza viruses can cause three types of infections: an uncomplicated upper respiratory infection (rhinotracheitis), viral pneumonia, and a respiratory viral infection followed by a bacterial infection. Influenza initially establishes upper airway infection. In doing this, the virus first targets and kills mucous-secreting, ciliated, and other epithelial cells, leaving holes between the underlying basal cells and allowing extracellular fluid to escape. This is the reason for the "runny nose" that is characteristic of this phase of the infection. If the virus spreads to the lower respiratory tract, the infection can cause severe shedding of bronchial and alveolar cells down to a single-cell–thick basal layer. Additionally, compromising the natural defenses of the respiratory tract, influenza infection promotes bacterial adhesion to epithelial cells. Pneumonia may result from a viral pathogenesis or from a secondary bacterial infection.

Clinical Manifestations

In the early stages, the symptoms of influenza are often indistinguishable from other viral infections. Influenza A or B results in an abrupt onset of fever and chills, rigors, malaise, muscle aching, headache, profuse, watery nasal discharge, nonproductive cough, and sore throat.[12] One distinguishing feature of an influenza viral infection is the rapid onset, sometimes in as little as 1 to 2 minutes, of profound malaise. The symptoms of uncomplicated rhinotracheitis usually peak by days 3 to 5 and disappear by days 7 to 10. Influenza C virus infection causes symptoms similar to the common cold.

Viral pneumonia occurs as a complication of influenza, most frequently in older adults or in people with cardiopulmonary disease but has been reported in healthy people. It typically develops within 1 day after onset of influenza and is characterized by rapid progression of symptoms. Adults with underlying comorbidities have exacerbations.[12] The clinical course of influenza pneumonia progresses rapidly. It can cause hypoxemia and death within a few days of onset. Survivors often develop diffuse pulmonary fibrosis.

Secondary complications typically include sinusitis, otitis media, bronchitis, bacterial pneumonia, and, in young children, croup; secondary complications may rarely include parotitis or bacterial tracheitis.[12] The most common causes of secondary bacterial pneumonia are *S. pneumoniae*, *S. aureus*, *H. influenzae*, and *Moraxella catarrhalis*. This form of pneumonia commonly produces less tachypnea and is usually milder than primary influenza pneumonia. Influenza-related deaths can result from pneumonia as well as exacerbations of cardiopulmonary conditions and other disease. Reye syndrome (fatty liver with encephalitis) is a rare complication of influenza, particularly in young children who have been given aspirin as an antipyretic agent.

Diagnosis and Treatment

Early diagnosis can reduce the inappropriate use of antibiotics and provide the opportunity for use of an antiviral drug. Rapid diagnostic tests allow accurate diagnosing of influenza, evaluation of treatment options, and monitoring the influenza type and its prevalence in the community.[13]

The goals of treatment for influenza are designed to limit the infection to the upper respiratory tract. The symptomatic approach for treatment of uncomplicated influenza rhinotracheitis focuses on rest, keeping warm, managing the fever, and keeping well hydrated. Analgesics and cough medications can also be used. Antiviral drugs are available for treatment of influenza.

Influenza Immunization

Because influenza is so highly contagious, prevention relies primarily on vaccination. All people aged 6 months and older in the United States are recommended to receive the annual influenza vaccine. The formulation of the vaccines must be changed yearly in response to antigenic changes in the influenza virus.[12,13] A higher dose of inactivated influenza vaccine is given to seniors older than 65 years.[12]

Avian Influenza (Bird Flu)

Avian influenza, or zoonotic influenza, is an infection caused by avian influenza viruses. The normal hosts for avian influenza viruses are birds and, occasionally, pigs. These influenza viruses occur naturally among birds.[12] Avian strains of the influenza virus do not usually cause outbreaks of disease in humans unless a reassortment of the virus genome has occurred within an intermediate mammalian host such as a pig. Zoonotic infections that cause a threat are subtypes H_5, H_7, and H_9.[12]

A highly pathogenic influenza A subtype, H5N1, occur after exposure to infected poultry or surfaces contaminated with poultry droppings. Because infection in humans is associated with a high mortality rate, there is considerable concern that the H5N1 strain might mutate and initiate a pandemic. People who contract avian flu generally complain of typical influenza symptoms along with eye infections, pneumonia, and acute RDS.[12]

There is currently no commercially available vaccine to protect humans against the bird flu. Current commercial rapid diagnostic tests are not optimally sensitive or specific for detection of the virus.

Swine Flu (H1N1)

In June 2009, the World Health Organization identified that influenza pandemic is caused by an influenza A flu, also known as the swine-origin influenza A flu (H1N1) or swine flu. H1N1 caused extremely high fevers and was especially serious in young adults less than 25 years of age. Older adults were not at higher risk for H1N1 because they tend to be for most infections such as seasonal influenza. This virus is spread from human to human. The majority of people affected by the virus did not experience severe illness, although there were some who needed hospitalization and who even died. The Centers for Disease Control and Prevention does recommend that most people be vaccinated against H1N1.

Pneumonias

The term *pneumonia* refers to inflammation of parenchymal structures of the lung in the lower respiratory tract, such as the alveoli and the bronchioles. It causes more than 1.25 million hospitalizations annually.[13] Pneumonia is the eighth leading cause of death in the United States and the most common cause of death from infectious disease.[2] Etiologic agents include infectious and noninfectious agents. Inhalation of irritating fumes or aspiration of gastric contents, although much less common than infectious causes, can result in severe pneumonia.

Although antibiotics have significantly reduced the mortality rate from pneumonias, these diseases remain an important immediate cause of death among older adults and in people with debilitating diseases.[13] There have been subtle changes in the spectrum of microorganisms that cause infectious pneumonias, including a decrease in pneumonias caused by *S. pneumoniae* and an increase in pneumonias caused by other microorganisms such as *Pseudomonas*, *Candida* and other fungi, and nonspecific viruses. Many of these pneumonias occur in people with impaired immune defenses, including those on immunosuppressant drugs or in people who frequently take anti-inflammatory drugs.

Because of the overlap in symptomatology and changing spectrum of infectious organisms involved, pneumonias are increasingly being classified according to the setting (community-acquired or hospital [nosocomial] in which it occurs).[13] People with compromised immune function constitute a special concern in both categories.

Pneumonias can also be classified according to the type of agent (typical or atypical) causing the infection and distribution of the infection (lobar pneumonia or bronchopneumonia). *Typical pneumonias* result from infection by bacteria that multiply extracellularly in the alveoli and cause inflammation and exudation of fluid into the air-filled spaces of the alveoli (Fig. 30-2). *Atypical pneumonias* are caused by viral and *Mycoplasma* infections that involve the alveolar septum and the interstitium of the lung. They produce less conspicuous symptoms and physical findings than bacterial pneumonia.

Acute bacterial pneumonias can be classified as lobar pneumonia or bronchopneumonia, based on their anatomic pattern of distribution (Fig. 30-3). In general, *lobar pneumonia* refers to consolidation of a part or all of a lung lobe, and *bronchopneumonia* signifies a patchy consolidation involving more than one lobe (see Fig. 30-4).

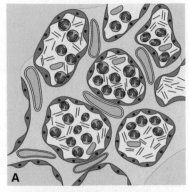

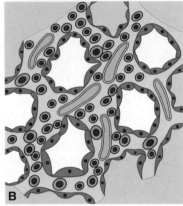

FIGURE 30-2. Location of inflammatory processes in (**A**) typical and (**B**) atypical forms of pneumonia.

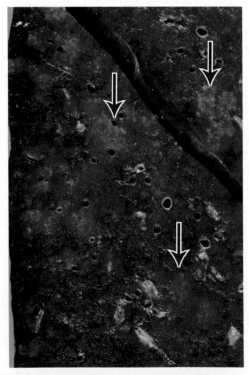

FIGURE 30-3. Bronchopneumonia. Scattered foci of consolidation (*arrows*) are centered on the bronchi and bronchioles. (From Strayer D. S., Rubin R. (Eds.). (2015). *Rubin's pathology: Clinicopathologic foundations of medicine* (7th ed., Fig. 18-12, p. 687). Philadelphia, PA: Lippincott Williams & Wilkins.)

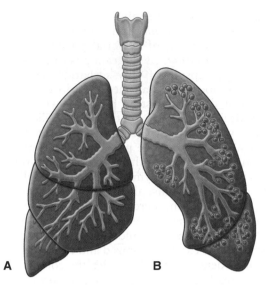

FIGURE 30-4. Distribution of lung involvement in (**A**) lobar pneumonia and (**B**) bronchopneumonia.

KEY POINTS

Pneumonias

- Pneumonias are respiratory disorders involving inflammation of the lung structures, such as the alveoli and bronchioles.

- Pneumonias caused by infectious agents are commonly classified according to the source of infection (community-acquired vs. hospital-acquired) and according to the immune status of the host (pneumonia in the immunocompromised person).

Community-Acquired Pneumonia

The term *community-acquired pneumonia* is used to describe infections from organisms found in the community rather than in the hospital or nursing home. It is defined as an infection that begins outside the hospital or is diagnosed within 48 hours after admission to the hospital in a person who has not resided in a long-term care facility for 14 days or more before admission.[14]

Community-acquired pneumonia may be either bacterial or viral. The most common cause of infection in all categories is *S. pneumoniae*.[13] Other common pathogens include *H. influenzae*, *S. aureus*, and gram-negative bacilli. Less common agents, although they are becoming more common, are *Mycoplasma pneumoniae*, *Legionella*,[13] *Chlamydia* species, and viruses, sometimes called *atypical agents*. Common viral causes of community-acquired pneumonia include the influenza virus, RSV, adenovirus, and parainfluenza virus.

In people younger than 65 years and without coexisting disease, diagnosis is usually based on history and physical examination, chest radiographs, and knowledge of the microorganisms currently causing infections in the community. Sputum specimens may be obtained for staining procedures and culture. Blood cultures may be done for people requiring hospitalization.

Treatment involves the use of appropriate antibiotic therapy.[13] Hospitalization and more intensive care may be required depending on the person's age, preexisting health status, and severity of the infection.

Hospital-Acquired Pneumonia

Hospital-acquired pneumonia is defined as a lower respiratory tract infection that was not present or incubating on admission to the hospital. Usually, infections occurring 48 hours or more after admission are considered hospital acquired.[13] Hospital-acquired pneumonia is the second most common cause of hospital-acquired infection and has a mortality rate of 30% to 50%.[13] People requiring airway instrumentation are particularly at risk. Others at risk include those with compromised immune function and chronic lung disease.

Most hospital-acquired infections are bacterial. The organisms are those present in the hospital environment and include *P. aeruginosa*, *S. aureus*, *Enterobacter* species, *Klebsiella* species, *Escherichia coli*, and *Serratia* species. The organisms that are responsible for hospital-acquired pneumonias differ from those responsible for community-acquired pneumonias, many of them having acquired antibiotic resistance.

Pneumonia in Immunocompromised People

Pneumonia in immunocompromised people remains a major source of morbidity and mortality. The term *immunocompromised host* is usually applied to people with a variety of underlying defects in host defenses.[15] It includes people with primary and acquired immunodeficiency states, those who have undergone bone marrow or organ transplantation, people with solid organ or hematologic cancers, and those on corticosteroid and other immunosuppressant drugs.

Although almost all types of microorganisms can cause pulmonary infection in immunocompromised people, certain types of immunologic defects tend to favor certain types of infections.[15] Defects in humoral immunity predispose to bacterial infections, whereas defects in cellular immunity predispose to infections caused by viruses, fungi, mycobacteria, and protozoa. Neutropenia and impaired granulocyte function predispose to infections caused by *S. aureus*, *Aspergillus*, gram-negative bacilli, and *Candida*. The time course of infection often provides a hint to the type of agent involved. A fulminant pneumonia is usually caused by bacterial infection, whereas an insidious onset is usually indicative of a viral, fungal, protozoal, or mycobacterial infection.

Acute Bacterial (Typical) Pneumonias

Bacterial pneumonias remain an important cause of mortality among older adults and people with debilitating illnesses. The lung below the main bronchi is normally sterile despite frequent entry of microorganisms into the air passages by inhalation during ventilation or has not been documented, and infection normally occurs when water that contains the pathogen is aerosolized into appropriately sized droplets and is inhaled or aspirated by a susceptible host.[16] The disease was first recognized and received its name after an epidemic of severe and, for some, fatal pneumonia that developed among delegates to the 1976 American Legion convention held in a Philadelphia hotel. The spread of infection was traced to a water-cooled air-conditioning system. Although healthy people can contract the infection, the risk is greatest among smokers, people with chronic diseases, and those with impaired cell-mediated immunity.[16]

Symptoms of the disease typically begin approximately 2 to 10 days after infection. Onset is usually abrupt, with malaise, weakness, lethargy, fever, and dry cough. Other manifestations include disturbances of central nervous system function, gastrointestinal tract involvement, arthralgias, and elevation in body temperature.[16] The presence of pneumonia along with diarrhea, hyponatremia, and confusion is characteristic of *Legionella* pneumonia. The disease causes consolidation of lung tissues and impairs gas exchange.

Diagnosis is based on clinical manifestations, radiologic studies, and specialized laboratory tests to detect the presence of the organism. Of these, the *Legionella* urinary antigen test is a relatively inexpensive, rapid test that detects antigens of *L. pneumophila* in the urine.[16] The test is available as both a radioimmunoassay and an enzyme immunoassay.

Treatment consists of administration of antibiotics that are known to be effective against *L. pneumophila*.[16]

Primary Atypical Pneumonia

The primary atypical pneumonias are caused by a variety of agents, the most common being *M. pneumoniae*. Mycoplasma infections are particularly common among children and young adults.[15] Other etiologic agents include viruses (*e.g.*, influenza virus, RSVs, adenoviruses, rhinoviruses, rubeola [measles], and varicella [chickenpox] viruses) and *Chlamydia cae*.[17] In some cases, the cause is unknown.

The atypical pneumonias are characterized by patchy involvement of the lung, largely confined to the alveolar septum and pulmonary interstitium. The term *atypical* denotes a lack of lung consolidation, production of moderate amounts of sputum, moderate elevation of white blood cell count, and lack of alveolar exudate.[15] The agents that cause atypical pneumonias damage the respiratory tract epithelium and impair respiratory tract defenses, thereby predisposing to secondary bacterial infections. The sporadic form of atypical pneumonia is usually mild with a low mortality rate. It may, however, assume epidemic proportions with intensified severity and greater mortality.

The clinical course among people with mycoplasmal and viral pneumonias varies widely from a mild infection (*e.g.*, influenza types A and B, adenovirus) that masquerades as a chest cold to a more serious and even fatal outcome. The symptoms may remain confined to fever, headache, and muscle aches and pains. Cough, when present, is characteristically dry, hacking, and nonproductive. The diagnosis is usually made based on history, physical findings, and chest x-rays.[18]

Tuberculosis

TB is the world's foremost cause of death from a single infectious agent. Approximately 10.4 million people are infected globally.[19] This does not include the millions of people who are thought to be latently infected with *Mycobacterium tuberculosis*. The World Health Organization estimates over 9 million new TB cases occur annually worldwide.[20] With the introduction of antibiotics in the 1950s, the United States and other Western countries enjoyed a long decline in the number of infections until the mid-1980s. Since that time, the rate of infection has increased, particularly among people infected with HIV. TB is more common among foreign-born people from countries with a high incidence of TB and among residents of high-risk congregate settings, such as correctional facilities, drug treatment facilities, and homeless shelters. Outbreaks of a drug-resistant form of TB have emerged, complicating the selection of drugs and affecting the duration of treatment.

TB is an infectious disease caused by *M. tuberculosis*. The mycobacteria are slender, rod-shaped aerobic bacteria that do not form spores. They are similar to other bacterial organisms except for an outer waxy capsule that makes them more resistant to destruction; the organism can persist in old necrotic and calcified lesions and remain capable of reinitiating growth. The waxy coat also causes the organism to retain red dye when treated with acid in acid-fast staining.[20] Thus, the mycobacteria are often referred to as *acid-fast bacilli*. Although *M. tuberculosis* can infect practically any organ of the body, the lungs are most frequently involved. The tubercle bacilli are strict aerobes that thrive in an oxygen-rich environment. This explains their tendency to cause disease in the upper lobe or upper parts of the lower lobe of the lung, where the ventilation and oxygen content are greatest.

Mycobacterium tuberculosis hominis is the most frequent form of TB that threatens humans. Other mycobacteria, including *Mycobacterium avium–intracellulare* (MAI) complex, are much less virulent than *M. tuberculosis hominis*. These mycobacteria rarely cause disease except in severely immunosuppressed people, such as those infected with HIV. Generally, MAI complex is transmitted from eating contaminated food or water.

Mycobacterium tuberculosis hominis is an airborne infection spread by minute, invisible particles, called *droplet nuclei* that are harbored in the respiratory secretions of people with active TB. Coughing, sneezing, and talking all create respiratory droplets. These droplets evaporate and leave organisms (droplet nuclei), which remain suspended in the air and are circulated by air currents. Thus, living under crowded and confined conditions increases the risk for spread of the disease.

Pathogenesis

The pathogenesis of TB in a previously unexposed immunocompetent person is centered on the development of a cell-mediated immune response that confers resistance to the organism and development of tissue hypersensitivity to the tubercular antigens.[20] The destructive features of the disease, such as caseating necrosis and cavitation, result from the hypersensitivity immune response rather than the destructive capabilities of the tubercle bacillus.

Macrophages are the primary cell infected with *M. tuberculosis*. Inhaled droplet nuclei pass down the bronchial tree without settling on the epithelium and are deposited in the alveoli. Soon after entering the lung, the bacilli are phagocytosed by alveolar macrophages but resist killing, apparently because cell wall lipids of *M. tuberculosis* block fusion of phagosomes and lysosomes. Although the macrophages that first ingest *M. tuberculosis* cannot kill the organisms, they initiate a cell-mediated immune response that eventually contains the infection. As the tubercle bacilli multiply, the infected macrophages degrade the mycobacteria and present their antigens to T lymphocytes. The sensitized T lymphocytes, in turn, stimulate the macrophages to increase their concentration of lytic enzymes and ability to kill the mycobacteria. When released, these lytic enzymes also damage lung tissue. The development of a population of activated T lymphocytes and related development of activated macrophages capable of ingesting and destroying the bacilli constitutes the cell-mediated immune response, a process that takes about 3 to 6 weeks to become effective.

In people with intact cell-mediated immunity, the cell-mediated immune response results in the development of a gray-white, circumscribed granulomatous lesion, called a *Ghon focus*, that contains the tubercle bacilli, modified macrophages, and other immune cells.[20] It is usually located in the subpleural area of the upper segments of the lower lobes or in the lower segments of the upper lobe. When the number of organisms is high,

the hypersensitivity reaction produces significant tissue necrosis, causing the central portion of the Ghon focus to undergo soft, caseous (cheese-like) necrosis. During this same period, tubercle bacilli, free or inside macrophages, drain along the lymph channels to the tracheobronchial lymph nodes of the affected lung, and there evoke the formation of caseous granulomas. The combination of the primary lung lesion and lymph node granulomas is called a *Ghon complex* (Fig. 30-7). The Ghon complex eventually heals, undergoing shrinkage, fibrous scarring, and calcification, the latter visible radiographically. However, small numbers of organisms may remain viable for years. Later, if immune mechanisms decline or fail, latent TB infection has the potential to develop into secondary TB.

Clinical Manifestations

Primary Tuberculosis

Primary TB is a form of the disease that develops in previously unexposed and therefore unsensitized people. It is typically initiated as a result of inhaling droplet nuclei that contain the tubercle bacillus (Fig. 30-8). Most people with primary TB go on to develop *latent infection* in which T lymphocytes and macrophages surround the organism in granulomas that limit their spread.[20] People with latent TB do not have active disease and cannot transmit the organism to others.

In small percentage of newly infected people, the immune response is inadequate. These people go on to develop progressive primary TB with continued

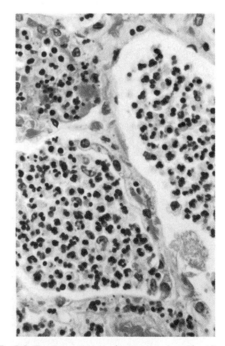

FIGURE 30-7. Pneumococcal pneumonia. Alveoli are packed with an exudate composed of polymorphonuclear leukocytes and occasional macrophages. (From Beasley M. B., Travis W. D., Rubin E. (2008). The respiratory system. In Strayer D. S., Rubin R. (Eds.), *Rubin's pathology: Clinicopathologic foundations of medicine* (7th ed., Fig. 18-14, p. 689). Philadelphia, PA: Lippincott Williams & Wilkins.)

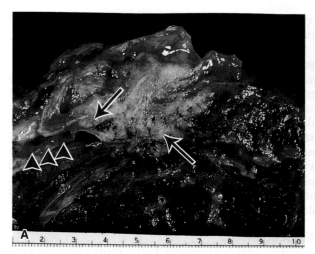
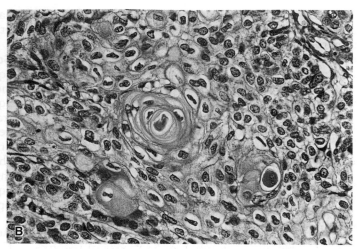

FIGURE 30-12. Squamous cell carcinoma of the lung. (**A**) The tumor (*large arrow*) grows within the lumen of a bronchus (*arrowheads* highlight the course of the bronchus) and invades the adjacent intrapulmonary lymph node (*small arrow*). (**B**) A photomicrograph shows well-differentiated squamous cell carcinoma with a keratin pearl composed of cells with brightly eosinophilic cytoplasm. (From Strayer D. S., Rubin R. (Eds.). (2015). *Rubin's pathology: Clinicopathologic foundations of medicine* (7th ed., Fig. 18-79, p. 737). Philadelphia, PA: Lippincott Williams & Wilkins.)

Clinical Manifestations

The manifestations of lung cancer can be divided into three categories:

1. Those due to involvement of the lung and adjacent structures
2. The effects of local spread and metastasis
3. Nonmetastatic paraneoplastic manifestations involving endocrine, neurologic, and connective tissue function

As with other cancers, lung cancer also causes nonspecific symptoms, such as anorexia and weight loss. Because its symptoms are similar to those associated with smoking and chronic bronchitis, they are often disregarded. Metastases already exist in many people presenting with evidence of lung cancer (see Fig. 30-13). The most common sites of these metastases are the brain, bone, and liver.

Many of the manifestations of lung cancers result from local irritation and obstruction of the airways and from invasion of the mediastinum and pleural space. The earliest symptoms are usually chronic cough, shortness of breath, and wheezing because of airway irritation and obstruction. Hemoptysis (*i.e.*, blood in the sputum) occurs when the lesion erodes blood vessels. Pain receptors in the chest are limited to the parietal pleura, mediastinum, larger blood vessels, and peribronchial afferent vagal fibers. Dull, intermittent, poorly localized retrosternal pain is common in tumors that involve the mediastinum. Pain becomes persistent, localized, and more severe when the disease invades the pleura.

Tumors that invade the mediastinum may cause hoarseness because of the involvement of the recurrent laryngeal nerve and cause difficulty in swallowing because of compression of the esophagus. An uncommon complication called the *superior vena cava syndrome* occurs in some people with mediastinal involvement. Interruption of blood flow in this vessel usually results

from compression by the tumor or involved lymph nodes. The disorder can interfere with venous drainage from the head, neck, and chest wall. Tumors adjacent to the visceral pleura often insidiously produce pleural effusion. This effusion can compress the lung and cause atelectasis and dyspnea.

Diagnosis and Treatment

The diagnosis of lung cancer is based on a careful history and physical examination and on other tests such as chest radiography, bronchoscopy, cytologic studies

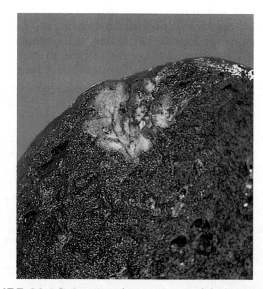

FIGURE 30-13. Invasive adenocarcinoma of the lung. A peripheral tumor of the upper right lobe has an irregular border and a tan or gray cut surface and causes puckering of the overlying pleura. (From Strayer D. S., Rubin R. (Eds.). (2015). *Rubin's pathology: Clinicopathologic foundations of medicine* (7th ed., Fig. 18-80, p. 738). Philadelphia, PA: Lippincott Williams & Wilkins.)

of the sputum or bronchial washings, percutaneous needle biopsy of lung tissue, and scalene lymph node biopsy.[32] CT scans, magnetic resonance imaging (MRI) studies, and ultrasonography are used to locate lesions and evaluate the extent of the disease. Positron emission tomography is a noninvasive alternative for identifying metastatic lesions in the mediastinum or distant sites. People with SCLC should also have a CT scan or MRI of the brain for detection of metastasis.

Like other cancers, lung cancer is classified according to extent of disease. NSCLCs are usually classified according to cell type and staged according to the Tumor, Node, Metastasis (TNM) international staging system.[32] SCLCs are not staged using the TNM system because micrometastases are assumed to be present at the time of diagnosis. Instead, they are usually classified as limited disease when the tumor is limited to the unilateral hemithorax, or extensive disease when it extends beyond these boundaries.[32]

Treatment methods for NSCLC include surgery, radiation therapy, and chemotherapy.[32] These treatments may be used singly or in combination. Surgery is used for the removal of small, localized NSCLC tumors. Radiation therapy can be used as a definitive or main treatment modality, as part of a combined treatment plan, or for palliation of symptoms. Because of the frequency of metastases, chemotherapy is often used in treating lung cancer. Combination chemotherapy, which uses a regimen of several drugs, is usually used.

Therapy for SCLC is based on the stage and currently includes chemotherapy and radiation therapy; however, this is changing because new therapies are developed.[32] Advances in the use of combination chemotherapy, along with thoracic irradiation, have improved the outlook for people with SCLC. Because SCLC may metastasize to the brain, prophylactic cranial irradiation is often indicated.

Management of Lung Cancer in Older Adults

Given the fact that most people are older than 65 years of age when diagnosed with lung cancer, it is important to understand management of lung cancer in older adults. Knowledge about the optimal treatment for older adults is limited because of underrepresentation in clinical trials and failure to evaluate younger versus older people in randomized clinical trials. At present, it is recommended that older adults should be treated based on their general physiologic rather than chronologic age. This includes an evaluation of functional status, coexisting medical conditions, nutritional status, cognition, psychological functioning, social support, and medication review. Those with good performance status and normal renal and hematologic parameters may be treated surgically or receive standard chemotherapy and radiation for limited-stage disease and combination chemotherapy for extensive-stage disease.

Surgery remains the mainstay for older adults with stages I to III NSCLC. Curative resection is feasible in older adults.

Radiation can be given with curative intent for older adults who are not surgical candidates. It may also be used for palliation of cancer-related symptoms. Older adults with good performance status may receive standard chemotherapy for limited disease and combination chemotherapy for extensive-stage disease. Some older adults may require dose reductions or be unable to complete the full chemotherapy course.

SUMMARY CONCEPTS

Cancer of the lung is a leading cause of death worldwide. Cigarette smoking is implicated in the majority of cases of lung cancer. The risk for lung cancer among cigarette smokers increases with duration of smoking and the number of cigarettes smoked per day. Industrial hazards, such as exposure to asbestos, increase the risk for development of lung cancer. Because lung cancer develops insidiously, it is often far advanced before it is diagnosed. This fact explains the poor 5-year survival rate. Carcinoma, which accounts for 95% of all primary lung cancers, can be subdivided currently into four major categories: squamous cell carcinoma, adenocarcinoma, large cell carcinoma, and small cell carcinoma. For purposes of staging and treatment, lung cancer is divided into SCLC and NSCLC. The main reason for this is that almost all SCLCs have metastasized at the time of diagnosis.

The manifestations of lung cancer can be attributed to the involvement of the lung and adjacent structures, the effects of local spread and metastasis, and paraneoplastic syndromes involving endocrine, neurologic, and hematologic dysfunction. As with other cancers, lung cancer causes nonspecific symptoms such as anorexia and weight loss. Treatment methods for lung cancer include surgery, irradiation, and chemotherapy. The current increase in lung cancer among older adults (those 65 years and older) has required a rethinking of the treatment strategies for this age group, with the trend being to base treatment on physiologic rather than chronologic age.

Respiratory Disorders in Children

Acute respiratory diseases are the most common cause of illness in infancy and childhood. This section focuses on the following:

- Lung development, with an emphasis on the developmental basis for lung disorders in children
- Respiratory disorders in the neonate
- Respiratory infections in children

require chest surgery. Medical procedures such as transthoracic needle aspirations, central line insertion, intubation, and positive-pressure ventilation occasionally may cause pneumothorax. Traumatic pneumothorax can also occur as a complication of cardiopulmonary resuscitation.

Tension Pneumothorax. Tension pneumothorax occurs when the intrapleural pressure exceeds atmospheric pressure. It is a life-threatening condition and occurs when injury to the chest or respiratory structures permits air to enter but not leave the pleural space (Fig. 31-7). This results in a rapid increase in pressure within the chest that causes compression atelectasis of the unaffected lung, a shift in the mediastinum to the opposite side of the chest, and compression of the vena cava, which results in a decrease in venous return to the heart and reduced cardiac output.[6] Although tension pneumothorax can develop in people with spontaneous pneumothoraces, it is seen most often in people with traumatic pneumothoraces. It may also result from barotrauma caused by mechanical ventilation due to high tidal volume on people on the ventilator.[8]

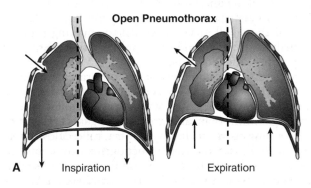

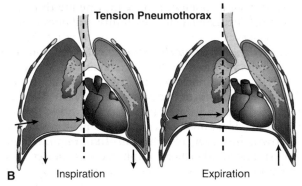

FIGURE 31-7. Open or communicating pneumothorax (**A**) and tension pneumothorax (**B**). In an open pneumothorax, air enters the chest during inspiration and exits during expiration. There may be slight inflation of the affected lung because of a decrease in pressure as air moves out of the chest. In tension pneumothorax, air can enter but not leave the chest. As the pressure in the chest increases, the heart and great vessels are compressed, and the mediastinal structures are shifted toward the opposite side of the chest. The trachea is pushed from its normal midline position toward the opposite side of the chest, and the unaffected lung is compressed.

Clinical Manifestations

The manifestations of pneumothorax depend on its size and the integrity of the underlying lung. In spontaneous pneumothorax, manifestations of the disorder sometimes include development of ipsilateral chest pain. There is an almost immediate increase in respiratory rate, often accompanied by dyspnea that occurs as a result of the activation of receptors that monitor lung volume. Asymmetry of the chest may occur because of the air being trapped in the pleural cavity on the affected side. This asymmetry may be evidenced during inspiration as a lag in the movement of the affected side, with inspiration delayed until the unaffected lung reaches the same level of pressure as the lung with the air trapped in the pleural space. Percussion of the chest produces a more hyperresonant sound, and breath sounds are decreased or absent over the area of the pneumothorax.

With tension pneumothorax, the structures in the mediastinal space shift toward the opposite side of the chest (see Fig. 31-7). When this occurs, the position of the trachea, normally located in the midline of the neck, deviates with the mediastinum. The position of the trachea can be used as a means of assessing for a mediastinal shift. Because of the increase in intrathoracic pressure, stroke volume is impaired to such an extent that cardiac output is decreased despite an increase in heart rate. There may be jugular neck vein distention, subcutaneous emphysema, and clinical signs of shock due to impaired cardiac function.

Hypoxemia usually develops immediately after a large pneumothorax, followed by vasoconstriction of the blood vessels in the affected lung, causing the blood flow to shift to the unaffected lung. In people with primary spontaneous pneumothorax, this mechanism usually returns oxygen saturation to normal within 24 hours. Hypoxemia is usually more serious in people with underlying lung disease in whom secondary spontaneous pneumothorax develops or in people with underlying heart disease who are unable to compensate with an increase in heart rate and stroke volumes. Regardless of etiology, the hypoxemia caused by the partial or total loss of lung function can be life-threatening. Without immediate intervention, the increased thoracic pressure will further impair both cardiac and pulmonary function, resulting in severe hypoxemia and hypotension, which often leads to respiratory and cardiac arrest.

Diagnosis and Treatment

Chest radiograph or CT scan confirms diagnosis of pneumothorax. Pulse oximetry and blood gas analysis are used to determine the effect on blood oxygen levels. Treatment of pneumothorax varies with the cause and extent of the disorder. In small spontaneous pneumothoraces, the air usually reabsorbs spontaneously. In larger pneumothoraces, the air is removed by needle aspiration or a closed drainage system to allow air to exit the pleural space and prevent it from reentering the chest.

Emergency treatment of tension pneumothorax involves the prompt insertion of a large-bore needle or chest tube into the affected side of the chest along with have asthma.[10] As adults are living longer, the prevalence of asthma in older adults is increasing.

The strongest risk factor for developing asthma is a genetic predisposition for the development of an immunoglobulin E (IgE)-mediated response to common allergens.[11] IgE is the antibody involved in causing allergic reactions and inflammation.[11] Other risk factors for childhood asthma include family history of asthma, allergies, antenatal exposure to tobacco smoke and pollution, and multiple potentially overlapping genetic predispositions.[12] Asthma severity is impacted by several factors including genetics, age of onset, pollution exposure, atopy, degree of exposure to triggers, environmental triggers such as tobacco smoke and dust mites, and the presence of gastroesophageal reflux disease or respiratory infections[10,11] (see the section "Severe or Refractory Asthma").

Etiology and Pathogenesis

The common denominator underlying asthma is an exaggerated hyperresponsiveness to a variety of stimuli. Airway inflammation manifested by the presence of inflammatory cells (particularly eosinophils, lymphocytes, and mast cells) and by damage to the bronchial epithelium contributes to the pathogenesis of the disease. T-helper 2 (T_2H) cells respond to allergens and helminths (intestinal parasites) by stimulating B cells to differentiate into IgE-producing plasma cells, produce growth factors for mast cells, and recruit and activate eosinophils. In people with allergic asthma, T-cell differentiation appears to be skewed toward a proinflammatory T_2H response. Although the molecular basis for this preferential differentiation is unclear, it seems likely that both genetic and environmental factors play a role.[11,13-16]

Cytokines also have an apparent role in the chronic inflammatory response and complications of asthma. Tumor necrosis factor (TNF)-α and interleukin 4 (IL-4) and IL-5 participate in the pathogenesis of bronchial asthma through their effects on the bronchial epithelial and smooth muscle cells.[17-19] Studies suggest that TNF-α, an inflammatory cytokine that is stored and released from mast cells, plays a critical role in the initiation and amplification of airway inflammation in people with asthma. TNF-α is credited with increasing the migration and activation of inflammatory cells (i.e., eosinophils and neutrophils) and contributing to all aspects of airway remodeling, including proliferation and activation of fibroblasts, increased production of extracellular matrix glycoproteins, and mucous cell hyperplasia.[19]

It has been determined that frequent viral respiratory infections predispose people with asthma to experience an exacerbation of their disease. In fact, frequent viral respiratory infections may also cause the development of asthma in some people.[14] When these respiratory infections are frequent at an early age, there is evidence that the T_2H response is exaggerated. When the CD4 T_2H cytokines IL-4, IL-5, and IL-13 are released, the airways are predisposed for an allergic response, which favors the production of IgE.[13-15]

The National Heart, Lung, and Blood Institute's Expert Panel Report 3 (NHLBI EPR 3): Guidelines for the Diagnosis and Management of Asthma defined asthma as a chronic inflammatory disorder of the airways. The immunologic aspects of asthma including the cascade of neutrophils, eosinophils, lymphocytes, and mast cells cause epithelial injury. This causes airway inflammation, which further increases hyperresponsiveness and decreased airflow.[11] There are multiple mediators and cell types that cause the inflammation and airway bronchoconstriction in asthma. When mast cells are activated, the release of histamine; prostaglandin D_2; cytokines such as IL-1 to IL-5, interferon, TNF, and granulocyte–macrophage colony-stimulating factor; and leukotrienes causes massive bronchoconstriction and inflammation of pulmonary vasculature endothelium. Mast cells can trigger multiple cytokine release, which causes major inflammation of the airway. The contraction of the airways and subsequent swelling leads to further airway obstruction.

The mast cell release may be linked to exercise-induced asthma (EIA), which is when people only experience wheezing and bronchospasm during exercise.[16,17] The cause of EIA is unclear. It is important to assess the type of air (polluted, cold, or warm), level of exercise, presence/absence of respiratory infectious process, and individual's asthma stability when identifying if a person has EIA.[16]

Eosinophils tend to be present in airways of people with asthma and generate inflammatory enzymes and release leukotrienes and many proinflammatory enzymes.[11,19] It is common to have increased neutrophils in sputum and airways of people experiencing asthma exacerbations.[19] The release of leukotrienes causes more mucus secretion, which often obstructs the airway further and causes more histamine release from the mast cells.[18]

This inflammatory process produces recurrent episodes of airway obstruction, characterized by wheezing, breathlessness, chest tightness, and a cough that is often worse at night and in the early morning. These episodes, which are usually reversible either spontaneously or with treatment, also cause an associated increase in bronchial responsiveness to a variety of stimuli.[14] Chronic inflammation can lead to airway remodeling, in which case airflow limitations may be only partially reversible.[11] This may be due to the long-term effects of the inflammation on the airway structures.[11]

There is a small group of people with the clinical triad of asthma, chronic rhinosinusitis with nasal polyps, and precipitation of asthma and rhinitis attacks in response to aspirin and other NSAIDs.[19] The mechanism of the hypersensitivity reaction is complex and not fully understood, but most evidence points toward an abnormality in arachidonic acid (AA) metabolism. Cyclooxygenase (COX), the rate-limiting enzyme in AA metabolism, exists in two main forms: COX-1 and COX-2. COX-1 is responsible for the synthesis of protective prostaglandins and COX-2 for the synthesis of mediators of inflammation and bronchoconstriction. It has been hypothesized that in people with aspirin-induced asthma, the inhibition of COX-1 shunts the metabolism of AA away from the production of protective prostaglandins and toward the generation of COX-2 and other mediators of

---

one-way valve drainage or continuous chest suction to aid in reinflating the affected lung. Sucking chest wounds, which allow air to pass in and out of the chest cavity, should be treated by promptly covering the area with an airtight bandage. Chest tubes are inserted as soon as possible to reexpand the lung.

> ### KEY POINTS
>
> #### Disorders of Lung Inflation
>
> - The pleura encases the lungs and is made up of two layers, which create the pleural cavity where pathology is often caused by air getting into the space, which is called a pneumothorax, or blood in the pleural space, which would cause a hemothorax.
> - Atelectasis is a partial expansion of the lung, which is caused by obstruction or compression of lung tissue.

Pleuritis

Pleuritis (also called *pleurisy*) refers to inflammation of the pleura. Pleuritis is common in infectious processes such as respiratory infections that extend to involve the pleura. Pain is a frequent symptom and most commonly is unilateral and abrupt in onset. When the central part of the diaphragm is irritated, the pain may be referred to the shoulder. Chest movements such as deep breathing and coughing that exaggerate pressure changes in the pleural cavity and increase movement of the inflamed or injured pleural surfaces usually make the pain worse. Because deep breathing is painful, tidal volumes are usually kept small, and breathing becomes more rapid to maintain minute volume. Reflex splinting of the chest muscles may occur, causing a lesser respiratory expansion on the affected side.

It is important to differentiate pleural pain from pain produced by other conditions, such as musculoskeletal strain of chest muscles, bronchial irritation, and myocardial disease. Musculoskeletal pain may occur as the result of frequent, forceful coughing. This type of pain is usually bilateral and located in the inferior portions of the rib cage, where the abdominal muscles insert into the anterior rib cage. Movements associated with contraction of the abdominal muscles make it worse. The pain associated with irritation of the bronchi is usually substernal and dull in character rather than sharp; it is often described as tightening. This type of pain is made worse with coughing but is not affected by deep breathing. Myocardial discomfort or pain is usually located in the substernal area and is not affected by respiratory movements.

Treatment of pleuritis consists of treating the underlying disease and inflammation. Analgesics and nonsteroidal anti-inflammatory drugs (NSAIDs) may be used for pleural pain.

Atelectasis

Atelectasis refers to an incomplete expansion of a lung or portion of a lung. It can be caused by airway obstruction, lung compression such as occurs in pneumothorax or pleural effusion, or increased recoil of the lung due to loss of pulmonary surfactant. The disorder may be present at birth (i.e., primary atelectasis) or develop during the neonatal period or later in life (i.e., acquired or secondary atelectasis).

Etiology and Pathogenesis

Primary atelectasis of the newborn implies that the lung has never been inflated. It is seen most frequently in premature and high-risk infants. A secondary form of atelectasis can occur in infants who established respiration and subsequently experienced impairment of lung expansion. Among the causes of secondary atelectasis in the newborn is respiratory distress syndrome associated with lack of surfactant, airway obstruction due to aspiration of amniotic fluid or blood, and bronchopulmonary dysplasia.

Acquired atelectasis occurs mainly in adults. It is caused most commonly by airway obstruction and lung compression (Fig. 31-8). A mucus plug in the airway or external compression by fluid, tumor mass, exudate, or other matter in the area surrounding the airway can cause obstruction. Portions of alveoli, a small segment of lung, or an entire lung lobe may be involved in obstructive atelectasis. Complete obstruction of an airway is followed by the absorption of air from the dependent alveoli and collapse of that portion of the lung. Breathing high concentrations of oxygen increases the rate at which gases are absorbed from the alveoli and predisposes to atelectasis. The danger of obstructive atelectasis increases after surgery. Administration of narcotics or anesthesia, pain, and immobility tend to promote retention of viscid bronchial secretions and can cause airway obstruction. The encouragement of coughing and deep breathing, frequent change of position, adequate hydration, and early ambulation decrease the likelihood of atelectasis developing.

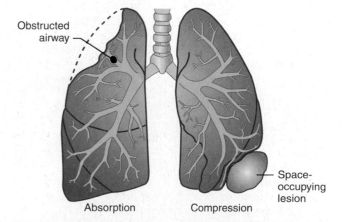

FIGURE 31-8. Atelectasis caused by airway obstruction and absorption of air from the involved lung area (**left**) and by compression of lung tissue (**right**).

Another cause of atelectasis is compression of lung tissue. It occurs when the pleural cavity is partially or completely filled with fluid, exudate, blood, a tumor mass, or air. It is observed most commonly in people with pleural effusion from congestive heart failure or cancer.

Clinical Manifestations

The clinical manifestations of atelectasis include tachypnea, tachycardia, dyspnea, cyanosis, signs of hypoxemia, diminished chest expansion, decreased breath sounds, and intercostal retractions. There may be *intercostal retraction* over the involved area during inspiration. Signs of respiratory distress are proportional to the extent of lung collapse. If the collapsed area is large, the mediastinum and trachea shift to the affected side. In compression atelectasis, the mediastinum shifts away from the affected lung.

Diagnosis and Treatment

The diagnosis of atelectasis is based on signs and symptoms. Chest radiographs are used to confirm the diagnosis. CT scans may be used to show the exact location of the obstruction.

Treatment depends on the cause and extent of lung involvement. It is directed at reducing the airway obstruction or lung compression and at reinflating the collapsed area of the lung. Ambulation, deep breathing, and body positions that favor increased lung expansion are used when appropriate. Administration of oxygen may be needed to correct the hypoxemia. There are new minimally invasive bronchoscopic procedures that may be used as both a diagnostic and treatment method.

SUMMARY CONCEPTS

Disorders of the pleura include pleural effusion, hemothorax, pneumothorax, and pleuritis. Pleural effusion refers to the abnormal accumulation of fluid in the pleural cavity. The fluid may be a transudate (*i.e.*, hydrothorax), exudate (*i.e.*, parapneumonic effusion, empyema), or chyle (*i.e.*, chylothorax). Hemothorax refers to the presence of blood in the pleural cavity. Pain is a common symptom of conditions that produce pleuritis or inflammation of the pleura. Characteristically, the pain is unilateral, abrupt in onset, and exaggerated by respiratory movements. Pneumothorax refers to an accumulation of air in the pleural cavity that causes partial or complete collapse of the lung. Pneumothorax can result from rupture of an air-filled bleb on the lung surface or from penetrating or nonpenetrating injuries. A tension pneumothorax is a life-threatening event in which air progressively accumulates in the thorax, collapsing the lung on the injured

side and progressively shifting the mediastinum to the opposite side of the thorax, producing severe cardiac and respiratory impairment.

Atelectasis refers to an incomplete expansion of the lung. Primary atelectasis occurs most often in premature and high-risk infants. Acquired atelectasis occurs mainly in adults and is caused most commonly by a mucus plug in the airway or by external compression by fluid, tumor mass, exudate, or other matter in the area surrounding the airway.

Obstructive Airway Disorders

Obstructive airway disorders are caused by disorders that limit expiratory airflow. Asthma refers to an acute and reversible form of airway disease caused by narrowing of airways due to bronchospasm, inflammation, and increased airway secretions. Chronic obstructive disorders include a variety of airway diseases, such as chronic bronchitis, emphysema, bronchiectasis, and CF.

KEY POINTS

Airway Disorders

■ Changes in airway patency involve changes in airway diameter due to bronchial smooth muscle hyperreactivity or changes in bronchial wall structure, injury to the mucosal lining of the airways, or excess respiratory tract secretions.

■ Bronchial asthma is a chronic disorder of the airways that causes episodes of airway obstruction due to bronchial smooth muscle hyperreactivity and airway inflammation. The episodes are usually reversible.

■ COPD represents a group of disorders that cause chronic and recurrent obstruction of the pulmonary airways. These disorders can affect patency of the bronchial structures (chronic bronchitis) or the gas-diffusing airspaces distal to the terminal bronchioles (emphysema) or a combination of both.

Asthma

Asthma is a chronic disorder of the airways that causes episodes of airway obstruction, bronchial hyperresponsiveness, airway inflammation, and, in some, airway remodeling.[9] More than 25 million people have asthma in the United States. An estimated 7.1 million children

---

Tubular Components of the Nephron

The nephron tubule is divided into four segments:

1. A highly coiled segment called the *proximal convoluted tubule*, which drains the Bowman capsule
2. A thin, looped structure called the *loop of Henle*
3. A distal coiled portion called the *distal convoluted tubule*
4. A *collecting tubule* (or *collecting duct*), which joins with several tubules to collect the filtrate[6]

The filtrate passes through each of these segments before reaching the pelvis of the kidney.

The proximal tubule dips toward the renal pelvis to become the descending limb of the loop of Henle. The ascending loop of Henle returns to the region of the renal corpuscle, where it becomes the distal tubule.[6] The distal convoluted tubule begins at the juxtaglomerular complex and is divided into two segments—the *diluting segment* and the *late distal tubule*. The late distal tubule fuses with the collecting tubule (or collecting duct). Like the distal tubule, the collecting duct is divided into two segments—the *cortical collecting tubule* and the *inner medullary collecting tubule*.[6]

Throughout its course, the tubule is composed of a single layer of epithelial cells resting on a basement membrane. The structure of the epithelial cells varies with tubular function. The cells of the proximal tubule have a fine, villous structure that increases the surface area for reabsorption. They are also rich in mitochondria, which support active transport processes. The epithelial layer of the thin segment of the loop of Henle has few mitochondria, indicating minimal metabolic activity and reabsorptive function.[6]

Urine Formation

Urine formation involves (a) the filtration of blood through the glomerulus to form an *ultrafiltrate of urine* and (b) the tubular reabsorption of electrolytes and nutrients needed to maintain the constancy of the internal environment while eliminating waste materials.

Glomerular Filtration

Urine formation begins with the filtration of essentially protein-free plasma through the glomerular capillaries into the Bowman space. The movement of fluid through the glomerular capillaries is determined by the same factors that facilitate fluid movement in all capillary beds: capillary hydrostatic pressure (filtration pressure), capillary colloidal osmotic pressure (reabsorptive pressure), and capillary permeability.[2] The glomerular filtrate has a chemical composition similar to plasma, but it contains almost no proteins because large molecules do not readily cross the glomerular wall. Approximately 125 mL of filtrate is formed each minute.[6] This is called the *glomerular filtration rate* (GFR). This rate can vary from a few milliliters per minute to as high as 200 mL/minute. The average adult has a GFR of 125 mL/minute or 180 L/day.[2]

The location of the glomerulus between two arterioles allows for maintenance of a high-pressure filtration

system. The capillary filtration pressure (approximately 60 mm Hg) in the glomerulus is approximately two to three times higher than that of other capillary beds in the body. The filtration pressure and the GFR are regulated by the constriction and relaxation of the afferent and efferent arterioles. Constriction of the efferent arteriole increases resistance to outflow from the glomeruli and increases the glomerular pressure and the GFR. Constriction of the afferent arteriole causes a reduction in renal blood flow (RBF), glomerular filtration pressure, and GFR.[2] The afferent and the efferent arterioles are innervated by the sympathetic nervous system and are sensitive to vasoactive hormones, such as angiotensin II, as well.[2]

Tubular Reabsorption and Secretion

From the Bowman capsule, the glomerular filtrate moves into the tubular segments of the nephron. While moving through the lumen of the tubular segments, the chemical composition of glomerular filtrate is changed considerably by the tubular transport of water and solutes. Tubular transport can result in reabsorption of substances from the tubular filtrate into the peritubular capillaries or secretion of substances from the peritubular capillaries into the tubular filtrate[2] (Fig. 32-6).

The basic mechanisms of transport across the tubular epithelial cell membrane are similar to those of other cell membranes in the body (including both active and passive transport mechanisms). Water and urea are passively absorbed along concentration gradients. Sodium (Na^+), potassium (K^+), chloride (Cl^-), calcium (Ca^{2+}),

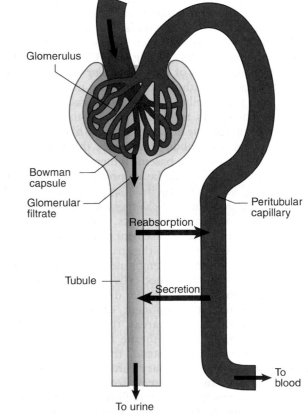

FIGURE 32-6. Reabsorption and secretion of substances between the renal tubules and peritubular capillaries.

and phosphate ions, as well as urate, glucose, and amino acids, are reabsorbed across the tubular epithelial cells and into the blood using primary or secondary active transport mechanisms. Some substances, such as hydrogen (H^+), K^+, and urate ions, are secreted from the blood, across the tubular epithelial cells, and into the tubular filtrate. Under normal conditions, only approximately 1 mL of the 125 mL of glomerular filtrate formed each minute is excreted in the urine.[2] The other 124 mL is reabsorbed in the tubules. This means that the average output of urine is approximately 60 mL/hour.

Renal tubular cells have two membrane surfaces through which substances must pass as they are reabsorbed from the tubular fluid. The outside membrane adjacent to the interstitial fluid is called the *basolateral membrane.* The side in contact with the tubular lumen and tubular filtrate is called the *luminal membrane.*[6] In most cases, substances move across the luminal membrane along a concentration gradient but require facilitated transport or active carrier systems to move across the basolateral membrane into the interstitial fluid, where the substances are absorbed into the peritubular capillaries.

The bulk of energy used by the kidney supports active transport mechanisms that facilitate Na^+ reabsorption with cotransport of other electrolytes and substances such as glucose and amino acids. This is called *secondary active transport* or *cotransport* (Fig. 32-7). Secondary active transport depends on the energy-dependent Na^+/K^+–adenosine triphosphatase (ATPase) pump on the basolateral side of renal tubular cells.[2] The pump maintains a low intracellular Na^+ concentration that facilitates the downhill (*i.e.,* from a higher to lower concentration) movement of Na^+ from the filtrate across the luminal membrane. Cotransport uses a carrier system in which the downhill movement of one substance, such as sodium, is coupled to the uphill movement (*i.e.,* from a lower to higher concentration) of another substance, such as glucose or an amino acid. A few substances, such as the H^+, are secreted into the tubule using countertransport, in which the movement of one substance, such as Na^+, enables the movement of a second substance in the opposite direction.[2]

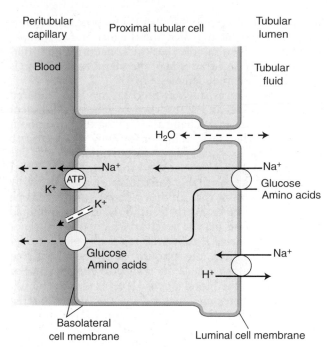

FIGURE 32-7. Mechanism for secondary active transport or cotransport of glucose and amino acids in the proximal tubule. The energy-dependent sodium–potassium pump on the basal lateral surface of the cell maintains a low intracellular gradient that facilitates the downhill movement of sodium and glucose or amino acids (cotransport) from the tubular lumen into the tubular cell and then into the peritubular capillary. ATP, adenosine triphosphate.

Proximal Tubule

Approximately 65% of all reabsorptive and secretory processes of the tubular system take place in the proximal tubule. Nutritionally, important substances (such as glucose, amino acids, lactate, and water-soluble vitamins) are almost completely reabsorbed, whereas electrolytes, such as Na^+, K^+, Cl^-, and bicarbonate (HCO_3^-), are 65% to 80% reabsorbed[2] (Fig. 32-8). As these solutes move into the tubular cells, their concentration in the tubular lumen decreases, providing a concentration gradient for

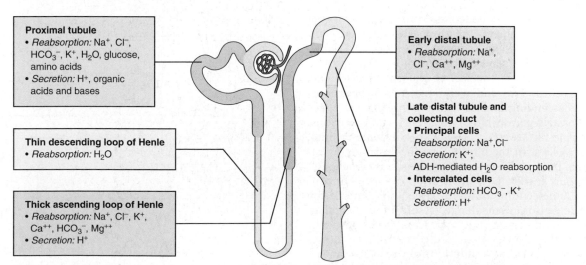

FIGURE 32-8. Sites of tubular water (H_2O), glucose, amino acids, Na^+ (sodium), Cl^- (chloride), HCO_3^- (bicarbonate), K^+ (potassium), Ca^{2+} (calcium), and Mg^{2+} (magnesium) reabsorption, and organic acids and bases, H^+ (hydrogen), and K^+ secretion. ADH, antidiuretic hormone.

the osmotic reabsorption of water. The proximal tubule is highly permeable to water, and the osmotic movement of water occurs so rapidly that the concentration difference of solutes on either side of the membrane seldom is more than a few milliosmoles.[2]

Many substances, such as glucose, are freely filtered in the glomerulus and reabsorbed by energy-dependent cotransport carrier mechanisms. The maximum amount of substance that these transport systems can reabsorb per unit time is called the *transport maximum*. The transport maximum is related to the number of carrier proteins that are available for transport and is usually sufficient to ensure that all of a filtered substance such as glucose can be reabsorbed rather than be eliminated in the urine. The plasma level at which the substance appears in the urine is called the *renal threshold*. Under some circumstances, the amount of substance filtered in the glomerulus exceeds the transport maximum. For example, when the blood glucose level is elevated in uncontrolled diabetes mellitus, the amount that is filtered in the glomerulus often exceeds the transport maximum (approximately 320 mg/minute), and glucose spills into the urine.[2]

In addition to *reabsorbing* solutes and water, cells in the proximal tubule also *secrete* organic cations and anions into the urine filtrate (see Figs. 32-6 and 32-8). Many of these organic anions and cations are end products of metabolism (*e.g.*, urate, oxalate) that circulate in the plasma. The proximal tubule also secretes exogenous organic compounds, many of which can be bound to plasma proteins and are not freely filtered in the glomerulus. Therefore, excretion by filtration alone eliminates only a small portion of these potentially toxic substances from the body.[2]

The Loop of Henle
The loop of Henle plays an important role in controlling the concentration of the urine. It does this by establishing a high concentration of osmotically active particles in the interstitium surrounding the medullary collecting tubules where the antidiuretic hormone (ADH) exerts its effects.

The loop of Henle is divided into three segments—the thin descending segment, the thin ascending segment, and the thick ascending segment. The loop of Henle, taken as a whole, always reabsorbs more Na^+ and Cl^- than water. This is in contrast to the proximal tubule, which reabsorbs Na^+ and water in equal proportions. The thin descending limb is highly permeable to water and moderately permeable to urea, Na^+, and other ions. As the urine filtrate moves down the descending limb, water moves out of the filtrate into the surrounding interstitium. Thus, the osmolality of the filtrate reaches its highest point at the elbow of the loop of Henle. In contrast to the descending limb, the ascending limb of the loop of Henle is impermeable to water.[2] In this segment, solutes are reabsorbed, but water cannot follow and remains in the filtrate. As a result, the tubular filtrate becomes more and more dilute, often reaching an osmolality of 100 mOsm/kg of water as it enters the distal convoluted tubule, compared with the 285 mOsm/kg of

water in plasma.[2] This allows for excretion of free water from the body. For this reason, it is often called the *diluting segment*.[2]

The thick segment of the loop of Henle begins in the ascending limb where the epithelial cells become thickened. As with the thin ascending limb, this segment is impermeable to water. The thick segment contains a $Na^+/K^+/2Cl^-$ cotransport system[6] (Fig. 32-9). This system involves the cotransport of a positively charged Na^+ and a positively charged K^+ ion accompanied by two negatively charged Cl^- ions. The gradient for the operation of this cotransport system is provided by the basolateral Na^+/K^+–ATPase pump, which maintains a low intracellular sodium concentration. Approximately 20% to 25% of the filtered load of Na^+, K^+, and Cl^- is reabsorbed in the thick loop of Henle. Movement of these ions out of the tubule leads to the development of a transmembrane potential that favors the passive reabsorption of small divalent cations such as Ca^{2+} and magnesium (Mg^{2+}).[6] The thick ascending loop of Henle is the site of action for the powerful "loop" diuretics (*e.g.*, furosemide [Lasix]), which exert their action by inhibiting the $Na^+/K^+/2Cl^-$ cotransporters.[7]

Distal and Collecting Tubules
Like the thick ascending loop of Henle, the distal convoluted tubule is relatively impermeable to water, and reabsorption of sodium chloride from this segment further dilutes the tubular fluid. Reabsorption of Na^+ occurs through a Na^+/Cl^- cotransport mechanism. Approximately 5% of filtered sodium chloride is reabsorbed in this section of the tubule. Unlike the thick ascending loop of Henle, neither Ca^{2+} nor Mg^{2+} is passively absorbed in this segment of the tubule. Instead,

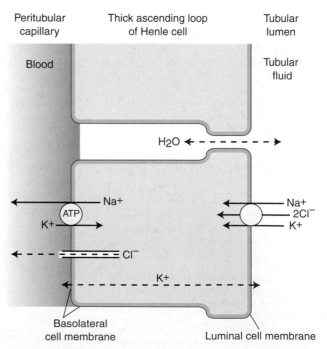

FIGURE 32-9. Sodium, chloride, and potassium reabsorption in the thick segment of the loop of Henle. ATP, adenosine triphosphate.

Ca^{2+} ions are actively reabsorbed in a process that is largely regulated by parathyroid hormone and possibly by vitamin D.[7]

The late distal tubule and the cortical collecting tubule are the sites where aldosterone exerts its action on Na^+ reabsorption and K^+ secretion and elimination. Although responsible for only 2% to 5% of sodium chloride reabsorption, this site is largely responsible for determining the final Na^+ concentration of the urine.[2] When the body is confronted with a K^+ excess, the amount of K^+ secreted at this site may exceed the amount filtered in the glomerulus.

The mechanism for Na^+ reabsorption and K^+ secretion in this section of the nephron is distinct from other tubular segments. This segment is composed of two types of cells, the *intercalated cells*, where K^+ is reabsorbed and H^+ is secreted, and the *principal cells*, where aldosterone exerts its action.[6] The secretion of H^+ into the tubular fluid by the intercalated cells is accompanied by the reabsorption of HCO_3^-. The intercalated cells can also reabsorb K^+. The principal cells reabsorb Na^+ and facilitate the movement of K^+ into the urine filtrate (Fig. 32-10). Under the influence of aldosterone, Na^+ moves from the urine filtrate into principal cells; from there, Na^+ moves into the surrounding interstitial fluid and peritubular capillaries. At the same time, K^+ moves in the opposite direction, from the peritubular capillaries into the principal cells and then into the urine filtrate.[6]

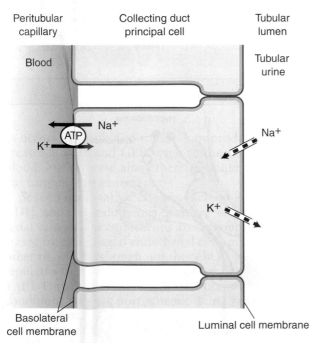

FIGURE 32-10. Mechanism of sodium reabsorption and potassium secretion by principal cells of the late distal and collecting tubules. Aldosterone exerts its action by increasing the activity of the Na^+/K^+–ATPase pump that transports sodium outward through the basolateral membrane of the cell and into the blood at the same time it pumps potassium into the cell. Aldosterone also increases the permeability of the luminal membrane for potassium. ATPase, adenosine triphosphatase.

Regulation of Urine Concentration

The kidney responds to changes in the osmolality of the extracellular fluid by producing either concentrated or dilute urine. The ability of the kidney to respond in this manner depends on the establishment of a high concentration of osmotically active particles in the interstitium of the kidney medulla and the action of ADH in regulating the water permeability of the surrounding medullary collecting tubules.[6]

In approximately one fifth of the juxtamedullary nephrons, the loops of Henle and special hairpin-shaped capillaries called the *vasa recta* descend into the medullary portion of the kidney. There, they form a countercurrent system that controls water and solute movement so that water is kept out of the area surrounding the tubule and solutes are retained.[6] The term *countercurrent* refers to a flow of fluids in opposite directions in adjacent structures. In this case, there is an exchange of solutes between the adjacent descending and ascending loops of Henle and between the ascending and descending sections of the vasa recta. Because of these exchange processes, a high concentration of osmotically active particles collects in the interstitium of the kidney medulla. The presence of these osmotically active particles in the interstitium surrounding the medullary collecting tubules facilitates the ADH-mediated reabsorption of water.[6]

ADH assists in maintenance of the extracellular fluid volume by controlling the permeability of the medullary collecting tubules. Osmoreceptors in the hypothalamus sense an increase in osmolality of extracellular fluids and stimulate the release of ADH from the posterior pituitary gland. In exerting its effect, ADH, also known as *vasopressin*, binds to receptors on the basolateral side of the tubular cells.[6] Binding of ADH to the vasopressin receptors causes water channels, known as *aquaporin-2 channels*, to move into the luminal side of the tubular cell membrane, producing a marked increase in water permeability. At the basolateral side of the membrane, water exits the tubular cell into the hyperosmotic interstitium of the medullary area, where it enters the peritubular capillaries for return to the vascular system.[6]

Regulation of Renal Blood Flow

In the adult, the kidneys are perfused with 1000 to 1300 mL of blood per minute, or 20% to 25% of the cardiac output. This large blood flow is mainly needed to ensure a sufficient GFR for the removal of waste products from the blood, rather than for the metabolic needs of the kidney. Feedback mechanisms, both intrinsic and extrinsic, normally keep blood flow and GFR constant despite changes in arterial blood pressure.[2]

Neural and Humoral Control Mechanisms

The kidney is richly innervated by the sympathetic nervous system. Increased sympathetic activity causes constriction of the afferent and efferent arterioles and thus a decrease in RBF. Intense sympathetic stimulation such

The Juxtaglomerular Complex

The juxtaglomerular complex is thought to represent a feedback control system that links changes in GFR with RBF. The juxtaglomerular complex is located at the site where the distal tubule extends back to the glomerulus and then passes between the afferent and efferent arterioles[2] (Fig. 32-11). The distal tubular site that is nearest to the glomerulus is characterized by densely nucleated cells called the *macula densa*.[2] In the adjacent afferent arteriole, the smooth muscle cells of the media are modified as special secretory cells called *juxtaglomerular cells*. These cells contain granules of inactive renin, an enzyme that functions in the conversion of angiotensinogen to angiotensin.[2]

Renin functions by means of angiotensin II to produce vasoconstriction of the efferent arteriole to prevent large decreases in the GFR. Angiotensin II also increases sodium reabsorption indirectly by stimulating aldosterone secretion from the adrenal gland and directly by increasing sodium reabsorption by the proximal tubule cells. The renin–angiotensin–aldosterone (RAA) mechanism is illustrated in Figure 32-12.

Because of its location between the afferent and efferent arterioles, the juxtaglomerular complex plays an essential role in linking RBF to both GFR and the composition of the distal tubular fluid. Specialized juxtaglomerular cells monitor the systemic arterial blood pressure by sensing the stretch of the afferent arteriole and also monitor the concentration of sodium chloride in the tubular filtrate as it passes through the macula densa. This information is then used in determining how much renin should be released to keep the arterial blood pressure within its normal range and maintain a relatively constant GFR.[2] It is thought that a decrease in the GFR slows the flow rate of the urine filtrate in the ascending loop of Henle, thereby increasing sodium and chloride reabsorption. This, in turn, decreases the delivery of sodium chloride to the macula densa. The decrease in delivery of sodium chloride to the macula densa has two effects: it decreases resistance in the afferent arterioles (which raises glomerular filtration pressure), and it increases the release of renin from the juxtaglomerular cells. The renin from these cells functions as an enzyme to convert angiotensinogen to angiotensin I, which is converted to angiotensin II.[2] Finally, angiotensin II acts to constrict the efferent arteriole as a means of producing a further increase in the glomerular filtration pressure and thereby returning the GFR toward a more normal range.

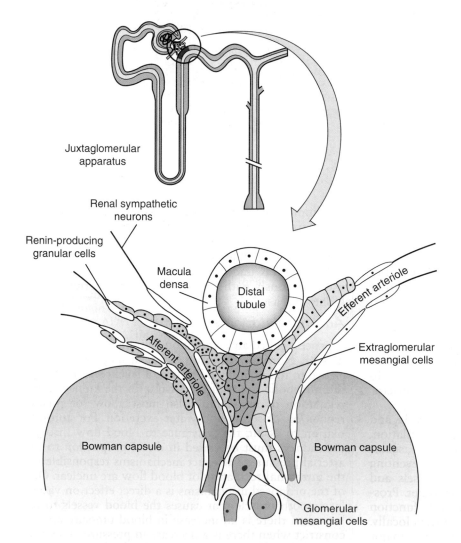

FIGURE 32-11. Juxtaglomerular apparatus and macula densa in tubuloglomerular feedback. The juxtaglomerular apparatus and macula densa cells at the beginning of the distal tubule are in close proximity. Chloride delivery is sensed by the N^+–K^+–$2Cl^-$ cotransporter in the thick ascending limb, and feedback regulates GFR. Renin release is also regulated at this site. GFR, glomerular filtration rate. (From Rennke H. G., Denker B. M. (2014). *Renal pathophysiology: The essentials* (4th ed., Fig. 1.9, p. 21). Philadelphia, PA: Lippincott Williams & Wilkins.)

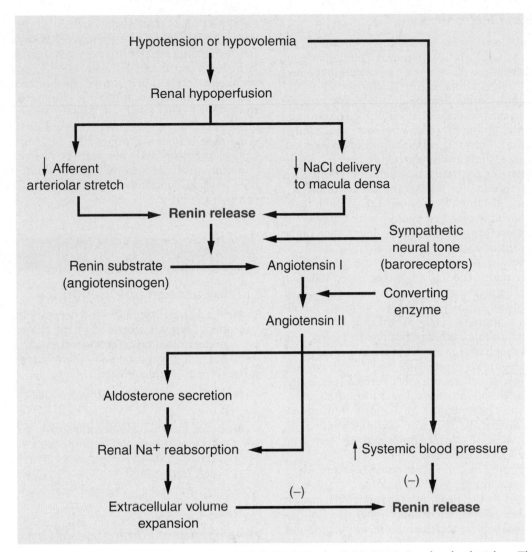

FIGURE 32-12. Pathway of angiotensin production. (From Rennke H. G., Denker B. M. (2014). *Renal pathophysiology: The essentials* (4th ed., Fig. 2.6, p. 49). Philadelphia, PA: Lippincott Williams & Wilkins.)

Effect of Increased Protein and Glucose Load

Although relatively stable under most conditions, both RBF and GFR increase in response to conditions of increased dietary protein and increased blood glucose. Within 1 to 2 hours after ingestion of a high-protein meal, RBF increases 20% to 30% within 1 to 2 hours. Although the exact mechanism for this increase is uncertain, it is thought to be related to the fact that amino acids and Na^+ are absorbed together in the proximal tubule (by secondary active transport). As a result, delivery of Na^+ to the macula densa is decreased, eliciting an increase in RBF through the juxtaglomerular complex feedback mechanism.[2] The resultant increase in RBF and GFR allows Na^+ excretion to be maintained at a near-normal level while increasing the excretion of the waste products of protein metabolism, such as urea. The same mechanism is thought to explain the large increases in RBF and GFR that occur with high blood glucose levels in people with uncontrolled diabetes mellitus.[2]

Elimination Functions of the Kidney

The primary functions of the kidney are elimination of water, waste products, excess electrolytes, and unwanted substances from the blood.[2]

Renal Clearance

Renal clearance is the volume of plasma that is completely cleared each minute of any substance that finds its way into the urine. It is determined by the ability of the substance to be filtered in the glomeruli and the capacity of the renal tubules to reabsorb or secrete the substance. Every substance has its own clearance rate, the units of which are always volume of plasma per unit time. It can be determined by measuring the amount of a substance that is excreted in the urine (*i.e.*, urine concentration × urine flow rate in milliliters per minute) and dividing by its plasma concentration.[9]

Regulation of Electrolytes

Elimination of electrolytes, particularly Na$^+$ and K$^+$, is regulated by the GFR and by humoral agents that control their reabsorption. Aldosterone functions in the regulation of Na$^+$ and K$^+$ elimination. Reabsorption of Na$^+$ in the distal tubule and collecting duct is highly variable and depends on the presence of aldosterone secretion by the adrenal gland. In the presence of aldosterone, almost all the sodium in the distal tubular fluid is reabsorbed, and the urine essentially becomes sodium free. In the absence of aldosterone, virtually, no sodium is reabsorbed from the distal tubule. The remarkable ability of the distal tubular and collecting duct cells to alter sodium reabsorption in relation to changes in aldosterone allows the kidneys to excrete urine with sodium levels that range from a few tenths of a gram to 40 g/day.[2]

Free filtration of K$^+$ also occurs at the glomerulus; however, K$^+$ is reabsorbed from and secreted into the tubular fluid. The secretion of K$^+$ into the tubular fluid occurs in the distal tubule and is also regulated by aldosterone. Only approximately 70 mEq of K$^+$ is delivered to the distal tubule each day, but the average person consumes this much and more K$^+$ in the diet. Excess K$^+$ that is not filtered in the glomerulus and delivered to the collecting tubule, therefore, must be secreted (*i.e.*, transported from the blood into the tubular filtrate) for elimination from the body.[2] In the absence of aldosterone, as in Addison disease, K$^+$ secretion becomes minimal. In these circumstances, K$^+$ reabsorption exceeds secretion, and blood levels of K$^+$ increase.

Also contributing to the excretion of Na$^+$ and water by the kidney are the *natriuretic peptides*, a group of peptides secreted by the heart in response to the stretch of cardiac muscle fibers. The primary renal effect of this group of chemicals is to increase the renal excretion of sodium (natriuresis), with a resultant osmotic increase in the excretion of water. This loss of sodium and water leads to a reduction in cardiac preload, which creates a negative feedback loop to decrease cardiac muscle stretch.[2] Atrial muscle cells release *atrial natriuretic peptide* (ANP) in response to muscle stretch. The primary effect of ANP is to inhibit sodium and water reabsorption, with action predominant in the collecting ducts. ANP also acts to disrupt the RAA cascade by inhibiting the renal secretion of renin. This disruption of the RAA cascade thus further decreases the reabsorption of sodium and water by the renal tubules.[2]

Regulation of pH

The kidneys regulate body pH by conserving HCO$_3^-$ and eliminating H$^+$. Most H$^+$ excreted in the urine is because of tubular secretory mechanisms. The lowest tubular fluid pH that can be achieved is 4.4 to 4.5.[10,11] The ability of the kidneys to excrete H$^+$ depends on buffers in the urine that combine with the H$^+$. The three major urine buffers are bicarbonate (HCO$_3^-$), phosphate, and ammonia. The combination of HCO$_3^-$ and H$^+$ in the renal tubule results in the formation of carbonic acid, which then dissociates into carbon dioxide and water. The carbon dioxide is then absorbed into the tubular

cells, and HCO$_3^-$ is regenerated inside the tubule cells through the action of the enzyme carbonic anhydrase. In the second renal buffering system, phosphate ions (which are produced by cells as end products of metabolic processes) join with H$^+$ in the renal tubules and then the resultant compound is eliminated in the urine. In the third renal buffering system, ammonia is synthesized in tubular cells by deamination of the amino acid glutamine (which is produced by the liver during amino acid metabolism and then transported to the kidneys). Ammonia diffuses into the tubular fluid, where it combines with H$^+$, and the compound molecule is eliminated through the urine.[2]

KEY POINTS

The Functions of the Kidney

- The kidney regulates the composition and pH of body fluids through the reabsorption and elimination or conservation of water and substances, particularly the electrolytes Na$^+$, K$^+$, H$^+$, Cl$^-$, and HCO$_3^-$.

- The kidney regulates the osmolality of the extracellular fluid through the action of ADH.

- The kidney plays a central role in blood pressure regulation through the influences of the RAA and ANP mechanisms on Na$^+$ and water elimination.

---

pH-Dependent Elimination of Organic Ions

The proximal tubule actively secretes large amounts of different organic anions. Foreign anions (*e.g.*, salicylates, penicillin) and endogenously produced anions (*e.g.*, bile acids, uric acid) are actively secreted into the tubular fluid. Most of the anions that are secreted use the same transport system, allowing the kidneys to rid the body of many different drugs and environmental agents.[2] Because the same transport system is shared by different anions, there is competition for transport such that elevated levels of one substance tend to inhibit the secretion of other anions. The proximal tubules also possess an active transport system for organic cations that is analogous to that for organic anions.

Uric Acid Elimination

Uric acid (an organic anion) is a product of purine metabolism. Excessively high blood levels (*i.e.*, hyperuricemia) can cause gout, and high levels of uric acid in the urine can cause kidney stones. Uric acid is freely filtered in the glomerulus and is reabsorbed and secreted in the proximal tubules.[5] Tubular reabsorption normally exceeds secretion, and the net effect is removal of uric acid from the filtrate. Although the rate of reabsorption exceeds secretion, the secretory process is homeostatically controlled to maintain a constant plasma level. Many people with elevated uric acid levels secrete less uric acid compared to those with normal uric acid levels.[5]

Urea Elimination

Urea is formed in the liver as a by-product of protein metabolism and is eliminated entirely by the kidneys. Healthy adults produce urea in the range of 25 to 30 g/day. Blood urea levels rise with a high-protein diet, excessive tissue breakdown, or gastrointestinal bleeding.[2] In gastrointestinal bleeding, the intestinal flora breaks down the blood to form ammonia, which is then absorbed into the portal venous circulation and transported to the liver, where it is converted to urea before being released into the bloodstream. The kidneys then regulate blood urea nitrogen (BUN) levels, maintaining a normal BUN in the range of 8 to 25 mg/dL (2.9 to 8.9 mmol/L).[2] During periods of dehydration, the blood volume and GFR drop, causing BUN levels to increase. This rise in BUN occurs because when GFR is reduced, the filtrate moves more slowly through the tubules, allowing more time for urea resorption. In contrast, when the GFR is high, only small amounts of urea are reabsorbed into the blood.[2]

Drug Elimination

Many drugs are eliminated in the urine. Only drugs that are not bound to plasma proteins are filtered in the glomerulus and, therefore, able to be eliminated by the kidneys.[7] Because uric acid competes for the same anion transport systems as some drugs (such as aspirin, sulfinpyrazone, and probenecid), these drugs can affect the blood levels of uric acid and, therefore, may not be indicated for use in person with gout. Thiazide and loop diuretics (*i.e.*, furosemide and ethacrynic acid) can also cause hyperuricemia and gout, presumably through a decrease in extracellular fluid volume and enhanced uric acid reabsorption.[6]

Endocrine Functions of the Kidney

In addition to regulating body fluids and electrolytes, the kidneys function as an endocrine organ by producing chemical mediators that travel through the blood to distant sites where they exert their actions. Endocrine functions of the kidneys include:

- Assisting with blood pressure regulation through the RAA mechanism
- Regulation of red blood cell production through the synthesis of erythropoietin
- Assisting with calcium homeostasis by activating vitamin D

The Renin–Angiotensin–Aldosterone Mechanism

As introduced earlier, the RAA mechanism plays an important part in short- and long-term regulation of blood pressure. Renin is an enzyme that is synthesized and stored in the juxtaglomerular cells of the kidney. This enzyme is thought to be released in response to a decrease in RBF or a change in the composition of the distal tubular fluid or as the result of sympathetic nervous system stimulation. Renin itself has no direct effect on blood pressure. Rather, it acts enzymatically to convert a circulating plasma protein called *angiotensinogen* to angiotensin I. Angiotensin I, which has few vasoconstrictor properties, leaves the kidneys and enters the circulation; as it is circulated through the lungs, *angiotensin-converting enzyme* catalyzes the conversion of angiotensin I to angiotensin II. Angiotensin II is a potent vasoconstrictor, and it acts directly on the kidneys to decrease salt and water excretion. Both mechanisms have relatively short periods of action. Angiotensin II also stimulates aldosterone secretion by the adrenal gland. Aldosterone acts on the distal tubule to increase sodium reabsorption and exerts a longer term effect on the maintenance of blood pressure. Renin also functions via angiotensin II to produce constriction of the efferent arteriole as a means of preventing a serious decrease in glomerular filtration pressure.[2]

Erythropoietin

Erythropoietin is a glycoprotein hormone that is produced by fibroblasts in the renal interstitium and regulates the production of red blood cells in the bone marrow. The synthesis of erythropoietin is stimulated by tissue hypoxia, which may be brought about by anemia, residence at high altitudes, or impaired oxygenation of tissues because of cardiac or pulmonary disease. Person with end-stage kidney disease is often anemic because of an inability of the kidneys to produce erythropoietin. This anemia is usually managed by the administration of a recombinant erythropoietin (epoetin alfa) produced through DNA technology to stimulate erythropoiesis.[12]

Vitamin D

Activation of vitamin D occurs in the kidneys. Vitamin D increases calcium absorption from the gastrointestinal tract and helps to regulate calcium deposition in the bone. It also has a weak stimulatory effect on renal calcium absorption. Although vitamin D is not synthesized and released from an endocrine gland, it is often considered a hormone because of its pathway of molecular activation and mechanism of action.

Vitamin D exists in two forms—natural vitamin D (cholecalciferol), produced in the skin from ultraviolet irradiation, and synthetic vitamin D (ergocalciferol), derived from irradiation of ergosterol. The active form of vitamin D is 1,25-dihydroxycholecalciferol. Cholecalciferol and ergocalciferol must undergo chemical transformation to become active: first to 25-hydroxycholecalciferol in the liver and then to 1,25-dihydroxycholecalciferol in the kidneys. People with end-stage renal disease are unable to transform vitamin D to its active form and may require pharmacologic preparations of the active vitamin (calcitriol) for maintaining mineralization of their bones.[6]

SUMMARY CONCEPTS

The kidneys perform excretory and endocrine functions. In the process of excreting wastes, the kidneys filter the blood and then selectively reabsorb those materials that are needed to maintain a stable internal environment. The kidneys rid the body of metabolic wastes, regulate fluid volume, regulate the concentration of electrolytes, assist in maintaining acid–base balance, aid in regulation of blood pressure (through the RAA mechanism and control of extracellular fluid volume), regulate red blood cell production through erythropoietin production, and aid in calcium metabolism by activating vitamin D.

The nephron is the functional unit of the kidney. It is composed of a glomerulus, which filters the blood, and a tubular component, where electrolytes and other substances needed to maintain the constancy of the internal environment are reabsorbed back into the bloodstream, whereas unneeded materials are secreted into the tubular filtrate for elimination. Urine concentration occurs in the collecting tubules under the influence of ADH. ADH maintains extracellular volume by returning water to the vascular compartment, producing concentrated urine by removing water from the tubular filtrate.

The GFR is the amount of filtrate that is formed each minute as blood moves through the glomeruli. It is regulated by the arterial blood pressure and RBF in the normally functioning kidney. The juxtaglomerular complex is thought to represent a feedback control system that links changes in the GFR with RBF. Renal clearance is the volume of plasma that is completely cleared each minute of any substance that finds its way into the urine. It is determined by the ability of the substance to be filtered in the glomeruli and the capacity of the renal tubules to reabsorb or secrete the substance.

Tests of Renal Function

The function of the kidneys is to filter the blood, selectively reabsorb those substances that are needed to maintain the constancy of body fluid, and excrete metabolic wastes. The composition of urine and blood provides valuable information about the adequacy of renal function. Radiologic tests, **endoscopy**, and renal biopsy provide means for viewing the gross and microscopic structures of the kidneys and urinary system.

Urine Tests

Urine is a clear, amber-colored fluid that is approximately 95% water and 5% dissolved solids. The kidneys normally produce approximately 1.5 L of urine each day. Normal urine contains metabolic wastes and few or no plasma proteins, blood cells, or glucose molecules. Urine tests can be performed on a single urine specimen or on a 24-hour urine specimen. First-voided morning specimens are useful for qualitative protein and specific gravity testing. A freshly voided specimen is the most reliable. Urine specimens that have been left standing may contain lysed red blood cells, disintegrating *casts*, and rapidly multiplying bacteria.[9] Table 32-1 describes urinalysis values for normal urine.

Casts are molds of the distal nephron lumen. A gel-like substance called *Tamm–Horsfall mucoprotein*, which is formed in the tubular epithelium, is the major protein constituent of urinary casts.[6] Casts composed of this gel but devoid of cells are called *hyaline casts*. These casts develop when the protein concentration of the urine is high (as in nephrotic syndrome), urine osmolality is high, and urine pH is low. The inclusion of granules or cells in the matrix of the protein gel leads to the formation of various other types of casts.[6]

Proteinuria is excessive protein excretion in the urine. Because of the glomerular capillary filtration barrier, less than 150 mg/L of protein is excreted in the urine over 24 hours in a healthy person. Urine tests for proteinuria are used to detect abnormal filtering of albumin in the glomeruli or defects in its reabsorption in the renal tubules. A protein reagent dipstick can be used as a rapid screening test for the presence of proteins in the urine. Once the presence of proteinuria has been detected, a 24-hour urine test is often used to quantify the amount of protein that is present.[9]

Albumin, which is the smallest of the plasma proteins, is filtered more readily than globulins or other plasma proteins. Thus, *microalbuminuria* tends to occur long before clinical proteinuria becomes evident. A dipstick test for microalbuminuria is available for screening purposes. The microalbuminuria dipstick method, however, only indicates an increase in urinary albumin that is below the detectable range of the standard proteinuria test. It does not specify the amount of albumin that is present in the urine. Therefore, a 24-hour urine collection is the standard method for detecting microalbuminuria (an albumin excretion >30 mg/day is abnormal).[9]

The *specific gravity* of urine varies with its concentration of solutes. Urine specific gravity provides a valuable index of the hydration status and functional ability of the kidneys. With a normal fluid intake, the usual range of urine specific gravity is 1.010 to 1.025. Healthy kidneys can produce concentrated urine with a specific gravity of 1.030 to 1.040. During periods of marked hydration, the specific gravity can approach 1.000. With diminished renal function, there is a loss of renal concentrating ability, and the urine specific gravity may fall to levels of 1.006 to 1.010.[9] *Urine osmolality*, which depends on the number of particles of solute in a unit of solution, is a more exact measurement of urine

TABLE 32-1. Normal Values for Routine Urinalysis

General Characteristics and Measurements	Chemical Determinations	Microscopic Examination of Sediment
Color: yellow amber Appearance: clear to slightly hazy Specific gravity: 1.005–1.025 with a normal fluid intake pH: 4.5–8.0; average person has a pH of about 5–6 Volume: 600–2500 mL/24 hour; average volume is 1200 mL/24 hour	Glucose: negative Ketones: negative Blood: negative Protein: negative Bilirubin: negative Urobilinogen: 0.5–4.0 mg/day Nitrate for bacteria: negative Leukocyte esterase: negative	Casts negative: occasional hyaline casts Red blood cells: negative or rare Crystals: negative (none) White blood cells: negative or rare Epithelial cells: few; hyaline casts 0–1/1pf (low-power field)

From Fischbach F., Dunning M. (2014). *A manual of laboratory and diagnostic tests* (9th ed., p. 192). Philadelphia, PA: Lippincott Williams & Wilkins.

concentration than specific gravity.[9] More information concerning renal function can be obtained if the serum and urine osmolality tests are done at the same time. The normal ratio between urine and serum osmolality is 3:1. A high urine-to-serum ratio is seen in concentrated urine. With poor concentrating ability, the ratio is low.[9]

Glomerular Filtration Rate

The GFR can be measured clinically by collecting timed samples of blood and urine. *Creatinine* is produced by muscles as a product of the metabolism of a molecule called creatine. The formation and release of creatinine are relatively constant and proportional to the amount of muscle mass present. Creatinine is freely filtered in the glomeruli, is not reabsorbed from the tubules into the blood, and is only minimally secreted into the tubules from the blood. Therefore, its blood values depend closely on the GFR. The comparison of creatinine levels in the blood and urine can provide a useful measure of GFR. The clearance rate for creatinine is the amount that is completely cleared by the kidneys in 1 minute. The formula is expressed as C = UV/P, where C is the clearance rate (mL/minute), U is the urine concentration (mg/dL), V is the urine volume excreted (mL/minute or 24 hours), and P is plasma concentration (mg/dL).[9]

Normal creatinine clearance is 115 to 125 mL/minute.[9] This value is corrected for body surface area, which reflects the muscle mass where creatinine production takes place. The test may be done on a 24-hour basis, with a blood creatinine level drawn at the completion of a 24-hour urine collection. In another method, two 1-hour urine specimens are collected, with a blood sample drawn in between.[9]

Although the creatinine clearance test is the traditional method of measuring GFR, most labs are now reporting a calculated "estimated GFR" (or eGFR) as part of various metabolic panels. The eGFR estimates the GFR using a measured plasma creatinine in a mathematical formula accounting for additional factors such as age, sex, and race.[12] Creatinine, which is a waste product of muscle metabolism, is filtered at the glomerulus, which allows serum creatinine levels to provide a good reflection of GFR. However, because creatinine is a molecule produced in the muscle and because muscle mass varies widely among different populations, creatinine levels can be less accurate as a GFR predictor among certain populations. Creatinine levels tend to increase among person with increased levels of physical activity, higher muscle mass, and diets higher in meat and in person with better health status.[13]

Additional biologic measures are being introduced into clinical practice to provide better assessment of GFR. The serum protein *cystatin C* has been demonstrated to serve as a useful marker of GFR because it is also filtered at the glomerulus but has a stable production rate across populations. An estimating equation for GFR that combines the effects of creatinine and cystatin C has been developed and demonstrated to perform better than eGFR equations based on either creatinine or cystatin C alone.[14]

Blood Tests

Blood tests can provide valuable information about the kidneys' ability to remove metabolic wastes and maintain normal electrolyte and pH composition of the blood. Normal blood values are listed in Table 32-2. Serum levels of K^+, phosphate, BUN, and creatinine increase in renal failure, whereas serum pH, Ca^{2+}, and HCO_3^- levels decrease in renal failure.[2]

Serum Creatinine

The normal creatinine value is approximately 0.7 mg/dL for a woman with a small frame, approximately 1.0 mg/dL for a normal adult man, and approximately 1.5 mg/dL (60 to 130 mmol/L) for a muscular man.[9] There is an age-related decline in creatinine clearance in many older adults because muscle mass and the GFR decline with age. A normal serum creatinine level usually indicates normal renal function. In addition to its use in calculating the GFR, the serum creatinine level is used in estimating the functional capacity of the kidneys (Fig. 32-13). If the value doubles, the GFR (and renal function) probably has fallen to one half of its normal state. A rise in the serum creatinine level to three times its normal value suggests that there is a 75% loss of renal function, and with creatinine values of 10 mg/dL

11. Zeisberg M., Kalluri R. (2015). Physiology of the renal interstitium. *Clinical Journal of the American Society of Nephrology* 10(10), 1831–1840.

12. American Association for Clinical Chemistry. (2016). Estimated glomerular filtration rate (eGFR). [Online]. Available: https://labtestsonline.org/understanding/analytes/gfr/tab/glance. Accessed May 23, 2019.

13. Shilpak M. G., Mattes M. D., Peralta C. A. (2013). Update on cystatin C: Incorporation into clinical practice. *American Journal of Kidney Disease* 62(3), 595–603.

14. Karger A. B., Inker L. A., Coresh J., et al. (2017). Novel filtration markers for GFR estimation. *Journal of the International Federation of Clinical Chemistry and Laboratory Medicine* 28(4), 277–288.

15. NIH National Institute of Diabetes and Digestive and Kidney Diseases. (2015). Cystoscopy and ureteroscopy. [Online]. Available: https://www.niddk.nih.gov/health-information/diagnostic-tests/cystoscopy-ureteroscopy. Accessed May 23, 2019.

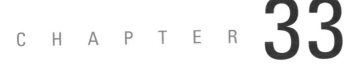

CHAPTER **33**

Disorders of Renal Function

Learning Objectives

After completing this chapter, the learner will be able to meet the following objectives:

1. Define the terms *agenesis*, *hypoplasia*, and *dysgenesis*, and discuss them as they refer to the development of the kidney.
2. Describe the inheritance, pathology, and manifestations of the different types of polycystic kidney disease.
3. List four common causes of urinary tract obstruction.
4. Define the term *hydronephrosis* and relate it to the destructive effects of urinary tract obstruction.
5. Describe the role of urine supersaturation, nucleation, and inhibitors of stone formation in the development of kidney stones.
6. List three physiologic mechanisms that protect against urinary tract infections (UTIs).

Disorders of Glomerular Function

Glomerulonephritis is an inflammatory process that involves glomerular structures. It is the second leading cause of kidney failure worldwide and ranks third, after diabetes and hypertension, as a cause of chronic kidney disease in the United States.[5] There are many causes of glomerular disease. The disease may occur as a primary condition in which the glomerular abnormality is the only disease present, or it may occur as a secondary condition in which the glomerular abnormality results from another disease, such as diabetes mellitus or SLE. See Figure 33-9 for an algorithm regarding primary versus secondary glomerulonephritis.

Etiology and Pathogenesis of Glomerular Injury

The causative agents or triggering events that produce glomerular injury include immunologic, nonimmunologic, and hereditary mechanisms. Most cases of primary and many cases of secondary glomerular disease probably have an immune origin.[5] Although many glomerular diseases are driven by immunologic events, a variety of nonimmunologic metabolic (*e.g.*, diabetes), hemodynamic (*e.g.*, hypertension), and toxic (*e.g.*, drugs, chemicals) stresses can induce glomerular injury, either alone or along with immunologic mechanisms. Hereditary glomerular diseases such as Alport syndrome, although relatively rare, are an important category of glomerular disease because of their association with progressive loss of renal function and transmission to future generations.

Two types of immune mechanisms have been implicated in the development of glomerular disease:

1. Injury resulting from antibodies reacting with fixed glomerular antigens or antigens planted within the glomerulus
2. Injury resulting from circulating antigen–antibody complexes that become trapped in the glomerular membrane (Fig. 33-10)

Antigens responsible for development of the immune response may be of endogenous origin, such as autoantibodies to deoxyribonucleic acid in SLE, or they may be of exogenous origin, such as streptococcal membrane antigens in poststreptococcal glomerulonephritis. Frequently, the source of the antigen is unknown.

The cellular changes that occur with glomerular disease include increases in glomerular or inflammatory cell number (proliferative or hypercellular), basement membrane thickening (membranous), and changes in noncellular glomerular components (sclerosis and fibrosis).[5,6] An increase in cell numbers is characterized by one or more of the following: proliferation of endothelial and mesangial cells, leukocyte infiltration (neutrophils, monocytes, and, in some cases, lymphocytes), and formation of crescents (half-moon–shaped collections of

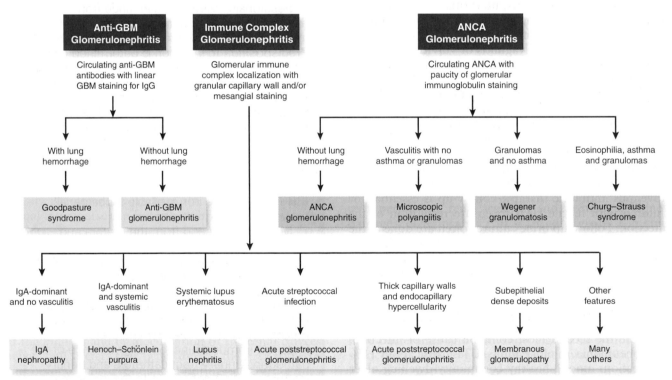

FIGURE 33-9. Algorithm demonstrating the integration of pathologic findings with clinical data to make a diagnosis of a specific form of primary or secondary glomerulonephritis. An important initial categorization is an anti-GBM immune complex or ANCA glomerulonephritis. Once this determination is made, more specific diagnoses depend on additional clinical or pathologic observations. ANCA, antineutrophil cytoplasmic autoantibody; GBM, glomerular basement membrane; IgA, immunoglobulin-A; IgB, immunoglobulin-B. (From Rubin R., Strayer D. (Eds.). (2015). *Rubin's pathology: Clinicopathologic foundations of medicine* (7th ed., p. 915, Fig. 22.15). Philadelphia, PA: Wolters Kluwer Health.)

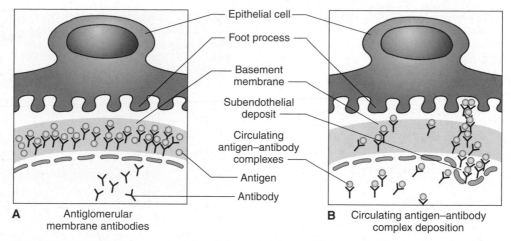

FIGURE 33-10. Immune mechanisms of glomerular disease. (**A**) Antiglomerular membrane antibodies leave the circulation and interact with antigens that are present in the basement membrane of the glomerulus. (**B**) Antigen–antibody complexes circulating in the blood become trapped as they are filtered in the glomerulus.

proliferating epithelial cells and infiltrating leukocytes) in the Bowman space.[5,6] *Basement membrane thickening* involves deposition of dense, noncellular material on the endothelial and epithelial sides of the basement membrane or within the membrane itself. Sclerosis refers to an increased amount of extracellular material in the mesangial, subendothelial, or subepithelial tissue of the glomerulus. Fibrosis refers to the deposition of collagen fibers. Glomerular changes can be *diffuse*, involving all glomeruli and all parts of the glomeruli; focal, in which only some glomeruli are affected and others are essentially normal; *segmental*, involving only a certain segment of each glomerulus; or *mesangial*, affecting only mesangial cells.[5,6] Figure 33-11 illustrates the location of lesions associated with various types of glomerular disease.

Types of Glomerular Disease

The clinical manifestations of glomerular disorders generally fall into one of five categories:

1. Nephritic syndromes
2. Rapidly progressive glomerulonephritis
3. The nephrotic syndrome
4. Asymptomatic disorders of urinary sediment (*i.e.*, -hematuria, prote inuria)
5. Chronic glomerulonephritis[5]

The nephritic syndromes produce a proliferative inflammatory response, whereas the nephrotic syndrome produces increased permeability of the glomerulus. Because most glomerular disorders can produce mixed nephritic

FIGURE 33-11. Schematic representation of three glomerular capillaries depicting the sites of immune complex formation. Subepithelial deposits are seen in postinfectious glomerulonephritis (*1*) and membranous nephropathy (*2*) and are likely to be assembled locally by an in situ mechanism. Subendothelial deposits (*3*) and mesangial deposits (*4*) may also form locally but are more often the result of passive entrapment of preformed circulating immune complexes. Anti-GBM antibodies bind in a linear pattern to the GBM (*5*), and because the specific antigen is part of the heavily cross-linked basement membrane, electron-dense deposits at the ultrastructural level are missing. EN, endothelial cell; EP, visceral epithelial cell or podocyte; GBM, glomerular basement membrane; MC, mesangial cell; MM, mesangial matrix. (From Rennke H. G., Denker B. M. (2014). *Renal pathophysiology: The essentials* (4th ed., p. 242). Philadelphia, PA: Lippincott Williams & Wilkins.)

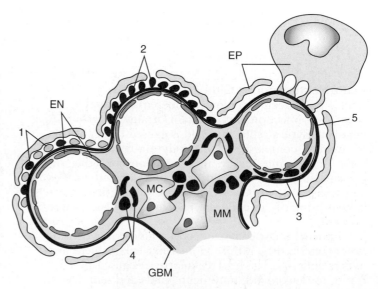

and nephrotic syndromes, a definitive diagnosis often requires renal biopsy.

Acute Nephritic Syndrome

The acute nephritic syndrome is the clinical correlate of acute glomerular inflammation. In its most dramatic form, the acute nephritic syndrome is characterized by a sudden onset of hematuria (either microscopic or grossly visible, with red cell casts), variable degrees of proteinuria, diminished GFR, oliguria, and signs of impaired renal function. Inflammatory processes that occlude the glomerular capillary lumen and damage the capillary wall cause it. This damage to the capillary wall allows RBCs to escape into the urine and produce hemodynamic changes that decrease the GFR. Extracellular fluid accumulation, hypertension, and edema develop because of the decreased GFR and enhanced tubular reabsorption of salt and water.

The acute nephritic syndrome may occur in such systemic diseases as SLE. Typically, however, it is associated with acute proliferative glomerulonephritis such as postinfectious glomerulonephritis.

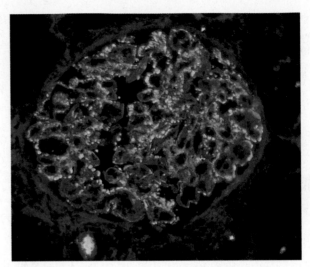

FIGURE 33-12. Acute postinfectious glomerulonephritis. An immunofluorescence micrograph demonstrates granular staining for complement C3 in capillary walls and the mesangium. (From Rubin R., Strayer D. (Eds.). (2015). *Rubin's pathology: Clinicopathologic foundations of medicine* (7th ed., p. 926, Fig. 22-37). Philadelphia, PA: Wolters Kluwer Health.)

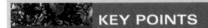

KEY POINTS

Glomerular Disorders

■ Glomerular disorders affect the semipermeable properties of the glomerular capillary membrane that allow water and small particles to move from the blood into the urine filtrate while preventing blood cells and plasma proteins from leaving the circulation.

■ The nephritic syndromes produce a decrease in glomerular permeability and manifestations related to a decrease in GFR, fluid retention, and nitrogenous waste accumulation.

■ The nephrotic syndrome produces an increase in glomerular permeability and manifestations of altered body function related to a massive loss of plasma proteins in the urine.

Acute Postinfectious Glomerulonephritis

Acute postinfectious glomerulonephritis usually occurs after infection with certain strains of group A beta-hemolytic streptococci and is caused by deposition of immune complexes of antibody and bacterial antigens.[5] It also may occur after infections by other organisms, including staphylococci, a viral agent (such as hepatitis), and various parasites.[3] Although the disease is seen primarily in children, people of any age can be affected.

The acute phase of postinfectious glomerulonephritis is characterized by diffuse glomerular enlargement and hypercellularity. The hypercellularity is caused by infiltration of leukocytes, both neutrophils and monocytes,

and proliferation of endothelial and mesangial cells.[5] There is also swelling of endothelial cells. The combination of proliferation, swelling, and leukocyte infiltration obliterates the glomerular capillary lumens. There may be interstitial edema and inflammation, and the tubules often contain RBCs. In the first weeks of disease, immunofluorescence microscopy typically reveals granular deposits of IgG and the complement component C3 in the mesangium and along the basement membrane (Fig. 33-12).

The classic case of poststreptococcal glomerulonephritis follows a streptococcal infection by approximately 7 to 12 days. This is the time needed for the development of antibodies. The primary infection usually involves the pharynx, but can be skin triggered. Oliguria, which develops as the GFR decreases, is one of the first symptoms. Proteinuria and hematuria follow because of increased glomerular capillary wall permeability. Materials in the urine degrade the RBCs, and cola-colored urine may be the first sign of the disorder. Sodium and water retention gives rise to edema (particularly of the face and hands) and hypertension. Important laboratory findings include an elevated antistreptococcal antibody (ASO) titer, a decline in serum concentrations of C3 and other components of the complement cascade, and cryoglobulins (*i.e.*, large immune complexes) in the serum.

Treatment of acute poststreptococcal glomerulonephritis includes elimination of the streptococcal infection with antibiotics and providing supportive care. The disorder carries an excellent prognosis and rarely causes chronic kidney disease.[5]

Rapidly Progressive Glomerulonephritis

Rapidly progressive glomerulonephritis is a clinical syndrome characterized by signs of severe glomerular injury that do not have a specific cause. As its name indicates, this type of glomerulonephritis is rapidly progressive, often within a matter of months. The disorder involves focal and segmental proliferation of glomerular cells and recruitment of monocytes and macrophages with formation of crescent-shaped structures that obliterate the Bowman space.[37] Rapidly proliferative glomerulonephritis may be caused by a number of immunologic disorders, some systemic and others restricted to the kidney. Among the diseases associated with this form of glomerulonephritis are immune complex disorders such as SLE, small-vessel vasculitides (*e.g.*, microscopic polyangiitis), and an immune disorder called *Goodpasture syndrome*.

Goodpasture Syndrome

Goodpasture syndrome is an uncommon and aggressive form of glomerulonephritis that is caused by antibodies to the alveolar and glomerular basement membrane (GBM). The anti-GBM antibodies cross-react with the pulmonary alveolar basement membrane to produce the syndrome of pulmonary hemorrhage associated with renal failure. The pathologic hallmark of anti-GBM glomerulonephritis is diffuse linear staining of GBMs for IgG (Fig. 33-13). The cause of the disorder is unknown, although influenza infection, exposure to hydrocarbon solvent (found in paints and dyes), various drugs, and cancer have been implicated in some people. There is some thought that Goodpasture syndrome has a genetic predisposition, but this is not conclusive.

Treatment includes plasmapheresis to remove circulating anti-GBM antibodies and immunosuppressive therapy (*i.e.*, corticosteroids and cyclophosphamide) to inhibit antibody production.[30]

Nephrotic Syndrome

The nephrotic syndrome is characterized by massive proteinuria (>3.5 g/day) and lipiduria (*e.g.*, free fat, oval bodies, fatty casts) along with an associated

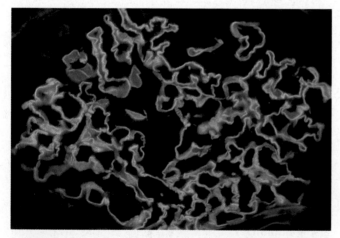

FIGURE 33-13. Anti-GBM glomerulonephritis. Linear immunofluorescence for IgG is seen along the GBM. Contrast this with the granular pattern of immunofluorescence typical of most types of immune complex deposition within the capillary wall. GBM, glomerular basement membrane; IgG, immunoglobulin-G. (From Rubin R., Strayer D. (Eds.). (2015). *Rubin's pathology: Clinicopathologic foundations of medicine* (7th ed., p. 933, Fig. 22-52). Philadelphia, PA: Wolters Kluwer Health.)

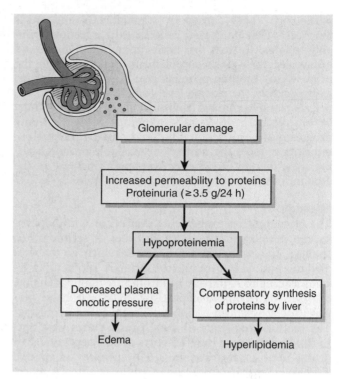

FIGURE 33-14. Pathophysiology of the nephrotic syndrome.

hypoalbuminemia (<3 g/dL), generalized edema, and hyperlipidemia (cholesterol > 300 mg/dL).[3] The nephrotic syndrome is not a specific glomerular disease but a constellation of clinical findings that result from an increase in glomerular permeability and loss of plasma proteins in the urine[5] (Fig. 33-14).

Pathogenesis

Any increase in glomerular membrane permeability allows proteins to escape from the plasma into the glomerular filtrate. Massive proteinuria results, leading to hypoalbuminemia. Generalized edema, which is a hallmark of the nephrotic syndrome, results from the loss of colloidal osmotic pressure of the blood with subsequent accumulation of fluid in the interstitial tissues.[5] There is also salt and water retention, which aggravates the edema. This appears to be due to several factors, including a compensatory increase in aldosterone, stimulation of the sympathetic nervous system, and a reduction in secretion of natriuretic factors. Initially, the edema presents in dependent parts of the body such as the lower extremities but becomes more generalized as the disease progresses. Dyspnea because of pulmonary edema, pleural effusions, and diaphragmatic compromise because of ascites can develop in people with nephrotic syndrome.

The hyperlipidemia that occurs in people with nephrosis is characterized by elevated levels of triglycerides and low-density lipoproteins (LDLs). Levels of high-density lipoproteins usually are normal. Because of the elevated LDL levels, people with nephrotic syndrome are at increased risk for development of atherosclerosis.

The largest proportion of protein lost in the urine is albumin, but globulins also may be lost. As a result, people with nephrosis may be vulnerable to infections, particularly those caused by staphylococci and pneumococci.[5] This decreased resistance to infection probably relates to loss of both immunoglobulins and low-molecular-weight complement components in the urine. Many binding proteins also are lost in the urine. Consequently, the plasma levels of many ions (iron, copper, zinc) and hormones (thyroid and sex hormones) may be low because of decreased binding proteins. Many drugs require protein binding for transport. Hypoalbuminemia reduces the number of available protein-binding sites, thereby producing a potential increase in the amount of free (active) drug that is available.

Etiology

The glomerular derangements that occur with nephrosis can develop as a primary disorder or secondary to changes caused by systemic diseases such as diabetes mellitus and SLE. Among the primary glomerular lesions leading to nephrotic syndrome are minimal change disease (MCD, lipoid nephrosis), focal segmental glomerulosclerosis, and membranous glomerulonephritis.[5] The relative frequency of these causes varies with age. In children younger than 15 years of age, nephrotic syndrome almost always is caused by primary idiopathic glomerular disease, whereas in adults, it often is a secondary disorder.[5]

Minimal Change Disease (Lipoid Nephrosis). MCD is characterized by diffuse loss (through fusion) of the foot processes of cells in the epithelial layer of the glomerular membrane. It is most commonly seen in children but may occasionally occur in adults. The cause of minimal change nephrosis is unknown. Although MCD does not progress to renal failure, it can cause significant complications, including predisposition to infection with gram-positive organisms, a tendency toward thromboembolic events, hyperlipidemia, and protein malnutrition.

Membranous Glomerulonephritis. Membranous glomerulonephritis is the most common cause of primary nephrosis in adults, most commonly those in the fifth and sixth decades of life and almost always after 30 years of age.[5] The disorder is caused by diffuse thickening of the GBM because of deposition of immune complexes. The disorder may be idiopathic or associated with a number of disorders, including autoimmune diseases such as SLE, infections such as chronic hepatitis B, and metabolic disorders such as diabetes mellitus. The presence of immunoglobulins and complement in the subendothelial deposits suggests that the disease represents a chronic immune complex–mediated disorder.

The disorder usually begins with an insidious onset of the nephrotic syndrome or, in a small percentage of people, with nonnephrotic proteinuria. Hematuria and mild hypertension may be present. The progress of the disease is variable. Some people experience a complete remission, others have repeated remissions and relapses, and still others progress to complete renal failure and even death. Spontaneous remissions and a relatively benign outcome occur more commonly in women and those with proteinuria in the nonnephrotic range. Treatment is controversial.

Focal Segmental Glomerulosclerosis. Focal segmental glomerulosclerosis is characterized by sclerosis (*i.e.*, increased collagen deposition) of some, but not all glomeruli, and in the affected glomeruli, only a portion of the glomerular tuft is involved.[5] It is a particularly common cause of nephrotic syndrome in Hispanic and African Americans.

Although focal segmental sclerosis often is an idiopathic syndrome, it may be associated with reduced oxygen in the blood (*e.g.*, sickle cell disease and cyanotic congenital heart disease), human immunodeficiency virus infection, or intravenous drug abuse, or it may occur as a secondary event reflecting glomerular scarring because of other forms of glomerulonephritis.[5] Impairment of autophagy (a repair process necessary to maintain homeostasis post cell injury) may be responsible for limited regenerative capacity of podocytes.[38]

The presence of hypertension and decreased renal function distinguishes focal sclerosis from MCD. In addition, research indicates that people with MCD (a manifestation of nephrotic syndrome diagnosed by renal biopsy) may later progress to focal segmental glomerulosclerosis.[39] The protein nephrin seems to be a marker for podocyte injury. People with MCD respond to varying degrees to corticosteroids. People who were treated and did not experience nephrin loss had a 96% remission rate compared with a 61% remission rate among those who experienced nephrin loss.[39] Most people with the disorder progress to kidney failure within 5 to 10 years.

Asymptomatic Hematuria or Proteinuria

Many cases of glomerulonephritis result in mild asymptomatic illness that is not recognized or brought to the attention of a health care professional and therefore remains undiagnosed. Population-based screening studies have shown that kidney damage as evidenced by proteinuria, hematuria, low GFR, or a combination of these features is present in the population. Disorders such as Henoch–Schönlein purpura often resolve without permanent kidney damage, whereas others such as IgA nephropathy and Alport syndrome can progress to chronic kidney disease and renal failure.

Immunoglobulin-A Nephropathy

Immunoglobulin-A nephropathy (IgAN) (*i.e.*, Berger disease) is a primary glomerulonephritis characterized by the presence of glomerular IgA immune complex deposits. It can occur at any age, but most commonly, the peak age of diagnosis is between 15 and 30 years of age.[5] The disease occurs more commonly in men than in women and is the most common cause of glomerular nephritis in Asians.

The disorder is characterized by the deposition of IgA-containing immune complexes in the mesangium of the glomerulus. Once deposited in the kidney, the immune complexes are associated with glomerular inflammation. The cause of the disorder is unknown, and there is a need for more specific classifications of the stages of IgA nephropathy so more information can be interpreted. Therefore, the International IgA Nephropathy Network is developing IgAN classifications to assist providers in diagnosing this disease. The classification system is based on biopsy findings in a minimum of eight glomeruli to yield a MEST-C score.[40] Some people with the disorder have elevated serum IgA levels.

Early in the disease, many people with the disorder have no obvious symptoms and are unaware of the problem. In these people, IgA nephropathy is suspected during routine screening or examination for another condition. In other people, the disorder presents with gross hematuria that is preceded by upper respiratory tract infection, gastrointestinal tract symptoms, or a flu-like illness. The hematuria usually lasts 2 to 6 days. Approximately one-half of the people with gross hematuria have a single episode, whereas the remainder experience a gradual progression in the disease with recurrent episodes of hematuria and mild proteinuria. Progression usually is slow, extending over several decades.

Immunofluorescence microscopy is essential for diagnosis of IgA nephropathy.[5] The diagnostic finding is mesangial staining for IgA more intense than staining for IgG or IgM (Fig. 33-15). At present, there are no satisfactory treatment measures for IgA nephropathy.

Henoch–Schönlein Purpura Nephritis

Henoch–Schönlein purpura is a small-vessel vasculitis that causes a purpuric rash largely of the lower extremities, arthritis or arthralgia, abdominal pain, and renal involvement identical to that of IgA nephropathy. Incidence has seasonal variation, with twice as many cases in the winter and fall.[41] The disease is seen most commonly in children but can also occur in adults. Renal involvement is not always present initially, but its incidence increases with time and is more common in older children, who have associated abdominal pain and a persistent rash. Although hematuria and proteinuria are the most common presentation, some people present with manifestations of acute nephritis, and others may present with combined nephritis and nephrotic manifestations. Most people recover fully over a period of several weeks. Some cases progress to end-stage renal

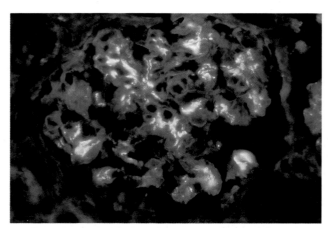

FIGURE 33-15. Immunoglobulin-A (IgA) nephropathy. An immunofluorescence micrograph shows deposits of IgA in the mesangial areas. (From Rubin R., Strayer D. (Eds.). (2015). *Rubin's pathology: Clinicopathologic foundations of medicine* (7th ed., p. 931, Fig. 22-48). Philadelphia, PA: Wolters Kluwer Health.)

disease. Corticosteroids are the most effective treatment and have been found to decrease the duration and intensity of abdominal and joint pain.[41]

Alport Syndrome

Alport syndrome represents a hereditary defect of the GBM that results in hematuria and may progress to chronic renal failure. It tends to be associated with defects in the ears or eyes.[5] The syndrome is caused by type IV collagen mutations. Approximately 85% of cases are inherited as an X-linked autosomal dominant trait, whereas others have autosomal dominant and recessive patterns of inheritance.[5] In X-linked pedigrees, boys are usually affected more seriously than girls. Affected boys usually progress to renal failure as adults, but progression may occur during adolescence. Although many girls never have more than mild hematuria with or without mild proteinuria, some have more significant disease and may even progress to kidney failure.

Diagnosis of Alport syndrome is often made after examination of the urine of a child from a family with multiple cases of hereditary nephritis. Children may initially present with heavy microscopic hematuria, followed by the development of proteinuria. Many, but not all, people with Alport syndrome have sensorineural deafness and various eye disorders, including lens dislocation, posterior cataracts, and corneal dystrophy. The hearing loss is bilateral and often is first detected during adolescence.

Chronic Glomerulonephritis

Chronic glomerulonephritis represents the chronic phase of a number of specific types of glomerulonephritis.[5] Some forms of acute glomerulonephritis (*e.g.*, poststreptococcal glomerulonephritis) undergo complete resolution, whereas others progress at variable rates to chronic glomerulonephritis. Some people who present with chronic glomerulonephritis have no history of glomerular disease. These cases may represent the end result of relatively asymptomatic forms of glomerulonephritis. Histologically, the condition is characterized by small kidneys with sclerosed glomeruli. In most cases, chronic glomerulonephritis develops insidiously and slowly progresses to chronic kidney disease over a period of years.

Glomerular Lesions Associated with Systemic Disease

Many immunologic, metabolic, or hereditary systemic diseases are associated with glomerular injury. In some diseases, such as SLE, diabetes mellitus, and hypertension, the glomerular involvement may be a major clinical manifestation.

Systemic Lupus Erythematosus Glomerulonephritis

Renal involvement is clinically evident in 40% to 85% of people with SLE and is seen more commonly in black women.[5] The pathogenesis of SLE is uncertain

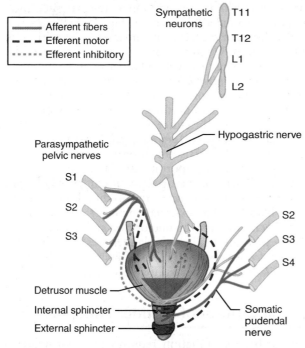

FIGURE 35-2. Nerve supply to the bladder and the urethra.

receptors in the bladder wall, the pudendal nerve carries sensory fibers from the external sphincter and pelvic muscles, and the hypogastric nerve carries sensory fibers from the trigone area.[1]

Pontine Micturition Center

The immediate coordination of the normal micturition reflex occurs in the micturition center in the pons, facilitated by descending input from the forebrain and ascending input from the reflex centers in the spinal cord[1-3] (Fig. 35-3). This center is thought to coordinate the activity of the detrusor muscle and the external sphincter. As bladder filling occurs, ascending spinal afferents relay this information to the micturition center, which also receives important descending information from the forebrain concerning behavioral cues for bladder emptying and urine storage. Descending pathways from the pontine micturition center produce coordinated inhibition or relaxation of the external sphincter. Disruption of pontine control of micturition, as in spinal cord injury, results in uninhibited spinal reflex–controlled contraction of the bladder without relaxation of the external sphincter, a condition known as *detrusor–sphincter dyssynergia*.[1]

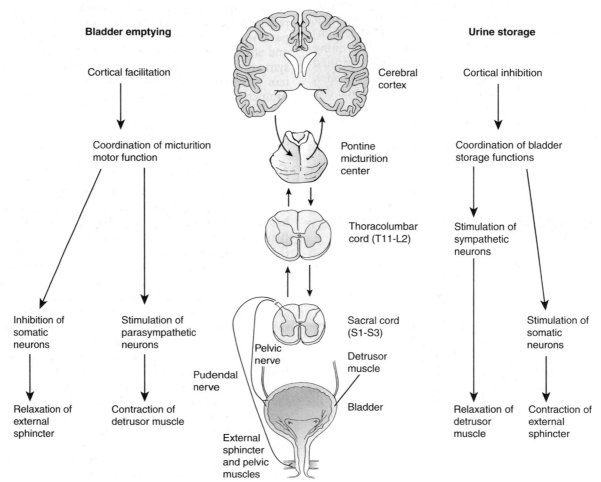

FIGURE 35-3. Pathways and CNS centers involved in the control of bladder emptying (**left**) and storage (**right**) functions. Efferent pathways for micturition (**left**) and urine storage (**right**) are also shown. CNS, central nervous system.

Cortical and Subcortical Centers

Cortical brain centers inhibit the micturition center in the pons and conscious control of urination. Neural influences from the subcortical centers in the basal ganglia modulate the contractile response. They delay the detrusor contractile response during filling and then modulate the expulsive activity of the bladder to facilitate complete emptying.

Micturition and Maintenance of Continence

To maintain continence, or retention of urine, the bladder must function as a low-pressure storage system, with the pressure in the bladder being lower than that in the urethra. Abnormal sustained elevations in intravesical pressures (>40 to 50 cm H_2O) are often associated with vesicoureteral reflux (*i.e.*, backflow of urine from the bladder into the ureter) and the development of ureteral dilation. Although the pressure in the bladder is maintained at low levels, sphincter pressure remains high (45 to 65 cm H_2O) as a means of preventing loss of urine as the bladder fills.

Micturition, or the act of bladder emptying, involves both sensory and motor functions associated with bladder emptying.[1] When the bladder is distended to 150 to 250 mL in the adult, the sensation of fullness is transmitted to the spinal cord and then to the cerebral cortex.[3] At approximately 400 to 500 mL, the person will sense fullness of the bladder.[3] During the act of micturition, the detrusor muscle of the bladder fundus and bladder neck contracts down on the urine; the ureteral orifices are forced shut; the bladder neck is widened and shortened because it is pulled up by the globular muscles in the bladder fundus; the resistance of the internal sphincter in the bladder neck is decreased; and the external sphincter relaxes as urine moves out of the bladder.[3]

Pharmacology of Micturition

The autonomic nervous system (ANS) and its neuromediators play a central role in micturition. Parasympathetic innervation of the bladder is mediated by the neurotransmitter acetylcholine. Two types of cholinergic receptors, nicotinic and muscarinic, affect various aspects of micturition. *Nicotinic* (N) receptors are found in the synapses between the preganglionic and postganglionic neurons of the sympathetic and the parasympathetic system, as well as in the neuromuscular end plates of the striated muscle fibers of the external sphincter and pelvic muscles. *Muscarinic* (M) receptors are found in the postganglionic parasympathetic endings of the detrusor muscle. Several subtypes of M receptors have been identified. Both M_2 and M_3 receptors appear to mediate detrusor muscle activity, with the M_3 subtype mediating direct activation of detrusor muscle contraction. The M_2 subtype appears to act indirectly by inhibiting sympathetically mediated detrusor muscle relaxation.[4] Although sympathetic innervation is not essential to the act of micturition, it allows the bladder to store a large volume without the involuntary escape of urine—a mechanism that is consistent with the fight-or-flight function served by the sympathetic nervous system. The bladder is supplied with α_1- and β_2-adrenergic receptors. The β_2-adrenergic receptors are found in the detrusor muscle. They produce relaxation of the detrusor muscle, increasing the bladder volume at which the micturition reflex is triggered. The α_1-adrenergic receptors are found in the trigone area, including the intramural ureteral musculature, bladder neck, and internal sphincter. The activation of α_1-adrenergic receptors produces contraction of these muscles. Sympathetic activity ceases when the micturition reflex is activated. During male ejaculation, which is mediated by the sympathetic nervous system, the musculature of the trigone area and that of the bladder neck and prostatic urethra contracts and prevents the backflow of seminal fluid into the bladder.

Because of their effects on bladder function, drugs that selectively activate or block ANS outflow or receptor activity can alter urine elimination.[5] Table 35-1 describes the action of drug groups that can impair bladder

TABLE 35-1 Action of Drug Groups on Bladder Function

Function	Drug Groups	Mechanism of Action
Detrusor Muscle		
Increased tone and contraction	Cholinergic drugs	Stimulate parasympathetic receptors that cause detrusor contraction
Inhibition of detrusor muscle relaxation during filling	β_2-Adrenergic blockers	Block β_2 receptors that produce detrusor muscle relaxation
Decreased tone	Anticholinergic drugs	Block the muscarinic receptors that cause detrusor muscle contraction
	Calcium channel blockers	May interfere with influx of calcium to support contraction of the detrusor smooth muscle
Internal Bladder Sphincter		
Increased tone	α_1-Adrenergic agonists	Activate α_1 receptors that produce contraction of the smooth muscle of the internal sphincter
Decreased tone	α_1-Adrenergic blockers	Block contraction of the smooth muscle of the internal sphincter
External Sphincter		
Decreased tone	Skeletal muscle relaxants	Decrease the tone of the external sphincter by acting at the level of the spinal cord or by interfering with the release of calcium in the muscle fibers

function or can be used in the treatment of micturition disorders.

Continence in Children

In infants and young children, micturition is an involuntary act that is triggered by a spinal cord reflex; when the bladder fills to a given capacity, the detrusor muscle contracts, and the external sphincter relaxes. As the child grows, the bladder gradually enlarges.[6,7] As the bladder grows and increases in capacity, the tone of the external sphincter muscle increases. Toilet training begins at about 2 to 3 years of age when the child becomes conscious of the need to urinate. Conscious control of bladder function depends on (1) normal bladder growth, (2) myelination of the ascending afferents that signal awareness of bladder filling, (3) development of cortical control and descending communication with the sacral micturition center, (4) ability to consciously tighten the external sphincter to prevent incontinence, and (5) motivation of the child to stay dry. Females typically achieve continence before males.

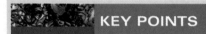

KEY POINTS

Bladder Function

■ The control of the storage and emptying functions of the bladder involves both the involuntary (ANS) and voluntary (somatic nervous system) control.

■ The striated muscles in the external sphincter and pelvic floor, which are innervated by the somatic nervous system, provide for the voluntary control of urination and maintenance of continence.

Diagnostic Methods of Evaluating Bladder Structure and Function

Bladder structure and function can be assessed by a number of methods.[8] Reports or observations of frequency, hesitancy, straining to urinate or void, and a weak or interrupted stream are suggestive of outflow obstruction. Palpation and percussion provide information about bladder distention.

Physical Examination

Postvoid residual (PVR) urine volume provides information about bladder emptying. It can be estimated by abdominal palpation and percussion. Catheterization and ultrasonography can be used to obtain specific measurements of PVR. A PVR value of less than 50 mL is considered adequate bladder emptying, and more than 200 mL indicates inadequate bladder emptying.[8]

Pelvic examination is used in females to assess perineal skin condition, perivaginal muscle tone, genital atrophy, pelvic prolapse, pelvic mass, or other conditions that may impair bladder function. Bimanual examination can be used to assess PVR volume. Rectal examination is used to test for perineal sensation, sphincter tone, fecal impaction, and rectal mass. It is also used to assess the contour of the prostate in males.

Laboratory and Radiologic Studies

Urine tests provide information about kidney function and urinary tract infections. Chapter 32 provides urine and radiologic studies to evaluate the function of the urinary system.

Ultrasonographic Bladder Scan

The ultrasonographic bladder scan provides a noninvasive method for estimating bladder volume, such as the PVR.[8] The device uses ultrasonic reflections to differentiate the urinary bladder from the surrounding tissue. The device can also be used to determine the need for catheterization, for evaluation and diagnosis of urinary retention, and for facilitating volume-dependent or time-dependent catheterization or toileting programs.

Urodynamic Studies

Urodynamic studies are used to study bladder function and voiding problems. Three aspects of bladder function can be assessed by urodynamic studies: bladder, urethral, and intra-abdominal pressure changes; characteristics of urine flow; and the activity of the striated muscles of the external sphincter and pelvic floor.[9]

Uroflowmetry

Uroflowmetry measures the flow rate (milliliters per minute) during urination.[9] As the person being tested voids, the weight of the commode receptacle unit increases. This weight change is electronically recorded and then analyzed as volume (weight converted to milliliters) versus time.

Cystometry

Cystometry is used to measure bladder pressure during filling and voiding. It provides valuable information about total bladder capacity, intravesical pressures during bladder filling, the ability to perceive bladder fullness and the desire to urinate, the ability of the bladder to contract and sustain a contraction, uninhibited bladder contractions, and the ability to inhibit urination.[9]

Urethral Pressure Profile

The urethral pressure profile is used to evaluate the intraluminal pressure changes along the length of the urethra with the bladder at rest.[9] It provides information about smooth muscle activity along the length of the urethra.

Sphincter Electromyography

Sphincter electromyography allows the activity of the striated (voluntary) muscles of the perineal area to be studied.[9] Activity is recorded using an anal plug electrode, a catheter electrode, adhesive skin electrodes, or needle electrodes.[8] Electrode placement is based on the muscle groups that need to be tested.

SUMMARY CONCEPTS

Although the kidneys function in the formation of urine and the regulation of body fluids, it is the bladder that stores and controls the elimination of urine. Micturition is a function of the peripheral ANS, subject to facilitation or inhibition from higher neurologic centers. The parasympathetic nervous system controls the function of the detrusor muscle and internal sphincter; its cell bodies are located in S1 through S3 of the spinal cord and communicate with the bladder through the pelvic nerve. Efferent sympathetic control originates at the thoracolumbar level (T11 through L2) of the spinal cord and produces relaxation of the detrusor muscle and contraction of the internal sphincter. Skeletal muscle found in the external sphincter and the pelvic muscles that support the bladder are supplied by the pudendal nerve, which exits at the sacral level (S2 through S4) of the spinal cord. The pontine micturition center coordinates the action of the detrusor muscle and the external sphincter, whereas cortical centers permit conscious control of micturition.

Bladder structure and function can be evaluated using physical examination; laboratory and radiologic studies; urodynamic studies that measure bladder, urethral, and abdominal pressures; urine flow characteristics; and skeletal muscle activity of the external sphincter.

Alterations in Bladder Function

Alterations in bladder function include urinary obstruction with retention or stasis of urine and urinary incontinence with involuntary loss of urine. Although the two conditions have almost opposite effects on urination, they can have similar causes. Both can result from structural changes in the bladder, urethra, or surrounding organs or from impairment of neurologic control of bladder function.

Lower Urinary Tract Obstruction and Stasis

Urinary tract obstructions are classified according to cause (congenital or acquired), degree (partial or complete), duration (acute or chronic), and level (upper or lower urinary tract).[10] In lower urinary tract obstruction and stasis, urine is produced normally by the kidneys but is retained in the bladder. Because it has the potential to produce vesicoureteral reflux and cause kidney damage, lower urinary tract obstruction and stasis are serious disorders.

The common sites of congenital obstructions are the external meatus (*i.e.*, meatal stenosis) in boys and just inside the external urinary meatus in girls. Another congenital cause of urinary stasis is the damage to sacral nerves that is seen in spina bifida and meningomyelocele.

The acquired causes of lower urinary tract obstruction and stasis are numerous. In males, the most important acquired cause of urinary obstruction is external compression of the urethra caused by the enlargement of the prostate gland. In males and females, gonorrhea and other sexually transmitted infections contribute to the incidence of infection-produced urethral strictures. Bladder tumors and secondary invasion of the bladder by tumors arising in structures that surround the bladder and urethra can compress the bladder neck or urethra and cause obstruction. Because of the proximity of the involved structures, constipation and fecal impaction can compress the urethra and produce urethral obstruction.

Compensatory and Decompensatory Changes

The body compensates for the obstruction of urine outflow with mechanisms divided into two stages: a compensatory stage and a decompensatory stage.[9]

During the early stage of obstruction, the bladder begins to hypertrophy and becomes hypersensitive to afferent stimuli arising from stretch receptors in the bladder wall. The ability to suppress urination is diminished, and bladder contraction can become so strong that it produces bladder spasm. There is urgency, sometimes to the point of incontinence, and frequency during the day and at night.[9]

The inner bladder surface forms smooth folds. With continued outflow obstruction, this smooth surface is replaced with coarsely woven structures (*i.e.*, hypertrophied smooth muscle fibers) called *trabeculae*. Small pockets of mucosal tissue, called *cellules*, commonly develop between the trabecular ridges.[9] These pockets form diverticula when they extend between the actual fibers of the bladder muscle (Fig. 35-4). Because the diverticula have no muscle, they are unable to contract and expel their urine into the bladder, and secondary infections caused by stasis are common.

Along with hypertrophy of the bladder wall, there is hypertrophy of the trigone area and the interureteric ridge, which is located between the two ureters. This causes back pressure on the ureters, the development of hydroureters (*i.e.*, dilated, urine-filled ureters), and, eventually, kidney damage. Stasis of urine predisposes an individual to urinary tract infections.[9]

When compensatory mechanisms are no longer effective, signs of decompensation begin to appear. The period of detrusor muscle contraction becomes too short to expel the urine completely, and residual urine remains in the bladder. The symptoms of obstruction—frequency of urination, hesitancy, need to strain to initiate urination, a weak and small stream, and termination of the stream before the bladder is completely emptied—become pronounced. With progressive decompensation,

UNDERSTANDING ➡ Intestinal Motility

Motility of the small intestine is organized to optimize the digestion and absorption of nutrients and the propulsion of undigested material toward the colon. Peristaltic movements mix the ingested foodstuffs with digestive enzymes and secretions and circulate the intestinal contents to facilitate contact with the intestinal mucosa. The regulation of motility results from an interplay of input from the **(1)** enteric and **(2)** ANSs and the intrinsic pacemaker activity of the **(3)** intestinal smooth muscle cells.

❶

Enteric Nervous System Innervation The GI system has its own nervous system, called the *enteric nervous system*. The enteric nervous system is composed mainly of two plexuses: (1) the outer *myenteric (Auerbach) plexus* that is located between the longitudinal and circular layers of smooth muscle cells and (2) an inner *submucosal (Meissner) plexus* that lies between the mucosal and circular muscle layers. The myenteric plexus controls mainly intestinal movements along the length of the gut, whereas the submucosal plexus is concerned mainly with controlling the function within each segment of the intestine. Fibers in the submucosal plexus also use signals originating from the intestinal epithelium to control intestinal secretion and local blood flow.

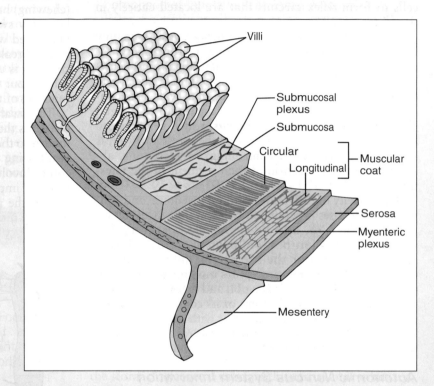

❷

Autonomic Nervous System Innervation The intestine is also innervated by the parasympathetic and sympathetic branches of the ANS (see Fig. 36-5). *Parasympathetic innervation* is supplied mainly by the vagus nerve with postganglionic neurons located primarily in the myenteric and submucosal plexuses. Stimulation of these parasympathetic nerves causes a general increase in both intestinal motility and secretory activity. *Sympathetic innervation* is supplied by nerves that run between the spinal cord and the prevertebral ganglia and between these ganglia and the intestine. Stimulation of the sympathetic nervous system is largely inhibitory, producing a decrease in intestinal motility and secretory activity.

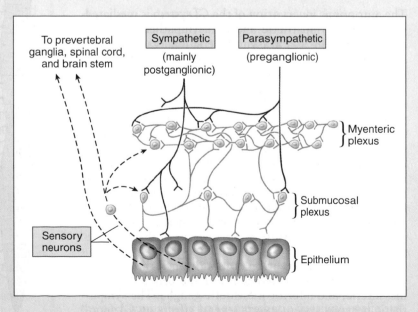

3

Intestinal Smooth Muscle

Intestinal smooth muscle has its own intrinsic slow-wave activity (described earlier), which varies from about 12 per minute in the duodenum to 8 or 9 per minute in the ileum. Slow waves are not action potentials, and they do not directly induce muscle contraction. Because action potentials occur at the peak of a smooth wave, slow-wave frequency determines the rate of smooth muscle contractions.

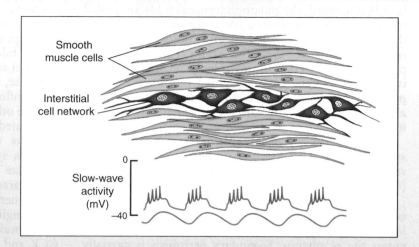

called the *swallowing center*. The motor impulses for the oral and pharyngeal phases of swallowing are carried in the trigeminal (V), glossopharyngeal (IX), vagus (X), and hypoglossal (XII) cranial nerves, and impulses for the esophageal phase are carried by the vagus nerve. Diseases that disrupt these brain centers or their cranial nerves disrupt the coordination of swallowing and

predispose a person to food and fluid lodging in the trachea and bronchi, which leads to risk of asphyxiation or aspiration pneumonia.

Swallowing consists of three phases—an oral or voluntary phase, a pharyngeal phase, and an esophageal phase (Fig. 36-6). During the *oral phase*, the bolus is collected at the back of the mouth so the tongue can

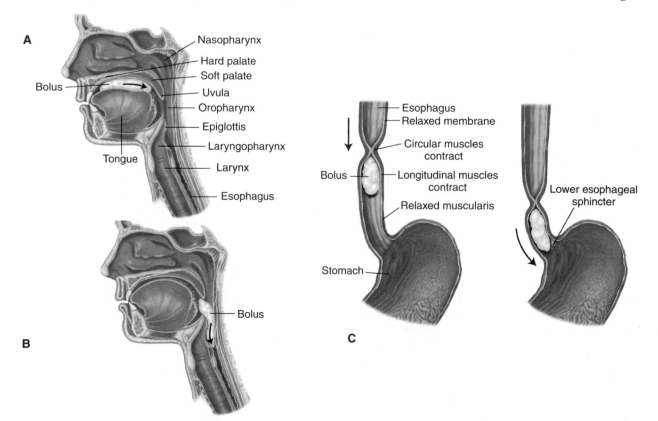

FIGURE 36-6. Steps in the swallowing reflex. (**A**) The *oral or voluntary phase* during which the bolus is collected at the back of the mouth so the tongue can lift the food upward and into the pharynx. (**B**) The *pharyngeal phase* during which food movement into the respiratory passages is prevented as the tongue is elevated and pressed against the soft palate closing the epiglottis, the upper esophageal sphincter relaxes, and the superior constrictor muscle contracts forcing food into the esophagus. (**C**) The *esophageal phase* during which peristalsis moves food through the esophagus and into the stomach.

in the stomach with the action of pepsin and is further facilitated in the intestine by the pancreatic enzymes, such as trypsin, chymotrypsin, carboxypeptidase, and elastase. Enzymes that break down proteins are released as proenzymes that are activated in the GI tract. The absorption of glucose and amino acids is facilitated by a sodium-dependent transport system. Fat in the diet is broken down by pancreatic lipase into triglycerides containing medium- and long-chain fatty acids. Bile salts form micelles that transport these substances to the surface of intestinal villi, where they are absorbed.

The Gastrointestinal Immunity

The GI system plays a central role in immune system homeostasis.[21] It is the main route of contact with the external environment and is overloaded every day with external stimuli. These stimuli are sometimes dangerous—pathogens (bacteria, protozoa, fungi, viruses) or toxic substances—and, in other cases, very useful—food or commensal flora. The crucial position of the GI system is testified by the huge amount of immune cells that reside within it.[22]

Immune Barrier

The surface area of the GI tract is estimated to be about 32 m², or about half a badminton court.[23] With such a large exposure, these immune components function to prevent pathogens from entering the blood and lymph circulatory systems.[24] Fundamental components of this protection are provided by the intestinal mucosal barrier, which is composed of physical, biochemical, and immune elements elaborated by the intestinal mucosa.[25]

Low pH (ranging from 1 to 4) of the stomach is fatal for many microorganisms that enter it.[26] Similarly, mucus (containing immunoglobulin A [IgA] antibodies) neutralizes many pathogenic microorganisms.[27]

Gut-associated lymphoid tissue (GALT) is a component of the mucosa-associated lymphoid tissue, which works in the immune system to protect the body from invasion in the gut.[28] The GALT lies throughout the intestine, covering an area of approximately 260 to 300 m²,[23] and consists of isolated or aggregated lymphoid follicles forming Peyer' patches.[29] The number of lymphocytes in the GALT is roughly equivalent to those in the spleen, and based on location, these cells are distributed in three basic populations.

Peyer Patches

These are lymphoid follicles similar in many ways to lymph nodes, located in the mucosa and extending into the submucosa of the small intestine, especially the ileum. In adults, B lymphocytes predominate in Peyer patches. Smaller lymphoid nodules can be found throughout the intestinal tract (see Fig. 36-15).

Lamina Propria Lymphocytes

The lamina propria is a thin layer of connective tissue that forms part of the moist linings known as mucous membranes or mucosa. The normal intestinal lamina propria contains B cells, T cells, and numerous innate immune cells, including dendritic cells, macrophages, eosinophils, and mast cells. IgA-producing plasma cells predominate throughout the length of the intestine.[30]

Intraepithelial Lymphocytes

These are lymphocytes that are positioned in the basolateral spaces between luminal epithelial cells, beneath the tight junctions. Unlike other T cells, intraepithelial lymphocytes do not need priming. Upon encountering antigens, they immediately release cytokines and cause killing of infected target cells.[31]

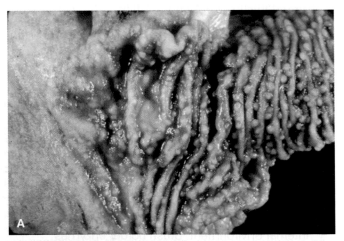
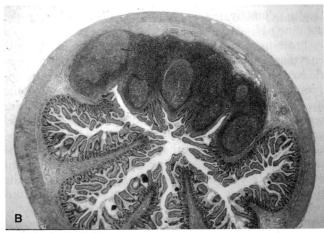

FIGURE 36-15. (A) **Peyer patches** are particularly prominent in the terminal ileum; they are small dome-shaped mucosal mounds. (B) The Peyer patch is composed of lymphoid tissue, often with prominent germinal centers, displacing the epithelial structure. (From Strayer D. S., Rubin E. (2015). *Rubin's pathology: Clinicopathologic foundations of medicine* (7th ed.). Philadelphia, PA: Wolters Kluwer (Fig. 19.38, p. 778).)

Microfold Cells

Another important component of the GI immune system is the M or microfold cell. M cells are a specific cell type in the intestinal epithelium over lymphoid follicles that endocytose a variety of protein and peptide antigens. Unlike their neighbor cells, M cells have the unique ability to take up antigen from the lumen of the small intestine via endocytosis, phagocytosis, or transcytosis and transport them into the underlying tissue, where they are taken up by local delivered to antigen-presenting cells (APCs), such as dendritic cells, B lymphocytes, and macrophages.[32]

Antigen-Presenting Cells

APCs, such as dendritic cells and macrophages, that receive antigens from M cells present them to T cells in the GALT, leading ultimately to appearance of IgA-secreting plasma cells in the mucosa. These antibodies are released into the gut mucosa, salivary glands, and lymph nodes. In females who are lactating, M cells recognize antigen, and IgA is directed from the gut to the mammary gland. IgA traveling from the gut to breast milk supply is controlled by hormones, chemokines, and cytokines. Thus, the mammary gland and breast milk have critical roles alongside M cells in mucosal immune system.[33]

T Cells

T cells exposed to antigen in Peyer patches also migrate into the lamina propria and the epithelium, where they mature to cytotoxic T cells, providing another mechanism for containing microbial assaults. In addition, lymph nodes that receive lymph draining from the mesenteric lymph nodes and intestinal macrophages play important roles in protecting the body against invasion.[21]

 SUMMARY CONCEPTS

The GI immunity system plays a vital role in protection against a host of pathogens. The size of the GI tract alone allows the pathogens to be exposed to a large area that serves as a barrier along with a vast number of immune cells. The Peyer patch, which is part of the lymphatic system formed by the GALT, has the ability to monitor and destroy pathogens. M cells have the ability to take up antigens from the small intestines, where they can be delivered to immune cells, producing an immune response. The T cell is another important cell type found in the Peyer patches; these mature into cytotoxic T cells and T helper cells, signaling the immune system to attack pathogens.

Review Exercises

1. People receiving chemotherapeutic agents, which interfere with mitosis of cancer cells as well as the cells of other rapidly proliferating tissues in the body, often experience disorders such as ulcerations in the mucosal tissues of the mouth and other parts of the GI tract. These disorders are resolved once the chemotherapy treatment has been completed.

   A. Explain.

2. People with gastroesophageal reflux (movement of gastric contents into the esophagus) often complain of heartburn that becomes worse as the pressure in the stomach increases.

   A. Use information on hormonal control of gastric emptying to explain why eating a meal that is high in fat content often exaggerates the problem.

3. Infections of the GI tract often cause profound diarrhea.

   A. Describe the neural mechanisms involved in the increase in GI motility that produces the diarrhea.
   B. Explain the rationale for using a "drink" that contains both glucose and sodium to treat the fluid deficit that often occurs with diarrhea.

4. Explain the physiologic mechanisms associated with the occurrence of diarrhea in people with:

   A. Lactase deficiency.
   B. Obstruction of bile flow into the intestine.
   C. Disruption of the normal intestinal flora because of antibiotic therapy.

REFERENCES

1. Binder H. J. (2016). Gastric function. In Boron F. W., Boulpaep E. L. (Eds.), *Medical physiology* (3rd ed., pp. 863–878). Philadelphia, PA: Saunders Elsevier.
2. Tortora G. J., Derrickson B. (2013). *Principles of anatomy and physiology* (14th ed., pp. 1004–1013). Hoboken, NJ: Wiley.
3. Patton K. T., Thibodeau G. A. (2015). *Anatomy & physiology* (9th ed., pp. 848–856). St. Louis, MO: Mosby Elsevier.
4. Ross M. H., Pawlina W. (2015). *Histology: A text and atlas* (7th ed., pp. 568–624). Philadelphia, PA: Lippincott Williams & Wilkins.
5. Hall J. E. (2015). *Guyton and Hall: Textbook of medical physiology* (13th ed., pp. 753–772). Philadelphia, PA: Saunders Elsevier.
6. Richerson G. B. (2016). The autonomic nervous system. In Boron F. W., Boulpaep E. L. (Eds.), *Medical physiology* (3rd ed., pp. 356–359). Philadelphia, PA: Saunders Elsevier.
7. Barrett K. M., Barman S. M., Boitano S., et al. (2015). *Ganong's review of medical physiology* (25th ed.). New York, NY: McGraw Hill. Available: http://www.accessmedicine.com. Accessed January 8, 2018.

8. Koeppen B. M., Stanton B. (Eds.). (2017). *Berne & Levy: Physiology* (7th ed., pp. 511–519). St. Louis, MO: Mosby.

9. Kapoor V. K. (2016). Gest. In Thomas R. (Ed.), *Upper GI tract anatomy*. Available: Medscape. WebMD LLC. Accessed June 26, 2016.

10. Hasler W. L. (2015). The physiology of gastric motility and gastric emptying. In Yamada T. (Ed.), *Textbook of gastroenterology* (6th ed., pp. 207–230). Hoboken, NJ: Wiley-Blackwell.

11. Glasgow R. E., Mulvihill S. J. (2015). Surgery for peptic ulcer disease and postgastrectomy syndromes. In Yamada T. (Ed.), *Textbook of gastroenterology* (6th ed., pp. 1060–1063). Hoboken, NJ: Wiley-Blackwell.

12. Howick K., Griffin B., Cryan J., et al. (2017). From belly to brain: Targeting the ghrelin receptor in appetite and food intake regulation. *International Journal of Molecular Sciences* 18, 273.

13. Del Valle J., Todisco A. (2015). Gastric secretion. In Yamada T. (Ed.), *Textbook of gastroenterology* (6th ed., pp. 284–329). Hoboken, NJ: Wiley-Blackwell.

14. Irwin N., Flatt P. R. (2013). Enteroendocrine hormone mimetics for the treatment of obesity and diabetes. *Current Opinion in Pharmacology* 13(6), 989–995.

15. Keely S. J., Montrose M. H., Barrett K. E. (2015). Electrolyte secretion and absorption: Small intestine and colon. In Yamada T. (Ed.), *Textbook of gastroenterology* (6th ed., pp. 330–367). Hoboken, NJ: Wiley-Blackwell.

16. de Graaf C., Donnelly D., Wootten D., et al. (2016). Glucagon-like peptide-1 and its class B G protein-coupled receptors: A long march to therapeutic successes. *Pharmacological Reviews* 68(4), 954–1013. doi:10.1124/pr.115.011395.

17. Turner J. R. (2014). The gastrointestinal tract. In Kumar V., Abbas A. K., Fausto N., et al. (Eds.), *Robbins and Cotran pathologic basis of disease* (9th ed., pp. 780–781). Philadelphia, PA: Saunders Elsevier.

18. Elena P. C. A., Andrés M., José G. M., et al. (2015). Colonization resistance of the gut microbiota against Clostridium difficile. *Antibiotics* 4(3), 337.

19. Keim N. L., Levin R. L., Havel P. J. (2012). Carbohydrates. In Shils M. E., Shike M., Ross A. K., et al. (Eds.), *Modern nutrition in health and disease* (12th ed., pp. 62–82). Baltimore, MD: Lippincott Williams & Wilkins.

20. Chernecky C. C., Berger B. J. (2012). *Laboratory test and diagnostic procedures* (6th ed.). Philadelphia, PA: Saunders Elsevier.

21. Mowat A. M., Agace W. W. (2014). Regional specialization within the intestinal immune system. *Nature Reviews Immunology* 14(10), 667–685.

22. Peterson L. W., Artis D. (2014) Intestinal epithelial cells: Regulators of barrier function and immune homeostasis. *Nature Reviews Immunology* 14, 141–153.

23. Helander H. F., Fändriks L. (2014). Surface area of the digestive tract-revisited. *Scandinavian Journal of Gastroenterology* 49(6), 681–689.

24. Flannigan K. L., Geem D., Harusato A., et al. (2015). Intestinal antigen-presenting cells: Key regulators of immune homeostasis and inflammation. *The American Journal of Pathology* 185(7), 1809–1819.

25. Sánchez de Medina F., Romero-Calvo I., Mascaraque C., et al. (2014). Intestinal inflammation and mucosal barrier function. *Inflammatory Bowel Diseases* 20(12), 2394–2404.

26. Schubert M. L. (2014). Gastric secretion. *Current Opinion in Gastroenterology* 30(6), 578–582.

27. Márquez M., Fernández Gutiérrez Del Álamo C., Girón-González J. A. (2016). Gut epithelial barrier dysfunction in human immunodeficiency virus-hepatitis C virus coinfected patients: Influence on innate and acquired immunity. *World Journal of Gastroenterology* 22(4), 1433–1448.

28. McGhee J. R., Fujihashi K. (2012). Inside the mucosal immune system. *PLoS Biology* 10(9), e1001397. doi:10.1371/journal.pbio.1001397.

29. Bonnardel J., Da Silva C., Henri S., et al. (2015). Innate and adaptive immune functions of Peyer's patch monocyte-derived cells. *Cell Reports* 11, 770–784. doi:10.1016/j.celrep.2015.03.067.

30. Society for Mucosal Immunology. (2012). Lymphocyte populations within the Lamina Propria. In Smith P. D., MacDonald T. T., Blumberg R. S. (Eds.), *Principles of mucosal immunology* (1st ed., Chapter 7, pp. 87–101). London, England: Garland Science.

31. Schuppan D., Dieterich W. (2016). Pathogenesis, epidemiology, and clinical manifestations of celiac disease in adults. In Gorver S. (Ed.), *UpToDate*. Available: https://www.uptodate.com/contents/pathogenesis-epidemiology-and-clinical-manifestations-of-celiac-disease-in-adults?source=history_widget. Accessed March 5, 2018.

32. Mabbott N. A., Donaldson D. S., Ohno H., et al. (2013). Microfold (M) cells: Important immunosurveillance posts in the intestinal epithelium. *Mucosal Immunology* 6, 666–677. doi:10.1038/mi.2013.30.

33. Milligan L. (2013). From mother's gut to milk. SPLASH! Milk science update. Available: http://milkgenomics.org/issue/splash-milk-science-update-september-2017. Accessed September, 2017.

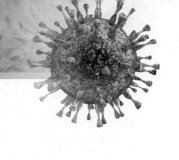
Disorders of Gastrointestinal Function

Learning Objectives

After completing this chapter, the learner will be able to meet the following objectives:

1. Characterize the relationship among anorexia, nausea, retching, and vomiting.
2. Describe the neural structures involved in vomiting and their mediators.
3. Describe the causes of dysphagia, odynophagia, and achalasia.
4. Relate the pathophysiology of gastroesophageal reflux to measures used in the diagnosis and treatment of the disorder in adults and children.
5. State the reason for the poor prognosis associated with esophageal cancer.
6. Differentiate between the causes and manifestations of acute and chronic gastritis.
7. Characterize the proposed role of *Helicobacter pylori* in the development of chronic gastritis and peptic ulcer as well as methods for diagnosis and treatment of the infection.
8. Describe the etiologic factors in ulcer formation related to Zollinger–Ellison syndrome and stress ulcer.
9. Compare the characteristics of Crohn disease and ulcerative colitis.
10. Describe the pathogenesis of the symptoms associated with appendicitis.

Gastrointestinal disorders do not receive the same publicity in the health-related media as do heart disease, cancer, and cerebrovascular disease. Colorectal cancer is the third leading cause of cancer mortality in men and in women. In 2019, 101,420 new cases of colon cancer and 44,180 new cases of rectal cancer are expected. Although the mortality rate from colorectal cancer has been dropping over the past several decades in both genders, 51,020 deaths are expected in 2019.[1] Health care expenditures for GI disease address more than that for heart or mental health. More people visit the emergency department for abdominal pain than for any other complaint.[2] Even more important is the fact that proper nutrition or a change in health practices could prevent or minimize many of these disorders.

Disruption in structure and function can occur at any level of the GI tract, from the esophagus to the colon and rectum. This chapter is divided into four sections:

1. Common manifestations of GI disorders
2. Disorders of the esophagus
3. Disorders of the stomach
4. Disorders of the small and large intestines

Disorders of the hepatobiliary system and exocrine pancreas are discussed in Chapter 38.

Common Manifestations of Gastrointestinal Disorders: Anorexia, Nausea, and Vomiting

Anorexia, nausea, and vomiting are physiologic responses that are common to many gastrointestinal (GI) disorders. These responses are protective to the extent that they signal the presence of disease and, in the case of vomiting, remove noxious agents from the GI tract. However, they also can contribute to impaired intake or loss of fluids and nutrients.

Anorexia

Anorexia represents a loss of appetite. Several factors influence appetite. One is hunger, which is stimulated by contractions of the empty stomach. The hypothalamus and other associated centers in the brain regulate appetite. Appetite can be stimulated or suppressed by the smell of food. Loss of appetite is associated with emotional factors, such as fear, depression, frustration, and anxiety. Many drugs and disease states cause anorexia. Anorexia often is a forerunner of nausea, and most conditions that cause nausea and vomiting also produce anorexia.

Many people refer to anorexia as anorexia nervosa, which is an eating disorder characterized by low weight, fear of gaining weight, and a strong desire to be thin, resulting in food restriction. People with anorexia nervosa perceive themselves as overweight even though they are underweight. They usually deny that they have a problem with low weight.[3]

Nausea

Nausea is the conscious sensation resulting from stimulation of the medullary vomiting center that often precedes or accompanies vomiting or anorexia. Nausea is an unpleasant, subjective, nonspecific symptom, which means that it has many possible causes. Some common causes of nausea are motion sickness, dizziness, migraine, fainting, low blood sugar, gastroenteritis, food poisoning, or severe pain. Nausea is a side effect of many medications and of morning sickness in early pregnancy.

A common cause of nausea is distension of the duodenum or upper small intestinal tract. Nausea frequently is accompanied by autonomic nervous system manifestations such as watery salivation and vasoconstriction with pallor, sweating, and tachycardia. Nausea also may function as an early warning signal of a pathologic process.

Retching and Vomiting

Retching consists of the rhythmic spasmodic movements of the diaphragm, chest wall, and abdominal muscles. It usually precedes or alternates with periods of vomiting. Vomiting or emesis is the sudden and forceful oral expulsion of the contents of the stomach. It usually is preceded by nausea. The contents that are vomited are called *vomitus*. Vomiting, as a basic physiologic protective mechanism, limits the possibility of damage from ingested noxious agents by emptying the contents of the stomach and portions of the small intestine. Nausea and vomiting may represent a total-body response to drug therapy, including overdose, cumulative effects, toxicity, and side effects.

Vomiting involves two functionally distinct medullary centers—the *vomiting center* and the *chemoreceptor trigger zone*.[4] The act of vomiting is thought to be a reflex that is integrated in the vomiting center, which is located in the dorsal portion of the reticular formation of the medulla near the sensory nuclei of the vagus (Fig. 37-1). The chemoreceptor trigger zone is located in a small area on the floor of the fourth ventricle, where it is exposed to both blood and cerebrospinal fluid. It is thought to mediate the emetic effects of blood-borne drugs and toxins.

The act of vomiting consists of taking a deep breath, closing the airways, and producing a strong, forceful contraction of the diaphragm and abdominal muscles along with relaxation of the gastroesophageal sphincter. Respiration ceases during the act of vomiting. Vomiting may be accompanied by dizziness, light-headedness, a decrease in blood pressure, and bradycardia.

The vomiting center receives input from the GI tract and other organs: from the cerebral cortex; from the vestibular apparatus, which is responsible for motion sickness; and from the chemoreceptor trigger zone, which is activated by many drugs and endogenous and exogenous toxins (see Fig. 37-1). Hypoxia exerts a direct effect on the vomiting center, producing nausea and vomiting. This direct effect probably accounts for the vomiting that occurs during periods of decreased cardiac output, shock, environmental hypoxia, and brain ischemia caused by increased intracranial pressure. Inflammation of any of the intra-abdominal organs, including the liver,

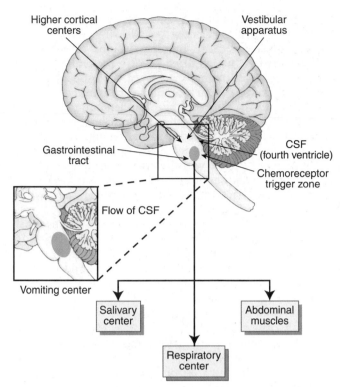

FIGURE 37-1. Physiologic events involved in vomiting. CSF, cerebrospinal fluid.

gallbladder, or urinary tract, can cause vomiting because of the stimulation of the visceral afferent pathways that communicate with the vomiting center. Distension or irritation of the GI tract also causes vomiting through the stimulation of visceral afferent neurons.

Several neurotransmitters and receptor subtypes are implicated as neuromediators in nausea and vomiting. Dopamine, serotonin, and opioid receptors are found in the GI tract and in the vomiting center and the chemoreceptor trigger zone. Motion sickness appears to be a central nervous system (CNS) response to vestibular stimuli. Norepinephrine and acetylcholine receptors are located in the vestibular center. The acetylcholine receptors are thought to mediate the impulses responsible for exciting the vomiting center. Norepinephrine receptors may have a stabilizing influence that resists motion sickness.

SUMMARY CONCEPTS

The signs and symptoms of many GI tract disorders are manifested by anorexia, nausea, and vomiting. Anorexia, or loss of appetite, may occur alone or may accompany nausea and vomiting. Nausea, which is an ill-defined unpleasant sensation, signals the stimulation of the medullary vomiting center. It often precedes vomiting and frequently is accompanied by autonomic responses, such as salivation and vasoconstriction with pallor, sweating, and tachycardia. The act of vomiting, which is integrated in the vomiting center, involves the forceful oral expulsion of the gastric contents. It is a basic physiologic mechanism that rids the GI tract of noxious agents.

Disorders of the Esophagus

The esophagus is a tube that connects the oropharynx with the stomach. It lies posterior to the trachea and larynx and extends through the mediastinum, intersecting the diaphragm at the level of the 11th thoracic vertebra.

The esophagus functions primarily as a conduit for passage of food and liquid from the pharynx to the stomach. The walls of the esophagus consist of the mucosal, submucosal, muscularis externa, and adventitial layers, reflecting the general structural organization of the GI tract. The inner mucosal layer contains nonkeratinized stratified epithelium. At the esophageal–stomach junction, the abrasion-resistant epithelium changes abruptly to the simple columnar epithelium of the stomach. The submucosal layer contains mucus-secreting glands that provide the mucin-containing fluids that lubricate the esophageal wall and aid in the passage of food. The muscularis externa layer consists of skeletal muscle progressing to skeletal and smooth muscle, and then entirely smooth muscle in its lower third. The outer fibrous adventitial layer of the esophagus is composed entirely of connective tissue.

There are sphincters at either end of the esophagus: an upper esophageal sphincter and a lower esophageal sphincter. The upper esophageal, or pharyngoesophageal, sphincter consists of a circular layer of striated muscle, the cricopharyngeal muscle. The lower esophageal, or gastroesophageal, sphincter is approximately 3 cm above the junction with the stomach. It acts as a valve, but the only structural evidence of a sphincter is a slight thickening of the circular smooth muscle, which normally remains tonically constricted, in contrast to the midportion of the esophagus, which normally remains relaxed.[5] The lower esophageal sphincter passes through an opening, or *hiatus*, in the diaphragm as it joins with the stomach, which is located in the abdomen. The portion of the diaphragm that surrounds the lower esophageal sphincter helps maintain the zone of high pressure needed to prevent reflux of stomach contents.

Congenital Anomalies

Congenital anomalies of the esophagus require early detection and correction because they are incompatible with life. Esophageal atresia (EA) and tracheoesophageal fistula (TEF) are common congenital anomalies of the esophagus, affecting approximately 1 in 45,000 neonates.[6] In the most common form of EA (85%),[7] the upper esophagus ends in a blind pouch and the TEF is connected to the trachea (Fig. 37-2). This defect now has a survival rate greater than 90% owing largely to early recognition and improved neonatal intensive care units. Infants weighing less than 1500 g have the greatest risk for mortality, especially when combined with a cardiac anomaly.[7]

The newborn infant with EA/TEF typically has frothing and bubbling at the mouth and nose and episodes of coughing, vomiting, cyanosis, and respiratory distress.

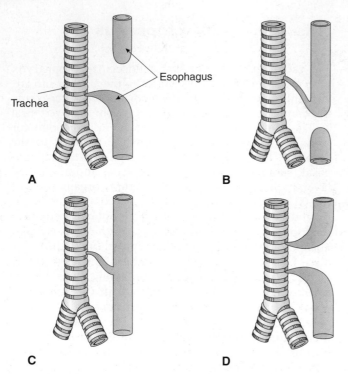

Trachea

Esophagus

A

B

C

D

FIGURE 37-2. Congenital tracheoesophageal fistulas. **(A)** The most common type (85% of cases) is a communication between the trachea and the lower portion of the esophagus. The upper segment of the esophagus ends in a blind sac. **(B)** In a few cases, the proximal esophagus communicates with the trachea. **(C)** H-type fistula without esophageal atresia, and **(D)** tracheal fistulas to both a proximal esophageal pouch and distal esophagus. (From Strayer D. S., Rubin R. (Eds.) (2015). *Rubin's pathophysiology: Clinicopathologic foundations of medicine* (7th ed., Figure 19-1, p. 753). Philadelphia, PA: Lippincott Williams & Wilkins.)

Feeding exacerbates these manifestations, causes regurgitation, and precipitates aspiration. The inability to pass a catheter into the stomach provides further evidence of the disorder. The infant with isolated TEF may develop respiratory symptoms at a later age.

Treatment of EA and TEF is surgical ligation of the TEF and end-to-end anastomosis of the esophagus, when possible. The main goal of preoperative management is to maintain the airway and prevent lung damage from aspiration of gastric contents. Prone positioning minimizes movement of gastric secretions into a distal fistula, and esophageal suctioning minimizes the risk of aspiration from a blind pouch.

Dysphagia

The act of swallowing depends on the coordinated action of the tongue and pharynx, which are innervated by cranial nerves V, IX, X, and XII. Dysphagia refers to difficulty in swallowing. If swallowing is painful, it is referred to as *odynophagia*. Dysphagia can result from neuromuscular or structural causes producing narrowing of the esophagus, lack of salivary secretion, weakness of the muscular structures that propel the food

bolus toward the stomach, or disruption of the neural networks coordinating the swallowing mechanism.[8] A neuromuscular cause involves lesions of the CNS, such as a stroke, which often involve the cranial nerves that control swallowing. Cancer of the esophagus and strictures resulting from scarring, a structural cause, can reduce the size of the esophageal lumen and make swallowing difficult. Scleroderma, an autoimmune disease that causes fibrous replacement of tissues throughout the body and in the GI tract, is another important cause of dysphagia.[9] People with dysphagia usually complain of choking, coughing, or an abnormal sensation of food sticking in the back of the throat or upper chest when they swallow.

In a condition called *achalasia*, the lower esophageal sphincter fails to relax because of a disruption in the input from the enteric neural plexus and the vagus nerve.[10] This results in difficulty passing food into the stomach, and the esophagus above the lower esophageal sphincter becomes enlarged. One or several meals may lodge in the esophagus and pass slowly into the stomach over time. There is danger of aspiration of esophageal contents into the lungs when the person lies down.

Endoscopy, barium esophagoscopy, and videoradiography may be used to determine the site and extent of a swallowing disorder. Esophageal **manometry**, a procedure in which a small pressure-sensing catheter is inserted into the esophagus, may be done to measure pressures in different parts of the esophagus. Treatment of swallowing disorders depends on the cause and type of altered function that is present. Treatment of dysphagia often involves a multidisciplinary team of health professionals, including a speech pathologist. Mechanical dilation or surgical procedures may be done to enlarge the lower esophageal sphincter in people with esophageal strictures.

Esophageal Diverticulum

A **diverticulum** of the esophagus is a herniation of the esophageal wall caused by a weakness of the muscularis layer.[11] An esophageal diverticulum tends to retain food. Complaints that the food stops before it reaches the stomach, gurgling, belching, coughing, and foul-smelling breath are common. The trapped food may cause esophagitis and ulceration. Because the condition usually is progressive, correction of the defect requires surgical intervention.

Tears (Mallory–Weiss Syndrome)

Longitudinal tears in the esophagus at the esophagogastric junction that often extend distally are termed *Mallory–Weiss tears*.[12] They are most often found in people with chronic alcoholism after a bout of severe retching or vomiting but may also occur during acute illness with severe vomiting. The presumed pathogenesis is inadequate relaxation of the esophageal sphincter during vomiting, with stretching and tearing of the esophageal junction at the moment of propulsive expulsion of gastric contents. Tears may involve only the mucosa or may penetrate the wall of the esophagus. Infection may lead to inflammatory ulcer or mediastinitis.

Healing is usually prompt, with minimal or no residual effects.

Hiatal Hernia

Hiatal hernia is characterized by a protrusion or herniation of the stomach through the esophageal hiatus of the diaphragm. There are two anatomic patterns of hiatal herniation: axial, or sliding, and nonaxial, or paraesophageal.[13] The sliding hiatal hernia is characterized by a bell-shaped protrusion of the stomach above the diaphragm (Fig. 37-3). Small sliding hiatal hernias are common and considered to be of no significance in asymptomatic people. However, in cases of severe erosive esophagitis where gastroesophageal reflux (GER) and a large hiatal hernia coexist, the hernia may retard esophageal acid clearance and contribute to the more severe esophagitis. In paraesophageal hiatal hernias, a separate portion of the stomach, usually along

the greater portion of the stomach, enters the thorax through a widened opening and then progressively enlarges. In extreme cases, most of the stomach herniates into the thorax. Large paraesophageal hiatal hernias may require surgical treatment.

Gastroesophageal Reflux

Normally, refluxed material is returned to the stomach by secondary peristaltic waves in the esophagus, and swallowed saliva neutralizes and washes away the refluxed acid. GER is the backward movement of gastric contents into the esophagus, a condition that causes heartburn or pyrosis. It probably is the most common disorder originating in the GI tract. The associated symptoms usually occur soon after eating, are short lived, and seldom cause more serious problems.

The lower esophageal sphincter regulates the flow of food from the esophagus into the stomach. The circular muscles of the distal esophagus constitute the intrinsic mechanisms to prevent reflux, and the portion of the diaphragm that surrounds the esophagus constitutes the extrinsic mechanism. The oblique muscles of the stomach, located below the lower esophageal sphincter, form a flap that contributes to the antireflux function of the internal sphincter. Relaxation of the lower esophageal sphincter is a brain stem reflex that is mediated by the vagus nerve in response to a number of afferent stimuli. Transient relaxation with reflux is common after meals. Gastric distension and meals high in fat increase the frequency of reflux.[14]

Gastroesophageal Reflux Disease

Gastroesophageal reflux disease (GERD) is defined as symptoms or mucosal damage produced by the abnormal reflux of gastric contents into the esophagus or into the oral cavity (including the larynx) or the lung.[15] It is thought to be associated with transient relaxations of a weak or an incompetent lower esophageal sphincter. This allows reflux to occur and, in addition, decreased clearance of the refluxed acid from the esophagus after it has occurred. It results in irritant effects of the refluxate.[16] In most cases, reflux occurs during transient relaxation of the esophagus. Delayed gastric emptying also may contribute to reflux by increasing gastric volume and pressure with greater chance for reflux. Esophageal mucosal injury is related to the destructive nature of the refluxate and the amount of time it is in contact with the mucosa. Acidic gastric fluids (pH < 4.0) are particularly damaging. Decreased salivation and salivary buffering capacity may contribute to impaired clearing of acid reflux from the esophagus.

GERD is a more serious and long-lasting form of GER that occurs more than twice a week for a few weeks and can lead to more serious health problems over time.[17] In the Western world, between 10% and 20% of the population are affected by the disease. GERD is broadly classified into two groups on the basis of endoscopy findings: having esophageal mucosal

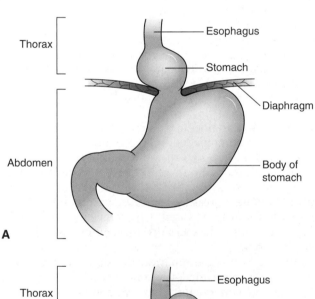
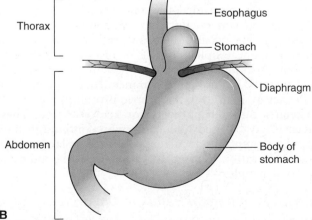

Thorax — Esophagus — Stomach — Diaphragm

Abdomen — Body of stomach

A

Thorax — Esophagus — Stomach — Diaphragm

Abdomen — Body of stomach

B

FIGURE 37-3. Hiatal hernia. (A) Sliding hiatal hernia. (B) Paraesophageal hiatal hernia.

damage (erosive esophagitis and Barrett esophagus) and no mucosal damage (endoscopy-negative reflux disease or nonerosive reflux disease).[18]

Clinical Manifestations

Heartburn and regurgitation are the characteristic symptoms of GERD. Heartburn is defined as a burning sensation in the retrosternal area. Regurgitation is defined as the perception of the flow of refluxed gastric contents into the mouth or hypopharynx. It frequently is severe, occurring 30 to 60 minutes after eating. It often is made worse by bending at the waist and recumbency and usually is relieved by sitting upright. The severity of heartburn is not indicative of the extent of mucosal injury. Often, the heartburn occurs during the night. Other symptoms include belching and chest pain located in the epigastric or retrosternal area that often radiates to the throat, shoulder, or back. Because of its location, the pain may be confused with angina. The reflux of gastric contents also may produce respiratory symptoms such as asthma, chronic cough, and laryngitis; however, these symptoms are often multifactorial in addition to the diagnosis of GERD.[18] The proposed mechanisms of reflux-associated asthma and chronic cough include microaspiration and macroaspiration, laryngeal injury, and vagal-mediated bronchospasm.

Reflux esophagitis involves mucosal injury to the esophagus, hyperemia, and inflammation. Complications, such as strictures and *Barrett esophagus*, can result from persistent reflux, which produces a cycle of mucosal damage that causes hyperemia, edema, and erosion of the luminal surface. Strictures are caused by a combination of scar tissue, spasm, and edema. They produce narrowing of the esophagus and cause dysphagia when the lumen becomes sufficiently constricted. Barrett esophagus (Fig. 37-4) refers to an abnormal change (metaplasia) in the cells of the lower portion of the esophagus characterized by a reparative process in which the squamous mucosa that normally lines the esophagus gradually is replaced by abnormal columnar epithelium resembling that in the stomach or intestines.[19] It is associated with increased risk of development of esophageal adenocarcinoma.

Diagnosis

Diagnosis of GER depends primarily on a history of reflux symptomatology and the use of optional diagnostic methods, including acid suppression trials, esophagoscopy, and ambulatory esophageal pH monitoring.[16] Acid suppression trials involve administering a proton pump inhibitor (PPI) medication for 7 to 14 days to determine whether the symptoms are alleviated. Esophagoscopy involves the passage of a flexible fiber-optic endoscope into the esophagus for the purpose of visualizing or obtaining a biopsy of the lumen of the upper GI tract. To monitor pH, an electrode is passed into the esophagus from which data are analyzed. The device allows the person to indicate position changes, meals, heartburn, or pain, which then can be correlated with episodes of acid reflux.

Treatment

The treatment of GER usually focuses on conservative measures that include avoidance of positions and conditions that increase gastric reflux.[16] Avoidance of large meals and foods that reduce lower esophageal sphincter tone (*e.g.*, caffeine, fats, and chocolate), alcohol, and smoking is recommended. It is recommended that meals be eaten sitting up and that the recumbent position be avoided for several hours after a meal. Bending for long periods should be avoided because it tends to increase intra-abdominal pressure and cause gastric reflux. Sleeping with the head elevated helps prevent reflux during the night. Weight loss usually is recommended in overweight people.

Antacids or a combination of antacids and alginic acid are recommended for mild disease. Alginic acid produces a foam when it comes in contact with gastric acid; if reflux occurs, the foam, rather than the acid, rises into the esophagus. Use of histamine-2 (H₂) receptor–blocking antagonists, which inhibit gastric acid production, is another recommended treatment. The PPIs act by inhibiting the gastric proton pump, which regulates the final pathway for acid secretion. These agents may be used for people who continue to have daytime symptoms, recurrent strictures, or large esophageal ulcerations. Surgical treatment may be indicated in some people.

Gastroesophageal Reflux in Children

GER occurs in more than two thirds of otherwise healthy infants. GER is considered a normal physiologic process that occurs several times a day in

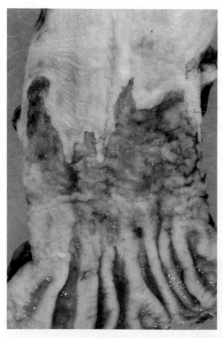

FIGURE 37-4. Barrett esophagus. The presence of the tan tongues of epithelium interdigitating with the more proximal squamous epithelium is typical of Barrett esophagus. (From Strayer D. S., Rubin R. (Eds.) (2015). *Rubin's pathophysiology: Clinicopathologic foundations of medicine* (7th ed., Figure 19-6A, p. 757). Philadelphia, PA: Lippincott Williams & Wilkins.)

healthy infants, children, and adults. Less is known about the normal physiology of GER in infants and children, but regurgitation or spitting up, the most visible symptom, is reported to occur daily in 50% of all infants.[20]

The small reservoir capacity of an infant's esophagus coupled with frequent spontaneous reductions in sphincter pressure contributes to reflux. At least one episode of regurgitation a day occurs in as much as half of infants aged 0 to 3 months.[21] It abates by 2 years of age[21] as the child's diet naturally advances and the child is able to maintain a more upright posture. Although many infants have minor degrees of reflux, complications can occur in children with more frequent or persistent episodes. The condition occurs more frequently in children with cerebral palsy, Down syndrome, cystic fibrosis, and other neurologic disorders.

Pathologic reflux is classified into three categories:

1. Regurgitation and malnutrition
2. Esophagitis
3. Respiratory problems

Clinical Manifestations

Symptoms of reflux vary depending on the child's age. Preadolescent children often experience heartburn, epigastric pain, abdominal pain, regurgitation, and intermittent vomiting. Infants and toddlers, however, more commonly experience regurgitation and feeding difficulties. If recurrent vomiting is accompanied by symptoms of poor weight gain, excessive crying, irritability, disturbed sleep, feeding, or respiratory problems, or if symptoms are persistent despite using a hypoallergenic formula or empirical acid suppression, then additional diagnostic tests may be required.[22] Tilting of the head to one side and arching of the back may be noted in children with severe reflux. The head positioning is thought to represent an attempt to protect the airway or reduce the pain-associated reflux. Sometimes regurgitation is associated with dental caries and recurrent otalgia. The ear pain is thought to occur through referral from the vagus nerve in the esophagus to the ear.

A variety of respiratory symptoms are caused by damage to the respiratory mucosa when gastric reflux enters the esophagus. Reflux may cause laryngospasm, apnea, and bradycardia. Asthma may co-occur with GERD in about 50% of children with asthma.[21] Such children, who are particularly likely to have GERD as a provocative factor, also have symptoms of reflux and have refractory or steroid-dependent asthma and nocturnal worsening of symptoms.[21]

Diagnosis and Treatment

Diagnosis of GER in infants and children often is based on parental and clinical observations.

Diagnostic testing is generally not necessary because it has not been found to be more reliable than the history and physical examination for diagnosing GER or GERD. Tests should be reserved for situations with atypical symptoms, warning signs, or doubts about the diagnosis; suspected complications of GERD or other conditions; or failure of initial therapies. The diagnosis may be confirmed by esophageal pH probe studies, barium fluoroscopic esophagography, and nuclear scintigraphy. In some cases, esophagoscopy may be used to demonstrate reflux and obtain a biopsy.[23]

Most infants, children, and adolescents who have reflux improve with conservative measures. In infants, feeding changes may reduce symptoms. For formula-fed infants, reducing feeding volumes in overfed infants, or offering smaller and more frequent feeds, may decrease reflux episodes and should be tried first. Adding thickening agents decreases observed regurgitation but does not reduce the reflux index and can lead to excess weight gain.[23] Changing the infant's body position while awake can be effective. The prone and left-side-down positions are associated with fewer reflux episodes but should be recommended only in awake, observed infants during the postprandial period. In older infants and children, raising the head of the bed and keeping the child upright may help. Medications usually are not added to the treatment regimen until pathologic reflux has been documented by diagnostic testing.[23]

Cancer of the Esophagus

Carcinoma of the esophagus accounts for approximately 1% of all diagnosed cancers.[24] It is more common in adults older than age 65 years. It occurs three times more frequently in men than in women, and its occurrence is equal between African Americans and whites.[24]

There are two types of esophageal cancer: squamous cell carcinoma and adenocarcinoma. Most squamous cell esophageal carcinomas are attributable to alcohol and tobacco use. Worldwide, squamous cell carcinomas are the most common type of esophageal cancers, but in the United States, there has been a significant increase in adenocarcinomas.[25] Barrett esophagus and GERD are the two most common risk factors for esophageal adenocarcinoma.[26]

Progressive dysphagia is the most frequent complaint in people with esophageal cancer. It is apparent first with ingestion of bulky food, later with soft food, and finally with liquids. Unfortunately, it is a late manifestation of the disease. Unintentional weight loss, anorexia, fatigue, and pain on swallowing also may occur.

Treatment of esophageal cancer depends on tumor stage. Surgical resection provides a means of cure when done in early disease and palliation when done in late disease. Radiation may be used as an alternative to surgery. Chemotherapy may be used before surgery to decrease the size of the tumor, or it may be used along with irradiation and surgery in an effort to increase survival.[27]

The prognosis for people with cancer of the esophagus, although poor, has improved. Even with modern forms of therapy, however, the long-term survival is limited because, in many cases, the disease has already metastasized by the time the diagnosis is made.

SUMMARY CONCEPTS

The esophagus is a tube that connects the oropharynx with the stomach; it functions primarily as a conduit for passage of food from the pharynx to the stomach. Although relatively uncommon, congenital anomalies (*i.e.*, EA and TEFs) must be corrected early because they cause aspiration of gastric and oral secretions and are incompatible with life. Dysphagia refers to difficulty in swallowing; it can result from altered nerve function or from disorders that produce narrowing of the esophagus. A diverticulum of the esophagus is an outpouching of the esophageal wall caused by a weakness of the muscularis layer. Longitudinal tears (Mallory–Weiss tears) at the esophagogastric junction can occur with severe bouts of retching or vomiting. They are most often encountered in people with chronic alcoholism, but may also occur during acute illness with severe vomiting. Hiatal hernia is characterized by a protrusion or herniation of the stomach through the esophageal hiatus of the diaphragm. There are two anatomic patterns of herniation: (1) the axial or sliding hiatal hernia, which is the most common type and is characterized by a bell-shaped protrusion of the stomach above the diaphragm and (2) the nonaxial or paraesophageal hernia, in which a portion of the stomach enters the thorax through a widened opening.

GER refers to the backward movement of gastric contents into the esophagus, a condition that causes heartburn. Although most people experience occasional GER and heartburn, persistent reflux can result in a cycle of mucosal damage that causes hyperemia, edema, erosion luminal surface, and Barrett esophagus. Reflux can cause respiratory symptoms, including chronic cough, and serve as a potential trigger for asthma. GER is a common problem in infants and children. Reflux commonly corrects itself with age, and symptoms abate in most children by 2 years of age. Although many infants have minor degrees of reflux, some infants and small children have significant reflux that interferes with feeding, causes esophagitis, and results in respiratory symptoms and other complications.

Carcinoma of the esophagus is more common in older adults and occurs more frequently in men than in women. There are two types of esophageal cancer: squamous cell carcinoma and adenocarcinoma. Most squamous cell carcinomas are attributable to alcohol and tobacco use. Adenocarcinomas are more closely linked to GER and Barrett esophagus.

Disorders of the Stomach

The stomach is a reservoir for contents entering the digestive tract. It lies in the upper abdomen, anterior to the pancreas, splenic vessels, and left kidney. Anteriorly, the stomach is bounded by the anterior abdominal wall and the left inferior lobe of the liver. While in the stomach, food is churned and mixed with hydrochloric acid and pepsin before being released into the small intestine. Normally, the mucosal surface of the stomach provides a barrier that protects it from the hydrochloric acid and pepsin contained in gastric secretions. Disorders of the stomach include gastritis, peptic ulcer, and gastric carcinoma.

Gastric Mucosal Barrier

The stomach lining usually is impermeable to the acid it secretes, a property that allows the stomach to contain acid and pepsin without having its walls digested. Several factors contribute to the protection of the gastric mucosa, including an exceptionally tight fitting and, therefore, impermeable epithelial cell surface covering of a hydrophobic lipid layer. This is coupled with the tenacious, thick mucus that is secreted by the cells, which creates a protective covering for the inner stomach wall that also contains bicarbonates that serve to maintain a neutral pH.[5,28] These mechanisms are collectively referred to as the *gastric mucosal barrier*. Prostaglandins, chemical messengers derived from cell membrane, are thought to exert their effect through improved mucosal blood flow, decreased acid secretion, increased bicarbonate ion secretion, and enhanced mucus production.[29]

Aspirin is able to cross the lipid layer and cause damage to the superficial cells, which can result in acute erosions.[30] Alcohol, which, like aspirin, is lipid soluble, also disrupts the mucosal barrier. When aspirin and alcohol are taken in combination, the permeability of the gastric mucosal barrier is significantly increased and cellular damage occurs.[31] Bile acids also attack the lipid components of the mucosal barrier and afford the potential for gastric irritation when there is reflux of duodenal contents into the stomach.

Normally, the secretion of hydrochloric acid by the parietal cells of the stomach is accompanied by secretion of bicarbonate ions (HCO_3^-). For every hydrogen ion (H^+) that is secreted, an HCO_3^- is produced, and as long as HCO_3^- production is equal to H^+ secretion, mucosal injury does not occur. Changes in gastric blood flow, as in shock, tend to decrease HCO_3^- production. This is particularly true in situations in which decreased blood flow is accompanied by acidosis. Aspirin and the nonsteroidal anti-inflammatory drugs (NSAIDs), also impair HCO_3^- secretion by way of inhibiting gastric cyclooxygenase (COX)-1, a fatty acid enzyme that synthesizes prostaglandins that mediate bicarbonate secretion.[29,32]

KEY POINTS

Disruption of the Gastric Mucosa and Ulcer Development

- Two of the major causes of gastric irritation and ulcer formation are aspirin or NSAIDs and infection with *H. pylori*.

Gastritis

Gastritis refers to inflammation of the gastric mucosa. There are many causes of gastritis, most of which can be grouped as either acute or chronic gastritis.

Acute Gastritis

Acute gastritis is characterized by an acute mucosal inflammatory process, usually transient in nature. The inflammation may be accompanied by emesis, pain, and, in severe cases, hemorrhage and ulceration.[33] This erosive form is an important cause of acute GI bleeding. The condition is most commonly associated with local irritants such aspirin or other NSAIDs, alcohol, or bacterial toxins. Oral administration of corticosteroids may also be complicated by acute hemorrhagic gastritis. Any serious illness or trauma that is accompanied by profound physiologic stress that requires substantial medical or surgical treatment renders the gastric mucosa more vulnerable to acute hemorrhagic gastritis because of mucosal injury (discussed under stress ulcers).[13] Uremia, treatment with cancer chemotherapy drugs, and gastric radiation are other causes of acute gastritis.

People with aspirin-related gastritis can be totally unaware of the condition or may complain only of heartburn or sour stomach. Gastritis associated with excessive alcohol consumption often causes transient gastric distress, which may lead to vomiting and, in more severe situations, to bleeding and hematemesis. Gastritis caused by the toxins of infectious organisms usually has an abrupt and violent onset, with gastric distress and vomiting ensuing approximately 5 hours after the ingestion of a contaminated food source. Acute gastritis usually is a self-limiting disorder, with complete regeneration and healing occurring within several days of removal of the inciting **agent**.

Chronic Gastritis

Chronic gastritis is characterized by the presence of grossly visible erosions and chronic inflammatory changes, leading eventually to atrophy of the glandular epithelium of the stomach. There are types of chronic gastritis: *H. pylori*, metaplastic atrophic gastritis, and chemical gastropathy.[13]

Helicobacter pylori Gastritis

H. pylori infection is the most common cause of chronic gastritis. The prevalence in the United States is associated with socioeconomic status, increased age, and Hispanic and African American ethnicity.[34] *H. pylori* is present in two thirds of the world's population.[34] It has been suggested that transmission in industrialized countries is largely person to person by vomitus, saliva, or feces, whereas additional transmission routes such as water may be important in developing countries. In industrialized countries, the rate of infection with *H. pylori* has decreased substantially over the past several decades owing to improved sanitation.

H. pylori gastritis is a chronic inflammatory disease of the antrum and body of the stomach. Chronic infection with *H. pylori* can lead to gastric atrophy and peptic ulcer and is associated with increased risk of gastric adenocarcinoma and the creation of mucosa-associated lymphoid tissue, which can progress to lymphoma.[33]

Pathogenesis. *H. pylori* are small, curved, or spiral shaped, gram-negative rods (proteobacteria) that can colonize the mucus-secreting epithelial cells of the stomach[33] (Fig. 37-5). *H. pylori* have multiple flagella, which allow them to move through the mucous layer of the stomach, and they secrete urease, which enables them to produce sufficient ammonia to buffer the acidity of their immediate environment. These properties help explain why the organism is able to survive in the acidic environment of the stomach. *H. pylori* produce enzymes and toxins that have the capacity to interfere with the local protection of the gastric mucosa against acid, produce intense inflammation, and elicit an immune response. There is increased production of proinflammatory cytokines (interleukin [IL]-6, IL-8) that serve to recruit and activate neutrophils.[35] Several *H. pylori* proteins are immunogenic, and they evoke an intense immune response in the mucosa.

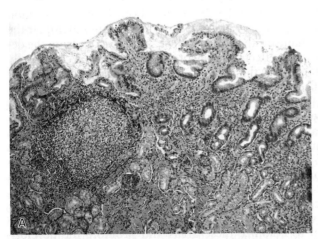 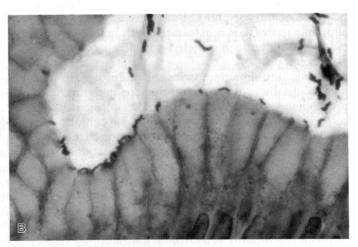

FIGURE 37-5. **(A)** A lymphoid aggregate; when present, these are highly suggestive of *Helicobacter*. **(B)** The Warthin–Starry stain highlights the small curvilinear organisms at the foveolar surface. (From Strayer D. S., Rubin R. (Eds.) (2015). *Rubin's pathophysiology: Clinicopathologic foundations of medicine* (7th ed., Figure 19-16B and D, p. 764). Philadelphia, PA: Lippincott Williams & Wilkins.)

endoscopic examination. The history should include careful attention to aspirin and NSAID use. Peptic ulcer should be differentiated from other causes of epigastric pain. X-ray studies with a contrast medium such as barium are used to detect the presence of an ulcer crater and to exclude gastric carcinoma.

Pharmacologic treatment focuses on eradicating *H. pylori*, relieving ulcer symptoms, and healing the ulcer crater. Acid-neutralizing, acid-inhibiting drugs and mucosa-protective agents are used to relieve symptoms and promote healing of the ulcer crater. There is no evidence that special diets are beneficial in treating peptic ulcer. Aspirin and NSAID use should be avoided when possible.

There are two pharmacologic methods for reducing gastric acid content. The first involves the neutralization of gastric acid through the use of antacids, and the second a decrease in gastric acid production through the use of H_2-receptor antagonists or PPIs.

Histamine is the major physiologic mediator for hydrochloric acid secretion. The H_2-receptor antagonists block gastric acid secretion stimulated by histamine, gastrin, and acetylcholine.[41] The PPIs block the final stage of hydrogen ion secretion by blocking the action of the gastric parietal cell proton pump.

Among the agents that enhance mucosal defenses are sucralfate and prostaglandin analogs. The drug sucralfate, which is a complex salt of sucrose-containing aluminum and sulfate, selectively binds to damaged ulcer tissue and serves as a barrier to acid, pepsin, and bile. Sucralfate also can directly absorb bile salts and initiate the secretion of bicarbonate and mucus.[41]

The current surgical management of peptic ulcer disease is largely limited to treatment of complications. It usually is performed using minimally invasive methods. With bleeding ulcers, hemostasis often can be achieved by endoscopic methods, and endoscopic balloon dilation often is effective in relieving outflow obstruction.

Zollinger–Ellison Syndrome

The Zollinger–Ellison syndrome is a rare condition caused by a gastrin-secreting tumor (gastrinoma), producing symptoms related to increased gastric acid secretions resulting in GERD or peptic ulcer disease.[42] The tumors may be single or multiple; duodenal tumors account for 40% to 50% of this type of gastrinoma.[43] Approximately 50% of gastrin-producing tumors are malignant.[44] Diarrhea may result from hypersecretion or from the inactivation of intestinal lipase and impaired fat digestion that occur with a decrease in intestinal pH.

Hypergastrinemia may also occur in an autosomal dominant disorder called the *multiple endocrine neoplasia type 1 (MEN 1) syndrome*, which is characterized by hyperparathyroidism and multiple endocrine tumors, including gastrinomas. Approximately 20% to 25% of gastrinomas are due to MEN 1.[42]

The diagnosis of the Zollinger–Ellison syndrome is based on elevated serum gastrin and basal gastric acid levels and elimination of the MEN 1 syndrome as a cause of the disorder. Computed tomography (CT), abdominal ultrasonography, and selective angiography are used to localize the tumor and determine whether metastatic disease is present.

Treatment of Zollinger–Ellison syndrome involves control of gastric acid secretion by PPIs and treatment of the malignant neoplasm.[44] Surgical removal is indicated when the tumor is malignant and has not metastasized.

Stress Ulcers

A stress ulcer refers to GI ulcerations that develop in relation to major physiologic stress.[13] People at high risk for development of stress ulcers include those with large surface area burns (Curling ulcer),[45] trauma, sepsis, acute respiratory distress syndrome, severe liver failure, and major surgical procedures. These lesions occur most often in the fundus and body of the stomach and are thought to result from ischemia to the mucosal tissue and alterations in the gastric mucosal barrier.[45] Another form of stress ulcer, called *Cushing ulcer*, consists of gastric, duodenal, and esophageal ulcers arising in people with intracranial injury, operations, or tumors. They are thought to be caused by hypersecretion of gastric acid resulting from stimulation of vagal nuclei by increased intracranial pressure.

People admitted to hospital intensive care units are at particular risk for development of stress ulcers.[46] PPIs are the first line of medications used in the prevention of stress ulcers.[45]

Cancer of the Stomach

According to the World Cancer Research Fund, in 2018, stomach cancer was the fifth most common cancer worldwide, with an estimated 1,033,701 new cases (6.1% of total cancer incidence) for both genders.[47]

Etiology and Pathogenesis

Factors thought to increase the risk of gastric cancer include genetic factors, carcinogenic factors in the diet (*e.g.*, N-nitroso compounds and benzopyrene found in smoked and preserved foods), autoimmune gastritis, and gastric adenomas or polyps. The incidence of stomach cancer in the United States has significantly decreased since 1930, presumably because of improved storage of food with decreased consumption of salted, smoked, and preserved foods.[48] Chronic infection with *H. pylori* appears to serve as a cofactor in some types of gastric carcinomas. The bacterial infection causes gastritis, followed by atrophy, intestinal metaplasia, and carcinoma. This sequence of cellular events depends on both the presence of the bacterial proteins and the host immune response, with the latter being influenced by the host genetic background. In addition to genetics, the likelihood of developing gastric cancer from an *H. pylori* infection is related to the strain of *H. pylori* infection, environmental factors, and the duration of infection.[49] Autoimmune gastritis, like *H. pylori* infection, increases the risk of gastric cancer, presumably due to chronic inflammation and intestinal metaplasia.[50]

Between 50% and 60% of gastric cancers occur in the pyloric region or adjacent to the antrum. Compared with a benign ulcer, which has smooth margins and is concentrically shaped, gastric cancers tend to be larger, are irregularly shaped, and have irregular margins.

Clinical Manifestations

Unfortunately, stomach cancer is often either asymptomatic or may cause only nonspecific symptoms in its early stages. By the time symptoms occur, one in five stomach cancers has often reached an advanced stage and may have metastasized.

Early cancers may be associated with indigestion or a burning sensation. However, less than 1 in every 50 people referred for endoscopy because of indigestion has cancer. Abdominal discomfort and loss of appetite, especially for meat, can occur.

Stomach cancers that have enlarged and invaded normal tissue can cause weakness, fatigue, bloating of the stomach after meals, abdominal pain in the upper abdomen, nausea and occasional vomiting, diarrhea, or constipation. Further enlargement may cause weight loss or bleeding with vomiting blood or having blood in the stool, the latter apparent as black discoloration (melena) and sometimes leading to anemia. Dysphagia suggests a tumor in the cardia or extension of the gastric tumor into the esophagus.

Diagnosis and Treatment

Diagnosis of gastric cancer is accomplished by a variety of techniques, including barium x-ray studies, endoscopic studies with biopsy, and cytologic studies (e.g., Papanicolaou smear) of gastric secretions.[51] Cytologic studies can prove particularly useful as routine screening tests for people with atrophic gastritis or gastric polyps. CT and endoscopic ultrasonography often are used to delineate the spread of a diagnosed stomach cancer.

Depending on the location and extent of the lesion, surgery in the form of radical subtotal gastrectomy usually is the treatment of choice. Irradiation and chemotherapy have not proved particularly useful as primary treatment modalities in stomach cancer. These methods usually are used for palliative purposes or to control metastatic spread of the disease. Molecular targeted therapy has attracted substantial attention to improve the specificity of anticancer efficacy and significantly reduce nonselective resistance and toxicity. An in-depth understanding of the mechanisms that underlie molecular targeted therapies will provide new insights into gastric cancer treatment.[52]

gastropathy. *H. pylori* is an "S"-shaped bacterium that colonizes the mucus-secreting epithelial cells of the stomach. Infection increases the risk of chronic gastritis, peptic ulcer, gastric carcinoma, and low-grade B-cell lymphoma. Treatment of *H. pylori* infection involves the use of multidrug therapy aimed at increasing the pH of gastric secretions and antimicrobial agents designed to eradicate the organism.

Peptic ulcer is a term used to describe a group of ulcerative disorders that occur in areas of the upper GI tract that are exposed to acid–pepsin secretions, most commonly in the duodenum and stomach. There are two main causes of peptic ulcer: *H. pylori* infection and aspirin or NSAID use. The treatment of peptic ulcer focuses on eradication of *H. pylori*, avoidance of gastric irritation from NSAIDs, and conventional pharmacologic treatment directed at symptom relief and ulcer healing.

The Zollinger–Ellison syndrome is a rare condition caused by a gastrin-secreting tumor in which gastric acid secretion reaches such levels that ulceration becomes inevitable. Stress ulcers, also called *Curling ulcers*, occur in relation to major physiologic stresses such as burns and trauma and are thought to result from ischemia, tissue acidosis, and bile salts entering the stomach in critically ill people with decreased GI tract motility. Another form of stress ulcer, Cushing ulcer, occurs in people with intracranial trauma or surgery and is thought to be caused by hypersecretion of gastric acid resulting from stimulation of vagal nuclei by increased intracranial pressure.

Although the incidence of cancer of the stomach has declined over the past 50 years in the United States, it remains the fifth leading cause of cancer death worldwide.[47] Because there are few early symptoms with this form of cancer, the disease often is far advanced at the time of diagnosis.

Disorders of the Small and Large Intestines

There are many similarities in conditions that disrupt the integrity and function of the small and large intestines. The walls of the small and large intestines consist of five layers:

1. An inner mucosal layer, which lines the lumen of the intestine
2. A submucosal layer
3. A circular muscularis layer
4. A layer of longitudinal muscle fibers
5. An outer serosal layer

Among the conditions that cause altered intestinal function are irritable bowel syndrome (IBS), inflammatory bowel disease (IBD), diverticulitis, appendicitis, disorders of bowel motility (i.e., diarrhea, constipation, and bowel obstruction), malabsorption syndrome, and cancers of the colon and rectum.

SUMMARY CONCEPTS

Disorders of the stomach include gastritis, peptic ulcer, and cancer of the stomach. Gastritis refers to inflammation of the gastric mucosa. Acute gastritis refers to a transient inflammation of the gastric mucosa; it is associated most commonly with local irritants such as bacterial endotoxins, caffeine, alcohol, and aspirin. Chronic gastritis is characterized by the absence of grossly visible erosions and the presence of chronic inflammatory changes leading eventually to atrophy of the glandular epithelium of the stomach. There are three main types of chronic gastritis: *H. pylori* gastritis, autoimmune gastritis and multifocal atrophic gastritis, and chemical

Irritable Bowel Syndrome

The term *irritable bowel syndrome* is used to describe a functional GI disorder characterized by a variable combination of chronic and recurrent intestinal symptoms not explained by structural or biochemical abnormalities. There is evidence to suggest that 10% to 15% of the US population have the disorder and one in four people worldwide.[53]

IBS is characterized by persistent or recurrent symptoms of abdominal pain; altered bowel function; and varying complaints of flatulence, bloating, nausea and anorexia, constipation or diarrhea, and anxiety or depression. A hallmark of IBS is abdominal pain that is relieved by defecation and associated with a change in consistency or frequency of stools. Abdominal pain usually is intermittent, cramping, and in the lower abdomen. It does not usually occur at night or interfere with sleep. The condition is believed to result from dysregulation of intestinal motor activity and central neural functions modulated by the CNS.[54] People with IBS tend to experience increased motility and abnormal intestinal contractions in response to psychological and physiologic stresses. The role that psychological factors play in the disease is uncertain. Although changes in intestinal activity are normal responses to stress, these responses appear to be exaggerated in people with IBS. Women tend to be affected more often than do men. **Menarche** often is associated with the onset of the disorder. Women frequently notice an exacerbation of symptoms during the premenstrual period, suggesting a hormonal component.

Clinical Manifestations and Diagnosis

Because IBS lacks anatomic or physiologic markers, diagnosis is usually based on signs and symptoms of abdominal pain or discomfort, bloating, and constipation or diarrhea, or alternating bouts of constipation and diarrhea. A commonly used set of diagnostic criteria require continuous or recurrent symptoms of at least 12 weeks' duration (which may be nonconsecutive) of abdominal discomfort or pain in the preceding 12 months, with two of three accompanying features: relief with defecation, onset associated with a change in bowel frequency, and onset associated with a change in form (appearance) of stool.[55]

Other symptoms that support the diagnosis of IBS include abnormal stool frequency (more than three times per day or less than three times per week), abnormal stool form (lumpy/hard or loose/watery), abnormal stool passage (straining, urgency, or feeling of incomplete evacuation), passage of mucus, and bloating or feeling of abdominal distension.[55] A history of lactose intolerance should be considered because intolerance to lactose and other sugars may be a precipitating factor in some people. The acute onset of symptoms raises the likelihood of organic disease, as does weight loss, anemia, fever, occult blood in the stool, nighttime symptoms, or signs and symptoms of malabsorption. These signs and symptoms require additional investigation of differential diagnoses.[56]

Treatment

The treatment of IBS focuses on methods of stress management, particularly those related to symptom production. Usually, no special diet is indicated, although adequate fiber intake usually is recommended. Avoidance of offending dietary substances by following specific elimination diets that omit such foods as fatty and gas-producing foods, alcohol, and caffeine-containing beverages may be beneficial.[57] Various pharmacologic agents, including antispasmodic and anticholinergic drugs, have been used with varying success in treatment of the disorder.

Inflammatory Bowel Disease

The term *inflammatory bowel disease* is used to designate two related inflammatory intestinal disorders: Crohn disease and ulcerative colitis. Over 1 million residents in the United States and 2.5 million in Europe are estimated to have IBD. Currently, the prevalence of IBD in the Western world is up to 0.5% of the general population.[58] Although the two diseases differ sufficiently to be distinguishable, they have many features in common. Both diseases produce inflammation of the bowel, lack confirming evidence of a proven causative agent, have a pattern of familial occurrence, and can be accompanied by systemic manifestations. Crohn disease most commonly affects the distal small intestine and proximal colon, but can affect any area of the GI tract from the esophagus to the anus, whereas ulcerative colitis is confined to the colon and rectum (Fig. 37-7). The distinguishing characteristics of Crohn disease and ulcerative colitis are summarized in Table 37-1.

Etiology and Pathogenesis

A remarkable feature of the GI tract is that the mucosal immune system is always ready to respond against ingested pathogens but is unresponsive to the normal intestinal microflora. According to the currently accepted hypothesis, this normal state of homeostasis is disrupted

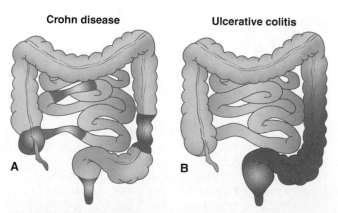

Crohn disease   **Ulcerative colitis**

A   B

FIGURE 37-7. Distribution patterns of disease with (**A**) skip lesions in Crohn disease and (**B**) continuous involvement of the colon, beginning with the rectum, in ulcerative colitis.

TABLE 37-1 Differentiating Characteristics of Crohn Disease and Ulcerative Colitis

Characteristic	Crohn Disease	Ulcerative Colitis
Types of inflammation	Granulomatous	Ulcerative and exudative
Level of involvement	Primarily submucosal	Primarily mucosal
Extent of involvement	Skip lesions	Continuous
Areas of involvement	Primarily ileum, secondarily colon	Primarily rectum and left colon
Diarrhea	Common	Common
Rectal bleeding	Rare	Common
Fistulas	Common	Rare
Strictures	Common	Rare
Perianal abscesses	Common	Rare
Development of cancer	Uncommon	Relatively common

in IBD, leading to unregulated and exaggerated immune responses. The question remains whether the response is an appropriate defense mechanism to a pathogen or is the immune system responding in an inappropriate manner. Thus, as in many other autoimmune disorders, the pathogenesis of Crohn disease and ulcerative colitis involves a failure of immune regulation, genetic predisposition, and an environmental trigger, especially microbial flora.[59]

Genetic Susceptibility

The genetic basis of IBD has long been suspected. First-degree relatives of people diagnosed with IBD have a 30 to 100 times greater incidence of IBD.[60] Genome-wide association studies have identified 163 distinct loci that confer risk of, or protection from, the development of Crohn disease and ulcerative colitis, with a substantial portion of these loci common to both diseases.[61] Family history remains the strongest predictor of IBD, although only 10% of people have an affected first-degree relative.[62] These associations clearly indicate that genetic susceptibility plays an important role in the development of IBD. However, classic mendelian inheritance patterns are not seen, and IBD therefore cannot be attributed to a single gene.

The most recent and largest genetic association study, which employed genome-wide association data for over 75,000 people with IBD and controls, identified 163 susceptibility loci for IBD, encompassing approximately 300 potential candidate genes.[63,64] Identified genetic factors account for only a small proportion of the disease variance: 13.1% for Crohn disease and 8.2% for ulcerative colitis. Overall, explainable susceptibility loci and

genetic risk factors discovered so far account for only 20% to 25% of the heritability (genetic risk).[63,65]

Role of Environmental Factors

Although family history is the strongest risk factor for IBD, and genes play an important role, considerable epidemiologic data supports a key role for the environment. The earliest and most consistently described environmental factor impacting Crohn disease and ulcerative colitis incidence is smoking.[66] Current smokers have a twofold increase in risk of Crohn disease, with a more modest association in former smokers. In contrast, former smoking is associated with substantial increase in risk of ulcerative colitis within 1 year of quitting, whereas current smoking appears to be protective.[67] The precise reason for this divergent effect is unclear. Smoking might contribute to the development of IBD by influencing the intestinal microbiome, because people with Crohn disease who smoke show a dysbiosis within their intestinal microbiota.[68]

Recent antibiotic use within 2 to 5 years of diagnosis was also associated with increased risk of adult-onset IBD, with increasing effect seen with greater number of antibiotic courses and exposure earlier in life.[69] Although it is unlikely that IBD is directly caused by microbes, it seems likely that microbes may provide the antigen trigger for an unregulated immune response.

Clinical Manifestations

The clinical manifestations of both Crohn disease and ulcerative colitis are ultimately the result of activation of inflammatory cells with elaboration of inflammatory mediators that cause nonspecific tissue damage. Both diseases are characterized by remissions and exacerbations of diarrhea, fecal urgency, and weight loss. Acute complications, such as intestinal obstruction, may develop during periods of fulminant disease (Fig. 37-8).

A number of systemic manifestations have been identified in people with Crohn disease and ulcerative colitis. These include axial arthritis affecting the spine and sacroiliac joints and oligoarticular arthritis affecting the large joints of the arms and legs; inflammatory conditions of the eye, usually uveitis; skin lesions, especially erythema nodosum; stomatitis; and autoimmune anemia, hypercoagulability of blood, and sclerosing cholangitis. Occasionally, these systemic manifestations may herald the recurrence of intestinal disease. In children, growth retardation may occur, particularly if the symptoms are prolonged and nutrient intake has been poor.

Crohn Disease

Crohn disease is a recurrent, granulomatous type of inflammatory response that can affect any area of the GI tract. The terminal ileum or cecum is the most common portion of the bowel where inflammation occurs.[60,70] It is a slowly progressive, relentless, and often disabling disease. The disease usually strikes people in their twenties or thirties, with women being affected slightly more often than men.

A characteristic feature of Crohn disease is the sharply demarcated, granulomatous lesions surrounded

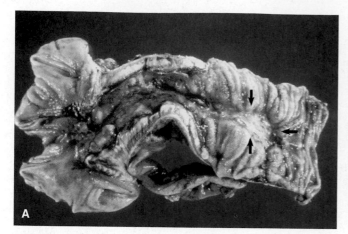
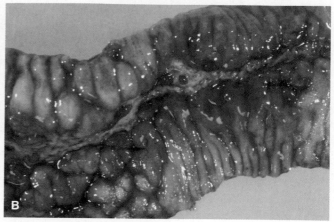

FIGURE 37-8. Crohn disease. (**A**) The terminal ileum shows striking thickening of the wall of the distal portion with distortion of the ileocecal valve. A longitudinal ulcer is present (*arrows*). (**B**) Another longitudinal ulcer is seen in this segment of the ileum. The large rounded areas of edematous damaged mucosa give a "cobblestone" appearance to the involved mucosa. A portion of the mucosa to the lower right is uninvolved. (From Rubin R., Strayer D. S. (Eds.) (2015). *Rubin's pathophysiology: Clinicopathologic foundations of medicine* (6th ed., Figure 19-52, p. 803). Philadelphia, PA: Lippincott Williams & Wilkins.)

by normal-appearing mucosal tissue. When the lesions are multiple, they often are referred to as *skip lesions* because they are interspersed between what appear to be normal segments of the bowel. All the layers of the bowel are involved, with the submucosal layer affected to the greatest extent. The surface of the inflamed bowel usually has a characteristic "cobblestone" appearance resulting from the fissures and crevices that develop, surrounded by areas of submucosal edema[13,70] (Fig. 37-9). There usually is a relative sparing of the smooth muscle layers of the bowel, with marked inflammatory and fibrotic changes of the submucosal layer. The bowel wall, after a time, often becomes thickened and inflexible. The adjacent mesentery may become inflamed, and the regional lymph nodes and channels may become enlarged.

Clinical Manifestations

The clinical course of Crohn disease is variable; often, there are periods of exacerbations and remissions, with symptoms being related to the location of the lesions. The principal symptoms, which are dependent on the area of the GI system that is affected, include diarrhea, abdominal pain, weight loss, fluid and electrolyte disorders, malaise, and low-grade fever.[70] Because Crohn disease affects the submucosal layer to a greater extent than does the mucosal layer, there is less bloody diarrhea than with ulcerative colitis. Ulceration of the perianal skin is common, largely because of the severity of the diarrhea. The absorptive surface of the intestine may be disrupted; nutritional deficiencies may occur, related to the specific segment of the intestine involved. When Crohn disease occurs in childhood, one of its major manifestations may be retardation of growth and significant malnutrition.[71]

Complications of Crohn disease include fistula formation, abdominal abscess formation, and intestinal obstruction. Fistulas are tubelike passages that form connections between different sites in the GI tract. They also may develop between other sites, including the bladder,

vagina, urethra, and skin. Perineal fistulas that originate in the ileum are relatively common.[58] Fistulas between segments of the GI tract may lead to malabsorption, syndromes of bacterial overgrowth, and diarrhea. They also can become infected and cause abscess formation.

Diagnosis

The diagnosis of Crohn disease requires a thorough history and physical examination. Sigmoidoscopy is used for direct visualization of the affected areas and to obtain biopsies. Stool cultures and examination of fresh stool specimens for ova and parasites evaluate infectious agents as the cause of the disorder. In people suspected of having Crohn disease, radiographic contrast studies provide a means for determining the extent of involvement of the small bowel and establishing the presence and nature of fistulas. CT scans may be used to detect an inflammatory mass or abscess.

Treatment

There is no cure for Crohn disease, and remission may not be possible or may be prolonged if achieved. Treatment methods focus on terminating the inflammatory response and promoting healing, maintaining adequate nutrition, and preventing and treating complications. Surgical resection of damaged bowel, drainage of abscesses, or repair of fistula tracts may be necessary.

Nutritional deficiencies are common in Crohn disease because of diarrhea, steatorrhea, and other malabsorption problems. A nutritious diet high in calories, vitamins, and proteins is recommended. Because fats often aggravate the diarrhea, it is recommended that they be avoided. Elemental diets, which are nutritionally balanced but are residue and bulk free, may be given during the acute phase of the illness. These diets are largely absorbed in the jejunum and allow the inflamed bowel to rest. Total parenteral nutrition consists of intravenous administration of hypertonic glucose solutions to which amino acids and fats may be added. This form of

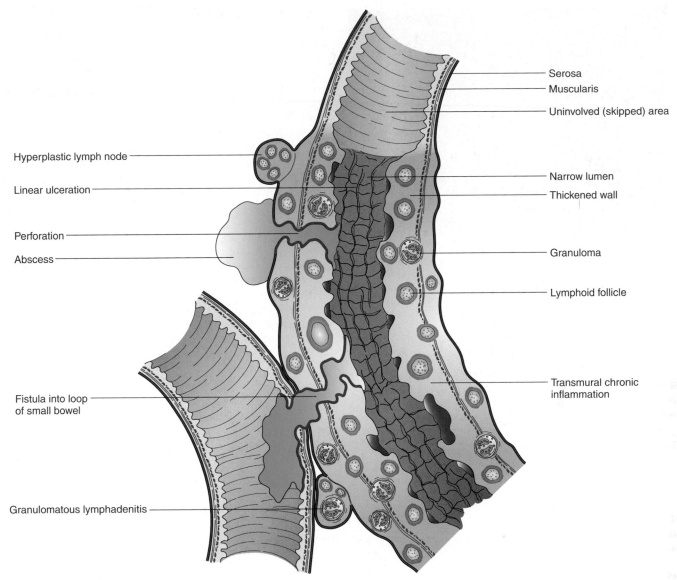

Serosa
Muscularis
Uninvolved (skipped) area

Narrow lumen
Thickened wall

Granuloma

Lymphoid follicle

Transmural chronic inflammation

Hyperplastic lymph node

Linear ulceration

Perforation

Abscess

Fistula into loop of small bowel

Granulomatous lymphadenitis

FIGURE 37-9. Crohn disease. A schematic representation of the major features of Crohn disease in the small intestines. (From Rubin R., Strayer D. S. (Eds.) (2015). *Rubin's pathophysiology: Clinicopathologic foundations of medicine* (7th ed., Figure 19-73, p. 805). Philadelphia, PA: Lippincott Williams & Wilkins.)

nutritional therapy may be needed when food cannot be absorbed from the intestine.

Ulcerative Colitis

Ulcerative colitis is a nonspecific inflammatory condition of the colon. The incidence and prevalence of ulcerative colitis vary greatly with geographic location.[72] In contrast to Crohn disease, which can affect various sites in the GI tract, the inflammatory response in ulcerative colitis is largely limited to the mucosa and submucosa and is confined to the rectum and colon so that colectomy is curative. The disease may arise at any age, with a peak incidence between 15 and 25 years of age.[60] The disease usually begins in the rectum and spreads proximally, affecting primarily the mucosal layer, although it can extend into the submucosal layer. The length of proximal extension varies. It may involve the rectum alone (ulcerative proctitis), the rectum and sigmoid colon (proctosigmoiditis), or the entire colon (pancolitis). The inflammatory process tends to be **confluent** and continuous instead of skipping areas, as it does in Crohn disease.

The cause of ulcerative colitis is unknown.[73] Characteristic of the disease are the lesions that form in the crypts of Lieberkühn in the base of the mucosal layer. The inflammatory process leads to the formation of pinpoint mucosal hemorrhages, which in time suppurate and develop into *crypt abscesses*. These inflammatory lesions may become necrotic and ulcerate. Although the ulcerations usually are superficial, they often extend, causing large denuded areas (Fig. 37-10). As a result of the inflammatory process, the mucosal layer often develops tonguelike projections that resemble polyps and therefore are called *pseudopolyps*. The bowel wall thickens in response to repeated episodes of colitis.

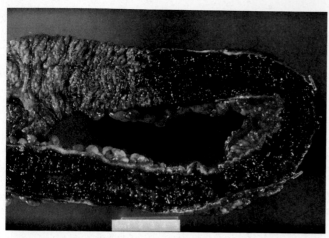

FIGURE 37-10. Ulcerative colitis. Prominent erythema and ulceration of the colon begin in and are the most severe in the rectosigmoid area and extend into the ascending colon. (From Strayer D. S., Rubin R. (Eds.) (2015). *Rubin's pathophysiology: Clinicopathologic foundations of medicine* (7th ed., Figure 19-74, p. 806). Philadelphia, PA: Lippincott Williams & Wilkins.)

Clinical Manifestations

Ulcerative colitis typically presents as a relapsing disorder marked by attacks of diarrhea. The diarrhea may persist for days, weeks, or months and then subside, only to recur after an asymptomatic interval of several months to years or even decades. Because ulcerative colitis affects the mucosal layer of the bowel, the stools typically contain blood and mucus. Nocturnal diarrhea usually occurs when daytime symptoms are severe. There may be mild abdominal cramping and fecal incontinence. Anorexia, weakness, and fatigability are common.

Depending on clinical and endoscopic findings, the disease is characterized by how much of the colon is affected and the extent of the inflammation. Severity is defined as mild, moderate, severe, or fulminant.[60] The most common form of the disease is the mild form, in which the person has less than four stools daily, with or without blood, no systemic signs of toxicity, and a normal erythrocyte sedimentation rate (ESR). People with moderate disease have more than four stools daily, but have minimal signs of toxicity. Severe disease is manifested by more than six bloody stools daily, and evidence of toxicity as demonstrated by fever, tachycardia, anemia, and elevated ESR (Fig. 37-11). People with

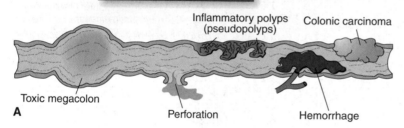

LOCAL COMPLICATIONS

Inflammatory polyps (pseudopolyps)

Colonic carcinoma

Toxic megacolon

Perforation

Hemorrhage

A

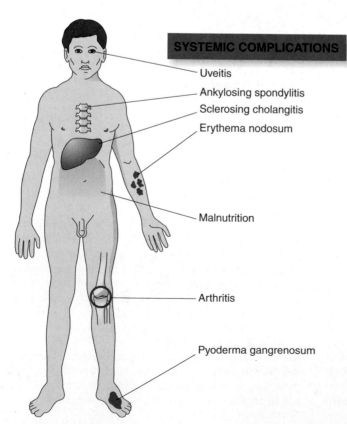

SYSTEMIC COMPLICATIONS

Uveitis

Ankylosing spondylitis

Sclerosing cholangitis

Erythema nodosum

Malnutrition

Arthritis

Pyoderma gangrenosum

B

FIGURE 37-11. Complications of ulcerative colitis. (**A**) A schematic representation of the major features of ulcerative colitis in the colon. (**B**) Systemic complications. (**A:** From Strayer D. S., Rubin R. (Eds.) (2012). *Rubin's pathophysiology: Clinicopathologic foundations of medicine* (6th ed., Figure 19-77, p. 807). Philadelphia, PA: Lippincott Williams & Wilkins; **B:** From Rubin R., Strayer D. S. (Eds.) (2012). *Rubin's pathophysiology: Clinicopathologic foundations of medicine* (6th ed., p. 658). Philadelphia, PA: Lippincott Williams & Wilkins.)

fulminant disease have features that include more than 10 bowel movements a day, continuous bleeding, fever and other signs of toxicity, abdominal tenderness and distension, need for blood transfusions, and colonic dilation on abdominal radiographs. These people are at risk for development of toxic megacolon, which is characterized by dilation of the colon and signs of systemic toxicity. It results from extension of the inflammatory response, with involvement of neural and vascular components of the bowel.

Ulcerative colitis is believed to have a systemic (*i.e.*, autoimmune) origin, so people may present with comorbidities leading to symptoms and complications outside the colon. The frequency of such extraintestinal manifestations has been reported as anywhere between 6% and 47% (Fig. 37-11).[74] The extraintestinal manifestations may include arthritis, uveitis, deep venous thrombosis, primary sclerosing cholangitis, or ankylosing spondylitis, and so on. The most common extraintestinal manifestation of IBD is arthritis. For some people, especially those with primary sclerosing cholangitis or ankylosing spondylitis, the extraintestinal manifestations may be more problematic than the bowel disease.[60]

Diagnosis and Treatment

Diagnosis of ulcerative colitis is based on history and physical examination. The diagnosis usually is confirmed by sigmoidoscopy, colonoscopy, biopsy, and by stool examinations for infectious or other causes that return negative results. Colonoscopy should not be performed on people with severe disease because of the danger of perforation, but may be performed after demonstrated improvement to determine the extent of disease and need for subsequent cancer surveillance.

Treatment depends on the extent of the disease and severity of symptoms. It includes measures to control the acute manifestations of the disease and to prevent recurrence. Some people with mild to moderate symptoms are able to control their symptoms simply by avoiding caffeine, lactose (milk), highly spiced foods, and gas-forming foods. Fiber supplements may be used to decrease diarrhea and rectal symptoms. Surgical treatment (*i.e.*, removal of the rectum and entire colon) with the creation of an ileostomy or ileoanal anastomosis may be required for people who do not respond to medications and conservative methods of treatment.

Cancer of the colon is one of the feared long-term complications of ulcerative colitis. Ulcerative colitis is characterized by deoxyribonucleic acid (DNA) damage with microsatellite instability in mucosa cells. More recently, genomic instability was detected in nondysplastic areas in people with ulcerative colitis, suggesting that these people have DNA repair deficiency and genomic instability throughout the intestinal tract.[75] In a meta-analysis focusing on studies involving people with ulcerative colitis, the cumulative risk of having colorectal cancer was 2% by 10 years, 8% by 20 years, and 18% by 30 years.[76,77] All people with the diagnosis should receive a colonoscopy for screening purposes within 8 years of them beginning to have symptoms.

The frequency of surveillance colonoscopies is often every 1 to 2 years and is dependent on the results of the examinations and biopsies obtained.[78]

Infectious Enterocolitis

A number of microbial agents, including viruses, bacteria, and protozoa, can infect the GI tract, causing diarrhea and sometimes ulcerative and inflammatory changes in the small or large intestine. Infectious enterocolitis is a global problem, causing more than 12,000 deaths per day among children in developing countries. Although far less common in industrialized countries, these disorders still have infection rates second only to the common cold. Most infections are spread by the oral–fecal route, often through contaminated water or food.

Viral Infection

Most viral infections affect the superficial epithelium of the small intestine, destroying these cells and disrupting their absorptive function. Repopulation of the small intestinal villi with immature enterocytes and preservation of crypt secretory cells lead to net secretion of water and electrolytes compounded by incomplete absorption of nutrients and osmotic diarrhea. Symptomatic disease is caused by several distinct viruses, including the rotavirus, which most commonly affects children 6 to 24 months of age; the norovirus (or Norwalk), which is responsible for the majority of nonbacterial food-borne epidemic gastroenteritis in all age groups; and enteric adenoviruses, which primarily affect children younger than 24 months.[79]

Rotavirus

Worldwide, rotavirus is the leading cause of severe diarrhea and is estimated to cause the death of 527,000 children younger than age 5 each year.[80]

The disease tends to be most severe in children 3 to 24 months of age. Infants younger than 3 months of age are relatively protected by transplacental antibodies and possibly by breast-feeding. The virus spreads via the fecal–oral route, and outbreaks are common in children in day care centers. The virus is shed before and for days after clinical illness. Very few infectious virions are needed to cause disease in a susceptible host.

Rotavirus infection typically begins after an incubation period of 1 to 3 days, with mild to moderate fever and vomiting, followed by the onset of frequent watery stools.[79] The fever and vomiting usually disappear on or about the second day, but the diarrhea continues for 5 to 7 days. Dehydration may develop rapidly, particularly in infants. Treatment is largely supportive. Avoiding and treating dehydration are the main goals.

Bacterial Infection

Infectious enterocolitis can be caused by a number of bacteria. There are several pathogenic mechanisms for bacterial enterocolitis: ingestion of preformed toxins that are present in contaminated food; infection by toxigenic organisms that proliferate in the gut lumen and produce an enterotoxin; and infection by entero-invasive organisms, which proliferate in the lumen and invade and destroy mucosal epithelial cells. The pathogenic effects of bacterial infections depend on the ability of the organism to adhere to the mucosal epithelial cells, elaborate enterotoxins, and then invade the mucosal epithelial cells.

In general, bacterial infections produce more severe effects than do viral infections. The complications of bacterial enterocolitis result from massive fluid loss or destruction of intestinal mucosa and include dehydration, sepsis, and perforation. Among the organisms that cause bacterial enterocolitis are *Staphylococcus aureus* (toxins associated with "food poisoning"), *Escherichia coli*, *Shigella* species, *Salmonella*, and *Campylobacter*.[81] Two particularly serious forms of bacterial enterocolitis are caused by *Clostridium difficile* and *E. coli* O157:H7.

Clostridium difficile Colitis

C. difficile colitis is associated with antibiotic therapy.[82-84] *C. difficile* is a gram-positive, spore-forming bacillus that is part of the normal flora in 1% to 3% of humans.[54] The spores are resistant to the acid environment of the stomach and convert to vegetative forms in the colon. Treatment with broad-spectrum antibiotics, especially those with activity against gram-negative enteric bacteria, predisposes to disruption of the normal protective bacterial flora of the colon, leading to colonization by *C. difficile* along with the release of toxins that cause mucosal damage and inflammation. After antibiotic therapy has made the bowel susceptible to infection, colonization by *C. difficile* occurs by the oral–fecal route. *C. difficile* infection usually is acquired in the hospital, where the organism is commonly encountered.

In general, *C. difficile* is noninvasive. Development of *C. difficile* colitis and diarrhea requires an alteration in the normal gut flora, acquisition and germination of the spores, overgrowth of *C. difficile*, and toxin production. The toxins bind to and damage the intestinal mucosa, causing hemorrhage, inflammation, and necrosis. The toxins also interfere with protein synthesis, attract inflammatory cells, increase capillary permeability, and stimulate intestinal peristalsis. The infection commonly manifests with diarrhea that is mild to moderate and sometimes is accompanied by lower abdominal cramping. Typically, symptoms begin within 4 to 9 days of an antibiotic treatment being started and, in most cases, systemic manifestations are absent, and the symptoms subside after the antibiotic has been discontinued.[85]

A more severe form of colitis, *Pseudomembranous colitis*, is characterized by an adherent inflammatory membrane overlying the areas of mucosal injury. It is a life-threatening form of the disease. People with the disease are acutely ill, with lethargy, fever, tachycardia, abdominal pain and distension, and dehydration. The smooth muscle tone of the colon may be lost, resulting in toxic dilation of the colon. Prompt therapy is needed to prevent perforation of the bowel.

The diagnosis of *C. difficile*–associated diarrhea requires a careful history, with particular emphasis on antibiotic use. Diagnostic findings include a history of antibiotic use and laboratory tests that confirm the presence of *C. difficile* toxins in the stool. Treatment includes the immediate discontinuation of antibiotic therapy. Specific treatment aimed at eradicating *C. difficile* is used when symptoms are severe or persistent. Metronidazole is the drug of choice, with vancomycin being reserved for people who cannot tolerate metronidazole, do not respond to the drug, or have severe symptoms.[86]

Escherichia coli O157:H7 Infection

E. coli O157:H7 has become recognized as an important cause of epidemic and sporadic colitis.[87] *E. coli* O157:H7 is a strain of *E. coli* found in the feces and contaminated milk of healthy dairy and beef cattle, but it also has been found in contaminated pork, poultry, and lamb. Infection usually is by food-borne transmission, often by ingesting undercooked hamburger. The organism also can be transferred to nonmeat products such as fruits and vegetables and unpasteurized milk. Transmission has also been reported in people swimming in a fecally contaminated lake as well as among visitors to farms and petting zoos, where children are in direct contact with animals. Person-to-person transmission may occur, particularly in nursing homes, day care settings, and hospitals. The very young and the very old are particularly at risk for the infection and its complications.

The infection may cause no symptoms or cause a variety of manifestations, including acute, nonbloody diarrhea; hemorrhagic colitis; hemolytic uremic syndrome (HUS); and thrombotic thrombocytopenic purpura. The infection often presents with abdominal cramping and watery diarrhea and subsequently may progress to bloody diarrhea. The diarrhea commonly lasts 5 to 10 days.[88]

Most strains of *E. coli* are harmless. However, entero-hemorrhagic *E. coli* can release *Shigella*-like toxins that attach to and damage the mucosal lining of the intestine. Subsequently, the *Shigella*-like toxins gain access to the circulatory system and travel in the plasma and on the surface of platelets and monocytes. The *Shigella*-like toxins bind to high-affinity galactose-containing receptors in the membranes of glomerular, cerebral, or microvascular endothelial cells; renal mesangial and tubular cells; and monocytes and platelets.[89] Two complications of the infection, HUS and thrombotic thrombocytopenic purpura, reflect the effects of the *Shigella*-like toxins. The HUS is characterized by hemolytic anemia, thrombocytopenia, and renal failure. It occurs predominantly in infants and young children and is the most common cause of acute renal failure in children. The prognosis of people with HUS is generally good, and most children recover fully without subsequent relapses. The mortality rate in children is less than 5% but is higher in adults (25%).[90] Thrombotic thrombocytopenic purpura is manifested by thrombocytopenia, renal failure, fever, and neurologic manifestations. It often is regarded as the severe end of the disease that leads to HUS plus neurologic problems.

No specific therapy is available for *E. coli* O157:H7 infection. Treatment is largely symptomatic and directed toward treating the effects of complications. The use of antibiotics or antimotility/antidiarrheal agents in the early stages of diarrhea has been shown to increase the risk of HUS because the gut is exposed to a greater amount of toxins for a longer time.

Because of the seriousness of the infection and its complications, educating the public about techniques for decreasing primary transmission of the infection from animal sources is important. Food handlers and consumers should be aware of the proper methods for handling uncooked meat to prevent cross-contamination of other foods. Particular attention should be paid to hygiene in day care centers and nursing homes, where the spread of infection to the very young and very old may result in severe complications.

Protozoan Infection

Amebiasis refers to an infection by *Entamoeba histolytica* involving the colon and, occasionally, the liver.[33] Humans are the only known reservoir for *E. histolytica*, which reproduce in the colon and pass in the feces. Although *E. histolytica* infection occurs worldwide, it is more common and more severe in tropical and subtropical areas, where crowding and poor sanitation prevail. Intestinal amebiasis ranges from completely asymptomatic infection to serious dysenteric disease.

Entamoeba histolytica has two distinct stages: the trophozoites (ameboid form) and cysts.[91] The trophozoites thrive in the colon and feed on bacteria and human cells. They may colonize any portion of the large bowel, but the area of maximum disease is usually the cecum. People with symptomatic disease pass both cysts and trophozoites in their feces, and these die when exposed to air outside of the body. Only the cysts are infectious because they survive gastric acidity, which destroys the trophozoites. Once established, the trophozoites invade the crypts of colonic glands and burrow down into the submucosa; the organism then fans out to create a flask-shaped ulcer. *Entamoeba histolytica* that have invaded into the submucosal veins of the colon enter the portal vein and embolize to the liver to produce solitary and, less often, multiple discrete hepatic abscesses.[92]

Acute onset of diarrhea can occur as early as 8 days (commonly 2 to 4 weeks) after infection.[93] Others may be asymptomatic or have only mild intestinal symptoms for months or several years. Manifestations include abdominal discomfort, tenderness, cramps, and fever, often accompanied by nausea, vomiting, and passage of malodorous **flatus**. There may be frequent passage of liquid stools containing bloody mucus, but the duration of diarrhea is not usually so prolonged as to cause dehydration. The infection often persists for months or years, causing emaciation and anemia. In severe cases, massive destruction of the colonic mucosa may lead to hemorrhage, perforation, or peritonitis. People with amebic liver abscesses often present with severe right upper quadrant pain, low-grade fever, and weight loss.[92]

Diagnostic methods include microscopic examination of the stool for *E. histolytica*, serum antibody tests, and colonoscopy with specimen collection or biopsy. Treatment includes use of the antimicrobial agents.

Diverticular Disease

A diverticulum is the outpouching of a hollow structure in the body. Diverticulosis is the condition of having diverticula in the colon that are not inflamed. Most people with diverticulosis do not have symptoms or problems. Diverticular disease is associated with symptoms such as left iliac fossa pain and alteration of bowel habit.[60] Diverticulosis commonly occurs on the distal descending and sigmoid colon, in which the mucosal layer of the colon herniates through the muscularis layer.[94] There are often multiple diverticula, most of which occur in the sigmoid colon (Fig. 37-12). Diverticular disease is common in Western society, affecting approximately 40% of the population by age 60 and 60% of the population by age 80.[94] Although the disorder is prevalent in the developed countries of the world, it is almost nonexistent in many African nations and underdeveloped countries. This suggests that factors such as lack of fiber in the diet, a decrease in physical activity, and poor bowel habits, along with the effects of aging, contribute to the development of the disease.

In the colon, the longitudinal muscle does not form a continuous layer, as it does in the small bowel. Instead, there are three separate longitudinal bands of muscle called the *teniae coli*. Bands of circular muscle constrict the large intestine, causing the lumen of the bowel to become almost occluded. The combined contraction of the circular muscle and the lack of a continuous longitudinal muscle layer cause the intestine to bulge outward

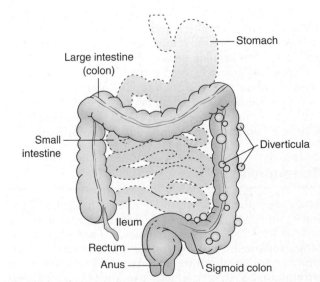

FIGURE 37-12. Location of diverticula in the sigmoid colon.

into pouches called *haustra*. Diverticula develop between the longitudinal muscle bands of the haustra. An increase in intraluminal pressure in the haustra provides the force for creating these herniations.

Diverticular disease often is found when x-ray studies are done for other purposes. When symptoms do occur, they often are attributed to IBS or to other causes. Ill-defined lower abdominal discomfort, a change in bowel habits, bloating, and flatulence are common.

Meckel diverticulum is an outpouching of all layers of the small intestine wall (usually in the ileum). It is the most common malformation of the GI tract and is present in approximately 2% of the population.[95] The majority of people with a Meckel diverticulum are asymptomatic (silent Meckel diverticulum).[96] If symptoms do occur, they typically appear before the age of 2 years. The most common presenting symptom is painless rectal bleeding followed by intestinal obstruction, volvulus, and intussusception. Treatment in those with symptoms is surgical resection.[97]

Diverticulitis is a complication of diverticulosis in which there is inflammation and gross or microscopic perforation of the diverticulum. One of the most common complaints of diverticulitis is pain and tenderness in the lower left quadrant, accompanied by nausea and vomiting, a slight fever, and an elevated white blood cell count.[98] These symptoms usually last for several days, unless complications occur. Complications include perforation with peritonitis, abscesses, hemorrhage, and bowel obstruction. Fistulas can form, involving the bladder (*i.e.*, vesicosigmoid fistula) but sometimes involving the skin, perianal area, vagina, or the small bowel. Pneumaturia (*i.e.*, air in the urine) is a sign of vesicosigmoid fistula.

The diagnosis of diverticular disease is based on history and presenting clinical manifestations. The disease may be confirmed by CT scans or ultrasonographic studies.[98] Flat abdominal radiographs may be used to detect complications associated with acute diverticulitis.

The usual treatment for diverticular disease is to prevent symptoms and complications by increasing the bulk in the diet and bowel retraining so that the person has at least one bowel movement each day. The increased bulk promotes regular defecation and increases colonic contents and colon diameter, thereby decreasing intraluminal pressure. Acute diverticulitis is treated by withholding solid food and administering a broad-spectrum antibiotic.[98] Surgical treatment is reserved for people experiencing nonresolving symptoms and complications.[94]

Appendicitis

Acute appendicitis is extremely common. In the United States, there is a 12% risk of developing appendicitis for males and a 25% risk for females.[99] The appendix becomes inflamed, swollen, and gangrenous, and it eventually perforates if not treated. Appendicitis is related to intraluminal obstruction with a fecalith (*i.e.*, hard piece of stool), gallstones, tumors, parasites, or lymphatic tissue.

Appendicitis usually has an abrupt onset, with pain referred to the epigastric or periumbilical area caused by stretching of the appendix during the early inflammatory process. Nausea usually accompanies the pain. Initially, the pain is vague, but over a period of 2 to 12 hours, it gradually increases and may become colicky. When the inflammatory process has extended to involve the serosal layer of the appendix and the peritoneum, the pain becomes localized to the lower right quadrant. There may be an elevated white blood cell count but not in all cases.[100] Palpation of the abdomen usually reveals a deep tenderness in the lower right quadrant, which is confined to a small area. Rebound tenderness, which is pain that occurs when pressure is applied to the area and then released, and spasm of the overlying abdominal muscles are common.

Diagnosis is usually based on symptoms and findings on physical examination. Ultrasonography or CT may be used to confirm the diagnosis in cases where alternative causes of abdominal pain are suspected.[101] Treatment consists of surgical removal of the appendix. Complications include peritonitis, localized periappendiceal abscess formation, and septicemia.

Alterations in Intestinal Motility

KEY POINTS

Disorders of Gastrointestinal Motility

- The luminal contents move down the GI tract as a result of peristaltic movements regulated by a complex interaction of electrical, neural, and hormonal control mechanisms.

- Local irritation and the composition and constituents of GI contents influence motility through the submucosal afferent neurons of the enteric nervous system. GI wall distension, chemical irritants, osmotic gradients, and bacterial toxins exert many of their effects on GI motility through these afferent pathways.

Diarrhea

Diarrhea is excessively frequent passage of loose or unformed stools. Diarrhea can be acute or chronic and can be caused by infectious organisms, food intolerance, drugs, or intestinal disease.

Acute Diarrhea

Diarrhea that is acute in onset and persists for less than 2 weeks is commonly caused by infectious agents (see previous discussion of Infectious Enterocolitis).[102] Acute diarrhea is commonly divided into noninflammatory and inflammatory diarrhea, depending on the characteristics of the diarrheal stool. Enteric organisms cause diarrhea by several ways. Some are noninvasive and do not cause inflammation, but secrete toxins that stimulate fluid secretion.[101] Others invade and destroy intestinal epithelial cells, thereby altering fluid transport so that secretory activity continues while absorption activity is halted.[103]

Noninflammatory diarrhea is associated with large-volume watery and nonbloody stools, periumbilical cramps, bloating, and nausea or vomiting. It is commonly caused by toxin-producing bacteria (*e.g.,* *S. aureus,*[104] enterotoxigenic *E. coli, Cryptosporidium parvum, Vibrio cholerae*) or other agents (*e.g.,* viruses, *Giardia*) that disrupt the normal absorption or secretory process in the small bowel.[105] Prominent vomiting suggests viral enteritis or *S. aureus* food poisoning. Although typically mild, the diarrhea (which originates in the small intestine) can be voluminous and result in dehydration with hypokalemia and metabolic acidosis. Because tissue invasion does not occur, leukocytes are not present in the feces.

Inflammatory diarrhea is usually characterized by the presence of fever and bloody diarrhea (dysentery). It is caused by invasion of intestinal cells (*e.g.,* *Shigella, Salmonella, Yersinia,* and *Campylobacter*) or the toxins associated with the previously described *C. difficile* or *E. coli* O157:H7 infection. Because infections associated with these organisms predominantly affect the colon, the diarrhea is frequent and small in volume[106] and is associated with left lower quadrant cramps, urgency, and *tenesmus.* Infectious dysentery must be distinguished from acute ulcerative colitis, which may present with bloody diarrhea, fever, and abdominal pain.

Chronic Diarrhea

Diarrhea is considered to be chronic when the symptoms persist for 4 weeks or greater.[102] Chronic diarrhea is often associated with conditions such as IBD, IBS, malabsorption syndrome, endocrine disorders (hyperthyroidism, diabetic autonomic neuropathy), or radiation colitis. There are four major causes of chronic diarrhea: presence of hyperosmotic luminal contents, increased intestinal secretory processes, inflammatory conditions, and infectious processes[102] (Chart 37-1). Factitious diarrhea is caused by indiscriminate use of laxatives or excessive intake of laxative-type foods.

In *osmotic diarrhea,* water is pulled into the bowel by the hyperosmotic nature of its contents in large quantities so that the colon is unable to reabsorb the excess fluid. It occurs when osmotically active particles are not absorbed. In people with lactase deficiency, lactose intolerance is due to the lack of the enzyme lactase in the small intestines to break lactose down into glucose and galactose.[107] Inadequate lactase activity allows lactose to reach the large intestine. There, the gut flora provides a salvage pathway for lactose digestion by cleaving lactose into short-chain fatty acids and gas, mainly hydrogen (H_2), carbon dioxide (CO_2), and methane (CH_4). Nondigested lactose can cause osmotic diarrhea; products of its bacterial digestion can lead to secretory diarrhea and gas distending the intestines. Lactose intolerance is characterized by abdominal symptoms (*e.g.,* nausea, bloating, and pain) after ingestion of dairy products. Another cause of osmotic diarrhea is decreased

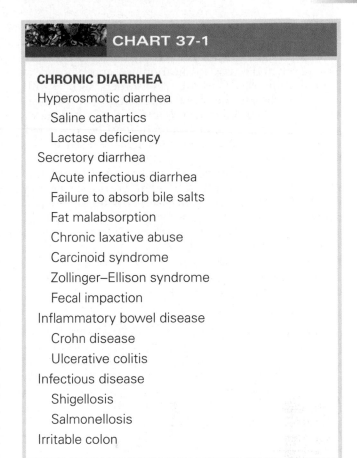

transit time, which interferes with absorption. Osmotic diarrhea usually disappears with fasting.[107,108]

Secretory diarrhea occurs when the secretory processes of the bowel are increased. Secretory diarrhea also occurs when excess bile acids remain in the intestinal contents as they enter the colon. This often happens with disease processes of the ileum because bile salts are absorbed there. It also may occur with bacterial overgrowth in the small bowel, which interferes with bile absorption. Some tumors, such as those of the Zollinger–Ellison syndrome and carcinoid syndrome, produce hormones that cause increased secretory activity of the bowel.[109]

Inflammatory diarrhea commonly is associated with acute or chronic inflammation or intrinsic disease of the colon, such as ulcerative colitis or Crohn disease. Inflammatory diarrhea usually is evidenced by frequency and urgency and colicky abdominal pain. It commonly is accompanied by **tenesmus,** fecal soiling of clothing, and awakening during the night with the urge to defecate.

Chronic parasitic infections may cause chronic diarrhea through a number of mechanisms. Pathogens most commonly associated with chronic diarrhea include the protozoans *Giardia, E. histolytica,* and *Cyclospora.* People who are immunocompromised are particularly susceptible to infectious organisms that can cause acute and chronic diarrhea, including *Cryptosporidium,* cytomegalovirus, and *Mycobacterium avium-intracellulare* complex.

Diagnosis and Treatment

The diagnosis of diarrhea is based on complaints of frequent stools and a history of accompanying factors such as concurrent illnesses, medication use, and exposure to potential intestinal pathogens. Disorders such as IBD and celiac disease should be considered.[102] If the onset of diarrhea is related to travel outside the United States, the possibility of traveler's diarrhea must be considered.

Although most acute forms of diarrhea are self-limited and require no treatment, diarrhea can be particularly serious in infants and small children, people with other illnesses, elderly people, and even previously healthy people if it continues for any length of time. Thus, the replacement of fluids and electrolytes is considered to be a primary therapeutic goal in the treatment of diarrhea.

Drugs used in the treatment of diarrhea include those that decrease GI motility and stimulate water and electrolyte absorption or adsorbents, which remove irritants and toxins from the bowel.

Acute Diarrheal Disease in Children

Despite global success in the reduction of diarrhea-specific mortality in the past 30 years, diarrhea remains the second leading cause of death because of infections among children younger than 5 years of age worldwide. Diarrhea is the second leading cause of death and malnutrition in children younger than age 5.[110] Although diarrheal diseases are less prevalent in the United States than they are in other countries, they place a burden on the health care system.[110]

The causes of acute diarrhea in children vary with location, time of year, and population studied.[111]

Rotaviruses and noroviruses are the frequently observed pathogens causing diarrheal illness. Other viruses that have been observed in the stools of children include astroviruses and enteric adenoviruses. Many of these pathogens are transmitted easily through food and water or from one person to another. Prevention remains the most vital measure in managing diarrheal disease in children, focusing on proper sanitation, hygiene, safe food handling, and exclusion of people with diarrhea from public recreational water.

The main objectives in the approach to a child with acute diarrhea are to assess the degree of dehydration, prevent spread of the infection, determine the nature of the etiologic agent, and provide specific therapy as needed. The hydration status of children can be assessed by oral intake, frequency and volume of stool output, general appearance and activity of the child, and frequency of urination. Thirst, dry mucous membranes, and decreased skin turgor are common symptoms of dehydration.[111] Day care attendance, recent travel to a diarrhea-endemic area, use of antimicrobial drugs, and exposure to contaminated water, unwashed fruits or vegetables, or improperly cooked meats may indicate the cause of the disorder.[111]

Infants in particular are more susceptible to dehydration because of their greater surface area, higher metabolic rate, and inability effectively to concentrate their urine. Oral replacement therapy is usually the method of choice for infants and children with uncomplicated diarrhea that can be treated at home.

Constipation

Constipation can be defined as the infrequent, incomplete, or difficult passage of stools.[102] The difficulty with this definition arises from the many individual variations of function that are normal. What is considered normal for one person (*e.g.*, two or three bowel movements per week) may be considered evidence of constipation by another. Constipation can occur as a primary disorder of intestinal motility, as a side effect of drugs, as a problem associated with another disease condition, or as a symptom of obstructing lesions of the GI tract. Some common causes of constipation are failure to respond to the urge to defecate, inadequate fiber in the diet, inadequate fluid intake, weakness of the abdominal muscles, inactivity and bed rest, pregnancy, and hemorrhoids. The pathophysiology of constipation can be classified into three broad categories: normal-transit constipation, slow-transit constipation, and disorders of defecatory or rectal evacuation. Normal-transit constipation (or functional constipation) is characterized by perceived difficulty in defecation and usually responds to increased fluid and fiber intake.[104] Slow-transit constipation, characterized by infrequent bowel movements, is often caused by alterations in the motor function of the colon.[112] Hirschsprung disease is an extreme form of slow-transit constipation in which the ganglion cells in the distal bowel are absent because of a defect that occurred during embryonic development; the bowel narrows at the area that lacks ganglionic cells.[113] Although most people with this disorder present in infancy or in early childhood, some with a relatively short segment of involved colon do not have symptoms until later in life. Defecatory disorders are most commonly due to deficiencies in muscle coordination involving the pelvic floor or anal sphincter.

Diseases associated with chronic constipation include neurologic diseases such as spinal cord injury, Parkinson disease, and multiple sclerosis; endocrine disorders such as hypothyroidism; and obstructive lesions in the GI tract. Drugs such as narcotics, anticholinergic agents, calcium channel blockers, diuretics, calcium (antacids and supplements), iron supplements, and aluminum antacids tend to cause constipation. Older adults with long-standing constipation and straining with defecation may develop dilation of the rectum, colon, or both. This condition allows large amounts of stool to accumulate with little or no sensation. Constipation, in the context of a change in bowel habits, may be a sign of colorectal cancer.

Diagnosis of constipation usually is based on a history of infrequent stools, straining with defecation, the passing of hard and lumpy stools, or the sense of incomplete evacuation with defecation. Rectal examination is used to determine whether fecal impaction, anal stricture, or rectal masses are present. Constipation as a sign of another disease condition should be ruled out. Tests that measure colon transit time and defecatory function are reserved for refractory cases.

The treatment of constipation usually is directed toward relieving the cause. A conscious effort should be made to respond to the defecation urge. A time should be set aside after a meal, when mass movements in the colon are most likely to occur, for a bowel movement. Mimicking a squatting position while sitting on the toilet may assist in promoting a bowel movement.[112] Adequate fluid intake and bulk in the diet should be encouraged. Moderate exercise is essential, and people on bed rest benefit from passive and active exercises. Laxatives and enemas should not be used on a regular basis to treat simple constipation because they interfere with the defecation reflex and actually may damage the rectal mucosa.

Fecal Impaction

Fecal impaction is the retention of hardened or putty-like stool in the rectum and colon, which interferes with normal passage of feces. If not removed, it can cause partial or complete bowel obstruction. It may occur in any age group but is more common in incapacitated older adults. Fecal impaction may result from painful anorectal disease, tumors, or neurogenic disease; use of constipating antacids or bulk laxatives; a low-residue diet; drug-induced colonic stasis; or prolonged bed rest and debility. In children, a habitual neglect of the urge to defecate in the school setting,[114] modesty, or play interference may promote impaction.

The manifestations may be those of severe constipation, but frequently there is a history of watery diarrhea, fecal soiling, and fecal incontinence caused by increased secretory activity of the bowel, representing the body's attempt to break up the mass so that it can be evacuated.[115] Abdominal distension and blood and mucus in the stool may occur. The fecal mass may compress the urethra, causing urinary incontinence.

Digital examination of the rectum is done to assess for the presence of a fecal mass. The mass may need to be broken up and dislodged manually or with the use of a sigmoidoscope. Oil enemas often are used to soften the mass before removal. The best treatment is prevention.

Intestinal Obstruction

Intestinal obstruction designates an impairment of movement of intestinal contents in a cephalocaudad direction. The causes can be categorized as mechanical or paralytic. Strangulation with necrosis of the bowel may occur and lead to perforation, peritonitis, and sepsis.

Mechanical obstruction can result from a number of conditions, intrinsic or extrinsic, that encroach on the patency of the bowel lumen (Fig. 37-13). Postoperative causes such as external hernia (*i.e.*, inguinal, femoral, or umbilical) and postoperative adhesions are responsible for 75% of intestinal obstruction occurrences.[116] Less common causes are strictures, tumors, foreign bodies, intussusception, and volvulus.

Intussusception involves the telescoping of the bowel into the adjacent segment (Fig. 37-14). It is the most common cause of intestinal obstruction in children younger than 2 years of age.[117] The most common form is intussusception of the terminal ileum into the right colon, but other areas of the bowel may be involved. About 2000 infants in the United States in the first year

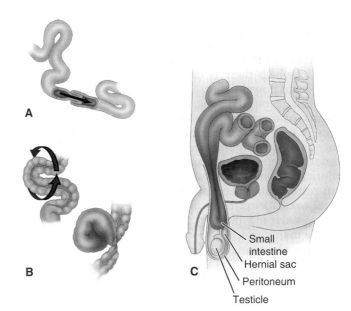

FIGURE 37-13. Three causes of intestinal obstruction. (**A**) Intussusception; invagination or shortening of the bowel caused by movement of one segment of the bowel into another. (**B**) Volvulus of the sigmoid colon; the twist is counterclockwise in most cases. Note the edematous section of bowel. (**C**) Hernia (inguinal). The sac of the hernia is a continuation of the peritoneum of the abdomen. The hernial contents are intestine, omentum, or other abdominal contents that pass through the hernial opening into the hernial sac. (From Hinkle J., Cheever, K. H. (Eds.) (2018). *Brunner and Suddarth's textbook of medical-surgical nursing* (14th ed., Figure 47-5, p. 1327). Philadelphia, PA: Lippincott Williams & Wilkins.)

of life are affected. In most cases, the cause of the disorder is unknown. The condition can also occur in adults when an intraluminal mass or tumor acts as a traction force and pulls the segment along as it telescopes into the distal segment. *Volvulus* refers to a complete twisting of the bowel on an axis formed by its mesentery (see Fig. 37-13B). It can occur in any portion of the GI tract,

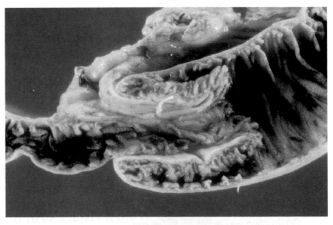

FIGURE 37-14. Intussusception. The proximal ileum has telescoped into the distal ileum in this case of intussusception; the anatomy is well seen in the cut section. (From Strayer D. S., Rubin R. (Eds.) (2012). *Rubin's pathophysiology: Clinicopathologic foundations of medicine* (7th ed., Figure 19-42B, p. 781). Philadelphia, PA: Lippincott Williams & Wilkins.)

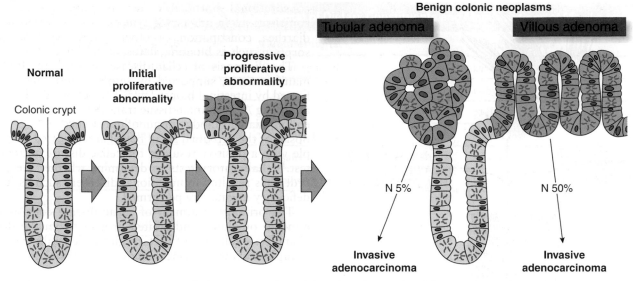

FIGURE 37-17. The histogenesis of adenomatous polyps of the colon. The initial proliferative abnormality of the colonic mucosa, the extension of the mitotic zone in the crypts, leads to accumulation of mucosal cells. The formation of adenomas may reflect epithelial–mesenchymal interactions. (From Rubin R., Strayer D. S. (Eds.) (2012). *Rubin's pathophysiology: Clinicopathologic foundations of medicine* (6th ed., p. 663). Philadelphia, PA: Lippincott Williams & Wilkins.)

to a large, sessile mass. They can be classified as tubular, villous, or tubulovillous adenomas.

Tubular adenomas, which constitute approximately 65% of benign large bowel adenomas, typically are smooth-surfaced spheres, usually less than 2 cm in diameter, that are attached to the mucosal surface by a stalk.[13] Although most tubular adenomas display little epithelial dysplasia, approximately 20% show a range of dysplastic changes, from mild nuclear changes to frank invasive carcinoma. *Villous adenomas* constitute 10% of adenomas of the colon.[13] They are found predominantly in the rectosigmoid colon. They typically are broad-based, elevated lesions, with an uneven, cauliflower-like surface. In contrast to tubular adenomas, villous adenomas are more likely to contain malignant cells. When invasive carcinoma develops, there is no stalk to isolate the tumor and invasion is directly into the wall of the colon. *Tubulovillous adenomas* manifest both tubular and villous architecture. They are intermediate between tubular and villous adenomas in terms of invasive carcinoma risk.

Most cases of colorectal cancer begin as benign adenomatous colonic polyps. The frequency of polyps increases with age, and the prevalence of adenomatous polyps significantly increases after 60 years of age.[132] Men and women are equally affected. The peak incidence of adenomatous polyps precedes by some years the peak for colorectal cancer. Follow-up for people with adenomatous polyps and removal of all suspect lesions have substantially reduced the incidence of colorectal cancer.[13]

Colorectal Cancer

The cause of cancer of the colon and rectum is largely unknown. The risk of colorectal cancer increases with age; the median age at diagnosis for colon cancer is 68

in men and 72 in women. Most cases (72%) occur in people who are in their 40s.[131] Its incidence is increased among people with a family history of cancer, people with Crohn disease or ulcerative colitis, and those with familial adenomatous polyposis of the colon. People with a familial risk—those who have two or more first- or second-degree relatives (or both) with colorectal cancer—make up approximately 20% of all people with colorectal cancer.[133] Familial adenomatous polyposis is a rare autosomal dominant trait linked to a mutation in the long arm of chromosome 5. People with the disorder develop multiple adenomatous polyps of the colon at an early age.[133] Carcinoma of the colon is inevitable, often by 40 years of age, unless a total colectomy is performed.

Diet also is thought to play a role.[131] Attention has focused on dietary fat intake, refined sugar intake, fiber intake, and the adequacy of such protective micronutrients as vitamins A, C, and E in the diet. It has been hypothesized that a high level of fat in the diet increases the synthesis of bile acids in the liver, which may be converted to potential carcinogens by the bacterial flora in the colon. Proliferation of bacteria is enhanced by a high dietary level of refined sugars. Dietary fiber is thought to increase stool bulk and thereby dilute and remove potential carcinogens. Refined diets often contain reduced amounts of vitamins A, C, and E, which may act as oxygen free radical scavengers.

Reports indicate that aspirin may protect against colorectal cancer.[134,135] Regular use of aspirin appears to reduce the risk of colorectal cancers that overexpress COX-2, but not the risk of colorectal cancers with weak or absent expression of COX-2.[136]

Usually, cancer of the colon and rectum is present for a long time before it produces symptoms. Bleeding is a highly significant early symptom and usually is the one that causes people to seek medical care. Other symptoms include a change in bowel habits, diarrhea or constipation, and sometimes a sense of urgency or incomplete emptying of the bowel. Pain usually is a late symptom.

Colorectal cancer commonly is classified into four TNM (tumor, node, and metastasis) stages. In this system, a stage I tumor is limited to invasion of the mucosal and submucosal layers of the colon and has a 5-year survival rate of 90% to 100%.[15] A stage II (lymph node–negative) tumor infiltrates into, but not through, the muscularis propria and has a 5-year survival rate of 80%.[15] With a stage III (lymph node–positive) tumor, in which there is invasion of the serosal layer and regional lymph node involvement, the 5-year survival rate is 30% to 50%.[14] Stage IV (metastatic) tumors penetrate the serosa or adjacent organs and have a much poorer prognosis.

Screening, Diagnosis, and Treatment

The single most important prognostic indicator of colorectal cancer is the extent (stage) of the tumor at time of diagnosis.[131] Therefore, the challenge is to discover the tumors at their earliest stages. Among the methods used for the detection of colorectal cancers are the digital rectal examination and the fecal occult blood test, usually done during routine physical examinations; x-ray studies using barium (*e.g.*, barium enema); and flexible sigmoidoscopy and colonoscopy.[131] The American Cancer Society recommends screening on the basis of age with a colonoscopy recommended whenever a screening test result is positive.[131]

Almost all cancers of the colon and rectum bleed intermittently, although the amount of blood is small and usually not apparent in the stools. It therefore is feasible to screen for colorectal cancers using commercially prepared tests for occult blood in the stool.[15,131] People with a positive fecal occult blood test result should be referred to their physician for further study. Usually, a physical examination, rectal examination, and flexible sigmoidoscopy or colonoscopy are done.

Flexible sigmoidoscopy involves examination of the rectum and sigmoid colon with a hollow, lighted tube that is inserted through the rectum. The procedure is performed without sedation and is well tolerated. Approximately 40% of cancers and polyps are out of the reach of the sigmoidoscope, emphasizing the need for fecal occult blood tests. Polyps can be removed or tissue can be obtained for biopsy during the procedure.

Colonoscopy provides a means for direct visualization of the rectum and colon. The colonoscope consists of a flexible, 4-cm-diameter glass fiber bundle that has a lens at either end to focus and magnify the image. Light from an external source is transmitted by the fiber-optic viewing bundle. This method is used for screening people at high risk for development of cancer of the colon and for those with symptoms. Colonoscopy also is useful for obtaining a biopsy and for removing polyps.

The only recognized treatment for cancer of the colon and rectum is surgical removal.[137] Preoperative radiation therapy may be used and has, in some cases, demonstrated increased 5-year survival rates. Postoperative adjuvant chemotherapy may be used. Radiation therapy and chemotherapy are used as palliative treatment methods.

SUMMARY CONCEPTS

Disorders of the small and large intestines include IBS, IBD, diverticular disease, disorders of motility (*i.e.*, diarrhea, constipation, fecal impaction, and intestinal obstruction), alterations in intestinal absorption, and colorectal cancer.

IBS is a functional disorder characterized by a variable combination of chronic and recurrent intestinal symptoms not explained by structural or biochemical abnormalities. The term *inflammatory bowel disease* is used to designate two inflammatory conditions: Crohn disease, which affects the small and large bowel, and ulcerative colitis, which affects the colon and rectum. Both are chronic diseases characterized by remissions and exacerbations of diarrhea, weight loss, fluid and electrolyte disorders, and systemic signs of inflammation.

Infectious forms of enterocolitis include viral (*e.g.*, rotavirus), bacterial (*e.g.*, *C. difficile* and *E. coli* O157:H7), and protozoal (*E. histolytica*) infections. Diverticular disease includes diverticulosis, which is a condition in which the mucosal layer of the colon herniates through the muscularis layer, and diverticulitis, in which there is inflammation and gross or microscopic perforation of the diverticulum.

Diarrhea and constipation represent disorders of intestinal motility. Diarrhea is characterized by excessively frequent passage of stools. It can be acute or chronic and can be caused by infectious organisms, food intolerance, drugs, or intestinal disease. Acute diarrheas that last less than 4 days are predominantly caused by infectious agents and follow a self-limited course. Chronic diarrhea persists beyond 3 to 4 weeks and is caused by the presence of hyperosmotic luminal contents, increased intestinal secretory processes, inflammatory conditions, and infectious processes. Constipation can be defined as the infrequent passage of stools; it commonly is caused by failure to respond to the urge to defecate, inadequate fiber or fluid intake, weakness of the abdominal muscles, inactivity and bed rest, pregnancy, hemorrhoids, and GI disease. Fecal impaction is the retention of hardened or putty-like stool in the rectum and colon, which interferes with normal passage of feces. Intestinal obstruction designates an impairment of movement of intestinal contents in a cephalocaudad direction as the result of mechanical or paralytic mechanisms. Peritonitis is an inflammatory response of the serous membrane that lines the abdominal cavity and covers the visceral organs. It can be caused by bacterial invasion or chemical irritation resulting from perforation of the viscera or abdominal organs.

Malabsorption results from the impaired absorption of nutrients and other dietary constituents from the intestine. It can involve a single dietary constituent, such as vitamin B_{12}, or extend to involve all of the substances absorbed in a particular part of the small intestine. Malabsorption can result from disease of the small bowel and disorders that impair digestion and, in some cases, obstruct the lymph flow by which fats are transported to the general circulation. Celiac disease is an immune-mediated disorder triggered by ingestion of gluten-containing grains (including wheat, barley, and rye).

Colorectal cancer, the second most common fatal cancer, is seen most commonly in people older than 50 years of age. Most, if not all, cancers of the colon and rectum arise in preexisting adenomatous polyps. Programs that provide careful follow-up for people with adenomatous polyps and removal of all suspect lesions have substantially reduced the incidence of colorectal cancer.

Review Exercises

1. A 40-year-old man reports to his health care provider complaining of "heartburn" that occurs after eating and also wakes him up at night. He is overweight, admits to enjoying fatty foods, and usually lies down on the sofa and watches TV after dinner. He also complains that lately he has been having a cough and some wheezing. A diagnosis of GERD was made.

   A. Explain the cause of heartburn and why it becomes worse after eating.
   B. People with GERD are advised to lose weight, avoid eating fatty foods, remain sitting after eating, and to sleep with their head slightly elevated. Explain the possible relationship between these situations and the occurrence of reflux.
   C. Explain the possible relationship between GERD and the respiratory symptoms this man is having.

2. A 36-year-old woman who has been taking aspirin for back pain experiences a sudden episode of tachycardia and feeling faint, accompanied by the vomiting of a coffee-ground emesis and the passing of a tarry stool. She relates that she has not had any signs of a "stomach ulcer" such as pain or heartburn.

   A. Relate the mucosal protective effects of prostaglandins to the development of peptic ulcer associated with aspirin or NSAID use.
   B. Explain the apparent suddenness of the bleeding and the fact that the woman did not experience pain as a warning signal.
   C. Among the results of her initial laboratory tests is an elevated blood urea nitrogen (BUN) level. Explain the reason for the elevated BUN.

3. A 29-year-old woman has been diagnosed with Crohn disease. Her medical history reveals that she began having symptoms of the disease at 24 years of age and that her mother died of complications of the disease at 54 years of age. She complains of diarrhea and chronic cramping abdominal pain.

   A. Define the term *inflammatory bowel disease* and compare the pathophysiologic processes and manifestations of Crohn disease and ulcerative colitis.
   B. One of the recommended treatments for stress incontinence is the use of Kegel exercises, which focus on strengthening the muscles of the pelvic floor. Explain how these exercises contribute to the control of urine leakage in women with stress incontinence.

REFERENCES

1. American Cancer Society. (2018). Cancer. How common is colorectal cancer? Available: https://www.cancer.org/cancer/colon-rectal-cancer/about/key-statistics.html. Accessed April 16, 2019.
2. Saltzman J. R. (October 23, 2018). Burden and cost of gastrointestinal disease in the U.S. Practice Watch Gastroenterology. Available: https://www.jwatch.org/na47723/2018/10/23/burden-and-costs-gastrointestinal-disease-us. Accessed April 16, 2019.
3. Nuckols C. C. (2013). *Diagnostic and statistical manual of mental disorders: DSM-5* (5th ed., pp. 338–345). Washington, DC: American Psychiatric Publishing.
4. Hasler W. L. (2014). Nausea, vomiting, and indigestion. In Kasper D., Fauci A., Hauser S., et al. (Eds.), *Harrison's principles of internal medicine* (19th ed.). New York, NY: McGraw-Hill. Available: http://accessmedicine.mhmedical.com/content.aspx?bookid=1130&sectionid=79726154. Accessed March 08, 2018.
5. Hall J. E. (2015). *Guyton and Hall: Textbook of medical physiology* (13th ed.). Philadelphia, PA: Saunders Elsevier.
6. Goyal A., Jones M. O., Couriel J. M., et al. (2017). Oesophageal atresia, tracheoesophageal fistula. *Archives of Disease in Childhood. Fetal and Neonatal Edition* 201, 381–384.
7. Teitelbaum J. E. (2017). Congenital abnormalities. In Kleinman R. E., Sanderson I. R., Goulet O., et al. (Eds.), *Walker's pediatric gastrointestinal disease: Physiology, diagnosis, management* (pp. 1–17). Hamilton, ON: BC Decker.
8. Devault K. R. (2016). Symptoms of esophageal disease. In Feldman M., Feldman L. S., Brandt L. J. (Eds.), *Sleisenger and Fordtran's gastrointestinal and liver disease: Pathophysiology, diagnosis, management* (10th ed., pp. 185–193). Philadelphia, PA: Saunders Elsevier.
9. Kumar V., Abbas A. K., Fausto N., et al. (Eds.). (2014). The gastrointestinal tract. In *Robbins and Cotran: Pathologic basis of disease* (9th ed., pp. 749–819). Philadelphia, PA: Saunders Elsevier.
10. Vaezi M. F., Pandolfino J. E., Vela M. F. (2013). ACG Clinical Guideline: Diagnosis and management of achalasia. *American Journal of Gastroenterology* 108(8), 1238–1249. DOI: 10.1038/ajg.2013.196. PMID: 23877351. Issn Print: 0002-9270. Publication Date: 2013/08/01. https://www.ncbi.nlm.nih.gov/pubmed/23877351

11. Kahrilas P. J., Pandolfino J. E. (2016). Esophageal neuromuscular function and motility disorders. In Feldman M., Feldman L. S., Brandt L. J. (Eds.), *Sleisenger and Fordtran's gastrointestinal and liver disease: Pathophysiology, diagnosis, management* (10th ed., pp. 701–732). Philadelphia, PA: Saunders Elsevier.

12. Savides T. J., Jensen D. M. (2016). Gastrointestinal bleeding. In Feldman M., Feldman L. S., Brandt L. J. (Eds.), *Sleisenger and Fordtran's gastrointestinal and liver disease: Pathophysiology, diagnosis, management* (10th ed., pp. 297–335). Philadelphia, PA: Saunders Elsevier.

13. Mitos F. A., Rubin E. (2015). The gastrointestinal tract. In Rubin R., Strayer D. S. (Eds.), *Rubin's pathophysiology: Clinicopathologic foundations of medicine* (7th ed., pp. 751–824). Philadelphia, PA: Lippincott Williams & Wilkins.

14. Martinucci I., de Bortoli N., Russo S., et al. (2016). Barrett's esophagus in 2016: From pathophysiology to treatment. *World Journal of Gastrointestinal Pharmacology and Therapeutics* 7(2), 190–206. doi:10.4292/wjgpt.v7.i2.190.

15. Badillo R., Francis D. (2014). Diagnosis and treatment of gastroesophageal reflux disease. *World Journal of Gastrointestinal Pharmacology and Therapeutics* 5(3), 105–112. doi:10.4292/wjgpt.v5.i3.105.

16. Roman S., Pandolfino J. E., Kahrilas P. J. (2015). Gastroesophageal reflux disease. In Yamada Y. (Ed.), *Textbook of Gastroenterology* (6th ed., pp. 906–928). Oxford, England: Wiley-Blackwell.

17. NIDDK. (November 13, 2014). Gastroesophageal reflux (GER) and gastroesophageal reflux disease (GERD) in adults.

18. Sylvester Chuks Nwokediuko. (2012). Current trends in the management of gastroesophageal reflux disease: A review. *ISRN Gastroenterology* 2012, 11. doi:10.5402/2012/391631.

19. Spechler J. S., Wang D. H., Souza R. F. (2016). Barrett esophagus and esophageal adenocarcinoma. In Yamada Y. (Ed.), *Textbook of gastroenterology* (6th ed., pp. 949–974). Oxford, England: Wiley-Blackwell.

20. Wu A. (2015). Gastroesophageal reflux disease management in pediatric patients. *US Pharmacist* 40(12), 28–32.

21. Rudolph C. D. (2011). Gastroesophageal reflux other causes of esophageal inflammation. In Rudolph C. D., Rudolph A. M., Lister G. E., et al. (Eds.), *Rudolph's pediatrics* (22nd ed., pp. 1405–1412). New York, NY: McGraw-Hill.

22. Tolia V., Gilger M. A., Barker P. N., et al. (2015). Healing of erosive esophagitis and improvement of symptoms of gastroesophageal reflux disease after esomeprazole treatment in children 12 to 36 months old. *Journal of Pediatrics Gastroenterology and Nutrition* 60(Suppl 1), S31–S36.

23. Baird D. C., Harker D. J., Karmes A. S., et al. (2015). Diagnosis and treatment of gastroesophageal reflux in infants and children. *American Family Physician* 92(8), 705–717.

24. Howlader N., Noone A. M., Krapcho M., et al. (Eds.). SEER cancer statistics review, 1975–2014, Bethesda, MD: National Cancer Institute. Available: https://seer.cancer.gov/csr/1975_2014/, based on November 2016 SEER data submission, posted to the SEER web site, updated on April 2017.

25. Gibson M. K., Tanabe K. K., Goldberg R. M., et al. Epidemiology, pathobiology, and clinical manifestations of esophageal cancer. Available: https://www.uptodate.com/contents/epidemiology-pathobiology-and-clinical-manifestations-of-esophageal-cancer

26. Wang H.-W., Kuo C.-J., Lin W.-R., et al. (2015). Barrett's esophagus and risk of esophageal adenocarcinoma: A retrospective analysis. *Advances in Digestive Medicine* 2(4), 135–140.

27. Patel N. C., Famirez F. C. (2016). Esophageal tumors. In Feldman M., Feldman L. S., Brandt L. J. (Eds.), *Sleisenger and Fordtran's gastrointestinal and liver disease: Pathophysiology,*

diagnosis, management (10th ed., pp. 773–791). Philadelphia, PA: Saunders Elsevier.

28. Ross M. H., Pawlina W. (2015). *Histology: A text and atlas: With correlated cell and molecular biology* (7th ed.). Baltimore, MD: Lippincott Williams & Wilkins.

29. Rang H. P., Dale M. M., Ritter J. M., et al. (2015). *Rang and Dale's pharmacology* (8th ed.). Philadelphia, PA: Elsevier

30. Cryer B., Mahaffey K. W. (2014). Gastrointestinal ulcers, role of aspirin, and clinical outcomes: Pathobiology, diagnosis, and treatment. *Journal of Multidisciplinary Healthcare* 7, 137–146. doi:10.2147/JMDH.S54324.

31. Zatorski H. (2017). Pathophysiology and risk factors in peptic ulcer disease. In Fichna J. (Ed.), *Introduction to gastrointestinal diseases* (Vol. 2, pp. 7–20). Berlin, Germany: Springer.

32. Kemmerly T., Kaunitz J. D. (2014). Gastroduodenal mucosal defense. *Current Opinion in Gastroenterology* 30(6), 583–588. doi:10.1097/MOG.0000000000000124.

33. Turner J. R. (2014). The gastrointestinal tract. In Kumar V., Abbas A. K., Fausto N., et al. (Eds.), *Robbins and Cotran: Pathologic basis of disease* (9th ed., pp. 763–831). Philadelphia, PA: Saunders Elsevier.

34. Santacroce L. (2017). Helicobacter pylori infection medscape medical news from WebMD. Available: https://emedicine.medscape.com/article/176938-overview. Accessed January 27, 2018.

35. Kumar P., Clark M. (2012). *Clinical medicine* (8th ed.). Philadelphia, PA: Saunders Elsevier.

36. Cover T. L., Blaser M. J. (2015). *Helicobacter pylori* and other gastric *Helicobacter* species. In Mandell G. L., Bennett J. E., Dolin R. (Eds.), *Mandell, Douglas and Bennett's principles and practice of infectious disease* (8th ed., pp. 2494–2505). Philadelphia, PA: Churchill Livingstone Elsevier.

37. Minalyan A., Benhammou J. N., Artashesyan A., et al. (2017). Autoimmune atrophic gastritis: Current perspectives. *Clinical and Experimental Gastroenterology* 10, 19–27.

38. Vakil N. (2016). Peptic ulcer disease. In Feldman M., Friedman L. S., Brandt L. J. (Eds.), *Sleisenger and Fordtran's gastrointestinal and liver disease: Pathophysiology, diagnosis and management* (10th ed., pp. 884–900). Philadelphia, PA: Saunders Elsevier.

39. Lanas A. (2016). *NSAIDs and Aspirin: Recent advances and implications for clinical management* (1st ed.). Cham, Switzerland: Springer International Publishing AG.

40. Lanas A., Chan F. K. L. (2017). Peptic ulcer disease. *The Lancet* 39(10094), 613–624. doi:10.1016/S0140-6736(16)32404-7.

41. Chan F. K., Lau J. Y. (2016). Treatment of peptic ulcer disease. In Feldman M., Friedman L. S., Brandt L. J. (Eds.), *Sleisenger and Fordtran's gastrointestinal and liver disease: Pathophysiology, diagnosis and management* (10th ed., pp. 888–891). Philadelphia, PA: Saunders Elsevier.

42. Jenson R. T., Norton J. A., Oberg K. (2016). Neuroendocrine tumors. In Feldman M., Friedman L. S., Brandt L. J. (Eds.), *Sleisenger and Fordtran's gastrointestinal and liver disease: Pathophysiology, diagnosis and management* (10th ed., pp. 501–541). Philadelphia, PA: Saunders Elsevier.

43. Bonheur J. L. eMedicine: Gastrinoma. [Online]. Available: https://emedicine.medscape.com/article/184332-overview. Accessed January 28, 2018.

44. Jensen R. T. (2015). Zollinger-Ellison syndrome. In Yamada T. (Ed.), *Textbook of gastroenterology* (6th ed., pp. 1078–1102). Hoboken, NJ: Wiley-Blackwell.

45. Del Valle J. (2014). Peptic ulcer disease and related disorders. In Kasper D., Fauci A., Hauser S., et al. (Eds.), *Harrison's principles of internal medicine* (19th ed.). New York, NY: McGraw-Hill. Available: http://accessmedicine.mhmedical.com/content.aspx?bookid=1130&sectionid=79747602. Accessed March 8, 2018.

112. Lembo A. J., Ullman S. P. (2016). Constipation. In Feldman M., Friedman L. S., Brandt L. J. (Eds.), *Sleisenger and Fordtran's gastrointestinal and liver disease: Pathophysiology, diagnosis and management* (10th ed., pp. 270–296). Philadelphia, PA: Saunders Elsevier.

113. Hanni Gulwani Hirschsprungs disease. PathologyOutlines.com website. Available: http://www.pathologyoutlines.com/topic/colonhirschsprung.html. Accessed January 31, 2018.

114. Sood M. R. (2011). Constipation and fecal incontinence. In Rudolph C. D., Rudolph A. M., Lister G. E., et al. (Eds.), *Rudolph's pediatrics* (22nd ed., pp. 1386–1389). New York, NY: McGraw Hill.

115. McQuaid K. R. (2017). Alimentary tract. In Tierney L. M., McPhee S. J., Papadakis M. (Eds.), *Current medical diagnosis and treatment* (56th ed., pp. 555, 567–585, 617–623, 652–658). New York, NY: Lange Medical Books/McGraw-Hill.

116. Gearhart S. L., Silen W. (2015). Acute intestinal obstruction. In Fauci A. S., Braunwald E., Kasper D. L., et al. (Eds.), *Harrison's principles of internal medicine* (19th ed., pp. 1912–1917). New York, NY: McGraw Hill.

117. Densmore J. C., Lal D. R. (2011). Intussusception. In Rudolph C. D., Rudolph A. M., Lister G. E., et al. (Eds.), *Rudolph's pediatrics* (22nd ed., pp. 1428–1429). New York, NY: McGraw Hill.

118. Turnage R. H., Heldmann M. (2016). Intestinal obstruction. In Feldman M., Friedman L. S., Brandt L. J. (Eds.), *Sleisenger and Fordtran's gastrointestinal and liver disease: Pathophysiology, diagnosis and management* (10th ed., pp. 2154–2170). Philadelphia, PA: Saunders Elsevier.

119. Allan P., Lal S. (2018). Intestinal failure: A review [version 1; referees: 2 approved]. *F1000Research* 7, 85. doi:10.12688/f1000research.12493.1.

120. Hogenauer C., Hammer H. F. (2016). Maldigestion and malabsorption. In Feldman M., Friedman L. S., Brandt L. J. (Eds.), *Sleisenger and Fordtran's gastrointestinal and liver disease: Pathophysiology, diagnosis and management* (10th ed., pp. 1788–1823). Philadelphia, PA: Saunders Elsevier.

121. Kannan A., Tilak V., Rai M., et al. (2016). Evaluation of clinical, biochemical and hematological parameters in macrocytic anemia. *International Journal of Research in Medical Sciences* 4(7), 2670–2678.

122. Rubio-Tapia A., Hill I. D., Kelly C. P., et al. (2013). ACG Clinical Guidelines: Diagnosis and management of celiac disease. *American Journal of Gastroenterology* 108, 656–676. doi:10.1038/ajg.2013.79.

123. Celiac.com. Celiac disease and gluten-free diet information. [Online]. Available: www.celiac.com. Accessed January 29, 2018.

124. Gujral N., Freeman H. J., Thomson A. B. (2012). Celiac disease: Prevalence, diagnosis, pathogenesis and treatment. *World Journal of Gastroenterology: WJG* 18(42), 6036–6059. doi:10.3748/wjg.v18.i42.6036.

125. Fasano A., Catassi C. (2012). Celiac disease. *New England Journal of Medicine* 367, 2419–2426. doi:10.1056/NEJMcp1113994.

126. Ludvigsson J. F., Card T. R., Kaukinen K., et al. (2015). Screening for celiac disease in the general population and in high-risk groups. *United European Gastroenterology Journal* 3(2), 106–120. doi:10.1177/2050640614561668.

127. Cecilio L. A., Bonatto M. W. (2015). The prevalence of HLA DQ2 and DQ8 in patients with celiac disease, in family and in general population. *Arquivos Brasileiros de Cirurgia Digestiva: ABCD = Brazilian Archives of Digestive Surgery* 28(3), 183–185. doi:10.1590/S0102-67202015000300009.

128. Binder H. J. (2014). Disorders of absorption. In Kasper D., Fauci A., Hauser S., et al. (Eds.), *Harrison's principles of internal medicine* (19th ed.). New York, NY: McGraw-Hill. http://accessmedicine.mhmedical.com/content.aspx?bookid=1130&sectionid=79747771. Accessed March 8, 2018.

129. Farrell R. J., Kelly C. P. (2016). Celiac disease and refractory celiac disease. In Feldman M., Friedman L. S., Brandt L. J. (Eds.), *Sleisenger and Fordtran's gastrointestinal and liver disease: Pathophysiology, diagnosis and management* (10th ed., pp. 1849–1872). Philadelphia, PA: Saunders Elsevier.

130. Hill I. D., Caicedo R. A. (2011). Disorders of absorption and absorption. In Rudolph C. D., Rudolph A. M., Lister G. E., et al. (Eds.), *Rudolph's pediatrics* (22nd ed., pp. 1438–1453). New York, NY: McGraw Hill.

131. American Cancer Society. (2017). Colorectal cancer facts and figures, 2016–2019. [Online]. Available: http://www.cancer.org. Accessed January 29, 2018.

132. Itzkowitz S. H., Potack J. (2016). Colonic polyps and polyposis syndromes. In Feldman M., Friedman L. S., Brandt L. J. (Eds.), *Sleisenger and Fordtran's gastrointestinal and liver disease: Pathophysiology, diagnosis and management* (10th ed., pp. 2213–2247). Philadelphia, PA: Saunders Elsevier.

133. American Cancer Society. (2017). American Cancer Society recommendations for colorectal cancer early detection. [Online]. Available: https://www.cancer.org/cancer/colon-rectal-cancer/detection-diagnosis-staging/acs-recommendations.html. Accessed January 29, 2018.

134. Ananthakrishnan A. N., Cheng S. C., Cai T., et al. (2014). Serum inflammatory markers and risk of colorectal cancer in patients with inflammatory bowel diseases. *Clinical Gastroenterology and Hepatology* 12(8), 1342.e1–1348.e1.

135. Friis S., Riis A. H., Erichsen R., et al. (2015). Low-dose aspirin or nonsteroidal anti-inflammatory drug use and colorectal cancer risk: A population-based, case–control study. *Annals of Internal Medicine* 163, 347–355. doi:10.7326/M15-0039.

136. Manzano A., Pérez-Segura P. (2012). Colorectal cancer chemoprevention: Is this the future of colorectal cancer prevention? *The Scientific World Journal* 2012, 8. doi:10.1100/2012/327341.

137. Bresalier R. S. (2016). Colorectal cancer. In Feldman M., Friedman L. S., Brandt L. J. (Eds.), *Sleisenger and Fordtran's gastrointestinal and liver disease: Pathophysiology, diagnosis and management* (10th ed., pp. 2248–2296). Philadelphia, PA: Saunders Elsevier.

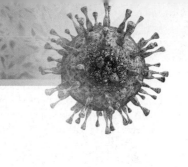

CHAPTER **38**

Disorders of Hepatobiliary and Exocrine Pancreas Function

Learning Objectives

**After completing this chapter, the learner
will be able to meet the following objectives:**

1. Describe the function of the liver in terms of carbohydrate, protein, and fat metabolism.
2. Relate the mechanism of bile formation and elimination to the development of cholestasis.
3. State the three ways by which drugs and other substances are metabolized or inactivated in the liver and provide examples of liver disease related to the toxic effects of drugs and chemical agents.
4. Compare hepatitis A, B, C, D, and E in terms of source of infection, incubation period, acute disease manifestations, development of chronic disease, and the carrier state.
5. Describe the physiologic basis for portal hypertension and relate it to the development of ascites, esophageal varices, and splenomegaly.
6. Explain the function of the gallbladder in regulating the flow of bile into the duodenum and relate it to the formation of cholelithiasis (gallstones).
7. Describe the clinical manifestations of acute and chronic cholecystitis.
8. Cite the possible causes and describe the manifestations and treatment of acute and chronic pancreatitis.

The liver, gallbladder, and exocrine pancreas are classified as accessory organs of the gastrointestinal tract. In addition to producing digestive secretions, the liver and the pancreas have other important functions. The endocrine pancreas, for example, supplies the insulin and glucagon needed for cell metabolism, whereas the liver synthesizes glucose, plasma proteins, and blood clotting factors and are responsible for the degradation and elimination of drugs and hormones, among other functions. This chapter focuses on functions and disorders of the liver, the biliary tract and gallbladder, and the exocrine pancreas.

The Liver and Hepatobiliary System

The liver is the largest visceral organ in the body, weighing approximately 1.3 kg (3 lb) in the adult. It is located below the diaphragm and occupies much of the right hypochondrium (Fig. 38-1). A tough fibroelastic capsule, called the Glisson capsule, surrounds the liver. The liver is anatomically divided into two large lobes (the right and left lobes) and two smaller lobes (the caudate and quadrate lobes). Except for the portion that is in the epigastric area, the liver is contained within the rib cage, and cannot normally be palpated in healthy people.

The liver receives 25% of the resting cardiac output.[1] The liver is unique among the abdominal organs in having a dual blood supply consisting of a venous (portal) supply through the hepatic portal vein and an arterial supply through the hepatic artery. Approximately 25% of blood per minute enters the liver through the hepatic artery; the remaining 75% enters by way of the valveless portal vein.[2] The venous blood delivered by the hepatic portal vein comes from the digestive tract and major abdominal organs, including the pancreas and spleen (Fig. 38-2). The portal blood supply carries nutrient and toxic materials absorbed in the intestine, blood cells and their breakdown products from the spleen, and insulin and glucagon from the pancreas. Although the blood from the portal vein is incompletely saturated with oxygen, it supplies approximately 75% of the oxygen needs of the liver.[1]

The venous outflow from the liver is carried by the valveless hepatic veins, which empty into the inferior vena cava just below the level of the diaphragm. The liver has the ability to store approximately 500 to 1000 mL of blood.[3] This blood can be shifted back into the general circulation during periods of hypovolemia and shock. In right heart failure in which the pressure in the vena cava increases, blood backs up and accumulates in the liver.

The *lobules* are the functional units of the liver. There are approximately 50,000 to 100,000 cylindrical lobules in the liver.[3] Each lobule is organized around a central vein that empties into the hepatic veins and from there into the vena cava. The terminal bile ducts and small branches of the portal vein and hepatic artery are located at the periphery of the lobule. Plates of hepatic cells radiate centrifugally from the central vein like spokes on a wheel (Fig. 38-3). These hepatic plates are separated by wide, thin-walled sinusoidal capillaries called *sinusoids*. The sinusoids are supplied by blood from the portal vein and hepatic artery. The sinusoids provide for the exchange of substances between the blood and liver cells. The sinusoids are lined with two types of cells: the typical capillary endothelial cells and Kupffer cells. *Kupffer cells* are reticuloendothelial cells that are capable of removing and phagocytizing old and defective blood cells, bacteria, and other foreign material from the portal blood as it flows through the sinusoid. This phagocytic action removes enteric bacilli and other harmful substances that filter into the blood from the intestine.

A major exocrine function of the liver is bile secretion. Small tubular channels, called *bile canaliculi*, supply the lobules. The bile produced by the hepatocytes

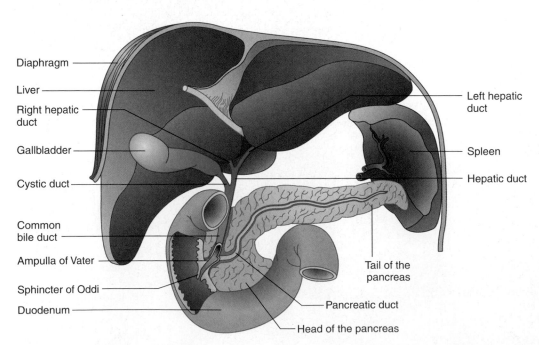

Diaphragm
Liver
Right hepatic duct
Gallbladder
Cystic duct
Common bile duct
Ampulla of Vater
Sphincter of Oddi
Duodenum

Left hepatic duct
Spleen
Hepatic duct
Tail of the pancreas
Pancreatic duct
Head of the pancreas

FIGURE 38-1. The liver and biliary system, including the gallbladder and bile ducts.

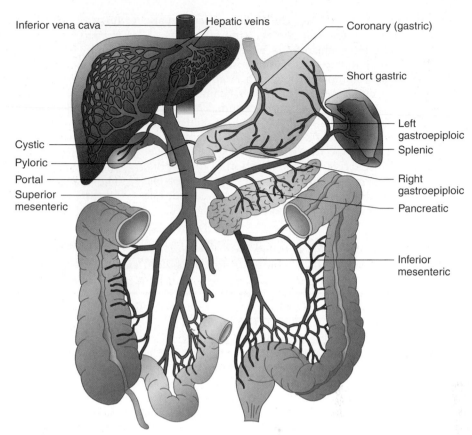

FIGURE 38-2. The portal circulation. Blood from the gastrointestinal tract, spleen, and pancreas travels to the liver through the portal vein before moving into the vena cava for return to the heart.

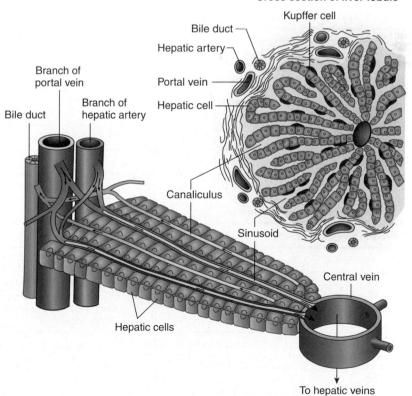

FIGURE 38-3. A section of liver lobule showing the location of the hepatic veins, hepatic cells, liver sinusoids, and branches of the portal vein and hepatic artery.

flows into the canaliculi into the right and left hepatic ducts. The intrahepatic and extrahepatic bile ducts often are collectively referred to as the *hepatobiliary tree*. These ducts unite to form the common duct (see Fig. 38-1). The common duct, which is approximately 10 to 15 cm long, descends and passes behind the pancreas and enters the descending duodenum. The pancreatic duct joins the common duct at a short dilated tube called the *hepatopancreatic ampulla* (ampulla of Vater), which empties into the duodenum through the duodenal papilla. Muscle tissue at the junction of the papilla, called the *sphincter of Oddi*, regulates the flow of bile into the duodenum. When this sphincter is closed, bile moves back into the common duct and gallbladder.

Metabolic Functions of the Liver

The liver is one of the most versatile and active organs in the body. It produces bile; metabolizes hormones and drugs; synthesizes proteins, glucose, and clotting factors; stores vitamins and minerals; changes ammonia produced by deamination of amino acids to urea; and converts fatty acids to ketones. The liver also degrades excess nutrients and converts them into substances essential to the body. In its capacity for metabolizing drugs and hormones, the liver serves as an excretory organ. The bile carries the end products of substances metabolized by the liver. The functions of the liver are summarized in Table 38-1.

TABLE 38-1 Functions of the Liver and Manifestations of Altered Function

Function	Manifestations of Altered Function
Production of bile salts	Malabsorption of fat and fat-soluble vitamins
Elimination of bilirubin	Elevation in serum bilirubin and jaundice
Metabolism of Steroid Hormones	
Sex hormones	Disturbances in gonadal function, including gynecomastia in the male
Glucocorticoids	
Aldosterone	Signs of increased cortisol levels (*i.e.*, Cushing syndrome)
Metabolism of drugs	Signs of hyperaldosteronism (*e.g.*, sodium retention and hypokalemia)
	Decreased drug metabolism
	Decreased plasma binding of drugs owing to a decrease in albumin production
Carbohydrate metabolism	Hypoglycemia may develop when glycogenolysis and gluconeogenesis are impaired
Stores glycogen and synthesizes glucose from amino acids, lactic acid, and glycerol	Abnormal glucose tolerance curve may occur because of impaired uptake and release of glucose by the liver
Fat Metabolism	
Formation of lipoproteins	Impaired synthesis of lipoproteins
Conversion of carbohydrates and proteins to fat	
Synthesis, recycling, and elimination of cholesterol	Altered cholesterol levels
Formation of ketones from fatty acid	
Protein Metabolism	
Deamination of proteins	
Formation of urea from ammonia	Elevated blood ammonia levels
Synthesis of plasma proteins	Decreased levels of plasma proteins, particularly albumin, which contributes to edema formation
Synthesis of clotting factors (fibrinogen, prothrombin, factors V, VII, IX, and X)	Bleeding tendency
Storage of minerals and vitamins	Signs of deficiency of fat-soluble and other vitamins that are stored in the liver
Filtration of blood and removal of bacteria and particulate matter by Kupffer cells	Increased exposure of the body to colonic bacteria and other foreign matter

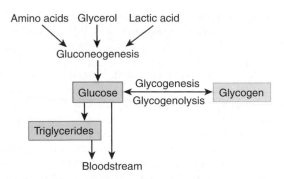

FIGURE 38-4. Hepatic pathways for storage and synthesis of glucose and conversion of glucose to fatty acids.

Carbohydrate Metabolism

The liver plays an essential role in carbohydrate metabolism and glucose homeostasis (Fig. 38-4). The liver cells have the ability to store large amounts of glucose as glycogen through a process called glycogenesis. When blood glucose levels are low, glycogen is converted back to glucose through glycogenolysis involving an enzyme phosphatase that is specific to liver cells. The liver also synthesizes glucose from amino acids, glycerol, and lactic acid as a means of maintaining blood glucose during periods of fasting or increased need. The liver converts excess carbohydrates to triglycerides for storage in adipose tissue.

Protein Synthesis and Conversion of Ammonia to Urea

The liver is an important site for protein synthesis and degradation, releasing secretory proteins into the circulation while producing proteins for its own cellular needs. The most important of these secretory proteins is albumin. Albumin contributes significantly to the plasma colloidal osmotic pressure and to the binding and transport of numerous substances, including some hormones, fatty acids, bilirubin, and other anions. The liver also produces other important proteins, such as fibrinogen and the blood clotting factors.

Through a variety of anabolic and catabolic processes, the liver is the major site of amino acid interconversion (Fig. 38-5). Hepatic catabolism and degradation involve two major reactions: transamination and deamination.[3] In *transamination*, an amino group (NH_2) is transferred to an acceptor substance. As a result of transamination, amino acids can participate in the intermediary metabolism of carbohydrates and lipids. During periods of fasting or starvation, amino acids are used for producing glucose (*i.e.*, gluconeogenesis). Most of the nonessential amino acids are synthesized in the liver by transamination. The process of transamination is catalyzed by *aminotransferases*, enzymes that are found in high amounts in the liver.

Oxidative *deamination* involves the removal of the amino groups from amino acids and conversion of amino acids to keto acids and ammonia by transamination, allowing the transfer of an amine group from one molecule to another. Because ammonia is very toxic to body tissues, particularly neurons, the ammonia that

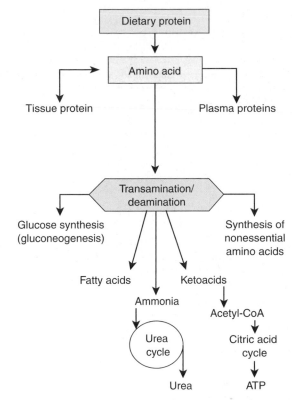

FIGURE 38-5. Hepatic pathways for conversion of amino acids to proteins, nucleic acids, keto acids, and glucose. The urea cycle converts ammonia generated by the deamination of amino acids to urea. Acetyl-CoA, acetyl-coenzyme A; ATP, adenosine triphosphate.

is released during deamination is rapidly removed from the blood by the liver and converted to urea. Essentially, all urea formed in the body is synthesized by the urea cycle in the liver and then excreted by the kidneys.[3] Although urea is mostly excreted by the kidneys, some of it diffuses into the intestine, where it is converted to ammonia by enteric bacteria. Ammonia produced in the intestine is absorbed into the portal circulation and transported to the liver, where it is converted to urea before being released into the systemic circulation. Intestinal production of ammonia is increased after ingestion of high-protein foods and gastrointestinal bleeding. In advanced liver disease, urea synthesis often is impaired, leading to an accumulation of blood ammonia.

Pathways of Lipid Metabolism

Although most cells of the body metabolize fat, certain aspects of lipid metabolism occur mainly in the liver, including the oxidation of free fatty acids to keto acids that supply energy for other body functions; synthesis of cholesterol, phospholipids, and lipoproteins; and formation of triglycerides from carbohydrates and proteins (Fig. 38-6). Because the liver cannot use all the acetyl-coenzyme A (CoA) that is formed from fatty acid oxidation, it converts the excess into acetoacetic acid, a highly soluble keto acid that is released into the bloodstream and transported to other tissues, where it is used for energy. During periods of starvation, ketones become

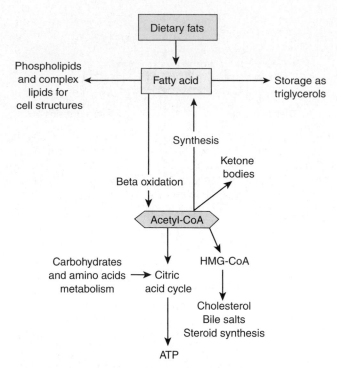

FIGURE 38-6. Hepatic pathways for fat metabolism. Beta oxidation breaks fatty acids into two-carbon acetyl-CoA units that are used in the citric acid cycle to generate ATP or are used in the synthesis of cholesterol of keto acids that are released into the blood for use by other tissues as an energy source. Acetyl-CoA, acetyl-coenzyme A; ATP, adenosine triphosphate; HMG-CoA, 3-hydroxy-3-methylglutaryl-CoA.

a major source of energy because fatty acids released from adipose tissue are converted to ketones by the liver.

Acetyl-CoA units from fat metabolism are used to synthesize cholesterol and bile acids in the liver. Cholesterol can be esterified and stored; exported bound to lipoproteins; or converted to bile acids. The rate-limiting step in cholesterol synthesis is that which is catalyzed by 3-hydroxy-3-methylglutaryl-coenzyme A reductase (HMG-CoA reductase). The HMG-CoA reductase inhibitors, or statins, are used to treat high cholesterol levels by inhibiting this step in cholesterol synthesis.

Almost all the fat synthesis in the body from carbohydrates and proteins occurs in the liver. Whenever a greater quantity of carbohydrates enters the body than can be immediately used, the excess is converted to triglycerides in the liver. The triglycerides formed in the liver are transported mainly in low-density lipoproteins to the adipose tissue, where they are stored.

Bile Production and Cholestasis

The secretion of bile is essential for digestion of dietary fats and absorption of fats and fat-soluble vitamins from the intestine. The liver produces approximately 500 to 600 mL of yellow-green bile daily.[4] Bile contains water, bile salts, bilirubin, cholesterol, and certain by-products of metabolism. Of these, only bile salts,

which are formed from cholesterol, are important in digestion. The other components of bile depend on the secretion of sodium, chloride, bicarbonate, and potassium by the bile ducts.

Bile salts serve an important function in digestion; they aid in **emulsifying** dietary fats, and they are necessary for the formation of the micelles that transport fatty acids and fat-soluble vitamins to the surface of the intestinal mucosa for absorption. Bile salts in excess of 90% that enter the intestine are reabsorbed into the portal circulation by an active transport process that takes place in the distal ileum.[4] From the portal circulation, the bile salts move into the liver cells and are recycled.

Cholestasis

Cholestasis represents a decrease in bile flow through the intrahepatic canaliculi and a reduction in secretion of water, bilirubin, and bile acids by the hepatocytes. As a result, the materials normally transferred to the bile, including bilirubin, cholesterol, and bile acids, accumulate in the blood.[5] The condition may be caused by intrinsic liver disease, in which case it is referred to as *intrahepatic cholestasis*, or by obstruction of the large bile ducts, a condition known as *extrahepatic cholestasis*.

Primary biliary cirrhosis (PBC) (an autoimmune disease) and primary sclerosing cholangitis (PSC) are caused by disorders of the small intrahepatic canaliculi and bile ducts. In the case of extrahepatic obstruction, which can be caused by conditions such as cholelithiasis, common duct strictures, or obstructing neoplasms, the effects begin with increased pressure in the large bile ducts. Genetic disorders that can result in cholestasis include benign recurrent cholestasis, Byler syndrome, and Alagille syndrome. Benign recurrent cholestasis involves the transport of bile into the canaliculi.[6] Byler syndrome is also known as progressive familial intrahepatic cholestasis type I, in which inadequate bile is produced, resulting in inadequate fat breakdown and absorption due to mutations in ATP8B1 protein.[7] Alagille syndrome is an autosomal dominant disease that involves the intrahepatic hypoplasia specifically of the interlobar bile ducts.[8,9] People with the syndrome present with cardiac and eye abnormalities along with skeletal abnormalities, specifically in the facial bones.[8,9]

The morphologic features of cholestasis depend on the underlying cause. Common to all types of obstructive and hepatocellular cholestasis is the accumulation of bile pigment in the liver. Elongated green-brown plugs of bile are visible in the dilated bile canaliculi. Prolonged obstructive cholestasis leads to fatty changes and possible rupture of the canaliculi leaking bile in the hepatocytes, destruction of the supporting connective tissue, and reservoirs of bile containing cellular debris and pigment.[10] Unrelieved obstruction leads to biliary tract fibrosis and ultimately to end-stage biliary cirrhosis.

Pruritus is the most common presenting symptom in people with cholestasis, probably related to an elevation in plasma bile acids. Skin xanthomas (focal accumulations of cholesterol) may occur, the result of hyperlipidemia and impaired excretion of cholesterol. An elevated serum alkaline phosphatase level is common. Other manifestations of reduced bile flow relate to intestinal absorption, including nutritional deficiencies of the fat-soluble vitamins A, D, and K.

Bilirubin Elimination and Jaundice

Bilirubin is the final product of the breakdown of heme contained in aged red blood cells. Bilirubin is the substance that gives bile its color. In the process of degradation, the hemoglobin from the red blood cell is broken down to form biliverdin, which is rapidly converted to free bilirubin (Fig. 38-7). Free bilirubin, which is insoluble in plasma, is transported in the blood attached to plasma albumin. Even when it is bound to albumin, this bilirubin is still called *free bilirubin*, to distinguish it from conjugated bilirubin. As it passes through the liver, free bilirubin is absorbed through the hepatocytes' cell membrane and released from its albumin carrier molecule. Inside the hepatocytes, free bilirubin is converted to conjugated bilirubin, making it soluble in bile. Conjugated bilirubin is secreted as a constituent of bile, and in this form it passes through the bile ducts into the small

intestine. In the intestine, approximately one half of the bilirubin is converted into a highly soluble substance called *urobilinogen* by the intestinal flora. Approximately one fifth of the urobilinogen produced is either absorbed into the portal circulation and the remaining is excreted in the feces.[10] Most of the urobilinogen that is absorbed is returned to the liver to be reexcreted into the bile.

The normal level of total serum bilirubin is less than 1.5 mg/dL (17 to 20.5 μmol).[11] Laboratory measurements of bilirubin usually measure the free and the conjugated bilirubin as well as the total bilirubin. These are reported as direct (conjugated) bilirubin and indirect (unconjugated or free) bilirubin.

Jaundice

Jaundice (*i.e.*, icterus) or a yellowish discoloration of the skin and deep tissues results from abnormally high levels of bilirubin in the blood. Jaundice occurs when there is an imbalance between the synthesis of bilirubin and the clearance of bilirubin. Jaundice becomes evident when the serum bilirubin levels rise above 2 to 2.5 mg/dL (34.2 to 42.8 μmol).[5,10] Because normal skin has a yellow cast, the early signs of jaundice often are difficult to detect, especially in people with dark skin. Bilirubin has a special affinity for elastic tissue. The sclera of the eye, which contains a high proportion of elastic fibers, usually is one of the first structures in which jaundice can be detected (Fig. 38-8).

The five major causes of jaundice are excessive destruction of red blood cells, impaired uptake of bilirubin by the liver cells, decreased conjugation of bilirubin, obstruction of bile flow in the canaliculi of the hepatic lobules or in the intrahepatic or extrahepatic bile ducts, and excessive extrahepatic production of bilirubin.[12] From an anatomic standpoint, jaundice can be categorized as prehepatic, intrahepatic, and posthepatic. Chart 38-1 lists the common causes of prehepatic, hepatic, and posthepatic jaundice.

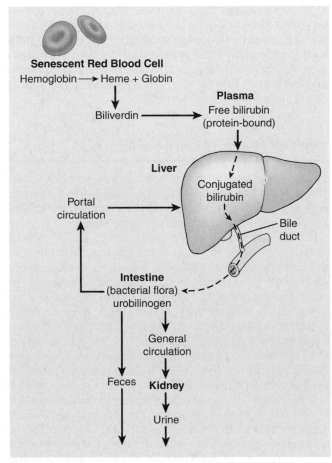

FIGURE 38-7. The process of bilirubin formation, circulation, and elimination.

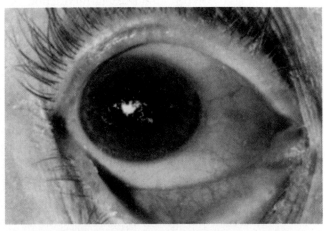

FIGURE 38-8. Jaundice. A person in hepatic failure displays *yellow sclera*. (From Strayer D., Rubin E. (2015). *Rubin's pathology: Clinicopathologic foundations of medicine* (7th ed., Fig. 20-4, p. 829). Philadelphia, PA: Lippincott Williams & Wilkins.)

CHART 38-1

CAUSES OF JAUNDICE

Prehepatic (Excessive Red Blood Cell Destruction)

Hemolytic blood transfusion reaction

Hereditary disorders of the red blood cell

  Sickle cell disease

  Thalassemia

  Spherocytosis

Acquired hemolytic disorders

Hemolytic disease of the newborn

Autoimmune hemolytic anemias

Intrahepatic

Decreased bilirubin uptake by the liver

Decreased conjugation of bilirubin

Hepatocellular liver damage

  Hepatitis

  Cirrhosis

  Cancer of the liver

Drug-induced cholestasis

Posthepatic (Obstruction of Bile Flow)

Structural disorders of the bile duct

Cholelithiasis

Congenital atresia of the extrahepatic bile ducts

Bile duct obstruction caused by tumors

The major cause of prehepatic jaundice is excessive hemolysis of red blood cells. Hemolytic jaundice occurs when red blood cells are destroyed at a rate in excess of the liver's ability to remove the bilirubin from the blood. It may follow a hemolytic blood transfusion reaction, because of the decreased lifespan of the donated red blood cells, or may occur in diseases such as hereditary spherocytosis, in which the red cell membranes are defective, or in hemolytic disease of the newborn. When internal hemorrhage occurs, there can also be excess bilirubin production with the reabsorption of the blood. In addition, diseases resulting in ineffective erythropoiesis can also increase bilirubin production.[10] Neonatal hyperbilirubinemia results from increased production of bilirubin in newborn infants and their limited ability to excrete it from 0 to 14 days old.[10] Premature infants are at particular risk because their red cells have a shorter life span and higher turnover rate. In prehepatic jaundice, there is mild jaundice, the unconjugated bilirubin is elevated, the stools are of normal color, and there is no bilirubin in the urine.

Intrahepatic or hepatocellular jaundice is caused by disorders that directly affect the ability of the liver to remove bilirubin from the blood or conjugate it so it can be eliminated in the bile. Gilbert disease is inherited as a dominant trait and results in a reduced removal of bilirubin from the blood. The disorder is benign and fairly common with a prevalence rate of approximately 8%.[12] Affected people have no symptoms other than a slightly elevated unconjugated bilirubin and mild jaundice. Conjugation of bilirubin is impaired whenever liver cells are damaged, when transport of bilirubin into liver cells becomes deficient, or when the enzymes needed to conjugate the bile are lacking. Liver diseases such as hepatitis and cirrhosis are the most common causes of intrahepatic jaundice. Drugs such as the anesthetic agent halothane, oral contraceptives, estrogen, anabolic steroids, isoniazid, rifampin, and chlorpromazine may also be implicated in this type of jaundice. Intrahepatic or hepatocellular jaundice usually interferes with all phases of bilirubin metabolism—uptake, conjugation, and excretion. Both conjugated and unconjugated bilirubin are elevated, the urine often is dark because of bilirubin in the urine, and the serum alkaline phosphatase is slightly elevated.

Posthepatic or obstructive jaundice, also called *cholestatic jaundice*, occurs when bile flow is obstructed between the liver and the intestine, with the obstruction located at any point between the junction of the right or left hepatic duct and the point where the bile duct opens into the intestine. Among the causes are strictures of the bile duct, gallstones, and tumors of the bile duct or the pancreas. Conjugated bilirubin levels usually are elevated; the stools are clay colored because of the lack of bilirubin in the bile; the urine is dark; the levels of serum alkaline phosphatase are markedly elevated; and the aminotransferase levels are slightly increased. Blood levels of bile acids often are elevated in obstructive jaundice. As the bile acids accumulate in the blood, pruritus develops. A history of pruritus preceding jaundice is common in obstructive jaundice.

Tests of Hepatobiliary Function

The history and physical examination provide clues about liver function. Diagnostic and laboratory tests help evaluate liver function and the extent of liver damage to confirm the diagnosis of liver disease.

Liver function tests, including serum levels of liver enzymes, are used to aid in the diagnosis of the disease, differentiate between different disorders, determine the severity of present disease, and monitor responses to established treatment.[13] Elevated serum enzyme test results usually indicate liver injury earlier than do other indicators of liver function. The key enzymes are alanine aminotransferase (ALT) and aspartate aminotransferase (AST), which are present in liver cells. ALT is found predominately in the liver, with lesser quantities found in the kidneys, heart, and skeletal muscle. As a result, ALT is a more specific indicator of liver inflammation than is AST, because AST may also be elevated in diseases affecting other organs, such as the heart or muscles. In most types of liver disease, ALT activity is higher than that of AST; exceptions include alcoholic hepatitis, hepatic cirrhosis, and hepatocellular carcinoma (HCC).[14] The reasons for the higher AST activity in alcoholic hepatitis is due to increased mitochondrial damage leading to increased release of mitochondrial AST in serum.[15] The most dramatic rise is seen in cases of acute hepatocellular injury, as occurs with viral hepatitis, hypoxic or ischemic injury, acute toxic injury, or Reye syndrome.

The liver's synthetic capacity is reflected in measures of serum protein levels and prothrombin time (*i.e.*, synthesis of coagulation factors). Hypoalbuminemia because of depressed synthesis may complicate severe liver disease. Deficiencies of coagulation factor V and vitamin K–dependent factors (II, VII, IX, and X) may occur.

Serum bilirubin, γ-glutamyltransferase (GGT), 5′-nucleotidase, and alkaline phosphatase measure hepatic excretory function. Alkaline phosphatase and 5′-nucleotidase are present in disorders affecting the bile duct.[13] GGT is located in the endoplasmic reticulum of the hepatocytes and in the bile duct epithelial cells. Measurement of GGT may be helpful in diagnosing alcohol abuse and is an indicator of hepatobiliary disease.[16]

Ultrasonography provides information about the size, composition, and blood flow of the liver. Computed tomography (CT) scanning and magnetic resonance imaging (MRI) have proved to be useful in some disorders. Selective angiography of the celiac, superior mesenteric, or hepatic artery may be used to visualize the hepatic or portal circulation. A liver biopsy affords a means of examining liver tissue without surgery to stage liver cancer.

SUMMARY CONCEPTS

The hepatobiliary system consists of the liver, gallbladder, and bile ducts. The liver is the largest and, in functions, one of the most versatile organs in the body. It is located between the gastrointestinal tract and the systemic circulation; venous blood from the intestine flows through the liver before it is returned to the heart. In this way, nutrients can be removed for processing and storage, and bacteria and other foreign matter can be removed by Kupffer cells before the blood is returned to the systemic circulation.

The liver synthesizes fats, glucose, and plasma proteins. Other important functions of the liver include the deamination of amino acids, conversion of ammonia to urea, and the interconversion of amino acids and other compounds that are important to the metabolic processes of the body. The liver produces approximately 500 to 600 mL of yellow-green bile daily. Bile serves as an excretory vehicle for bilirubin, cholesterol, and certain products of organic metabolism, and it contains bile salts that are essential for digestion of fats and absorption of fat-soluble vitamins. The liver also removes, conjugates, and secretes bilirubin into the bile. Jaundice occurs when bilirubin accumulates in the blood. It can occur because of excessive red blood cell destruction, failure of the liver to remove and conjugate the bilirubin, or obstructed biliary flow.

Liver function tests, including serum aminotransferase levels, are used to assess injury to liver cells. Serum bilirubin, GGT, 5′-nucleotidase, and alkaline phosphatase are used as measures of hepatic excretory function. Ultrasonography, CT scans, and MRI are used to evaluate liver structures. Angiography may be used to visualize the hepatic or portal circulation, and a liver biopsy obtains tissue specimens for microscopic examination.

Disorders of Hepatic and Biliary Function

The structures of the hepatobiliary system are subject to many of the same pathologic conditions that affect other body systems: injury from drugs and toxins; infection, inflammation, and immune responses; metabolic disorders; and neoplasms. This section focuses on alterations in liver function because of drug-induced injury; viral and autoimmune hepatitis (AIH); intrahepatic biliary tract disorders; alcohol-induced liver disease; cirrhosis, portal hypertension, and liver failure; and cancer of the liver.

Hepatotoxic Disorders

By virtue of its many enzyme systems that are involved in biochemical transformations and modifications, the liver has an important role in the metabolism of many drugs and chemical substances. The liver is particularly important in terms of metabolizing lipid-soluble substances that cannot be directly excreted by the kidneys. The liver is central to the metabolic disposition of virtually all drugs and foreign substances. Therefore, drug-induced liver toxicity is a potential complication of many medications.

Drug and Hormone Metabolism

Three major types of reactions are involved in the hepatic detoxification and metabolism of drugs and other chemicals:

1. Phase 1 reactions, which involve chemical modification or inactivation of a substance
2. Phase 2 reactions, which involve conversion of lipid-soluble substances to water-soluble derivatives
3. Phase 3 reactions, which involve the substance, its metabolites, or conjugates being secreted as bile[17]

All three types of reactions may be linked, depending on the composition of the substance being eliminated. For example, many phase 1 reactants are not water soluble and must therefore undergo a subsequent phase 2 reaction to be eliminated. These reactions, which are called *biotransformations*, are important considerations in drug therapy.

Phase 1 Reactions
Phase 1 reactions result in chemical modification of reactive drug groups by oxidation, reduction, hydroxylation,

well-being, return of appetite, and disappearance of jaundice. The acute illness usually subsides gradually over 2 to 12 weeks, with complete clinical recovery in 1 to 4 months depending on the type of hepatitis.[26] Infection with HBV and HCV can produce a *carrier state* in which the person does not have symptoms but harbors the virus and can therefore transmit the disease.[28] Evidence also indicates a carrier state for HDV infection. There is no carrier state for HAV infection. There are two types of carriers: healthy carriers who have few or no ill effects and those with chronic disease who may or may not have symptoms. Factors that increase the risk of becoming a carrier are age at time of infection and immune status.[26] People at high risk of becoming carriers are infants of HBV-infected mothers, those with impaired immunity, those who have received multiple transfusions or blood products, those who are on hemodialysis, and drug addicts.

Hepatitis A

Hepatitis A is caused by the HAV, a small, unenveloped, single-stranded ribonucleic acid (RNA) virus. It usually is a benign, self-limited disease, although it can cause acute fulminant hepatitis and death or need for transplantation in 0.15% to 0.2% of cases.[29]

Etiology and Pathogenesis

Hepatitis A is contracted primarily by the fecal–oral route.[30] It has a brief incubation period of 14 to 28 days.[31] The virus replicates in the liver, is excreted in the bile, and is shed in the stool. The fecal shedding of HAV occurs during the first 2 weeks of the illness.[30] The disease often occurs sporadically or in epidemics. Drinking contaminated milk or water and eating shellfish from infected waters are fairly common routes of transmission. At special risk are people traveling abroad who have not previously been exposed to the virus. Because young children are asymptomatic, they play an important role in the spread of the disease. Institutions housing large numbers of people (usually children) sometimes are stricken with an epidemic of hepatitis A. Oral behavior and lack of toilet training promote viral infection among children attending preschool day care centers, who then carry the virus home to older siblings and parents. Hepatitis A usually is not transmitted by transfusion of blood or plasma derivatives, presumably because its short period of viremia usually coincides with clinical illness, so that the disease is apparent and blood donations are not accepted.

Clinical Manifestations

The onset of symptoms usually is abrupt and includes fever, malaise, nausea, anorexia, abdominal discomfort, dark urine, and jaundice. The presentation of symptoms is dependent on age, with the severity of symptoms increasing in older age groups.[32] Children younger than 6 years often are asymptomatic, and few develop jaundice. The illness in older children and adults usually is symptomatic and jaundice occurs in approximately 70% of cases.[32] Symptoms usually last approximately 2 months but can last longer. HAV does not cause chronic hepatitis or induce a carrier state.

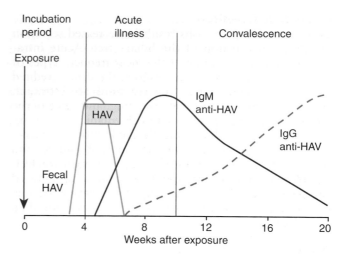

FIGURE 38-9. The sequence of fecal shedding of the HAV, HAV viremia, and HAV antibody (IgM and IgG anti-HAV) changes in hepatitis A. HAV, hepatitis A virus; Ig, immunoglobulin.

Serologic Markers

Antibodies to HAV (anti-HAV) appear early in the disease and tend to persist in the serum (Fig. 38-9). The immunoglobulin (Ig) M antibodies usually appear during the first week of symptomatic disease and slowly decline over a period of 3 to 4 months. Their presence coincides with a decline in fecal shedding of the virus. Peak levels of IgG antibodies occur after 1 month of illness and may persist for life; they provide long-term protective immunity against reinfection.[30] The presence of IgM anti-HAV is indicative of acute hepatitis A, whereas IgG anti-HAV merely documents past infection.

Immunization

A hepatitis A vaccine is available.[32] Immunization is intended for international travelers to regions where sanitation is poor and endemic HAV infections are high, children living in communities with high rates of HAV infection, homosexually active men, and users of illicit drugs. People with preexisting chronic liver disease also may benefit from immunization. A public health benefit also may be derived from vaccinating people with increased potential for transmitting the disease (*e.g.*, food handlers). The Centers for Disease Control and Prevention (CDC) has recently recommended vaccination of children in states, counties, and communities with high rates of infection.[33] Because the vaccine is of little benefit in prevention of hepatitis in people with known HAV exposure, IgG is recommended for these people.

Hepatitis B

Hepatitis B is caused by the HBV, a double-stranded deoxyribonucleic acid (DNA) virus.[34] The complete virion, also called a *Dane particle*, consists of an outer envelope and an inner nucleocapsid that contains HBV DNA and DNA polymerase (Fig. 38-10).[35] HBV infection can produce acute hepatitis, chronic hepatitis, progression of chronic hepatitis to cirrhosis, fulminant hepatitis with massive hepatic necrosis, and the carrier state. It also participates in the development of hepatitis D (delta hepatitis).

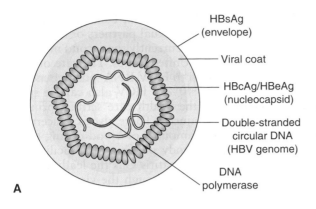

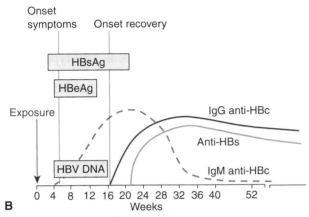

FIGURE 38-10. (A) The HBV. (B) The sequence of HBV viral antigens (HBsAg, HBeAg), HBV DNA, and HBV antibody (IgM, IgG, anti-HBc, and anti-HBs) changes in acute resolving hepatitis B. DNA, deoxyribonucleic acid; HBcAg, hepatitis B core antigen; HBeAg, hepatitis B envelop antigen; HBsAg, hepatitis B surface antigen; HBV, hepatitis B virus; Ig, immunoglobulin.

Worldwide, 350 million people have long-term hepatitis B infections.[36] In the United States, acute hepatitis B has been declining in incidence since 1990, mainly because of effective vaccination strategies.[37] The number of reported cases of acute hepatitis B has remained relatively stable since 2009. In 2016, 3218 cases of HBV were reported to the CDC. In the United States, 850,000 to 2.2 million people are estimated to be living with HBV infection,[38,39] many of whom are unaware of their infection status.[40] To improve health outcomes for these people, the CDC recommended HBV testing for populations at risk for HBV infection and public health management of people living with chronic HBV infection.[41]

Hepatitis B has a longer incubation period and represents a more serious health problem than does hepatitis A. The virus usually is transmitted through inoculation with infected blood or serum. However, the viral antigen can be found in most body secretions and can be spread by oral or sexual contact. In the United States, most people with hepatitis B acquire the infection as adults or adolescents. The disease is highly prevalent among injecting drug users, heterosexuals with multiple sex partners, and men who have sex with men.[42,43] Health care workers are at risk owing to blood exposure and accidental needle injuries. Although the virus

can be spread through transfusion or administration of blood products, routine screening methods have appreciably reduced transmission through this route. The risk of hepatitis B in infants born to HBV-infected mothers ranges from 10% to 85%, depending on the mother's HBV status. Infants who become infected have a 90% risk of becoming chronic carriers, and up to 25% will die of chronic liver disease as adults.[43,44]

Serologic Markers

Three well-defined antigens are associated with the virus: a core antigen, HBcAg, which is contained in the nucleocapsid; a longer polypeptide transcript with precore and core regions, designated HBeAg; and a surface antigen, HBsAg, which is found in the outer envelope of the virus. The precore region directs the HBeAg polypeptide toward the blood, whereas the HBcAg remains in the hepatocytes to direct the assembly of new virions.

The HBV antigens evoke specific antibodies: anti-HBs, anti-HBc, and anti-HBe. These antigens and their antibodies serve as serologic markers for following the course of the disease[45] (see Fig. 38-10). The *HBsAg* is the viral antigen measured most routinely in blood. It appears before the onset of symptoms, peaks during overt disease, and then declines to undetectable levels in 3 to 6 months. Persistence beyond 6 months indicates continued viral replication, infectivity, and risk of chronic hepatitis. HBeAg appears in the serum soon after HBsAg and signifies active viral replication. IgM anti-HBc becomes detectable shortly before the onset of symptoms, concurrent with the onset of an elevation in serum transaminases. Over the months, the IgM antibody is replaced by IgG anti-HBc. Anti-HBe is detectable shortly after the disappearance of HBeAg, and its appearance signals the onset of resolution of the acute illness. IgG anti-HBs, a specific antibody to HBsAg, occurs in most people after clearance of HBsAg. The time between the removal of the HBsAg and the appearance of anti-HBs is called the *window period*. Development of anti-HBs signals recovery from HBV infection, noninfectivity, and protection from future HBV infection. Anti-HBs is the antibody present in people who have been successfully immunized against HBV.

The presence of HBV DNA in peripheral blood is a reliable marker of active HBV replication.

HBV DNA is detectable within a few days of infection. It generally increases to reach a peak at the time of acute hepatitis, before progressively decreasing and disappearing when the infection resolves spontaneously. In cases of acute viral hepatitis, testing for HBV DNA in serum may be a useful adjunct in the diagnosis of acute HBV infection, because HBV DNA can be detected approximately 21 days before HBsAg typically appears in the serum.[46] Polymerase chain reaction (PCR) tests have been developed to detect and measure the amount of HBV DNA, called the viral load, in clinical specimens. These tests are used to assess a person's infection status and to monitor treatment.[47]

Immunization

Hepatitis B vaccine provides long-term protection (up to 20 years in some cases) against HBV infection.[37] HBsAg is the antigen used for hepatitis B vaccines. A hepatitis

The late manifestations of cirrhosis are related to portal hypertension and liver cell failure. Splenomegaly, ascites, and portosystemic shunts (*i.e.*, esophageal varices, hemorrhoids, and caput medusae) result from portal hypertension.[10] Other complications include bleeding because of decreased clotting factors, thrombocytopenia because of splenomegaly, gynecomastia and a feminizing pattern of pubic hair distribution in men because of testicular atrophy, spider angiomas, palmar erythema, and encephalopathy with asterixis and neurologic signs.

Portal Hypertension

Portal hypertension is characterized by increased resistance to flow in the portal venous system and sustained portal vein pressure. Normally, venous blood returning to the heart from the abdominal organs collects in the portal vein and travels through the liver before entering the vena cava. Portal hypertension can be caused by a variety of conditions that increase resistance to hepatic blood flow, including prehepatic, posthepatic, and intrahepatic obstructions (with *hepatic* referring to the liver lobules rather than the entire liver). Prehepatic causes of portal hypertension include portal vein thrombosis and external compression because of cancer or enlarged lymph nodes that produce obstruction of the portal vein before it enters the liver.

Posthepatic obstruction refers to any obstruction to blood flow through the hepatic veins beyond the liver lobules, either within or distal to the liver. It is caused by conditions such as thrombosis of the hepatic veins, veno-occlusive disease, and severe right-sided heart failure that impede the outflow of venous blood from the liver. *Budd–Chiari syndrome* refers to a congestive disease of the liver caused by occlusion of multiple hepatic veins or the hepatic portion of the inferior vena cava.[10] The principal cause of the Budd–Chiari syndrome is thrombosis of the hepatic veins, in association with diverse conditions such as polycythemia vera, hypercoagulability states associated with malignant tumors, pregnancy, bacterial infection, metastatic disease of the liver, and trauma. *Sinusoidal obstruction syndrome* or *hepatic veno-occlusive disease* is a variant of the Budd–Chiari syndrome seen most commonly in people treated with certain cancer chemotherapeutic drugs, hepatic irradiation, or bone marrow transplantation.[80,81]

Intrahepatic causes of portal hypertension include conditions that cause obstruction of blood flow within the liver. In alcoholic cirrhosis, which is the major cause of portal hypertension, bands of fibrous tissue and fibrous nodules distort the architecture of the liver and increase the resistance to portal blood flow, which leads to portal hypertension.

Complications of portal hypertension arise from the increased pressure and dilation of the venous channels behind the obstruction (Fig. 38-14). In addition, collateral channels that connect the portal circulation with the systemic circulation open. The major complications of the increased portal vein pressure and the opening of collateral channels are ascites, splenomegaly, hepatic encephalopathy, and the formation of portosystemic shunts with bleeding from esophageal varices.[10]

KEY POINTS

Portal Hypertension

■ Venous blood from the gastrointestinal tract empties into the portal vein and travels through the liver before moving into the general venous circulation.

■ Obstruction of blood flow in the portal vein produces an increase in the hydrostatic pressure within the peritoneal capillaries, contributing to the development of ascites, splenic engorgement with sequestration and destruction of blood cells and platelets, and shunting of blood to collateral venous channels causing varicosities of the hemorrhoidal and esophageal veins.

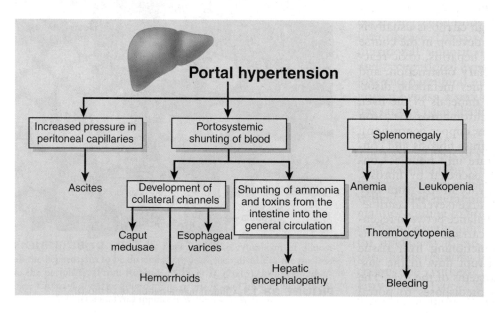

FIGURE 38-14. Mechanisms of disturbed liver function related to portal hypertension.

Ascites

Ascites occurs when the amount of fluid in the peritoneal cavity is increased and is a late-stage manifestation of cirrhosis and portal hypertension.[82] It is not uncommon for people with advanced cirrhosis to present with an accumulation of 15 L or more of ascitic fluid. These people often experience abdominal discomfort, dyspnea, and insomnia. They may also have difficulty walking or living independently.

Although the mechanisms responsible for the development of ascites are not completely understood, portal hypertension is one of the leading causes. Nitric oxide–induced splanchnic vasodilation, low albumin levels resulting in low **oncotic** pressure, sodium retention, and activation of the renin–angiotensin–aldosterone system also appear to contribute to ascites.

Treatment of ascites usually focuses on dietary restriction of sodium and administration of diuretics. Water intake also may need to be restricted. Because of the many limitations in sodium restriction, the use of diuretics has become the mainstay of treatment for ascites. Oral potassium supplements often are given to prevent hypokalemia.[83]

Large-volume paracentesis (removal of 5 L or more of ascitic fluid) may be done in people with massive ascites and pulmonary compromise. Because the removal of fluid produces a decrease in vascular volume along with increased plasma renin activity and aldosterone-mediated sodium and water reabsorption by the kidneys, a volume expander such as albumin usually is administered to maintain the effective circulating volume.[84] A transjugular intrahepatic portosystemic shunt (TIPS) may be inserted in people with refractory ascites.[84]

Spontaneous bacterial peritonitis is a complication in people with both cirrhosis and ascites. The infection is serious and carries a high mortality rate even when treated with antibiotics. Presumably, the peritoneal fluid is seeded with bacteria from the blood or lymph or from the passage of bacteria through the bowel wall. Symptoms include fever, altered mental status, and abdominal pain. Other symptoms include worsening of hepatic encephalopathy, diarrhea, hypothermia, and shock. It is diagnosed by a neutrophil count of 250/mm^3 or higher.[85]

Splenomegaly

The spleen enlarges progressively in portal hypertension because of shunting of blood into the splenic vein. The enlarged spleen often gives rise to sequestering of significant numbers of blood elements and development of a syndrome known as *hypersplenism*. Hypersplenism is characterized by a decrease in the lifespan of all the formed elements of the blood and a subsequent decrease in their numbers, leading to anemia, thrombocytopenia, and leukopenia.[85] The decreased lifespan of the blood elements is thought to result from an increased rate of removal because of the prolonged transit time through the enlarged spleen.

Portosystemic Shunts

With the gradual obstruction of venous blood flow in the liver, the pressure in the portal vein increases, and large collateral channels develop between the portal and systemic veins that supply the lower rectum and esophagus and the umbilical veins of the falciform ligament that attaches to the anterior wall of the abdomen. The collaterals between the inferior and internal iliac veins may give rise to hemorrhoids. In some people, the fetal umbilical vein is not totally obliterated; it forms a channel on the anterior abdominal wall. Dilated veins around the umbilicus are called *caput medusae*.[86] Portopulmonary shunts also may develop and cause blood to bypass the pulmonary capillaries, interfering with blood oxygenation and producing cyanosis.

Clinically, the most important collateral channels are those connecting the portal and coronary veins that lead to reversal of flow and formation of thin-walled varicosities in the submucosa of the esophagus[87] (Fig. 38-15). These thin-walled *esophageal varices* are subject to rupture, producing massive and sometimes fatal hemorrhage. Impaired hepatic synthesis of coagulation factors and decreased platelet levels (*i.e.*, thrombocytopenia) because of splenomegaly may further complicate the control of esophageal bleeding. Esophageal varices are present in nearly 30% to 40% of people with compensated cirrhosis and in 60% of those with decompensated cirrhosis. Variceal hemorrhage is perhaps the most devastating portal hypertension-related complication in people with cirrhosis, occurring in up to 30% of such people during the course of their illness. Although mortality rates of variceal hemorrhage in people with cirrhosis have been falling over the past few decades because of the implementation of effective treatments and improvements in general medical care, it still carries a

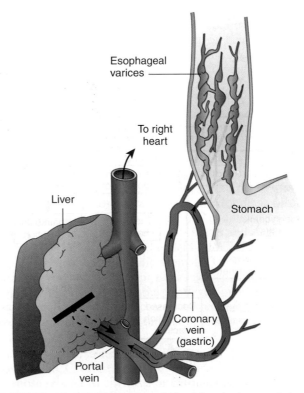

FIGURE 38-15. Obstruction of blood flow in the portal circulation, with portal hypertension and diversion of blood flow to other venous channels, including the gastric and esophageal veins.

The cholesterol found in bile has no known function. It is assumed to be a by-product of bile salt formation, and its presence is linked to the excretory function of bile.[100] Normally insoluble in water, cholesterol is rendered soluble by the action of bile salts and lecithin, which combine with it to form micelles. In the gallbladder, water and electrolytes are absorbed from the liver bile, causing the bile to become more concentrated. Because neither lecithin nor bile salts are absorbed in the gallbladder, their concentration increases along with that of cholesterol; in this way, the solubility of cholesterol is maintained.

Entrance of food into the intestine causes the gallbladder to contract and the sphincter of the bile duct to relax, such that bile stored in the gallbladder moves into the duodenum. The stimulus for gallbladder contraction is primarily hormonal. Products of food digestion, particularly lipids, stimulate the release of a gastrointestinal hormone called *cholecystokinin* from the mucosa of the duodenum. Cholecystokinin provides a strong stimulus for gallbladder contraction. The role of other gastrointestinal hormones in bile release is less clearly understood.

Pressure in the common duct largely is responsible for regulating passage of bile into the intestine. Normally, the gallbladder regulates this pressure. It collects and stores bile as it relaxes and the pressure in the common bile duct decreases, and it empties bile into the intestine as the gallbladder contracts, producing an increase in common duct pressure. After gallbladder surgery, the pressure in the common duct changes, causing the common duct to dilate. The sphincters in the common duct then regulate the flow of bile.

Two common disorders of the biliary system are cholelithiasis (*i.e.*, gallstones) and inflammation of the gallbladder (cholecystitis) or common bile duct (cholangitis). In adult Western populations, 15% of people have gallstones.[101] In both circumstances, hypersecretion of biliary cholesterol appears to play a major role.

Cholelithiasis

Cholelithiasis or gallstones is caused by precipitation of substances contained in bile, mainly cholesterol and bilirubin. Approximately 80% of gallstones are composed primarily of cholesterol; the other 20% are black or brown pigment stones composed of mucin glycoproteins and calcium salts.[102] Many stones have a mixed composition. Figure 38-18 shows a gallbladder with numerous cholesterol gallstones.

Two primary factors contribute to the formation of gallstones: abnormalities in the composition of bile (particularly increased cholesterol) and the stasis of bile.[102] The formation of cholesterol stones is associated with obesity and occurs more frequently in women, especially women who have had multiple pregnancies or who are taking oral contraceptives. All of these factors cause the liver to excrete more cholesterol into the bile. Estrogen reduces the synthesis of bile acid in women. Gallbladder sludge (thickened gallbladder mucoprotein with tiny trapped cholesterol crystals) is thought to be a precursor of gallstones. Sludge frequently occurs with pregnancy, starvation, and rapid weight loss. Drugs that lower serum cholesterol levels also cause increased

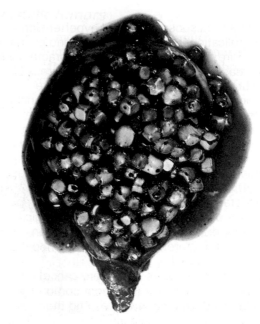

FIGURE 38-18. Cholesterol gallstones. The gallbladder has been opened to reveal numerous yellow cholesterol gallstones. (From Rubin R., Strayer D. (2015). *Rubin's pathology: Clinicopathologic foundations of medicine* (7th ed., Fig. 20-71, p. 881). Philadelphia, PA: Lippincott Williams & Wilkins.)

cholesterol excretion into the bile. Malabsorption disorders stemming from ileal disease or intestinal bypass surgery tend to interfere with the absorption of bile salts, which are needed to maintain the solubility of cholesterol. Inflammation of the gallbladder alters the absorptive characteristics of the mucosal layer, allowing excessive absorption of water and bile salts. Cholesterol gallstones are extremely common among Native Americans and Chilean Indians and Chilean Hispanics, which suggests that a genetic component may have a role in gallstone formation.[103] Pigment stones containing bilirubin are seen in people with hemolytic disease (*e.g.*, sickle cell disease) and hepatic cirrhosis.

Clinical Manifestations

Many people with gallstones have no symptoms. Gallstones cause symptoms when they obstruct bile flow or cause inflammation.[102] Small stones (*i.e.*, <8 mm in diameter) pass into the common duct, producing symptoms of indigestion and biliary colic. Larger stones are more likely to obstruct flow and cause jaundice. The pain of biliary colic is usually located in the upper right quadrant or epigastric area and may be referred to the upper back, the right shoulder, or midscapular region. Typically, the pain is abrupt in onset, increases steadily in intensity, persists for 30 minutes to 5 hours, and is followed by soreness in the upper right quadrant.

Acute and Chronic Cholecystitis

Acute cholecystitis is a diffuse inflammation of the gallbladder, usually secondary to obstruction of the gallbladder outlet. Most cases of acute cholecystitis (85% to 90%) are associated with the presence of gallstones (calculous cholecystitis).[103] The remaining cases (acalculous cholecystitis) are associated with sepsis, severe trauma, or infection of the gallbladder. It has been theorized that obstruction of the cystic duct by a gallstone leads to the release of phospholipase from the epithelium of the gallbladder. In turn, this enzyme may hydrolyze lecithin and release lysolecithin, a membrane-active toxin.[103] At the same time, disruption of the normally protective mucous lining of the epithelium renders the mucosal cells vulnerable to damage by the detergent action of concentrated bile salts. Acute acalculous cholecystitis occurs with no apparent cause in 50% of cases, trauma, burns, biliary sludge, and vasculitis have been possible causative factors.[102] Acute acalculous cholecystitis can rapidly progress to gangrene and perforation because the process appears to involve a transmural infarction, rather than inflammatory changes associated with stones.

Chronic cholecystitis results from repeated episodes of acute cholecystitis or chronic irritation of the gallbladder by stones. It is characterized by varying degrees of chronic inflammation. Gallstones almost always are present. Cholelithiasis with chronic cholecystitis may be associated with acute exacerbations of gallbladder inflammation, common duct stone, pancreatitis, and, rarely, carcinoma of the gallbladder.

Clinical Manifestations
People with acute cholecystitis usually experience an acute onset of upper right quadrant or epigastric pain, frequently associated with mild fever, anorexia, nausea, and vomiting. In biliary colic the cystic duct obstruction is transient, whereas in acute cholecystitis it is persistent. People with calculus cholecystitis usually, but not always, have experienced previous episodes of biliary pain. The pain may appear with remarkable suddenness and constitute a surgical emergency. In the absence of medical attention, the attack usually subsides in 7 to 10 days. In people who recover, recurrence is common. The onset of acalculous cholecystitis tends to be more insidious because the manifestations are obscured by the underlying conditions precipitating the attack. In the severely ill person, early recognition is crucial because a delay in treatment can prove life-threatening. People with acute cholecystitis usually have an elevated white blood cell count, and many have mild elevations in AST, ALT, alkaline phosphatase, and bilirubin.

The manifestations of chronic cholecystitis are more vague than those of acute cholecystitis. There may be intolerance to fatty foods, belching, and other indications of discomfort. Often, there are episodes of colicky pain with obstruction of biliary flow caused by gallstones. The gallbladder, which in chronic cholecystitis usually contains stones, may be enlarged, shrunken, or of normal size.

Diagnosis and Treatment
The methods used to diagnose gallbladder disease include ultrasonography, cholescintigraphy (nuclear scanning), and CT scans.[103] Ultrasonography is widely used in diagnosing gallbladder disease and has largely replaced the oral cholecystogram in most medical centers. It can detect stones as small as 1 to 2 cm, and its overall accuracy in detecting gallbladder disease is high. In addition to stones, ultrasonography can detect wall thickening, which indicates inflammation. It also can

rule out other causes of right upper quadrant pain such as tumors. Cholescintigraphy, also called a *gallbladder scan*, relies on the ability of the liver to extract a rapidly injected radionuclide, technetium-99m, bound to one of several iminodiacetic acids, that is excreted into the bile ducts. The gallbladder scan is highly accurate in detecting acute cholecystitis. Although CT is not as accurate as ultrasonography in detecting gallstones, it can show thickening of the gallbladder wall or pericholecystic fluid associated with acute cholecystitis.

Gallbladder disease usually is treated by removing the gallbladder. The gallbladder stores and concentrates bile, and its removal usually does not interfere with digestion. Laparoscopic cholecystectomy has become the treatment of choice for symptomatic gallbladder disease.[104]

Choledocholithiasis and Cholangitis
Choledocholithiasis refers to stones in the common duct and *cholangitis* to inflammation of the common duct. Common duct stones usually originate in the gallbladder but can form spontaneously in the common duct.

Clinical Manifestations
The manifestations of choledocholithiasis are similar to those of gallstones and acute cholecystitis. There is a history of acute biliary colic and right upper abdominal pain, with chills, fever, and jaundice associated with episodes of abdominal pain. Bilirubinuria and an elevated serum bilirubin are present if the common duct is obstructed. Complications include acute suppurative cholangitis accompanied by purulent fluid in the common duct. It is characterized by the presence of an altered sensorium, lethargy, and septic shock.[10] Acute suppurative cholangitis represents an endoscopic or surgical emergency. Common duct stones also can obstruct the outflow of the pancreatic duct, causing a secondary pancreatitis.

Diagnosis and Treatment
Ultrasonography, CT scans, and radionuclide imaging may be used to demonstrate dilation of bile ducts and impaired blood flow. Endoscopic ultrasonography and magnetic resonance cholangiography are used for detecting common duct stones. Both percutaneous transhepatic cholangiography (PTC) and endoscopic retrograde cholangiopancreatography (ERCP) provide a direct means for determining the cause, location, and extent of obstruction. PTC involves the injection of dye directly into the biliary tree. ERCP involves the passage of an endoscope into the duodenum and the passage of a catheter into the hepatopancreatic ampulla. ERCP can be used to enlarge the opening of the sphincter of the hepatopancreatic ampulla, which may allow the lodged stone to pass, or an instrument may be inserted into the common duct to remove the stone.

Common duct stones in people with cholelithiasis usually are treated by stone extraction followed by laparoscopic cholecystectomy. Antibiotic therapy, with an agent that penetrates the bile, is used to treat the infection. Emergency decompression of the common duct, usually by ERCP, may be necessary for people with sepsis or fail to improve with antibiotic treatment.

Cancer of the Gallbladder

Gallbladder cancers (GBCs) are cancers arising from the gallbladder mucosa. The incidence of GBC in the United States is 1 to 2 per 100,000. The incidence of GBC increases with age, with the greatest incidence in people aged 65 or older. GBC affects women three to four times more often than it does men, and is more common in Caucasians than in African Americans. Risk factors for GBC include genetic characteristics, gallstone disease, bile composition, calcification of the gallbladder wall, congenital biliary cysts or ductal anatomy, some infections, environmental carcinogens, and drugs. People with GBC are often asymptomatic, and the diagnosis may be made at the time of imaging or cholecystectomy for other indications. When symptoms are present, they are nonspecific.[105] The onset of symptoms usually is insidious, and they resemble those of cholecystitis. The diagnosis often is made unexpectedly at the time of gallbladder surgery. About 70% to 80% of people with GBC have cholelithiasis.[106] Because of its ability to produce chronic irritation of the gallbladder mucosa, it is believed that cholelithiasis plays a role in the development of GBC. It is generally considered to confer a poor prognosis because this tumor typically remains dormant until an advanced and often noncurative stage. Five-year survival rates are 80% in stage 0 disease, 50% in stage I, 28% in stage II, 7% to 8% in stage III, and 2% to 4% in stage IV.[107]

Disorders of the Exocrine Pancreas

The pancreas lies transversely in the posterior part of the upper abdomen (see Fig. 38-1). The head of the pancreas is at the right of the abdomen; it rests against the curve of the duodenum in the area of the hepatopancreatic ampulla and its entrance into the duodenum. The body of the pancreas lies beneath the stomach. The tail touches the spleen. The pancreas is virtually hidden because of its posterior position; unlike many other organs, it cannot be palpated. Because of the position of the pancreas and its large functional reserve, symptoms from conditions such as cancer of the pancreas do not usually appear until the disorder is far advanced.

The pancreas is both an endocrine and exocrine organ. The exocrine pancreas is made up of lobules that consist of acinar cells, which secrete digestive enzymes into a system of microscopic ducts. These ducts empty into the main pancreatic duct, which extends from left to right through the substance of the pancreas. The main pancreatic duct and the bile duct unite to form the hepatopancreatic ampulla, which empties into the duodenum. The sphincter of the pancreatic duct controls the flow of pancreatic secretions into duodenum (see Fig. 38-17).

The pancreatic secretions contain proteolytic enzymes that break down dietary proteins, including trypsin, chymotrypsin, carboxypolypeptidase, ribonuclease, and deoxyribonuclease. The pancreas also secretes pancreatic amylase, which breaks down starch, and lipases, which hydrolyze neutral fats into glycerol and fatty acids. The pancreatic enzymes are secreted in the inactive form and become activated in the intestine.[108] This is important because the enzymes would digest the tissue of the pancreas itself if they were secreted in the active form. The acinar cells secrete a trypsin inhibitor, which prevents trypsin activation. Because trypsin activates other proteolytic enzymes, the trypsin inhibitor prevents subsequent activation of the other enzymes.

Two types of pancreatic disease are discussed in this chapter: acute and chronic pancreatitis and cancer of the pancreas.

Acute Pancreatitis

Acute pancreatitis represents a reversible inflammatory process of the pancreatic acini brought about by premature activation of pancreatic enzymes.[109,110] Although the disease process may be limited to pancreatic tissue, it also can involve peripancreatic tissues or those of more distant organs. In the United States, up to 220,000 people are admitted to the hospital each year with acute pancreatitis.[110] Acute pancreatitis is best defined clinically by a people presenting with two of the following three criteria[111,112]: (1) symptoms (e.g., epigastric pain) consistent with pancreatitis, (2) a serum amylase or lipase level greater than three times the laboratory's upper limit of normal, and (3) radiologic imaging consistent with pancreatitis, usually using CT or MRI.

The pathogenesis of acute pancreatitis involves the autodigestion of pancreatic tissue by inappropriately activated pancreatic enzymes. The process is thought to begin with the activation of trypsin. Once activated, trypsin can then activate a variety of digestive enzymes that cause pancreatic injury, resulting in an intense inflammatory response. The acute inflammatory response itself causes substantial tissue damage and may progress beyond the pancreas to produce a systemic inflammatory response syndrome and multiorgan failure.[110] Although a number of factors are associated with the development of acute pancreatitis, most cases result from gallstones (stones in the common duct) or alcohol abuse.[110] In the case of biliary tract obstruction because of gallstones, pancreatic duct obstruction or biliary reflux is believed to activate the enzymes in the pancreatic duct system. The precise mechanisms whereby alcohol exerts its action are largely unknown. The capacity for oxidative and nonoxidative metabolism of ethanol by the pancreas and the harmful by-products that result have been related to the disease process.[110] Acute pancreatitis also is associated with hyperlipidemia, hypercalcemia, infections (particularly viral), abdominal and surgical trauma, and drugs such as thiazide diuretics.[110]

Clinical Manifestations

The manifestations of acute pancreatitis can range from mild with minimal organ dysfunction to severe and life-threatening. Overall, about 20% of people with acute pancreatitis have a severe course.[113] Abdominal pain is a cardinal manifestation of acute pancreatitis. The pain is usually located in the epigastric or periumbilical region and may radiate to the back, chest, or flank areas. Physical examination findings are variable and include fever, tachycardia, hypotension, severe abdominal tenderness, respiratory distress, and abdominal distension. Recognized markers of severe disease include laboratory values that measure the inflammatory response (*e.g.*, C-reactive protein), scoring systems that assess inflammation or organ failure, and findings on imaging studies. Clinical findings such as thirst, poor urine output, progressive tachycardia, tachypnea, hypoxemia, agitation, confusion, a rising hematocrit level, and lack of improvement in symptoms within the first 48 hours are warning signs of impending severe disease. Complications include the systemic inflammatory response, acute respiratory distress syndrome, acute tubular necrosis, and organ failure. An important disturbance related to acute pancreatitis is the loss of a large volume of fluid into the retroperitoneal and peripancreatic spaces and the abdominal cavity.

Diagnosis and Treatment

The diagnosis of acute pancreatitis requires two of the following three features: (1) abdominal pain characteristic of acute pancreatitis; (2) serum amylase and/or lipase three or more times the upper limit of normal; and (3) characteristic findings of acute pancreatitis on transabdominal ultrasound, contrast-enhanced CT scan, or MRI. This definition allows for the possibility that an amylase and/or lipase might be less than three times the upper limit of normal in acute pancreatitis. In a person with abdominal pain characteristic of acute pancreatitis and serum enzyme levels that are lower than three times the upper limit of normal, a CT scan must be performed to confirm a diagnosis of acute pancreatitis.

Once the diagnosis of acute pancreatitis is established, people are classified on the basis of disease severity. The Atlanta Criteria revision[112] of 2012 classifies severity as mild, moderately severe, or severe. Mild acute pancreatitis, the most common form, has no organ failure, no local or systemic complications, and usually resolves in the first week. Moderately severe acute pancreatitis is defined by the presence of transient organ failure (lasting <48 hours) and/or local complications. Severe acute pancreatitis is defined by persistent organ failure (lasting >48 hours). Local complications include peripancreatic fluid collections, pancreatic and peripancreatic necrosis (sterile or infected), pseudocyst, and walled-off necrosis (sterile or infected). The white blood cell count may be increased, and hyperglycemia and an elevated serum bilirubin level may be present. Determination of the cause is important in guiding the immediate management and preventing recurrence. Abdominal ultrasonography is usually performed to assess for gallstones. CT scans and dynamic contrast-enhanced CT of the pancreas are used to detect necrosis and fluid accumulation. Recent research has focused on potential biomarkers for predicting the severity and prognosis of pancreatitis. One study has examined trypsinogen-2 and pancreatic proteases, enzymes involved in the autodigestive processes.[114] Other investigational serologic markers include tumor necrosis factor, C-reactive protein, procalcitonin,

phospholipase A$_2$, and the cytokines interleukin-6 (IL-6), IL-8, and IL-10.[115]

Treatment measures depend on the severity of the disease. People who present with persistent or severe pain, vomiting, dehydration, or signs of impending severe acute pancreatitis require hospitalization. Treatment measures are directed at pain relief, withholding oral foods and fluids, and restoration of lost plasma volume. Gastric suction is instituted to treat distension of the bowel and prevent further stimulation of the secretion of pancreatic enzymes. Intravenous fluids and electrolytes are administered to replace those lost from the circulation and to combat hypotension and shock. Intravenous colloid solutions are given to replace the fluid that has become sequestered in the abdomen and retroperitoneal space.

Complications

Sequelae in people surviving an episode of severe acute pancreatitis include fluid collections and infection.[113] In people with acute necrotizing pancreatitis, the necrotic debris becomes infected, usually by gram-negative organisms from the alimentary canal, further complicating the condition.[116] Fluid collections with a high level of pancreatic enzymes are usually associated with pancreatic duct disruptions and may eventually form pseudocysts (a collection of pancreatic fluid enclosed in a layer of inflammatory tissue). A pseudocyst most often is connected to a pancreatic duct, so that it continues to increase in mass. The symptoms depend on its location; for example, jaundice may occur when a cyst develops near the head of the pancreas, close to the common duct. Pseudocysts may resolve or, if they persist, may require surgical intervention.

Chronic Pancreatitis

Chronic pancreatitis is characterized by progressive destruction of the exocrine pancreas, by fibrosis, and, in the later stages, by destruction of the endocrine pancreas. Most factors that cause acute pancreatitis can also cause chronic pancreatitis. However, the chief distinction between the two conditions is the irreversibility of pancreatic function that is characteristic of chronic pancreatitis.[117] By far the most common cause of chronic pancreatitis in Western countries is long-term alcohol abuse.[113] Less common causes are long-standing obstruction of the pancreatic duct by pseudocysts, calculi, or neoplasms; autoimmune chronic pancreatitis, which occurs in association with autoimmune disorders such as Sjögren syndrome, PSC, and inflammatory bowel disease; idiopathic chronic pancreatitis, associated with cystic fibrosis; and hereditary pancreatitis, a rare autosomal dominant disorder that is associated with both acute and chronic pancreatitis.

Clinical Manifestations

Chronic pancreatitis is manifested in episodes that are similar but less severe than acute pancreatitis. People with chronic pancreatitis have persistent, recurring episodes of epigastric and upper left quadrant pain; the attacks often are precipitated by alcohol abuse or overeating.

Anorexia, nausea, vomiting, constipation, and flatulence are common. Eventually, the disease progresses to the extent that endocrine and exocrine pancreatic functions become deficient. At this point, signs of diabetes mellitus and the malabsorption syndrome (*e.g.*, weight loss and fatty stools [steatorrhea]) become apparent.

Treatment

Treatment consists of measures to treat coexisting biliary tract disease. A low-fat diet usually is prescribed. The signs of malabsorption may be treated with pancreatic enzymes. When diabetes is present, it is treated with insulin. Alcohol is forbidden because it frequently precipitates attacks. Frequent pain is treated with narcotics or may require surgical intervention and focuses on relieving any obstruction that may be present. In advanced cases, a subtotal or total pancreatectomy may be necessary.[113]

Cancer of the Pancreas

There are a number of types of pancreatic cancer. The most common, pancreatic adenocarcinoma, accounts for about 85% of cases, and the term *pancreatic cancer* is sometimes used to refer only to that type.[118] In 2019, approximately 56,770 people (29,940 men and 26,830 women) will be diagnosed with pancreatic cancer. Another 45,750 people (23,800 men and 21,950 women) are expected to die of pancreatic cancer. It is the cause of 7% of all cancer deaths. It ranks fourth as a cause of cancer death in both men and women in the United States each year. Early-stage pancreatic cancer usually has no symptoms and spreads quickly throughout the body, making it difficult to detect and harder to treat when it is found in its later stages.[119] For all stages combined, the 5-year survival rate is about 7% to 8%. The 5-year survival rate for people with stage I, II, III, and IV are about 13%, 6%, 3%, and 1%, respectively.[120] One to two percent of cases of pancreatic cancer are neuroendocrine tumors, which arise from the hormone-producing cells of the pancreas. Pancreatic neuroendocrine tumors are a diverse group of benign or malignant tumors and are generally less aggressive than is pancreatic adenocarcinoma.[118]

Etiology

The cause of pancreatic cancer is unknown. Age, smoking, alcohol, obesity, diabetes mellitus, male gender, chronic pancreatitis, and hereditary factors have been found to be risk factors.[113] Pancreatic cancer rarely occurs in people younger than 50 years of age, and the risk increases with age. The most significant and reproducible environmental risk factor is cigarette smoking.[109,121] The incidence of pancreatic cancer is twice as high among smokers than nonsmokers. Overweight or obesity during early adulthood has been associated with a greater risk of pancreatic cancer. A younger age of disease onset and onset at an older age were associated with lower overall survival in people with pancreatic cancer. According to the American Cancer Society, 56,770 people (29,940 men and 26,830 women) will be diagnosed with pancreatic cancer in 2019.[122] Hereditary pancreatitis and familial atypical mole multiple melanoma syndrome are two other causes linked to pancreatic cancer.[113]

Clinical Manifestations

Most pancreatic cancers are adenocarcinomas of the ductal epithelium, and symptoms are primarily caused by mass effect rather than disruption of exocrine or endocrine function. The clinical manifestations depend on the size and location of the tumor as well as its metastasis. Pain, jaundice, and weight loss constitute the classic presentation of the disease. The most common pain is a dull epigastric pain often accompanied by back pain, often worse in the supine position, and relieved by sitting forward. Although the tumor can arise anywhere in the pancreas, the most frequent site is the head (60%), followed by the body (10%), and tail (5%). The pancreas is diffusely involved in the remaining 25%.[118] Because of the proximity of the pancreas to the common duct and the hepatopancreatic ampulla, cancer of the head of the pancreas tends to obstruct bile flow. Jaundice frequently is the presenting symptom of a person with cancer of the head of the pancreas, and it usually is accompanied by complaints of pain and pruritus.[123] Cancer of the body of the pancreas usually impinges on the celiac ganglion, causing pain. The pain usually worsens with ingestion of food or assumption of the supine position. Cancer of the tail of the pancreas usually has metastasized before symptoms appear.

Migratory thrombophlebitis (deep vein thrombosis) develops in about 10% of people with pancreatic cancer, particularly when the tumor involves the body or tail of the pancreas.[109] Thrombi develop in multiple veins, including the deep veins of the legs, the subclavian vein, the inferior and superior mesentery veins, and even the vena cava. It is not uncommon for the migratory thrombophlebitis to provide the first evidence of pancreatic cancer, although it may present in other cancers as well. The mechanism responsible for the hypercoagulable state is largely unclear, but it may relate to activation of clotting factors by proteases released from the tumor cells.[109]

Diagnosis and Treatment

Personal history, physical examination, and elevated serum bilirubin and alkaline phosphate levels may suggest the presence of pancreatic cancer, but are not diagnostic.[123] The serum cancer antigen (CA 19-9), a Lewis blood group antigen, may help confirm the diagnosis in symptomatic people and may help predict prognosis and recurrence after resection. However, CA 19-9 has a sensitivity and specificity of 80% to 90%, so it does not confirm the diagnosis.[123]

Ultrasonography and CT scanning are the most frequently used diagnostic methods to confirm the disease. Percutaneous fine-needle aspiration cytology of the pancreas has been one of the major advances in the diagnosis of pancreatic cancer. Unfortunately, the smaller and more curable tumors are most likely to be missed by this procedure. ERCP may be used for evaluation of people with suspected pancreatic cancer and obstructive jaundice.

Surgical resection of the tumor is done when the tumor is localized. However, this only occurs in 15% to 20% of people because most cancers of the pancreas have metastasized by the time of diagnosis.[124] Otherwise, surgical resection is reserved for palliative measures. Radiation therapy may be useful when the disease is not resectable but appears to be localized. The use of irradiation and chemotherapy for pancreatic cancer continues to be investigated. Pain control is one of the most important aspects in the management of people with end-stage pancreatic cancer. Ultimately, prognosis for pancreatic cancer remains poor, even after potentially curative surgery in appropriately selected people. Five-year survival rates after resection remain approximately 25%.[125]

SUMMARY CONCEPTS

The biliary tract serves as a passageway for the delivery of bile from the liver to the intestine. This tract consists of the bile ducts and gallbladder. The most common causes of biliary tract disease are cholelithiasis and cholecystitis. Three factors contribute to the development of cholelithiasis: abnormalities in the composition of bile, stasis of bile, and inflammation of the gallbladder. Cholelithiasis predisposes to obstruction of bile flow, causing biliary colic and acute or chronic cholecystitis. Cancer of the gallbladder, which has a poor 5-year survival rate, occurs in 2% of people with biliary tract disease.

The pancreas is an endocrine and exocrine organ. The exocrine pancreas produces digestive enzymes that are secreted in an inactive form and transported to the small intestine through the main pancreatic duct, which usually empties into the hepatopancreatic ampulla and then into the duodenum through the sphincter of the pancreatic duct. The most common diseases of the exocrine pancreas are acute and chronic forms of pancreatitis, and cancer. Acute and chronic pancreatitis are associated with biliary reflux and chronic alcoholism. Acute pancreatitis is an inflammatory condition of the pancreas because of inappropriate activation of pancreatic enzymes, with manifestations that can range from mild to severe and life threatening. Chronic pancreatitis causes progressive destruction of the endocrine and exocrine pancreas. It is characterized by episodes of pain and epigastric distress that are similar to but less severe than those that occur with acute pancreatitis. Cancer of the pancreas is the fourth leading cause of cancer death in the United States. It usually is far advanced at the time of diagnosis, and the 5-year survival rate is 5%.

Review Exercises

1. A 24-year-old woman reports to her health care professional with complaints of a yellow discoloration of her skin, loss of appetite, and a feeling of upper gastric discomfort. She denies use of intravenous drugs and has not received blood products. She cannot recall eating uncooked shellfish or drinking water that might have been contaminated. She has a daughter who attends day care.

   A. What tests could be done to confirm a diagnosis of hepatitis A?
   B. What is the most common mode of transmission for hepatitis A? It is suggested that the source might be through the day care center that her daughter attends. Explain.
   C. What methods could be used to protect other family members from getting the disease?

2. A 56-year-old man with a history of heavy alcohol consumption and a previous diagnosis of alcoholic cirrhosis and portal hypertension is admitted to the emergency department with acute gastrointestinal bleeding because of a tentative diagnosis of bleeding esophageal varices and signs of circulatory shock.

   A. Relate the development of esophageal varices to portal hypertension in people with cirrhosis of the liver.
   B. Many people with esophageal varices have blood coagulation problems. Explain.

3. A 40-year-old woman presents in the emergency department with a sudden episode of vomiting and severe right epigastric pain that developed after eating a fatty evening meal. Although there is no evidence of jaundice in her skin, the sclera of her eyes is noted to have a yellowish discoloration. Palpation reveals tenderness of the upper right quadrant with muscle splinting and rebound pain. Right upper quadrant abdominal ultrasonography confirms the presence of gallstones. The woman is treated conservatively with pain and antiemetic medications. She is subsequently scheduled for a laparoscopic cholecystectomy.

   A. Relate this woman's signs and symptoms to gallstones and their effect on gallbladder function.
   B. Explain the initial appearance of jaundice in the eyes as opposed to the skin. Which of the two laboratory tests for bilirubin would you expect to be elevated—direct (conjugated) or indirect (unconjugated or free)?
   C. What effect will removal of the gallbladder have on the storage and release of bile into the intestine, particularly as it relates to meals?

REFERENCES

1. Segal S. S. (2017). Special circulations. In Boron W. F., Boulpaep E. L. (Eds.), *Medical physiology* (3rd ed., pp. 556–571). Philadelphia, PA: Saunders Elsevier.
2. Suchy F. J. (2017). Hepatobiliary function. In Boron W. F., Boulpaep E. L. (Eds.), *Medical physiology* (3rd ed., pp. 944–971). Philadelphia, PA: Saunders Elsevier.

3. Hall J. E. (2015). *Guyton and Hall textbook of medical physiology* (13th ed., pp. 881–886). Philadelphia, PA: Saunders Elsevier.

4. Dawson P. A. (2016). Bile secretion and enterohepatic circulation. In Feldman M., Friedman L. S., Brandt L. J. (Eds.), *Sleisenger and Fordtran's gastrointestinal and liver disease* (10th ed., pp. 1085–1099). Philadelphia, PA: Saunders Elsevier.

5. Rubin R., Rubin E. (2014). The liver and biliary system. In Rubin R., Strayer D. S. (Eds.), *Rubin's pathophysiology: Clinicopathologic foundations of medicine* (7th ed., pp. 825–886). Philadelphia, PA: Lippincott Williams & Wilkins.

6. Jameson J. L. (2018). Jaundice. In Jameson J. L., Fauci A. S., Kasper D. L., et al. (Ed.), *Harrison's principles of internal medicine* (20th ed., pp. 276–280). New York, NY: McGraw Hill.

7. Deng B.-C., Lv S., Cui W., et al. (2012). Novel ATP8B1 mutation in an adult male with progressive familial intrahepatic cholestasis. *World Journal of Gastroenterology* 18(44), 6504–6509. doi:10.3748/wjg.v18.i44.6504

8. Patel K. R. Alagille syndrome. PathologyOutlines.com. [Online]. Available: http://www.pathologyoutlines.com/topic/liveralagillessyndrome.html. Accessed January 31, 2018

9. Suchy F. J. (2016). Anatomy, histology, embryology, developmental anomalies, and pediatric disorders of the biliary tract. In Feldman M., Friedman L. S., Brandt L. J. (Eds.), *Sleisenger and Fordtran's gastrointestinal and liver disease* (10th ed., pp. 1055–1077). Philadelphia, PA: Saunders Elsevier.

10. Theise N. D., Crawford J. M., Lui C. (2015). The liver and bile ducts. In Kumar V., Abbas A. K., Aster J. C. (Eds.), *Robbins and Cotran pathologic basis of disease* (9th ed., pp. 821–881). Philadelphia, PA: Saunders Elsevier.

11. Chernecky C. C., Berger B. J. (2012). *Laboratory tests and diagnostic procedures* (6th ed.). Philadelphia, PA: Saunders Elsevier.

12. Jameson, J. L. (2018). Hyperbilirubinemias. In Jameson J. L., Fauci A. S., Kasper D. L., et al. (Ed.), *Harrison's principles of internal medicine* (20th ed., pp. 2342–2346). New York, NY: McGraw Hill.

13. Jameson J. L. (2018). Evaluation of liver function. In Jameson J. L., Fauci A. S., Kasper D. L., et al. (Ed.), *Harrison's principles of internal medicine* (20th ed., pp. 2338–2341). New York, NY: McGraw Hill.

14. Laura P., Kampfrath T. (2017). Chapter 8: Enzymes. In Larson D. (Ed.), *Clinical chemistry: Fundamentals and laboratory techniques*. St. Louis, MO: Elsevier. ISBN 9781455742141

15. Botros M., Sikaris K. A. (2013). The de ritis ratio: The test of time. *The Clinical Biochemist Reviews* 34(3), 117–130.

16. Torruellas C., French S. W., Medici V. (2014). Diagnosis of alcoholic liver disease. *World Journal of Gastroenterology* 20(33), 11684–11699. doi:10.3748/wjg.v20.i33.11684

17. Teoh N. C., Chitturi S., Farrell G. C. (2016). Hepatic drug metabolism and liver disease caused by drugs. In Feldman M., Friedman L. S., Brandt L. J. (Eds.), *Sleisenger and Fordtran's gastrointestinal and liver disease* (10th ed., pp. 1442–1477). Philadelphia, PA: Saunders Elsevier.

18. Katzung B. G. (2014). *Basic and clinical pharmacology* (13th ed., pp. 50–63). New York, NY: McGraw-Hill Medical.

19. Farrell S. E. (2018). Acetaminophen toxicity treatment & management. Medscape Medical News. Available: https://emedicine.medscape.com/article/820200-treatment. Accessed January 31, 2018

20. Chalasani N., Bonkovsky H. L., Fontana R., et al. (2015). Features and outcomes of 899 patients with drug-induced liver injury: The DILIN prospective study. *Gastroenterology* 148(7):1340–1352.e7

21. Lee W. M. (2013). Drug-induced acute liver failure. *Clinics in Liver Disease* 17(4), 575–586. doi:10.1016/j.cld.2013.07.001

22. Pandit A., Sachdeva T., Bafna P. (2012). Drug-induced hepatotoxicity: A review. *Journal of Applied Pharmaceutical Science* 02(05), 233–243.

23. Harshad D. (2012). An update on drug-induced liver injury. *Journal of Clinical and Experimental Hepatology* 2(3), 247–259.

24. Feld J. J., Heathcote E. J. (2016). Hepatitis caused by other viruses. In Feldman M., Friedman L. S., Brandt L. J. (Eds.), *Sleisenger and Fordtran's gastrointestinal and liver disease* (10th ed., pp. 1366–1373). Philadelphia, PA: Saunders Elsevier.

25. Stapleton J. T., Williams C. F., Xiang J. (2004). GB virus C: A beneficial infection? *Journal of Clinical Microbiology* 42, 3915–3919.

26. Jameson J. L. (2018). Acute viral hepatitis. In Jameson J. L., Fauci A. S., Kasper D. L., et al. (Ed.), *Harrison's principles of internal medicine* (20th ed., pp. 2347–2365). New York, NY: McGraw Hill.

27. World Health Organization. (2017). Hepatitis C: Fact sheet. [Online]. Available: https://www.who.int/en/news-room/fact-sheets/detail/hepatitis-c. Accessed January 31, 2019

28. Dudley T. (2016). Viral hepatitis. In Sargent S. (Ed.), *Liver diseases: An essential guide for nurses and healthcare professionals*. Hoboken, NJ: Wiley-Blackwell.

29. Lai M., Chopra S. (2016). Hepatitis A virus infection in adults: Epidemiology, clinical manifestations, and diagnosis. *UpToDate*. Available: https://www.uptodate.com/contents/hepatitis-a-virus-infection-in-adults-epidemiology-clinical-manifestations-and-diagnosis. Accessed January 12, 2018

30. Sjogren M. H., Basssett J. T. (2015). Hepatitis A. In Feldman M., Friedman L. S., Brandt L. J. (Eds.), *Sleisenger and Fordtran's gastrointestinal and liver disease* (10th ed., pp. 1302–1308). Philadelphia, PA: Saunders Elsevier.

31. World Health Organization. (2017). Hepatitis A: Fact sheet. [Online]. Available: http://www.who.int/mediacentre/factsheets/fs328/en/. Accessed January 31, 2018

32. World Health Organization. (2017). Hepatitis A: Vaccine. [Online]. Available: http://www.who.int/ith/vaccines/hepatitisA/en/. Accessed January 31, 2018

33. Centers for Disease Control and Prevention. (2015). Hepatitis A. [Online]. Available: https://www.cdc.gov/vaccines/pubs/pinkbook/hepa.html. Accessed January 31, 2018

34. Wells J. T., Perillo R. (2016). Hepatitis B. Hepatitis D. In Feldman M., Friedman L. S., Brandt L. J. (Eds.), *Sleisenger and Fordtran's gastrointestinal and liver disease* (10th ed., pp. 1309–1331; 1353–1359). Philadelphia, PA: Saunders Elsevier.

35. Hu J., Liu K. (2017). Complete and incomplete Hepatitis B virus particles: Formation, function, and application. *Viruses* 9(3), 56. [Online]. Available: http://www.mdpi.com/1999-4915/9/3/56/pdf

36. World Health Organization. (2017). Hepatitis B: Fact sheet. [Online]. Available: http://www.who.int/mediacentre/factsheets/fs204/en/. Accessed January 31, 2018

37. Centers for Disease Control and Prevention. (2018). Hepatitis B FAQs for health professionals. [Online]. Available: https://www.cdc.gov/hepatitis/hbv/hbvfaq.htm. Accessed January 31, 2018

38. Roberts H., Kruszon-Moran D., Ly K. N., et al. (2016). Prevalence of chronic hepatitis B virus (HBV) infection in U.S. households: National Health and Nutrition Examination Survey (NHANES), 1988–2002. *Hepatology* 63(2), 388–973.

39. Kowdley K. V., Wang C. C., Welch S., et al. (2012). Prevalence of chronic hepatitis B among foreign-born persons living in the United States by country of origin. *Hepatology* 56(2), 422–433.

40. Spradling P. R., Rupp L., Moorman A. C., et al. (2012). Hepatitis B and C virus infection among 1.2 million persons with

access to care: Factors associated with testing and infection prevalence. *Clinical Infectious Diseases* 55(8), 1047–1055.

41. Centers for Disease Control and Prevention. (2018). Viral hepatitis. [Online]. Available: https://www.cdc.gov/hepatitis/hbv/testingchronic.htm. Accessed January 31, 2018

42. Centers for Disease Control and Prevention. (2017). Surveillance for viral hepatitis–United States, 2015. [Online]. Available: https://www.cdc.gov/hepatitis/statistics/2015surveillance/index.htm. Accessed January 31, 2018

43. Schillie S., Vellozzi C., Reingold A., et al. (2018). Prevention of hepatitis B virus infection in the United States: Recommendations of the Advisory Committee on Immunization Practices. *Morbidity and Mortality Weekly Report. Recommendations and Reports* 67(RR-1), 1–31. doi:10.15585/mmwr.rr6701a1

44. Terrault N. A., Bzowej N. H., Chang K.-M., et al. (2015). AASLD guidelines for treatment of chronic hepatitis B. [Online]. Available: https://www.aasld.org/sites/default/files/guideline_documents/hep28156.pdf. Accessed January 18, 2018

45. Al-Joudi F. S., Mohd Arif M. B., Mohamed Z. B., et al. (2014). Testing for hepatitis B virus core antigen and e antigen may confer additional safety of donors' blood negative for hepatitis B virus surface antigen. *Asian Journal of Transfusion Science* 8, 63–64.

46. Mansouri N., Movafagh A., Sayad A., et al. (2014). Hepatitis B virus infection in patients with blood disorders: A concise review in pediatric study. *Iranian Journal of Pediatric Hematology and Oncology* 4(4), 178–187.

47. Hepatitis B Foundation. (2016). HBV viral load test. [Online]. Available: http://www.hepb.org/blog/tag/hbv-viral-load-test/. Accessed February 1, 2018

48. Center for Disease Control. (2018). Hepatitis C questions and answer for health professionals. Available: https://www.cdc.gov/hepatitis/hcv/hcvfaq.htm. Accessed April 23, 2019

49. National Academies of Sciences, Engineering, and Medicine. (2016). *Eliminating the public health problem of hepatitis B and C in the United States: Phase one report*. Washington, DC: The National Academies Press. doi:10.17226/23407

50. Lee M.-H., Yang H.-I., Yuan Y., et al. (2014). Epidemiology and natural history of hepatitis C virus infection. *World Journal of Gastroenterology* 20(28), 9270–9280. doi:10.3748/wjg.v20.i28.9270

51. Huffman M. M., Mounsey A. L. (2014). Hepatitis C for primary care physicians. *Journal of the American Board of Family Medicine* 27, 284–291. doi:10.3122/jabfm.2014.02.130165

52. Akamatsu N., Sugawara Y. (2012). Liver transplantation and hepatitis C. *International Journal of Hepatology* 2012, 22. doi:10.1155/2012/686135

53. Horsley-Silva J. L., Vargas H. E. (2017). New therapies for hepatitis C virus infection. *Gastroenterology & Hepatology* 13(1), 22–31.

54. Wedeyer H. (2016). Hepatitis C. In Feldman M., Friedman L. S., Brandt L. J. (Eds.), *Sleisenger and Fordtran's gastrointestinal and liver disease* (10th ed., pp. 1332–1352). Philadelphia, PA: Saunders Elsevier.

55. Nouroz F., Shaheen S., Mujtaba G., et al. (2015). An overview on hepatitis C virus genotypes and its control. *Egyptian Journal of Medical Human Genetics* 16, 291–298.

56. Centers for Disease Control and Prevention. (2017). Hepatitis C FAQs for health professionals. [Online]. Available: https://www.cdc.gov/hepatitis/hcv/hcvfaq.htm. Accessed January 31, 2018

57. Centers for Disease Control and Prevention. (2015). Hepatitis D. [Online]. Available: https://www.cdc.gov/hepatitis/hdv/index.htm. Accessed January 31, 2018

58. de Alencar Arrais Guerra J. A., Kampa K. C., Morsoletto D. G. B., et al. (2017). Hepatitis E: A literature review. *Journal of Clinical and Translational Hepatology* 5(4), 376–383. doi:10.14218/JCTH.2017.00012

59. Patrick B., Steinmann E., Manns M. P., et al. (2014). The impact of hepatitis E in the liver transplant setting. *Journal of Hepatology* 61(6), 1418–1429.

60. Zhou X., de Man R. A., de Knegt R. J., et al. (2013). Epidemiology and management of chronic hepatitis E infection in solid organ transplantation: A comprehensive literature review. *Reviews in Medical Virology* 23(5), 295–304.

61. John S. Mackenzie, Patrick Drury, Ray R. Arthur, Michael J. Ryan, Thomas Grein, Raphael Slattery, Sameera Suri, Christine Tiffany Domingo & Armand Bejtullahu (2014) The Global Outbreak Alert and Response Network, *Global Public Health*, 9:9, 1023-1039, DOI: 10.1080/17441692.2014.951870

62. Centers for Disease Control and Prevention. (2015). Hepatitis E: FAQs for health professionals. [Online]. Available: https://www.cdc.gov/hepatitis/hev/hevfaq.htm. Accessed January 31, 2018

63. Friedman L. S. (2018). Liver, biliary tract, & pancreas disorders. In Papadakis M. A., McPhee S. J., Rabow M. W. (Eds.), *Current medical diagnosis & treatment 2017*. New York, NY: McGraw-Hill. Available: http://accessmedicine.mhmedical.com.ezproxy.uthsc.edu/content.aspx?bookid=1843&sectionid=135711381. Accessed March 5, 2018

64. Fialho A., Fialho A., Carey W. D. (2015). Autoimmune hepatitis. [Online]. Cleveland Clinic–Center for Continuing Education. Available: http://www.clevelandclinicmeded.com/medicalpubs/diseasemanagement/hepatology/chronic-autoimmune-hepatitis/. Accessed August 2017

65. Hubscher S. G., Burt A. D., Portmann B. C., et al. (2017). *MacSween's pathology of the liver* (7th ed.). Philadelphia, PA: Elsevier.

66. Czaja A. J. (2016). Autoimmune hepatitis. In Feldman M., Friedman L. S., Brandt L. J. (Eds.), *Sleisenger and Fordtran's gastrointestinal and liver disease* (10th ed., pp. 1493–1551). Philadelphia, PA: Saunders Elsevier.

67. Angulo P., Lindor K. D. (2015). Primary biliary cirrhosis. In Feldman M., Friedman L. S., Brandt L. J. (Eds.), *Sleisenger and Fordtran's gastrointestinal and liver disease* (10th ed., pp. 1477–1487). Philadelphia, PA: Saunders Elsevier.

68. Raszeja-Wyszomirska J., Miazgowski T. (2014). Osteoporosis in primary biliary cirrhosis of the liver. *Przegląd Gastroenterologiczny* 9(2), 82–87. doi:10.5114/pg.2014.42502

69. Yamagiwa S., Kamimura H., Takamura M., et al. (2014). Autoantibodies in primary biliary cirrhosis: Recent progress in research on the pathogenetic and clinical significance. *World Journal of Gastroenterology* 20(10), 2606–2612. doi:10.3748/wjg.v20.i10.2606

70. Pietro I., Floreani A., Carbone M., et al. (2017). Primary biliary cholangitis: Advances in management and treatment of the disease. *Digestive and Liver Disease* 49(8), 841–846.

71. Mathurin P., Bataller R. (2015). Trends in the management and burden of alcoholic liver disease. *Journal of Hepatology* 62(1 Suppl), S38–S46. doi:10.1016/j.jhep.2015.03.006

72. Cederbaum A. I. (2012). Alcohol metabolism. *Clinics in Liver Disease* 16(4), 667–685. doi:10.1016/j.cld.2012.08.002

73. Carithers R. L., McClain C. J. (2016). Alcoholic liver disease. In Feldman M., Friedman L. S., Brandt L. J. (Eds.), *Sleisenger and Fordtran's gastrointestinal and liver disease* (10th ed., pp. 1409–1427). Philadelphia, PA: Saunders Elsevier.

74. Rahimi E., Pan J.-J. (2015). Prognostic models for alcoholic hepatitis. *Biomarker Research* 3, 20. doi:10.1186/s40364-015-0046-z

75. Shaker M., Tabbaa A., Albeldawi M., et al. (2014). Liver transplantation for nonalcoholic fatty liver disease: New

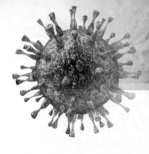

Alterations in Nutritional Status

Learning Objectives

After completing this chapter, the learner will be able to meet the following objectives:

1. State the number of calories derived from the oxidation of 1 g of protein, fat, or carbohydrate.
2. Describe four types of energy expenditure.
3. Discuss the different dietary standards that are utilized to formulate uniform diet guidelines for calories, proteins, fats, carbohydrates, fiber, vitamins, and minerals.
4. Differentiate between hunger, appetite, and satiety.
5. State the interactions between neurohormones in both short-term and long-term mechanisms to control food intake.
6. Explain the use of body mass index (BMI) in evaluating body weight.
7. Define and discuss the causes and types of obesity and health risks associated with obesity.
8. Discuss the treatment of obesity in terms of diet, behavior modification, exercise, social support, pharmacotherapy, and surgical methods.
9. Differentiate between protein–calorie starvation (*i.e.*, **marasmus**) and protein malnutrition (*i.e.*, **kwashiorkor**).
10. Explain the effect of malnutrition on muscle mass, respiratory function, acid–base balance, wound healing, immune function, bone mineralization, the menstrual cycle, and testicular function.
11. Compare the eating disorders of anorexia nervosa (AN) and bulimia nervosa (BN) and the complications associated with each.

Nutritional status describes the condition of the body with respect to the availability and use of nutrients. Nutrients that are taken into the body can be used to provide the energy needed to perform various body functions, or they can be stored for future use. The stability and composition of body weight over time require that a person's energy intake be balanced with energy expenditure. When a person is overfed and nutrient intake consistently exceeds expenditure, most of the nutrients are stored and body weight increases. Conversely, when energy expenditure exceeds nutrient intake, energy stores are lost and body weight decreases.

Also, because different foods contain different amounts of proteins, fats, carbohydrates, vitamins, and minerals, appropriate amounts of these dietary elements must be maintained to ensure that all parts of the body's metabolic systems can be supplied with requisite materials. This chapter discusses the regulation of energy expenditure and storage, nutritional needs, overnutrition and obesity, and undernutrition and eating disorders.

Nutritional Status

The nutrients that the body uses to maintain its nutritional status are derived from the digestive tract through the ingestion of foods or, in some cases, through liquid feedings that are delivered directly into the gastrointestinal tract by a synthetic tube. The exception occurs in people with certain illnesses in which the digestive tract is bypassed and the nutrients are infused directly into the circulatory system. Once inside the body, nutrients are used for energy or as the building blocks for tissue growth and repair. When excess nutrients are available, they frequently are stored for future use. If the required nutrients are unavailable, the body adapts by conserving and using its nutrient stores.

Energy Metabolism

Energy is measured in heat units called *calories*. A calorie (c), also called a *gram calorie*, is the amount of heat or energy required to raise the temperature of 1 g of water by 1°C. A *kilocalorie* (kcal) or *large Calorie* (C), which is equivalent to 1000 calories, is the amount of energy needed to raise the temperature of 1 kg of water by 1°C.[1] Because a gram calorie is so small, the kilocalorie or large Calorie is often used when discussing energy metabolism. The oxidation of proteins provides 4 kcal/g; fats, 9 kcal/g; carbohydrates, 4 kcal/g; and alcohol, 7 kcal/g.

Metabolism is the organized process through which nutrients such as carbohydrates, fats, and proteins are broken down, transformed, or otherwise converted into cellular energy. The process of metabolism is unique in that it enables the continual release of energy, and it couples this energy with physiologic functioning. Because most of our energy sources come from the nutrients in the food that is eaten, the ability to store energy and control its release is important.

Anabolism and Catabolism

There are two phases of metabolism: anabolism and catabolism. *Anabolism* is the phase of metabolic storage and synthesis of cell constituents. Anabolism does not provide energy for the body; it requires energy. *Catabolism* involves the breakdown of complex molecules into substances that can be used in the production of energy. The chemical intermediates for anabolism and catabolism are called metabolites. Both anabolism and catabolism are catalyzed by enzyme systems located in body cells. A *substrate* is a substance on which an enzyme acts. Enzyme systems selectively transform fuel substrates into cellular energy and facilitate the use of energy.

Because body energy cannot be stored as heat, the cellular oxidative processes that release energy are low-temperature reactions that convert food components to chemical energy that can be stored or dissipated. The body transforms carbohydrates, fats, and proteins into the intermediary compound, *adenosine triphosphate* (ATP).[1] ATP is called the *energy currency of the cell* because almost all body cells store and use ATP as their energy source. The metabolic events involved in ATP formation allow cellular energy to be stored, used, and replenished. However, under some circumstances, decreasing metabolic efficiency can increase energy expenditure. This process may have relevance to obesity (the more energy "wasted" as heat loss, the less weight gain) but is also important in maintaining body warmth in newborns.

Energy Storage

Adipose Tissue

More than 90% of body energy is stored in the adipose tissues of the body. *Adipocytes*, or fat cells, occur singly or in small groups in loose connective tissue. In many parts of the body, they cushion body organs such as the kidneys. In addition to isolated groups of fat cells, entire regions of fat tissue are committed to fat storage. Collectively, fat cells are metabolically active in the uptake, synthesis, storage, and mobilization of lipids, which are the main source of stored fuel for the body. Some tissues, such as liver cells, are able to store small amounts of lipids, but when these lipids accumulate (so-called ectopic deposition, as occurs in fatty liver), they begin to interfere with normal cell function. Adipose tissue not only serves as a storage site for body fuels but also provides insulation for the body, fills body crevices, and protects body organs.

Adipocytes that are fully differentiated cells do not divide but have a long life span. Anyone born with large numbers of adipocytes runs the risk of becoming obese. Some immature adipocytes (termed *preadipocytes*) capable of division are present in postnatal life.[2] Fat deposition can result from proliferation of these existing immature adipocytes. Some medications can also have an important effect on fat cell numbers. The thiazolidinedione class of antidiabetic drugs can also stimulate the formation of new fat cells from preadipocytes, allowing increased uptake of glucose into these cells (and storage as fat) and resulting in the desired reduction in serum glucose levels, but with unwanted weight gain. In contrast, some drugs can cause loss of fat cells, resulting in lipodystrophy. This occurs in human immunodeficiency virus (HIV)-associated lipodystrophy in people treated with highly active antiretroviral therapy. The mechanism of fat loss is unknown. However, it may be due to increased programmed cell death of the adipocytes (*i.e.*, increased apoptosis).

There are two types of adipose tissue: white fat and brown fat. White fat is the prevalent form of adipose tissue in postnatal life. It constitutes 10% to 20% of body weight in adult men and 15% to 25% in adult women. At body temperature, the lipid content of fat cells exists

Food and supplement labels use *daily values* (DVs), which are set by the U.S. Food and Drug Administration (FDA). Percent daily value (%DV) tells the consumer what percentages of the DV one serving of a food or supplement supplies.

Nutritional Needs

Proteins, fats, carbohydrates, vitamins and minerals, and fiber each have their own function in providing the body with what it needs to maintain life and health.

Calories

Energy requirements are greater during growth periods. A person requires approximately 115 kcal/kg of body weight at birth, 105 kcal/kg at 1 year of age, and 80 kcal/kg from 1 to 10 years of age. During adolescence, boys require 45 kcal/kg of body weight and girls require 38 kcal/kg. During pregnancy, a woman needs an extra 300 kcal/day above her usual requirement, and during the first 3 months of breast-feeding, she requires an additional 500 kcal.[7]

Proteins

Proteins are required for growth and maintenance of body tissues, enzymes and antibody formation, fluid and electrolyte balance, and nutrient transport. Proteins are composed of amino acids, nine of which are essential to the body. These are leucine, isoleucine, methionine, phenylalanine, threonine, tryptophan, valine, lysine, and histidine. Complete protein foods are those that provide these essential amino acids in adequate amounts and are derived from animal sources that include milk, eggs, meat, fish, and poultry. However, there are a few vegetable-derived complete protein sources, including soy and quinoa. Other vegetable proteins, including dried peas and beans, nuts, seeds, and grains, contain all the essential amino acids but in less than adequate proportions. The average daily protein requirement is 30 to 50 g, provided the protein is of good quality, and the diet contains adequate carbohydrates and fats.[9] Diets that are adequate in calories but inadequate in protein can result in **kwashiorkor**. If both calories and protein are inadequate, protein–calorie malnutrition occurs (see "Protein–Energy Malnutrition" section).

Fats

Fat is the most concentrated source of energy. The Food and Nutrition Board has set an AMDR for fat of 20% to 35% of daily caloric intake in adults, 25% to 35% in children between 4 and 18 years of age, and 30% to 40% in children between 1 and 3 years of age.[9] The daily dietary recommendation for cholesterol is less than 300 mg. Cholesterol is a waxy lipid contained in every body cell, which is produced in the liver. It is necessary for numerous body functions, including hormone production, metabolism of many vitamins, nerve function, and cell permeability. Excess cholesterol in the body can cause significant harm and risk to the cardiovascular system. Careful monitoring of

blood levels and reduction of dietary intake of cholesterol help to keep cholesterol levels in balance.

Dietary fats are composed primarily of triglycerides (*i.e.*, a mixture of fatty acids and glycerol). The fatty acids are saturated (*SFA*), monounsaturated (*MUFA*), or polyunsaturated (*PUFA*). The SFAs elevate blood cholesterol, whereas the MUFAs and PUFAs lower blood cholesterol. Saturated fats usually are from animal sources and remain solid at room temperature. With the exception of coconut and palm oils (which are saturated), unsaturated fats are found in plant oils and usually are liquid at room temperature. *Trans fatty acids* (*TFAs*) are produced when unsaturated oils are partially hydrogenated and are called *artificial trans fats*. They are found primarily in vegetable shortenings, some margarines, and in foods containing either of these. Natural sources of TFAs include dairy products, some meats, and other animal-based foods. TFAs increase low-density lipoprotein (LDL) cholesterol ("bad cholesterol") and decrease high-density lipoprotein (HDL) cholesterol ("good cholesterol"). However, the naturally occurring trans fats may have a beneficial effect. Dietary fats provide energy, function as carriers for the fat-soluble vitamins, serve as precursors of prostaglandins, and are a source of fatty acids.

PUFAs, including linoleic acid (an omega-6 fatty acid) and alpha-linolenic acid (an omega-3 fatty acid), are examples of essential fatty acids. An AI has been set for both linoleic and alpha-linolenic acids.[9] Because certain vegetable oils are rich sources of alpha-linolenic and linoleic acid, the AI can be met by including two teaspoons per day of vegetable oil in the diet. Deficiency of linoleic acid results in dermatitis, and deficiency of alpha-linolenic acid can result in neurologic abnormalities and poor growth.

Omega-3 and omega-6 fatty acids have been found to contribute to both formation and treatment of many disease states.[1] Much is still unknown about the effects of this group of nutrients. Omega-3 acids are primarily found in cold water fish, walnuts, and flaxseeds. Omega-6 fatty acids are found in seeds and nuts. In general, omega-6 fatty acids promote inflammation, blood clotting, and cell proliferation, whereas omega-3 fatty acids decrease these functions. A diet with a balanced intake of both is often recommended.

Carbohydrates

Dietary carbohydrates are composed of simple sugars, complex carbohydrates, and indigestible carbohydrates (*i.e.*, fiber). Because of their vitamin, mineral, and fiber content, it is recommended that the bulk of the carbohydrate content in the diet be in the complex form rather than as simple sugars that contain few nutrients.

Although some tissues, such as the nervous system, require glucose as an energy source, this need can be met through the conversion of amino acids and the glycerol part of the triglyceride molecule to glucose. The fatty acids from triglycerides are converted to ketones and used for energy by other body tissues. A carbohydrate-deficient diet usually results in the loss of tissue proteins and the development of ketosis. Because protein and fat metabolism increase the production of osmotically active metabolic wastes that must be eliminated through the kidneys, there is a danger of dehydration and electrolyte imbalances. The amount of carbohydrate needed to prevent tissue wasting and ketosis is 50 to 100 g/day.

Carbohydrates should supply most of the daily energy requirement because many protein sources also are high in fat and more expensive. The AMDR indicates that carbohydrate intake should consist of 45% to 65% of the daily calories in the diet.[9] Carbohydrates should be in the form of whole grains, vegetables, and fruits, which have higher fiber content compared to refined flour and sugar products.

Vitamins and Minerals

Vitamins

Vitamins are a group of organic compounds that act as **catalysts** in various chemical reactions. A compound cannot be classified as a vitamin unless it is shown that a deficiency of it causes disease. Contrary to popular belief, vitamins do not provide energy directly. As catalysts, they are part of the enzyme systems required for the release of energy from protein, fat, and carbohydrates. Vitamins are also necessary for the formation of red blood cells, hormones, genetic materials, and the nervous system. They are essential for normal growth and development.

There are two types of vitamins: fat soluble and water soluble. The four fat-soluble vitamins are vitamins A, D, E, and K. The nine required water-soluble vitamins are thiamine, riboflavin, niacin, pyridoxine (vitamin B_6), pantothenic acid, vitamin B_{12}, folic acid, biotin, and vitamin C. Fat-soluble vitamins are stored in the body and may reach toxic levels if ingested in amounts greater than what is required by the body. Because the water-soluble vitamins are excreted in the urine, they are less likely to accumulate in the body to toxic levels. Table 39-1 lists the major food sources of vitamins.

Minerals

Minerals serve many functions. They are involved in acid–base balance and in the maintenance of osmotic pressure in body compartments. Minerals are components of vitamins, hormones, and enzymes. They maintain normal hemoglobin levels, play a role in nervous system function, and are involved in muscle contraction and skeletal development and maintenance. Minerals that are present in relatively large amounts in the body are called *macrominerals*. These include calcium, phosphorus, sodium, chloride, potassium, magnesium, and sulfur. Other minerals are classified as *trace minerals* and include iron, manganese, copper, iodine, zinc, cobalt, fluorine, and selenium. Over- or underingestion of recommended levels of minerals can result in illness or toxicity. Table 39-2 provides a list of mineral sources and their functions.

Fiber

Total fiber, which has physiologic benefits, includes dietary fiber, the non-digestible carbohydrates found in plants such as fruits, vegetables, beans, nuts, and whole grains; functional fiber, and isolated non-digestible carbohydrates. Functional fibers are synthetic or extracted from plant sources and added to food. Examples include psyllium and methylcellulose, and they are commonly found in processed foods. Dietary fiber provides increased bulk, viscosity, and fermentation. Bulking slows gastric emptying, therefore increasing satiety, and increases the rate of transport through the gastrointestinal tract, thereby increasing stool bulk and facilitating normal bowel movements. Viscosity thickens the lining of the intestinal track, helps moderate blood glucose levels, and lowers cholesterol levels. Fermentation contributes to growth of healthy intestinal bacteria and to immune system functioning. Recommendations for fiber in males and females who are young adults are 34 and 28 g, respectively, of fiber daily, whereas those older than 50 years should have 28 and 22 g, respectively, each day.[8,9]

TABLE 39-1 Major Food Sources of Vitamins	
Vitamin	**Major Food Sources**
Vitamin A (retinol, provitamin, carotenoids)	Retinol: liver, butter, whole milk, cheese, egg yolk; provitamin A: carrots, green leafy vegetables, sweet potatoes, pumpkin, winter squash, apricots, cantaloupe, fortified margarine
Vitamin D (calciferol)	Fortified dairy products, fortified margarine, fish oils, egg yolk
Vitamin E (tocopherol)	Vegetable oil, margarine, shortening, green and leafy vegetables, wheat germ, whole-grain products, egg yolk, butter, liver
Vitamin C (ascorbic acid)	Broccoli, sweet and hot peppers, collards, Brussels sprouts, kale, potatoes, spinach, tomatoes, citrus fruits, strawberries
Thiamin (vitamin B_1)	Pork, liver, meat, whole grains, fortified grain products, legumes, nuts
Riboflavin (vitamin B_2)	Liver, milk, yogurt, cottage cheese, meat, fortified grain products
Niacin (nicotinamide, nicotinic acid)	Liver, meat, poultry, fish, peanuts, fortified grain products
Folacin (folic acid)	Liver, legumes, green leafy vegetables
Vitamin B_6 (pyridoxine)	Meat, poultry, fish, shellfish, green and leafy vegetables, whole-grain products, legumes
Vitamin B_{12}	Meat, poultry, fish, shellfish, eggs, dairy products
Biotin	Kidney, liver, milk, egg yolk, most fresh vegetables
Pantothenic acid	Liver, kidney, meats, milk, egg yolk, whole-grain products, legumes

TABLE 39-2 Sources and Functions of Minerals

Mineral	Major Sources	Functions
Calcium	Milk and milk products, fish with bones, greens	Bone formation and maintenance; tooth formation, vitamin B absorption, blood clotting, nerve and muscle function
Chloride	Table salt, meats, milk, eggs	Regulates pH of stomach, acid–base balance, osmotic pressure of extracellular fluids
Cobalt	Organ meats, meats	Aids in maturation of red blood cells (as part of B_{12} molecule)
Copper	Cereals, nuts, legumes, liver, shellfish, grapes, meats	Catalyst for hemoglobin formation, formation of elastin and collagen, energy release (cytochrome oxidase and catalase), formation of melanin, formation of phospholipids for myelin sheath of nerves
Fluoride	Fluorinated water	Strengthens bones and teeth
Iodine	Iodized salt, fish	Thyroid hormone synthesis and its function in maintenance of metabolic rate
Iron	Meats, heart, liver, clams, oysters, lima beans, spinach, dates, dried nuts, enriched and whole-grain cereals	Hemoglobin synthesis, cellular energy release (cytochrome pathway), killing bacteria (myeloperoxidase)
Magnesium	Milk, green vegetables, nuts, bread, cereals	Catalyst of many intracellular nerve impulses, retention of reactions, particularly those related to intracellular enzyme reactions; low magnesium levels produce an increase in irritability of the nervous system, vasodilation, and cardiac arrhythmias
Phosphorus	Meats, poultry, fish, milk and cheese, cereals, legumes, nuts	Bone formation and maintenance; essential component of nucleic acids and energy exchange forms such as ATP
Potassium	Oranges, dried fruits, bananas, meats, potatoes, peanut butter, coffee	Maintenance of intracellular osmolality, acid–base balance, transmission of nerve impulses, catalyst in energy metabolism, formation of proteins, formation of glycogen
Sodium	Table salt, cured meats, meats, milk, olives	Maintenance of osmotic pressure of extracellular fluids, acid–base balance, neuromuscular function; absorption of glucose
Zinc	Whole-wheat cereals, eggs, legumes	Integral part of many enzymes, including carbonic anhydrase, which facilitates combination of carbon dioxide with water in red blood cells; component of lactate dehydrogenase, which is important in cellular metabolism; component of many peptidases; important in digestion of proteins in gastrointestinal tract

Regulation of Food Intake and Energy Storage

Stability of body weight and composition over time requires that energy intake matches energy utilization. Environmental, cultural, genetic, and psychological factors all influence food intake and energy expenditure. In addition, body weight is tightly controlled by various physiologic feedback control systems that contribute to the regulation of hunger, food intake, and energy expenditure.[1]

Hunger, Appetite, and Control Mechanisms of Food Intake

The sensation of *hunger* is associated with several sensory perceptions, such as the rhythmic contractions of the stomach and that "empty feeling" in the stomach that stimulates a person to seek food. A person's *appetite* is the desire for a particular type of food. *Satiety* is the feeling of fullness or decreased desire for food.

Two centers in the brain interact with various hormones and neurotransmitters to help control food intake and energy output. The arcuate nucleus of the hypothalamus has been identified as the center for hunger and satiety.[10] Other centers in the brain receive neural input from the gastrointestinal tract that provides information about stomach filling, chemical signals from nutrients (glucose, amino acids, and fatty acids) in the blood, and input from the cerebral cortex regarding the smell, sight, and taste of the food. Centers in the hypothalamus also control the secretion of several hormones (*e.g.*, thyroid and adrenocortical hormones) that regulate energy balance and metabolism.

Neurohormones are responsible for the short-term regulation of food intake either by increasing feeding considered to be orexigenic or decreasing feeding classified as anorexigenic.[11] Figure 39-2 lists several of these neural messengers and the overall effects they promote. More than 30 gastrointestinal hormone genes that play a role in regulating hunger and satiety have been identified.[12]

Three main short-term messengers that promote orexigenic effects include ghrelin, produced mainly in the stomach, and neuropeptide Y and agouti-related protein, both produced in the hypothalamus. Many of the other gut hormones have anorexigenic effects by signaling satiety to the neural centers. All of these messengers send

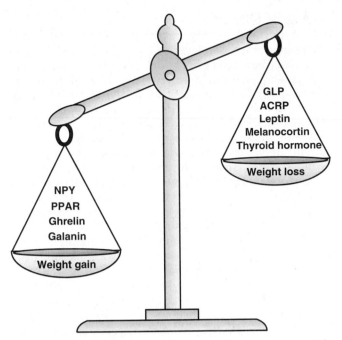

include recommendations for calories, proteins, fats, carbohydrates, vitamins, and minerals. Hunger and satiety are controlled by a complex group of neurohormones, many of which are produced in the gastrointestinal tract. These messengers function to either stimulate hunger or signal satiety to control both short- and long-term effects. Although much information has been revealed through research in recent years, there is still much to be learned effectively manage the complex process more effectively.

FIGURE 39-2. The balance of chemical mediators impacting weight gain and loss. ACRP, adipocyte complement–related protein; GLP, glucagon-like peptide; NPY, neuropeptide Y; PPAR, peroxisome proliferator–activated receptor. (From Strayer D., Rubin R. (Ed.). (2015). *Rubin's pathology: Clinicopathologic foundations of medicine* (7th ed., Fig. 13-1, p. 517). Philadelphia, PA: Lippincott Williams & Wilkins.)

messages of satiety that ultimately help decrease food intake.[10]

The intermediate- and long-term regulation of food intake is determined by the amount of nutrients that are in the blood and in storage sites. It has long been known that a decrease in blood glucose causes hunger. In contrast, an increase in breakdown products of lipids such as ketoacids produces a decrease in appetite. A ketogenic weight-loss diet (*e.g.*, the Atkins diet) relies partly on the appetite-suppressant effects of ketones in the blood.

Adipocytes release leptin in proportion to the amount of fat stores. The stimulation of leptin receptors in the hypothalamus produces a decrease in appetite and food intake as well as an increase in metabolic rate and energy consumption. It also produces a decrease in insulin release from the beta cells, which decreases energy storage in fat cells.[13]

Overweight and Obesity

Obesity is defined as having excess body fat accumulation with multiple organ-specific pathologic consequences. Overweight and obesity have become global health problems. In 2016, 1.9 billion people were classified as overweight; 650 million were further classified as obese.

In the United States, more than 65% of adults are currently either overweight or obese, and more than 36.5% of the population is obese, with obesity having an even higher prevalence in minority groups such as non-Hispanic blacks and those of Hispanic ethnicity.[14] The prevalence of overweight and obesity is even more alarming in children and adolescents. Approximately 17% of children between 2 and 19 years of age are obese—a percentage that has tripled since 1980.[15]

Body Mass Index

Clinically, obesity and overweight have been defined in terms of the BMI. The BMI is based on height and weight measurements (see Fig. 39-3) and has a correlation with body fat. In 1997, the World Health Organization defined the various classifications of overweight (BMI ≥ 25) and obesity (BMI ≥ 30). The National Institutes of Health (NIH) subsequently adopted this classification.[16] The use of a BMI cutoff of 25 as a measure of overweight raised some concern that the BMI of some men might be a function of muscle rather than of fat weight. However, it has been shown that a BMI cutoff of 25 can sensitively detect most people with overweight and does not erroneously detect people with overlean.

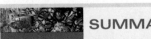
SUMMARY CONCEPTS

The body requires more than 40 nutrients on a daily basis. Nutritional status reflects the continued daily intake of nutrients over time and the deposition and use of these nutrients in the body. The DRIs classify the amounts of essential nutrients considered to be adequate to meet the known nutritional needs of healthy people. The DRIs have 22 age and sex classifications and

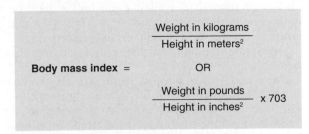

$$\text{Body mass index} = \frac{\text{Weight in kilograms}}{\text{Height in meters}^2}$$
$$\text{OR}$$
$$\frac{\text{Weight in pounds}}{\text{Height in inches}^2} \times 703$$

FIGURE 39-3. Body mass index equation.

The definition for obesity in children is a BMI at or above the sex- and age-specific 95th percentile, whereas a BMI between the 85th and 95th percentiles is defined as being overweight.[6] These criteria have been selected because they correspond to adult BMIs of 30 and 25, respectively.

Causes of Obesity

Although overweight and obesity ultimately result from an energy imbalance of eating too many calories and not getting enough physical activity, many factors contribute to both the development of obesity and the body's response to attempts to control it. Commonly acknowledged contributing causes include genetics, metabolism, behavior, environment, culture, and socioeconomic status.[17] Medical conditions such as thyroid disorder, Cushing syndrome, and polycystic ovarian syndrome can also contribute to weight gain and obesity, as do many medications.

The relationship between genetics and weight gain is complex. The most recent update of the human obesity gene map, completed in 2005, suggests that there are 100 chromosomal locations relevant to obesity.[18] Many of these relate to known brain–gut controls of hunger and satiety, metabolism, and the body's storage mechanisms. Identification of these genetic influences may allow for more targeted treatment interventions in the future. It is yet unknown how genes and mutations may directly or indirectly interact with environmental causes of obesity.[19]

There is new evidence that behavior-based interventions may help keep genetic influence in check.[17]

Environmental influence remains the major contributor to obesity worldwide.[17,18] Obesity rates have reached epidemic proportions in populations with high availability of calorie-rich foods and decreased physical activity.[18] Influences such as family eating patterns, time spent on the computer, watching television, reliance on the automobile for transportation, easy access to food, higher energy density of food, increased consumption of sugar-sweetened beverages, and increasing portion sizes have all been cited as contributing factors to overweight trends. More recent epidemiologic studies indicate that although decreased physical activity plays a role in increasing rates of overweight and obesity, diet changes because of increased availability of inexpensive, tasty, highly promoted, obesogenic types of food appear to have caused a much more steep rise in obesity.[20]

Psychological factors are another area of influence on behavior related to weight gain. Eating may be a way to cope with stress, mood, or anxiety.[21] Grazing, emotional eating, and binge eating disorder (BED) have been noted to be predictors for classifying obese patients.[22]

Culture and socioeconomic status are also believed to be contributing factors in the increased rates of overweight and obesity. It is clear that interventions will need to be developed to address the needs of different cultures, as well as to address the socioeconomic barriers to improved dietary choices.[17]

Types of Obesity

Two types of obesity, based on distribution of fat, have been described: upper body and lower body obesity (see Fig. 39-4). *Upper body obesity* is also referred to as *central, abdominal, visceral*, or *male ("android")* obesity. Lower body obesity is also known as *peripheral, gluteal–femoral*, or *female ("gynoid")* obesity. Subjects with upper body obesity are often referred to as being shaped like an "apple" compared with lower body obesity, which is more "pear" shaped. In general, men have more intra-abdominal fat and women more subcutaneous fat. As men age, the proportion of intra-abdominal fat to subcutaneous fat increases. After menopause, women tend to acquire more central fat distribution.

The obesity type is determined by dividing the waist by hip circumference. Comparison of the waist measurement and hip measurement can identify the type of obesity. A waist–hip ratio greater than 1.0 in men and 0.8 in women also indicates upper body or central obesity. Central obesity can be further differentiated into intra-abdominal adipose tissue (visceral fat) and subcutaneous abdominal adipose tissue by the use of computed tomography or magnetic resonance imaging scans.[23] Waist circumference, which is a measure of central fat distribution, measures both subcutaneous abdominal adipose tissue and intra-abdominal adipose tissue. One of the characteristics of visceral fat is the release of adipokines (such as TNF-α and adiponectin) and fatty acids directly to the liver before entering the systemic circulation, having a potentially greater impact on hepatic function (*e.g.*, the increased fatty acids are deposited in the liver, causing fatty liver, resulting in insulin resistance in the liver). Higher levels of these adipokines and circulating free fatty acids in people who are obese, particularly those with upper body obesity, are thought to be associated with many of the adverse effects of obesity.[24]

The presence of excess fat in the abdomen out of proportion to total body fat is an independent predictor of risk factors and mortality. Both BMI and waist circumference are positively correlated with total body adipose tissue, but waist circumference is a better predictor of abdominal or visceral fat content than is BMI.[25] A waist

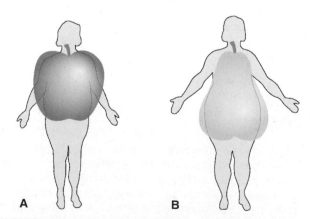

FIGURE 39-4. Distribution of adipose tissue in (**A**) upper body or central (visceral) obesity and (**B**) lower body or peripheral (subcutaneous) obesity. People with upper body obesity are often described as having an "apple-shaped" body and those with lower body obesity as having a "pear-shaped" body.

TABLE 39-3 Classification of Overweight and Obesity by BMI, Waist Circumference, and Associated Disease Risk*

	BMI (kg/m²)	Obesity Class	Disease Risk* Relative to Normal Weight and Waist Circumference	
			Men ≤ 102 cm (≤40 in) *Women ≤ 88 cm (≤35 in)*	*Men > 102 cm (>40 in)* *Women > 88 cm (>35 in)*
Underweight	<18.5		–	–
Normal†	18.5–24.9		–	–
Overweight	25.0–29.9		Increased	High
Obesity	30.0–34.9	I	High	Very high
	35.0–39.9	II	Very high	Very high
Extreme obesity	≥40	III	Extremely high	Extremely high

*Disease risk for type 2 diabetes, hypertension, and cardiovascular disease.
†Increased waist circumference also can be a marker for increased risk, even in people of normal weight.
BMI, body mass index.
From National Heart, Lung, and Blood Institute. (n.d.). Clinical guidelines on the identification, evaluation, and treatment of overweight and obesity in adults. [Online]. Available: https://www.nhlbi.nih.gov/health/educational/lose_wt/BMI/bmi_dis.htm. Accessed April 16, 2018.

circumference 88 cm (35 in) or greater in women and 102 cm (40 in) or greater in men has been associated with increased health risk[26] (see Table 39-3).

Weight loss causes a preferential loss of visceral fat (because of higher turnover of visceral fat cells than of subcutaneous) and can result in improvements in metabolic and hormonal abnormalities. Although peripheral obesity is associated with varicose veins in the legs and mechanical problems, it is not as strongly associated with cardiometabolic risk.

Health Risks Associated with Obesity

The excess body fat of obesity often significantly impairs health. Obesity puts many people at risk for the some of the leading causes of death in the United States including stroke, cancer, diabetes, kidney disease, heart disease, and respiratory diseases.[27] It has been predicted that the health effects of obesity will result in a shorter life expectancy for today's youth.[28] Adults with a BMI greater than 40 have a shorter life expectancy by 6 to 13 years.[29]

Obesity affects nearly every body system (see Fig. 39-5). Cardiac disease is increased, as well as hypertension, hypertriglyceridemia, and decreased HDL cholesterol. Significant weight gain increases the risk of developing type 2 diabetes, obstructive sleep apnea, gastric reflux, urinary stress incontinence, and gallbladder disease. Limited mobility and increased joint disorders are functional results of increased weight on the body's skeletal system. In women, obesity can contribute to infertility, higher risk pregnancy, gestational diabetes, maternal hypertension, and difficulty in labor and delivery. Infants who are born to obese mothers are more likely to be high birth weight, contributing to an increased rate of cesarean section delivery. Several types of cancer are seen in higher frequency in people who are obese, including endometrial, colon, gallbladder, prostate, kidney, and postmenopausal breast cancer. Obesity also causes nonalcoholic steatohepatitis and fatty liver disease.[16,19]

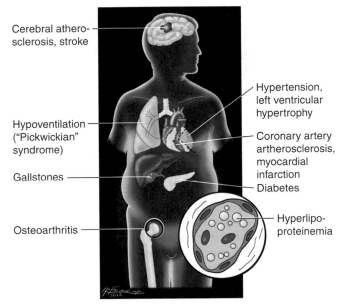

FIGURE 39-5. Medical complications of obesity. (From Strayer D., Rubin R. (Ed.). (2015). *Rubin's pathology: Clinicopathologic foundations of medicine* (7th ed., Fig. 13-5, p. 521). Philadelphia, PA: Lippincott Williams & Wilkins.)

Prevention and Treatment of Obesity

Prevention

Obesity in epidemic proportions has led to much discussion on methods of prevention. Most interventions involve modification of lifestyle behaviors to promote healthy food choices and more physical activity. Public debate is also focused on policy methods to regulate availability of less desirable food choices, such as high-calorie snacks and sweetened drinks.[17,18]

Major public education and policy efforts are now being undertaken by federal agencies. *We Can!* is a national educational program developed by the NIH to help studies. *PLoS Medicine* 11(7), e1001673. doi:10.1371/journal.pmed.1001673.

30. Flament M. F., Bissada H., Spettigue W. (2012). Evidence-based pharmacotherapy of eating disorders. *International Journal of Neuropsychopharmacology* 15(2), 189–207, doi:10.1017/S1461145711000381.

31. Rubino F., Nathan D., Eckel R., et al. (2017). Metabolic surgery in the treatment algorithm for type 2 diabetes: A joint statement by international diabetes organizations. *Obesity Surgery* 27(1), 2–21.

32. FAO, IFAD, UNICEF, WFP and WHO. (2017). *The state of food security and nutrition in the world: Building resilience for peace and food security*. Rome: FAO.

33. Roser M., Ritchie H. (2018). Hunger and undernourishment. [Online]. Available: https://ourworldindata.org/hunger-and-undernourishment. Accessed March 25, 2018.

34. Morley J. (2012). Undernutrition in older adults. *Family Practice* 29, 89–93.

35. Guyton A. C., Hall J. E. (2011). *Textbook of medical physiology* (12th ed., pp. 807–810, 859–866, 880–887). Philadelphia, PA: Elsevier Saunders.

36. Trehan I., Manary M. J. (2015). Management of severe acute malnutrition in low-income and middle-income countries. *Archives of Disease in Childhood* 100, 283–287.

37. Nigam P. K., Nigam P. (2017). Premature greying of hair (premature canities): A concern for parent and child. *Pigmentary Disorders* 4, 261.

38. Mehta N., Corkins M., Lyman B. (2013). Defining pediatric malnutrition: A paradigm shift toward etiology-related definitions. *Journal of Parenteral and Enteral Nutrition* 4(37), 460–481.

39. Bharadwaj S., Ginoya S., Tandon P., et al. (2016). Malnutrition: Laboratory markers vs nutritional assessment. *Gastroenterology Report* 4(4), 272–280. doi:10.1093/gastro/gow013.

40. National Eating Disorders Association. (2018). [Online]. Available: https://www.nationaleatingdisorders.org/learn. Accessed March 9, 2018.

41. National Institute of Mental Health. Eating disorders. (2016). [Online]. Available: https://www.nimh.nih.gov/health/topics/eating-disorders/index.shtml. Accessed March 9, 2018.

42. National Association of Anorexia Nervosa and Associated Disorders. Statistics on eating disorders. (2016). [Online]. Available: http://www.anad.org/get-information/about-eating-disorders/eating-disorders-statistics/. Accessed March 9, 2018.

43. American Psychiatric Association. (2013). *Diagnostic and statistical manual of mental disorders* (5th ed.). Arlington, VA: American Psychiatric Publishing.

44. Fonville L., Giampietro V., Williams S., et al. (2014). Alterations in brain structure in adults with anorexia nervosa and the impact of illness duration. *Psychological Medicine* 44(9), 1965–1975. doi:10.1017/S0033291713002389.

45. O'Brien P., MacDonald L., Anderson M., et al. (2013). Long-term outcomes after bariatric surgery: Fifteen-year follow-up of adjustable gastric banding and a systematic review of the bariatric surgical literature. *Annals of Surgery* 257(1), 87–94.

46. American Psychiatric Association. (2012). Guideline watch (August 2012): Practice guideline for the treatment of patients with eating disorders (3rd ed.). [Online]. Available: https://psychiatryonline.org/pb/assets/raw/sitewide/practice:guidelines/guidelines/eatingdisorders-watch.pdf. Accessed March 9, 2018.

Mechanisms of Endocrine Control

The Endocrine System

Hormones
 Hormonal Actions
 Structural Classification
 Synthesis and Release
 Transport
 Metabolism and Elimination
 Mechanisms of Action
Control of Hormone Levels
 Hypothalamic–Pituitary Regulation
 Feedback Regulation
Diagnostic Tests
 Blood Tests
 Urine Tests
 Hormone Stimulation and Suppression
  Tests
 Genetic Testing
 Imaging

Learning Objectives

**After completing this chapter, the learner
will be able to meet the following objectives:**

1. Describe the function of a hormone receptor
   that differentiates between cell surface hormone
   receptors and intracellular hormone receptors.
2. Describe the role of the hypothalamus in
   regulating pituitary control of endocrine function.
3. State the major difference between positive and
   negative feedback control mechanisms.

The endocrine system is involved in all of the integrative
aspects of life, including growth, sex differentiation,
metabolism, and adaptation to an ever-changing environment. This chapter focuses on the general aspects of

endocrine function, organization of the endocrine system,
hormone receptors and hormone actions, and regulation
of hormone levels.

The Endocrine System

The endocrine system uses chemical substances called
hormones as a means of regulating and integrating body
functions. The endocrine system participates in many
essential body functions, including the regulation of digestion, the usage and storage of nutrients, growth and
development, electrolyte and water metabolism, and reproductive functions. The endocrine network is closely
integrated with the central and peripheral nervous systems as well as with the immune systems. Therefore, the
terms "neuroendocrine" and "neuroendocrine–immune"
are often used to describe these interactions.[1,2]

Hormones

Hormones are chemical messengers that are transported
in body fluids. They are highly specialized organic molecules produced by endocrine cells that exert their action on specific target cells. The word *hormone* is from
the Greek word for "arouse to activity."[2] Hormones
do not perform reactions themselves, but instead hormones function as modulators of cellular and systemic
responses. Most hormones are present in body fluids
at all times, in greater or lesser amounts depending on
the needs of the body.[3,4] Hormones are released from
various organs that are "endocrine glands," including
the pituitary gland, thyroid gland, adrenal glands, and
pancreas. Many other organs and tissues throughout
the body also actively secrete hormonal substances that

Cell Surface Receptors. Peptide hormones and catecholamines tend to be water-soluble molecules that are electrically charged (polar) molecules. Because of their low lipid solubility and high electrical charge, peptide hormones and catecholamines cannot readily cross the lipid cellular membrane.[2,3] Instead, these hormones interact with surface receptors to generate an intracellular signal through a *second messenger* signaling system, with the hormone acting as the first messenger. The first messenger hormone signals the need for action; however, the hormone itself never enters the cell. It is the second messenger molecules inside the cell that interact directly with the intracellular control mechanisms to effect the change.[2,3] For example, the first messenger hormone glucagon binds to surface receptors on liver cells to send a second intracellular message for glycogen breakdown.[2,3]

Intracellular Receptors. Lipid-soluble hormones (such as steroid hormones and the thyroid hormones) are typically nonpolar and can pass freely through cell membranes to bind with intracellular receptors.[2,3] The intracellular hormone–receptor complex can then directly exert the hormonal effects by entering the cell nucleus to bind with hormone response elements that activate or suppress intracellular mechanisms of protein synthesis.[2,3]

Control of Hormone Levels

Hormone secretion varies widely over a 24-hour period. Some hormones, such as GH and adrenocorticotropic hormone (ACTH), have diurnal fluctuations that vary with the sleep–wake cycle.[2] Others, such as the female sex hormones, are secreted in a complicated cyclic manner. The levels of hormones, such as insulin and ADH, are regulated by feedback mechanisms that monitor substances such as glucose (insulin) and water (ADH) in the body. The levels of many of the hormones are regulated by feedback mechanisms that involve the hypothalamic–pituitary target cell system.[3]

Hypothalamic–Pituitary Regulation

The hypothalamus and pituitary gland form a functional unit that exerts control over the activities of several endocrine glands and thus a wide range of physiologic functions. The hypothalamus is located centrally in the brain and serves as the coordinating center of the brain for endocrine, behavioral, and autonomic nervous system function. It is at the level of the hypothalamus that emotion, pain, body temperature, and other neural inputs are communicated to the endocrine system.[3]

The pituitary gland is connected to the floor of the hypothalamus by the pituitary stalk, with the main structural portion of the pituitary gland encased in a bony structure called the sella turcica. The opening to the sella turcica is bridged over by the diaphragma sellae, which protects the pituitary gland from the transmission of the pressures from the cerebrospinal fluid.[6] The pituitary gland is also called the "hypophysis." The pituitary consists of two structurally different sections (Fig. 40-2):

1. The *anterior pituitary*, also called the adenohypophysis because of its glandular structure. The hypothalamus and anterior pituitary are connected by blood flow through the hypophyseal portal venous system, which begins in the hypothalamus and drains into the anterior pituitary gland.
2. The *posterior pituitary*, also called the neurohypophysis. The hypothalamus and posterior pituitary are connected through nerve axons from neurons that originate in the hypothalamus and connect the supraoptic and paraventricular nuclei of the hypothalamus with the posterior pituitary gland.
3. Melanocyte-stimulating hormones (MSH) are produced in the intermediate part of the pituitary gland. MSH regulates the production of melanin which provides protection against harmful ultraviolet rays from the sun.

Hypothalamic Hormones

The hypothalamus produces hormones that act upon the anterior pituitary to regulate the synthesis and release of anterior pituitary hormones. These hypothalamic hormones are called releasing hormones (RHs) or inhibiting hormones, based on the response sent to the anterior pituitary. RHs signal for the anterior pituitary to increase the synthesis and release of a particular hormone, whereas inhibiting hormones have the reverse effect—decreased hormonal release by the anterior pituitary. These RHs and inhibiting hormones travel to the anterior pituitary through a localized portal venous system[2,3] (Fig. 40-2). The hypothalamic hormones that regulate the secretion of anterior pituitary hormones include GH-releasing hormone (GHRH), somatostatin, dopamine, TRH, corticotropin-releasing hormone (CRH), and gonadotropin-releasing hormone (GnRH).[2,3]

The hypothalamus also sends regulatory signals to the posterior pituitary; however, the route through which the message is conducted is through nerve tracts instead of through release of hormones into the blood. The posterior pituitary is called the neurohypophysis because it contains a series of neurons whose cell bodies are located in the hypothalamus and axons extend down into the posterior pituitary. The posterior pituitary can essentially be thought of as an extension of the hypothalamus. The posterior pituitary hormones, ADH and oxytocin, are synthesized in the cell bodies of neurons in the hypothalamus that have axons that travel to the posterior pituitary.[2,3]

The activity of the hypothalamus is regulated by both hormonally mediated signals (*e.g.*, negative feedback signals) and neuronal input from a number of sources. Neuronal signals are mediated by neurotransmitters, such as acetylcholine, dopamine, norepinephrine, serotonin, γ-aminobutyric acid, and opioids. Cytokines that are involved in immune and inflammatory responses, such as the interleukins, are also involved in the regulation of hypothalamic function. This is particularly true of the hormones involved in the hypothalamic–pituitary–adrenal axis. Thus, the hypothalamus can be viewed as a bridge by which signals from multiple systems are relayed to the pituitary gland.[2,3] (Fig. 40-3).

Pituitary Hormones

The pituitary gland has been called the *master gland* because its hormones control the functions of many target glands and cells.[2] Hormones produced by the anterior

Understanding ➡ Hormone Receptors

Hormones bring about their effects on cell activity by binding to specific cell receptors. There are two general types of receptors: **(1)** cell surface receptors that exert their actions through cytoplasmic second messenger systems and **(2)** intracellular nuclear receptors that modulate gene expression by binding to DNA or promoters of target genes.

1

Cell Surface Receptors Water-soluble peptide hormones (such as parathyroid hormone and glucagon) cannot penetrate the lipid layer of the cell plasma membrane and, therefore, exert their effects through intracellular second messengers. They bind to a portion of a membrane receptor that protrudes through the surface of the cell. This produces a structural change in the receptor molecule itself, causing activation of a hormone-regulated signal system located on the inner aspect of the cell membrane. This system allows the cell to sense extracellular events and pass this information to the intracellular environment. There are several types of cell surface receptors, including G-protein–coupled receptors, which mediate the actions of catecholamines, prostaglandins, TSH, and others. Binding of the hormone to the receptor activates a G-protein, which, in turn, acts on an effector such as adenyl cyclase to generate a second messenger, such as cyclic adenosine monophosphate. The second messenger, in turn, activates other enzymes that participate in cellular secretion, gene activation, or other target cell responses.

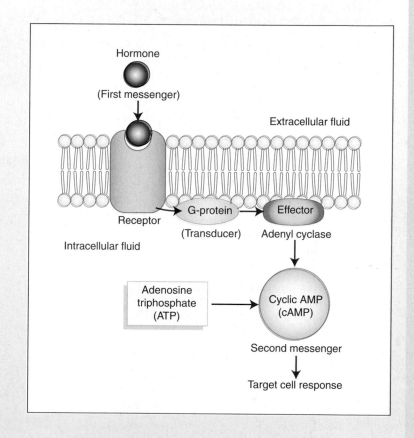

②

Nuclear Receptors Steroid hormones, vitamin D, thyroid hormones, and other lipid-soluble hormones diffuse across the cell membrane into the cytoplasm of the target cell. Once inside the cell, these hormones bind to an intracellular receptor that is activated by the binding and then moves to the nucleus, where the hormone binds to a hormone response element in the promoters on a target gene or to another transcription factor. This binding results in transcription of a specific messenger RNA, which moves into the cytoplasm, where the "transcribed message" is translated by cytoplasmic ribosomes to produce new cellular proteins or to change the production of existing proteins. This hormone-directed change in protein synthesis leads to cellular responses, such as the promotion of a specific intracellular response or the synthesis of specific proteins to be secreted from the cell.

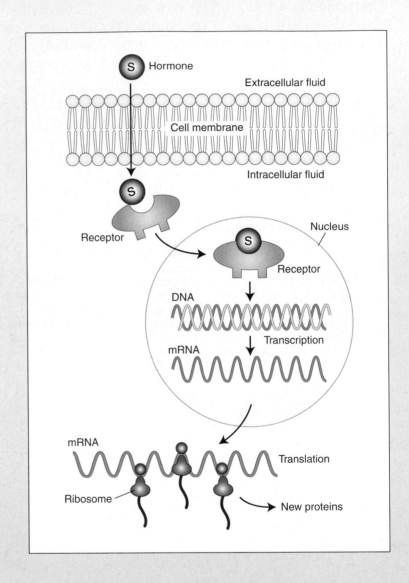

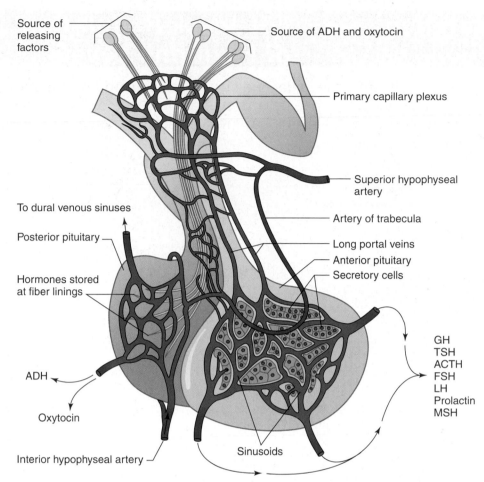

Source of releasing factors

Source of ADH and oxytocin

Primary capillary plexus

Superior hypophyseal artery

Artery of trabecula

To dural venous sinuses

Long portal veins

Posterior pituitary

Anterior pituitary

Secretory cells

Hormones stored at fiber linings

ADH

Oxytocin

GH
TSH
ACTH
FSH
LH
Prolactin
MSH

Interior hypophyseal artery

Sinusoids

FIGURE 40-2. The hypothalamus and the anterior and posterior pituitary. The hypothalamic releasing or inhibiting hormones are transported to the anterior pituitary through the portal vessels. ADH and oxytocin are produced by nerve cells in the supraoptic and paraventricular nuclei of the hypothalamus and then transported through the nerve axon to the posterior pituitary, where they are released into the circulation. ACTH, adrenocorticotropic hormone; ADH, antidiuretic hormone; FSH, follicle-stimulating hormone; GH, growth hormone; LH, luteinizing hormone; TSH, thyroid-stimulating hormone.

pituitary control body growth and metabolism (GH), function of the thyroid gland (TSH), glucocorticoid hormone levels (ACTH), function of the gonads (FSH and luteinizing hormone [LH]), and breast growth and milk production (prolactin). Hypothalamic RHs regulate most of the pituitary hormones. GH secretion is stimulated by GHRH, TSH by TRH, ACTH by CRH, and LH and FSH by GnRH.[2,3]

Feedback Regulation

The level of many of the hormones in the body is regulated by negative feedback mechanisms.[2,3] In the endocrine system, sensors detect a change in the hormone level and adjust hormone secretion so that body levels are maintained within an appropriate range. When the sensors detect a decrease in hormone levels, they initiate changes that cause an increase in hormone production. When hormone levels rise above the set point of the system, the sensors cause the production and release of hormones decrease. The feedback loops for the hypothalamic–pituitary feedback mechanisms are illustrated in Figure 40-3.

In positive feedback control, rising levels of a hormone cause another gland to release a hormone that is stimulating to the first.[3] An example is increased estradiol production during the follicular stage of the menstrual cycle causes increased gonadotropin (FSH) production by the anterior pituitary gland. This stimulates further increases in estradiol levels until the demise of the follicle, which is the source of estradiol, results in a fall in gonadotropin levels.[3]

Diagnostic Tests

Many techniques are available for assessing endocrine function and hormone levels. Diagnostic assessments include blood tests, urine tests, hormone stimulation and suppression tests, genetic testing, and diagnostic imaging studies.

Blood Tests

Blood tests for endocrine disorders encompass a wide variety of strategies to assess endocrine function. Hormones

Understanding ➔ Feedback Regulation of Hormone Levels

Like many physiologic systems, the endocrine system is regulated by feedback mechanisms that enable the endocrine cells to change their rate of hormone secretion. Feedback can be negative or positive and may involve complex feedback loops, involving hypothalamic–pituitary regulation.

1 **Negative Feedback** With negative feedback, the most common mechanism of hormone control, some feature of hormone action directly or indirectly inhibits further hormone secretion so that the hormone level returns to an ideal level or set point. In the simple negative feedback loop, the amount of hormone or its effect on a physiologic mechanism regulates the response of the endocrine gland.

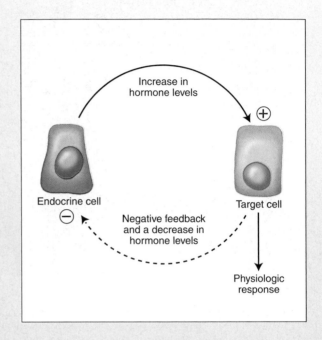

2 **Hypothalamic–Pituitary Target Cell Feedback** Hormones of the thyroid, adrenal cortex, and the gonads are regulated by more complex loops involving the hypothalamus and anterior pituitary gland. The hypothalamus produces a RH that stimulates the production of a tropic hormone by the anterior pituitary. The tropic hormone then stimulates the peripheral target gland to secrete its hormone, which acts on target cells to produce a physiologic response. A rise in blood levels of the target gland hormone also feeds back to the hypothalamus and anterior pituitary gland, resulting in a decrease in tropic hormone secretion and a subsequent reduction in hormone secretion by the target gland. As a result, blood levels of the hormone vary only within a narrow range.

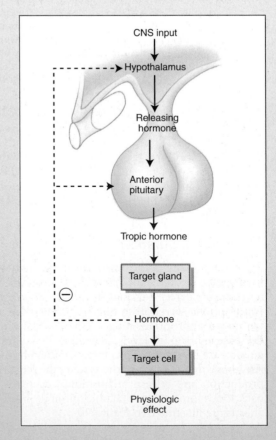

③ Positive Feedback A small number of hormones are regulated by positive feedback. In this type of regulation, a hormone stimulates continued secretion until appropriate levels are reached.

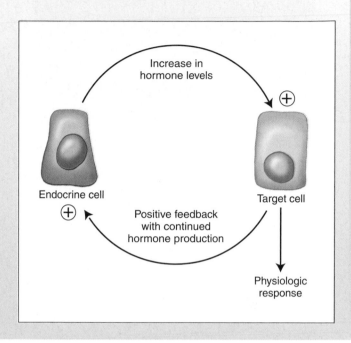

can be measured directly or, very commonly, physiologic indicators of hormone function can be measured to indirectly reflect hormone levels. Blood hormone levels provide information about hormone levels at a specific time under specific conditions.

Hormone levels in plasma are measured using radioimmunoassay (RIA) methods based on the competitive binding of hormones.[3] This method uses a radiolabeled form of the hormone and a hormone antibody that has been prepared by a purified form of the hormone. The limitations of RIA include a lack of specificity because of cross-reactivity with more than one hormone.[3] The immunoradiometric assay (IRMA) uses the same principle of antibody recognition with two antibodies instead of one. These two antibodies are directed against two different parts of the molecule; therefore, IRMA is more specific.[9]

Enzyme-linked immunosorbent assay (ELISA) assesses endocrine function and does not require the use of radioisotopes. ELISA testing combines the use of antibody testing using two antibodies that use different antigen-binding sites (which allows higher specificity) with an enzyme testing approach (which has high sensitivity). The ELISA test method is widely used and has been demonstrated to be both cost-effective and accurate.[3] Other blood tests that are routinely measured in endocrine disorders include tests for various autoantibodies.[10,11]

Urine Tests

Measurements of urinary hormone or hormone metabolite excretion are often done on a 24-hour urine sample and provide a better measure of hormone levels during that period compared to hormones measured in an isolated blood sample. In particular, a 24-hour urine sample for urinary cortisol levels is frequently performed in the diagnostic workup for Cushing syndrome.[12]

Hormone Stimulation and Suppression Tests

Hormone stimulation tests are used when hypofunction of an endocrine organ is suspected. A tropic or stimulating hormone can be administered to test the capacity of an endocrine organ to increase hormone production. The capacity of the target gland to respond is measured by an increase in the appropriate hormone.[2]

Suppression tests are used when hyperfunction of an endocrine organ is suspected. When an organ or a tissue is functioning autonomously, a suppression test may be useful to confirm the situation.

Genetic Testing

Genetic testing is rapidly becoming an important approach for the diagnosis of selected endocrine disorders. Some endocrine-related disorders for which specific genetic pathophysiologic markers have been identified include X-linked hypophosphatemic rickets, epithelial thyroid carcinoma, hypopituitarism, familial pheochromocytoma and paraganglioma, multiple endocrine neoplasia types I and II, and certain disorders of short stature, including Turner syndrome.[2] A drawback to genetic testing is the cost, which, at this point in the development of the technology, can still be quite expensive.[2]

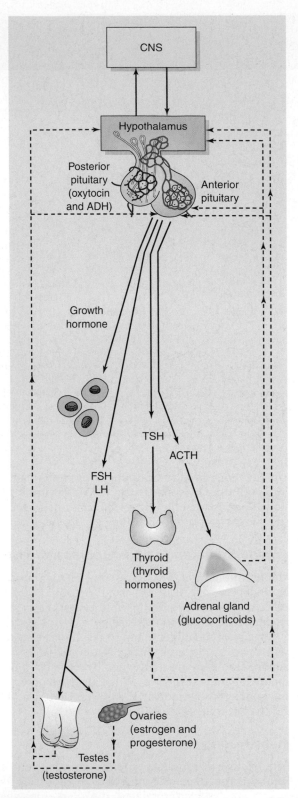

FIGURE 40-3. Control of hormone production by the hypothalamic–pituitary target cell feedback mechanism. Hormone levels from the target glands regulate the release of hormones from the anterior pituitary through a negative feedback system. The *dashed line* represents feedback control. ACTH, adrenocorticotropic hormone; ADH, antidiuretic hormone; CNS, central nervous system; FSH, follicle-stimulating hormone; LH, luteinizing hormone; TSH, thyroid-stimulating hormone.

Imaging

Imaging studies are important in the diagnosis and follow-up of endocrine disorders. Imaging modalities related to endocrinology can be divided into nonisotopic and isotopic types.

Nonisotopic imaging includes magnetic resonance imaging (MRI) and computed tomography (CT) scanning, both of which provide important information about structural changes within solid tissue. An advantage of MRI is that it does not require the use of ionizing radiation (which is required for CT scanning). An issue that must be considered with CT scanning is the use of contrast agents. Nonradioactive iodine is often used as a contrast agent to enhance the quality of CT images. Iodine contrast preparations must be used with caution with a person with renal disease and allergies.[2]

Ultrasonographic scanning provides good structural imaging and has the advantages of providing a "real-time" image that does not use radioactive elements. Therefore, ultrasonography is frequently used to aid in visualization of a lesion for biopsy.[2] Dual-electron x-ray absorptiometry is used routinely for the diagnosis and monitoring of osteoporosis and metabolic bone diseases.[13]

Isotopic imaging includes nuclear medicine imaging studies performed after administering a radioisotope, which is selectively taken up by the tissue being investigated.[2] Positron emission tomography (PET) scanning is another isotopic method, which is being used more widely in evaluating selected endocrine disorders, such as detecting the presence of metastatic thyroid cancers. PET scanning involves the administration of a short-lived radionuclide emitter of positrons in a form that is taken up by body tissues.[2] PET scanning has expanded to PET/CT imaging, in which both types of images are acquired almost simultaneously for enhanced detail and identification of previously difficult structures. The advantage of PET/CT is that the CT component allows a good examination of the tissue structure, whereas the PET component provides information about tissue function.[14] PET/CT has been demonstrated to be useful in managing thyroid cancers.[15]

SUMMARY CONCEPTS

The endocrine system acts as a communication system that uses chemical messengers, or hormones, for the transmission of information from cell to cell and from organ to organ. Hormones act by binding to receptors that are specific for the different types of hormones. Many of the endocrine glands are under the regulatory control of other parts of the endocrine system. The hypothalamus and the pituitary gland form a complex integrative network that interconnects the nervous system and the endocrine system; this central network controls the output from many of the other glands in the body.

Endocrine function can be assessed directly by measuring hormone levels or indirectly by assessing the effects that a hormone has on the body (*e.g.*, assessment of insulin function through blood glucose). Imaging techniques are used to visualize endocrine structures, and genetic techniques are used to determine the presence of genetic markers specific for selected endocrine disorders.

Review Exercises

1. Thyroid hormones are transported in the serum bound to transport proteins such as thyroid-binding globulin and albumin.

   A. Explain why free thyroxine (T_4) levels are usually used to assess thyroid function rather than total T_4 levels.

2. People who are being treated with exogenous forms of corticosteroid hormones often experience diminished levels of ACTH and endogenously produced cortisol.

   A. Explain, using information regarding the hypothalamic–pituitary feedback, control of cortisol production by the adrenal cortex.

REFERENCES

1. Verburg-van Kemenade B. M. L., Cohen N., Chadzinska M. (2017). Neuroendocrine-immune interaction: Evolutionarily conserved mechanisms that maintain allostasis in an ever-changing environment. *Developmental and Comparative Immunology* 66, 2–23. doi:10.1016/j.dci.2016.05.015.

2. Neal J. M. (2016). *How the endocrine system works* (2nd ed.). West Sussex: John Wiley & Sons.

3. Hall J. E. (2015). *Guyton and Hall textbook of medical physiology* (13th ed.). Philadelphia, PA: Elsevier.

4. Saladin K. S. (2015). *Anatomy & physiology: The unity of form and function* (7th ed.). New York: McGraw Hill Education.

5. Fruhbeck G., Mendez-Gimenez L., Fernandez-Formoso J. A., et al. (2014). Regulation of adipocyte lipolysis. *Nutrition Research Reviews* 27, 63–93. doi:10.1017/S095442241400002X.

6. Rubin R., Strayer D. S., Saffitz J. E., et al. (Eds.). (2015). *Rubin's pathology: Clinicopathologic foundations of medicine* (7th ed.) Philadelphia, PA: Wolters Kluwer.

7. Styne D. M. (2016). *Pediatric endocrinology: A clinical handbook*. Switzerland: Springer.

8. Ildrose A. M. (2015). Acute and emergency care for thyrotoxicosis and thyroid storm. *Acute Medicine and Surgery* 2, 147–157. doi:10.1002/ams2.104.

9. Government of India Department of Atomic Energy Board of Radiation and Isotope Technology. (2016). Frequently asked questions: Medical & biological products. [Online]. Available: http://www.britatom.gov.in/htmldocs/faqs_ec3.html. Accessed June 21, 2019.

10. American Association for Clinical Chemistry. (2014). Autoantibodies. Available: https://labtestsonline.org/tests/autoantibodies. Accessed June 21, 2019.

11. Kemp E. H., Weetman A. P. (2015). Autoimmune hypoparathyroidism. In Brandi M., Brown E. (Eds.), *Hypoparathyroidism*. Milano: Springer.

12. American Association for Clinical Chemistry. (2016). Cushing syndrome. [Online]. Available: https://labtestsonline.org/conditions/cushing-syndrome. Accessed June 21, 2019.

13. The Royal Australian and New Zealand College of Radiologists. (2018). Bone mineral density scan (Bone Densitometry or DXA Scan). [Online]. Available: https://www.insideradiology.com.au/bone-mineral-density-scan-hp/. Accessed June 21, 2019.

14. The American Board of Nuclear Medicine. (2017). What is PET/CT? [Online]. Available: https://www.abnm.org/index.php/sample-page-2/what-is-petct/. Accessed June 21, 2019.

15. Marcus C., Whitworth P. W., Surasi D. S., et al. (2014). PET/CT in the management of thyroid cancers. *American Journal of Roentgenology* 202, 1316–1329. doi:10.2214/AJR.13.11673.

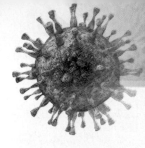

Disorders of Endocrine Control of Growth and Metabolism

Complications of Diabetes Mellitus

Acute Complications of Diabetes
Diabetic Ketoacidosis
Hyperosmolar Hyperglycemic State
Hypoglycemia
**Diabetic Complications Related to
Counter-Regulatory Mechanisms**
The Somogyi Effect
The Dawn Phenomenon
Chronic Complications of Diabetes Mellitus
Microvascular Complications
Macrovascular Complications
Diabetic Foot Ulcers
Infections

Learning Objectives

**After completing this chapter, the learner
will be able to meet the following objectives:**

1. Describe the mechanisms of endocrine hypofunction, hyperfunction, and hormone resistance.
2. Differentiate among primary, secondary, and tertiary endocrine disorders.
3. Describe the clinical features and causes of hypopituitarism.
4. Analyze the effects of a deficiency in growth hormone (GH).
5. Relate the functions of GH to the manifestations of acromegaly and adult-onset GH deficiency.
6. Characterize the synthesis, transport, and regulation of thyroid hormone.
7. Describe the various tests in the diagnosis and management of thyroid disorders.
8. Describe the function of the adrenal cortical hormones and their feedback regulation.
9. Relate the functions of the adrenal cortical hormones to Addison disease (*i.e.*, adrenal insufficiency) and Cushing syndrome (*i.e.*, glucocorticoid excess).
10. Discuss the functions of glucose, fats, and proteins in meeting the energy needs of the body.
11. Discuss the actions of insulin with respect to glucose, fat, and protein metabolism.
12. Explain what is meant by *counter-regulatory hormones*, and describe the actions of glucagon, epinephrine, GH, and the glucocorticoid hormones in regulation of blood glucose levels.
13. Discuss the statistics of incidence and prevalence of diabetes mellitus (DM).
14. Differentiate the types of blood and urine testing used in the diagnosis and management of DM.
15. Differentiate the distinguishing features of the four classifications of DM (type 1, type 2, gestational, and diabetes due to other causes).
16. Discuss the metabolic syndrome and its relationship with type 2 DM.
17. Differentiate among common acute complications of diabetes: diabetic ketoacidosis, hyperosmolar hyperglycemic state, and hypoglycemia.
18. Discuss the complications of diabetes related to counter-regulatory hormones: the Somogyi effect and the dawn phenomenon.
19. Differentiate among common chronic complications of diabetes: microvascular effects, macrovascular effects, diabetic foot ulcers, and infections.

The endocrine system affects all aspects of body function, including growth and development, energy metabolism, muscle and adipose tissue distribution, sexual development, fluid and electrolyte balance, and inflammation and immune responses. This chapter focuses on the disorders of pituitary function, growth and growth hormone (GH), thyroid function, and adrenal cortical function. This chapter also addresses the increasingly prevalent conditions of diabetes mellitus (DM) and the metabolic syndrome.

General Aspects of Altered Endocrine Function

Hypofunction, Hyperfunction, and Hormone Resistance

Disturbances of endocrine function usually are related to either hypofunction or hyperfunction of an endocrine gland or to hormone resistance of the target cells. Hypofunction of an endocrine gland can occur for a variety of reasons, such as the absence or impaired development of a gland or deficiency of an enzyme needed for hormone synthesis. The gland may be destroyed by a disruption in blood flow, infection, inflammation, autoimmune responses, or neoplastic growth. Decline in function may occur with aging, or an endocrine gland may atrophy as a result of drug therapy or for unknown reasons. A gland may produce a biologically inactive hormone, or circulating antibodies may destroy an active hormone before it can exert its action.[1-3]

Endocrine hyperfunction usually is due to excessive hormone production. This can result from excessive stimulation and hyperplasia of the endocrine gland or from a hormone-producing tumor. A tumor can produce hormones that are not normally secreted by the tissue from which the tumor is derived (ectopic hormone production).[1-3]

Endocrine dysfunction because of hormone resistance may be associated with receptor defects at the target cells. Hormone receptors may be absent or the receptor binding of hormones may be defective. Laron syndrome is a type of dwarfism that is caused by abnormalities in the receptors for GH in target tissues. Another mechanism associated with hormone resistance is an impaired intracellular responsiveness to stimulation by the hormone. This impaired cellular responsiveness occurs in congenital adrenal hyperplasia (CAH) in which the adrenal gland is receiving stimulation by adrenocorticotropic hormone (ACTH) but cannot respond appropriately because of a defect in the intracellular pathways within the adrenal cortex for production of cortisol.[1-3]

Primary, Secondary, and Tertiary Disorders

Endocrine disorders can be considered as primary, secondary, and tertiary disorders, related to the cascade of hormonal responses regulated through the hypothalamic–pituitary–target endocrine gland axis. *Primary disorders* of endocrine function originate in the target endocrine gland responsible for producing the hormone.[1,2]

In *secondary disorders* of endocrine function, the target endocrine gland is essentially normal; however, the gland is not producing appropriate levels of hormone because it is not receiving appropriate stimulation from the pituitary gland. The actual source of dysfunction is at the level of the pituitary gland. An example of a secondary endocrine disorder is a pituitary adenoma that results in increased secretion of pituitary hormones and excessive stimulation of target endocrine glands such as the adrenal glands and thyroid gland.[1,2] A *tertiary disorder* results from hypothalamic dysfunction (as may occur with craniopharyngiomas or cerebral irradiation). Thus, both the pituitary and target organ are understimulated.[3]

SUMMARY CONCEPTS

Endocrine disorders typically occur as the result of either hypofunction or hyperfunction of an endocrine gland or as a result of hormone resistance by target cells. Endocrine disorders can be classified as a primary disorder (because of a dysfunction of a target endocrine gland of the hypothalamic–pituitary axis, such as the thyroid gland or the adrenal glands), a secondary disorder (because of dysfunction of the pituitary gland), or a tertiary disorder (resulting from a defect in the hypothalamus).

Pituitary and Growth Disorders

The pituitary gland, or *hypophysis*, is a pea-sized gland located at the base of the brain, where it lies in a saddle-shaped depression in the sphenoid bone called the *sella turcica*. A short funnel-shaped stalk, the *infundibulum*, connects the pituitary gland with the hypothalamus. The pituitary gland has two components—a posterior lobe that is the neural component (neurohypophysis) and an anterior glandular lobe (adenohypophysis).[4,5]

The anterior lobe of the pituitary gland produces ACTH, thyroid-stimulating hormone (TSH), GH, the gonadotrophic hormones (follicle-stimulating hormone [FSH] and luteinizing hormone [LH]), and prolactin. Four of these, ACTH, TSH, LH, and FSH, control the secretion of hormones from other endocrine glands:

- ACTH controls the release of cortisol from the adrenal gland.
- TSH controls the secretion of thyroid hormone from the thyroid gland.
- LH regulates sex hormones in the ovaries and testes.
- FSH regulates fertility in the ovaries and testes.[4,5]

Assessment of Hypothalamic–Pituitary Function

A general overview of the various strategies available for assessing endocrine function is provided in Chapter 40. Assessment of the baseline status of the hypothalamic–pituitary and target cell hormones may include measuring the following (ideally the laboratory specimens are obtained before 8:00 AM because of circadian variations):

- Serum cortisol
- Serum prolactin
- Serum thyroxine and TSH
- Serum testosterone (male), serum estrogen (female), and serum LH/FSH
- Serum GH and serum insulin-like growth factor-1 (IGF-1, also known as somatomedin C)
- Plasma osmolality and urine osmolality

Additional diagnostic methods include dynamic testing of hypothalamic–pituitary–adrenal (HPA) axis function, as well as the insulin tolerance test, glucagon stimulation test, and short Synacthen (corticotropin) test.[6]

Pituitary Tumors

Pituitary tumors can be divided into primary and secondary tumors. Tumors of the pituitary can be further divided into functional tumors that secrete pituitary hormones and nonfunctional tumors that do not secrete hormones. They can range in size from small lesions that do not enlarge the gland (microadenomas <10 mm) to large, expansive tumors (macroadenomas >10 mm) that erode the sella turcica and impinge on surrounding cranial structures. Small, nonfunctioning tumors are found in up to 27% of adult autopsies.[1] Benign adenomas account for most of the functioning anterior pituitary tumors. Carcinomas of the pituitary are less common tumors. Functional adenomas can be subdivided according to cell type and the type of hormone secreted (Table 41-1).[1]

Hypopituitarism

Hypopituitarism is characterized by a decreased secretion of pituitary hormones and is associated with increased morbidity and mortality. The cause may be

TABLE 41-1 Frequency of Adenomas of the Anterior Pituitary

Cell Type	Hormone	Frequency (%)
Lactotrope	Prolactin	26
Somatotrope	Growth hormone	14
Corticotrope	Adrenocorticotropic hormone	15
Gonadotrope	Follicle-stimulating hormone, luteinizing hormone	8
Thyrotrope	Thyroid-stimulating hormone	1

Adapted from Strayer D., Rubin E., Saffitz J. E., Schiller A. L. (Eds.). (2015). Rubin's pathology: Clinicopathologic foundations of medicine (7th ed., Table 27.1, p. 1177). Philadelphia, PA: Wolters Kluwer, with permission.)

congenital or may result from a variety of acquired abnormalities (Chart 41-1).[2]

Typically, approximately 75% of the anterior pituitary must be destroyed before hypopituitarism becomes clinically evident.[2] The clinical manifestations of hypopituitarism usually occur gradually but can present as an acute and life-threatening condition. People usually complain of being chronically unfit, with weakness, fatigue, loss of appetite, impairment of sexual function,

---

CHART 41-1

CAUSES OF HYPOPITUITARISM

- Tumors and mass lesions—pituitary adenomas, cysts, metastatic cancer, and other lesions
- Pituitary surgery or radiation
- Infiltrative lesions and infections—hemochromatosis and lymphocytic hypophysitis
- Pituitary infarction—infarction of the pituitary gland after substantial blood loss during childbirth (Sheehan syndrome)
- Pituitary apoplexy—sudden hemorrhage into the pituitary gland
- Genetic diseases—rare congenital defects of one or more pituitary hormones
- Empty sella syndrome—an enlarged sella turcica that is not entirely filled with pituitary tissue
- Hypothalamic disorders—tumors and mass lesions (*e.g.*, craniopharyngiomas and metastatic malignancies), hypothalamic radiation, infiltrative lesions (*e.g.*, sarcoidosis), trauma, and infections

---

and cold intolerance. ACTH deficiency (secondary adrenal insufficiency) is the most serious endocrine deficiency, leading to weakness, nausea, anorexia, fever, and postural hypotension.[3]

Anterior pituitary hormone loss tends to follow a typical sequence, especially with progressive loss of pituitary reserve because of tumors or previous pituitary radiation therapy. The sequence of loss of pituitary hormones can be remembered by the mnemonic "*Go Look For The Adenoma*":

- GH (GH secretion typically is first to be lost)
- LH (results in sex hormone deficiency)
- FSH (causes infertility)
- TSH (leads to secondary hypothyroidism)
- ACTH (usually the last to become deficient, results in secondary adrenal insufficiency)[7]

Treatment of hypopituitarism includes treating any identified underlying cause. Hormone deficiencies should be treated as dictated by baseline hormone levels and more sophisticated pituitary testing where appropriate. Cortisol replacement is started when ACTH deficiency is present, thyroid replacement is started when TSH deficiency is detected, and sex hormone replacement is started when LH and FSH are deficient. GH replacement is indicated for pediatric GH deficiency and may also be used to treat GH deficiency in adults.[1-3]

Growth and Growth Hormone Disorders

Several hormones are essential for normal body growth and maturation, including GH, insulin, thyroid hormone, and androgens. In addition to its actions on carbohydrate and fat metabolism, insulin plays an essential role in growth processes. Children with diabetes, particularly those who have difficulty with balancing blood sugar, often fail to grow normally even though GH levels are normal. When levels of thyroid hormone are lower than normal, bone growth and epiphyseal closure are delayed. Androgens such as testosterone and dihydrotestosterone exert anabolic growth effects through their actions on protein synthesis. Glucocorticoids at excessive levels inhibit growth, apparently because of their antagonistic effect on GH secretion.[4,8,9]

Growth Hormone

GH, also called *somatotropin*, is a 191-amino acid polypeptide hormone synthesized and secreted by special cells in the anterior pituitary called *somatotropes*. It is now known that the rate of GH production in adults is almost as great as it is in children. GH is necessary for growth and contributes to the regulation of metabolic functions (Fig. 41-1). GH stimulates all aspects of cartilage growth. One of the most obvious effects of GH is on linear bone growth, resulting from its action on the epiphyseal growth plates of long bones. The width of bone increases because of enhanced periosteal growth. Visceral and endocrine organs, skeletal and cardiac muscle, skin, and connective tissue all undergo increased growth in response to GH.[1,4]

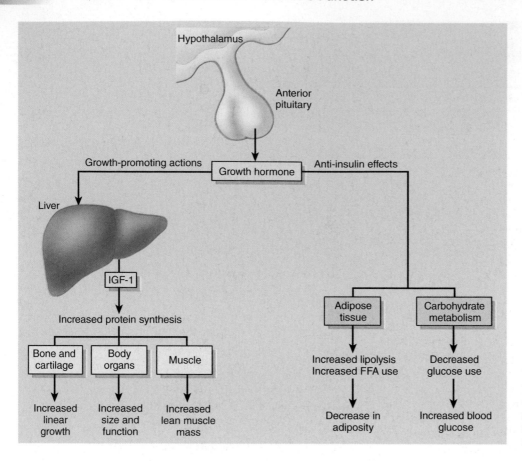

FIGURE 41-1. Growth-promoting and anti-insulin effects of growth hormone. FFA, free fatty acids; IGF-1, insulin-like growth factor-1.

Additionally, GH facilitates the rate of protein synthesis in the body. It enhances fatty acid mobilization, increases the use of fatty acids for fuel, and maintains or increases blood glucose levels by decreasing the use of glucose for fuel.[4] GH has an initial effect of increasing insulin levels. However, the predominant effect of prolonged GH excess is to increase glucose levels despite an insulin increase. This is because GH induces a resistance to insulin in the peripheral tissues, inhibiting the uptake of glucose by muscle and adipose tissues.[4]

Many of the effects of GH depend on *IGFs*, also called *somatomedins*, which are produced mainly by the liver. GH cannot directly cause bone growth. Instead, it acts indirectly by causing the liver to produce IGF. These IGF peptides act on cartilage and bone to promote their growth. At least four IGFs have been identified. Of these, IGF-1 (somatomedin C) appears to be the more important in terms of growth. It is also the most frequently measured IGF in laboratory tests. The IGFs have been sequenced and have structures similar to those of proinsulin. This explains the insulin-like activity of the IGFs and the weak action of insulin on growth. IGF levels are themselves influenced by a family of six-binding factors called *IGF-binding proteins* (IGFBPs).[4]

GH is carried unbound in the plasma and has a half-life of less than 50 minutes.[4] Two hypothalamic hormones regulate the secretion of GH:

- GH-releasing hormone (GHRH) that increases GH release
- Somatostatin that inhibits GH release

The secretion of GH fluctuates over a 24-hour period, with peak levels occurring 1 to 4 hours after onset of sleep. GH secretion is stimulated by hypoglycemia, fasting, starvation, increased blood levels of amino acids (particularly arginine), and decreased blood levels of fatty acids. Stress conditions such as trauma, excitement, emotional stress, and heavy exercise also increase GH, as does secretion of the hormone ghrelin by the stomach and the hormones estrogen and testosterone. GH is inhibited by increased glucose levels, levels of free fatty acids (FFAs) in the blood, cortisol, and obesity. GH levels also decrease with aging.[4]

KEY POINTS

Growth Hormone

- Growth hormone (GH), which is produced by somatotropes in the anterior pituitary, is necessary for linear bone growth in children. It also increases the rate at which cells transport amino acids across their cell membranes, and it increases the rate at which they use fatty acids and decreases the rate at which they use carbohydrates.

- The effects of GH on linear growth are dependent upon IGFs, which are produced mainly by the liver.

Short Stature in Children

Short stature is a condition in which height is less than the third percentile on the appropriate growth curve.[10,11] Short stature, or growth retardation, may have a variety of endocrine causes, including GH deficiency, hypothyroidism, and panhypopituitarism (*i.e.*, deficiency of *all* pituitary-derived hormones). A variety of other genetic and chromosomal causes of short stature have been noted, including Turner syndrome, Noonan syndrome, achondroplasia, and various types of skeletal dysplasias.[12] Other conditions known to cause short stature include protein–calorie malnutrition, chronic diseases such as chronic kidney disease and poorly controlled DM, malabsorption syndromes (including celiac disease), and certain pharmacologic therapies such as steroids, anticonvulsants, and drugs for attention deficit and hyperactivity. Emotional disturbances can lead to functional endocrine disorders, causing psychosocial dwarfism, which is also referred to as psychosocial short stature. The causes of short stature are summarized in Chart 41-2.[1,2,10,11]

A thorough physical and history, including developmental history, is important in diagnosing growth disorders. Accurate measurement of height and weight is an important part of the physical examination of children, with careful evaluation and tracking on growth curves. Diagnosis of short stature is not made on a single measurement but is based on sequential height measurements, velocity of growth, and parental height.[11,13]

The diagnostic procedures for children with short stature include tests to exclude nonendocrine causes. Suggested tests for conditions that may cause short stature include: complete blood count (anemia), comprehensive metabolic panel (renal and hepatic disease), C-reactive protein (CRP) and erythrocyte sedimentation rate (inflammatory bowel disease), FSH and karyotyping (Turner syndrome and other chromosomal abnormalities), IGF-1 (GH deficiency), TSH and free thyroxine (hypothyroidism), tissue transglutaminase and immunoglobulin-A (celiac disease), and urinalysis (renal disease).[11] Test for IGFBP-3 may also be useful to assess for GH deficiency and chronic disease.[11] Radiologic films are used to assess bone age, which often is delayed.[14] Magnetic resonance imaging (MRI) of the hypothalamic–pituitary area is recommended if a lesion is clinically suspected.[9] After the cause of short stature has been determined, treatment with recombinant DNA GH is approved for certain disorders, including GH deficiency, certain genetic problems (such as Prader–Willi syndrome and Noonan syndrome), chronic renal disease, and idiopathic short stature.[11]

Familial and Constitutional Short Stature

Two forms of short stature, genetic (familial) short stature and constitutional delay of growth and puberty, are not disease states but variations from population norms. These conditions require monitoring but not treatment. Genetically, short children tend to be well proportioned and to have a height close to the midparental height of their parents. The bone age and chronologic age of these children are equivalent. Children who have constitutional delay of growth have bone age that is less than

---

CHART 41-2

CAUSES OF SHORT STATURE

Variants of Normal

Genetic or "familial" short stature

Constitutional short stature

Low Birth Weight (*e.g.*, Intrauterine Growth Retardation)

Endocrine Disorders

GH deficiency

Primary GH deficiency

Idiopathic GH deficiency

Pituitary agenesis

Secondary GH deficiency (panhypopituitarism)

Biologically inactive GH production

Deficient IGF-1 production in response to normal or elevated GH (Laron-type dwarfism)

Hypothyroidism

Diabetes mellitus in poor control

Glucocorticoid excess

Endogenous (Cushing syndrome)

Exogenous (glucocorticoid drug treatment)

Abnormal mineral metabolism (*e.g.*, pseudohypoparathyroidism)

Chronic Illness and Malnutrition

Chronic organic or systemic disease (*e.g.*, asthma, especially when treated with glucocorticoids; heart or renal disease)

Nutritional deprivation

Malabsorption syndrome (*e.g.*, celiac sprue)

Functional Endocrine Disorders (Psychosocial Dwarfism)

Chromosomal Disorders (*e.g.*, Turner Syndrome)

Skeletal Abnormalities (*e.g.*, Achondroplasia)

GH, growth hormone; IGF, insulin-like growth factor.

---

the chronologic age, with the absence of other causes of decreased growth.[11,13]

Psychosocial Dwarfism (Psychosocial Short Stature)

Psychosocial dwarfism involves a functional hypopituitarism and is seen in some emotionally deprived children. These children usually present with poor growth, potbelly, and poor eating and drinking habits. Typically, there is a history of disturbed family relationships in which the child has been severely neglected or disciplined. Often, the neglect is confined to one child in the family. GH function usually returns to normal after the child is removed from the constraining environment.

The prognosis depends on improvement in behavior and catch-up growth.[15]

Growth Hormone Deficiency in Children

Several forms of GH deficiency present in childhood. Children with GH deficiency often present with physical findings of short stature (pituitary dwarfism), increased subcutaneous fat in the abdominal area, immature facial features with frontal bossing, delayed dentition, and an underdeveloped nasal bridge.[14] Several genetic mutations have been identified in the gene that codes for GH; however, some children present with idiopathic GH deficiency in which none of the known mutations are found. Childhood GH deficiency can also occur as a result of pituitary tumors. When short stature is caused by a GH deficiency, replacement therapy with GH produced by recombinant DNA technology is the treatment of choice. GH is administered by daily subcutaneous injection during the period of active growth and can be continued into adulthood.[4,11,16]

In a rare condition called *Laron syndrome (or Laron dwarfism)*, the pathophysiologic problem is hormone resistance because of abnormal GH receptors. GH levels are normal or elevated; however, levels of IGF-1 are low. Laron syndrome can be treated with IGF-1 replacement. Transmission of Laron syndrome is through autosomal recessive inheritance, with over 30 different mutations of GH receptors identified.[1]

Growth Hormone Deficiency in Adults

There are two categories of GH deficiency in adults:

1. GH deficiency that was present in childhood
2. GH deficiency that developed during adulthood, mainly as the result of hypopituitarism resulting from a pituitary tumor or its treatment

Some of the differences between childhood and adult-onset GH deficiency are described in Table 41-2.

TABLE 41-2 Differences between Childhood and Adult-Onset Growth Hormone Deficiency

Characteristic	Childhood Onset	Adult Onset
Adult height	↓	NL
Body fat	↑	↑
Lean body mass	↓↓	↓
Bone mineral density	↓	NL, ↓
IGF-1	↓↓	NL, ↓
IGF binding protein-3	↓	NL
Low-density lipoprotein cholesterol	↑	↑
High-density lipoprotein cholesterol	NL, ↓	↓

IGF, insulin-like growth factor; NL, normal.

The diagnosis of GH deficiency in adults is made by finding subnormal serum GH responses to provocative stimuli. A low IGF-1 level in the presence of low levels of three or more pituitary hormones indicates GH deficiency. Either the insulin tolerance test or the combination of the GHRH and arginine test is used as stimulation tests to detect GH deficiency.[17]

Treatment with recombinant GH replacement is indicated for adults with documented GH deficiency, with serum IGF-1 levels used to guide treatment.[17] The risk of atherosclerosis has been shown to be increased in children with GH deficiency. Treatment with GH has been demonstrated to improve the lipid profile and reduce the thickness of the intimal layer of the carotid artery in this population.[18] GH levels can also decline with aging, and there has been interest in the effects of declining GH levels in older adults (described as *somatopause*). GH replacement is obviously important in the growing child.[19,20]

Tall Stature in Children

Height that is greater than the 97th percentile norms for age and sex is considered tall stature in children.[11] As with short stature, normal variants of tall stature include familial tall stature and constitutional advancement of growth. Other causes of tall stature are genetic or chromosomal disorders such as Marfan syndrome, Klinefelter (XXY) syndrome, Fragile X syndrome, and Beckwith-Wiedemann syndrome. Treatment is not usually indicated for these non–GH-related causes of tall stature, or with the normal variants.[11]

Growth Hormone Excess in Children

GH excess occurring before puberty and the fusion of the epiphyses of the long bones result in pituitary *gigantism*. All body tissues grow rapidly, including the bones.[4] Excessive secretion of GH by somatotrope adenomas causes gigantism in the prepubertal child. It occurs when the epiphyses are not fused and high levels of IGF-1 stimulate excessive skeletal growth. The individual often has other complications because of the larger body mass and possible excessive secretion of other pituitary hormones. Fortunately, the condition is rare because of early recognition and treatment of the adenoma.[3] Treatment for GH excess typically consists of administration of the medications octreotide and pegvisomant to decrease GH levels.[11]

Growth Hormone Excess in Adults

When GH excess occurs in adulthood or after the epiphyses of the long bones have fused, the condition is referred to as *acromegaly*. The annual incidence of acromegaly is three to four cases per 1 million people, with a prevalence of 30 to 60 cases per million.[21]

Etiology and Pathogenesis
Clinical manifestations of acromegaly result from the effects on body cells from excess circulating blood levels of GH and IGF-1.[21] The most common cause of acromegaly is a GH-secreting somatotrope adenoma in the pituitary gland. Approximately 75% of people with acromegaly

have a somatotrope macroadenoma at the time of diagnosis, and most of the remainder has microadenomas.[1] The other causes of acromegaly are hypothalamic tumors that result in excess secretion of GHRH, ectopic secretion of GHRH by nonendocrine tumors (such as carcinoid tumors or small-cell lung cancers), or, more rarely, GH secretion from nonendocrine tumors. The binding of the excess circulating GH with the GH receptors in hepatic cells triggers an excess secretion of IGF-1 from hepatic cells. Then, it is the circulating IGF-1 molecules that bind with the IGF-1 receptor molecules in peripheral tissues, which directly act to stimulate the tissue growth that produces the clinical manifestations of acromegaly.[21]

Clinical Manifestations

The disorder usually has an insidious onset, with symptoms often present for a considerable period before a diagnosis is made. Because acromegaly is the production of excessive GH in adulthood, after the epiphyses of the long bones have closed, the person cannot grow taller; however, the soft tissues continue to grow. Enlargement of the small bones of the hands and feet and of the membranous bones of the face and skull results in a pronounced enlargement of the hands and feet, a broad and bulbous nose, a protruding lower jaw, and a slanting forehead (Fig. 41-2). The teeth become splayed, causing a disturbed bite and difficulty in chewing. The cartilaginous structures in the larynx and respiratory tract also become enlarged, resulting in a deepening of the voice and tendency to develop bronchitis. Vertebral changes often lead to kyphosis or hunchback. Bone overgrowth often leads to arthralgias and degenerative arthritis of the spine, hips, and knees. Virtually, every organ of the body is increased in size. Enlargement of the heart, the development of hypertension, and accelerated atherosclerosis can produce significant morbidity and mortality.[1,2,21,22]

The metabolic effects of excess levels of GH and IGF-1 include alterations in fat and carbohydrate metabolism. GH causes lipolysis, with the increased release of FFAs from adipose tissue leading to increased concentration of FFAs in body fluids. In addition, GH enhances the formation of ketones and the use of FFAs for energy in preference to use of carbohydrates and proteins. GH exerts multiple effects on carbohydrate metabolism, including decreased glucose uptake by tissues such as skeletal muscle and adipose tissue, increased glucose production by the liver, and increased insulin secretion.[4] Each of these changes results in GH-induced insulin resistance. This leads to glucose intolerance, which stimulates the beta cells of the pancreas to produce additional insulin. Long-term elevation of GH results in overstimulation of the beta cells, which may cause them literally to "burn out." The net result of these metabolic changes is impaired glucose regulation that often leads to the development of DM.[22]

Plasma levels of IGF-1 have been demonstrated to be more predictive of the risk for developing DM than are plasma GH levels. Higher plasma levels of IGF-1 have been associated with an increased risk for the development of diabetes in people with acromegaly; however,

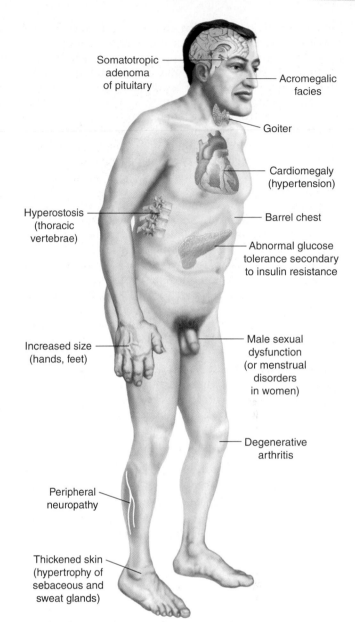

FIGURE 41-2. Clinical manifestations of acromegaly.

plasma concentrations of GH have not demonstrated the same correlation. Reported prevalence of DM in people with acromegaly ranges from 12% to 37.6%. When other forms of glucose dysregulation are considered (such as impaired fasting glucose [IFG] and impaired glucose tolerance), the reported prevalence rates for glucose dysregulation in people with acromegaly rise to 16% to 54%.[22]

Additional clinical manifestations associated with acromegaly are related to pituitary adenomas, as this is the etiologic cause of most cases of acromegaly. As the pituitary adenoma grows, it causes further dysfunction of the pituitary gland and surrounding brain structures. The pituitary gland is located in the pituitary fossa of the sphenoid bone (i.e., sella turcica), which lies directly below the optic nerve. Enlargement of the pituitary gland eventually causes erosion of the surrounding bone, and because of its location, this can lead to headaches, visual field defects resulting from compression of the optic nerve (classically, bitemporal hemianopia), and palsies of cranial nerves III, IV, and VI. Compression of other pituitary structures can cause secondary hypothyroidism, hypogonadism, and adrenal insufficiency. Hypogonadism can result from direct damage to the hypothalamic or pituitary system or indirectly because of hyperprolactinemia owing to prevention of the prolactin inhibitory factor (dopamine) from reaching pituitary lactotropes (cells that secrete prolactin) because of damage by the pituitary tumor.[1-3]

Other manifestations include excessive sweating with an unpleasant odor, oily skin, heat intolerance, moderate weight gain, muscle weakness and fatigue, menstrual irregularities, and decreased libido. Hypertension is relatively common. Sleep apnea syndrome is present in up to 90% of people. The pathogenesis of sleep apnea syndrome is obstructive in the majority of people because of increased pharyngeal soft tissue accumulation. Paresthesias may develop because of nerve entrapment and compression caused by excess soft tissue and accumulation of subcutaneous fluid (especially carpal tunnel syndrome). Acromegaly is also associated with an increased risk of colonic polyps and colorectal cancer.[1,21,22] The mortality rate of people with acromegaly is higher than the general population; however, advances in treatment have reduced the mortality rate from the previous two to three times the general population, to the current mortality rate that is less than two times the expected rate.[21] Mortality in people with acromegaly is primarily due to cardiovascular disease (60%), respiratory disease (25%), and cancer (15%).[21] The cardiovascular disease results from the combination of cardiomyopathy, hypertension, insulin resistance and hyperinsulinemia, and hyperlipidemia.[21,22]

Diagnosis

Acromegaly often develops insidiously, with an estimated 20% of people already having developed DM at the time of the acromegaly diagnosis.[22] The diagnosis of acromegaly is made via combination of a clinical examination revealing the typical physical features of the disorder (including enlargement of the hands and feet and coarsening of facial features) and diagnostic laboratory studies. Serum IGF-1 testing is the recommended initial laboratory test in evaluating a suspected diagnosis of acromegaly, and a finding of normal plasma IGF-1 levels essentially rules out the diagnosis. If the serum IGF-1 is elevated or equivocal, then the confirmatory test is a glucose challenge test. If serum GH levels are not suppressed by a glucose load, then the diagnosis of acromegaly is confirmed. MRI scanning is the recommended first-line imaging approach to detect and localize pituitary lesions, with computed tomography (CT) scanning as the alternative if MRI is contraindicated. Visual field testing is also recommended because of the anatomic proximity of the pituitary gland to the optic chiasm.[21]

Treatment

Treatment for acromegaly focuses on the correction of metabolic abnormalities, normalization of IGF-1 levels to age- and sex-matched control levels, removal or reduction of the tumor mass, relieving the central pressure effects, and improvement of adverse clinical features. Pituitary tumors are removed surgically using the transsphenoidal approach. Medical therapy is inoperable. Somatostatin is a hormone that can be effective in the medical management of acromegaly by producing feedback inhibition of GH secretion. Pegvisomant is a pegylated recombinant DNA analogue that incorporates nine different mutations, making the drug molecule different than the endogenous GH molecule. Pegvisomant can bind with the GH receptor sites and block GH binding; therefore, although GH levels remain elevated, the GH action on the target cells is reduced. A third class of drugs used in the treatment of acromegaly are the dopamine agonists, which exert their action by binding to dopamine receptors in the pituitary gland, thereby reducing pituitary secretion of both GH and prolactin. Radiotherapy is useful if surgical treatment is not possible and medical therapy is not well tolerated. Radiotherapy has demonstrated success with lowering serum GH levels; however, radiotherapy has not been as effective in lowering serum IGF-1 levels.[21]

Precocious Puberty

Precocious puberty is defined as early activation of the hypothalamic–pituitary–gonadal axis, resulting in the early development of sexual characteristics and fertility. The American Academy of Pediatrics (in 2015) and the American Academy of Family Physicians (in 2017) both recommend a diagnosis of precocious puberty if signs of pubertal changes are noted before the age of 8 years for girls and 9 years for boys.[23,24] Both organizations recognize recent research indicating that the population may be shifting toward a new normal of earlier ages of puberty, with black girls entering puberty earlier than white girls and children who are obese entering puberty at earlier ages than children of normal body weight for age.[23,24]

Precocious sexual development may be idiopathic or may be caused by gonadal, adrenal, or hypothalamic disease. Benign and malignant tumors of the central nervous system (CNS) can cause precocious puberty. These tumors are thought to remove the inhibitory influences normally exerted on the hypothalamus during childhood. Diagnosis of precocious puberty is based on physical findings of early **thelarche, adrenarche**, and *menarche* in girls. The most common sign in boys is early genital enlargement. Radiologic findings may indicate advanced bone age. People with precocious puberty are usually tall for their age as children but short as adults because of the early closure of the epiphyses. MRI or CT may be used to exclude intracranial lesions. Depending on the cause of precocious puberty, the treatment may involve surgery, medication, or no treatment. Administration of a long-acting GnRH agonist results in a decrease in pituitary responsiveness to GnRH, leading to decreased secretion of gonadotropic hormones and sex steroids. Administration of GnRH may also help with reducing the incidence of short stature.[23,24]

SUMMARY CONCEPTS

Pituitary tumors can result in deficiencies or excesses of pituitary hormones. Hypopituitarism, which is characterized by a decreased secretion of pituitary hormones, is a condition that affects many of the other endocrine systems. Depending on the extent of the disorder, it can result in decreased levels of GH, thyroid hormones, adrenal corticosteroid hormones, and testosterone in the male and estrogens and progesterone in the female.

A number of hormones are essential for normal body growth and maturation, including GH, insulin, thyroid hormone, and androgens. GH exerts its growth effects through IGF-1. GH also exerts an effect on metabolism and is produced in the adult and in the child. Its metabolic effects include a decrease in peripheral use of carbohydrates and an increased mobilization and use of fatty acids.

In children, alterations in growth include short stature, tall stature, and precocious puberty. Short stature is a condition in which the attained height is below the third percentile on the appropriate growth curve for a child's age and sex. Short stature can occur as a variant of normal growth (*i.e.*, familial short stature or constitutional delay of growth and puberty) or can occur as the result of endocrine disorders, chronic illness, malnutrition, emotional disturbances, or chromosomal disorders. Short stature resulting from GH deficiency can be treated with human GH preparations. In adults, GH deficiency represents a deficiency carried over from childhood or one that develops during adulthood as the result of a pituitary tumor or its treatment. GH levels also can decline with aging, and there has been interest in the effects of declining GH levels with aging.

Tall stature refers to the condition in which children are tall for their age and gender. It can occur as a variant of normal growth (*i.e.*, familial tall stature or constitutional advancement of growth), as the result of a genetic or chromosomal abnormality or GH excess. GH excess in adults results in acromegaly, which involves proliferation of bone, cartilage, and soft tissue along with the metabolic effects of excessive hormone levels. Precocious puberty defines a condition of early activation of the hypothalamic–pituitary–gonadal axis, resulting in the development of appropriate sexual characteristics and fertility. It is associated with tall stature during childhood but may lead to short stature in adulthood because of the early closure of the epiphyses.

Thyroid Disorders

Control of Thyroid Function

The thyroid gland is a shield-shaped structure located immediately below the larynx in the anterior middle portion of the neck (Fig. 41-3A). It is composed of a large number of tiny, saclike structures called *follicles* (see Fig. 41-3B). These are the functional units of the thyroid. Each follicle is formed by a single layer of epithelial (follicular) cells and is filled with a secretory substance called *colloid*, which consists largely of a glycoprotein–iodine complex called *thyroglobulin*.[4,9]

The thyroglobulin that fills the thyroid follicles is a large glycoprotein molecule that contains about 100 tyrosine amino acid residues.[4] It is these tyrosine molecules to which iodine is attached to create thyroid hormone. This process of thyroid synthesis occurs within the follicles of the thyroid gland.[4]

In the process of removing the iodine from the blood and storing it for future use, iodide is pumped into the follicular cells against a concentration gradient. Iodide (I^-) is transported across the basement membrane of the thyroid cells by an intrinsic membrane protein called the Na^+/I^- *symporter* (NIS).[4] At the apical border, a second I^- transport protein called *pendrin* moves iodine into the colloid, where it is involved in hormonogenesis.[4] The NIS derives its energy from Na^+/K^+-ATPase, which drives the process. As a result, the concentration of iodide in the normal thyroid gland is approximately 30 times than that in the blood.[4]

Once inside the follicle, most of the iodide is oxidized by the enzyme thyroid peroxidase (TPO) in a reaction that facilitates combination with a tyrosine molecule to form monoiodotyrosine (MIT) and then diiodotyrosine (DIT).[4] Two DIT residues are coupled to form thyroxine (T_4), or a MIT and a DIT are coupled to form triiodothyronine (T_3).[4] Only T_4 (93%) and T_3 (7%) are released into the circulation[4] (see Fig. 41-3C). Although T_3 is significantly more potent in its activity, T_4 has a much longer half-life in the blood (7 days) than T_3 (1 day); therefore, T_4 serves as an effective storage molecule. The circulating T_4 is converted to T_3 when needed.[9]

Stimulation by TSH from the pituitary gland serves as the stimulus for the thyroid gland to secrete the T_3 and T_4 thyroid hormones into the blood.[9] Thyroid hormones are bound to thyroxine-binding globulin (TBG) and other plasma proteins for transport in the blood. Only the free T_3 or T_4 hormone can enter target cells to exert the hormonal effect; the protein-bound forms cannot enter the cells. Protein-bound thyroid hormone forms a large reservoir that is slowly drawn on as free thyroid hormone is needed. There are three major thyroid-binding proteins: TBG, transthyretin (also known as thyroxine-binding prealbumin [TBPA]), and albumin. More than 99% of T_4 and T_3 is carried in these bound forms.[4,25]

A number of disease conditions and pharmacologic agents can decrease the amount of binding protein in the plasma or influence the binding of hormone.

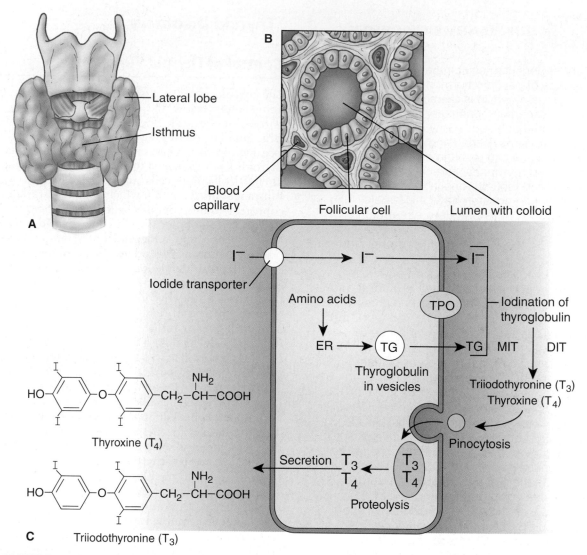

FIGURE 41-3. (A) The thyroid gland. (B) Microscopic structure of thyroid follicles. (C) Cellular mechanisms for transport of iodide (I⁻), oxidation of I⁻ by thyroid peroxidase (TPO), coupling of oxidized I⁻ with thyroglobulin to form thyroid hormones, and movement of T_3 and T_4 into the follicular cell by pinocytosis and release into the blood. DIT, diiodotyrosine; MIT, monoiodotyrosine.

Several genetic alterations of TBG function have been identified, including an X-linked TBG deficiency associated with a gene on the long arm of the X chromosome.[25] Glucocorticoid medications and systemic disease conditions such as protein malnutrition, nephrotic syndrome, and cirrhosis can decrease TBG concentrations of the thyroid-binding proteins. A variety of drugs, such as phenytoin, salicylates, and diazepam, can affect the binding of thyroid hormone to normal concentrations of binding proteins or disrupt thyroid metabolism in other ways.[26]

The secretion of thyroid hormone is regulated by the hypothalamic–pituitary–thyroid feedback system (see Chapter 40, Fig. 40-3). In this system, thyrotropin-releasing hormone (TRH), which is produced by the hypothalamus, controls the release of TSH from the anterior pituitary gland. TSH increases the overall activity of the thyroid gland by increasing thyroglobulin breakdown and the release of thyroid hormone from follicles into

the bloodstream, activating the iodide pump (by increasing NIS activity), increasing the oxidation of iodide and the coupling of iodide to tyrosine, and increasing the number and the size of the follicle cells.[4,9]

Increased plasma levels of thyroid hormone lead to feedback inhibition of TRH or TSH. High levels of iodide also cause a temporary decrease in thyroid activity that lasts for several weeks, probably through a direct inhibition of TSH on the thyroid. Cold exposure is one of the strongest stimuli for increased thyroid hormone production and probably is mediated through TRH from the hypothalamus. Various emotional reactions can also affect the output of TRH and TSH.[4]

Actions of Thyroid Hormone

Altered levels of thyroid hormone affect all the major organs in the body. Thyroid hormone has two major functions—it increases metabolism and protein synthesis and it is necessary for growth and development in children, including mental development and attainment of sexual maturity. These actions are mainly mediated by T_3. In the cell, T_3 binds to a nuclear receptor, resulting in transcription of specific thyroid hormone response genes.[4]

Metabolic Rate

Thyroid hormone increases the metabolism of target cells throughout the body. The basal metabolic rate can increase by 60% to 100% above normal when large amounts of T_4 are present.[4] As a result of this higher metabolism, the rate of glucose, fat, and protein use increases. Lipids are mobilized from adipose tissue, and the catabolism of cholesterol by the liver is increased. Blood levels of cholesterol are decreased in hyperthyroidism and increased in hypothyroidism. Muscle proteins are broken down and used as fuel, probably accounting for some of the muscle fatigue that occurs with hyperthyroidism. The absorption of glucose from the gastrointestinal tract is increased.[4]

Cardiovascular Function

Cardiovascular and respiratory functions are strongly affected by thyroid function. With an increase in metabolism, there is a rise in oxygen consumption and production of metabolic end products, with an accompanying increase in vasodilation. Blood flow to the skin, in particular, is augmented as a means of dissipating the body heat that results from the higher metabolic rate. Blood volume, cardiac output, and ventilation are all increased as a means of maintaining blood flow and oxygen delivery to body tissues. Heart rate and cardiac contractility are enhanced as a means of maintaining the needed cardiac output. Blood pressure is likely to change little because the increase in vasodilation tends to offset the increase in cardiac output.[4]

Gastrointestinal Function

Thyroid hormone enhances gastrointestinal function, causing an increase in motility and production of gastrointestinal secretions that often result in diarrhea. An increase in appetite and food intake accompanies the higher metabolic rate that occurs with increased thyroid hormone levels. At the same time, weight loss occurs because of the increased use of calories.[4]

Neuromuscular Effects

Thyroid hormone has marked effects on neural control of muscle function and tone. Slight elevations in hormone levels cause skeletal muscles to react more vigorously, and a drop in hormone levels causes muscles to react more sluggishly. In the hyperthyroid state, a fine muscle tremor is present. The cause of this tremor is unknown, but it may represent an increased sensitivity of the neural synapses in the spinal cord that controls muscle tone. In the infant, thyroid hormone is necessary for normal brain development. The hormone enhances cerebration; in the hyperthyroid state, it causes extreme nervousness, anxiety, and difficulty in sleeping.[4]

Evidence suggests a strong interaction between the thyroid hormone and the sympathetic nervous system.[4]

Many of the signs and symptoms of hyperthyroidism suggest overactivity of the sympathetic division of the autonomic nervous system, such as tachycardia, palpitations, and sweating. Tremor, restlessness, anxiety, and diarrhea may also reflect autonomic nervous system imbalances. Drugs that block sympathetic activity have proved to be valuable adjuncts in the treatment of hyperthyroidism because of their ability to relieve some of these undesirable symptoms.[2]

KEY POINTS

Thyroid Hormone

- Thyroid hormone increases the metabolism and protein synthesis in nearly all of the tissues of the body.

- When hypothyroidism occurs in older children or adults, it produces a decrease in metabolic rate, an accumulation of a hydrophilic mucopolysaccharide substance (myxedema) in the connective tissues throughout the body, and an elevation in serum cholesterol.

- Hyperthyroidism has an effect opposite to that of hypothyroidism. It produces an increase in metabolic rate and oxygen consumption, increased use of metabolic fuels, and increased sympathetic nervous system responsiveness.

Tests of Thyroid Function

Various tests aid in the diagnosis of thyroid disorders. Measures of T_3 (total and free), T_4 (total and free), and TSH have been made available through immunoassay methods. The total T_3 and T_4 tests measure both the protein-bound and free components of each hormone. The free T_3 and T_4 tests measure the fractions that are not bound to plasma proteins, which are therefore free to enter cells to produce effects. TSH levels are used to differentiate between primary thyroid disorders (which originate at the thyroid gland) and secondary thyroid disorders (which originate at the pituitary gland). T_3 and T_4 levels (bound and free) are low in primary hypothyroidism; however, the TSH level is elevated. The assessment of thyroid autoantibodies (*e.g.*, anti-TPO antibodies in Hashimoto thyroiditis) is also important in the diagnostic workup and follow-up of people with thyroid disorders.[2,9]

The radioiodine (^{123}I) uptake test measures the ability of the thyroid gland to concentrate and retain iodine from the blood. Thyroid scans (^{123}I, ^{99m}Tc-pertechnetate) can be used to detect thyroid nodules and determine the functional activity of the thyroid gland. Ultrasonography can be used to differentiate cystic from solid thyroid lesions, and CT and MRI scans are used to demonstrate tracheal compression or impingement on other neighboring structures. Fine-needle aspiration biopsy of a thyroid nodule has proved to be the best method for differentiation of benign from malignant thyroid disease.[2,9]

Alterations in Thyroid Function

An alteration in thyroid function can represent a hypofunctional or a hyperfunctional state. The manifestations of these two altered states are summarized in Table 41-3. Disorders of the thyroid may be due to a congenital defect in thyroid development, or they may develop later in life, with a gradual or sudden onset.

Goiter is an increase in the size of the thyroid gland (Fig. 41-4). It can occur in hypothyroid, euthyroid, and hyperthyroid states. Goiters may be diffuse, involving the entire gland without evidence of nodularity, or they may contain nodules. Diffuse goiters usually become nodular. Goiters may be toxic, producing signs

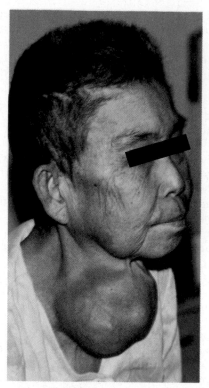

FIGURE 41-4. Nontoxic goiter. In a middle-aged woman with nontoxic goiter, the thyroid has enlarged to produce a conspicuous neck mass. (From Strayer D., Rubin E. (Eds.). (2015). *Rubin's pathology: Clinicopathologic foundations of medicine* (7th ed., Figure 27-11A, p. 1183). Philadelphia, PA: Wolters Kluwer.)

TABLE 41-3 Manifestations of Hypothyroid and Hyperthyroid States		
Level of Organization	**Hypothyroidism**	**Hyperthyroidism**
Basal metabolic rate	Decreased	Increased
Sensitivity to catecholamines	Decreased	Increased
General features	Myxedematous features	Exophthalmos (in Graves disease)
	Deep voice	Lid lag
	Impaired growth (child)	Accelerated growth (child)
Blood cholesterol levels	Increased	Decreased
General behavior	Intellectual disability (infant)	Restlessness, irritability, anxiety
	Mental and physical sluggishness	Hyperkinesis
	Somnolence	Wakefulness
Cardiovascular function	Decreased cardiac output	Increased cardiac output
	Bradycardia	Tachycardia and palpitations
Gastrointestinal function	Constipation	Diarrhea
	Decreased appetite	Increased appetite
Respiratory function	Hypoventilation	Dyspnea
Muscle tone and reflexes	Decreased	Increased, with tremor and twitching
Temperature tolerance	Cold intolerance	Heat intolerance
Skin and hair	Decreased sweating	Increased sweating
	Coarse and dry skin and hair	Thin and silky skin and hair
Weight	Gain	Loss

of extreme hyperthyroidism, or thyrotoxicosis, or they may be nontoxic. Diffuse nontoxic and multinodular goiters are the result of compensatory hypertrophy and hyperplasia of follicular epithelium from some derangement that impairs thyroid hormone output.[1,2,4]

The degree of thyroid enlargement is usually proportional to the extent and duration of thyroid deficiency. Multinodular goiters produce the largest thyroid enlargements. When sufficiently enlarged, they may compress the esophagus and trachea, causing difficulty in swallowing, a choking sensation, and inspiratory stridor. Such lesions may also compress the superior vena cava, producing distention of the veins of the neck and upper extremities, edema of the eyelids and conjunctiva, and syncope with coughing.[1,2,4]

Hypothyroidism

Hypothyroidism can occur as a congenital or an acquired defect. Congenital hypothyroidism develops prenatally and is present at birth. Acquired hypothyroidism develops because of primary disease of the thyroid gland or secondary to disorders of hypothalamic or pituitary origin.

Congenital Hypothyroidism

Congenital hypothyroidism is a common cause of preventable intellectual disability. Hypothyroidism in the infant may result from a congenital lack of the thyroid gland or from abnormal biosynthesis of thyroid hormone or deficient TSH secretion. With congenital lack of the thyroid gland, the infant usually appears normal and functions normally at birth because hormones have been supplied in utero by the mother.[1,2,4]

Thyroid hormone is essential for normal growth and brain development, almost half of which occurs during the first 6 months of life. If untreated, congenital hypothyroidism causes intellectual disability and impairs physical growth. The manifestations of untreated congenital hypothyroidism are referred to as cretinism. However, the term does not apply to the normally developing infant in whom replacement thyroid hormone therapy was instituted shortly after birth.[1,2,4]

Many countries throughout the world now routinely perform neonatal screening to detect congenital hypothyroidism during early infancy.[27] Premature or sick newborn infants need to be screened with a comprehensive serum thyroid profile to prevent missing primary hypothyroidism in these infants.

Transient congenital hypothyroidism (characterized by high TSH levels with low or normal thyroid hormone levels) has been recognized more frequently since the introduction of neonatal screening. The fetal and infant thyroid gland is sensitive to iodine excess. Iodine can cross the placenta, be excreted in breast milk, and is also readily absorbed by infant skin. Transient hypothyroidism may be caused by maternal or infant exposure to substances such as povidone–iodine used as a disinfectant (i.e., vaginal douche or skin disinfectant). Antithyroid drugs such as propylthiouracil and methimazole can also cross the placenta and block fetal thyroid function.[1,2,4,27]

Congenital hypothyroidism is treated by thyroid hormone replacement. Evidence indicates that it is important to normalize T_4 levels as rapidly as possible because a delay is accompanied by poorer psychomotor and mental development. When early and adequate thyroid hormone replacement treatment is implemented for congenital hypothyroidism, the risk of intellectual disability is very low.[1,2,4,27]

Acquired Hypothyroidism and Myxedema

Hypothyroidism in older children and adults causes a general slowing down of metabolic processes and myxedema. Myxedema implies the presence of a nonpitting mucus type of edema caused by an accumulation of a hydrophilic mucopolysaccharide substance in the connective tissues throughout the body. The hypothyroid state may be mild, with only a few signs and symptoms, or it may progress to a life-threatening condition with angioedema.[1,2,4]

Etiology and Pathogenesis

Acquired hypothyroidism can result from destruction or dysfunction of the thyroid gland (i.e., primary hypothyroidism), or it can be a secondary disorder caused by impaired pituitary function or as a tertiary disorder caused by a hypothalamic dysfunction.

Primary hypothyroidism is much more common than secondary (and tertiary) hypothyroidism. It may result from thyroidectomy (i.e., surgical removal) or ablation of the gland with radiation for treatment of hyperthyroidism. Certain goitrogenic agents, such as lithium carbonate, and the antithyroid drugs propylthiouracil and methimazole in continuous dosage can block hormone synthesis and produce hypothyroidism with goiter. Large amounts of iodine can also block thyroid hormone production and cause hypothyroidism, particularly in people with autoimmune thyroid disease. Iodine deficiency, which can cause goiter and hypothyroidism, is uncommon in the United States because of the widespread use of iodized salt and other iodide sources. However, iodine deficiency continues to occur in less developed areas of the world.[1,2,4] Subacute thyroiditis, which can occur in postpartum women, is another cause of hypothyroidism.[28]

The most common cause of acquired hypothyroidism is Hashimoto thyroiditis, an autoimmune disorder in which the thyroid gland may be totally destroyed by an immunologic process. It is the major cause of acquired hypothyroidism in children and adults.[1,27] Hashimoto thyroiditis is predominantly a disease of women. The course of the disease varies. At the onset, only a goiter may be present. In time, hypothyroidism usually becomes evident. Although the disorder usually causes hypothyroidism, a hyperthyroid state may develop midcourse in the disease. The transient hyperthyroid state may be related to leakage of preformed thyroid hormone from damaged cells of the gland.[1,2,4]

Clinical Manifestations

Hypothyroidism may affect almost all body functions. The manifestations of the disorder are related largely to two factors: the hypometabolic state resulting from thyroid hormone deficiency and myxedematous involvement of body tissues. The hypometabolic state associated with hypothyroidism is characterized by a gradual onset of weakness and fatigue, a tendency to gain weight despite a loss of appetite, and cold intolerance (Fig. 41-5). As the condition progresses, the skin becomes dry and rough and the hair becomes coarse and brittle. The face becomes puffy with edematous eyelids, and there is thinning of the outer third of the eyebrows. Gastrointestinal motility is decreased, producing constipation, flatulence, and abdominal distention. Delayed relaxation of deep tendon reflexes and bradycardia are sometimes noted. CNS involvement is manifested in mental dullness, lethargy, and impaired memory.[1,2,4]

Although the myxedematous fluid is usually most obvious in the face, it can collect in the interstitial spaces of almost any body structure and is responsible for many of the manifestations of the severe hypothyroid state. The tongue is often enlarged and the voice becomes hoarse and husky. Carpal tunnel and other entrapment syndromes are common, as is impairment of muscle function with stiffness, cramps, and pain. Mucopolysaccharide deposits in the heart cause generalized cardiac dilation, bradycardia, and other signs of altered cardiac function. The signs and symptoms of hypothyroidism are summarized in Table 41-3.[1,2,4]

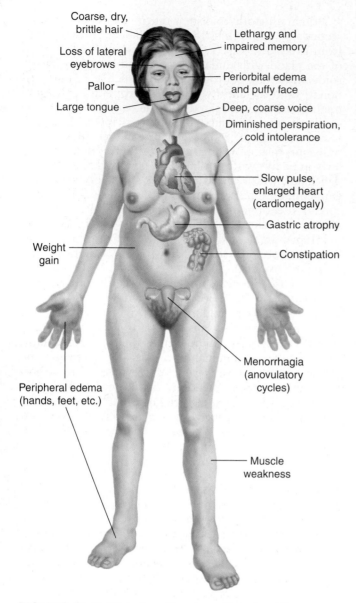

Coarse, dry, brittle hair

Loss of lateral eyebrows

Pallor

Large tongue

Weight gain

Peripheral edema (hands, feet, etc.)

Lethargy and impaired memory

Periorbital edema and puffy face

Deep, coarse voice

Diminished perspiration, cold intolerance

Slow pulse, enlarged heart (cardiomegaly)

Gastric atrophy

Constipation

Menorrhagia (anovulatory cycles)

Muscle weakness

FIGURE 41-5. Clinical manifestations of hypothyroidism.

Diagnosis and Treatment

Diagnosis of hypothyroidism is based on history, physical examination, and laboratory tests. A low serum T_4 and elevated TSH levels are characteristic of primary hypothyroidism. The tests for antithyroid antibodies should be done when Hashimoto thyroiditis is suspected.[1,2,4]

Hypothyroidism is treated by replacement therapy with synthetic preparations of T_3 or T_4. Most people are treated with T_4. Serum TSH levels are used to estimate the adequacy of T_4 replacement therapy. When the TSH level is normalized, the T_4 dosage is considered satisfactory (for primary hypothyroidism only). A "go low and go slow" approach should be considered in the treatment of older people with hypothyroidism because of the risk of inducing acute coronary syndromes in the susceptible individual. It is also important that people consistently take the form of T_4 prescribed, so that their laboratory values are the most representative of their thyroid state. Therefore, people should remain on generic forms of T_4 and, similarly, if people are put on brand names of T_4, they should stay on the same drug.[1,2,4,29]

Myxedematous Coma

Myxedematous coma is a life-threatening, end-stage expression of hypothyroidism. Long-standing hypothyroidism leads to a crisis state with severely reduced cellular metabolism that affects all organ systems throughout the body. Hypothermia also develops and is a strong predictor of mortality. The condition is associated with cardiovascular collapse, hypoventilation, and severe metabolic disorders that include hyponatremia, hypoglycemia, and lactic acidosis.[8,30]

Treatment includes aggressive management of precipitating factors; supportive therapy such as management of cardiorespiratory status, hyponatremia, and hypoglycemia; and thyroid replacement therapy. If hypothermia is present, active rewarming of the body is contraindicated because it may induce vasodilation and vascular collapse. Prevention is preferable to treatment and entails special attention to high-risk populations, such as women with a history of Hashimoto thyroiditis. These people should be informed about the signs and symptoms of severe hypothyroidism and the need for early medical treatment.[8,30]

Hyperthyroidism

Thyrotoxicosis is the clinical syndrome that results when tissues are exposed to high levels of circulating thyroid hormone.[4]

Etiology and Pathogenesis

In most instances, thyrotoxicosis is due to hyperactivity of the thyroid gland, or hyperthyroidism. The most common cause of hyperthyroidism is Graves disease, which is accompanied by ophthalmopathy, dermopathy, and diffuses goiter. Other causes of hyperthyroidism are multinodular goiter, adenoma of the thyroid, and thyroiditis. Iodine-containing agents can induce hyperthyroidism as well as hypothyroidism. Thyroid crisis, or storm, is an acutely exaggerated manifestation of the thyrotoxic state.[1,8]

Clinical Manifestations

Many of the manifestations of hyperthyroidism are related to the increase in oxygen consumption and use of metabolic fuels associated with the hypermetabolic state, as well as to the increase in sympathetic nervous system activity that occurs. Hyperthyroidism resembles those of excessive sympathetic nervous system activity, suggesting that thyroid hormone may heighten the sensitivity of the body to the catecholamines or that it may act as a pseudocatecholamine. With the hypermetabolic state, there are frequent complaints of nervousness, irritability, and fatigability (Fig. 41-6). Weight loss is common despite a large appetite. Other manifestations include

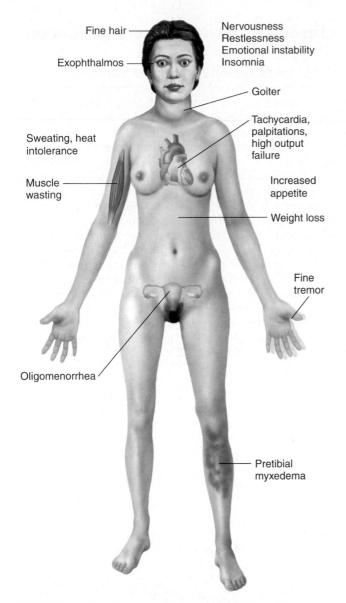

Fine hair

Exophthalmos

Nervousness
Restlessness
Emotional instability
Insomnia

Goiter

Tachycardia,
palpitations,
high output
failure

Sweating, heat
intolerance

Muscle
wasting

Increased
appetite

Weight loss

Fine
tremor

Oligomenorrhea

Pretibial
myxedema

FIGURE 41-6. Clinical manifestations of hyperthyroidism.

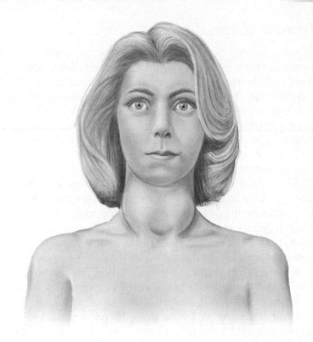

FIGURE 41-7. Graves disease. A patient with Graves disease may show symptoms of an enlarged thyroid (goiter) and protrusion of one or both eyeballs (exophthalmos). (Asset provided by Anatomical Chart Co.)

tachycardia, palpitations, shortness of breath, excessive sweating, muscle cramps, and heat intolerance. The person appears restless and has a fine muscle tremor. Even in people without *exophthalmos*, there is an abnormal retraction of the eyelids and infrequent blinking such that they appear to be staring. The hair and skin are usually thin and have a silky appearance.[1,8,31] Atrial fibrillation occurs in 10% to 15% of adults with hyperthyroidism.[32] The signs and symptoms of hyperthyroidism are summarized in Table 41-3.

The treatment of hyperthyroidism is directed toward reducing the level of thyroid hormone. This can be accomplished with eradication of the thyroid gland with radioactive iodine, through surgical removal of part or all of the gland, or the use of drugs that decrease thyroid function and thereby the effect of thyroid hormone on the peripheral tissues. Antithyroid drugs prevent the thyroid gland from converting iodine to its organic form or block the conversion of T_4 to T_3 in the tissues.[1,8,31,33]

Graves Disease

Graves disease is a state of hyperthyroidism, goiter, and ophthalmopathy. It affects approximately 0.5% to 1% of the population under 40 years of age.[1] Graves disease is an autoimmune disorder characterized by abnormal stimulation of the thyroid gland by thyroid-stimulating antibodies (TSH receptor antibodies) that act through the normal TSH receptors. It may be associated with other autoimmune disorders such as myasthenia gravis. The disease is associated with a major histocompatibility complex class 1 chain–related gene A (MICA), with genotypes MICA A5 correlated with Graves disease and MICA A6/A9 being preventive for Graves disease.[1]

The ophthalmopathy, which occurs in up to one-third of people with Graves disease, is thought to result from accumulation of T lymphocytes sensitized to antigens along thyroid follicular cells and orbital fibroblasts that secrete cytokines.[1] The ophthalmopathy of Graves disease can cause severe eye problems, including tethering of the extraocular muscles resulting in diplopia; involvement of the optic nerve, with some visual loss; and corneal ulceration because the lids do not close over the protruding eyeball (because of the **exophthalmos**). The ophthalmopathy usually tends to stabilize after treatment of the hyperthyroidism. However, ophthalmopathy can worsen acutely after radioiodine treatment. Some physicians prescribe glucocorticoids for several weeks surrounding the radioiodine treatment if the person had signs of ophthalmopathy. Ophthalmopathy can also be aggravated by smoking, which should be strongly discouraged.[34] Figure 41-7 shows a woman with Graves disease.

Thyroid Storm

Thyroid storm, or thyrotoxic crisis, is an extreme and life-threatening form of thyrotoxicosis rarely seen today because of improved diagnosis and treatment methods. When it does occur, it is seen most often in undiagnosed cases or in people with hyperthyroidism who have not been adequately treated. It is often precipitated by stress, such as an infection, by physical or emotional trauma, or by manipulation of a hyperactive thyroid gland during thyroidectomy. Thyroid storm is manifested by a very high fever, extreme cardiovascular effects (*i.e.*, tachycardia, congestive failure, and angina), and severe CNS effects (*i.e.*, agitation, restlessness, and delirium). The mortality rate is high.[35-37]

Thyroid storm requires rapid diagnosis and implementation of treatment. Initially, the person must be hemodynamically stabilized. The thyroid hormones can be removed by plasmapheresis, dialysis, or hemoperfusion adsorption. Peripheral cooling is initiated with cold packs and a cooling mattress. For cooling to be effective, the shivering response must be prevented. General supportive measures to replace fluids, glucose, and electrolytes are essential during the hypermetabolic state. A β-adrenergic blocking drug, such as propranolol, is given to block the undesirable effects of T_4 on cardiovascular function. Glucocorticoids are used to correct the relative adrenal insufficiency resulting from the stress imposed by the hyperthyroid state and to inhibit the peripheral conversion of T_4 to T_3. Propylthiouracil or methimazole may be given to block thyroid synthesis. Aspirin increases the level of free thyroid hormones by displacing the hormones from their protein carriers and should not be used during thyroid storm.[35-37]

SUMMARY CONCEPTS

Thyroid hormones play a role in the metabolic process of almost all body cells and are necessary for normal physical and mental growth in the infant and young child. Alterations in thyroid function can manifest as a hypothyroid or a hyperthyroid state. Hypothyroidism can occur as a congenital or an acquired defect. Congenital hypothyroidism leads to intellectual disability and impaired physical growth unless treatment is initiated during the first month of life. Acquired hypothyroidism leads to a decrease in metabolic rate and an accumulation of a mucopolysaccharide substance in the intercellular spaces; this substance attracts water and causes a mucous type of edema called *myxedema*. Hyperthyroidism causes an increase in metabolic rate and alterations in body function similar to those produced by enhanced sympathetic nervous system activity. Graves disease is characterized by the triad of hyperthyroidism, goiter, and ophthalmopathy. A life-threatening complication of hyperthyroidism is *thyroid storm*.

Disorders of Adrenal Cortical Function

Control of Adrenal Cortical Function

The adrenal glands are small, bilateral structures that weigh approximately 5 g each and lie retroperitoneally at the apex of each kidney (Fig. 41-8). The medulla or inner portion of the gland (which constitutes approximately 20% of each adrenal) secretes epinephrine and norepinephrine and is part of the sympathetic nervous system.[4] The cortex forms the bulk of the adrenal gland (approximately 80%) and is responsible for secreting three types of hormones—the glucocorticoids, the mineralocorticoids, and the adrenal androgens.[4] Because the sympathetic nervous system also secretes epinephrine and norepinephrine, adrenal medullary function is not essential for life, but adrenal cortical function is. The total loss of adrenal cortical function is fatal in a few days to a few weeks if untreated.[4] This section of the chapter describes the synthesis and function of the adrenal cortical hormones and the effects of adrenal cortical insufficiency and excess.

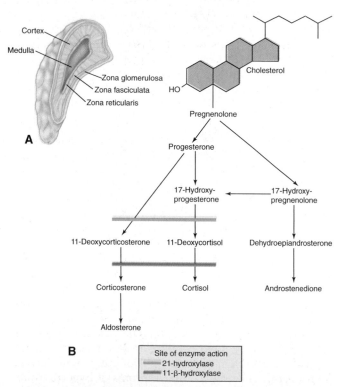

FIGURE 41-8. (A) The adrenal gland showing the medulla and the three layers of the cortex. The outer layer of the cortex (zona glomerulosa) is primarily responsible for mineralocorticoid production and the middle layer (zona fasciculata) and the inner layer (zona reticularis) produce the glucocorticoids and the adrenal androgens. (B) Predominant biosynthetic pathways of the adrenal cortex. Critical enzymes in the biosynthetic process include 11-β-hydroxylase and 21-hydroxylase. A deficiency in one of these enzymes blocks the synthesis of hormones dependent on that enzyme and routes the precursors into alternative pathways.

Biosynthesis, Transport, and Metabolism

More than 30 hormones are produced by the adrenal cortex. Of these hormones, aldosterone is the principal mineralocorticoid, cortisol (hydrocortisone) is the major glucocorticoid, and androgens are the chief sex hormones. All of the adrenal cortical hormones have a similar structure in which all are steroids and are synthesized from acetate and cholesterol. Each of the steps involved in the synthesis of the various hormones requires a specific enzyme (see Fig. 41-8). The ACTH secreted by the anterior pituitary gland controls the secretion of the glucocorticoids and the adrenal androgens.[4,9]

Cortisol, aldosterone, and the adrenal androgens are secreted in an unbound state and bind to plasma proteins for transport in the circulatory system.[4,9]

The main site for metabolism of the adrenal cortical hormones is the liver, where they undergo a number of metabolic conversions before being conjugated and made water-soluble. They are then eliminated in either the urine or the bile.[4,9]

KEY POINTS

Adrenal Cortical Hormones

■ The manifestations of primary adrenal cortical insufficiency are related mainly to mineralocorticoid deficiency (impaired ability to regulate salt and water elimination) and glucocorticoid deficiency (impaired ability to regulate blood glucose and control the effects of the immune and inflammatory responses).

■ Adrenal cortical excess results in derangements in glucose metabolism, disorders of sodium and potassium regulation (increased sodium retention and potassium loss), impaired ability to respond to stress because of inhibition of inflammatory and immune responses, and signs of increased androgen levels such as hirsutism.

Adrenal Androgens

The adrenal androgens are synthesized primarily by the zona reticularis and the zona fasciculata of the cortex (see Fig. 41-8A).[4] These sex hormones probably exert little effect on normal sexual function. There is evidence, however, that the adrenal androgens (the most important of which is dehydroepiandrosterone and its dehydroepiandrosterone sulfate [DHEAS]) contribute to the pubertal growth of body hair, particularly pubic and axillary hair in women. They may also play a role in steroid hormone economy of the pregnant woman and the fetal–placental unit. The levels of DHEAS and other adrenal hormones decline with age, a process referred to as the *adrenopause*. DHEAS levels may represent another aging marker because it is involved with cardiovascular, immunologic, and endocrine systems and may be a trend indicator for prevention of specific problems with aging.[38-40]

Mineralocorticoids

The mineralocorticoids play an essential role in regulating potassium and sodium levels and water balance. They are produced in the zona glomerulosa, the outer layer of cells of the adrenal cortex. Aldosterone secretion is regulated by the renin–angiotensin mechanism and by blood levels of potassium. Increased levels of aldosterone promote sodium retention by the distal tubules of the kidney while increasing urinary losses of potassium.[4]

Aldosterone is significant for balancing sodium, chloride, and potassium as well as maintaining the total body volume. To understand the importance of aldosterone, consider that both aldosterone and cortisone provide mineralocorticoid function; however, approximately 90% of mineralocorticoid function is provided through aldosterone. Although aldosterone is responsible for about 3000 times greater the amount of mineralocorticoid activity than cortisol, there is nearly 2000 times more serum cortisol than aldosterone.[4] Because of the potency of aldosterone, it is crucial that the body does not have excess or deficiency of this potent steroid. The consequences of excess aldosterone are low potassium and muscle weakness, although low amounts of aldosterone cause high potassium and cardiac toxicity.[4]

Glucocorticoids

The glucocorticoid hormones, mainly cortisol, are synthesized in the zona fasciculata and the zona reticularis of the adrenal gland.[4] The blood levels of these hormones are regulated by negative feedback mechanisms of the HPA system (Fig. 41-9). Just as other pituitary hormones are controlled by releasing factors from the hypothalamus, corticotropin-releasing hormone (CRH) is important in controlling the release of ACTH. Cortisol levels increase as ACTH levels rise and decrease as ACTH levels fall. There is considerable diurnal variation in ACTH levels, which reach their peak in the early morning (around 6 to 8 AM) and decline as the day progresses. This appears to be due to rhythmic activity in the CNS, which causes bursts of CRH secretion and, in turn, ACTH secretion. This diurnal pattern is reversed in people who work during the night and sleep during the day. The rhythm may also be changed by physical and psychological stresses, endogenous depression, manic-depressive psychosis, and liver disease or other conditions that affect cortisol metabolism.[4]

The glucocorticoids perform a necessary function in response to stress and are essential for survival. When produced as part of the stress response, these hormones aid in regulating the metabolic functions of the body and in controlling the inflammatory response. The actions of cortisol are summarized in Table 41-4. Many of the anti-inflammatory actions attributed to cortisol result from the administration of pharmacologic levels of the hormone.[4]

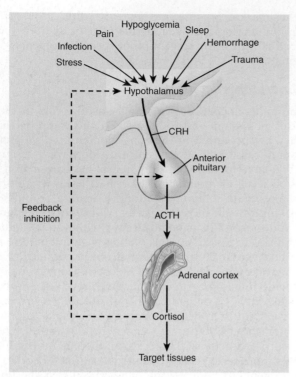

FIGURE 41-9. The HPA feedback system that regulates glucocorticoid (cortisol) levels. Cortisol release is regulated by ACTH. Stress exerts its effects on cortisol release through the HPA system and CRH, which controls the release of ACTH from the anterior pituitary gland. Increased cortisol levels incite a negative feedback inhibition of ACTH release. ACTH, adrenocorticotropic hormone; CRH, corticotropin-releasing hormone; HPA, hypothalamic–pituitary–adrenal.

TABLE 41-4	Actions of Cortisol
Major Influence	**Effect on Body**
Glucose metabolism	Stimulates gluconeogenesis
	Decreases glucose use by the tissues
Protein metabolism	Increases breakdown of proteins
	Increases plasma protein levels
Fat metabolism	Increases mobilization of fatty acids
	Increases use of fatty acids
Anti-inflammatory action (pharmacologic levels)	Stabilizes lysosomal membranes of the inflammatory cells, preventing the release of inflammatory mediators
	Decreases capillary permeability to prevent inflammatory edema
	Depresses phagocytosis by white blood cells to reduce the release of inflammatory mediators
	Suppresses the immune response
	Causes atrophy of lymphoid tissue
	Decreases eosinophils
	Decreases antibody formation
	Decreases the development of cell-mediated immunity
	Reduces fever
	Inhibits fibroblast activity
Psychic effect	May contribute to emotional instability
Permissive effect	Facilitates the response of the tissues to humoral and neural influences, such as that of the catecholamines, during trauma and extreme stress

Metabolic Effects

Cortisol stimulates glucose production by the liver, promotes protein breakdown, and causes mobilization of fatty acids. As body proteins are broken down, amino acids are mobilized and transported to the liver, where they are used in the production of glucose. Mobilization of fatty acids converts cell metabolism from the use of glucose for energy to the use of fatty acids instead. As glucose production by the liver rises and peripheral glucose use falls, a moderate resistance to insulin develops. In people with diabetes and those who are diabetes prone, this has the effect of raising the blood glucose level.[4,9]

Psychological Effects

The glucocorticoid hormones appear to be involved directly or indirectly in emotional behavior. Receptors for these hormones have been identified in brain tissue, which suggests that they play a role in the regulation of behavior. People treated with adrenal cortical hormones have been known to display behavior ranging from mildly aberrant to psychotic.[41]

Immunologic and Inflammatory Effects

Cortisol influences multiple aspects of immunologic function and inflammatory responsiveness. Large quantities of cortisol are required for an effective anti-inflammatory action. This is achieved by the administration of pharmacologic rather than physiologic doses of synthetic cortisol. The increased cortisol blocks inflammation at an early stage by decreasing capillary permeability and stabilizing the lysosomal membranes, so that inflammatory mediators are not released. Cortisol suppresses the immune response by reducing humoral and cell-mediated immunity. With this lessened inflammatory response comes a reduction in fever. During the healing phase, cortisol suppresses fibroblast activity and thereby lessens scar formation. Cortisol also inhibits prostaglandin synthesis, which may account in large part for its anti-inflammatory actions.[4]

Pharmacologic Suppression of Adrenal Function

A highly significant aspect of long-term therapy with pharmacologic preparations of the glucocorticoids is adrenal insufficiency on withdrawal of drugs. The deficiency results from suppression of the HPA system. Chronic suppression causes atrophy of the adrenal gland, and the abrupt withdrawal of drugs can cause acute adrenal insufficiency. Recovery to a state of normal adrenal function may be prolonged, requiring 6 to 12 months or more.[42]

Tests of Adrenal Function

Several diagnostic tests can be used to evaluate adrenal cortical function and the HPA system. Blood levels of cortisol, aldosterone, and ACTH can be measured using immunoassay methods. A 24-hour urine specimen measuring the excretion of various metabolic end products of adrenal hormones provides information about alterations in the biosynthesis of the adrenal cortical hormones. The 24-hour urinary free cortisol, late-night (between 11 PM and midnight) serum or salivary cortisol levels, and the overnight 1-mg dexamethasone suppression test are excellent screening tests for Cushing syndrome.[39,43,44]

Suppression and stimulation tests afford a means of assessing the state of the HPA feedback system. CRH tests can be used to diagnose a pituitary ACTH-secreting tumor (i.e., Cushing disease). Corticotropin (cosyntropin) stimulation testing is the most frequently used diagnostic test to assess testing responsiveness of the HPA axis.[39,43,44]

Congenital Adrenal Hyperplasia

CAH, or the adrenogenital syndrome, describes a congenital disorder caused by an autosomal recessive trait in which a deficiency exists in any of the enzymes necessary for the synthesis of cortisol (see Fig. 41-8). A common characteristic of all types of CAH is a defect in the synthesis of cortisol that results in increased levels of ACTH and adrenal hyperplasia.[1] The increased levels of ACTH overstimulate the pathways for production of adrenal androgens. Mineralocorticoids may be produced in excessive or insufficient amounts, depending on the precise enzyme deficiency. Infants of both sexes are affected. Boys are seldom diagnosed at birth unless they have enlarged genitalia or lose salt and manifest adrenal crisis.[1] In female infants, an increase in androgens is responsible for creating the virilization syndrome of ambiguous genitalia with an enlarged clitoris, fused labia, and urogenital sinus (Fig. 41-10). In male and female children, other secondary sex characteristics are normal, and fertility is unaffected if appropriate therapy is instituted.[1]

A spectrum of 21-hydroxylase deficiency state exists, ranging from simple virilizing CAH to a complete salt-losing enzyme deficiency. Simple virilizing CAH impairs the synthesis of cortisol, and steroid synthesis is shunted to androgen production. People with these deficiencies usually produce sufficient aldosterone or aldosterone intermediates to prevent signs and symptoms of mineralocorticoid deficiency. The salt-losing form is accompanied by deficient production of aldosterone and its intermediates, resulting in fluid and electrolyte disorders (including hyponatremia, vomiting, dehydration, and shock). Hyperkalemia is not always present, so it should not be considered a major screening diagnostic parameter.[1,45]

The 11-β-hydroxylase deficiency is rare and manifests a spectrum of severity. Affected people have excessive androgen production and impaired conversion of 11-deoxycorticosterone to corticosterone. The overproduction of 11-deoxycorticosterone, which has mineralocorticoid activity, is responsible for the hypertension that accompanies this deficiency. Diagnosis of

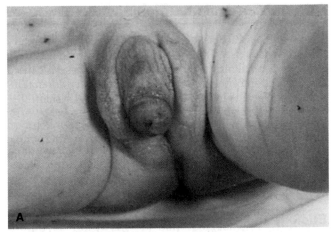

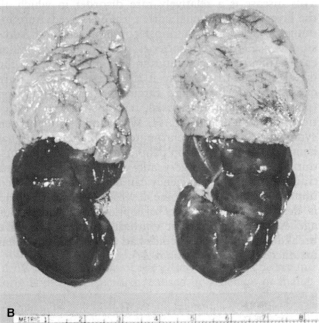

FIGURE 41-10. (A) A female infant is markedly virilized with hypertrophy of the clitoris and partial fusion of labioscrotal folds with CAH demonstrating virilization of the genitalia with hypertrophy of the clitoris and partial fusion of labioscrotal folds. (B) A 7-week-old male died of severe salt-wasting CAH. At autopsy, both adrenal glands were markedly enlarged. (From Strayer D., Rubin E. (Eds.). (2015). *Rubin's pathology: Clinicopathologic foundations of medicine* (7th ed., Figure 27.31, p. 1203). Philadelphia, PA: Wolters Kluwer.). CAH, congenital adrenal hyperplasia.

CAH depends on the precise biochemical evaluation of metabolites in the cortisol pathway and on clinical signs and symptoms. Genetic testing is also invaluable. However, correlation between the phenotype and genotype is not always straightforward.[45]

Medical treatment of CAH includes oral or parenteral glucocorticoid replacement. Fludrocortisone acetate, a mineralocorticoid, may also be given to children who are salt losers. Depending on the degree of virilization, reconstructive surgery during the first year of life may be indicated to reduce the size of the clitoris, separate the labia, and exteriorize the vagina. Women with CAH who are experiencing unwanted hair growth or androgenic hair loss may be prescribed antiandrogen drugs.[45]

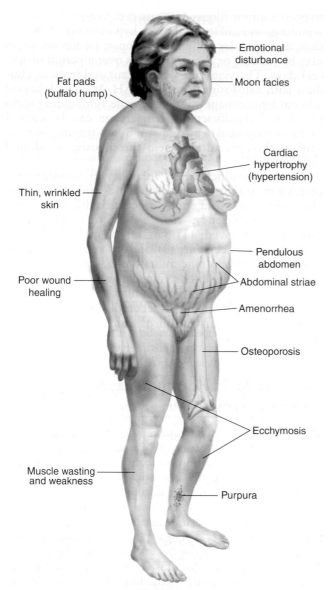

Emotional disturbance

Moon facies

Fat pads (buffalo hump)

Cardiac hypertrophy (hypertension)

Thin, wrinkled skin

Poor wound healing

Pendulous abdomen

Abdominal striae

Amenorrhea

Osteoporosis

Ecchymosis

Muscle wasting and weakness

Purpura

FIGURE 41-12. Clinical features of Cushing syndrome.

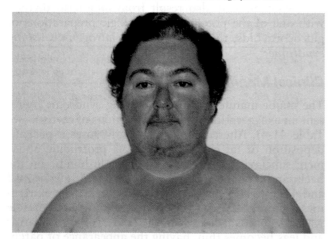

FIGURE 41-13. Cushing syndrome. A woman who had a pituitary adenoma that produced adrenocorticotropic hormone exhibits a moon face, buffalo hump, increased facial hair, and thinning of the scalp hair. (From Strayer D., Rubin E. (Eds.). (2015). *Rubin's pathology: Clinicopathologic foundations of medicine* (7th ed., Figure 27-37, p. 1209). Philadelphia, PA: Wolters Kluwer.)

resulting in back pain, compression fractures of the vertebrae, and rib fractures. As calcium is mobilized from bone, renal calculi may develop.[1,2,8]

The glucocorticoids possess mineralocorticoid properties. This causes hypokalemia, as a result of excessive potassium excretion, and hypertension, resulting from sodium retention. Inflammatory and immune responses are inhibited, resulting in increased susceptibility to infection. Cortisol increases gastric acid secretion, which may provoke gastric ulceration and bleeding. An accompanying increase in androgen levels causes hirsutism, mild acne, and menstrual irregularities in women. Excess levels of the glucocorticoids may give rise to extreme emotional lability, ranging from mild euphoria and absence of normal fatigue to grossly psychotic behavior.[1,2,8]

Diagnosis and Treatment

Diagnosis of Cushing syndrome is a two-step process: the first step is the diagnosis of hypercortisolism and the second step is testing to determine the cause of the cortisol hypersecretion. The tests most commonly used for diagnosis are the 24-hour urinary free cortisol level, the midnight plasma and late-night salivary cortisol measurements, and the low-dose dexamethasone suppression test. After a diagnosis of Cushing syndrome has been made, the following tests can be used to help determine the cause: CRH stimulation test, high-dose dexamethasone suppression test, radiologic imaging of the pituitary and adrenal glands, and petrosal sinus sampling.[50]

Untreated, Cushing syndrome produces serious morbidity and even death. The choice of surgery, irradiation, or pharmacologic treatment is determined largely by the cause of the hypercortisolism. The goal of treatment for Cushing syndrome is to remove or correct the source of hypercortisolism without causing permanent pituitary or adrenal damage. Transsphenoidal removal of a pituitary adenoma or a hemihypophysectomy is the preferred method of treatment for Cushing disease. This allows removal of only the tumor rather than the entire pituitary gland.[50,51]

Incidental Adrenal Mass

An incidentaloma is a mass found unexpectedly in an adrenal gland by an imaging procedure (done for other reasons), most commonly CT. Incidentalomas can also occur in other organs, and it is important to determine if they are malignant or hormonally active. Primary adrenal carcinoma is quite rare, but other cancers, particularly lung cancers, commonly metastasize to the adrenal gland (other cancers include breast, stomach, pancreas, colon, kidney, melanomas, and lymphomas). The size and imaging characteristics of the mass may help determine whether the tumor is benign or malignant. Appropriate screening to exclude a hormonally active lesion includes tests to rule out pheochromocytoma, Cushing syndrome, and Conn syndrome (mineralocorticoid excess).[1]

SUMMARY CONCEPTS

The adrenal cortex produces three types of hormones: mineralocorticoids, glucocorticoids, and adrenal androgens. The mineralocorticoids, along with the renin–angiotensin mechanism, aid in controlling body levels of sodium and potassium. The glucocorticoids have anti-inflammatory actions and aid in regulating glucose, protein, and fat metabolism during periods of stress. These hormones are under the control of the HPA system. The adrenal androgens exert little effect on daily control of body function, but they probably contribute to the development of body hair in women. CAH is caused by a genetic defect in the cortisol pathway resulting from a deficiency of one of the enzymes needed for its synthesis. Depending on the enzyme involved, the disorder causes virilization of female infants and, in some instances, fluid and electrolyte disturbances because of impaired mineralocorticoid synthesis.

Chronic adrenal insufficiency can be caused by destruction of the adrenal gland (Addison disease) or by dysfunction of the HPA system. Adrenal insufficiency requires replacement therapy with adrenal cortical hormones. Acute adrenal insufficiency is a life-threatening situation. Cushing syndrome refers to the manifestations of excessive glucocorticoid levels. This syndrome may be a result of pharmacologic doses of glucocorticoids, a pituitary or adrenal tumor, or an ectopic tumor that produces ACTH. The clinical manifestations of Cushing syndrome reflect the very high level of glucocorticoid that is present.

An incidental adrenal mass is a mass found unexpectedly in an adrenal gland by an imaging procedure done for other reasons. They are being recognized with increasing frequency, emphasizing the need for correct diagnosis and treatment.

General Aspects of Altered Glucose Regulation

 Hormonal Control of Glucose, Fat, and Protein Metabolism

The body uses glucose, fatty acids, and other substrates as fuel to satisfy its energy needs. Although the pulmonary and circulatory systems combine efforts to furnish the body with the oxygen needed for metabolic purposes, it is the liver, in response to hormones from the endocrine pancreas, which controls the body's fuel supply (Fig. 41-14).

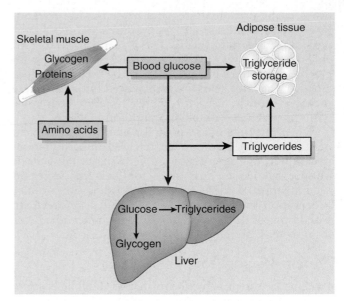

FIGURE 41-14. Hormonal and hepatic regulation of blood glucose.

Glucose Metabolism

Glucose is a six-carbon molecule. It is an efficient fuel that, when metabolized in the presence of oxygen, breaks down to form carbon dioxide and water. Although many tissues and organ systems are able to use other forms of fuel (such as fatty acids and ketones), the brain relies almost exclusively on glucose as a fuel source. Because the brain can neither synthesize nor store more than a few minutes' supply of glucose, normal cerebral function requires a continuous supply from the circulation. Severe and prolonged hypoglycemia can cause brain death, and even moderate hypoglycemia can result in substantial brain dysfunction.[4]

Body tissues obtain glucose from the blood. In people without diabetes, fasting blood glucose levels are usually tightly regulated between 80 and 90 mg/dL. After a meal, blood glucose levels rise from 100 to 120 mg/dL and the normal hormonal regulatory mechanisms return the blood levels to the control range within approximately 2 hours.[4] Insulin is secreted in response to this rise in glucose. The hormone insulin facilitates the entry of glucose into body cells (to be discussed in greater depth later). Most of the glucose that is ingested with a meal is removed from the blood and stored in the liver as glycogen, with the remaining glucose used for cellular metabolic needs. Between meals, the liver releases glucose from the stored glycogen as a means of maintaining the blood glucose within its normal range. Some glycogen can also be stored within muscle for use within muscle cells by energy. The process of breaking down glycogen to release glucose is called *glycogenolysis*.[4] In addition to mobilizing its glycogen stores, the liver can also synthesize new glucose from amino acids, glycerol, and lactic acid in a process called *gluconeogenesis*. This newly formed glucose may be released directly into the circulation or stored as glycogen.[4]

Fat Metabolism

Fat is the most dense form of fuel storage, providing 9 kcal/g of stored energy, compared with the 4 kcal/g provided by carbohydrates and proteins. The metabolism of triglycerides from fats produces a glycerol molecule and three fatty acids. The glycerol molecule can enter the glycolytic pathway and be used along with glucose to produce energy, or it can be used to produce glucose. The fatty acids are transported to tissues where they may also be used for energy by most body cells, with the previously noted exception of the brain.[4]

When fatty acids are used for energy, organic acid molecules called ketones are released into the bloodstream, creating a situation of *ketosis*. During periods of excessive use of fatty acids for fuels, the increased accumulation of these organic keto acids can produce a condition of metabolic acidosis called *ketoacidosis*. Conditions of decreased availability of either glucose or insulin create an increased risk of ketoacidosis.[4]

Protein Metabolism

Proteins are essential for the formation of all body structures, including genes, enzymes, contractile structures in muscle, matrix of bone, and hemoglobin of red blood cells.[4] Amino acids are the building blocks of proteins. Unlike glucose and fatty acids, excess amino acids can be stored in only a limited capacity in the body. Amino acids in excess of those needed for protein synthesis are converted to fatty acids, ketones, or glucose.[4] Because fatty acids cannot be converted to glucose, the body must break down proteins and use the amino acids as a major substrate for gluconeogenesis during periods when the metabolic needs for glucose exceed glucose intake.[4]

Glucose-Regulating Hormones

The hormonal control of blood glucose resides largely with the endocrine pancreas. The pancreas is made up of two major tissue types—the acini and the islets of

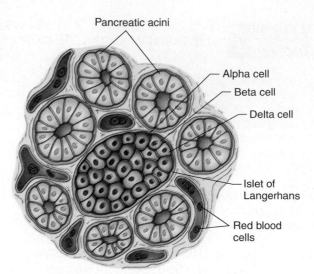

FIGURE 41-15. Islet of Langerhans in the pancreas.

Langerhans (Fig. 41-15). The acini secrete digestive juices into the duodenum; the islets of Langerhans secrete hormones into the blood.[4] Each islet is composed of beta cells (which secrete insulin and amylin), alpha cells (which secrete glucagon), and a small number of delta cells (which secrete somatostatin).[4]

Insulin

Although several hormones increase blood glucose levels, insulin is the only hormone that acts to lower blood glucose levels. The active form of insulin is produced in the beta cells of the pancreas from a larger molecule called *proinsulin* (Fig. 41-16). Insulin is formed by cleaving away the C-peptide of the proinsulin molecule, leaving the A and B polypeptide chains, which form the active insulin molecule.[4] The insulin molecule itself has

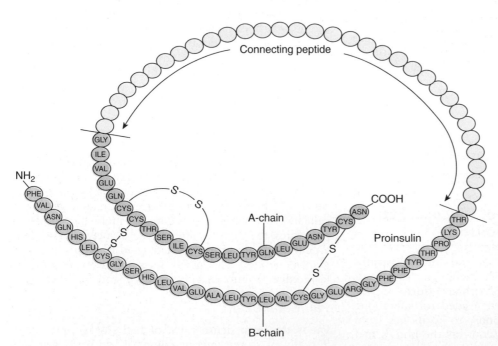

FIGURE 41.16. Structure of proinsulin. With removal of the connecting peptide (C-peptide), proinsulin is converted to insulin.

a short plasma half-life of approximately 6 minutes, with clearance from the body primarily through hepatic mechanisms and the action of the enzyme *insulinase*.[4] However, circulating blood levels of the C-peptide molecule can be measured and are used as a proxy measure to reflect pancreatic insulin production.[4,52]

The actions of insulin include:

1. Promoting glucose uptake by target cells and storage of glucose as glycogen (in liver and muscles) or fat (in adipose tissue)
2. Inhibiting fat and glycogen breakdown
3. Inhibiting gluconeogenesis and increasing protein synthesis[1,2,4] (Table 41-6)

Target cells for insulin include fat cells; therefore, insulin acts to promote fat storage by increasing the transport of glucose into fat cells. Within the fat cells, insulin facilitates the synthesis of triglycerides from glucose and inhibits the intracellular breakdown of stored triglycerides. Insulin increases protein synthesis and inhibits protein breakdown by increasing the active transport of amino acids into body cells. When sufficient glucose and insulin are present, protein breakdown is minimal because the body uses glucose and fatty acids for energy.[4]

Blood glucose levels regulate the release of insulin from the pancreatic beta cells. Insulin levels increase as blood glucose levels rise and decrease as blood glucose levels decline. Insulin binds to specific insulin receptor molecules embedded within the plasma membranes of the target cells for insulin. The insulin molecule itself does not enter the target cells; instead, the binding of insulin to its receptor causes several actions to occur within the cell, including the activation of the glucose transport proteins (described in the next paragraph). Other cellular actions triggered by the binding of insulin with its receptor include increasing the cellular permeability to amino acids and to potassium ions and phosphate ions, which increase the rate of transfer of these molecules into the cell.[4]

The binding of insulin with its cell surface receptors triggers the insertion into the cell membrane of specific glucose transporter proteins. The liver does most of the processing of glucose. When a glucose molecule enters hepatic cells through the glucose transporter protein, the glucose molecule is phosphorylated by the enzyme *glucokinase*, which creates a molecule that cannot diffuse through the cell membrane, thus effectively "trapping" the glucose inside the liver.[4] Insulin also activates the enzyme *glycogen synthase*, which then catalyzes the intrahepatic process transformation of glucose into glycogen.[4]

Because cell membranes are impermeable to glucose, a family of glucose transporters mediates the movement of glucose from the blood into the cells. These glucose transporters (named *GLUT-1*, *GLUT-2*, etc.) each have

TABLE 41-6 Actions of Insulin and Glucagon on Glucose, Fat, and Protein Metabolism

	Insulin	Glucagon
Glucose		
Glucose transport	Increases glucose transport into skeletal muscle and adipose tissue	
Glycogen synthesis	Increases glycogen synthesis	Promotes glycogen breakdown
Gluconeogenesis	Decreases gluconeogenesis	Increases gluconeogenesis
Fats		
Fatty acid and triglyceride synthesis	Promotes fatty acid and triglyceride synthesis by the liver	
Fat storage in adipose tissue	Increases the transport of fatty acids into adipose cells	
	Increases conversion of fatty acids to triglycerides by increasing the availability of α-glycerol phosphate through increased transport of glucose in adipose cells	
	Maintains fat storage by inhibiting breakdown of stored triglycerides by adipose cell lipase	Activates adipose cell lipase, making increased amounts of fatty acids available to the body for use as energy
Proteins		
Amino acid transport	Increases active transport of amino acids into cells	Increases amino acid uptake by liver cells and their conversion to glucose by gluconeogenesis
Protein synthesis	Increases protein synthesis by increasing transcription of messenger RNA and accelerating protein synthesis by ribosomal RNA	
Protein breakdown	Decreases protein breakdown by enhancing the use of glucose and fatty acids as fuel	

their own unique tissue distribution. This process is shown in Figure 41-17.

Glucagon

Glucagon is a polypeptide molecule produced in the pancreas by the alpha cells of the islets of Langerhans in response to a decrease in blood glucose. The actions of glucagon maintain blood glucose levels between meals and during periods of fasting. Glucagon levels also increase during strenuous exercise to prevent a decrease in blood glucose. After release from the pancreas, glucagon travels through the portal vein to the liver to initiate hepatic breakdown of glycogen (glycogenolysis), which rapidly raises blood glucose (see Table 41-6). Glucagon also increases the transport of amino acids into the liver and stimulates protein conversion into new glucose through the previously described process of gluconeogenesis. Because liver glycogen stores are limited, gluconeogenesis is important in maintaining blood glucose levels over time.[4]

Somatostatin, Amylin, and Gut-Derived Hormones

Somatostatin is a pancreatic polypeptide hormone containing only 14 amino acids. It has an extremely short plasma half-life of 3 minutes; however, it acts locally in the islets of Langerhans to decrease secretion of insulin and also of glucagon. Somatostatin secretion is triggered by multiple characteristics related to the ingestion of food, including the release of certain gastrointestinal hormones as well as increased blood levels of glucose, fatty acids, and amino acids. In addition to the local pancreatic effects to reduce insulin and glucagon secretion, somatostatin also decreases gastrointestinal motility and slows the absorption of food. The overall role of somatostatin appears to be to increase the time in which nutrients are available in the bloodstream for use by the body cells.[4]

Islet amyloid polypeptide, or *amylin*, is another hormone secreted by the pancreatic beta cells. Plasma levels of amylin increase after a meal or a glucose infusion.[3] Amylin appears to work with insulin to regulate plasma glucose concentrations by suppressing postprandial secretion of glucagon and slowing gastric emptying.[4,53] Several *gut-derived hormones* have been identified as having what is termed an *incretin effect*, meaning that they increase insulin release and decrease glucagon release when the plasma glucose is elevated.[4]

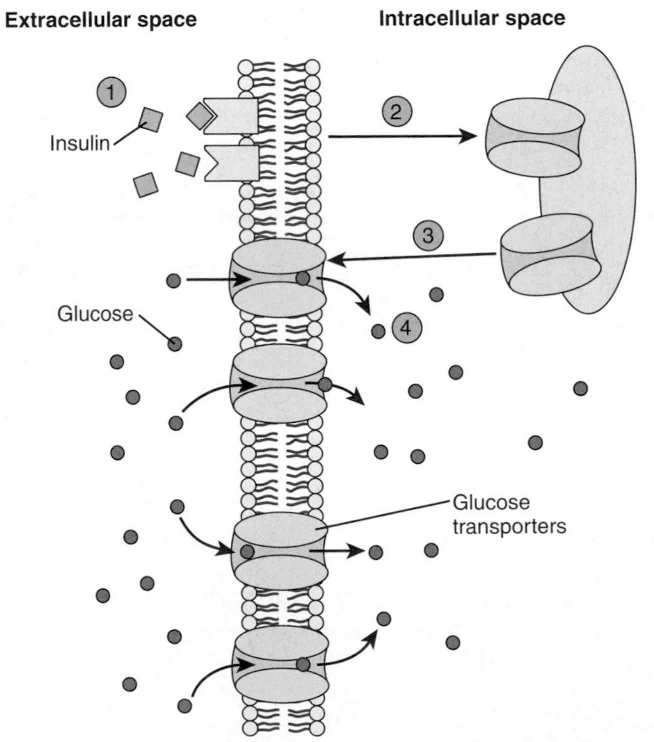

Counter-Regulatory Hormones

Other hormones that can affect blood glucose include the catecholamines, GH, and the glucocorticoids. These hormones, along with glucagon, are sometimes called *counter-regulatory hormones* because they counteract the storage functions of insulin to regulate blood glucose levels during periods of fasting, exercise, and other situations that either limit glucose intake or deplete glucose stores.[1,2,4]

Epinephrine

Epinephrine, a catecholamine from the adrenal medulla, helps to maintain blood glucose levels during periods of stress by stimulating glycogenolysis in the liver, thus causing large quantities of glucose to be released into the blood. Epinephrine also inhibits insulin release from pancreatic beta cells, which decreases movement of glucose into muscle cells and increases the breakdown of muscle glycogen stores. Although the glucose released from muscle glycogen does not enter the blood, the use of these internal energy stores by muscles conserves blood glucose for use by tissues such as the brain. Epinephrine also has a direct lipolytic effect on adipose cells, increasing the availability of fatty acids for use as an energy source. The blood glucose–elevating effect of epinephrine is also an important homeostatic mechanism during periods of hypoglycemia.[1,2,4]

Growth Hormone

In addition to the previously described effects on growth, GH has metabolic effects, which include increasing cellular protein synthesis, stimulating release of fatty acids from adipose tissue, and antagonizing the effects of insulin. Secretion of GH is normally inhibited by insulin and by increased levels of blood glucose. During periods of fasting, when both blood glucose levels and insulin secretion fall, GH levels increase. Exercise, such as running and cycling, and various stresses, including anesthesia, fever, and trauma, increase GH levels. Chronic

FIGURE 41-17. Insulin-dependent glucose transporter (GLUT-4). (*1*) Binding of insulin-to-insulin receptor on the surface of the cell membrane, (*2*) generation of intracellular signal, (*3*) insertion of GLUT-4 receptor from its inactive site into the cell membrane, and (*4*) transport of glucose across the cell membrane.

hypersecretion of GH, as occurs in acromegaly, can lead to glucose intolerance and the development of DM. The production of GH increases during childhood, peaks at puberty, and decreases with aging.[1,2,4]

Glucocorticoid Hormones

The glucocorticoid hormones, synthesized in the adrenal cortex, are critical to survival during periods of fasting and starvation, with hypoglycemia a potent stimulus of glucocorticoid release. These hormones stimulate gluconeogenesis by the liver, thus increasing hepatic glucose production. Glucocorticoids also suppress the inflammatory phase of the immune response. The pharmacotherapeutic use of glucocorticoids is a common treatment for inflammatory diseases, with hyperglycemia a potential side effect of these drugs.[1,2,4]

SUMMARY CONCEPTS

The body can use glucose, fatty acids, and proteins as fuel to satisfy its energy needs; however, the brain neurons are exclusively dependent on glucose for energy. The liver stores excess glucose as glycogen and can convert amino acids, lactate, and glycerol into glucose through the process of gluconeogenesis during periods of fasting or when glucose intake does not keep pace with demand. Blood glucose levels reflect the difference between the amount of glucose released into the circulation by the liver and the amount of glucose removed from the blood by body tissues. Fats, which serve as an efficient source of fuel for the body, are stored in adipose tissue as triglycerides (which consist of three fatty acids linked to a glycerol molecule). In conditions that favor fat breakdown, such as fasting or DM, the triglycerides in adipose tissue are broken down through the process of lipolysis. The fatty acids that are produced through lipolysis are either used as energy by body tissues or converted to ketones by the liver. Proteins, composed of amino acids, are essential for the formation of all body structures. Unlike glucose and fatty acids, excess amino acids can be stored in only a limited capacity in the body. Because fatty acids cannot be converted to glucose, the body must break down proteins and use the amino acids for gluconeogenesis during conditions in which there is insufficient glucose available to support metabolic energy needs.

A number of hormones, including insulin, glucagon, epinephrine, GH, and the glucocorticoids, control energy metabolism. Of these hormones, only insulin has the effect of lowering the blood glucose level. Insulin lowers blood glucose by increasing the transport of glucose into body cells and decreasing the hepatic production and release of glucose. Insulin also has the effect of decreasing the use of fats as an energy source by decreasing lipolysis. Other hormones—glucagon, epinephrine, GH, and the glucocorticoids—act to maintain or increase blood glucose concentrations; these hormones are referred to as *counter-regulatory hormones*. Glucagon and epinephrine promote glycogenolysis (the breakdown of glycogen stores). Glucagon and the glucocorticoids increase gluconeogenesis (the production of new glucose from nonglucose substrates, primarily amino acids). GH decreases the peripheral use of glucose. Epinephrine and glucagon also increase the use of fat for energy by increasing the release of fatty acids from adipose cells.

 ## Diabetes Mellitus and the Metabolic Syndrome

Overview, Incidence, and Prevalence

DM refers to a group of common metabolic disorders characterized by hyperglycemia resulting from imbalances between insulin secretion and cellular responsiveness to insulin. A person with uncontrolled diabetes is unable to transport glucose into cells. As a result, body cells are starved, and the breakdown of fat and protein is increased to generate cellular energy.[1,2] DM is classified into four types, as described in Chart 41-3.

DM is a chronic health problem, with the United States Centers for Disease Control and Prevention reporting 30.3 million people have diabetes (9.4% of the U.S. population).[54] Of the total number of adults with diagnosed diabetes, only 5% had type 1 diabetes, with the majority of people having type 2 diabetes. In addition, another 84.1 million adults aged 18 years or older (33.9%) have been classified as having "prediabetes," based on laboratory findings of elevations in either the fasting glucose or hemoglobin A1C levels (both to be discussed later in this chapter). Prediabetes and diabetes affect people across genders, ages, races, and ethnicity. Among U.S. adults, DM is more prevalent among American Indians/Alaska Natives (14.9% of men; 15.3% of women), non-Hispanic African Americans (12.2% of men; 13.2% of women), and Hispanic Americans (12.6% of men; 11.7% of women).[54] Type 1 diabetes is the more prevalent form in children, with the childhood incidence of new cases of type 1 diabetes highest in non-Hispanic whites. The incidence of type 2 diabetes in children is also increasing, with the incidence of new childhood cases of type 2 diabetes highest in minority populations.[54]

DM, and the resulting impact of short-term and long-term blood glucose fluctuations, can lead to a variety of complications, ranging from acute medical

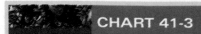

CHART 41-3

CLASSIFICATIONS OF DM

Prediabetes

- This classification is used when the blood glucose levels are elevated but do not meet the diagnostic criteria for diabetes.

Type 1 DM

- Characterized by insufficient insulin production, typically because of autoimmune destruction of pancreatic beta cells and frequently leading to absolute insulin deficiency. There is also a subtype that is idiopathic in which no autoimmune antibodies are detected.

Type 2 DM

- Characterized by a state of insulin resistance and progressive decline in pancreatic beta-cell secretion of insulin. Commonly accompanied by co-occurring clinical manifestations called the "metabolic syndrome."

Gestational DM

- Abnormalities of glucose regulation presenting initially during pregnancy, primarily during the second or third trimester.

Diabetes due to other causes

- Includes monogenic diabetic syndromes (such as neonatal diabetes and maturity-onset diabetes of the young [MODY]), as well as diabetes related to conditions such as cystic fibrosis and organ transplantation.

Adapted from American Diabetes Association. (2018). Classification and diagnosis of diabetes: Standards of medical care in diabetes—2018. *Diabetes Care* 41(Suppl 1), S13–S27.

CHART 41-4

CRITERIA FOR THE DIAGNOSIS OF DIABETES

Fasting plasma glucose ≥126 mg/dL (7.0 mmol/L). Fasting is defined as no caloric intake for at least 8 hours.

OR

2-h PG ≥ 200 mg/dL (11.1 mmol/L) during OGTT.

OR

Hemoglobin A1C ≥ 6.5% (48 mmol/L) tested using a laboratory method that is NGSP certified (National Glycohemoglobin Standardization Program) and standardized to the Diabetes Control and Complications Trial (DCCT) assay. Repeat testing should be done to confirm the results in the absence of unequivocal hyperglycemia.

OR

A random plasma glucose of ≥200 mg/dL (11.1 mmol/L) in a person with classic symptoms of hyperglycemia or hyperglycemic crisis.

Adapted from American Diabetes Association (2018). Classification and diagnosis of diabetes: Standards of medical care in diabetes—2018. *Diabetes Care* 41(Suppl 1), S15.

Blood Tests

Blood tests that are useful in the diagnosis and management of DM include the fasting blood glucose test, the random (or casual) blood glucose test, the oral glucose tolerance test (OGTT), capillary whole blood glucose testing, and glycated hemoglobin levels.

Fasting Plasma Glucose Test

The fasting plasma glucose (FPG) test is a measure of plasma glucose after a period of at least 8 hours with no caloric intake.[55] An FPG level below 100 mg/dL (5.6 mmol/L) is considered normal (see Table 50-2). A level between 100 and 125 mg/dL (5.6 and 6.9 mmol/L) is significant and is defined as IFG. The diagnostic FPG level for diabetes is 126 mg/dL (7.0 mmol/L) or higher.[55]

Random Blood Glucose Test

A random (or casual) plasma glucose is one that is done without regard to the time of the last meal. A random plasma glucose concentration that is unequivocally elevated (≥200 mg/dL [11.1 mmol/L]) in a person with classic symptoms of diabetes (such as polydipsia, polyphagia, polyuria, and blurred vision) or in a person in hyperglycemic crisis is diagnostic of DM.[55]

Oral Glucose Tolerance Test

The OGTT is an important screening test for diabetes, measuring the body's ability to remove glucose from the

---

emergencies to disability and death. DM is a significant risk factor in coronary heart disease and stroke, and it is the leading cause of blindness and chronic kidney disease as well as a common cause of lower extremity amputations. Optimizing glycemic control, through a variety of interventions, minimizes the complications associated with diabetes.[1,2]

Testing for Diagnosis and Management

The diagnosis of DM is confirmed through the use of laboratory tests that measure blood glucose levels. The diagnostic criteria for each type of DM are described in Chart 41-4. Both blood glucose measurements and tests for urinary glucose and ketones are useful in the management of diabetes.

TABLE 41-7 Correlation between Hemoglobin A1C Level and Mean Plasma Glucose Levels

Hemoglobin A1C (%)	Mean Plasma Glucose	
	In mg/dL	In mmol/L
6	126 (100–152)	7.0 (5.5–8.5)
7	154 (123–185)	8.6 (6.8–10.3)
8	183 (147–217)	10.2 (8.1–12.1)
9	212 (170–249)	11.8 (9.4–13.9)
10	240 (193–282)	13.4 (10.7–15.7)
11	269 (217–314)	14.9 (12.0–17.5)
12	298 (240–347)	16.5 (13.3–19.3)

Adapted from American Diabetes Association. (2018). Glycemic targets: Standards of medical care in diabetes—2018. Diabetes Care 48 (Suppl 1), S55–S64.

blood. In both men and women, the test measures the plasma glucose response to 75 g of a concentrated glucose solution at selected intervals, usually 1 and 2 hours. In people with normal glucose tolerance, blood glucose levels return to normal within 2 to 3 hours after ingestion of a glucose load, in which case it can be assumed that sufficient insulin is present to allow glucose to leave the blood and enter body cells. Because a person with diabetes lacks the ability to respond to an increase in blood glucose by releasing adequate insulin to facilitate storage, blood glucose levels rise above those observed in people with normal glucose tolerance and remain elevated for longer periods. For diagnostic purposes, the 2-hour plasma glucose value during an OGTT is used as an indicator, with levels ≥200 mg/dL (11.1 mmol/L) serving as a threshold criteria for diagnosis of DM (see Table 41-7).[55,56]

Capillary Whole Blood Glucose Monitoring

Technologic advances have provided the means for monitoring blood glucose levels by using a drop of capillary blood.[57,58]

Continuous glucose monitoring systems are becoming available to fine-tune glucose management. The various systems have small catheters implanted in the subcutaneous tissue to provide frequent samples. Endocrine centers are increasingly using this technology in selected people to achieve optimal glycemic management. However, capillary glucose monitoring remains the standard of care.[59]

Glycated Hemoglobin Testing (Hemoglobin A1C)

Hemoglobin A1C is a test that measures the quantity of a subtype of hemoglobin that has been glycated, meaning glucose molecules have become bound to the hemoglobin molecule.[60] When red blood cells are released from the bone marrow, hemoglobin normally does not contain glucose; however, during the 120-day life span of the red blood cell, hemoglobin normally becomes glycated. Because glucose entry into red blood cells is not insulin-dependent, the rate at which glucose becomes attached to the hemoglobin molecule reflects blood glucose levels. Glycosylation is essentially irreversible; therefore, the *level of A1C present in the blood provides an index of blood glucose levels over the approximate 120-day life span of red blood cells.* In conditions of hyperglycemia, the A1C level is increased. Table 41-7 lists A1C values with correlations of mean plasma glucose levels.

Urine Tests

Urine tests for glucose indicate that the renal threshold for reabsorption of glucose has been exceeded, which is typically accompanied by hyperglycemia. Renal tests for ketones indicate that the body is producing excessive ketone bodies, typically because of the use of nonglucose energy substrates for fuel.[61,62]

Classifications and Pathophysiology

An overview of the classification scheme of DM is shown in Chart 41-3. The pathophysiologic characteristics and clinical manifestations of each type are described in the following sections.

Prediabetes

Prediabetes is the diagnostic term used when the blood glucose is elevated but does not yet meet the threshold criteria for the diagnosis of DM. Detection of the prediabetic state is more common in people at risk for type 2 DM. If prediabetes is detected, lifestyle modifications of diet, exercise, and weight loss can help to prevent the progression to type 2 DM.[1,2,52]

Type 1 Diabetes Mellitus

Type 1 DM is characterized by destruction of the pancreatic beta cells. Approximately 5% of the cases of DM are type 1.[55] Most instances of type 1 DM are immune mediated, as reflected by the detection of specific autoantibodies. A small minority of people with type 1 DM are considered to have an idiopathic form of type 1 DM in which no autoantibodies are detected. This idiopathic form is more likely in people of Asian or African ancestry.[55]

Immune-mediated type 1 DM was formerly called *juvenile-onset diabetes* or *insulin-dependent diabetes.*[55] It occurs more commonly in young people but can occur at any age. The rate of beta-cell destruction is quite variable. The rapidly progressive form is not only commonly observed in children but also may occur in adults. Adults with type 2 DM sometimes also present with a slowly progressive form of insulin-dependent DM with autoimmune findings similar to type 1 DM. This slowly progressive adult form is sometimes referred to as *latent autoimmune diabetes in adults.*[52] Immune-mediated type 1 DM is often related to a genetic predisposition (*i.e.,* diabetogenic genes). Susceptibility to type 1A DM involves multiple genes; however, the major susceptibility gene for type 1A DM is located in the human leukocyte antigen gene related to antigen presentation to T cells.[63]

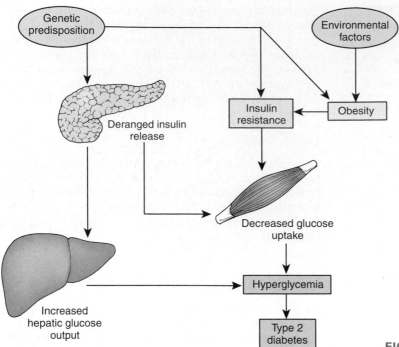

FIGURE 41-18. Pathogenesis of type 2 diabetes mellitus.

Type 1 diabetes is a catabolic disorder characterized by an absolute lack of insulin, an elevation in blood glucose, and a breakdown of body fats and proteins. The absolute lack of insulin in people with type 1 DM means that they are particularly prone to the development of ketoacidosis. One of the actions of insulin is the inhibition of *lipolysis* (*i.e.*, fat breakdown) and release of FFAs from fat cells. In the absence of insulin, ketosis develops when these fatty acids are released from fat cells and converted to ketones in the liver. Because of the loss of insulin response, *all people with immune-mediated type 1 diabetes require exogenous insulin replacement* to reverse the catabolic state, control blood glucose levels, and prevent ketosis.[1,2,52,55,63]

Type 2 Diabetes Mellitus and the Metabolic Syndrome

Type 2 DM accounts for the majority of cases of diabetes, approximately 90% to 95%.[55] It is a heterogeneous condition that describes the presence of hyperglycemia in association with *relative* insulin deficiency. Many people with type 2 diabetes are adults and overweight; however, recent trends indicate that type 2 diabetes has become a more common occurrence in adolescents and children with obesity, a condition termed *MODY*.[52] Although autoimmune destruction of the beta cells does not occur, people with type 2 diabetes eventually may require insulin. Therefore, the previous terms related to type 2 diabetes, such as *adult-onset diabetes* and *non–insulin-dependent diabetes*, can generate confusion and are thus obsolete.[55] Type 2 diabetes has a strong genetic component. A number of genetic and acquired pathogenic factors have been implicated in the progressive impairment of beta-cell function in people with prediabetes and type 2 diabetes.[52,63]

The metabolic abnormalities associated with type 2 diabetes are illustrated in Figure 41-18. These abnormalities include:

1. Insulin resistance
2. Deranged secretion of insulin by the pancreatic beta cells
3. Increased glucose production by the liver[52,55,63]

In contrast to type 1 diabetes, where *absolute* insulin deficiency is present, people with type 2 diabetes can have high, normal, or low insulin levels. Insulin resistance is the decreased ability of insulin to act effectively on target tissues, especially muscle, liver, and fat. It is the predominate characteristic of type 2 diabetes and results from a combination of factors such as genetic susceptibility and obesity.[52,55,63] Table 41-8 compares the characteristics of type 1 and type 2 DM.

Insulin resistance initially stimulates an increase in insulin secretion, often to a level of modest hyperinsulinemia, as the beta cells attempt to maintain a normal blood glucose level. In time, the increased demand for insulin secretion leads to beta-cell exhaustion and failure. This results in elevated postprandial blood glucose levels and an eventual increase in glucose production by the liver. Because people with type 2 DM do not have an absolute insulin deficiency, they are less prone to ketoacidosis compared to people with type 1 diabetes.[52,55,63]

In type 2 DM, the basal hepatic insulin resistance is manifested by a hepatic overproduction of glucose despite a fasting hyperinsulinemia, with the rate of glucose production being the primary determinant of the elevated FPG in people with type 2 diabetes. Although the insulin resistance seen in people with type 2 diabetes can be caused by a number of factors, it is strongly associated with obesity and physical inactivity.[1,2,52,55,63] Specific causes of beta-cell dysfunction in type 2 DM are unclear; however, it appears that in both type 1 DM and type 2

TABLE 41-8 Comparison of Type 1 and Type 2 DM

	Type 1 Diabetes	Type 2 Diabetes
Age of onset	Usually childhood	Usually adulthood
Type of onset	Abrupt; symptomatic (polyuria, polydipsia, dehydration) often with severe ketoacidosis	Gradual; usually subtle; often asymptomatic
Usual body weight	Normal; recent weight loss is common	Overweight
Family history	Occurs, but less common	Very common
Human leukocyte antigen associations	+	No
Islet lesions	Early—inflammation	Late—fibrosis, amyloid
	Late—atrophy and fibrosis	
Beta-cell mass	Markedly reduced	Normal or slightly reduced
Circulating insulin level	Markedly reduced	Elevated or normal
Clinical management	Insulin absolutely required	Insulin usually not needed initially; insulin supplementation may be needed at later stages; weight loss typically improves the condition

DM, there may be an increased apoptosis of pancreatic beta cells in response to the stress of hyperglycemia.[63]

Insulin Resistance and the Metabolic Syndrome

Increasing evidence indicates that insulin resistance not only contributes to the hyperglycemia in people with type 2 diabetes, but it also may play a role in other metabolic abnormalities. These include obesity, high levels of plasma triglycerides and low levels of high-density lipoproteins (HDL), hypertension, systemic inflammation (as detected by CRP and other mediators), abnormal fibrinolysis, abnormal function of the vascular endothelium, and macrovascular disease (coronary artery, cerebrovascular, and peripheral arterial disease). This constellation of abnormalities is often referred to as the *insulin resistance syndrome*, *syndrome X*, or, the preferred term, *metabolic syndrome*.[1,2,52,55,63] The clinical signs, laboratory abnormalities, and associated illnesses associated with this syndrome are described in Chart 41-5.

A major factor in people with metabolic syndrome that leads to type 2 diabetes is obesity. People with obesity have increased resistance to the action of insulin and impaired suppression of glucose production by the liver, resulting in both hyperglycemia and hyperinsulinemia. The type of obesity is an important consideration in the development of type 2 diabetes. People with upper body (or central) obesity are at greater risk for developing type 2 diabetes and metabolic disturbances than people with lower body (or peripheral) obesity. Waist circumference and waist–hip ratio, which are both surrogate measures of central obesity, have been shown to correlate well with insulin resistance. A loss of 5% to 10% of body weight has the potential to improve insulin resistance and lower blood glucose levels.[1,2,55]

The increased adipose tissue and/or dense distribution of central adiposity challenge the vascular perfusion of that tissue, leading to chronic underperfusion with areas

CHART 41-5

FREQUENTLY OBSERVED CONCOMITANTS OF THE METABOLIC SYNDROME

Clinical Signs
- Central (upper body) obesity with increased waist circumference
- Acanthosis nigricans (hypertrophic, hyperpigmented skin changes)

Laboratory Abnormalities
- Elevated fasting and/or postprandial glucose
- Insulin resistance with hyperinsulinemia
- Dyslipidemia characterized by increased triglycerides and low HDL cholesterol
- Abnormal thrombolysis
- Hyperuricemia
- Endothelial and vascular smooth muscle dysfunction
- Albuminuria

Comorbid Illnesses
- Hypertension
- Atherosclerosis
- Hyperandrogenism with polycystic ovary syndrome

Adapted from Rubin R., Strayer D. S. (2015). *Rubin's pathology: Clinicopathologic foundations of medicine* (7th ed., Table 13-1, p. 521). Philadelphia, PA: Lippincott Williams & Wilkins.

of tissue hypoxia and necrosis in the adipose tissue. Tissue macrophages respond to the hypoxic–ischemic cellular damage that induces a condition of chronic inflammation. This inflammatory state begins in the adipose tissue and progresses to other areas of the body to foster a chronic systemic inflammatory response state with oxidative stress that contributes to the development of atherosclerotic plaque and atherothrombosis.[64]

In type 2 DM, adipose tissues are among the tissues that demonstrate inadequate response to insulin, contributing to the pancreatic response of hyperinsulinemia to attempt to reduce the hyperglycemia. Overexpression of insulin receptors also may occur. Normally, cellular response to insulin binding stimulates two intracellular pathways—the phosphoinositide 3-kinase (P13K) pathway and the mitogen-activated protein (MAP) pathway. In type 2 DM, the P13K pathway does not maintain its function; this P13K functional decline contributes to decreased nitric oxide production from endothelial cells and to a decrease in the translocation of the GLUT-4 proteins that facilitate glucose entry into cells.[64] Nitric oxide is a powerful endothelial-derived relaxing factor, which promotes vasodilation.[4] Therefore, the decline in nitric oxide production contributes to vasoconstriction and increased vascular resistance. In type 2 DM, the MAP pathway that is also stimulated by the binding of insulin to cellular insulin receptors continues to function. The actions of stimulation of the MAP pathway include stimulation of the vasoconstriction molecule endothelin-1, along with increased expression of adhesion molecules and smooth muscle stimulation, all of which further contribute to the increased risk of development of atherosclerosis in type 2 DM.[64]

Insulin also normally signals the inhibition of lipolysis; however, the insulin resistance in type 2 DM causes increased lipolysis with increased release of FFAs. The liver transforms these FFAs into triglycerides and very-low-density lipoproteins. The net results of the combined systemic inflammation, increased oxidative stress, endothelial dysfunction, and increased blood lipids all contribute to the constellation of metabolic alterations that are present in the metabolic syndrome—including dyslipidemia, hypertension, vascular pathology, and abnormal coagulation.[64]

KEY POINTS

Diabetes Mellitus

- DM is a disorder of carbohydrate, fat, and protein metabolism brought about by impaired beta-cell synthesis or release of insulin, or the inability of tissues to use insulin.

- Type 1 DM results from loss of beta-cell function and an absolute insulin deficiency.

- Type 2 DM results from impaired ability of the tissues to use insulin (insulin resistance) accompanied by a relative lack of insulin or impaired release of insulin in relation to blood glucose levels (beta-cell dysfunction).

Gestational Diabetes

Gestational diabetes mellitus (GDM) is any degree of glucose intolerance that occurs initially during pregnancy, particularly presenting during the second and third trimesters. Diagnosis and careful medical management are essential because women with GDM are at higher risk for complications of pregnancy, mortality, and fetal abnormalities. Fetal abnormalities include macrosomia (*i.e.*, large body size), hypoglycemia, hypocalcemia, polycythemia, and hyperbilirubinemia. Women with GDM have an increased risk of developing type 2 DM; therefore, women in whom GDM is diagnosed should be followed after delivery to detect diabetes early in its course.[55,65]

Diabetes due to Other Causes

A small percentage of the overall number of cases of diabetes consist of specific types of diabetes associated with certain other conditions and syndromes. Such diabetes can occur with pancreatic disease or the removal of pancreatic tissue and with endocrine diseases, such as acromegaly, Cushing syndrome, or pheochromocytoma. Endocrine disorders that produce hyperglycemia do so by increasing the hepatic production of glucose or decreasing the cellular use of glucose. Several specific types of diabetes are associated with monogenetic defects in beta-cell function. Other causes for diabetes can be genetic defects in beta-cell function or insulin secretion, drug treatment, or chemicals.[1,2,52,55]

Clinical Manifestations of Diabetes Mellitus

In type 1 DM, signs and symptoms often arise suddenly. Type 2 DM usually develops more insidiously, often existing for years without detection until diagnosed during a routine medical examination or care for other conditions.

The most commonly identified signs and symptoms of diabetes are referred to as the *three polys*:

1. Polyuria (*i.e.*, excessive urination)
2. Polydipsia (*i.e.*, excessive thirst)
3. Polyphagia (*i.e.*, excessive hunger)

These three symptoms are closely related to the hyperglycemia and glycosuria of diabetes. Glucose is a small, osmotically active molecule. When blood glucose levels are sufficiently elevated, the amount of glucose filtered by the glomeruli of the kidney exceeds the amount that can be reabsorbed by the renal tubules. This results in glycosuria accompanied by osmotic large volume losses of water in the urine. Thirst results from the intracellular dehydration that occurs as blood glucose levels rise causing an osmotic movement of water out of body cells, including cells in the hypothalamic thirst center. This early symptom of increased thirst may be easily overlooked in people with type 2 DM, particularly in those who have had a gradual increase in blood glucose levels. Polyphagia is usually not present in people with type 2 diabetes. In type 1 diabetes, polyphagia probably results from cellular starvation and the depletion of cellular stores of carbohydrates, fats, and proteins.[1,2,4,52,63]

Weight loss despite normal or increased appetite is a common occurrence in people with uncontrolled type 1 diabetes. The cause of weight loss is twofold. First, loss of body fluids results from osmotic diuresis. Vomiting may exaggerate fluid loss in ketoacidosis. Second, body tissue is lost because the lack of insulin forces the body to use fat stores and cellular proteins for energy. Although weight loss is a frequent phenomenon in people with uncontrolled type 1 DM, type 2 DM is associated with obesity. However, some people with undiagnosed type 2 DM may experience unexplained weight loss as cellular resistance to circulating insulin reduces energy availability.[1,2,4,52,63]

Other signs and symptoms of hyperglycemia include recurrent blurred vision, fatigue, and skin infections. In type 2 DM, these are often the symptoms that prompt a person to seek medical treatment. Blurred vision develops as the lens and retina are exposed to hyperosmolar fluids. Lowered plasma volume produces weakness and fatigue. Chronic skin infections often occur in people with type 2 DM. Hyperglycemia and glycosuria also favor the growth of yeast organisms. *Candida* infections are common initial complaints in women with diabetes.[1,2,4,52,63]

Treatment

The desired management outcome in both type 1 and type 2 DM is normalization of blood glucose with the goal of preventing short-term and long-term complications. Treatment plans involve medical nutrition therapy, exercise, and antidiabetic agents. People with type 1 diabetes require insulin therapy from the time of diagnosis. Weight loss and dietary management may be sufficient to control blood glucose levels in some people with type 2 diabetes who adopt lifestyle changes long term. However, follow-up care is also important for type 2 diabetes because insulin secretion from the beta cells may decrease or insulin resistance may persist or worsen. If this is the case, medications to treat insulin resistance are prescribed. Pancreas transplantation methods are also increasingly being used as a method of diabetic control.[1,2,55,65]

 SUMMARY CONCEPTS

DM is a disorder of carbohydrate, protein, and fat metabolism resulting from an imbalance between insulin availability and insulin need. The disease can be classified as type 1 DM in which there is destruction of beta cells and an absolute insulin deficiency, or type 2 DM in which there is a lack of insulin availability or effectiveness. GDM develops during pregnancy, and although glucose tolerance often returns to normal after childbirth, it indicates an increased risk for the development of diabetes. The metabolic syndrome represents a constellation of metabolic abnormalities characterized by obesity, insulin resistance, high triglyceride levels and low HDL levels, hypertension, cardiovascular disease, insulin resistance, and increased risk for development of type 2 DM.

The most commonly identified symptoms of type 1 DM are polyuria, polydipsia, polyphagia, and weight loss despite normal or increased appetite. Although people with type 2 DM may present with one or more of these symptoms, they are often asymptomatic initially. The diagnosis of DM is based on clinical signs of the disease, fasting blood glucose levels, random plasma glucose measurements, and results of the glucose tolerance test. Glycation involves the irreversible attachment of glucose to the hemoglobin molecule; the measurement of A1C provides an index of blood glucose levels over several months. Self-monitoring provides a means of maintaining near-normal blood glucose levels through frequent testing of blood glucose and adjustment of insulin dosage.

Complications of Diabetes Mellitus

Acute Complications of Diabetes

The three major acute complications of diabetes are diabetic ketoacidosis (DKA), hyperosmolar hyperglycemic state (HHS), and hypoglycemia. All are life-threatening conditions that demand immediate recognition and treatment. These complications account for a significant number of hospitalizations and consumption of health care resources.[1,2,4]

Diabetic Ketoacidosis

DKA most commonly occurs in a person with type 1 diabetes in whom the lack of insulin leads to increased release of fatty acids from adipose tissue because of the unsuppressed adipose cell lipase activity that breaks down triglycerides into fatty acids and glycerol. The increase in fatty acid levels leads to ketone production by the liver (Fig. 41-19). DKA can occur at the onset of the disease, often before diagnosis, and can occur as a complication during the course of the disease.

Stress increases the release of gluconeogenic hormones and predisposes the person to the development of ketoacidosis. DKA is often preceded by physical or emotional stress, such as infection or inflammation, pregnancy, or extreme anxiety. Ketoacidosis also occurs with the omission or inadequate use of insulin.[1,2,4]

Etiology and Pathogenesis
The three major metabolic derangements in DKA are hyperglycemia, ketosis, and metabolic acidosis. Hyperglycemia leads to osmotic diuresis, dehydration, and a critical loss of electrolytes. Hyperosmolality of

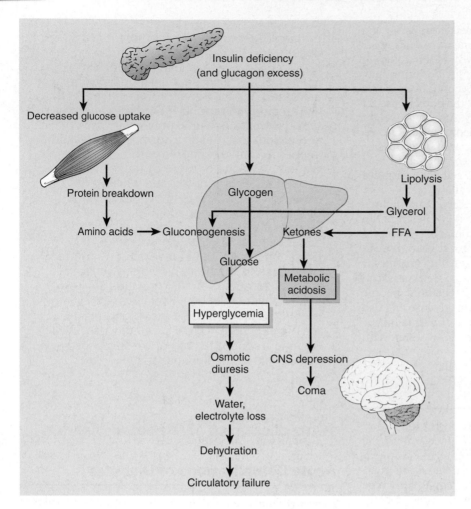

FIGURE 41-19. Mechanisms of diabetic ketoacidosis (DKA). DKA is associated with very low insulin levels and extremely high levels of glucagon, catecholamines, and other counter-regulatory hormones. Increased levels of glucagon and the catecholamines lead to mobilization of substrates for gluconeogenesis and ketogenesis by the liver. Gluconeogenesis in excess of that needed to supply glucose for the brain and other glucose-dependent tissues produces a rise in blood glucose levels. Mobilization of free fatty acid (FFA) from triglyceride stores in adipose tissue leads to accelerated ketone production and ketosis. CNS, central nervous system.

extracellular fluid because of hyperglycemia leads to a shift of water from the intracellular to the extracellular compartment. Extracellular sodium concentration is frequently low or normal despite increased urinary water losses because of the intracellular–extracellular fluid shift. This dilutional effect is referred to as *pseudohyponatremia*. Serum potassium levels may be normal or elevated despite total potassium depletion resulting from protracted polyuria and vomiting. Metabolic acidosis is caused by the excess keto acids that require buffering by bicarbonate ions. This leads to a marked decrease in serum bicarbonate levels. The severity of DKA is classified on the severity of the metabolic acidosis.[1,2,4]

Clinical Manifestations
A day or more of polyuria, polydipsia, nausea, vomiting, and marked fatigue, with eventual stupor that can progress to coma commonly precedes DKA. Abdominal pain and tenderness may be experienced without abdominal disease. The breath has a characteristic fruity smell because of the presence of the volatile keto acids. Hypotension and tachycardia may be present because of a decrease in blood volume. A number of the signs and symptoms that occur in DKA are related to compensatory mechanisms. The heart rate increases as the body compensates for a decrease in blood volume, and the rate and depth of respiration increase (*i.e.*, Kussmaul

respiration) as a compensatory mechanism to prevent further decrease in pH.[1,2,4]

Treatment
The goals in treating DKA are to improve circulatory volume and tissue perfusion, decrease blood glucose, correct the metabolic acidosis, and correct electrolyte imbalances. These objectives are usually accomplished through the administration of insulin along with intravenous fluid and electrolyte replacement solutions. Because insulin resistance accompanies severe acidosis, low-dose insulin therapy may be used.[1,2,65]

Hyperosmolar Hyperglycemic State

HHS is characterized by hyperglycemia, hyperosmolarity with dehydration, the absence of ketoacidosis, and depression of the sensorium. HHS occurs frequently in people with type 2 diabetes.[1,2,4]

Etiology and Pathogenesis
A partial or relative insulin deficiency may initiate HHS by reducing glucose utilization while increasing glucagon release and hepatic glucose output. The hyperglycemia leads to large volume water loss through osmotic diuresis. Dehydration is usually more severe in HHS than in DKA. As the plasma volume contracts, renal insufficiency develops. The resultant decrease in renal

elimination of glucose further elevates blood glucose levels, which increases the severity of the hyperosmolar state. In hyperosmolar states, the increased serum osmolarity has the effect of pulling water out of body cells, including brain cells. HHS may also be complicated by thromboembolic events related to the contraction of plasma volume with increased coagulability because of stasis.[1,2,4]

Clinical Manifestations and Treatment

The most prominent manifestations of HHS are weakness, dehydration, polyuria, neurologic alterations, and excessive thirst. Neurologic alterations include hemiparesis, seizures, and coma; these symptoms may be mistaken for a stroke. Successful treatment of HHS involves careful patient monitoring and correction of dehydration, hyperglycemia, and electrolyte imbalance. Close observation and care is particularly important as water moves back into brain cells, posing a threat of cerebral edema.[1,2,65]

Hypoglycemia

Hypoglycemia is generally defined as any blood glucose concentration of less than 70 mg/dL, with or without symptoms.[65] It occurs most commonly in people treated with insulin injections, but prolonged hypoglycemia can also result from some oral antidiabetic agents.[1,2,65]

Etiology and Pathogenesis

Many factors can precipitate hypoglycemia in a person with type 1 DM, including error in insulin dose, failure to eat, increased exercise, decreased insulin need after removal of a stress situation, medication changes, and a change in insulin injection site. Alcohol decreases liver gluconeogenesis; therefore, people with diabetes need to be cautioned about the potential for alcohol ingestion to cause hypoglycemia, particularly if consumed in large amounts or on an empty stomach.[1,2,65]

Clinical Manifestations

Hypoglycemia usually has a rapid onset and progression of symptoms. The signs and symptoms of hypoglycemia can be divided into two categories: (a) those caused by altered brain function and (b) those related to activation of the autonomic nervous system. Because the brain relies on blood glucose as its main energy source, hypoglycemia produces behaviors related to altered brain function. Headache, difficulty in problem solving, disturbed or altered behavior, coma, and seizures may occur. At the onset of the hypoglycemic episode, activation of the parasympathetic nervous system often causes hunger. The initial parasympathetic response is followed by activation of the sympathetic nervous system; this causes anxiety, tachycardia, sweating, and constriction of the skin vessels (*i.e.*, the skin is cool and clammy).[1,2,4]

The signs and symptoms of hypoglycemia are highly variable, and not everyone manifests all or even most of the symptoms. The signs and symptoms are particularly variable in children and in older adults. Older adults may not display the typical autonomic responses associated with hypoglycemia but frequently develop signs of impaired function of the CNS, including mental confusion. Some people develop hypoglycemic unawareness. Unawareness of hypoglycemia should be suspected in people who do not report symptoms when their blood glucose concentrations are <50 to 60 mg/dL (2.8 to 3.3 mmol/L). This occurs most commonly in people who have a longer duration of diabetes and A1C levels within the normal range. Some medications, such as β-adrenergic blocking drugs, interfere with the sympathetic response normally seen in hypoglycemia.[1-3,65]

Treatment

Recommended treatment of an insulin reaction is the immediate oral administration of a rapidly absorbed form of glucose, which can be repeated as necessary. For people who are unconscious or unable to swallow, glucagon may be given intramuscularly or subcutaneously to raise blood glucose through hepatic glycogenolysis.[65]

Diabetic Complications Related to Counter-Regulatory Mechanisms

The counter-regulatory mechanisms described above are associated with several patterns of diabetic complications, known as the Somogyi effect and the dawn phenomenon.

The Somogyi Effect

In people with DM, the insulin-induced hypoglycemia produces a compensatory increase in blood levels of counter-regulatory hormones such as catecholamines, glucagon, cortisol, and GH, known as the Somogyi effect. These counter-regulatory hormones cause blood glucose to become elevated and produce some degree of insulin resistance. The cycle begins when the increase in blood glucose and insulin resistance is treated with larger insulin doses. The Somogyi phenomenon is less common than the dawn phenomenon, which is described below.[66]

Clinically, high blood glucose levels in the morning can complicate medical treatment of diabetes if not fully understood to be a counter-regulatory result of hypoglycemia. The hypoglycemic episode often occurs during the night or at a time when it is not recognized, rendering the diagnosis of the phenomenon more difficult. Without proper evaluation, an increase in medication can exacerbate the situation. When a Somogyi situation is suspected, people may be asked to test blood sugars in the middle of the night to identify possible hypoglycemia.[66]

The Dawn Phenomenon

The dawn phenomenon is characterized by increased fasting blood glucose and/or insulin requirements during the early morning hours that are *not* triggered by a preceding hypoglycemic event (in contrast with the Somogyi effect described above). The dawn phenomenon is the result of circadian variations in hormone secretion, with glucagon secretion to release energy stores in preparation for the activity of the day. High fasting blood glucose levels are common in people with type 2 DM because of the dawn phenomenon.[67]

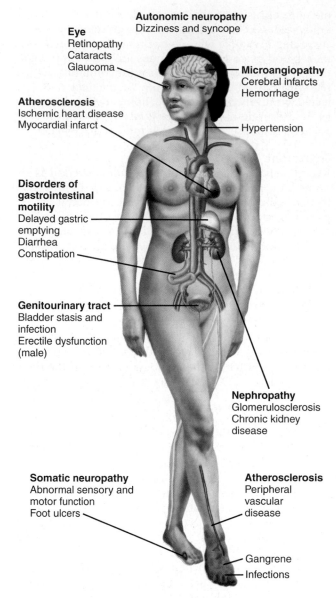

FIGURE 41-20. Long-term complications of diabetes mellitus.

Chronic Complications of Diabetes Mellitus

The chronic complications of diabetes include disorders of the microvasculature (*i.e.*, neuropathies, nephropathies, and retinopathies), disorders of gastrointestinal motility, macrovascular complications (*i.e.*, coronary artery, cerebral vascular, and peripheral vascular disease), and foot ulcers (Fig. 41-20). People with diabetes are also more susceptible to infections. The level of chronic hyperglycemia is the best predictive factor for diabetic complications; therefore, glycemic control is a primary goal of diabetic treatment.[55,65,68]

Microvascular Complications

The microvascular complications of DM are related to the production of advanced glycation end products (AGEs), as reflected in the hemoglobin A1C measure. AGEs induce vascular damage by stimulating an increased production of reactive oxygen species (ROS). These ROS are thought to damage endothelial cells by decreasing the production of the vascular endothelial relaxing factor NO, thus leading to endothelial dysfunction.[69]

In type 2 DM, this damage from AGEs may be compounded by the increased oxidative stress, chronic systemic inflammation, and dyslipidemia associated with the metabolic syndrome (as described previously). The types of microvascular complications that occur in DM can include neuropathy, retinopathy, nephropathy, and disorders of gastrointestinal motility. In the United States, diabetes is a leading cause of vision loss and blindness as well as chronic kidney disease.[1,2]

Macrovascular Complications

Because of the previously discussed vascular damage owing to hyperglycemia and the metabolic syndrome, people with DM are at increased risk of macrovascular complications such as coronary artery disease, cerebrovascular disease and stroke, and peripheral vascular disease.

KEY POINTS

Chronic Complications of Diabetes

- The chronic complications of diabetes result from elevated blood glucose levels and associated impairment of lipid and other metabolic pathways.

- Macrovascular disorders such as coronary heart disease, stroke, and peripheral vascular disease reflect the combined effects of unregulated blood glucose levels, elevated blood pressure, and hyperlipidemia.

- The chronic complications of diabetes are best prevented by measures aimed at tight control of blood glucose levels, maintenance of normal lipid levels, and control of hypertension.

Diabetic Foot Ulcers

Foot problems are common among people with diabetes and may become severe enough to cause ulceration, infection, and, eventually, the need for amputation. In people with diabetes, lesions of the feet represent the effects of neuropathy and vascular insufficiency. People with sensory neuropathies have impaired pain sensation and are often unaware of the constant trauma to the feet caused by poorly fitting shoes, improper weight bearing, hard objects or pebbles in the shoes, or infections such

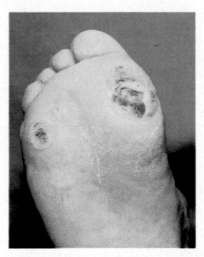

FIGURE 41-21. Peripheral neuropathies, most common in people with diabetes mellitus and chronic hyperglycemia, are classified as somatic or autonomic. Somatic neuropathies typically affect lower extremities. Paresthesia, burning sensations, and numbness may occur along with decreased senses of vibration, pain, temperature, and proprioception. These symptoms increase risk for tissue injury and falls. Daily foot assessment is critical because these people may not feel a break in the skin or a burn and develop subsequent foot lesions, which are challenging to heal. For some people, peripheral neuropathies cause chronic lower extremity pain. Pain assessment and management are crucial to their quality of life. A pharmacologic approach to management is often employed. (From Marks R. (1987). *Skin disease in old age*. Philadelphia, PA: JB Lippincott.)

as athlete's foot; thus, injuries and infections often go undetected. Motor neuropathy can lead to weakness of the intrinsic muscles of the foot and may result in foot deformities with focal areas of high pressure. When this abnormal focus of pressure is coupled with loss of sensation, a foot ulcer can occur. Common sites of trauma are the back of the heel, the plantar metatarsal area, or the great toe, where weight is borne during walking[1,2,55,65] (Fig. 41-21).

Infections

Infections are a primary concern to people with diabetes, with certain types of infections occurring with increased frequency (including soft tissue infections of the extremities, osteomyelitis, urinary tract infections and pyelonephritis, candida infections of the skin and mucous surfaces, dental caries, and periodontal disease). The presence of chronic vascular complications contributes to suboptimal response to infection in a person with diabetes, as do hyperglycemia and altered neutrophil function. Sensory deficits may cause a person with diabetes to ignore minor trauma and infection. Vascular disease may impair circulation and delivery of blood cells and other necessary substances for promotion of adequate inflammatory response and effective healing. Hyperglycemia and glycosuria may influence the growth of microorganisms and increase severity of infections.[1,2,4]

SUMMARY CONCEPTS

The metabolic disturbances associated with diabetes affect almost every body system. The acute complications of diabetes include DKA, hyperglycemic hyperosmolar state, and hypoglycemia in people with insulin-treated diabetes. Complications also occur because of compensatory changes by counter-regulatory hormones. The chronic complications of diabetes affect the microvascular system (including the retina, kidneys, and peripheral nervous system) and the macrovascular system (coronary, cerebrovascular, and peripheral arteries). Microvascular and macrovascular dysfunctions contribute to diabetic foot ulcers. Infection is a significant concern because of the alterations in the healing process associated with the physiologic changes in diabetes. Chronic hyperglycemia plays a key role in complications, and people should receive significant education and support to learn to control blood sugar and minimize complications.

Review Exercises

1. A 59-year-old man was referred to a neurologist for evaluation of headaches. Subsequent MRI studies revealed a large suprasellar mass (2.5 × 2.4 cm), consistent with a pituitary tumor. His history is positive for hypertension, and on direct inquiry, he believes that his hands are slightly larger than previously, and he is experiencing increased sweating. Family history is negative, as are weight change, polyuria and polydipsia, visual disturbance, and erectile dysfunction. Subsequent laboratory findings reveal a baseline serum GH of 8.7 ng/mL (normal is 0 to 5 ng/mL), which is unsuppressed after oral glucose tolerance testing, glucose intolerance, and increased IGF-1 on two occasions (1044 and 1145 µg/L [upper limit of normal is 480 µg/L]). Other indices of pituitary function are within the normal range.

   A. What diagnosis would this man's clinical features, MRI, and laboratory findings suggest?
   B. What is the reason for asking the person about weight change, polyuria and polydipsia, visual disturbance, and erectile dysfunction?
   C. How would you explain his impaired glucose tolerance?
   D. What are the possible local effects of a large pituitary tumor?

2. A 76-year-old woman presents with weight gain, subjective memory loss, dry skin, and cold intolerance. On examination, she is found to have a multinodular goiter. Laboratory findings reveal a low serum T_4 and elevated TSH.

   A. What diagnosis would this woman's history, physical, and laboratory tests suggest?
   B. Explain the possible relationship between the diagnosis and her weight gain, dry skin, cold intolerance, and subjective memory loss.

3. A 45-year-old woman presents with a history of progressive weakness, fatigue, weight loss, nausea, and increased skin pigmentation (especially of creases, pressure areas, and nipples). Her blood pressure is 120/78 mm Hg when supine and 105/52 mm Hg when standing. Laboratory findings reveal a serum sodium of 120 mEq/L (normal is 135 to 145 mEq/L), a potassium level of 5.9 mEq/L (normal is 3.5 to 5 mEq/L), and low plasma cortisol and high ACTH levels.

   A. What diagnosis would this woman's clinical features and laboratory findings suggest?
   B. Would her diagnosis be classified as a primary or secondary endocrine disorder?
   C. What is the significance of her darkened skin?

4. A 6-year-old boy is admitted to the emergency department with nausea, vomiting, and abdominal pain. He is very lethargic; his skin is warm, dry, and flushed; his pulse is rapid; and he has a sweet smell to his breath. His parents relate that he has been very thirsty during the past several weeks, his appetite has increased, and he has been urinating frequently. His initial plasma glucose is 420 mg/dL (23.1 mmol/L) and a urine test for ketones is strongly positive.

   A. What is the most likely cause of this boy's elevated blood glucose and ketonuria?
   B. Explain his presenting signs and symptoms in terms of the elevated blood glucose and metabolic acidosis.
   C. What are the priorities of treatment?
   D. What associated electrolyte disturbances would you expect and why?

5. A 53-year-old accountant presents for his routine yearly examination. His history indicates that he was found to have a FPG of 120 mg/dL (6.7 mmol/L) on two prior occasions. Currently, he is asymptomatic. He has no other medical problems and does not use any medications. He neither smokes nor drinks alcohol. His father had type 2 diabetes at age 60 years. His physical examination reveals a blood pressure of 125/80 mm Hg, a body mass index of 32 kg/m², and a waist circumference of 45 inches (114 cm). Laboratory study results are as follows: complete blood count, TSH, and alanine aminotransferase are within normal limits. The lipid panel shows that his HDL cholesterol (30 mg/dL [0.8 mmol/L]) and low-density lipoproteins cholesterol (136 mg/dL [3.5 mmol/L]) are within the normal range, and triglycerides are elevated (290 mg/dL [2.3 mmol/L]; normal is <165 mg/dL [1.9 mmol/L]).

   A. What is this man's probable diagnosis?
   B. Based on this man's blood glucose level and the American Diabetes Association classification system, what diabetic status would you place this man in? Does he need a 75-g OGTT for further assessment of his IFG?
   C. His OGTT test result reveals a 2-hour glucose value of 175 mg/dL (9.63 mmol/L). What is the diagnosis?

REFERENCES

1. Rubin R., Strayer D. S., Saffitz J. E., et al. (Eds.). (2015). *Rubin's pathology: Clinicopathologic foundations of medicine* (7th ed.). Philadelphia, PA: Wolters Kluwer.
2. Kumar V., Abbas A. K., Aster J. C. (Eds.). (2015). *Robbins and Cotran pathologic basis of disease* (9th ed.). Philadelphia, PA: Elsevier.
3. Capriotti T., Frizzell J. P. (2016). *Pathophysiology: Introductory concepts and clinical perspectives*. Philadelphia, PA: F.A. Davis.
4. Hall J. E. (2015). *Guyton and Hall textbook of medical physiology* (13th ed.). Philadelphia, PA: Elsevier.
5. Saladin K. S. (2015). *Anatomy & physiology: The unity of form and function* (7th ed.). New York, NY: McGraw Hill Education.
6. Garrahy A., Agha A. (2016). How should we interrogate the hypothalamic-pituitary-adrenal axis in patients with suspected hypopituitarism? *BMC Endocrine Disorders* 16(1), 36. doi:10.1186/s12902-016-0117-7.
7. Skugor M., Hamrahian A. H. (2012). Pituitary disorders. Cleveland Clinic for Continuing Education. [Online]. Available: https://knowmedge.com/blog/medical-mnemonics-go-look-for-the-adenoma-please/. Accessed June 20, 2019.
8. Hammer G. D., McPhee S. J. (Eds.). (2014). *Pathophysiology of disease: An introduction to clinical medicine* (7th ed.). New York, NY: McGraw Hill Education.
9. Neal J. M. (2016). *How the endocrine system works* (2nd ed.). West Sussex, UK: John Wiley & Sons.
10. Braun L. R., Marino R. Disorders of growth and stature. *Pediatrics in Review* 38(7), 293–304.
11. Barstow C., Rerucha C. (2015). Evaluation of short and tall stature in children. *American Family Physician* 92(1), 43–50.
12. Dauber A., Rosenfeld R. G., Hirschhorn J. N. (2014). Genetic evaluation of short stature. *Journal of Clinical Endocrinology and Metabolism* 99(9), 3080–3092. doi:10.1210/jc.2014-1506.
13. Rogol A. D., Hayden G. F. (2014). Etiologies and early diagnosis of short stature and growth failure in children and adolescents. *The Journal of Pediatrics* 164(5 Suppl), 1–14. doi:10.1016/j.jpeds.2014.02.027.
14. Cohen L. E. (2014). Idiopathic short stature: A clinical review. *Journal of the American Medical Association* 311(17), 1787–1796. doi:10.1001/jama.2014.3970.

15. Sirotnak A. P., Pataki C. (2015). Psychosocial short stature. Emedicine Medscape. [Online]. Available: https://emedicine.medscape.com/article/913843-overview#a5. Accessed June 20, 2019.

16. Calabria A. (2017). Growth hormone deficiency in children (pituitary dwarfism). Merck Manual Professional. [Online]. Available at: https://www.merckmanuals.com/professional/pediatrics/endocrine-disorders-in-children/growth-hormone-deficiency-in-children. Accessed June 20, 2019.

17. Eledrisi M. S., Griffing G. T. (2018). Growth hormone deficiency in adults. Emedicine Medscape. [Online]. Available: https://emedicine.medscape.com/article/120767-overview. Accessed June 20, 2019.

18. Binay C., Simsek E., Yıldırım A., et al. (2015). Growth hormone and the risk of atherosclerosis in growth hormone-deficient children. *Growth Hormone and IGF Research* 25(6), 294–297.

19. Sonksken P. (2013). Idiopathic growth hormone deficiency in adults, Ben Johnson, and the somatopause. *The Journal of Clinical Endocrinology and Metabolism* 98(6), 2270–2273.

20. Gentili A., Griffing G. T. (2015). Growth hormone replacement in older men. Emedicine Medscape. [Online]. Available: https://emedicine.medscape.com/article/126999-overview. Accessed June 20, 2019.

21. Dineen R., Stewart P. M., Sherlock M. (2015). Acromegaly. *QJM: An International Journal of Medicine* 110(7), 411–420. doi:10.1093/qjmed/hcw004.

22. Hannon A. M., Thompson C. J., Sherlock M. (2017). Diabetes in patients with acromegaly. *Current Diabetes Reports* 17(8), 1–8. doi:10.1007/s11892-017-0838-7.

23. Kaplowitz P., Bloch C. (2015). Evaluation and referral of children with signs of early puberty. *Pediatrics* 137(1), e20153732. Available: http://pediatrics.aappublications.org/content/early/2015/12/11/peds.2015-3732.

24. Klein D. A., Emerick J. E., Sylvester J. E., et al. (2017). Disorders of puberty: An approach to diagnosis and management. *American Family Physician* 96(9), 590–599. Available: https://www.aafp.org/afp/2017/1101/p590.html.

25. Sarlis N. J., Griffing G. T. (2017). Thyroxine-binding globulin deficiency. Emedicine Medscape. [Online]. Available: https://emedicine.medscape.com/article/125764-overview. Accessed June 20, 2019.

26. Procopiou M., Meyer C. A. (2017). Effects of drugs on thyroid function tests. Renal and Urology News. [Online]. Available: https://www.renalandurologynews.com/endocrinology-metabolism/effects-of-drugs-on-thyroid-function-tests/article/595483/. Accessed June 20, 2019.

27. Nierengarten M. B., Bauer A. J. (2016). Hypothyroidism in children. *Contemporary Pediatrics* 33(5), 29–33.

28. American Thyroid Association. (2014). Postpartum thyroiditis. [Online]. Brochure available: https://www.thyroid.org/postpartum-thyroiditis/. Accessed June 20, 2019.

29. Orlander P. R., Griffing G. T. (2018). Hypothyroidism treatment & management. Emedicine Medscape. [Online]. Available: https://emedicine.medscape.com/article/122393-treatment. Accessed June 20, 2019.

30. Eledrisi M. S., Griffing G. T. (2017). Myxedema coma or crisis. Emedicine Medscape. [Online]. Available: https://emedicine.medscape.com/article/123577-overview#a1. Accessed June 20, 2019.

31. Lee S. L., Khardori R. (2017). Hyperthyroidism and thyrotoxicosis. Emedicine Medscape. [Online]. Available: https://emedicine.medscape.com/article/121865-overview. Accessed June 20, 2019.

32. Osuna P. M., Udovcic M., Sharma M. D. (2017). Hyperthyroidism and the heart. *Methodist Debakey Cardiovascular Journal* 13(2), 60–63.

33. Felicilda-Reynaldo R. F. D., Kenneally M. (2016). Antithyroid drugs for hyperthyroidism. *Medsurg Nursing* 25(1), 50–54.

34. Ing E., Roy H. (2016). Thyroid-associated orbitopathy. Emedicine Medscape. [Online]. Available: https://emedicine.medscape.com/article/1218444-overview. Accessed June 20, 2019.

35. Idrose A. M. (2015). Acute and emergency care for thyrotoxicosis and thyroid storm. *Acute Medicine and Surgery* 2, 147–157.

36. Misra M., Hoffman R. P. (2018). Thyroid storm. Emedicine Medscape. [Online]. Available: https://emedicine.medscape.com/article/925147-overview. Accessed June 20, 2019.

37. Schraga E. D., Khardori R. (2017). Hyperthyroidism, thyroid storm, and Graves disease. Emedicine Medscape. [Online]. Available: https://emedicine.medscape.com/article/767130-overview. Accessed June 20, 2019.

38. Turcu A., Smith J. M., Auchus R., et al. (2014). Adrenal androgens and androgen precursors: Definition, synthesis, regulation, and physiologic actions. *Comprehensive Physiology* 4(4), 1369–1381.

39. National Institute of Diabetes and Digestive and Kidney Diseases. (2014). Adrenal Insufficiency and Addison's Disease. [Online]. Available: https://www.niddk.nih.gov/health-information/endocrine-diseases/adrenal-insufficiency-addisons-disease. Accessed June 20, 2019.

40. Papierska L. (2017). The adrenopause: Does it really exist? *Menopause Review* 16(2), 57–60.

41. Judd L. L., Schettler P. J., Brown E. S., et al. (2014). Adverse consequences of glucocorticoid medication: Psychological, cognitive, and behavioral effects. *American Journal of Psychiatry* 171(10), 1045–1051. doi:10.1176/appi.ajp.2014.13091264.

42. Younes A. J., Younes N. K. (2017). Recovery of steroid induced adrenal insufficiency. *Translational Pediatrics* 6(4), 269–273. doi:10.21037/tp.2017.10.01.

43. American Association for Clinical Chemistry. (2017). Adrenal insufficiency and Addison disease. [Online]. Available: https://labtestsonline.org/conditions/adrenal-insufficiency-and-addison-disease. Accessed June 20, 2019.

44. Elhomsy G., Staros E. B. (2014). Dexamethasone suppression test. Emedicine Medscape. [Online]. Available: https://emedicine.medscape.com/article/2114191-overview. Accessed June 20, 2019.

45. Witchel S. F. (2017). Congenital adrenal hyperplasia. *Journal of Pediatric and Adolescent Gynecology* 30(2017), 520–534.

46. Charmandari E., Nicolaides N. C., Chrousos G. P. (2014). Adrenal insufficiency. *The Lancet* 383, 2152–2167.

47. Pramono L., Purnamasari D., Tarigan T. J. E., et al. (2015). Generalized hyperpigmentation caused by Addison's disease in a patient with HIV/AIDS and multiple opportunistic infections. *Journal of the ASEAN Federation of Endocrine Societies* 30(2), 169–173.

48. Griffing G. T., Khardori R. (2018). Addison disease. Emedicine Medscape. [Online]. Available: https://emedicine.medscape.com/article/116467-overview. Accessed June 20, 2019.

49. Kirkland L., Griffing G. T. (2018). Adrenal Crisis. Emedicine Medscape. [Online]. Available: https://emedicine.medscape.com/article/116716-overview. Accessed June 20, 2019.

50. National Institute of Diabetes and Digestive and Kidney Diseases. (2012). Cushing's syndrome. [Online]. Available: https://www.niddk.nih.gov/health-information/endocrine-diseases/cushings-syndrome. Accessed June 20, 2019.

51. Nguyen H. C. T., Khardori R. (2017). Endogenous Cushing syndrome. Emedicine Medscape. [Online]. Available: https://emedicine.medscape.com/article/2233083-overview. Accessed June 20, 2019.

52. Leslie R. D., Palmer J., Schloot N. C., et al. (2016). Diabetes at the crossroads: Relevance of disease classification to pathophysiology and treatment. *Diabetologia* 59, 13–20. doi:10.1007/s00125-015-3789-z.

53. Hay D. L., Chen S., Lutz T. A., et al. (2015). Amylin: Pharmacology, physiology, and clinical potential. *Pharmacological Reviews* 67, 564–600. doi:10.1124/pr.115.010629.

54. Centers for Disease Control and Prevention. (2018). *National diabetes statistics report*. Atlanta, GA: Centers for Disease Control and Prevention, U.S. Department of Health and Human Services. Available: https://www.cdc.gov/diabetes/data/statistics/statistics-report.html. Accessed April 26, 2019.

55. American Diabetes Association. (2018). Classification and diagnosis of diabetes: Standards of medical care in diabetes—2018. *Diabetes Care* 41(Suppl 1), S13–S27.

56. Lin J. L. J., Papantonlou L. G. C., Staros E. B. (2016). Glucose tolerance testing. Emedicine Medscape. [Online]. Available: https://emedicine.medscape.com/article/2049402-overview#a4. Accessed June 20, 2019.

57. Breslin Diabetes Center of Harvard Medical School. (2018). Plasma glucose meters and whole blood meters. [Online]. Available: http://www.joslin.org/info/plasma_glucose_meters_and_whole_blood_meters.html. Accessed June 20, 2019.

58. Breslin Diabetes Center of Harvard Medical School. (2018). Blood glucose testing delivers tight control. [Online]. Available: http://www.joslin.org/info/blood-glucose-testing-delivers-tight-control.html. Accessed June 20, 2019.

59. Breslin Diabetes Center of Harvard Medical School. (2018). The facts about continuous glucose monitoring. [Online]. Available: http://www.joslin.org/info/the_facts_about_continuous_glucose_monitoring.html. Accessed June 20, 2019.

60. Horowitz G. L., Wheeler T. M. (2015). Hemoglobin A1C testing. Emedicine Medscape. [Online]. Available: https://emedicine.medscape.com/article/2049478-overview#a3. Accessed June 20, 2019.

61. American Association of Clinical Chemistry. (2014). Glucose tests. Lab Tests Online. [Online]. Available: https://labtestsonline.org/tests/glucose-tests. Accessed June 20, 2019.

62. Breslin Diabetes Center of Harvard Medical School. (2018). Ketone testing: What you need to know. [Online]. Available: http://www.joslin.org/info/ketone_testing_what_you_need_to_know.html. Accessed June 20, 2019.

63. Skyler J. S., Bakris G. L., Bonifacio E., et al. (2017). Differentiation of diabetes by pathophysiology, natural history, and prognosis. *Diabetes* 66, 241–255.

64. Bokhari A. S., Alshaya M. M., Badghaish M. M. O., et al. (2018). Metabolic syndrome: Pathophysiology and treatment. *The Egyptian Journal of Hospital Medicine* 70(8), 1388–1392. doi:10.12816/0044654.

65. Handelsma Y., Bloomgarden Z. T., Grunberger G., et al. (2015). American Association of Clinical Endocrinologists and American College of Endocrinology—Clinical practice guidelines for developing a diabetes mellitus comprehensive care plan–2015—Executive summary. *Endocrine Practice* 21(4), 413–437.

66. Cooperman M., Griffing G. (2016). Somogyi phenomenon. Emedicine Medscape. [Online]. Available: https://emedicine.medscape.com/article/125432-overview. Accessed June 20, 2019.

67. American Diabetes Association. (2017). Dawn phenomenon. [Online]. Available: http://www.diabetes.org/living-with-diabetes/treatment-and-care/blood-glucose-control/dawn-phenomenon.html. Accessed June 20, 2019.

68. American Diabetes Association. (2018). Glycemic targets: Standards of medical care in diabetes—2018. *Diabetes Care* 48(Suppl 1), S55–S64.

69. Yang S. L., Zhu L., Han R., et al. (2017). Pathophysiology of peripheral arterial disease in diabetes mellitus. *Journal of Diabetes* 9, 133–140. doi:10.1111/1753-0407.12474.

C H A P T E R *42*

Structure and Function of the Male Genitourinary System

Structure of the Male Reproductive System

Embryonic Development
Testes and Scrotum
Genital Duct System
Accessory Organs
Penis

Spermatogenesis and Hormonal Control of Male Reproductive Function

Spermatogenesis
Hormonal Control of Male Reproductive Function
Testosterone and Other Male Sex Hormones
Action of the Hypothalamic and Anterior Pituitary Hormones
Hypogonadism

Neural Control of Sexual Function and Changes with Aging

Neural Control
Changes with Aging

Objectives

After completing this chapter, the learner will be able to meet the following objectives:

1. Characterize the embryonic development of the male reproductive organs and genitalia.
2. Describe the structure and function of the testes and scrotum, the genital ducts, accessory organs, and penis.
3. Describe the process of spermatogenesis.
4. State the functions of testosterone.
5. Draw a diagram illustrating secretion, site of action, and feedback control of gonadotropin-releasing hormone, luteinizing hormone, follicle-stimulating hormone, and inhibin.
6. Describe the autonomic and peripheral nervous systems' control of erection, emission, and ejaculation.
7. Describe changes in the male reproductive system that occur with aging.

The male genitourinary system consists of paired gonads (testes), genital ducts, accessory organs, and a penis (Fig. 42-1). The testes produce male sex hormones and germ cells. Internal accessory organs produce the fluid constituents of semen, and ductile systems facilitate storage and transport of spermatozoa. The penis is important for urine elimination and sexual function.

Structure of the Male Reproductive System

Embryonic Development

A region in the arm of the Y chromosome determines the sex of the embryo.[1] Until the seventh week of gestation, male and female genital tracts both consist of two wolffian ducts, from which male genitalia develop, and two müllerian ducts, from which female genital structures develop. In early gestational weeks, the gonads (ovaries and testes) are also undifferentiated.[1]

Between the sixth and eighth weeks of gestation, the testes begin developing under the influence of the Y chromosome. If the *SRY* gene is present, undifferentiated gonads differentiate into testes. If the *SRY* gene is absent, the gonads develop into ovaries. As a result,

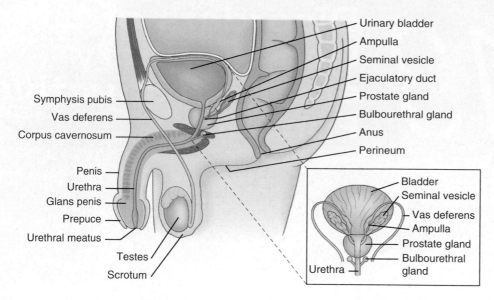

FIGURE 42-1. The structures of the male reproductive system. (From Jensen S. (2015). *Nursing health assessment: A best practice approach* (2nd ed., p. 703). Philadelphia, PA: Lippincott Williams & Wilkins.)

male and female reproductive organs and structures share many homologies.

During gestation, the testicular cells produce anti-müllerian hormone (AMH) and testosterone.[1] AMH suppresses the müllerian ducts and prevents development of the uterus and fallopian tubes. Testosterone stimulates the wolffian ducts to develop into the epididymis, vas deferens, and seminal vesicles.[1] Testosterone is the precursor of dihydrotestosterone (DHT), which allows formation of the male urethra, prostate, and external genitalia. The enzyme 5α-reductase converts testosterone to DHT, predominantly in peripheral tissues.[1] Although testosterone and DHT share the same nuclear androgen receptor, they have differences in tissue activity. DHT exerts most of its effects on external genitalia, including the prostate, and is important for the development of facial and body hair. If testosterone and DHT are absent in gestation, development of müllerian ducts will not be inhibited, and an XY embryo will develop female external genitalia.[1,2]

Testes and Scrotum

The testes are located outside the abdominal cavity in the scrotum.[3] The adult testes are 15 to 25 mL. Approximately 80% of this volume is for cells involved in spermatogenesis, and 20% for testosterone production. The testes develop in the abdominal cavity and descend through the inguinal canal into a pouch of peritoneum in the scrotum.[4] Descent occurs in two stages. The first stage is between the 7th and 12th weeks of gestation, with AMH responsible for the descent to the inguinal region. The second stage occurs in the 26th week of gestation, with testosterone responsible for the descent into the scrotum.[1] As they descend, the testes pull arteries, veins, lymphatics, nerves, and excretory ducts with them, which are encased by the cremaster muscle and fascia that constitute the spermatic cord.[4] After the descent, the inguinal canal closes. Failure of closure increases the risk of an inguinal hernia, a protrusion of parietal peritoneum and part of the intestine through an abnormal opening from the abdominal cavity. A loop of small bowel may become incarcerated (strangulated hernia), and its lumen may be obstructed and vascular supply compromised.

Testes have a double-layered membrane (tunica vaginalis).[4] An outer covering (tunica albuginea) is a tough, white, fibrous sheath that protects the testes and gives them shape. Cremaster muscles, skeletal muscle arising from the internal oblique muscles, elevate the testes. Testes receive arterial blood supply from long testicular arteries that branch from the abdominal artery. Testicular veins drain the testes and arise from the *pampiniform plexus* that surrounds the testicular artery. Autonomic nervous system fibers innervate the testes.[4] Sensory nerves transmit pain impulses, resulting in pain when hit.

The scrotum (homologous to the female labia majora), which houses the testes and is composed of a thin outer layer of skin that forms rugae, is continuous with the perineum and outer skin of the groin. Under the outer skin lies a thin layer of fascia and smooth muscle, the dartos muscle. This layer contains a septum that separates the two testes. The dartos muscle responds to temperature[3]: When cold, the muscle contracts, bringing the testes closer to the body, and when warm, the muscle relaxes, allowing the scrotum to fall away from the body.

The location of the testes in the scrotum is important for sperm production, which is optimal at 2°C to 3°C below body temperature. Two systems maintain the temperature of the testes: the pampiniform plexus of testicular veins absorbs heat from the arterial blood, cooling it as it enters the testes, and the cremaster muscles respond to decreases in testicular temperature by moving the testes closer to the body.[4] Prolonged exposure to elevated temperatures, as a result of prolonged fever or dysfunction of thermoregulatory mechanisms, may impair spermatogenesis. Cryptorchidism, the failure of the testes to descend into the scrotum, also exposes the testes to the higher temperature of the body.

Genital Duct System

The testes consist of several hundred lobules (Fig. 42-2), each containing one or more coiled seminiferous tubules, the site of sperm production. As the tubules lead into efferent ducts, they become the rete testis, which are multiple interconnecting channels.[1] From the rete testis, 10,000 to 20,000 efferent ducts emerge to join the epididymis, the final site for sperm maturation. Because spermatozoa are not motile at this stage, peristaltic movements of the epididymis ductal walls aid movement. The spermatozoa continue their migration through the ductus deferens (*vas deferens*).[1]

The ampulla of the vas deferens stores sperm until they are released through the penis during ejaculation (Fig. 42-3). Surgical disconnection of the vas deferens (*e.g.*, vasectomy) is an effective method of male contraception. Because sperm are stored in the ampulla, men can remain fertile for 4 to 5 weeks after a vasectomy.

Human testes can produce up to 300 million sperm cells/day.[1] Mature spermatozoa are about 60 μm long.[1]

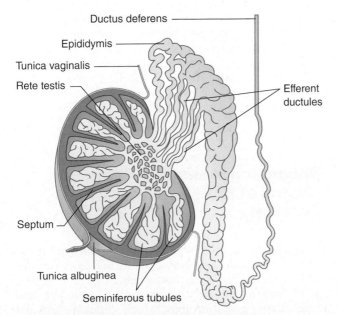

FIGURE 42-2. The parts of the testes and epididymis.

Ductus deferens

Epididymis

Tunica vaginalis

Rete testis

Efferent ductules

Septum

Tunica albuginea

Seminiferous tubules

Approximately 3 mL of semen is expelled with each ejaculate (about 45 million sperm).[5] However, a large percentage of sperm in ejaculate may be immobile or dead.[1]

Accessory Organs

The male accessory organs consist of seminal vesicles, a prostate gland, and bulbourethral glands. Seminal fluid combines with secretions from genital ducts and accessory organs. Spermatozoa plus the secretions make up semen.[1]

The seminal vesicles are two tortuous tubes that secrete fluid for semen. They are lined with secretory epithelium containing an abundance of fructose, prostaglandins, and other proteins. Fructose secreted by the seminal vesicles provides energy for sperm motility. Prostaglandins are thought to assist in fertilization by making the cervical mucus more receptive to sperm and by causing peristaltic contractions to move the sperm toward the ovaries.[1]

A seminal vesicle joins a vas deferens to form the ejaculatory duct, which enters the posterior part of the prostate and continues through until it ends in the prostatic portion of the urethra.[1] During emission, vesicles empty fluid into the ejaculatory duct, adding bulk to the semen.

The prostate is a fibromuscular, glandular organ inferior to the bladder. It secretes thin, alkaline fluid with citric acid, calcium, acid phosphate, a clotting enzyme, and profibrinolysin. During ejaculation, the prostate capsule contracts, adding fluid to semen.[1] Vaginal secretions and vas deferens fluid are strongly acidic. Sperm mobilization occurs at pH 6.0 to 6.5, so alkaline prostatic secretions are essential for ovum fertilization.[4] Bulbourethral (Cowper glands) lie on either side of the urethra and secrete alkaline mucus, neutralizing acids from urine in the urethra.[4]

The prostate gland eliminates urine through the *prostatic urethra*. This region consists of a thin, fibrous capsule that encloses the circularly oriented smooth muscle fibers and collagenous tissue that surround the urethra where it joins the bladder. The prostatic urethra traverses the prostate gland, where it is lined by a thin, longitudinal layer of smooth muscle that is continuous with the bladder wall. The smooth muscle that surrounds the prostate gland is derived primarily from the longitudinal bladder musculature and is the true involuntary sphincter of the male posterior urethra. Because the prostate surrounds the urethra, enlargement can cause urinary obstruction.[1]

The prostate gland is made up of secretory glands arranged in three concentric areas surrounding the prostatic urethra, into which they open. They include the small mucosal glands associated with the urethral mucosa, the intermediate submucosal glands that lie peripheral to the mucosal glands, and the large main prostatic glands that are situated toward the outside of the gland.[1] Overgrowth of the mucosal glands causes benign prostatic hyperplasia (BPH) in older men.

Penis

The penis is the external genital organ through which the urethra passes. The external penis is a shaft that ends in a tip (the *glans*, homologous to the female clitoris) (Fig. 42-4). The loose skin of the shaft covers the glans,

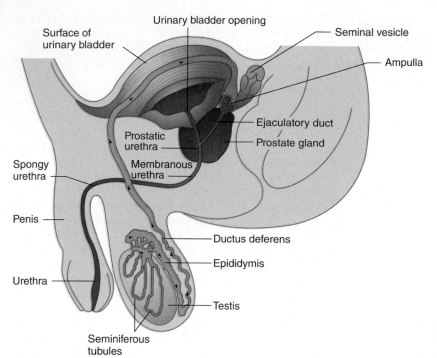

FIGURE 42-3. The excretory ducts of the male reproductive system and the path that sperm follows as it leaves the testis and travels to the urethra.

forming the prepuce (foreskin). The glans contains sensory nerves and is the most sensitive portion of the penile shaft. Foreskin is removed during circumcision.

The shaft of the penis (cylindrical body) consists of three masses of erectile tissue, held together by fibrous strands and covered with a skin layer. Two lateral masses are the *corpora cavernosa*, and the ventral mass is the *corpus spongiosum*, where the spongy part of the urethra is found.[1] These three masses are cavernous sinuses and are engorged with blood during penile erection.

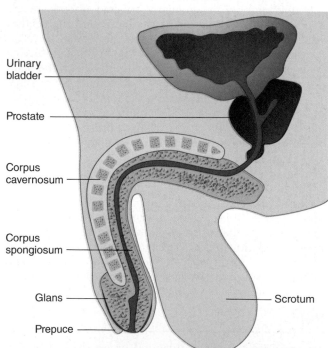

FIGURE 42-4. Sagittal section of the penis, showing the prepuce, glans, corpus cavernosum, and corpus spongiosum.

SUMMARY CONCEPTS

The male reproductive system consists of a pair of gonads (*i.e.*, testes), a system of excretory ducts (*i.e.*, seminiferous tubules and efferent ducts), the accessory organs (*i.e.*, epididymis, seminal vesicles, prostate, and Cowper glands), and the penis. During the seventh week of gestation, the XY chromosome pattern and the *SRY* gene in the male embryo are responsible for the development of the testes; the subsequent production of AMH and testosterone results in the development of the internal and external male genital structures. Before this period of embryonic development, the tissues from which the male and female reproductive structures develop are undifferentiated. In the absence of testosterone production and its derivative, DHT, a male embryo with an XY chromosomal pattern will develop female external genitalia.

Spermatogenesis and Hormonal Control of Male Reproductive Function

During childhood, gonads are essentially **quiescent.** At puberty, the male gonads begin to mature and carry out spermatogenesis and hormone production. At 10 or 11 years of age, the anterior pituitary, under control of the hypothalamus, secretes gonadotropins, which stimulates testicular function and causes interstitial Leydig cells to produce testosterone. At the same time, hormonal stimulation induces mitotic activity of the germ cells that develop into sperm. The testes enlarge as individual tubules grow. Males attain full maturity and spermatogenesis by 16 years of age.

Spermatogenesis

Spermatogenesis is the generation of spermatozoa or sperm. It begins at 13 years and continues throughout the reproductive years. It occurs in the seminiferous tubules (see Fig. 42-2). These tubules, if placed end to end, would measure about 750 feet. The outer layer of the seminiferous tubules is connective tissue and smooth muscle. The inner lining is Sertoli cells, with sperm in various stages of development (Fig. 42-5A). Sertoli cells secrete a fluid with nutrients to bathe and nourish immature germ cells and provide digestive enzymes that play a role in spermiation (converting spermatocytes to sperm).[1] Sertoli cells secrete several hormones, including AMH, which is secreted *in utero* to inhibit development of fallopian tubes; estradiol, the principal feminizing sex hormone, which seems to be required for spermatogenesis; and inhibin, which controls Sertoli cell function through feedback inhibition of follicle-stimulating hormone (FSH) from the anterior pituitary gland.[1,4] For spermatogenesis to occur, FSH binds to receptors in Sertoli cells. This process requires a high concentration of intratesticular testosterone.[1]

In the first stage of spermatogenesis, unspecialized **diploid** germinal cells (*spermatogonia*) are located adjacent to the tubular wall. Spermatogonia undergo rapid mitotic division and provide a continuous source of new germinal cells. Mature spermatogonia divide into two daughter cells, which become primary spermatocytes—the precursors of sperm.[1] Over several weeks, primary spermatocytes divide by *meiosis* to form two smaller secondary spermatocytes. Meiosis consists of two consecutive nuclear divisions with formation of four daughter cells, each with a single set of 23 chromosomes (rather than a pair of 46 chromosomes, as with mitotic division in somatic cells). Secondary spermatocytes divide to form two spermatids, each with 23 chromosomes.

The spermatid elongates into a spermatozoon (the mature sperm cell) with a head and a tail (Fig. 42-5B). The anterior two thirds of the head, the *acrosome*, contains enzymes for penetration and fertilization of the ovum.[1] Flagellar motion of the tail moves the sperm. The mitochondria in the midpiece supply energy for movement. A sperm moves in a straight line at 1 to 4 mm/minute. As the sperm grows to full size, it moves to the epididymis to mature further and gain motility. The epididymis can store a small quantity of sperm, but the ampulla of the vas deferens stores most of the sperm. Sperm can live for many weeks in the male genital tract but can survive in the female genital tract for only 1 to 2 days.[1] Spermatogenesis and sperm maturation take approximately 90 days. Infertility may occur when insufficient numbers of motile, healthy sperm are present. A "fertile sample" on seminal fluid analysis has a count greater than 15 million/mL, greater than 40% motility, normal morphology, and a volume of 1.5 or more.[5]

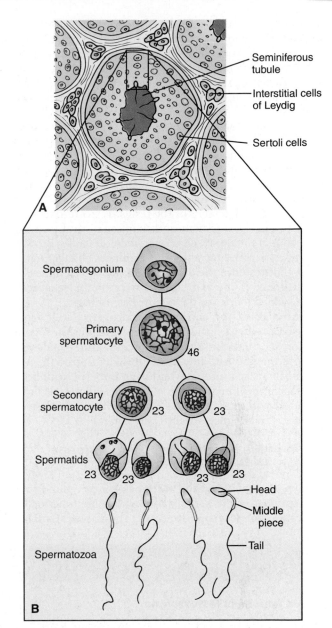

FIGURE 42-5. The various stages of spermatogenesis. **(A)** Cross section of the seminiferous tubule. **(B)** Stages of development of spermatozoa.

Hormonal Control of Male Reproductive Function

Testosterone and Other Male Sex Hormones

The testes secrete several male sex hormones (androgens), including *testosterone, DHT,* and *androstenedione.* The adrenal cortex produces less than 5% of the total male androgens. Testosterone, the most abundant of the androgens, is considered the main testicular hormone.[4] The testes also secrete small quantities of estradiol and estrone.[1,4]

The interstitial Leydig cells in the testes produce and secrete testosterone under the influence of luteinizing hormone (LH) producing approximately 6 mg/day of testosterone.[1] Testosterone is metabolized in the liver and excreted by the kidneys. In the bloodstream, testosterone exists in an unbound or a bound form. The bound form is attached to plasma proteins, including albumin and the sex hormone–binding globulin produced by the liver. Only 2% of circulating testosterone is unbound and able to enter the cell. Much of the testosterone that becomes fixed to the tissues is converted to DHT by 5α-reductase, especially in certain target tissues such as the prostate gland. Testosterone can be aromatized or converted to estradiol in the peripheral tissues.

Testosterone and DHT exert a variety of biologic effects in the male (Chart 42-1). In the male embryo, testosterone is essential for differentiation of internal and external genitalia descent of the testes. Testosterone is essential to the development and maintenance of primary and secondary male sex characteristics.[1] It causes growth of pubic, chest, and facial hair; it produces changes in the larynx that result in the male bass voice; and it increases the thickness of the skin and activity of the sebaceous glands, which increases the occurrence of acne.

Almost all of the actions of androgens result from increased protein synthesis in target tissues. Androgens function as anabolic agents in males and females to promote metabolism and musculoskeletal growth. Androgens increase musculature during puberty, with boys averaging approximately a 50% increase in muscle mass compared with girls. Chart 42-2 describes the abuse of androgens to enhance athletic performance.

Action of the Hypothalamic and Anterior Pituitary Hormones

The hypothalamus and the anterior pituitary gland promote spermatogenic activity and endocrine function of the testes. gonadotropin-releasing hormone (GnRH),

---

CHART 42-1

Main Actions of Testosterone

Induces differentiation of the male genital tract during fetal development

Induces development of primary and secondary sex characteristics

  Gonadal function

  External genitalia and accessory organs

  Male voice timbre

  Male skin characteristics

  Male hair distribution

Anabolic effects

  Promotes protein metabolism

  Promotes musculoskeletal growth

  Influences subcutaneous fat distribution

Promotes spermatogenesis (in FSH-primed tubules) and maturation of sperm

Stimulates erythropoiesis

CHART 42-2

Abuse of Androgens to Enhance Athletic Performance

- Athletes use synthetic androgens to improve their skill and endurance by bulking up their muscles.

- Athletes have taken virtually all androgens produced for human and veterinary purposes.

- Occasionally, athletes take several medications simultaneously in an attempt to increase the overall effect on performance, which can cause potentially more deleterious side effects.

- Hormones are frequently taken in doses that far exceed physiologic levels.

- There are potential harmful effects to taking these supplements including acne, decreased testicular size, and azoospermia.

- The detrimental effects may persist for months after use of the agents has ceased, depending on the type and dose administered.

- Because testosterone can be aromatized to estradiol in the peripheral tissues, androgens can also produce gynecomastia (breast enlargement).

---

which is synthesized by the hypothalamus and secreted into the hypophysial portal blood stream, regulates synthesis and release of gonadotropic hormones from the anterior pituitary (Fig. 42-6).[1]

The anterior pituitary secretes two gonadotropic hormones: LH regulates the production of testosterone by the interstitial Leydig cells (Fig. 42-6), and FSH binds selectively to Sertoli cells and functions in the initiation of spermatogenesis. Under the influence of FSH, the Sertoli cells produce androgen-binding protein, plasminogen activator, and inhibin. Androgen-binding protein binds testosterone and serves as a carrier of testosterone in Sertoli cells and as a storage site for testosterone.[1] Although FSH is necessary for initiating spermatogenesis, full maturation of the spermatozoa requires testosterone (intratesticular testosterone concentration is 100-fold greater than are serum levels). Androgen-binding protein also serves as a carrier of testosterone from the testes to the epididymis. Plasminogen activator, which converts plasminogen to plasmin, functions in the final detachment of mature spermatozoa from Sertoli cells.

High levels of testosterone suppress LH secretion through a direct action on the pituitary and an inhibitory effect on the hypothalamus. *Inhibin* is produced by Sertoli cells and suppresses FSH release from the pituitary gland. The pituitary gonadotropic hormones and Sertoli cells in the testes form a classic negative feedback loop in which FSH stimulates inhibin and inhibin suppresses FSH.[1,4] In males, FSH, LH, and testosterone secretion and spermatogenesis occur at relatively unchanging rates during adulthood.[1]

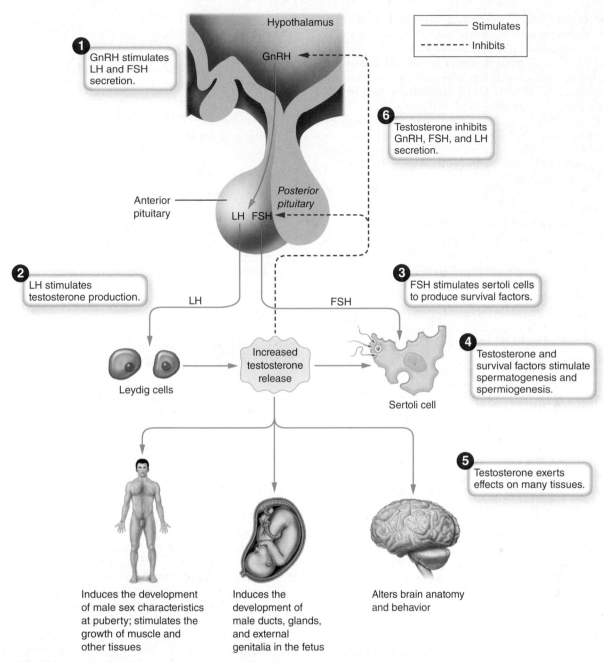

FIGURE 42-6. Hypothalamic–pituitary feedback control of spermatogenesis and testosterone levels in the male. FSH, follicle-stimulating hormone; GnRH, gonadotropin-releasing hormone; LH, luteinizing hormone. (From McConnell T., Hull K. (2011). *Human form human function: Essentials of anatomy & physiology* (p. 675). Philadelphia, PA: Lippincott Williams & Wilkins.)

Hypogonadism

Hypogonadism is the reduced function of the gonads. Primary hypogonadism is due to a problem in the testes, secondary hypogonadism is due to the lack of secretion of LH and FSH from the anterior pituitary, and tertiary hypogonadism is due to the lack of stimulation of LH and FSH secretion from the anterior pituitary due to decreased/absent GnRH secretion from the hypothalamus.[1] Primary hypogonadism in males is low androgens and sperm count due to lack of negative feedback at the hypothalamic–pituitary level, and high levels of gonadotropins (low testosterone and high LH and FSH).[6] Secondary and tertiary hypogonadisms are described by low androgens and sperm count due to lack of secretion of gonadotropins at the hypothalamic–pituitary level and low levels of gonadotropins (low testosterone and low LH and FSH).

Clinical Manifestations

Primary hypogonadism occurs when the testes do not function normally. Mumps and Klinefelter syndrome are often the cause. Sperm counts are often lower than normal. Secondary hypogonadism is caused by failure of the hypothalamus or pituitary gland, resulting in decreased testosterone levels.[6] Onset occurring in the adult is associated with fatigue, depression, decreased libido, erectile dysfunction, loss of secondary sex characteristics, changes in body composition (including loss of muscle mass and increase in fat mass), and decreased bone density or osteoporosis.[6] When hypogonadism is diagnosed, clinicians should follow up with a comprehensive cardiovascular examination, because hypogonadism, along with erectile dysfunction and type II diabetes mellitus, are predictors of cardiac disease.[7]

It is more challenging to identify the correct etiology and complete pathophysiology of hypogonadism in adolescents. However, there are multiple treatment options to induce puberty and to manage the adolescent's symptoms of hypogonadism.[8]

Diagnosis

Diagnosis of hypogonadism includes measurement of total testosterone levels (ideally between 7 AM and 11 AM, when the testosterone level is usually at its peak) in the ambulatory man. If the initial total testosterone level is low, the clinician should confirm diagnosis of hypogonadism with either a repeat measure of total testosterone or a measure of free (bioavailable) testosterone. Once the clinician establishes a diagnosis of hypogonadism, LH and FSH levels should be measured. High LH and FSH indicates primary hypogonadism (hypergonadotropic hypogonadism), and low or normal LH and FSH indicates a secondary or tertiary hypogonadism (hypogonadotropic hypogonadism). Seminal fluid analyses should be considered if a person has concerns about fertility. Clinicians should assess pituitary hormones and conduct a pituitary magnetic resonance imaging scan with hypogonadotropic hypogonadism. In hypergonadotropic hypogonadism, clinicians should conduct a karyotype analysis because Klinefelter syndrome is the most common chromosomal abnormality associated with male hypogonadism. The usual karyotype in Klinefelter syndrome is 47,XXY, although mosaicism or variants can present with a similar phenotype.[6] Males with Klinefelter syndrome characteristically have small, firm testes (unlike many other cases of hypogonadism, in which the testicular consistency is soft).[9] Other common causes of primary hypogonadism are listed in Chart 42-3.

Treatment

Testosterone therapy is available for treatment of androgen deficiency to men with confirmed hypogonadism. The principal goal of testosterone therapy is to restore the serum testosterone concentration to the normal range while keeping in mind the risks and benefits especially with men diagnosed or at risk for BPH and/or prostate cancer.

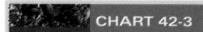

CHART 42-3

Common Causes of Primary Gonadal Failure

Chromosomal abnormalities (*e.g.*, Klinefelter syndrome)

Disorders of androgen biosynthesis

Cryptorchidism

Alkylating and antineoplastic agents

Other medications (*e.g.*, ketoconazole and glucocorticoids)

Infections—mumps orchitis (gonadal failure is a much more common manifestation when mumps occurs after puberty)

Radiation (direct and indirect testicular radiation)

Environmental toxins

Trauma

Testicular torsion

Autoimmune damage

Chronic systemic diseases (many of these can result in both primary and secondary hypogonadism, *e.g.*, cirrhosis, hemochromatosis, chronic renal failure, and acquired immunodeficiency syndrome)

Idiopathic

SUMMARY CONCEPTS

The function of the male reproductive system is under the negative feedback control of the hypothalamus and anterior pituitary gonadotropic hormones: FSH initiates spermatogenesis, and LH regulates production of testosterone. Testosterone is produced by the interstitial Leydig cells in the testes. In addition to its role in the differentiation of internal and external genitalia in the male embryo, testosterone is essential for development of secondary male characteristics during puberty, maintenance of these characteristics during adult life, and spermatozoa maturation.

Hypogonadism is a decrease in testicular function. Primary hypogonadism originates in the testes, secondary hypogonadism arises from lack of stimulation from the pituitary gonadotropins, and tertiary hypogonadism is due to decreased or absent GnRH secretion from the hypothalamus.

Neural Control of Sexual Function and Changes with Aging

In the male, the stages of the sexual act are erection, emission, ejaculation, and detumescence. The physiology involves a complex interaction between spinal cord reflexes, higher neural centers, the vascular system, and the endocrine system.

Neural Control

The impulse stimulation for initiating the male sexual act is the glans penis. Afferent impulses from sensory receptors in the glans penis pass through the pudendal nerve to ascending fibers in the spinal cord by way of the sacral plexus. Stimulation of other perineal areas, such as the anal epithelium, the scrotum, and the testes, can transmit signals to higher brain centers, such as the limbic system and cerebral cortex, through the cord, adding to sexual arousal.[1]

The psychological element to sexual stimulation, such as thinking sexual thoughts, can cause erection and ejaculation.[1] Although psychological involvement and higher center functions contribute, they are not necessary for sexual performance. Genital stimulation can produce erection and ejaculation in some males with complete transection of the spinal cord.

Erection involves shunting blood into the corpus cavernosum. It is controlled by the sympathetic, parasympathetic, and nonadrenergic–noncholinergic (NANC) systems. Nitric oxide is the locally released NANC mediator that produces relaxation of vascular smooth muscle. In the flaccid or detumescent state, sympathetic discharge through α-adrenergic receptors maintains contraction of the arteries that supply the penis and vascular sinuses of the corpora cavernosa and corpus spongiosum (Fig. 42-7). Parasympathetic stimulation produces erection by inhibiting sympathetic neurons that cause detumescence and by stimulating release of nitric oxide to effect a rapid relaxation of the smooth muscle in the sinusoidal spaces of the corpus cavernosum. During sexual stimulation, parasympathetic impulses cause urethral and bulbourethral glands to secrete mucus to aid in lubrication. Parasympathetic innervation is effected through the pelvic nerve and sacral segments of the spinal cord. Sympathetic innervation exits the spinal cord at L1 and L2.

Emission and ejaculation are a function of the sympathetic nervous system. Spinal cord reflexes regulate both emission and ejaculation. With increasing intensity of the stimulus, reflex centers of the spinal cord emit sympathetic impulses that leave the cord at the L1 and L2 levels and pass through the hypogastric plexus to the genital organs to initiate emission. Emission causes sperm to move from the epididymis to the urethra. Efferent impulses from the spinal cord produce contraction of smooth muscle in the vas deferens and ampulla that move sperm forward and close the internal urethral sphincter to prevent retrograde ejaculation into the bladder.[1]

Ejaculation is the expulsion of the sperm from the urethra. It involves contraction of the seminal vesicles and prostate gland, which add fluid to the ejaculate and propel it forward. Ejaculation is accompanied by contraction of the ischiocavernosus and bulbocavernosus muscles located at the base of the penis. The filling of the internal urethra elicits signals that are transmitted through the pudendal nerves from the spinal cord, giving the sudden feeling of fullness of the genital organs. Rhythmic increases in pressure in the urethra cause the semen to be propelled, resulting in ejaculation. Simultaneously, rhythmic contractions of pelvic and trunk muscles produce thrusting movements of the pelvis and penis, which help propel the ejaculate into the vagina.

The period of emission and ejaculation is defined as the male orgasm. After ejaculation, erection ceases within 1 to 2 minutes. A male usually ejaculates 3 mL of semen (but can range from 2 to 5 mL). Volume may be less with frequent ejaculations and may increase to four times its normal amount during periods of abstinence. Ejaculate is approximately 98% fluid and 2% sperm.[1]

Changes with Aging

The declining physiologic efficiency of male reproductive function with age occurs gradually and involves the endocrine, circulatory, and neuromuscular systems. Age does not directly result in gonadal and reproductive failure, so males may remain fertile into advanced age; 80- and 90-year-old men have been known to father children.[1]

The reproductive system becomes measurably different in structure and function with age. Male sex hormone levels, particularly of testosterone, decrease with age, but the rate varies per person and is affected by multiple variables.[10] Beginning at 25 to 30 years of age in healthy, nonobese males, testosterone levels gradually decrease at 10% per decade. *Andropause* describes an ill-defined collection of symptoms in aging males, generally older than 50 years, who have some degree of hypogonadism associated with aging.[10] The existence and significance of andropause has important public health implications given the current number of males older than 65 years of age.

Sex hormones affect protein synthesis, salt and water balance, bone growth, and cardiovascular function. Low testosterone levels have an atherogenic effect that may be part of the etiology of the higher incidence of cardiovascular disease in androgen-deficient males.[7,10] Decreasing levels of testosterone affect sexual energy, muscle strength, and genital tissues. Testes become smaller and lose their firmness. Seminiferous tubules thicken and begin a degenerative process that finally inhibits sperm production. The prostate gland enlarges, and its contractions become weaker. The force of ejaculation decreases due to reduced volume and viscosity of seminal fluid. The seminal vesicle changes little from childhood to puberty. Pubertal increases in fluid capacity of the gland decline after 60 years of age. After this, the walls of the seminal vesicles thin, the epithelium shrinks, and the muscle layer is replaced by connective tissue. Age-related changes in the penis consist of fibrotic changes in the trabecula in the corpus spongiosum, with progressive sclerotic changes in arteries and veins. Sclerotic changes also follow in the corpora

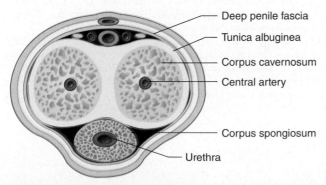

- Deep penile fascia
- Tunica albuginea
- Corpus cavernosum
- Central artery
- Corpus spongiosum
- Urethra

FIGURE 42-7. Erectile tissue of the penis.

cavernosa, with the condition becoming generalized in 55- to 60-year-old men.

Erectile dysfunction is common in older males with type II diabetes mellitus, cardiovascular disease, and hyperlipidemia.[7] *Erectile dysfunction* is the persistent inability to achieve and maintain an erection sufficient to permit satisfactory sexual intercourse. Aging is a major etiologic factor. Secondary impotence may be related to cardiovascular, respiratory, hormonal, neurologic, and hematologic disorders (*e.g.,* vascular disease may impair blood flow, resulting in loss of blood volume with subsequent poor distention of the vascular spaces of erectile tissue). Certain medications can also affect sexual function.

A great inhibitor of sexual functioning in older males is loss of self-esteem and development of a negative self-image. Many older men live in environments that are not sensitive to the importance of helping them maintain a positive self-image. Premature cessation of esteem-building activities can contribute to loss of libido.

Clinicians may use testosterone and other synthetic androgens in older males with low androgen levels to improve muscle strength and vigor. Testosterone replacement therapy should be accompanied by screening for prostate cancer.[7,11] Side effects may include acne, gynecomastia, and reduced high-density lipoprotein cholesterol levels.[6,7,11] At present, the routine treatment of older males with testosterone is not recommended.

SUMMARY CONCEPTS

The sex act involves erection, emission, ejaculation, and detumescence. The physiology of these functions involves a complex interaction between autonomic-mediated spinal cord reflexes, higher neural centers, and the vascular system. Erection is mediated by the parasympathetic nervous system and emission and ejaculation by the sympathetic nervous system. Like other body systems, the male reproductive system undergoes changes as a result of the aging process. The changes occur gradually and involve parallel changes in endocrine, circulatory, and neuromuscular function. Testosterone levels decrease (andropause), the size and firmness of the testes decrease, sperm production declines, and the prostate gland enlarges. There is usually a decrease in frequency of intercourse, intensity of sensation, speed of attaining erection, and force of ejaculation. However, sexual thought, interest, and activity usually continue into old age.

Review Exercises

1. In the absence of the *SRY* gene on the Y chromosome, a developing embryo with an XY genotype will develop female genitalia.

    A. Explain.

2. Males who have had a vasectomy often remain fertile for 4 to 5 weeks after the procedure has been done.

    A. Explain.

3. A 55-year-old male presents with various vague symptoms (fatigue, depression). On examination, he is noted to have small testes (8 mL bilaterally), marked gynecomastia, and scanty body hair. He is obese at 122 kg, with a body mass index of 34.2. Investigations reveal low testosterone and elevated gonadotropin (LH and FSH) levels.

    A. What endocrine diagnosis is related to this phenotype and these biochemical manifestations?

REFERENCES

1. Ross M. H., Pawlina W. (2015). *Histology: A text and atlas* (7th ed.). Philadelphia, PA: Lippincott Williams & Wilkins.
2. Rubin R., Strayer D. (2015). *Rubin's pathology: Clinicopathologic foundations of medicine* (6th ed.). Philadelphia, PA: Lippincott Williams & Wilkins.
3. Scanlon V. C., Sanders T. (2014). *Essentials of anatomy and physiology.* Philadelphia, PA: FA Davis.
4. Boron W. F., Boulpaep E. L. (2016). *Medical physiology* (3rd ed.). Philadelphia, PA: Elsevier Health Sciences.
5. World Health Organization. (2010). WHO laboratory manual for the examination and processing of human semen (5th ed.). [Online]. Available: http://apps.who.int/iris/bitstream/10665/44261/1/9789241547789_eng.pdf?ua=1. Accessed June 10, 2019.
6. Sandher R. K., Aning J. (2017). Diagnosing and managing androgen deficiency in men. *The Practitioner* 261(1803), 19–22.
7. Phe V., Roupret M. (2012). Erectile dysfunction and diabetes: A review of the current evidence-based medicine and a synthesis of the main available therapies. *Diabetes & Metabolism* 38(1), 1–13.
8. Simoni M., Huhtaniemi I. T. (Eds.). (2017). *Endocrinology of the testis and male reproduction.* New York, NY: Springer International Publishing.
9. NIH U.S. National Library of Medicine. (2017). Klinefelter syndrome. [Online]. Available: https://ghr.nlm.nih.gov/condition/klinefelter-syndrome. Accessed June 10, 2019.
10. Cunningham G. (2013). Andropause or male menopause? Rationale for testosterone replacement therapy in older men with low testosterone levels. *Endocrine Practice* 19(5), 847–852.
11. Lunenfeld B., Arver S., Moncada I., et al. (2012). How to help the aging male? Current approaches to hypogonadism in primary care. *The Aging Male* 15(4), 187–197.

Disorders of the Male Reproductive System

Learning Objectives

After completing this chapter, the learner will be able to meet the following objectives:

1. Describe the anatomic changes, signs, and symptoms that occur with various penile disorders, both acquired and congenital.
2. Explain the physiology of penile erection and relate it to erectile dysfunction and priapism.
3. List the signs of penile cancer.
4. Compare the cause, appearance, and significance of hydrocele, hematocele, spermatocele, and varicocele.
5. Describe the symptoms of epididymitis.
6. State the cell types involved in seminoma, embryonal carcinoma, teratoma, and choriocarcinoma tumors of the testes.
7. Compare the pathology and symptoms of acute bacterial prostatitis, chronic bacterial prostatitis, and chronic prostatitis/pelvic pain syndrome.
8. Describe the urologic manifestations and treatment of benign prostatic hyperplasia.

The male genitourinary system is subject to structural defects, inflammation, and neoplasms, all of which can affect urine elimination, sexual function, and fertility. This chapter discusses disorders of the penis, the scrotum and testes, and the prostate.

Disorders of the Penis

The penis is the external male genital organ through which the urethra passes to the exterior of the body. It is involved in urinary and sexual function.

Congenital and Acquired Disorders

Hypospadias and Epispadias

Hypospadias and epispadias are congenital disorders resulting from embryologic defects in the development of the urethral groove and penile urethra (Fig. 43-1). In hypospadias, which affects 1 in 350 male infants, the urethral opening or meatus may be along the underside of the shaft of the penis, the scrotum, or the perineum.[1] Proximal hypospadias are more severe and associated with more negative psychological effects than distal hypospadias.[2] Hypospadias is a result of abnormal fusion of urethral tissue. During weeks 8 to 14 of fetal development, fetal testes release androgens that stimulate male sexual differentiation. Inactivity or deficiency of these androgens is believed to be responsible for the development of hypospadias. The majority of cases involve multifactorial causes, including family history of hypospadias and maternal factors (*e.g.*, older maternal age, multiple pregnancies, high body mass index, health conditions such as hypertension or preeclampsia). Testes are undescended in 10% of males born with hypospadias, and chordee (*i.e.*, ventral bowing of the penis) and inguinal hernia may accompany the disorder.

In the newborn with severe hypospadias and cryptorchidism (undescended testes), differential diagnosis should consider ambiguous genitalia and masculinization that is seen in females with congenital adrenal hyperplasia. Common treatment intervention for hypospadias is surgical repair.[3] In severe cases, repair becomes essential for normal sexual and urinary functioning and to prevent the psychological sequelae of having malformed genitalia. The goal of surgery is the construction of a urethral meatus at the tip of the glans that allows for easy passage of urine and semen. If chordee is present, straightening of the penis is also an indication for surgery. The recommended timing of surgery involving the male genitalia is between the ages of 6 and 18 months.[4] Surgical and anesthetic risk and the psychological impact of surgery are factors that influence surgery timing.

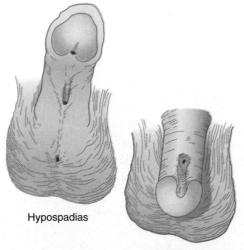

FIGURE 43-1. Hypospadias and epispadias.

Hypospadias

Epispadias

In cases of minor hypospadias with no functional impairment, there are concerns that surgery should be delayed until the person can give informed consent for the procedure.[2] *Epispadias*, in which the opening of the urethra is on the dorsal or upper surface of the penis, is less common than hypospadias. Although epispadias may occur as a separate entity, it is often associated with exstrophy of the bladder, where the bladder protrudes through a weakness in the abdominal wall.[1] Treatment depends on the extent of the developmental defect.

Phimosis and Paraphimosis

Phimosis is tightening of the prepuce or penile foreskin that prevents retraction over the glans.[4] The foreskin develops during the 8th week of gestation as a fold at the distal edge of the penis that grows over the base of the glans.[1] By the 16th week of gestation, the prepuce and the glans are adherent. A small percentage of newborns have a fully retractable foreskin. With growth, a space develops between the glans and the foreskin, and most males have retractable foreskins.[4]

Because the foreskin cannot be fully retracted in early childhood, a thorough cleaning is important. People with phimosis may seek medical care when signs and symptoms of infection develop, including pain and swelling of the foreskin or purulent discharge from the penile meatus.[5] Forcible retraction of the foreskin could lead to infection, scarring, or paraphimosis.[2] As the child grows, the foreskin becomes retractable, and the glans and foreskin should be cleaned routinely. If symptomatic phimosis occurs after childhood, such as with uncircumcised males with multiple infections, it can cause difficulty with voiding or sexual activity. Circumcision is then the treatment of choice. Phimosis is an important predisposing factor for penile cancer.[2]

In *paraphimosis*, the foreskin is so constricted that it cannot cover the glans. A tight foreskin can constrict blood supply and lead to ischemia and necrosis. Many cases are due to the foreskin being retracted for an extended period, as in the case of catheterized uncircumcised males.[2] Paraphimosis can present as a swollen, tender penis with multiple skin folds under the glans.[5]

Balanitis and Balanoposthitis

Balanitis is chronic or acute inflammation of the glans penis, and posthitis is inflammation of the prepuce. Often, both the glans penis and the prepuce are affected, resulting in *balanoposthitis*.[6] This condition may be characterized by erythema of the glans and prepuce, itching, soreness, blisters, ulcers, painful urination, and foul-smelling discharge.[7] Males with poor hygiene, immunosuppression, or diabetes are prone to balanoposthitis.[2] It is often encountered in males with phimosis or a large, redundant prepuce that interferes with cleanliness and predisposes to bacterial growth in accumulated secretions and smegma (debris from desquamated epithelia). It is uncommon in circumcised males.[7] Complications include permanent scarring of the glans and/or prepuce, phimosis, urethral stenosis or narrowing, sexual dysfunction, and malignant transformation.[7] Causes include infection, trauma, or irritation.

Infective balanoposthitis may be caused by *Candida albicans*, *Chlamydia trachomatis*, streptococci, staphylococci, herpes simplex virus, human papillomavirus (HPV), and *Mycoplasma genitalium*.[7] Although inflammation is common across all forms of balanoposthitis, treatment will vary depending on the cause.[7] If the suspected cause is a microorganism, treatment requires identification of that microorganism through microbial smears and cultures. Treatment will be tailored to the results. People with balanoposthitis caused by *Candida* are treated commonly with oral and topical antifungal medications. Balanoposthitis caused by Lichen sclerosis, an inflammatory skin condition that may be an autoimmune disease, are treated with topical steroids used to suppress the overactive immune system contributing to the balanoposthitis.[7] For some with balanoposthitis, no causative agent can be identified, yet the person is chronically symptomatic. This is *nonspecific balanoposthitis*. Circumcision is curative in these situations.

Because certain causes of balanoposthitis are potentially cancerous or precancerous, biopsy is often included in the care of people with balanoposthitis.[7] The goals of management are to reduce sexual dysfunction, minimize urinary dysfunction, exclude penile cancer, treat premalignant disease, and diagnose and treat sexually transmitted infections (STIs).[7]

Peyronie Disease

Peyronie disease is localized and progressive fibrosis of unknown origin that affects the tunica albuginea of the penis. Approximately 1% of males are impacted, most commonly after 40 years of age.[2] It is characterized initially by inflammation resulting in dense fibrous plaque formation. The plaque is usually on the dorsal midline of the shaft, causing upward bowing of the shaft during erection (Fig. 43-2). Some males may develop scarring on both the dorsal and ventral aspects of the shaft, causing the penis to be straight but shortened or have a lateral bend.[2] Fibrous tissue prevents lengthening of the involved area during erection, making intercourse difficult and painful.

Manifestations of Peyronie disease include painful erection, bent erection, and a hard mass at the site of fibrosis. Two thirds of males complain of pain, which usually disappears as inflammation resolves. During the first year after formation of the plaque, while the scar tissue is undergoing remodeling, penile distortion may increase, remain static, or resolve and disappear.[8] In some cases, the scar tissue may progress to calcification and formation of bonelike tissue.

Diagnosis is based on history and physical examination. Doppler ultrasonography may be used to assess causation. Surgical intervention can be used to correct the disorder. Indications for surgery include penile shortening, persistent pain, severe curvature, and penile narrowing or indentation.

Disorders of Erectile Function

Erection is a neurovascular process involving the autonomic nervous system, neurotransmitters and endothelial relaxing factors, vascular smooth muscle of the arteries and veins supplying the penile tissue, and trabecular smooth muscle of the sinusoids of the corpora cavernosa (Fig. 43-3). The penis is innervated by both the autonomic and somatic nervous systems.[8] In the pelvis, the sympathetic and parasympathetic components of the autonomic nervous systems merge to form the cavernous nerves.[8] Erection is under the control of the parasympathetic nervous system, and ejaculation and

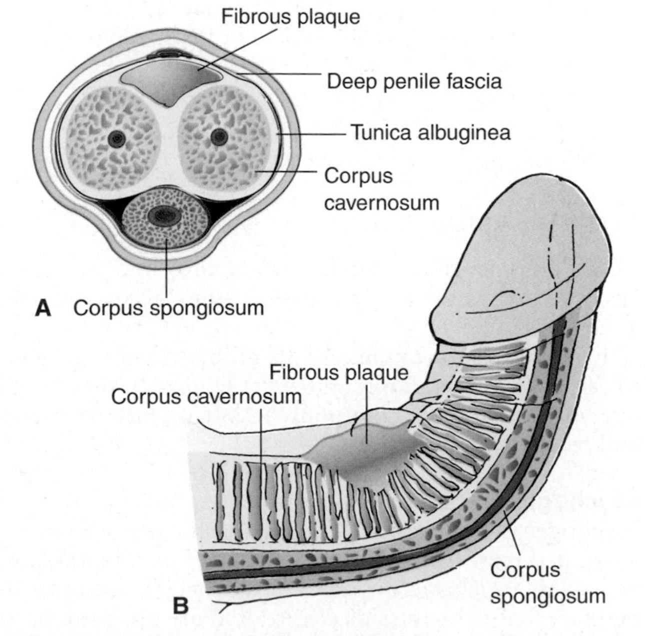

FIGURE 43-2. Peyronie disease. **(A)** Penile cross section showing plaque between the corpora. **(B)** Penile curvature.

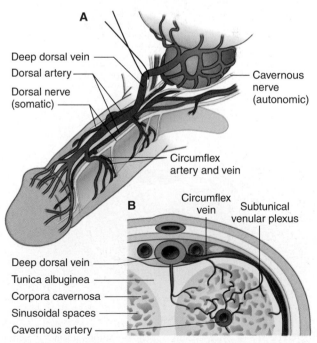

FIGURE 43-3. Anatomy and mechanism of penile erection. **(A)** Innervation and arterial and venous blood supply to the penis. **(B)** Cross section of the sinusoidal system of the corpora cavernosa.

detumescence are under sympathetic nervous system control.[8] Somatic innervation through the pudendal nerve is responsible for penile sensation and contraction and relaxation of the extracorporeal striated muscles.

Penile erection is the first effect of male sexual stimulation (Fig. 43-4). It requires dilation of penile vasculature, relaxation of smooth muscle, increased intracavernosal blood flow, and normal veno-occlusive function. It involves increased blood flow into the corpora cavernosa due to relaxation of smooth muscle that surrounds the sinusoidal spaces and compression of veins controlling outflow of blood from the venous plexus. Erection is mediated by parasympathetic impulses passing from sacral segments of the spinal cord to the penis. Parasympathetic stimulation results in release of nitric oxide, a nonadrenergic–noncholinergic neurotransmitter, which

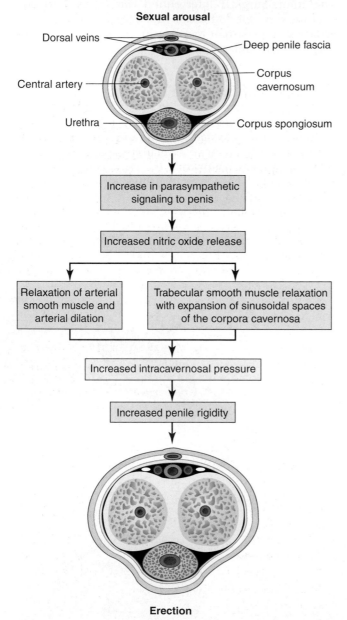

Sexual arousal

- Dorsal veins
- Central artery
- Urethra
- Deep penile fascia
- Corpus cavernosum
- Corpus spongiosum

Increase in parasympathetic signaling to penis

↓

Increased nitric oxide release

↓

Relaxation of arterial smooth muscle and arterial dilation

Trabecular smooth muscle relaxation with expansion of sinusoidal spaces of the corpora cavernosa

↓

Increased intracavernosal pressure

↓

Increased penile rigidity

↓

Erection

FIGURE 43-4. Mechanisms of penile erection and sites of action of drugs, vacuum suction, and penile prosthesis used in the treatment of erectile dysfunction.

causes relaxation of trabecular smooth muscle of the corpora cavernosa.[2] This permits inflow of blood to the cavernosa sinuses. Because erectile tissues of the cavernosa are surrounded by a nonelastic fibrous covering, high pressure in the sinusoids causes ballooning of the tissue to such an extent that the penis becomes hard and elongated. Contraction of ischiocavernosus muscles also forcefully compresses the blood-filled corpora cavernosa, producing a further rise in intercavernous pressures. During this phase, inflow and outflow of blood cease.

Parasympathetic innervation must be intact and nitric oxide synthesis active for erection to occur. Nitric oxide activates guanylyl cyclase, which increases cyclic guanosine monophosphate (cGMP), which causes relaxation of smooth muscle. Other smooth muscle relaxants (e.g., prostaglandin E_1 analogs and α-adrenergic antagonists) can cause sufficient cavernosal relaxation to result in erection. Many drugs developed to treat erectile dysfunction (ED) act at these mediators.[9]

Detumescence is largely a sympathetic nervous system response. It can result from a cessation of neurotransmitter release, breakdown of second messengers such as cGMP, or sympathetic discharge during ejaculation. Contraction of the trabecular smooth muscle opens the venous channels so that the trapped blood can be expelled and penile flaccidity can return.

KEY POINTS

Disorders of Penile Erection

- Erection is a neurovascular process involving the autonomic nervous system, the somatic nervous system by way of the pudendal nerve, the vascular system, and the sinusoidal spaces of the corpora cavernosa.

- Erectile failure can result from disorders in one or a combination of the neural, vascular, or chemical pathways that produce an erection.

Erectile Dysfunction

ED is the persistent inability to achieve and maintain an erection sufficient to permit satisfactory sexual intercourse.[10]

ED affects approximately 30 million males aged 40 to 70 years in the Unites States.[11] ED has a physical etiology for most men, commonly involving blood flow to and from the penis.

Psychogenic Causes

Psychogenic causes of ED include performance anxiety, a strained relationship with a sexual partner, depression, and overt psychotic disorders. Psychogenic factors can be exacerbated by the side effects of many therapies used to treat these disorders, which can themselves cause ED.

Organic Causes

Organic causes of ED include neurogenic, hormonal, vascular, drug-induced, and penile-related etiologies. The most common cause involves the penile arteries and/or veins.[11] Arterial issues are usually caused by arteriosclerosis, although sometimes they are due to trauma to arteries.[11] Risk factors for arteriosclerosis include obesity, physical inactivity, high cholesterol levels, high blood pressure, and cigarette smoking. These risk factors can result in ED before the heart is ever affected.[11] Another proposed vascular cause is partial or complete atrophy of smooth muscle in the penis (cavernous smooth muscle) or growth of excessive smooth muscle tissue (fibrosis). This atrophy or fibrosis can contribute to impaired ability to maintain an erection.

There are many neurologic causes of ED, including Parkinson disease, multiple sclerosis, heavy metal poisoning, stroke, cerebral trauma, and spinal cord and nerve injuries. In spinal cord injury, the extent of neural impairment depends on the level, location, and extent of the lesion.

ED is common in people with diabetes. An estimated 10.9 million adult males in the United States have diabetes, and 35% to 50% of these males have ED. The process involves premature and severe hardening of the arteries, and peripheral neuropathy involving the nerves controlling erection. Extensive pelvic surgery is a common cause of ED due to both direct and indirect nerve damage.

Endocrine disorders—such as hypogonadism, hyperprolactinemia, and thyroid disease—play a significant role in ED physiology. Testosterone regulates cavernosal nerve structure and function, nitric oxide synthesis, and corporal smooth muscle cell growth and differentiation. Prolactin inhibits release of gonadotropin-releasing hormone (GnRH) from the hypothalamus.

For people with hypertension, erectile function is impaired by associated arterial lesions caused by high pressure that narrows the vessel lumen (stenosis). Focal stenosis of the common penile artery most often occurs in males who sustained blunt pelvic or perineal trauma (e.g., from bicycling accidents). Failure of the veins to close completely during an erection (veno-occlusive dysfunction) may occur in males with large venous channels that drain the corpora cavernosa.

Many drugs are reported to cause ED, including antidepressants, antipsychotics, antiandrogens, glaucoma eye drops, chemotherapy drugs, and antihypertensive medications.[11] Cigarettes can induce vasoconstriction and penile venous leakage due to effects on cavernous smooth muscle and can double the risk of ED.[12] Alcohol in small amounts may increase libido and improve erection, but in large amounts, can cause central sedation, decreased libido, and transient ED.

Aging increases the risk of ED.[10] Many pathologic processes that contribute to ED, including diabetes, hyperlipidemia, vascular disease, and the long-term effects of cigarette smoking, are more common in older men. Age-related testosterone decline may also play a role (andropause).

Diagnosis and Treatment

A diagnosis requires a careful history (medical, sexual, and psychosocial), physical examination, and laboratory tests to rule out organic causes. Because many medications can cause ED, an accurate drug history is needed.

When a person presents with multiple metabolic conditions simultaneously, the likelihood of developing cardiovascular disease is greater than if he or she had a single metabolic disorder.[13] The association between ED and metabolic syndrome may be related to the underlying endothelial dysfunction seen in both conditions.[12] A person with ED should be evaluated for coexisting vascular disease and type 2 diabetes mellitus. Any cardiovascular risk factors should be modified or treated (e.g., smoking, diabetes, hypertension, physical inactivity, and hyperlipidemia).

Many people experience a combination of psychogenic and organic ED. Organic ED may be associated with progressively worsening performance anxiety, which further worsens function. To treat males holistically, the physician and psychotherapist may need to collaborate and combine counseling with one or more treatment options.

The treatment selected depends on multiple factors, such as severity of ED, underlying cause, and patient and partner choice. Evidence suggests that the only lifestyle modification that may make a difference in ED incidence is maintaining or initiating physical exercise.[12]

Treatments should consider the partner's attitude about the problem and the likely response to effective treatment. Methods include psychosexual counseling, androgen replacement therapy, oral and intracavernous drug therapy, vacuum constriction devices, and surgical treatment.[9]

Psychosexual therapy for ED varies among individuals due to varying sources of anxiety. Stress in a relationship, depression, guilt, problems with intimacy, and lack of sexual experience may all increase anxiety, which may present as ED. Psychosexual treatments can include sex education, strategies to improve partner communication, and/or cognitive behavioral therapy. These are often combined with ED pharmacotherapy.[12] Results of psychosexual therapy are relatively good in the short term, but long-term results are more difficult to sustain.[14]

Most people with ED respond to oral pharmacologic interventions. Phosphodiesterase-5 inhibitors (PDE5 inhibitors) are a common treatment. PDE5 inhibitors selectively inhibit PDE5 and increase cGMP available for smooth muscle relaxation, inducing vasodilatation, increased corporal blood flow, and erection. The concurrent use of PDE5 inhibitors and nitrates (used in ischemic heart disease) is contraindicated because of the risk of profound hypotension.[12]

Patient-administered intracavernosal injection (ICI) therapy with vasodilator drugs is an effective ED treatment. This prostaglandin E_1 analog relaxes arterial and trabecular smooth muscle. It is injected directly into one cavernosa (with diffusion into the opposite cavernosa) or placed in the urethra as a mini-suppository. Phentolamine (α_2-adrenergic receptor antagonist) and papaverine (smooth muscle relaxant) are also administered ICI. ICI therapy is especially useful in males who fail to respond to oral pharmacologic agents. Other physical treatments, such as vacuum devices and intracavernosal drugs, are used "on demand"; however, the rates of discontinuation are high due to side effects, dislike of needles, and unwillingness of the partner to participate.[12]

The vacuum constriction device involves application of a vacuum to the penis in a vacuum cylinder, causing tumescence and rigidity, which is sustained using a constricting ring at the base of the penis. The penile physiologic changes differ from a normal erection in that trabecular smooth muscle relaxation does not occur, and blood is trapped in both the intracorporeal and extracorporeal compartments of the penis distal to the ring. Vacuum constriction devices require a motivated patient and partner. They are more popular in middle-aged and older group couples.

Surgical treatment of ED is reserved for patients in whom more conservative therapy has failed or for whom conservative therapy is contraindicated. Most surgical patients have significant arterial or venous disease, penile corpus cavernosum fibrosis, or Peyronie disease. Although the outcome of surgical intervention may be more reliable in certain people, the incidence of morbidity and complications is significantly greater than with other treatment options.

Malleable or multicomponent inflatable penile implants are reserved for patients in whom more conservative therapy has failed and are associated with high satisfaction rates.

Peyronie Disease and Erectile Dysfunction

Peyronie disease is penis curvature due to fibrosis within the tunica albuginea. Affected corpora cavernosa cannot lengthen on erection. ED occurs in 30% to 40% of males with Peyronie disease. Although the mechanism of their ED is not understood, many have a vascular problem.

If a person has ED and Peyronie disease, he may be advised to undergo insertion of a penile implant because surgical straightening of the penis alone is unlikely to overcome the ED.

Priapism

Priapism is an involuntary, persistent (>4 hours) penile erection that continues hours beyond, or is unrelated to, sexual stimulation. Typically, only the corpora cavernosa are affected. Priapism is a true urologic emergency because prolonged erection can result in ischemia and fibrosis of erectile tissue with risk of impotence. It can occur at any age, and sickle cell disease or neoplasms are the most common cause in males between the ages of 5 and 10 years. Subtypes of priapism include ischemic (veno-occlusive, low-flow) priapism, a nonsexual, persistent erection characterized by little or no cavernous blood flow and abnormal cavernous blood gases (hypoxic, hypercapnic, and acidotic). The corpora cavernosa are rigid and tender to palpation. Patients typically report pain. Ischemic priapism is an emergency. Nonischemic (arterial, high flow) priapism is

a nonsexual, persistent erection caused by unregulated cavernous arterial inflow. Cavernous blood gases are not hypoxic or acidotic. Typically, the penis is neither fully rigid nor painful. Preceding trauma is the most common etiology. Stuttering (intermittent) priapism is a recurrent form in which unwanted painful erections occur with periods of detumescence.

Although not all forms of priapism require immediate intervention, ischemic priapism is associated with progressive fibrosis of the cavernosal tissues and ED.[15] Thus, all people with priapism should be evaluated emergently to intervene as early as possible. The goal of management of people with priapism is to achieve detumescence and preserve erectile function.

Priapism can occur secondary to a disease or drug effect. Secondary causes include hematologic conditions such as leukemia, sickle cell disease, and thrombocytopenia; neurologic conditions such as stroke, spinal cord injury, and other central nervous system lesions; and renal failure. Males with sickle cell disease are frequently affected by priapism. The relative deoxygenation and stasis of cavernosal blood during erection is thought to increase sickling. Medications, such as antihypertensive drugs, anticoagulant drugs, antidepressant drugs, alcohol, and marijuana, can contribute to development. ICI therapy for ED is a common cause of priapism.

Diagnosis is based on clinical findings. Doppler studies of penile blood flow, ultrasonography, and computed tomography (CT) scans may be used to determine intrapelvic pathology. Initial treatment measures include analgesics, sedation, and hydration. Urinary retention may necessitate catheterization. Local measures include ice packs and cold saline enemas, aspiration and irrigation of the corpus cavernosum with plain or heparinized saline, or instillation of α-adrenergic drugs. If less aggressive treatment does not produce detumescence, a temporary surgical shunt may be established between the corpus cavernosum and the corpus spongiosum.

Cancer of the Penis

The average age of diagnosis of squamous cell cancer of the penis is 60 years. It is most common in uncircumcised men and in developing countries, where it may account for 10% of cancers in males.[2] When it is diagnosed early, penile cancer is highly curable.

The cause of penile cancer is unknown. Risk factors exist, including age, poor hygiene, smoking, HPV types 16 and 18 infections, ultraviolet radiation exposure, and immunosuppression.[2] There is an association between penile cancer and poor genital hygiene and phimosis. Males treated for psoriasis with ultraviolet A radiation have increased incidence of genital squamous cell carcinomas. Squamous cell carcinoma of the penis is thought to progress from an in situ lesion to an invasive carcinoma. Lesions with histologic features of carcinoma in situ require follow-up because of their potential to progress to invasive carcinoma.

Invasive carcinoma of the penis begins as a small lump or ulcer. If phimosis is present, there may be painful swelling, purulent drainage, or difficulty urinating. Palpable lymph nodes may be present in the inguinal region. Diagnosis is usually based on physical examination and biopsy results. Cavernosography, urethroscopy, CT scans, and magnetic resonance imaging (MRI) may be used for diagnosis.

Treatment options depend on stage, size, location, and invasiveness. Surgery is the mainstay of treatment for invasive carcinoma. Superficial primary lesions that are freely movable, do not invade the corpora, and show no evidence of metastatic disease can be resected. Partial or total penectomy with appropriate lymph node dissection is indicated for invasive lesions.

SUMMARY CONCEPTS

Disorders of the penis can be congenital or acquired. Hypospadias and epispadias are congenital defects in which there is malpositioning of the urethral opening: it is located on the ventral surface in hypospadias and on the dorsal surface in epispadias. Phimosis is the condition in which the opening of the foreskin is too tight to permit retraction over the glans. Balanitis is an acute or chronic inflammation of the glans penis, and balanoposthitis is an inflammation of the glans and prepuce. Peyronie disease is the growth of a band of fibrous tissue on top of the penile shaft. ED is the inability to achieve and maintain an erection sufficient to permit satisfactory sexual intercourse due to psychogenic factors, organic disorders, or mixed psychogenic and organic conditions. Priapism is a prolonged, painful erection that can lead to thrombosis with ischemia and necrosis of penile tissue. Cancer of the penis accounts for less than 1% of male genital cancers in developed countries. The tumor is slow growing and highly curable when diagnosed early, but the greatest hindrance to successful treatment is a delay in medical attention.

Disorders of the Scrotum and Testes

The scrotum is a skin-covered pouch that contains the testes and their accessory organs (Fig. 43-6A).

Congenital and Acquired Disorders

Cryptorchidism

Cryptorchidism (undescended testes) occurs when one or both testicles fail to move down into the scrotal sac. Undescended testes may remain in the lower abdomen, at a point of descent in the inguinal canal, or in the upper scrotum (Fig. 43-5).[2] Chapter 42 describes testicular descent.

Cryptorchidism is the most common congenital disorder of the genitourinary system affecting male infants.[16] The incidence is 2% to 4%, but as many as one third of premature newborn males are affected.[14] The pathophysiology of cryptorchidism is not fully understood. Uncorrected cryptorchidism may have extreme implications, particularly on fertility potential and malignant transformation of some testicular cell lines.[14] Clinically, the presence of unilateral cryptorchidism is more common than bilateral cryptorchidism. Approximately 80% of cases are unilateral, and the remaining 20% represent bilateral cryptorchidism.[17]

Cryptorchidism can be divided into primary or secondary types. In primary cryptorchidism, the testis fails to complete migration from the pararenal embryologic origin to the scrotum. It may be located in a nonpalpable intra-abdominal position or may be palpable in an intracanalicular position, suprascrotal position, or an ectopic position (outside the normal path of descent). In secondary cryptorchidism, a testis that had previously been in a scrotal position can be pulled into a suprascrotal position as a result of scarring, often after surgical repair of an inguinal hernia.[18] Identified risk factors for cryptorchidism remain elusive. The strongest risk factor is believed to be prematurity; the incidence of cryptorchidism among premature neonates is reported to be greater than 30%.[19] Many cases of cryptorchidism spontaneously descend postnatally. Because spontaneous descent after 6 months is less likely, clinical guidelines recommend referral to a specialist if the testis is not completely descended by 6 months of age.[17]

Clinical Manifestations and Complications

The major clinical manifestation of cryptorchidism is the absence of one or both testes from the scrotum. The testis either is not palpable or can be felt external to the inguinal ring.

Histologic abnormalities of the testes reflect intrinsic defects in the testicle or adverse effects of the extrascrotal environment. There is a delay in germ cell development, changes in spermatic tubules, and reduced Leydig cells. Changes are progressive if the testes remain undescended.

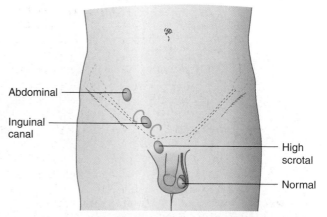

FIGURE 43-5. Possible locations of undescended testes.

Diagnosis and Treatment

Diagnosis is based on examination. Undescended testes due to cryptorchidism should be differentiated from retractable testes that retract into the inguinal canal in response to an exaggerated cremasteric muscle reflex. Retractable testes are usually palpable at birth but become nonpalpable later. They can be brought down with palpation in a warm room. Retractable testes usually assume a scrotal position during puberty. Techniques for testicular localization include ultrasonography, gonadal venography and arteriography, and laparoscopy.

The only definitive management for an undescended testis is surgical intervention. Hormonal treatments with human chorionic gonadotropin (hCG) and GnRH may encourage descent. Hormonal therapies appear more appropriate for low-level cryptorchidism and retractile testes, but success rates are poor.[20] Consequences of cryptorchidism include infertility, malignancy (20- to 40-fold higher risk), testicular torsion (10-fold increased risk), and possible psychological effects of an empty scrotum.[1] Therefore, definitive and corrective surgical therapy is the mainstay of treatment, and hormonal therapies are no longer recommended.[17]

Treatment of males with undescended testes should include lifelong follow-up. Parents need to be aware of increased risks of infertility and testicular cancer. After puberty, males should be instructed on testicular self-examination.

Hydrocele

Hydrocele is a collection of fluid in the scrotum without an obvious inguinal hernia. The testes and epididymis are surrounded by tunica vaginalis, derived from the peritoneum during fetal descent of the testes. The tunica vaginalis has an outer parietal layer and a deeper visceral layer that adheres to the tunica albuginea. A space exists between the two layers that contain a few milliliters of fluid. Hydrocele forms when excess fluid collects between the layers (Fig. 43-6C).[9] Typically, hydrocele is seen shortly after birth as a unilateral or bilateral swelling in the scrotum, and may vary in size. The scrotum appears swollen with fluid and may be bluish in color. The scrotum may be tense and is usually not tender. Transillumination of the scrotum (*i.e.*, shining a light through the scrotum to visualize its internal structures) or ultrasonography may determine whether the mass is solid or cystic and whether the testicle is normal. A dense hydrocele that does not illuminate should be differentiated from a testicular tumor. Management of hydrocele is observation in the first 1 to 2 years of life, unless the diagnosis of a hernia cannot be excluded. Hydroceles that persist or appear beyond that age are unlikely to resolve spontaneously and should undergo surgical repair. Prevalence of congenital hydroceles is 6% at birth and 1% in adulthood.[21] Acute hydrocele may develop after local injury, testicular torsion, epididymitis or orchitis, gonorrhea, lymph obstruction, germ cell testicular tumor, or radiation therapy. Chronic hydrocele is more common, with fluid collecting around the testis and a gradually growing mass.

Most cases of hydrocele in male infants and children are caused by a patent processus vaginalis, which is an outpouching of peritoneum through the internal inguinal ring that normally closes spontaneously following testicular descent. Incomplete closure may result in an abnormal communication between the abdominal cavity and inguinal region.[21] Hydrocele that develops in a young male without apparent cause requires exclusion of cancer or infection. In an adult male, a hydrocele is often asymptomatic, and no treatment is necessary. Symptoms may include a feeling of heaviness in the scrotum or pain in the lower back. If it is painful or cosmetically undesirable, surgical correction is indicated, which may be done inguinally or transscrotally.

Hematocele

A hematocele is an accumulation of blood in the space between the parietal and visceral tunica vaginalis, which causes the scrotal skin to become dark red or purple. Hematocele is often associated with hydrocele. It may develop as a result of an abdominal surgical procedure, scrotal trauma, a bleeding disorder, or a testicular tumor.

Spermatocele

A spermatocele is a painless, sperm-containing cyst that forms at the end of the epididymis. It is located above

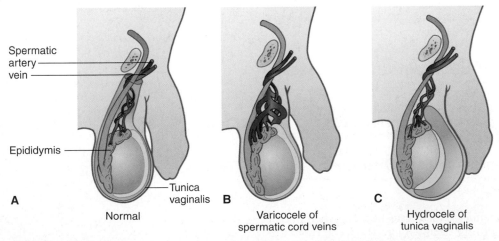

FIGURE 43-6. (**A**) Normal testis and appendages, (**B**) varicocele, and (**C**) hydrocele.

and posterior to the testis, is attached to the epididymis, and is separate from the testes.[2] Spermatoceles may be solitary or multiple and are usually less than 1 cm in diameter. They are freely movable and should transilluminate. Spermatoceles rarely cause problems, but a large one may become painful and require removal.

Varicocele

A varicocele is varicosities of the pampiniform plexus, a network of veins supplying the testes (see Fig. 43-6B). The left side is more commonly affected. The left internal spermatic vein inserts into the left renal vein at a right angle, whereas the right spermatic vein enters the inferior vena cava.[9] Incompetent valves are common in the left internal spermatic veins, causing a reflux of blood into pampiniform plexus veins. The force of gravity from the upright position contributes to venous dilation. If it persists, there may be damage to the elastic fibers and hypertrophy of the vein walls. Sperm concentration and motility are decreased with varicocele. It can result from a number of conditions, but most cases are idiopathic. Unilateral varicocele in older males may indicate a renal tumor that has invaded the renal vein and occluded spermatic vein drainage.[21]

Varicoceles are rarely found before puberty. Symptoms include abnormal feeling of heaviness in the left scrotum, although many are asymptomatic. Usually, it is diagnosed on physical examination in the standing and recumbent positions. Typically, the varicocele disappears in the lying position because of venous decompression into the renal vein.[9] Scrotal palpation of a varicocele is compared to feeling a "bag of worms."[9] Small varicoceles may be difficult to identify. The Valsalva maneuver may be used to accentuate small varicosities. If the varicocele is present, retrograde blood flow to the scrotum can be detected by Doppler ultrasonography.

Treatment options include surgical ligation or sclerosis using a percutaneous transvenous catheter under fluoroscopic guidance. Aside from improving fertility, other reasons for surgery include relief of the sensation of "heaviness" and cosmetic improvement.

Testicular Torsion

Testicular torsion is twisting of the spermatic cord and loss of the blood supply to the ipsilateral testicle (Fig. 43-7). Considered a urologic emergency, early diagnosis and treatment are critical to preserving the testicle and fertility.[22] Viability decreases rapidly after 6 hours from the onset of symptoms.[23] It is the most common acute scrotal disorder in the pediatric and young adult population, occurring in 1 in 4000 males under 25 years.[9] Depending on the level of spermatic cord involvement, testicular torsion can be divided into intravaginal or extravaginal torsion.[24]

Intravaginal Torsion
Typically, the tunica vaginalis is attached securely to the posterior lateral side of the testicle. If attachment to the testicle is too high, the spermatic cord can rotate, resulting in intravaginal torsion. This occurs in about 17%

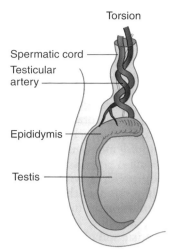

FIGURE 43-7. Testicular torsion with twisting of the spermatic cord that suspends the testis and the spermatic vessels that supply the testis with blood.

of males and is bilateral in 40%.[25] Intravaginal torsion commonly occurs in adolescents. Increased weight of the testicle after puberty and sudden contraction of the cremaster muscles may be catalysts for acute torsion in this population.[25] Intravaginal torsion is more common than extravaginal torsion. Patients usually present in severe distress within hours of onset and often have nausea, vomiting, and tachycardia. The affected testis is large and tender, with pain radiating to the inguinal area. Intravaginal testicular torsion is a true surgical emergency, and early recognition and treatment are necessary.

Extravaginal Torsion
Extravaginal torsion occurs almost exclusively in neonates. In neonates, the testicle frequently has not yet descended into the scrotum, where it becomes attached within the tunica vaginalis. Mobility of the testicle predisposes it to torsion. Inadequate fusion of the testicle to the scrotal wall is typically diagnosed within the first 7 to 10 days of life. At birth or shortly thereafter, a firm, smooth, painless scrotal mass is identified. The scrotal skin appears red, and some edema is present. Differential diagnosis is straightforward: Testicular tumors, epididymitis, and orchitis are rare in neonates; a hydrocele is softer and can be transilluminated; and physical examination can exclude the presence of hernia. Surgical treatment is controversial.[24] The testicle is often high in the scrotum and in an abnormal orientation. This is caused by twisting and shortening of the spermatic cord. The degree of scrotal swelling and redness depends on the duration of symptoms. The testes are firm and tender. The cremasteric reflex is frequently absent.[26]

Infection and Inflammation

Epididymitis

Epididymitis is an acute or chronic inflammation of the epididymis.[1] There are approximately 600,000 cases of epididymitis per year in the United States.[27]

cell cancers. Radical surgery and radiation therapy are both curative with more advanced cancers. When there is upper vaginal involvement, radical surgery may be required, including a total hysterectomy, pelvic lymph node dissection, and partial vaginectomy. Ovaries usually are preserved unless they are diseased. Extensive lesions and those located in the middle or lower vaginal area usually are treated by radiation therapy. Prognosis depends on stage of the disease, involvement of lymph nodes, and degree of mitotic activity of the tumor.[22]

 SUMMARY CONCEPTS

The surface of the vulva is affected by disorders that affect the skin on other parts of the body. Bartholin cysts are the result of occluded ducts in Bartholin glands. They often are painful and can become infected. Nonneoplastic epithelial disorders are characterized by thinning or hyperplastic thickening of vulvar tissues. Vulvodynia is a chronic vulvar pain syndrome with several classifications and variable treatment results. Cancer of the vulva is associated with HPV infections in younger women and lichen sclerosus in older females.

Normal vaginal ecology depends on the balance of hormones and bacterial flora. Disruptions predispose to vaginal infections. Vaginitis is characterized by vaginal discharge and burning, itching, redness, and swelling of vaginal tissues. It may be caused by chemical irritants, foreign bodies, or infectious agents. Primary cancers of the vagina account for about 1% of all cancers of the female reproductive system. Daughters of females treated with DES to prevent miscarriage are at increased risk for development of adenocarcinoma of the vagina.

Disorders of the Cervix and Uterus

Disorders of the Uterine Cervix

The cervix is composed of two types of tissue. The exocervix, the visible portion, has stratified squamous epithelium, which also lines the vagina.[1] The endocervix, the canal that leads to the endometrial cavity, is lined with columnar epithelium that has large, branched mucus-secreting glands.[1] During a menstrual cycle, cervical glands undergo functional changes. The mucus secreted by the gland cells vary under the influence of ovarian hormones, and blockage of the glands results in trapping of mucus in the deeper glands, leading to formation of dilated benign cysts in the cervix (*nabothian cysts*). These may grow to one centimeter or more.[6]

The junction of squamous and mucus-secreting columnar epithelium (squamocolumnar junction) appears at various locations over a lifetime (Fig. 45-2).[6] During the reproductive years, the cervix everts or turns outward, exposing the columnar epithelium to the vaginal environment. The combination of hormonal and pH changes, long-term inflammation, and mechanical irritation lead to a gradual transformation from columnar to squamous epithelium—a process called *metaplasia*. This area of continuous change is called the *transformation zone*.[6]

The transformation zone is a critical area in the development of cervical cancer. During metaplasia, newly developed squamous epithelial cells are vulnerable to development of dysplasia (disordered growth or development of cells) and genetic changes if exposed to cancer-producing agents. Although initially reversible, untreated dysplasia can develop into carcinoma. The transformation zone is sampled in a Pap smear. If the Pap smear is abnormal, the transformation zone is carefully examined during colposcopy, a vaginal examination using a *colposcope*.[6]

Cervicitis and Cervical Polyps

Acute cervicitis may result from direct infection of the cervix or may be secondary to a vaginal or uterine infection. It may be caused by infective agents including *Streptococcus, Staphylococcus, Enterococcus, C. albicans, T. vaginalis, Neisseria gonorrhoeae, Gardnerella vaginalis, Chlamydia trachomatis, Ureaplasma urealyticum*, and herpes simplex virus type 2.[1] *C. trachomatis* is most commonly associated with mucopurulent cervicitis. With acute cervicitis, the cervix becomes reddened and edematous. Irritation from infection results in mucopurulent drainage and leukorrhea.[1] Depending on the cause, acute cervicitis is treated with appropriate antibiotic therapy. Untreated cervicitis may extend to include the development of pelvic cellulitis, dyspareunia, cervical stenosis, and ascending infection of the uterus or fallopian tubes.

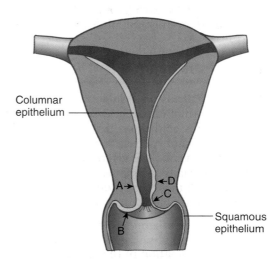

FIGURE 45-2. Location of the squamocolumnar junction (transformation zone) in menarchial, menstruating, menopausal, and postmenopausal women. (*A*, menarchial; *B*, menstruating; *C*, menopausal; *D*, postmenopausal.)

Polyps are the most common lesions of the cervix. Incidence is higher during reproductive years.[1] They are soft, velvety, red lesions, usually pedunculated and found protruding through the cervical os. They usually develop due to inflammatory hyperplasia of endocervical mucosa. They typically are asymptomatic but may be associated with postcoital bleeding. Most are benign but should be removed and examined to exclude possibility of malignant change.[23]

Cancer of the Cervix

Cervical cancer is readily detected and, if detected early, is the most easily cured of all female reproductive system cancers. Approximately 13,170 new cases of invasive cervical cancer will be diagnosed in the United States in 2019, with 4250 predicted deaths.[24] In the past 40 years, cervical cancer deaths have decreased by 50%, indicating the importance of early detection and treatment.[24]

Risk Factors

Risk factors include early age at first intercourse, multiple sexual partners, smoking, and a history of sexually transmitted infections (STIs). Homosexual and heterosexual females should follow the same guidelines for Pap smear screening.[23] HPV is an STI passed through genital or skin-to-skin contact. At least 50% of people contract HPV in their lifetime.[24] HPV type 16 and HPV type 18 have been associated with cervical cancer.[1] Other HPV types linked with cervical cancer include HPV types 31, 33, 35, 39, 45, 51, 52, 56, 58, 59, and 68.[1] Other factors such as smoking, nutrition, and coexisting sexual infections such as *C. trachomatis*, herpes simplex virus type 2, and HIV may contribute to whether an HPV infection develops into cervical cancer.[24]

Preventing Cervical Cancer

The HPV vaccine has decreased the risk of cervical cancer by 97%.[1] Gardasil is an HPV vaccine that prevents infection with HPV subtypes 16, 18, 6, and 11. It is approved for females and males between 9 and 26 years of age (before sexual activity) to prevent HPV 6 and HPV 11 genital warts. HPV 16 and 18 are responsible for 70% of cervical cancer, and the two most common benign strains (HPV 6 and 11) account for up to 90% of genital warts. The vaccine is safe and effective in inducing a sustained immunity response to HPV.[24,25]

Gardasil 9 vaccine offers the same protection as Gardasil and protects against HPV types 31, 33, 45, 52, and 58. These nine strains contribute to 90% of cervical cancers.[24] The other U.S. Food and Drug Administration-approved HPV vaccine is Cervarix, which is recommended for females between 9 and 25 years of age, before becoming sexually active. Cervarix protects against HPV 16 and 18.[26]

Pathogenesis

Pap smear cytological screening allows precancerous lesions to be detected and treated before cancer develops. Atypical cells may display changes in the nuclear and cytoplasmic parts of the cell and variation in cell size and shape (*i.e.*, dysplasia). These precancerous changes represent a continuum of changes with indistinct boundaries that may gradually progress to cancer *in situ* and then to invasive cancer or may spontaneously regress.[1]

A system of grading to describe the histopathologic findings of dysplastic changes of cancer precursors uses the term *cervical intraepithelial neoplasia* (CIN),[18] which describes premalignant changes in the epithelial tissue. CIN I is defined as dysplasia or atypical changes in the cervical epithelium, CIN II is moderate dysplasia, and CIN III is severe dysplasia.[25]

Diagnosis

Abnormal Pap smear results will return as atypical squamous cells of undetermined origin (ASC-US); atypical squamous cells of undetermined origin that cannot exclude high-grade squamous intraepithelial lesion (ASC-H); low-grade squamous intraepithelial lesion (LGSIL); high-grade squamous intraepithelial lesion (HGSIL); or squamous cell cancer. If abnormal results are detected, a colposcopy may be done. Biopsies are taken of potential abnormal lesions or areas of increased vascularity, as well as a curettage of the endocervical canal that may not be fully seen on colposcopy. The abnormal Pap smear finding of LGSIL is often CIN I on biopsy, whereas HGSIL on a Pap smear is likely CIN II or CIN III on a biopsy[27] (Fig. 45-3).

Recommendations for screening include HPV testing and cytology in females over 30 years of age. Results dictate the next steps in disease management. Cytology (Pap smear) alone is recommended beginning at 21 years of age and then every 3 years until age 29. For females over 30, a Pap smear alone should be performed every 3 years or cotesting every 5 years.[25]

False-negative Pap smears occur,[28] and care must be taken to obtain a smear from the transformation zone that includes endocervical cells. The presence of normal endometrial cells in a cervical cytologic sample during the luteal phase or during the postmenopausal period is associated with endometrial disease and warrants evaluation with endometrial biopsy. This demonstrates that shedding of normal cells at an inappropriate time may indicate disease. Because adenocarcinoma of the cervix is detected more frequently, a Pap smear result of atypical glandular cells warrants evaluation by endocervical or endometrial curettage, hysteroscopy, or, ultimately, a cone biopsy if the abnormality cannot be identified through other means.[21]

Cone biopsy involves removal of a cone-shaped wedge of cervix, including the entire transformation zone and at least 50% of the endocervical canal. Postoperative hemorrhage, infection, cervical stenosis, infertility, and incompetent cervix are possible, and this procedure should be avoided unless necessary. LEEP is the first-line management for CIN II/III.[21] This outpatient procedure allows for simultaneous diagnosis and treatment of dysplastic lesions found on colposcopy. It uses a thin, rigid, wire loop electrode attached to a generator that blends high-frequency, low-voltage current for cutting and a modulated higher voltage for coagulation. It can remove the entire transformation zone, providing adequate treatment for the lesion and obtaining a specimen for histologic evaluation.

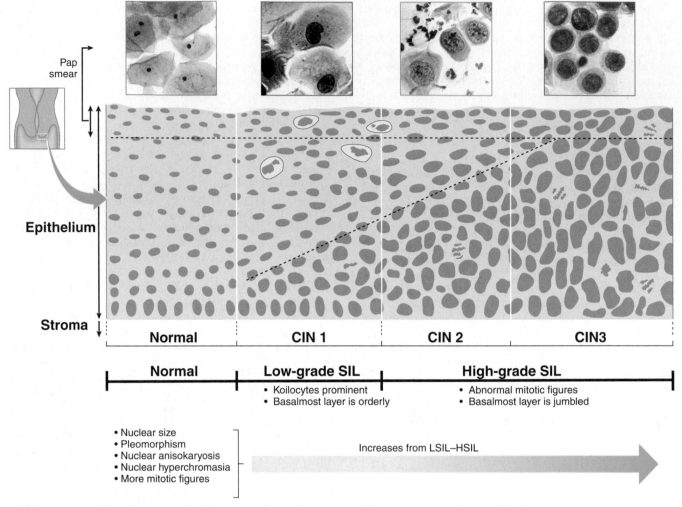

FIGURE 45-3. The Bethesda system for designation of premalignant cervical disease as squamous intraepithelial lesions (SILs). This chart integrates multiple aspects across the normal–LGSIL (low-grade squamous intraepithelial lesion), and LSIL–HSIL (high-grade squamous intraepithelial lesion) interfaces, which correspond to therapeutic thresholds. It lists the qualitative and quantitative features that distinguish low-cancer-risk (LSIL) from high-cancer-risk (HSIL) lesions, which are generally caused by different subtypes of HPV. It also illustrates approximate counterparts for the legacy cervical intraepithelial neoplasia (CIN) system, which was based on a model of continuous progression rather than on dichotomous viral subtypes. Finally, the scheme illustrates the corresponding cytologic smear resulting from exfoliation of the most superficial cells, indicating that even in the mildest disease state, abnormal cells reach the surface and are shed. (From Strayer D. S., Rubin R. (Eds.). (2015). *Rubin's pathology: Clinicopathologic foundations of medicine* (7th ed., Fig. 24-18, p. 1012). Philadelphia, PA: Lippincott Williams & Wilkins.)

Clinical Manifestations and Treatment

In its early stages, cervical cancer is often a poorly defined lesion of the endocervix. Frequently, females will present with abnormal vaginal bleeding, spotting, and discharge. Bleeding is reported most frequently after intercourse. More advanced disease may present with pelvic or back pain that may radiate down the leg, hematuria, fistulas (rectovaginal or vesicovaginal), or evidence of metastatic disease to supraclavicular or inguinal lymph node areas.

Early treatment involves removal of the lesion. Biopsy or local cautery may be therapeutic in and of itself. Electrocautery, cryosurgery, or carbon dioxide laser therapy may treat moderate to severe dysplasia that is limited to the exocervix (*i.e.*, squamocolumnar

junction clearly visible). Therapeutic conization is necessary if the lesion extends into the endocervical canal and can be done surgically or with LEEP in the physician's office.

Invasive cancer is treated with radiation therapy, surgery, or both. External-beam irradiation and intracavitary irradiation or *brachytherapy* (*i.e.*, insertion of radioactive materials into the body) can be used.[29,30] Intracavitary radiation provides direct access to the central lesion and increases the tolerance of the cervix and surrounding tissues, permitting curative levels of radiation. External-beam radiation eliminates metastatic disease in pelvic lymph nodes and other structures, and shrinks the cervical lesion to optimize the effects of intracavitary radiation. Surgery can include trachelectomy (removal of cervix) in females with early-stage cancer desiring fertility, radical hysterectomy (includes uterus, cervix, parametria, and upper portion of the vagina) with pelvic lymph node dissection,[29] or pelvic exenteration (removal of all pelvic organs, including the bladder, rectum, vulva, and vagina).

Disorders of the Uterus

Disorders of the uterus include endometritis, endometriosis, and endometrial cancer. There is also a high frequency of leiomyomas, including uterine fibroid tumors that are benign neoplasms, and adenomyosis, which is uterine thickening due to tissue from the endometrium being displaced in the outer muscular wall of the uterus.

Endometritis

The endometrium and myometrium are resistant to infections primarily because the endocervix forms a barrier to ascending infections. Endometritis is inflammation of the endometrium. Acute endometritis can occur after an abortion or delivery of a newborn when the cervical barrier is compromised.[1] Thus, prophylactic antibiotics are given before and after an abortion. There is an increased risk of endometritis after delivery if the female had chorioamnionitis during labor, a cesarean section, or needed manual or instrumented removal of the placenta. Treatment includes antibiotics, and a curettage if there are retained products of conception or placenta.[1]

Chronic endometritis can occur with PID, after instrumentation of the uterus (*e.g.*, after endometrial biopsy or intrauterine device [IUD] insertion), and with unrecognized retained products of conception after delivery or abortion. The presence of plasma cells is required for diagnosis.[1] The clinical picture is variable, but often includes mild to severe uterine tenderness, fever, malaise, and foul-smelling discharge. Treatment involves oral or intravenous antibiotic therapy, depending on severity.

Endometriosis

In endometriosis, functional endometrial tissue is found in ectopic sites outside the uterus. It is estrogen dependent. It is unclear whether it is an inflammatory disease or an immune disorder. Implants of endometriosis are functional and can lead to scarring, adhesions, and ovarian cysts (*endometriomas*).[31] Sites may include ovaries, posterior broad ligaments, uterosacral ligaments, pouch of Douglas, pelvis, vagina, vulva, perineum, or intestines[32] (Fig. 45-4).

Etiology and Pathogenesis
The cause is unknown. Its incidence has increased in Western countries in the past five decades. Approximately 10% of premenopausal women have some degree of endometriosis, causing infertility and chronic pain, and 24% to 50% of infertile women have some degree of endometriosis.[33]

Clinical Manifestations
Endometriosis usually becomes apparent in the reproductive years when ovarian hormones stimulate both the lesions and normal endometrium. Lesions become proliferative, secretory, and undergo menstrual breakdown. Bleeding into surrounding structures can cause pain and development of pelvic adhesions. Symptoms tend to be strongest premenstrually, subsiding after menstruation. Pelvic pain is the most common symptom. Others include back pain, dyspareunia, and pain on defecation and micturition. Endometriosis is associated with infertility because of adhesions that distort the pelvic anatomy and cause impaired ovum release and transport.[33]

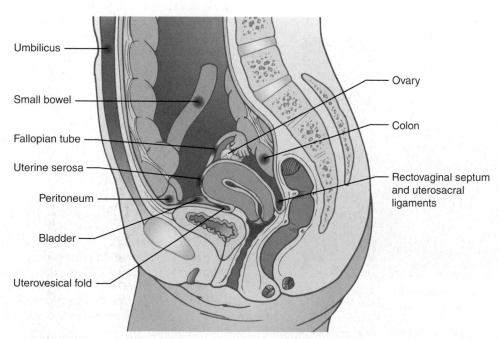

FIGURE 45-4. Common locations of endometriosis in the pelvis and abdomen.

Gross pathologic changes differ with location and duration. In the ovary, endometrial tissue may form endometriomas. Rupture of these cysts, which are filled with old blood, can cause peritonitis and adhesions. Elsewhere in the pelvis, the tissue may be small hemorrhagic lesions, usually appearing as red-blue nodules (Fig. 45-5). Lesions may be surrounded by scar tissue.[31,33]

Diagnosis and Treatment

Endometriosis may be difficult to diagnose: its symptoms mimic other pelvic disorders, and the symptoms do not always reflect the extent of the disease. Treatment may be initiated on the basis of clinical presentation because definitive diagnosis can be accomplished only through laparoscopy and confirmed with histology.[34,35] This minimally invasive surgery allows visualization of pelvic organs to determine presence and extent of endometrial lesions. Imaging, including ultrasonography and magnetic resonance imaging (MRI), is useful in evaluating endometriomas and deep endometriosis.[33]

Treatments are pain relief, endometrial suppression, and surgery. In young females, observation and analgesics (nonsteroidal anti-inflammatory drugs [NSAIDs]) may be sufficient. Use of hormones to induce physiologic amenorrhea is based on the observation that pregnancy and menopause relieve pain by inducing atrophy of endometrial tissue. This can be accomplished via oral contraceptive pills (OCPs) or continuous progestogen agents. In severe endometriosis, long-acting gonadotropin-releasing hormone (GnRH) analogs that inhibit the pituitary gonadotropins and suppress ovulation may be used short term, but is limited in its time course because of the side effects of prolonged artificial menopause (decreased bone density).[36]

Surgery may offer definitive therapy with large or symptomatic endometriomas, or individuals who have failed medical therapy for endometriosis. The goal is to restore normal anatomy, remove visible lesions, and slow progression of the disease in a way that minimizes development of pelvic adhesions and avoids injury to surrounding structures. Laparoscopy is the preferred surgical approach aimed at repairing adhesions and ablation of lesions. Even with extensive surgery, the risk of continued symptoms and disease recurrence is great. Hormone suppression with OCPs or other suppressive therapy before and after surgery can aid in suppression of the disease.[36] Definitive treatment involves total hysterectomy and bilateral salpingo-oophorectomy when the symptoms are unbearable or the woman's childbearing is completed.

Adenomyosis

In adenomyosis, endometrial glands and stroma are found within the myometrium, interspersed between smooth muscle fibers.[1] It is typically found in multiparous females, perhaps due to repeated pregnancies, deliveries, and uterine involution causing endometrium displacement throughout the myometrium.[1] Adenomyosis frequently coexists with uterine myomas or endometrial hyperplasia. Diagnosis often occurs as an incidental finding in a uterus removed for symptoms of myoma or hyperplasia. Heavy, painful periods (with clots) and painful intercourse are common. MRI is the diagnostic tool. Conservative medical therapy with OCPs and NSAIDs is the first choice for treatment. Severe adenomyosis will ultimately require a hysterectomy (with preservation of the ovaries in premenopausal females) for full resolution.

Endometrial Cancer

Endometrial cancer is the most common cancer in the female pelvis, occurring over twice as often as cervical cancer. Most cases are adenocarcinomas, and fewer than 1% are sarcomas.[37] The American Cancer Society estimates that in 2019 approximately 61,880 females will be diagnosed with endometrial cancer and 12,170 will die. The average age for endometrial cancer is older than 60 years, and it is less common in females younger than 45.[38]

Approximately 5% of endometrial cancer can develop as part of a hereditary cancer syndrome.[39] Females with a family history of hereditary nonpolyposis colorectal cancer may have an inherited disorder in deoxyribonucleic acid (DNA) mismatch repair genes that predisposes to cancers, including colorectal and endometrial.

Pathogenesis

Two general groups of endometrial cancer can be identified. The first develops on a background of prolonged estrogen stimulation and endometrial hyperplasia, whereas the second is less commonly associated with hyperestrogenism and endometrial hyperplasia.

About 85% of endometrial cancers are moderately well-differentiated adenocarcinomas that develop on a background of endometrial hyperplasia. These tumors, *type 1 endometrial cancers*, are typically hormone sensitive, low grade, and have a favorable prognosis.[1] They are associated with long-duration unopposed estrogen

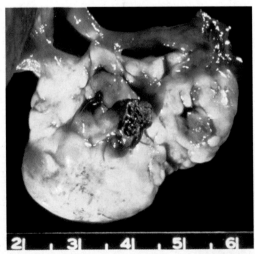

FIGURE 45-5. Endometriosis. Implants of endometrium on the ovary appear as red-blue nodules. (From Strayer D. S., Rubin R. (Eds.). (2015). *Rubin's pathology: Clinicopathologic foundations of medicine* (7th ed., Fig. 24-73A, p. 1049). Philadelphia, PA: Lippincott Williams & Wilkins.)

stimulation and tend to be well differentiated, mimicking normal endometrial glands in histologic appearance, or display altered differentiation.

The endometrium undergoes structural modification and cellular changes during the menstrual cycle. Prolonged unopposed estrogen leads to endometrial hyperplasia, which increases the chance of atypical hyperplasia and type 1 endometrial cancer. Although the molecular basis for this is still unknown, anovulatory cycles, disorders of estrogen metabolism, unopposed estrogen therapy, estrogen-secreting granulosa cell tumor, and obesity increase risk of endometrial cancer.

Ovulatory dysfunction that causes infertility or occurs with declining ovarian function in perimenopausal females can result in unopposed estrogen and increase the risk of endometrial cancer. In the 1970s, a sharp rise in endometrial cancer was seen in middle-aged females who had received unopposed estrogen therapy (estrogen without progesterone) for menopausal symptoms. Progesterone in the second half of the menstrual cycle matures the endometrium, and withdrawal of progesterone results in endometrial sloughing. Long-term unopposed estrogen without progesterone allows for continued endometrial growth and hyperplasia, which increases the chance of development of atypical cells. Hyperplasia usually regresses after treatment with cyclic progesterone. Combination oral contraceptives (estrogen and progestin in each pill) prevent hyperplasia and decrease the risk of cancer by 50%.[21] Tamoxifen, a drug that blocks estrogen receptor sites and is used in treatment of breast cancer, exerts a weak estrogenic effect on the endometrium and represents another exogenous risk factor for endometrial cancer.

Diabetes mellitus, hypertension, and polycystic ovary syndrome (PCOS) are conditions that alter estrogen metabolism and elevate estrogen levels. Excessive fat consumption and being overweight are important risk factors. In premenopausal females, overweight causes insulin resistance, ovarian androgen excess, anovulation, and chronic progesterone deficiency. In postmenopausal females, estrogens are synthesized in body fats from adrenal and ovarian androgen precursors. Because of its effect on insulin-like growth factor-1 (IGF-1) and its binding protein, obesity can be a risk factor even when circulating estrogen levels are normal. Estrogen receptor transcriptional activity can be induced by IGF-1 signaling even without estrogen.

A second subset of endometrial cancers (about 10%) is high-grade tumors with high recurrence, even in early stages. These *type 2 endometrial cancers* are not estrogen driven, typically occur in females who acquire the disease at older ages, and are mostly associated with endometrial atrophy rather than with hyperplasia.[40] Type 2 endometrial cancers usually have a poorer prognosis than that associated with prolonged estrogen stimulation and endometrial hyperplasia.

Clinical Manifestations

The major symptom of endometrial hyperplasia or overt endometrial cancer is abnormal, painless bleeding. In menstruating females, this is bleeding between periods or excessive, prolonged menstrual flow. In postmenopausal females, any bleeding is abnormal and is an early warning sign of the disease. Because it tends to grow slowly in the early stages, the chances of cure are good if prompt medical care is sought. Later signs may include cramping, pelvic discomfort, postcoital bleeding, lower abdominal pressure, and enlarged lymph nodes.

Diagnosis and Treatment

Endometrial biopsy (tissue sample obtained by direct aspiration of the endometrial cavity) is far more accurate than a Pap smear. Dilation and curettage (D&C), which consists of dilating the cervix and scraping the uterine cavity, is the definitive procedure for diagnosis because it provides a more thorough evaluation.

Prognosis depends on the clinical stage when it is discovered and its histologic grade and type. Surgery and radiation therapy are the most successful methods of treatment. When used alone, radiation therapy has a 20% lower cure rate than does surgery for stage I disease. It may be the best option in females who are not good surgical candidates. Total abdominal hysterectomy with bilateral salpingo-oophorectomy plus sampling of regional lymph nodes and peritoneal washings for cytologic evaluation of occult disease is the treatment of choice when possible. The 5-year relative survival rates of early-diagnosed endometrial cancers are 96%. The survival rate for all endometrial cancers (diagnosed early and late stage) is 83%.[37]

Leiomyomas

Uterine leiomyomas (or *fibroids*) are benign neoplasms of smooth muscle origin. These are the most common form of pelvic tumor and occur in one of every four or five females over 35 years of age. Leiomyomas usually develop as submucosal, subserosal, or intramural tumors in the corpus of the uterus (Fig. 45-6). Intramural fibroids are embedded in the myometrium. They are the most common type of fibroid and present as a symmetric enlargement of the nonpregnant uterus. Subserosal tumors are located beneath the perimetrium of the uterus. These tumors are irregular projections on the uterine surface. They may become pedunculated, displacing or impinging on other genitourinary structures and causing hydroureter or bladder problems. Submucosal fibroids displace endometrial tissue and are more likely to cause bleeding, necrosis, and infection.

Leiomyomas are asymptomatic approximately half of the time and may be discovered during a routine pelvic examination, or may cause menorrhagia, anemia, urinary frequency, rectal pressure/constipation, abdominal distension, and, infrequently pain. Rate of growth is variable, but they may increase in size during pregnancy or with exogenous estrogen stimulation (*i.e.*, OCPs or menopausal estrogen replacement therapy). Interference with pregnancy is rare unless the tumor is submucosal and interferes with implantation or obstructs the cervical outlet. Tumors may outgrow their blood supply, become infarcted, and undergo degenerative changes.

Most leiomyomas regress with menopause, but if bleeding, pressure on the bladder, pain, or other problems persist, hysterectomy may be required. Myomectomy (removal of the tumors) can preserve the uterus for

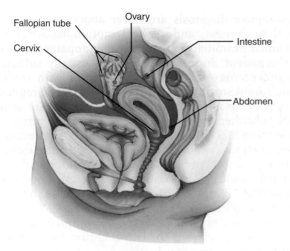

Fallopian tube
Ovary
Cervix
Intestine
Abdomen

FIGURE 45-8. Ectopic pregnancy. (From Jensen S. (2015). *Nursing health assessment: A best practice approach* (2nd ed., p. 778). Philadelphia, PA: Lippincott Williams & Wilkins.)

and a tubal lesion or abnormality.[44] Smoking, current IUD, history of PID or therapeutic abortion, and use of fertility drugs to induce ovulation have also been associated with an increased risk.

Clinical Manifestations

The site of implantation may determine onset of symptoms and timing of diagnosis. As the tubal pregnancy progresses, surrounding tissue is stretched. The pregnancy eventually outgrows its blood supply, at which point the pregnancy terminates or the tube ruptures.

Symptoms include lower abdominal discomfort—diffuse or localized to one side—that progresses to severe pain caused by rupture, spotting, syncope, referred shoulder pain from bleeding into the abdominal cavity, and amenorrhea. Physical examination usually reveals adnexal tenderness; an adnexal mass is found in about half of cases.

Diagnosis and Treatment

Diagnostic tests include a urine pregnancy test, ultrasonography, and β-human chorionic gonadotropin (hCG; a hormone produced by placental cells) levels. Serial hCG tests may detect lower than expected hCG rise. Transvaginal ultrasonographic studies after 5 weeks of gestation may reveal an empty uterine cavity or presence of the gestational sac outside the uterus.[44] Definitive diagnosis may require laparoscopy. Differential diagnosis for this pelvic pain includes ruptured ovarian cyst, threatened/incomplete abortion, PID, acute appendicitis, and degenerating fibroid.

Treatment aims to resolve the problem with minimal morbidity and protecting future fertility. Early ectopic pregnancies can be treated medically with methotrexate to stop the pregnancy followed by serial hCG to ensure that it has been effectively treated. Surgical removal of the pregnancy is required when it is unlikely that medical management will be effective (large ectopic pregnancy, presence of a fetal heartbeat, noncompliance), rupture

is imminent or has already occurred, or when the patient is hemodynamically unstable.[12,44,45] Laparoscopic treatment is well tolerated and more cost-effective than is laparotomy because of shorter convalescence and the reduced need for postoperative analgesia. Laparotomy, which involves an open incision into the abdominopelvic cavity, is necessary when there is uncontrolled internal bleeding or when the ectopic site cannot be visualized through the laparoscope.

Methotrexate (an antimetabolite used in treatment of chronic inflammatory diseases and cancer) eliminates residual ectopic pregnancy tissue after laparoscopy. It is a primary treatment in cases where the pregnancy is diagnosed early and tubal rupture has not occurred, or when the pregnancy is not in a common location, such as when the pregnancy occurs in the cornua of the uterus or in the cervix. This folic acid antagonist interferes with DNA and ribonucleic acid synthesis, thus inhibiting growth of trophoblastic cells at the placental implantation site. Adverse effects include bone marrow depression, transient elevation of liver enzymes, anemia, and stomatitis.[44]

Cancer of the Fallopian Tube

The fallopian tube is the primary site of cancer in a large majority of ovarian cancer cases.[1,46] Metastasis from the uterus and/or ovaries is also observed. When primary fallopian tube cancer is diagnosed, it is usually an adenocarcinoma.[1] Symptoms are uncommon, but intermittent serosanguineous vaginal discharge, abnormal vaginal bleeding, and colicky low abdominal pain have been reported. Management usually includes total hysterectomy, bilateral salpingo-oophorectomy, pelvic lymph node dissection, and chemotherapy, depending on the type of cancer cells. The staging of ovarian, fallopian tube, and peritoneal cancer has been integrated, potentially allowing for better treatment options.[1,46]

Ovarian Cysts and Tumors

Ovaries produce germ cells (ova) and synthesize female sex hormones. Disorders often cause menstrual and fertility problems. Benign conditions can present as primary lesions of ovarian structures or as secondary disorders related to hypothalamic, pituitary, or adrenal dysfunction.

Ovarian Cysts

Cysts are the most common form of ovarian tumor. Many are benign. A follicular cyst results from occlusion of the duct of the follicle. Each month, several follicles develop. The dominant follicle normally ruptures to release the egg (ovulation), but occasionally persists and continues growing. A luteal cyst is a persistent cystic enlargement of the corpus luteum formed after ovulation and does not regress in the absence of pregnancy. Functional cysts are asymptomatic unless there is substantial enlargement or bleeding into the cyst. This can cause discomfort or a dull, aching sensation on the affected side. These cysts usually regress spontaneously. Occasionally, a cyst may become twisted or may rupture into the intra-abdominal cavity (Fig. 45-9).

Polycystic Ovary Syndrome

PCOS is a common endocrine disorder affecting 6% to 15% of females of reproductive age and is a frequent source of chronic anovulation. Diagnosis is made after other endocrine diseases are ruled out and the person has oligomenorrhea (irregular infrequent periods), signs of hyperandrogenism (acne and excess body hair [hirsutism]), elevated testosterone levels on blood testing, or polycystic-appearing ovaries in which there are numerous small cysts at the periphery of the ovary.[47]

Etiology and Pathogenesis

About 50% of females diagnosed with PCOS are obese. People with PCOS will have irregular menses due to anovulation that can lead to infertility. Because of the hyperandrogenism associated with PCOS, many individuals with PCOS suffer from hirsutism and acne.[47]

The etiology of PCOS is probably multifactorial. A genetic basis has been suggested, with an autosomal dominant mode of inheritance. The disorder may begin before adolescence.[48] Because many of the symptoms, such as excess hair, acne, and obesity, can be detrimental to a teenage girl's health and self-esteem, early detection and treatment in adolescents are essential.

The underlying mechanisms of PCOS remain unclear. Chronic anovulation may underlie the amenorrhea or irregular menses, and the enlarged, "polycystic" ovaries. Most individuals with PCOS have elevated

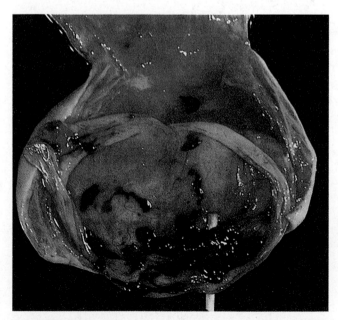

FIGURE 45-9. Follicular cyst of the ovary. The rupture of this thin-walled follicular cyst (*dowel stick*) led to intra-abdominal hemorrhage. (From Strayer D. S., Rubin R. (Eds.). (2015). *Rubin's pathology: Clinicopathologic foundations of medicine* (7th ed., Fig. 24-44, p. 1033). Philadelphia, PA: Lippincott Williams & Wilkins.)

luteinizing hormone (LH) levels with normal estrogen and follicle-stimulating hormone (FSH) levels. Elevated circulating total testosterone, free testosterone, and dehydroepiandrosterone sulfate (DHEAS) are not uncommon, along with occasional hyperprolactinemia or hypothyroidism. Persistent anovulation results in an estrogen environment that alters hypothalamic release of GnRH, causing increased LH secretion and suppression of FSH release. This altered LH/FSH ratio often is used as a diagnostic criterion, but it is not universally present. Although the presence of FSH allows for new follicular development, full maturation is not attained, and ovulation does not occur. An elevated LH level results in increased androgen production, which prevents follicular development and contributes to anovulation.[49]

There is an association between hyperandrogenism and hyperinsulinemia. The frequency and degree of hyperinsulinemia in PCOS are often amplified by obesity. Insulin may cause hyperandrogenism in several ways. The ovary possesses insulin receptors, and there is evidence that insulin may act directly on the ovary.[50]

Long-term health problems including cardiovascular disease and diabetes are linked to PCOS. There is concern that females with PCOS who are anovulatory do not produce progesterone. Although there is a reported association with breast, endometrial, and ovarian cancer, PCOS has not been conclusively shown to be an independent risk factor for these malignancies.[47]

Diagnosis and Treatment

Diagnosis can be suspected from clinical presentation. Commonly, laboratory evaluation is used to exclude hyperprolactinemia, late-onset adrenal hyperplasia, and androgen-secreting tumors of the ovary and adrenal gland. Although a fasting blood glucose, 2-hour oral glucose tolerance test, and insulin levels are often measured to evaluate for hyperinsulinemia, this testing is not required before treatment because insulin resistance is almost universal in women with PCOS. Confirmation with ultrasonography of the ovaries is often done, but not required.[51]

The overall goal of treatment is directed toward symptom relief, prevention of potential malignant endometrial sequelae, and reduction in risk for development of diabetes and cardiovascular disease. The most effective treatment for PCOS is lifestyle modification. Weight loss may be beneficial in restoring normal ovulation when obesity is present. Treatment choice depends on the most bothersome manifestations and the individual's goals. Combined oral contraceptive agents ameliorate menstrual irregularities and improve hirsutism and acne.

Metformin, an insulin-sensitizing drug, is an important component of PCOS treatment.[51] In addition to improvements in insulin sensitivity and glucose metabolism, it is associated with reduced androgen and LH levels, and restoring normal menstrual regularity and ovulatory cycles.

When fertility is desired, PCOS usually is treated by the administration of the hypothalamic-pituitary–stimulating drug clomiphene citrate or injectable gonadotropins to induce ovulation. These drugs must be used carefully because they can induce extreme enlargement of the ovaries.

Benign and Functioning/Endocrine Active Ovarian Tumors

Ovarian tumors are common, and most are benign. They can arise from any of the ovarian tissue types—serosal epithelium, germ cell layers, or gonadal stroma tissue[21] (Fig. 45-10).

Serous and mucinous cystadenomas are common benign ovarian neoplasms. Endometriomas develop secondary to ovarian endometriosis. Ovarian fibromas are connective tissue tumors composed of collagen, ranging in size from 15 to 30 cm. Cystic teratomas, or dermoid cysts, are derived from primordial germ cells and composed of well-differentiated ectodermal, mesodermal, and endodermal elements. They can contain sebaceous material, hair, or teeth.[1]

Hormonally active tumors can impact the body either with an excess or a decrease in reproductive hormone excretion. The granulosa cell tumor is associated with excess estrogen production. Most granulosa cell tumors occur after menopause. When they develop during the reproductive period, uncontrolled production of estrogen interferes with the normal menstrual cycle. In addition, when present in young females, early puberty and an associated loss of oocytes occur.[1] Androgen-secreting tumors (Sertoli–Leydig cell tumor or androblastoma) inhibit ovulation and estrogen production. They may cause hirsutism and development of masculine characteristics, such as baldness, acne, oily skin, breast atrophy, and deepening of the voice.[1]

Treatment for ovarian tumors includes surgical excision, chemotherapy, and/or radiation. Tissue, lymph nodes, and fluid are analyzed. If metastasis has occurred, the goal is to remove as much of the cancer as possible and, when combined with chemotherapy, provides the best results.[46]

Ovarian Cancer

Ovarian cancer is often lethal. It is the fifth leading cause of female cancer deaths. The rate of ovarian cancer has declined slowly over the past 20 years. In 2019, there will be an estimated 22,530 new cases of ovarian cancer in the United States, and 13,980 deaths.[52] It is difficult to

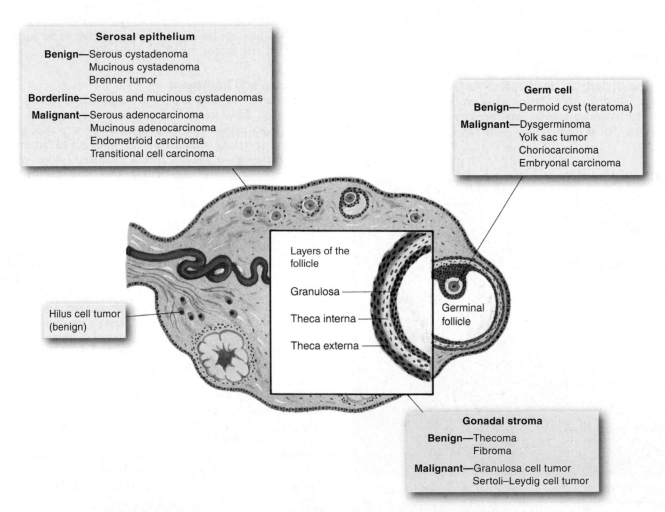

Serosal epithelium

Benign—Serous cystadenoma
Mucinous cystadenoma
Brenner tumor

Borderline—Serous and mucinous cystadenomas

Malignant—Serous adenocarcinoma
Mucinous adenocarcinoma
Endometrioid carcinoma
Transitional cell carcinoma

Germ cell

Benign—Dermoid cyst (teratoma)

Malignant—Dysgerminoma
Yolk sac tumor
Choriocarcinoma
Embryonal carcinoma

Hilus cell tumor
(benign)

Layers of the follicle

Granulosa

Theca interna

Theca externa

Germinal follicle

Gonadal stroma

Benign—Thecoma
Fibroma

Malignant—Granulosa cell tumor
Sertoli–Leydig cell tumor

FIGURE 45-10. Classification of ovarian neoplasms based on cell of origin. (From Strayer D. S., Rubin R. (Eds.). (2015). *Rubin's pathology: Clinicopathologic foundations of medicine* (7th ed., Fig. 24-48, p. 1035). Philadelphia, PA: Lippincott Williams & Wilkins.)

diagnose because symptoms mimic other benign health issues. Because of this, the disease often spreads before the time of discovery.[53]

Risk Factors

The most significant risk factor appears to be ovulatory age: the length of time during a female's life when her ovarian cycle is not suppressed by pregnancy, lactation, or oral contraceptive use. The incidence is much lower in **parous** versus nulliparous women.[54] Family history also is a significant risk factor. A female with two or more first- or second-degree relatives who have had *site-specific ovarian cancer* have up to a 50% risk for development of the disease. There are two other types of inherited risk for ovarian cancer: *breast–ovarian cancer syndrome*, where both breast and ovarian cancer occur among first- and second-degree relatives, and *family cancer syndrome* or *Lynch syndrome II*, in which male or female relatives have a history of colorectal, endometrial, ovarian, pancreatic, or other types of cancer.[21] The breast cancer susceptibility genes, *BRCA1* and *BRCA2*, which are tumor suppressor genes, are linked to approximately 10% of hereditary ovarian cancers.[29] Susceptibility to ovarian cancer is transmitted as an autosomal dominant characteristic. A high-fat Western diet and use of powders containing talc in the genital area are other factors that have been linked to the development of ovarian cancer.

Prevention

Chemoprevention strategies include long-term oral contraceptive use, acetaminophen, and aspirin. Additional clinical trials are needed to support the effectiveness of these agents. Surgical strategies that reduce the risk of developing ovarian cancer include prophylactic removal of both fallopian tubes and ovaries.[55]

Types of Ovarian Cancer

Cancer of the ovary is a complex neoplasm because of the diversity of tissue types that originate in the ovary. As a result, there are several types of ovarian cancers. Malignant neoplasms of the ovary can be divided into epithelial tumors, germ cell tumors, and gonadal stromal tumors (Fig. 45-10). Epithelial tumors account for approximately 90% of cases.[21]

Clinical Manifestations

Different types of ovarian cancers display various degrees of virulence, depending on the type of tumor and degree of differentiation involved. A well-differentiated cancer may produce symptoms for many months and still be operable at the time of surgery. A poorly differentiated tumor may have been clinically evident for only a few days but be found to be widespread and inoperable. Often, no correlation exists between duration of symptoms and extent of the disease.

Ovarian cancer is often diagnosed at an advanced stage because many symptoms are nonspecific and therefore difficult to distinguish from other problems. Symptoms believed to have a strong correlation to ovarian cancer include abdominal or pelvic pain, increased abdominal size or bloating, and difficulty eating or feeling full quickly after ingesting food. Many self-treat with antacids and other remedies for a time before seeking treatment, and health care providers may dismiss the complaints as being caused by other conditions. Recent onset (<12 months) and frequent occurrence (>12 times per month) of these symptoms suggest the need for further evaluation.[21] It is not fully understood why initial symptoms of ovarian cancer are manifested as gastrointestinal disturbances. It is thought that biochemical changes in peritoneal fluids may irritate the bowel, or pain originating in the ovary may be referred to the abdomen and be interpreted as a gastrointestinal disturbance. Clinically evident ascites is seen in approximately one fourth of females with malignant ovarian tumors and is associated with a worse prognosis.

Diagnosis and Treatment

There are no good screening tests or early methods of detection. Transvaginal sonography (TVS) can evaluate ovarian masses for malignant potential, but its cost precludes its use as a universal screening method. The serum tumor marker CA-125 is a cell surface antigen and is detectable in the serum of about half of epithelial tumors confined to the ovary and 90% of those that have spread. The specificity of this is highest when combined with TVS.[1] Screening with CA-125 is not recommended for asymptomatic women. It can be used in monitoring therapy and recurrences when preoperative levels have been elevated. Despite its role in diagnostic evaluation and follow-up, CA-125 is not cancer or tissue specific for ovarian cancer. Levels also are elevated in other cancers and some benign conditions.[56]

When ovarian cancer is suspected, surgical evaluation is required for diagnosis, complete and accurate staging, and cytoreduction and debulking procedures to reduce the size of the tumor. The most common surgery involves removal of uterus, fallopian tubes, ovaries, and omentum. The liver, diaphragm, retroperitoneal and aortic lymph nodes, and peritoneal surface are examined and biopsies are taken as needed. Cytologic washings test for cancerous cells in the peritoneal fluid. Individuals with early cancer who may wish to become pregnant may have only the affected ovary removed. Recommendations for treatment beyond surgery and prognosis depend on the stage of the disease.[21] The lack of accurate screening tools and the resistant nature of ovarian cancers significantly affect the success of treatment and survival.

SUMMARY CONCEPTS

PID is an inflammation of the upper reproductive tract that involves the uterus (endometritis), fallopian tubes (salpingitis), or ovaries (oophoritis). It is commonly caused by *N. gonorrhoeae* or *C. trachomatis*. Accurate diagnosis and therapy aim to prevent complications such as pelvic adhesions, infertility, ectopic pregnancy, chronic abdominal pain, and tubo-ovarian abscesses.

Ectopic pregnancy occurs when a fertilized ovum implants outside the uterine cavity; the most common site is the fallopian tube. Causes of ectopic pregnancy are delayed ovum transport resulting from complications of PID, therapeutic abortion, tubal ligation or tubal reversal, previous ectopic pregnancy, or other conditions such as use of fertility drugs to induce ovulation. It represents a true gynecologic emergency, often necessitating surgical intervention. Cancer of the fallopian tube is rare; diagnosis is difficult and the condition usually is advanced at diagnosis.

Disorders of the ovaries include benign cysts, functioning ovarian tumors, and cancer of the ovary; they usually are asymptomatic unless there is substantial enlargement or bleeding into the cyst, or the cyst becomes twisted or ruptured. PCOS is characterized by anovulation with varying degrees of menstrual irregularity and infertility; hyperandrogenism with hirsutism, acne, male pattern of hair loss, and obesity; polycystic ovaries; and hyperinsulinemia with insulin resistance. Benign ovarian tumors consist of endometriomas (chocolate cysts that develop secondary to ovarian endometriosis), ovarian fibromas (connective tissue tumors composed of fibrocytes and collagen), and cystic teratomas or dermoid cysts (germ cell tumors composed of various combinations of ectodermal, mesodermal, and endodermal elements). Functioning ovarian tumors may be benign or malignant and are of three types: estrogen secreting, androgen secreting, and mixed estrogen–androgen secreting. Because ovarian cancer has vague symptoms until the disease has progressed, it is among the most lethal of female cancers. It can be divided into epithelial tumors, germ cell tumors, and gonadal stromal tumors. There are no effective screening methods for ovarian cancer, and often the disease is well advanced at diagnosis.

KEY POINTS

Gynecologic Cancers

- Cancers of the vulva, cervix, endometrium, and ovaries are a spectrum of malignancies.

- Ovarian cancer often goes undiagnosed until in advanced stages; therefore, it is often lethal. The most significant risk factors for ovarian cancer are the length of time that ovarian cycles are not suppressed by pregnancy, lactation, or oral contraceptive use, and family history.

Disorders of Pelvic Support and Uterine Position

Disorders of Pelvic Support

The uterus and the pelvic structures are maintained in position by the uterosacral ligaments, round ligaments, broad ligaments, and cardinal ligaments. The two cardinal ligaments maintain the cervix in position. The uterosacral ligaments hold the uterus in a forward position and the broad ligaments suspend the uterus, fallopian tubes, and ovaries. The vagina is encased in the semirigid structure of strong supporting fascia (Fig. 45-11A). The muscular floor of the pelvis is a strong, slinglike structure that supports the uterus, vagina, urinary bladder, and rectum (Fig. 45-12). The pelvic viscera must be supported against the force of gravity and increases in intra-abdominal pressure associated with coughing, sneezing, defecation, and laughing while allowing for urination, defecation, and reproductive tract function. The bony pelvis provides support and protection for parts of the digestive tract and genitourinary structures, and the peritoneum holds the pelvic viscera in place. The main support for the viscera is the pelvic diaphragm, made up of muscles and connective tissue that stretch across the bones of the pelvic outlet. Openings for the urethra, rectum, and vagina cause an inherent weakness in the pelvic diaphragm. Congenital or acquired weakness of the pelvic diaphragm results in widening of these openings, particularly the vagina, with the possible herniation of pelvic viscera through the pelvic floor (*i.e.*, prolapse).[57]

Relaxation of the pelvic outlet is usually due to over-stretching of perineal supporting tissues during pregnancy and childbirth. Although the tissues are stretched only during these times, there may be no difficulty until the fifth or sixth decade, when further loss of elasticity and muscle tone occurs. The combination of aging and postmenopausal changes may give rise to problems related to relaxation of the pelvic support structures regardless of a history of pregnancy. The most common conditions associated with this relaxation are cystocele, rectocele, and uterine prolapse. These may occur separately or together.[58,59]

Cystocele

Cystocele is a herniation of the bladder into the vagina. It occurs when muscle support for the bladder is weakened, and the bladder sags below the uterus. This causes the anterior vaginal wall to stretch and bulge downward, allowing the bladder to herniate into the vagina due to gravity and pressures from coughing, lifting, or straining (Fig. 45-11B). The symptoms of cystocele include a bearing-down sensation, difficulty in emptying the bladder, frequency and urgency of urination, and cystitis. Stress incontinence may occur at times of increased abdominal pressure, such as during squatting, straining, coughing, sneezing, laughing, or lifting.[57–59]

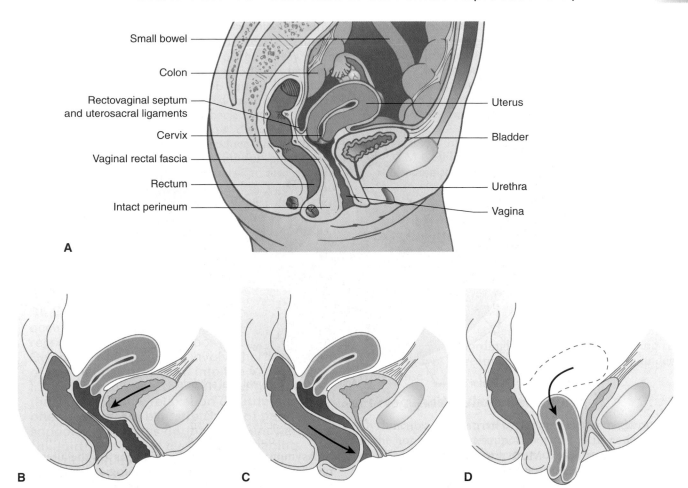

Small bowel

Colon

Rectovaginal septum
and uterosacral ligaments

Cervix

Vaginal rectal fascia

Rectum

Intact perineum

Uterus

Bladder

Urethra

Vagina

A

B   **C**   **D**

FIGURE 45-11. **(A)** Normal support of the uterus and vagina, **(B)** cystocele, **(C)** rectocele, and **(D)** uterine prolapse.

Rectocele and Enterocele

Rectocele is the herniation of the rectum into the vagina. It occurs when the posterior vaginal wall and underlying rectum bulge forward, protruding through the introitus because the pelvic floor and perineal muscles are weakened. Symptoms include discomfort because of the protrusion of the rectum and difficulty in defecation (Fig. 45-11C). Digital pressure (*i.e.*, splinting) on the bulging posterior wall of the vagina may be necessary for defecation. The area between the uterosacral ligaments posterior to the cervix may weaken and form a hernial sac into which the small bowel protrudes when standing. This defect, an *enterocele*, may extend into the rectovaginal septum. It may be congenital or acquired through birth trauma. Enterocele can be asymptomatic or cause a dull, dragging sensation and, occasionally, low backache.[57–59]

Uterine Prolapse

Uterine prolapse is bulging of the uterus into the vagina that occurs when the primary supportive ligaments (*i.e.*, cardinal ligaments) are stretched (Fig. 45-11D). Prolapse is ranked as first, second, or third degree, depending on uterus protrusion through the introitus. First-degree prolapse shows some descent, but the cervix has not reached the introitus. In second-degree prolapse, the cervix or part of the uterus has passed through the introitus.

The entire uterus protrudes through the vaginal opening in third-degree prolapse (*i.e.*, procidentia).[57,59]

Symptoms associated with uterine prolapse result from irritation of exposed mucous membranes of the cervix and vagina and discomfort of the protruding mass.[56] There may be incontinence along with discomfort from the pelvic floor prolapse. Prolapse often is accompanied by perineal relaxation, cystocele, or rectocele. Like cystocele, rectocele, and enterocele, it occurs most commonly in multiparous females because childbearing is accompanied by injuries to pelvic structures and uterine ligaments. It also may result from pelvic tumors and neurologic conditions, which interrupt the innervation of pelvic muscles. Generally, it is a benign condition, but problems can arise with infection, obstruction, and skin irritation, leading to skin breakdown.[59]

A pessary may be inserted to hold the uterus in place and may stave off surgical intervention in females who want to have children or in older females for whom surgery may pose a significant risk. Pelvic floor physical therapy is suitable for females who wish to preserve their uterus.[60]

Treatment of Pelvic Support Disorders

Kegel exercises, which strengthen the pubococcygeus muscle, may be helpful in cases of mild cystocele or rectocele (or after surgical repair to help maintain the is beginning to decline, and, commonly, in obese women with PCOS.

Dysfunctional menstrual cycles can originate as a primary disorder of the ovaries or as a secondary defect in ovarian function related to hypothalamic–pituitary stimulation. The latter can be initiated by emotional stress, marked variation in weight (*i.e.*, sudden gain or loss), or nonspecific endocrine or metabolic disturbances. Nonhormonal causes of irregular menstrual bleeding include endometrial polyps, submucosal myoma (*i.e.*, fibroid), bleeding disorder (*e.g.*, von Willebrand disease, platelet dysfunction), infection, endometrial cancer, and pregnancy.[62]

Treatment

Treatment is based on the probable cause. Evaluation should include a history with emphasis on bleeding pattern and physical examination. Endocrine studies (*e.g.*, FSH/LH ratio, prolactin, testosterone, DHEAS levels), β-hCG pregnancy test, endometrium ultrasonography, endometrial biopsy, D&C with or without hysteroscopy, and progesterone withdrawal tests may be needed for diagnosis. Nonhormonal causes may require surgical intervention. D&C can be therapeutic and diagnostic. Endometrial ablation (thinning or elimination of the basal layer of endometrium from which the monthly buildup generates) is a primary treatment for heavy bleeding.[55] If alterations in hormone levels are the primary cause, treatment may include oral contraceptives, cyclic progesterone therapy, or long-acting progesterone via injection or IUD.

Amenorrhea

Primary amenorrhea is failure to menstruate by 15 years of age, or by 13 years of age if accompanied by absence of secondary sex characteristics. Secondary amenorrhea is the cessation of menses for at least 6 months in an individual with established normal menstrual cycles.[62]

Etiology

Primary amenorrhea usually is caused by gonadal dysgenesis, congenital müllerian agenesis, testicular feminization, or a hypothalamic–pituitary–ovarian axis disorder. Causes of secondary amenorrhea include pregnancy; ovarian, pituitary, or hypothalamic dysfunction; intrauterine adhesions; chronic conditions or infections; pituitary tumor; anorexia nervosa; or strenuous physical exercise, which can alter the body fat–muscle ratio needed for menses to occur.[63]

Diagnosis and Treatment

Diagnosis resembles that for AUB, with the possible addition of a computed tomographic scan or an MRI to exclude a pituitary tumor. Treatment is based on correcting the underlying cause and inducing menstruation with cyclic progesterone or combined estrogen–progesterone.[62]

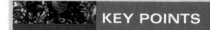

KEY POINTS

Dysfunctional Menstrual Cycles

- The pattern of menstrual bleeding tends to be fairly consistent in most healthy women with regard to frequency, duration, and amount of flow.

- AUB in postpubertal women can take the form of absent or scanty periods, infrequent periods, excessive and irregular periods, excessive bleeding during periods, and bleeding between periods.

Dysmenorrhea

Dysmenorrhea is pain or discomfort with menstruation that causes some degree of monthly disability for a significant number of individuals. Primary dysmenorrhea is menstrual pain not associated with physical abnormality or pathology.[64] It occurs with ovulatory menstruation beginning 6 months to 2 years after menarche. Symptoms begin 1 to 2 days before menses, peak on the first day of flow, and subside within several hours to days. Severe dysmenorrhea may be associated with systemic symptoms such as headache, nausea, vomiting, diarrhea, fatigue, irritability, dizziness, and syncope.[65] The pain is dull, lower abdominal aching or cramping, spasmodic or colicky in nature, often radiating to the lower back, labia majora, or upper thighs.

Secondary dysmenorrhea is menstrual pain caused by specific organic conditions, such as endometriosis, uterine fibroids, adenomyosis, pelvic adhesions, IUDs, or PID. Laparoscopy often is required for diagnosis if medication for primary dysmenorrhea is ineffective.

Treatment for primary dysmenorrhea aims for symptom control. Although analgesic agents (aspirin, acetaminophen) may relieve minor uterine cramping or low back pain, prostaglandin synthetase inhibitors (ibuprofen, naproxen, mefenamic acid, and indomethacin) are specific for dysmenorrhea and treatment of choice if contraception is not desired. Ovulation suppression and symptomatic relief of dysmenorrhea can be used simultaneously with oral contraceptives. Relief of secondary dysmenorrhea depends on the cause, and medical or surgical intervention may be needed.[57]

Premenstrual Symptom Disorders

Approximately 80% of females experience some type of premenstrual emotional or physical changes, and 20% indicate that these mild to moderate monthly symptoms cause some difficulty, sometimes enough to present for medical assistance.[66] How many have symptoms that are severe enough to warrant treatment is unknown because of the multiple symptoms associated with premenstrual syndrome (PMS).[61]

The spectrum of premenstrual symptom disorders ranges from mild to severe and includes the following:

- *PMS*: mild to moderate physical and psychological symptoms limited to within 14 days preceding menstruation and relieved by onset of the menses
- *Premenstrual dysphoric disorder* (PMDD): the most severe form of premenstrual distress and generally is associated with mood disorders

The incidence of PMS seems to increase with age. It is less common in teens and those in the 20s, and most individuals seeking help are in their mid-30s. The disorder is not culturally distinct.[62]

Etiology

The causes of PMS and PMDD are unknown but likely multifactorial. Previously, they were linked to endocrine imbalances such as hyperprolactinemia, estrogen excess, and alteration in estrogen–progesterone ratios. Recent studies suggest females may have normal hormone levels but react abnormally to changes in levels. Other hypotheses suggest alterations in the renin–angiotensin–aldosterone system and/or prostaglandin excess may contribute to symptoms.[62]

One theory suggests a relationship between normal gonadal fluctuations and central neurotransmitter activity, particularly serotonin. It is unclear as to whether decreased levels of serotonin are present during the luteal phase, and only susceptible women respond with varying degrees of PMS, or if women with PMDD have a neurotransmitter abnormality.[67–69]

Clinical Manifestations

Physical symptoms of PMS include painful and swollen breasts, bloating, abdominal pain, headache, and backache. Psychologically, there may be depression, anxiety, irritability, and behavioral changes. Females with PMS may report one or several symptoms, and symptoms vary between and within individuals[67,68] (Table 45-1). It can affect normal daily performance.

TABLE 45-1 Symptoms of Premenstrual Syndrome by System

Body System	Symptoms
Cerebral	Irritability, anxiety, nervousness, fatigue, exhaustion, increased physical and mental activity, lability, crying spells, depression, inability to concentrate
Gastrointestinal	Craving for sweets or salt, lower abdominal pain, bloating, nausea, vomiting, diarrhea, constipation
Vascular	Headache, edema, weakness, fainting
Reproductive	Swelling and tenderness of the breasts, pelvic congestion, ovarian pain, altered libido
Neuromuscular	Trembling of the extremities, changes in coordination, clumsiness, backache, leg aches
General	Weight gain, insomnia, dizziness, acne

Diagnosis

A history and physical examination are necessary to exclude other causes. Blood studies, including thyroid hormones, glucose, and prolactin assays, may be done. Psychosocial evaluation is helpful to exclude mental illness that is exacerbated premenstrually. The American College of Obstetricians and Gynecologists (ACOG) has clinical management guidelines for PMS that include diagnostic criteria similar to what the American Psychiatric Association did for PMDD in the *Diagnostic and Statistical Manual of Mental Disorders, Fifth Edition* (DSM-5).[61] Diagnosis focuses on identification of symptoms by a daily calendar on which symptoms are recorded for 2 to 3 consecutive months. PMDD is a psychiatric diagnosis that distinguishes those whose symptoms are severe enough to interfere significantly with daily activities. It requires prospective symptom charting, and a minimum of 5 of the 11 symptom groups as described in the DSM. Presence of one symptom is sufficient for PMS diagnosis.[66]

Treatment

Management of PMS/PMDD has been largely symptomatic and includes education and support directed toward lifestyle changes for females with mild symptoms. Treatment includes diuretics to reduce fluid retention, analgesics for pain, and anxiolytic drugs to treat mood changes. An integrated program of personal assessment by diary, regular exercise, avoidance of caffeine, and a diet low in simple sugars and high in lean proteins is often beneficial. Additional therapeutic regimens include vitamin or mineral supplements (particularly pyridoxine, vitamin E, and magnesium), evening primrose oil (which contains linoleic acid, a precursor of prostaglandin E_1), natural progesterone supplements, low-dose oral monophasic contraceptives, GnRH agonists, bromocriptine for prolactin suppression, danazol (a synthetic androgen), and spironolactone (an aldosterone antagonist and inhibitor of adrenal androgen synthesis).[66] Although a variety of therapeutic choices exist, few treatments have been adequately evaluated in randomized, controlled clinical trials. Selective serotonin reuptake inhibitor antidepressants demonstrate significant improvement in overall symptoms compared with placebo, whether used continuously or only in the luteal phase, and are recommended by ACOG as first-line therapy for severe PMS or PMDD.[61,68]

SUMMARY CONCEPTS

Menstrual disorders include dysfunctional menstrual cycles, dysmenorrhea, and PMS. Dysfunctional menstrual cycles, which involve amenorrhea, oligomenorrhea, metrorrhagia, or menorrhagia, occur when hormonal support of the endometrium is altered. Estrogen deprivation causes retrogression of a previously built-up endometrium and bleeding. A lack of progesterone can cause abnormal menstrual needle aspiration, stereotactic needle biopsy (*i.e.*, core biopsy), and excisional biopsy (Fig. 45-14). Breast cancer is often a solitary, painless, firm, fixed lesion with poorly defined borders. It can be found anywhere in the breast, but it is most common in the upper outer quadrant. Because of the variability, any suspect change in breast tissue warrants investigation. The diagnostic use of mammography enables additional definition of the clinically suspect area and may lead to early detection. A wire marker under radiographic guidance can ensure accurate surgical biopsy of nonpalpable suspect areas. Ultrasonography is useful as a diagnostic adjunct to differentiate cystic from solid tissue in females with nonspecific thickening.[82]

Fine-needle aspiration is an in-office procedure that can be performed repeatedly in multiple sites and with minimal discomfort. A palpable mass is stabilized between two fingers or in conjunction with handheld sonography to define cystic masses or fibrocystic changes. Fine-needle aspiration can identify malignant cells but cannot differentiate *in situ* from infiltrating cancers. Stereotactic needle biopsy is an outpatient procedure done with the guidance of a mammography machine. After the lesion is localized, a large-bore needle is inserted quickly, removing a core of tissue. Discomfort is mild, and healing occurs rapidly. Histologic evaluation provides 96% accuracy in detecting cancer. This procedure is less costly than is excisional biopsy. However, excisional biopsy to remove the entire lump provides the only definitive diagnosis of breast cancer, and often is therapeutic without additional surgery. MRI, positron emission tomography, and computer-based or digital mammography are additional diagnostic modalities for breast cancer, and may supplement conventional mammography in females with radiographically dense breasts or a strong family history of cancer, or who are known carriers of *BRCA1* or *BRCA2*.[83]

Tumors are classified according to tissue characteristics and staged clinically according to size, nodal involvement, and metastasis. Estrogen and progesterone receptor analysis should be performed on surgical specimens, because the presence or absence of these receptors can predict tumor responsiveness to hormonal manipulation. High levels of both receptors improve prognosis and increase likelihood of remission.

Treatment

Treatment methods include surgery, chemotherapy, radiation, and hormonal manipulation. Radical mastectomy (*i.e.*, removal of the entire breast, underlying muscles, and all axillary nodes) is rarely the primary surgical therapy unless cancer is advanced at diagnosis. Modified surgical techniques (mastectomy plus axillary dissection or lumpectomy for breast conservation) plus chemotherapy or radiation therapy have comparable outcomes and are preferred.

Prognosis is related more to the extent of nodal involvement than to breast involvement. Greater nodal involvement requires more aggressive postsurgical treatment, and a diagnosis is not complete until dissection and testing of axillary lymph nodes. Evaluating lymph node involvement can be done via sentinel lymph node (SLN) biopsy. If the SLN biopsy is positive, more nodes are removed. If it is negative, further lymph node evaluation may not be needed.

Systemic therapy is administration of chemotherapy, biologic therapy, or hormonal therapy. Neoadjuvant therapy is given before surgery to shrink the tumor and make surgical removal more effective. Adjuvant therapy is given after surgery to females with and without detectable metastatic disease. The goal of this therapy depends on nodal involvement, menopausal status, and hormone receptor status. Systemic adjuvant therapy has benefits in reducing rates of recurrence and death from breast cancer.[83] Biologic therapy, using trastuzumab, is used to stop growth of breast tumors that express the HER2/neu receptor on the cell surface. The HER2/neu receptor binds an epidermal growth factor that contributes to cancer cell growth.

Hormone therapy can block the effects of estrogen on breast cancer cell growth. Tamoxifen is a nonsteroidal antiestrogen that binds to estrogen receptors and blocks

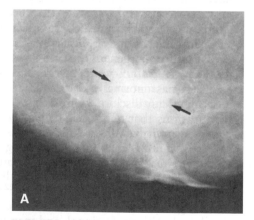
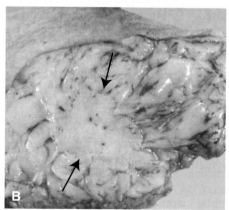

FIGURE 45.14. Carcinoma of the breast. (**A**) Mammogram. An irregularly shaped, dense mass (*arrows*) is seen in this otherwise fatty breast. (**B**) Mastectomy specimen. The irregular white, firm mass in the center is surrounded by fatty tissue. (From Strayer D. S., Rubin R. (Eds.). (2015). *Rubin's pathology: Clinicopathologic foundations of medicine* (7th ed., Fig. 25-35A and B, p. 1071). Philadelphia, PA: Lippincott Williams & Wilkins.)

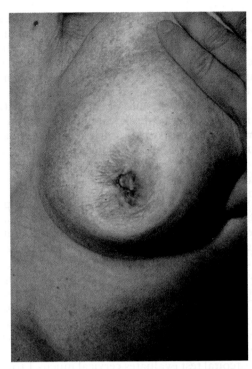

FIGURE 45-15. Paget disease of the nipple. (From Strayer D. S., Rubin R. (Eds.). (2015). *Rubin's pathology: Clinicopathologic foundations of medicine* (7th ed., Fig. 25-30A, p. 1069). Philadelphia, PA: Lippincott Williams & Wilkins.)

the effects of estrogens on growth of malignant breast cells. Decreased cancer recurrence and mortality rates, and increased 5-year survival rates, have been found in females with estrogen receptor–positive tissue samples treated with tamoxifen. Aromatase inhibitors block the enzyme that converts androstenedione and testosterone to estrogen in peripheral tissues. This reduces circulating estrogen levels in postmenopausal females and is an effective adjuvant therapy for early-stage breast cancer.[84]

Paget Disease

Paget disease accounts for 1% of all breast cancers. It presents as an eczematoid lesion of nipple and areola (Fig. 45-15). It usually is associated with infiltrating, intraductal carcinoma. Complete examination includes a mammogram and biopsy. Treatment depends on the extent of spread.[85]

 SUMMARY CONCEPTS

The breasts are subject to benign and malignant diseases. Mastitis is inflammation of the breast, occurring most frequently during lactation. Galactorrhea is an abnormal secretion of milk that may occur as a symptom of increased prolactin secretion. Ductal ectasia and intraductal papilloma

cause abnormal drainage from the nipple. Fibroadenoma and fibrocystic changes are abnormal masses in the breast that are benign. Breast cancer is a significant cause of death of females. Clinical breast examination and mammography afford the best protection against breast cancer. They provide the means for early detection and allow early treatment and cure.

Infertility

Infertility is the inability to conceive a child after 1 year of unprotected intercourse. Primary infertility refers to situations in which there has been no prior conception. Secondary infertility occurs after one or more previous pregnancies. Sterility is the inability to father a child or to become pregnant because of congenital anomalies, disease, or surgical intervention. In the United States, approximately 6% to 12% of females ages 15 to 44 are affected by infertility.[86]

For pregnancy to occur, three things must be available: (a) oocytes or eggs, (b) spermatozoa or sperm, and (c) a place for oocytes and spermatozoa to fertilize and implant.

There are several contributing factors to infertility. Male and female factors each make up about one third. Approximately 20% of couples suffer from unexplained infertility. Roughly 10% of infertility is caused by a combination of both male and female factors.[87] Although a full discussion of the diagnosis and treatment of infertility is beyond the scope of this book, an overview is presented.

Male Factors

For pregnancy to occur, the man must provide sperm in sufficient quantity, delivered to the upper end of the vagina, with adequate motility. This is assessed by a semen analysis, which evaluates volume (normally 1.5 mL), sperm density (15 to 39 million/mL), motility (>32% good progressive), viability (58%), morphology (4% normal), and viscosity (full liquefaction within 20 minutes).[88] The specimen is best collected by masturbation into a sterile container after 3 days of abstinence. Because of variability, abnormal results should lead to a repeat test before the need for treatment is presumed. *Azoospermia* is the absence of sperm, *oligospermia* refers to decreased numbers of sperm, and *asthenospermia* refers to poor motility of sperm.[89]

Causes include varicocele, ejaculatory dysfunction, hyperprolactinemia, hypogonadotropic hypogonadism, infection, immunologic problems, obstruction, and congenital anomalies. Risk factors include a history of mumps orchitis, cryptorchidism, testicular torsion, hypospadias, previous urologic surgery, and history of

3. A 45-year-old woman makes an appointment to see her physician because of a painless lump in her breast that she discovered while doing her routine monthly BSE.

   A. What tests should be done to confirm the presence or absence of breast cancer?

   B. During the removal of breast cancer, an SLN biopsy is often done to determine whether the cancer has spread to the lymph nodes. Explain how this procedure is done and its value in determining lymph node spread.

   C. After surgical removal of breast cancer, an aromatase inhibitor may be used as an adjuvant systemic therapy for women without detectable metastatic disease. The presence or absence of estrogen receptors in the cytoplasm of tumor cells is important in determining the selection of an agent for use in adjuvant therapy. Explain.

REFERENCES

1. Strayer D., Rubin R. (Eds.). (2015). *Rubin's pathology: Clinicopathologic foundations of medicine* (7th ed.). Philadelphia, PA: Lippincott Williams & Wilkins.
2. Gorrol A. H., Mulley A. G. (2014). *Primary care medicine: Office evaluation and management of the adult patient* (7th ed.). Philadelphia, PA: Lippincott Williams & Wilkins.
3. Krissi H., Shmuely A., Aviram A., et al. (2016). Acute Bartholin's abscess: Microbial spectrum, patient characteristics, clinical manifestation, and surgical outcomes. *European Journal Clinical Microbial Infectious Disease* 35, 443–446.
4. Cash J. C., Glass C. A. (2014). *Family practice guidelines* (3rd ed.). New York, NY: Springer Publishing Company, LLC.
5. Chan M. P., Zimarowski M. J. (2015). Vulvar dermatoses: A histopathologic review and classification of 183 cases. *Journal of Cutaneous Pathology* 42, 510–518.
6. Girardi F., Reich O., Tamussino K., et al. (2015). *Burghardt's colposcopy and cervical pathology: Textbook and atlas* (4th ed.). Stuttgart, New York, Delhi, Rio de Janeiro: Thieme.
7. Lee A., Bradford J., Fischer G. (2015). Long-term management of adult vulvar lichen sclerosus a prospective cohort study of 507 women. *Journal of American Medical Association Dermatology* 151(10), 1061–1067.
8. De Andres J., Sanchis-Lopez N., Marcos Ansensio-Samper J. M., et al. (2016). Vulvodynia—an evidence-based literature review and proposed treatment algorithm. *World Institute of Pain* 16(2), 204–236.
9. International Society for the Study of Vulvovaginal Disorders. (2015). Vulvovaginal disorders. [Online]. Available: https://www.issvd.org/issvd-terminology-classification-of-vulvar-diseases/. Accessed October 26, 2017.
10. Basson R., Driscoll M., Correia S. (2016). When sex is always painful: Provoked vestibulodynia. *British Columbia Medical Journal* 58(2), 77–81.
11. CerVigni M., Natale F. (2014). Gynecological disorders in bladder pain syndrome/interstitial cystitis patients. *International Journal of Urology* 21(suppl 1), 85–88.
12. IsHak W. W. (Ed.). (2017). *The textbook of clinical sexual medicine* (1st ed.). New York, NY: Springer Publishing Company, LLC.
13. National Cancer Institute. (2019). Surveillance, epidemiology, and end results cancer statistics review: Vulva cancer. [Online]. Available: http://seer.cancer.gov/statfacts/html/vulva.html. Accessed May 11, 2019.
14. Reyes M. C., Cooper K. (2014). An update on vulvar intraepithelial neoplasia: Terminology and a practical approach to diagnosis. [abstract]. *Journal of Clinical Pathology* 67(4), 290–294.
15. American College of Obstetrics and Gynecology and American Society for Colposcopy and Cervical Pathology. (2017). Management of vulvar intraepithelial lesions. Committee opinion. [Online]. Available: https://www.acog.org/-/media/Committee-Opinions/Committee-on-Gynecologic-Practice/co675.pdf?dmc=1&ts=20180312T0238240039. Accessed March 11, 2018.
16. Ramirez P. D., Gershenson D. M., Salvo G. (2018). Vulvar cancer. Merck Manual Professional. [Online]. Available: https://www.merckmanuals.com/professional/gynecology-and-obstetrics/gynecologic-tumors/vulvar-cancer. Accessed March 4, 2018.
17. International Federation of Gynecology and Obstetrics. (2009). Vulvar cancer. [Online]. Available: http://www.ncbi.nlm.nih.gov/pmc/articles/PMC2757555/. Accessed November 6, 2017.
18. Khanna N., Raug L. A., Lachiewicz M. P., et al. (2016). Margins for cervical and vulvar cancer. *Journal of Surgical Oncology* 113, 304–309.
19. Rhoads J., Murphy M. (2014). *Differential diagnosis for the advanced practice nurse.* New York, NY: Springer Publishing Company, LLC.
20. American Cancer Society. (2017). What are the key statistics about vaginal cancer? [Online]. Available: https://www.cancer.org/cancer/vaginal-cancer/about/key-statistics.html. Accessed June 22, 2019.
21. Yarbro C. H., Wujcik D., Gobel B. H. (2018). *Cancer nursing: Principles and practice* (8th ed.). Burlington, MA: Jones & Bartlett.
22. Jentschke M., Hoffmeister V., Soergel P., et al. (2016). Clinical presentation, treatment and outcome of vaginal intraepithelial neoplasia. *Archives of Gynecology and Obstetrics* 293, 415–419. doi:10:1007/s0040-015-3835-6.
23. Carcio H. N., Secor M. (2015). *Advanced health assessment of women: Clinical skills and procedures* (3rd ed). New York, NY: Springer Publishing Company, LLC.
24. American Cancer Society. (2018). Cervical cancer. [Online]. Available: https://www.cancer.org/content/dam/cancer-org/research/cancer-facts-and-statistics/annual-cancer-facts-and-figures/2018/cancer-facts-and-figures-2018.pdf. Accessed May 5, 2018.
25. American Cancer Society. (2016). Tests for cervical cancer. [Online]. Available: https://www.cancer.org/cancer/cervical-cancer/detection-diagnosis-staging/how-diagnosed.html. Accessed October 29, 2017.
26. United States Federal Drug Administration. (2017). Cervarix. [Online]. Available: https://www.fda.gov/BiologicsBloodVaccines/Vaccines/ApprovedProducts/ucm186957.htm. Accessed October 29, 2017.
27. Nayar R., Wilbur D. C. (2015). The pap test and Bethesda 2014. *Acta Cytologica* 59, 121–132. doi:10.1159/000381842.
28. Baker E. (2013). HPV and Pap: Shifting roles in cervical cancer screening. Medical Laboratory Observer. [Online]. Available: https://www.mlo-online.com/hpv-and-pap-shifting-roles-in-cervical-screening.php. Accessed October 29, 2017.
29. Medlin E. E., Kushner D. M., Barroilhet L. (2016). Robotic surgery for early stage cervical cancer: Evolution and current trends. *Journal of Surgical Oncology* 112, 772–781.
30. Marnitz S., Budach V., Weiber F., et al. (2012). Rectum separation in patients with cervical cancer for treatment planning in primary chemo-radiation. *Radiation Oncology* 7, 109.

31. Ahn S. H., Monsanto S. P., Miller C., et al. (2015). Pathophysiology and Immune dysfunction in endometriosis. *Biomed Research International* 2015, 795976. doi:10.1155/2015/795976.

32. Morotti M., Vincent K., Brawn J., et al. (2014). Peripheral changes in endometriosis-associated pain. *Human Reproduction Update* 20(5), 717–736.

33. American Society for Reproductive Medicine. (2012). *Endometriosis a guide for patients [pamphlet]*. Birmingham, AL: American Society for Reproductive Medicine under the direction of the Patient Education Committee and the Publications Committee.

34. Sinervo K. R. (2015). The case for surgery for endometriosis. *Contemporary OB/GYN* 60(10), 51–54.

35. Mishra V. V., Gaddagi R. A., Aggarwal R., et al. (2015). Prevalence; characteristics and management of endometriosis amongst infertile women: A one year retrospective study. *Journal of Clinical and Diagnostic Research* 9(6), 1–3.

36. Fraser I. (2016). Current trends in the medical management of endometriosis "available therapies in perspective". *Indian Obstetrics and Gynaecology* 6(1), 8–17.

37. American Cancer Society. (2017). Endometrial cancer. [Online]. Available: https://www.cancer.org/cancer/endometrial-cancer/about/key-statistics.html. Accessed October 29, 2017.

38. American Cancer Society. (2017). What are key statistics about uterine sarcoma? [Online]. Available: https://www.cancer.org/cancer/uterine-sarcoma/about/key-statistics.html. Accessed October 31, 2017.

39. Folkins A. K., Longmore T. A. (2013). Hereditary gynaecological malignancies: Advances in screening and treatment. *Histopathology* 62(2), 2–30.

40. American Cancer Society. (2017). What is endometrial cancer. [Online]. Available: https://www.cancer.org/cancer/endometrial-cancer/about/what-is-endometrial-cancer.html. Accessed October 29, 2017.

41. Tang Y., Chen C., Duan H., et al. (2015). Low vascularity predicts favourable outcomes in leiomyoma patients treated with uterine artery embolization. *European Radiology* 26, 3571–3579.

42. Centers for Disease Control and Prevention. (2015). STI pelvic inflammatory disease. [Online]. Available: https://www.cdc.gov/std/tg2015/pid.htm. Accessed November 1, 2017.

43. Gradison M. (2012). Pelvic inflammatory disease. *American Family Physician*. 85(8), 791–796.

44. Taran F. A., Kagan K. O., Hubner M., et al. (2015). The diagnosis and treatment of ectopic pregnancy. *Deutsches Aerzteblatt International* 112, 693–704.

45. Epee-Bekima M., Overton C. (2013). Diagnosis and treatment of ectopic pregnancy. *The Practitioner* 257(1759), 15–17.

46. American Society of Clinical Oncology. (2017). Ovarian, fallopian tube, and peritoneal cancer: Statistics. [Online]. Available: https://www.cancer.net/cancer-types/ovarian-fallopian-tube-and-peritoneal-cancer/statistics. Accessed April 17, 2018.

47. Fauser B. C., Tarlatzis B. C., Rebar R. W., et al. (2012). Consensus on women's health aspects of polycystic ovary syndrome (PCOS): The Amsterdam ESHRE/ASRM-sponsored 3rd PCOS consensus workshop group. *Fertility and Sterility* 97(1), 28.e25–36.e25. doi:10.1016/j.fertnstert.2011.09.024.

48. Franks S., Berga S. L. (2012). Does PCOS have developmental origins? *Fertility and Sterility* 97(1), 1–6.

49. Tsai Y., Wang T., Wei H., et al. (2013). Dietary intake, glucose metabolism and sex hormones in women with polycystic ovary syndrome (PCOS) compared with women with non-PCOS-related infertility. *British Journal of Nutrition* 109(12), 2190–2198.

50. Dumitrescu R., Mehedintu C., Briceag I., et al. (2015). The polycystic ovary syndrome: An update on metabolic and hormonal mechanisms. *Journal of Medicine and Life* 8(2), 142–145.

51. Legro R. S., Arsianian S. A., Ehrmann D. A., et al. (2013). Diagnosis and treatment of polycystic ovary syndrome: An endocrine society clinical practice guideline. *Journal of Clinical Endocrinology & Metabolism* 98(12), 4565–4592.

52. American Cancer Society. (2017). Ovarian cancer. [Online]. Available: https://www.cancer.org/cancer/ovarian-cancer/about/key-statistics.html. Accessed October 31, 2017.

53. American Cancer Society. (2016). Can ovarian cancer be found early? [Online]. Available: https://www.cancer.org/cancer/ovarian-cancer/detection-diagnosis-staging/detection.html. Accessed October 31, 2017.

54. Wentzensen N., Poole E. M., Trabert B., et al. (2016). Ovarian cancer risk factors by histologic subtype: An analysis from the ovarian cancer cohort consortium. *Journal of Clinical Oncology* 34(24), 2888–2897.

55. American Cancer Society. (2018). What are the risk factors for ovarian cancer? [Online]. Available: https://www.cancer.org/cancer/ovarian-cancer/causes-risks-prevention/risk-factors.html. Accessed April 17, 2018.

56. King G. G. T., Leighton J. C. (2015). CA 125. Medscape Drugs and Diseases/Laboratory Medicine. [Online]. Available: https://emedicine.medscape.com/article/2087557-overview#a2. Accessed March 5, 2018.

57. Hacker N. F., Gambone J. C., Moore C. J. (2016). *Hacker and Moore's essentials of obstetrics and gynecology* (6th ed.). Philadelphia, PA: Elsevier.

58. McNeely S. G. (2017). Cystoceles, urethroceles, enteroceles, and rectoceles. Merck Manual Professional version. [Online]. Available: https://www.merckmanuals.com/professional/gynecology-and-obstetrice/pelvic-relaxation-syndromes/cystoceles-urethroceles-enteroceles-and-rectoceles. Accessed March 5, 2018.

59. McNeely S. G. (2018). Uterine and vaginal prolapse. Merck manual professional version. [Online]. Available: https://www.merckmanuals.com/professional/gynecology-and-obstetrics/pelvic-relaxation-syndromes/uterine-and-vaginal-prolapse#v1064484. Accessed March 17, 2018.

60. Kow N., Goldman H. B., Ridgeway B. (2013). Management options for women with utcrine prolapse interested in uterine preservation. *Current Urology Reports* 14, 395–402.

61. U.S. National Library of Medicine. (2017). Premenstrual syndrome: Overview. PubMed Health. [Online]. Available: https://www.ncbi.nlm.nih.gov/pubmedhealth/PMH0072449/. Accessed March 4, 2018.

62. Callahan T. (2018). *Blueprints obstetrics gynecology* (7th ed.) Philadelphia, PA: Wolters Kluwer.

63. Fothergill D. (2012). Causes of primary and secondary amenorrhea. *Practice Nursing* 23(9), 465–469.

64. American Congress of Obstetrics and Gynecology. (2015). Dysmenorrhea, painful periods. [Online]. Available: https://www.acog.org/Patients/FAQs/Dysmenorrhea-Painful-Periods#are. Accessed November 1, 2017.

65. Hawkins J. W., Roberto-Nichols D. M., Stanley-Haney J. L. (2016). *Guidelines for nurse practitioners in gynecological settings* (11th ed.). New York, NY: Springer Publishing Company, LLC.

66. Hantsoo L., Epperson C. N. (2015). Premenstrual dysphoric disorder: Epidemiology and treatment. *Current Psychiatry* 17, 87. doi:10.1007/s11920-015-0628-3.

67. Patient education: Premenstrual syndrome (PMS) and premenstrual dysphoric disorder (PMDD) (beyond the basics). [Online]. Available: https://www.uptodate.com/contents/premenstrual-syndrome-pms-and-premenstrual-dysphoric-disorder-pmdd-beyond-the-basics. Accessed June 22, 2019.

68. American College of Obstetrics and Gynecology. (2015). Frequently askcd questions gynecological problems premenstrual syndrome. [Online]. Available: https://www.acog.org/Patients/

Sexually transmitted infections (STIs) encompass a broad range of infectious diseases that are spread by sexual contact. The incidence of STIs is increasing as is the technology's ability to screen STIs.[1] The Centers for Disease Control and Prevention (CDC; 2014) requires reporting of chlamydia, syphilis, and gonorrhea and, therefore, tracks these three STIs most specifically.[1] However, the actual figures of total STIs are probably much higher because many STIs are not reportable or not reported.

There are many factors that contribute to the increased prevalence and the continued spread of STIs. One key factor is that STIs are frequently asymptomatic, which promotes the spread of infection by people who are unaware they are carrying the infection.[2] Furthermore, partners of infected people are often difficult to notify and treat. In addition, there currently are no cures for viral STIs (e.g., human immunodeficiency virus [HIV], herpes simplex virus [HSV]). Although there are drugs available that may help to manage the infections, they do not entirely control the spread.[3] Also, drug-resistant microorganisms are rapidly emerging, making treatment of many STIs more difficult.

Sexual contact transmission has been identified in over 30 bacteria.[2] There are currently four curable infections: trichomoniasis, syphilis, gonorrhea, and chlamydia. Four of the infections are viral and considered incurable: hepatitis B, HSV, HIV, and human papillomavirus (HPV).[2] Portals of entry include the mouth, genitalia, urinary meatus, rectum, and skin. The rates of many STIs are highest among adolescents. All STIs are more common in people who have more than one sexual partner. Furthermore, it is not uncommon for a person to be concurrently infected with more than one type of STI.[2] STIs can result in stillbirth, death of the neonate, prematurity and low-birth weight, sepsis, pneumonia, and congenital deformities.[2]

This chapter discusses the manifestations of STIs in men and women in terms of infections of the external genitalia, vaginal infections, and infections that have genitourinary as well as systemic manifestations.

Infections of the External Genitalia

STIs can selectively infect the mucocutaneous tissues of the external genitalia, cause vaginitis in women, or produce both genitourinary and systemic effects. Some STIs may be transmitted by an infected mother to the fetus, causing congenital defects or death of the child or the newborn.[2] The discussion in this section of the chapter focuses on STIs that affect the mucocutaneous tissues of the oropharynx and external genitalia and anorectal tissues. These infections include condylomata acuminata, genital herpes, molluscum contagiosum, chancroid, granuloma inguinale, and lymphogranuloma venereum.

Condylomata Acuminata (Genital Warts)

Condylomata acuminata, or genital warts, are caused by the HPV (Fig. 46-1). Although recognized for centuries, HPV-induced genital warts have become the most

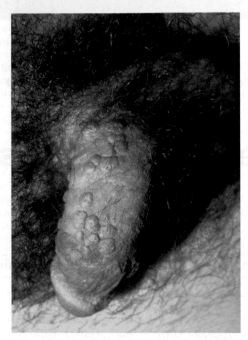

FIGURE 46-1. Condylomata of the penis. Raised circumscribed lesions are seen on the shaft of the penis. (From Rubin R., Strayer D. (Eds.) (2015). *Rubin's pathology: Clinicopathologic foundations of medicine* (7th ed., p. 975). Philadelphia, PA: Lippincott Williams & Wilkins.)

common STI, and there are over 40 different types of the HPV virus. The CDC estimates that 20 million Americans carry the virus and up to 6 million new cases are diagnosed each year.[4] Risk factors for acquiring HPV include young age (<25 years), early age of first intercourse (<16 years), increased number of sex partners, and having a male partner with multiple sex partners. HPV infection can occur with any type of vaginal or anal penetration, or, more rarely, oral sex.

Most HPV infections are asymptomatic and transient and resolve spontaneously within 2 years without treatment if the person has an intact immunologic system.[4] However, infection with some HPV types results in genital warts, cervical dysplasia, and cervical cancer.[4]

Types of Human Papillomavirus

HPVs are **nonenveloped**, double-stranded deoxyribonucleic acid (DNA) viruses that cause proliferative lesions of the squamous epithelium.[5] More than 100 distinct HPV subtypes have been identified, with some affecting the mouth and throat.[5] These subtypes have been divided into three categories on the basis of their likelihood of inducing dysplasia and carcinoma. For example, HPV types 16 and 18 are strongly associated with cervical dysplasia and anogenital cancers and are considered high risk.[5] However, only a small percentage of women infected with HPV go on to develop cervical cancer. Over 90% of infections clear within 2 years.[5] This suggests that even the most virulent HPV strains may vary in terms of their oncogenic potential. Cofactors that may increase the risk for cervical cancer include smoking, immunosuppression, and exposure to hormonal alteration (e.g., pregnancy, oral contraceptives).[5]

Pathogenesis and Clinical Manifestations

HPV infection begins with viral inoculation into a stratified squamous epithelium, where infection stimulates replication of the squamous epithelium, producing the various HPV-proliferative lesions.[5] The incubation period for HPV-induced genital warts ranges from 3 weeks to several months; for cervical abnormalities, the incubation period is several months, and for cervical cancer, the incubation period is decades.[5] Genital warts typically present as soft, raised, fleshy lesions on the external genitalia, including the penis (Fig. 46-2), vulva, scrotum, perineum, and perianal skin. External warts may appear as small bumps, or they may be flat, rough surfaced, or pedunculated. Less commonly, they can appear as smooth reddish or brown raised papules or as dome-shaped lesions on keratinized skin. Internal warts are cauliflower-shaped lesions that affect the mucous membranes of the vagina, urethra, anus, or mouth.

Subclinical infection occurs more frequently than visible genital warts. Both spontaneous resolution and infection with new HPV types are common. Approximately, 70% of women with HPV become HPV DNA negative within 1 year, and as much as 90% become negative within 2 years.[5] Many women with transient HPV infections develop atypical squamous cells of undetermined significance (ASC-US) or low-grade squamous intraepithelial lesions (LSILs) of the cervix as detected on a Pap test, colposcopy, or biopsy. In men, transient HPV infection may be associated with intraepithelial neoplasia of the penis and anus. Development of an effective immune response helps clear the infection, but the virus can remain dormant for years and reactivate at a later time.

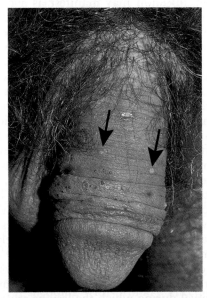

FIGURE 46-2. Herpes simplex virus (HSV) types 1 and 2 HSV-1 and HSV-2 are epidermotropic viruses. Transmission is limited to direct contact with active lesions or a virus-containing fluid such as saliva. Incubation period is 2 to 14 days. HSV-1 is associated with infection of the lips, face, buccal mucosa, and throat. HSV-2 is associated with genitalia. There may be an overlap in site of infection; type 1 strains can be recovered from the genital tract, and type 2 strains can be recovered from the pharynx following oral–genital activity. The usual sequence is painful papules followed by vesicles, ulceration, crusting, and healing. (From Jensen S. (2015). *Nursing health assessment: A best practice approach* (2nd ed., p. 730). Philadelphia, PA: Lippincott Williams & Wilkins.)

Diagnosis

The association with premalignant and malignant changes has increased the concern regarding the diagnosis and treatment of this viral infection. Lack of regular cervical cancer screening (Pap test) is the primary risk factor for development of invasive cervical cancer.[5] There are no approved serologic tests for HPV or routine methods for culturing the virus. The only test that is currently approved by the US Food and Drug Administration (FDA) is a solution hybridization method to test for high-risk HPV DNA.[5] The HPV DNA test detects whether one or more of the high-risk types of HPV are present. It does not identify the individual HPV type. HPV DNA testing is warranted with equivocal (ASC-US) Pap test results and is now recommended to determine which women older than 30 years of age need annual Pap smear screening.

Genital condylomata should be considered in any woman who presents with the primary complaint of vulvar pruritus or who has had an abnormal Pap smear result. Microscopic examination of a wet-mount slide preparation and cultures are used to exclude associated vaginitis. Careful inspection of the vulva, with magnification as needed, generally reveals the characteristic lesions, and specimens for biopsy can be taken from questionable areas. Colposcopic examination of the cervix and vagina may be advised as a follow-up measure when there is an abnormal Pap smear result or when HPV lesions are identified on the vulva.

Prevention and Treatment

There are three vaccines currently available to protect against specific HPV strains: Gardasil, Gardasil 9, and Cervarix.[6] In 2016, the CDC changed the vaccine recommendation to two doses if given before the adolescent's 15th birthday and spaced out by 6 to 12 months.[6] The recommendation at age 15 to 26 is still three doses. Both protect against types 16 and 18, which cause 70% of cervical cancers,[6] and Gardasil also protects against types 6 and 11, which are known to lead to genital warts. Currently, however, there is no treatment to eradicate the virus once a person has become infected. Prevention of HPV transmission through condom use has not been adequately demonstrated, but circumcision has been shown to decrease acquisition of some STIs, including HPV.[7] Treatment goals are aimed at elimination of symptomatic warts, surveillance for malignancy and premalignant changes, and education and counseling to decrease psychosocial distress.

Genital Herpes

Genital herpes is one of the most common causes of genital ulcers in the United States. Because herpesvirus infection is not reportable in all states, reliable data on its true incidence (estimated number of new cases every year) and prevalence (estimated number of people currently infected) are lacking. Recent estimates in the United States indicate a 16.2% prevalence of genital herpes.[8] Women have a greater mucosal surface area exposed in the genital area and therefore are at greater risk of acquiring the infection.[8]

most frequently in tropical areas such as India, Brazil, the West Indies, and parts of China, Australia, and Africa.[10]

Granuloma inguinale causes ulceration of the genitalia, beginning with an innocuous papule. The papule progresses through nodular or vesicular stages until it begins to break down as pink, granulomatous tissue. At this final stage, the tissue becomes thin and friable and bleeds easily. There are complaints of swelling, pain, and itching. Extensive inflammatory scarring may cause late sequelae, such as lymphatic obstruction with the development of enlarged and elephantoid external genitalia. The liver, bladder, bone, joint, lung, and bowel tissue may become involved. Genital complications include tubo-ovarian abscess, fistula, vaginal stenosis, and occlusion of vaginal or anal orifices. Lesions may become neoplastic.

Diagnosis is made through the identification of Donovan bodies (*i.e.*, large mononuclear cells filled with intracytoplasmic gram-negative rods) in tissue smears, biopsy samples, or culture.[10] A minimum 3-week period of treatment with doxycycline, azithromycin, ciprofloxacin, or erythromycin is used in treating the disorder.[10]

Lymphogranuloma Venereum

Lymphogranuloma venereum (LGV) is an acute and chronic venereal disease caused by *Chlamydia trachomatis* types L1, L2, and L3.[10,11] The disease, although found worldwide, has a low incidence outside the tropics. Most cases reported in the United States are in men.

The lesions of LGV can incubate for a few days to several weeks and thereafter cause small, painless papules or vesicles that may go undetected. An important characteristic of the infection is the early (1 to 4 weeks later) development of large, tender, and sometimes fluctuant inguinal lymph nodes called *buboes*.[10,11] There may be flulike symptoms with joint pain, rash, weight loss, pneumonitis, tachycardia, splenomegaly, and proctitis.[10,11] In later stages of the disease, a small percentage of affected people develop elephantiasis of the external genitalia, caused by lymphatic obstruction or fibrous strictures of the rectum or urethra from inflammation and scarring. Urethral involvement may cause pyuria and dysuria. Cervicitis is a common manifestation of primary LGV and could extend to perimetritis or salpingitis, which are known to occur in other chlamydial infections.[12] Anorectal structures may be compromised to the point of incontinence. Complications of LGV may be minor or extensive, involving compromise of whole systems or progression to a cancerous state.

Diagnosis is usually accomplished by a complement fixation test for LGV-specific *Chlamydia* antibodies. High titers for this antibody differentiate this group from other chlamydial subgroups.[10,11] Treatment involves 3 weeks of doxycycline or erythromycin.[10,11] Surgery may be required to correct sequelae such as strictures or fistulas or to drain fluctuant lymph nodes.

SUMMARY CONCEPTS

STIs that primarily affect the external genitalia include HPV-induced genital warts, genital herpes, molluscum contagiosum, chancroid, granuloma inguinale, and LGV. The lesions of these infections occur on the external genitalia of male and female sexual partners. Of concern is the relation between HPV and genital neoplasms. Genital herpes is caused by a neurotropic HSV (HSV-2 and, sometimes, HSV-1) that ascends through the peripheral nerves to reside in the sacral dorsal root ganglia. The herpesvirus can be reactivated, producing recurrent lesions in genital structures that are supplied by the peripheral nerves of the affected ganglia. There is no permanent cure for herpes infections. Molluscum contagiosum is a benign and self-limiting infection that is contagious. Chancroid, granuloma inguinale, and LGV produce external genital lesions with various degrees of inguinal lymph node involvement. These last three diseases are uncommon in the United States.

KEY POINTS

Sexually Transmitted Infections

■ In general, STIs because of bacterial pathogens can be successfully treated and the pathogen eliminated by antimicrobial therapy. However, many of these pathogens are developing antibiotic resistance.

■ STIs because of viral pathogens such as genital herpes simplex virus infections (HSV-1 and HSV-2) are not eliminated by current treatment modalities and persist with risk of recurrence (HSV infections).

Vaginal Infections

Candidiasis, trichomoniasis, and bacterial vaginosis are vaginal infections that may be associated with sexual activity. Trichomoniasis is the only form of vaginitis that is known to be sexually transmitted and requires partner treatment. The male partner is usually asymptomatic.

Candidiasis

Also called *yeast infection*, *thrush*, and *moniliasis*, *candidiasis* is the second leading cause of vulvovaginitis in the United States. Approximately, 75% of reproductive-age women in the United States experience one episode in their lifetime: 40% to 45% experience two or more infections.[13]

Candida albicans is the most commonly identified organism in vaginal yeast infections. However, other *Candida* species, such as *Candida glabrata* and *Candida tropicalis*, may also be present and be responsible for complicated candidiasis.[13] Although vulvovaginal candidiasis is usually not transmitted sexually, it is included in the CDC STI treatment guidelines because it is often diagnosed in women being evaluated for STIs.[3] The possibility of sexual transmission has been recognized for many years. However, candidiasis requires a favorable environment for growth of the organism. The gastrointestinal tract also serves as a reservoir for this organism, and candidiasis can develop through autoinoculation in women who are not sexually active. Although studies have documented the presence of *Candida* on the penis of male partners of women with vulvovaginal candidiasis (Fig. 46-4), few men develop balanoposthitis that requires treatment.[13]

Etiology and Clinical Manifestations

Reported risk factors for the overgrowth of *C. albicans* include recent antibiotic therapy, which suppresses the normal protective bacterial flora; high hormone levels owing to pregnancy or the use of oral contraceptives, which cause an increase in vaginal glycogen stores; and uncontrolled diabetes mellitus or HIV infection, because they compromise the immune system.[2] Women with vulvovaginal candidiasis commonly complain of vulvovaginal pruritus accompanied by irritation, erythema, swelling, dysuria, and dyspareunia. The characteristic discharge, when present, is usually thick, white, and odorless. In obese people, *Candida* may grow in skin

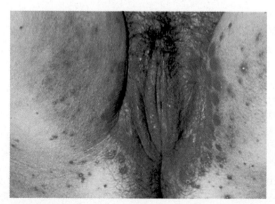

FIGURE 46-4. Candidiasis—Women will have vaginal pruritus and usually thick, white, curdlike secretions, but the secretions could be thin. (From Jensen S. (2015). *Nursing health assessment: A best practice approach* (2nd ed., p. 770). Philadelphia, PA: Lippincott Williams & Wilkins.)

folds underneath the breast tissue, the abdominal flap, and the inguinal folds.

 Concept Mastery Alert

The person with vulvovaginal candidiasis will have redness, swelling, and painful urination. Discharge will be thick and white because of yeast overgrowth and will be odorless.

Diagnosis and Treatment

Accurate diagnosis is made by identification of budding yeast filaments (*i.e.*, hyphae) or spores on a wet-mount slide using 20% potassium hydroxide. The pH of the discharge, which is checked with litmus paper, is typically less than 4.5. When the wet-mount technique is negative but the clinical manifestations are suggestive of candidiasis, a culture may be necessary.

Antifungal agents such as clotrimazole, miconazole, butoconazole, and terconazole, in various forms, are effective in treating candidiasis. These drugs, with the exception of terconazole, are available without prescription for use by women who have had a previously confirmed diagnosis of candidiasis. Oral fluconazole has been shown to be as safe and effective as the standard intravaginal regimen.[3]

Trichomoniasis

Trichomoniasis is credited with being a far more prevalent STI than gonorrhea infection, and almost as common as chlamydia.[13-15] In the United States, it has been estimated that 7.4 million new cases of trichomoniasis appear annually.[14] Epidemiologically, *Trichomonas vaginalis* infections are commonly associated with other STIs and are therefore a marker for high-risk sexual behavior. An anaerobic protozoan that can be transmitted sexually, *T. vaginalis* is shaped like a turnip and has three or four anterior flagella (see Fig. 46-5). Trichomonads can reside in the paraurethral glands of both sexes.

Clinical Manifestations and Complications

Men harbor the organism in the urethra and prostate and are asymptomatic. Although 10% to 25% of women are asymptomatic, trichomoniasis is a common cause of vaginitis when some imbalance allows the protozoan to proliferate.[15] This extracellular parasite feeds on the vaginal mucosa and ingests bacteria and leukocytes. The infection causes a copious, frothy, malodorous, green or yellow discharge. There is commonly erythema and edema of the affected mucosa, with occasional itching and irritation. Sometimes, small hemorrhagic areas, called *strawberry spots*, appear on the cervix.

Trichomoniasis can cause a number of complications.[13] It is a risk factor for HIV transmission and infectivity in both men and women. In women, it increases the risk of tubal infertility and atypical pelvic inflammatory disease (PID), and it is associated with adverse outcomes such as premature birth in pregnant women.[13] Trichomonads attach easily to mucous membranes. They may serve as vectors for the spread of other organisms, carrying pathogens attached to their surface into the fallopian tubes. In men, it is a common cause of nongonococcal urethritis and is a risk factor for infertility.[14]

Diagnosis and Treatment

Diagnosis is made microscopically by identification of the motile protozoan on a wet-mount slide preparation. The pH of the discharge is usually greater than 6.0. Because the organism resides in other urogenital structures besides the vagina, systemic treatment is recommended. The treatment of choice is oral metronidazole or tinidazole, medications that are effective against anaerobic protozoans.[13] Sexual partners should be treated to avoid reinfection, and abstinence is recommended until the full course of therapy is completed.

Bacterial Vaginosis

Bacterial vaginosis is the most prevalent form of vaginal infection seen by health care professionals.[16] The prevalence for bacterial vaginosis is approximately 21.2 million people per year in the 14 to 49 age group.[16] The disorder is associated with having multiple sex partners, a new sex partner, douching, and a lack of vaginal lactobacilli. Its relation to sexual activity is not clear. Sexual activity is believed to be a catalyst rather than a primary mode of transmission, and endogenous factors may play a role in the development of symptoms.

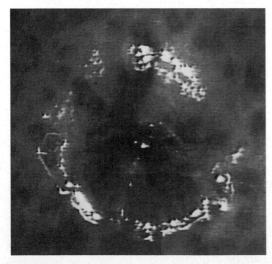

FIGURE 46-5. Trichomoniasis—Women will have vaginal pruritus, thin or thick secretions, a foul vaginal odor, and possibly dysuria. (From Jensen S. (2015). *Nursing health assessment: A best practice approach* (2nd ed., p. 771, Table 24.3). Philadelphia, PA: Lippincott Williams & Wilkins.)

Pathogenesis

The pathogenesis of bacterial vaginosis is poorly understood. It is a complex polymicrobial disorder characterized by a shift in the vaginal flora from one dominated by hydrogen peroxide–producing lactobacilli to one with greatly reduced numbers of *Lactobacillus* species and an overgrowth of other organisms, including *Gardnerella vaginalis*, *Mobiluncus* species, *Mycoplasma hominis*, and numerous anaerobes.[16,17] The massive overgrowth of vaginal anaerobes is associated with increased conversion of vaginal peptides to a variety of amines that, in high pH, become volatile and malodorous. The amines are associated with increased vaginal transudation and squamous epithelial cell **exfoliation**, creating the typical discharge. In conditions of elevated pH, *G. vaginalis* more efficiently adhere to the exfoliating epithelial cells, creating clue cells (squamous epithelial cells covered with masses of coccobacilli, often with large clumps of organisms floating free from the cell). Amines further provide a suitable substrate for *M. hominis* growth.

Clinical Manifestations

The predominant symptom of bacterial vaginosis is a thin, grayish-white discharge that has a foul, fishy odor. Burning, itching, and erythema are usually absent because the bacteria have only minimal inflammatory potential. Because of the lack of inflammation, the term *vaginosis* rather than *vaginitis* is used to describe the condition. The organisms associated with bacterial vaginosis may be carried asymptomatically by men and women.

In addition to causing bothersome symptoms, bacterial vaginosis is associated with an increased risk of PID, preterm labor, premature rupture of membranes, chorioamnionitis, and postpartum endometritis linked to the organisms associated with bacterial vaginosis. Postoperative infections, including postabortion PID, posthysterectomy cuff cellulitis, and postcesarean endometritis, have been shown to be associated with asymptomatic bacterial vaginosis.

Diagnosis and Treatment

The diagnosis of bacterial vaginosis is made when at least three of the following characteristics are present:

- Homogeneous, thin, white discharge
- Production of a fishy, amine odor when a saline solution is dropped onto the secretions
- Vaginal pH above 4.5 (usually 5.0 to 6.0)
- Appearance of characteristic "clue cells" on wet-mount microscopic studies

When indicated, treatment is aimed at relieving the vaginal symptoms and signs of infection and reducing the risk of infectious complications after abortion or hysterectomy. The CDC recommends treatment by oral metronidazole, metronidazole vaginal gel, or clindamycin vaginal cream.[16]

SUMMARY CONCEPTS

Candidiasis, trichomoniasis, and bacterial vaginosis are common vaginal infections that become symptomatic because of changes in the vaginal ecosystem. Only trichomoniasis is spread through sexual contact. Candidiasis, also called a *yeast infection*, is a frequent cause of vulvovaginitis. *Candida* can be present without producing symptoms; usually some host factor, such as altered immune status, contributes to the development of vulvovaginitis. It can be treated with over-the-counter medications. The infection, which is caused by the anaerobic protozoan *T. vaginalis*, incites the production of a copious, frothy, yellow or green, malodorous discharge. It is a risk factor for HIV transmission and infectivity in both men and women. In women, it increases the risk of tubal infertility and atypical PID and it is associated with adverse outcomes such as premature birth in pregnant women. Bacterial vaginosis is the most common cause of vaginal discharge. It is a complex polymicrobial disorder characterized by a shift in the vaginal flora from one dominated by hydrogen peroxide–producing lactobacilli to one with greatly reduced numbers of lactobacilli and an overgrowth of other organisms, including *G. vaginalis*, *Mobiluncus* species, *M. hominis*, and numerous anaerobes. The predominant symptom of bacterial vaginosis is a thin, grayish-white discharge that has a foul, fishy odor. Because it does not produce inflammation, it is referred to as *vaginosis* rather than *vaginitis*.

Vaginal–Urogenital–Systemic Infections

Some STIs infect male and female genital and extragenital structures. Among the infections of this type are chlamydial infections, gonorrhea, and syphilis. Many of these infections also pose a risk to infants born to infected mothers. Some infections, such as syphilis, may be spread to the infant while in utero, whereas others, such as chlamydial and gonorrheal infections, can be spread to the infant during the birth process.

Chlamydial Infections

Chlamydial infection is the most prevalent STI in the United States, with an incidence estimated to be more than twice that of gonorrhea. As of 2015, chlamydial infections are reportable in all 50 states and the District of Columbia. According to the CDC, in 2017, 1,708,569 chlamydial infections were reported to CDC in the 50 states and the District of Columbia. Rates were highest in females ages 19 and 20 years. The CDC estimates about twice the reported rate of people are actually infected with chlamydia.[18] Rates for chlamydial infections have risen significantly over the past 15 years because of an increase in screening programs, improved sensitivity of diagnostic tests, and improved surveillance and reporting systems.

C. trachomatis is an obligate intracellular bacterial pathogen that tends to be much smaller than most bacteria.[18] It resembles a virus in that it requires tissue culture for isolation, but like bacteria, it has ribonucleic acid (RNA) and DNA and is susceptible to some antibiotics. *C. trachomatis* causes a wide variety of genitourinary infections, including nongonococcal urethritis in men and PID in women. The closely related organisms *Chlamydia pneumoniae* and *Chlamydia psittaci* cause mild and severe pneumonia, respectively. *C. trachomatis* is the most common sexually transmitted disease in North America.[18] It can be serologically subdivided into types A, B, and C, which are associated with trachoma and chronic keratoconjunctivitis; types D through K, which are associated with genital infections and their complications; and types L1, L2, and L3, which are associated with LGV. *C. trachomatis* can cause significant ocular disease in neonates. It is a leading cause of blindness in underdeveloped countries. In these countries, the organism is spread primarily by flies, fomites, and nonsexual personal contact. In industrial countries, the organism is spread almost exclusively by sexual contact and therefore affects primarily the genitourinary structures.

Chlamydiae exist in two forms: elementary and reticulate bodies.[18] The 48-hour growth cycle starts with attachment of the elementary body to the susceptible host cell, after which it is ingested by a process that resembles phagocytosis. Once inside the cell, the elementary body is organized into the reticulate body, the metabolically active form of the organism that is capable of reproduction. The reticulate body is not infectious and cannot survive outside the body. The reticulate bodies divide in the cell for up to 36 hours and then condense to form new elementary bodies, which are released when the infected cell bursts.

Clinical Manifestations

The signs and symptoms of chlamydial infection resemble those produced by gonorrhea. The most significant difference between chlamydial and gonococcal salpingitis is that chlamydial infections may be asymptomatic or clinically nonspecific. If there are symptoms in women, the most common symptom is a mucopurulent cervical discharge (Fig. 46-6). The cervix itself frequently hypertrophies and becomes erythematous, edematous, and extremely friable. This can lead to greater fallopian tube damage and increase the reservoir for further chlamydial infections.

In men, chlamydial infections, if there are symptoms, cause urethritis, including meatal erythema and

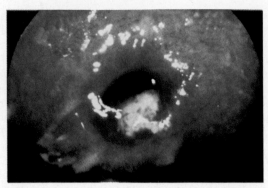

FIGURE 46-6. Chlamydia—In women there may be no symptoms or manifestation. Occasionally there are clear or white secretions. (From Jensen S. (2015). *Nursing health assessment: A best practice approach* (2nd ed., p. 770). Philadelphia, PA: Lippincott Williams & Wilkins.)

tenderness, a purulent penile discharge, and urethral itching[18] (Fig. 46-7). Prostatitis and epididymitis with subsequent infertility may develop.

The most serious complication of untreated chlamydial infection is the development of Reiter syndrome. This triad of symptoms includes urethritis, conjunctivitis, and arthritis of weight-bearing joints, such as the knee, sacroiliac, and vertebral joints.[18] Women can also develop reactive arthritis, but the male-to-female ratio for this complication is 5:1. The arthritis begins 1 to 3 weeks after the onset of chlamydial infection. The joint involvement is asymmetric, with multiple affected joints and a predilection for the lower extremities. Mucocutaneous lesions also occur and are papulosquamous eruptions that tend to be located on the palms of the hands and soles of the feet of both genders. The US Preventive Services Task Force (USPSTF) has suggested annual screening for sexually active adolescents and young female adults in an effort to minimize infection.[19]

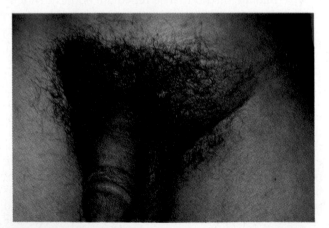

FIGURE 46-7. Chlamydia—*Chlamydomonas trachomatis* is a bacterium with a variable incubation period, usually 1 week of exposure. There is a mucopurulent discharge in men. (From Jensen S. (2015). *Nursing health assessment: A best practice approach* (2nd ed., p. 728). Philadelphia, PA: Lippincott Williams & Wilkins.)

Diagnosis and Treatment

Diagnosis of chlamydial infections takes several forms. The identification of polymorphonuclear leukocytes on Gram stain of penile discharge in the man or cervical discharge in the woman provides presumptive evidence. The direct fluorescent antibody test and the enzyme-linked immunosorbent assay that use antibodies against an antigen in the *Chlamydia* cell wall are rapid tests that are highly sensitive and specific. The positive predictive value of these tests is excellent among high-risk groups, but false-positive results occur more often in low-risk groups. The methodologic challenges of culturing this organism have led to the development of non–culture-based tests that amplify and detect *C. trachomatis*–specific DNA and RNA sequences.[18] One of the newest sets of nonculture techniques, the nucleic acid amplification tests (NAATs), does not require viable organisms for detection and can produce a positive signal from as little as a single copy of the target DNA or RNA.[18] These amplification methods are highly sensitive and, if properly monitored, very specific. NAATs can be performed on urine or self-collected swab specimens from the distal vagina as well as the traditional endocervical and urethral specimens. Most NAATs in use today detect both *C. trachomatis* and *Neisseria gonorrhoeae* in a single test.

The CDC recommends the use of azithromycin or doxycycline in the treatment of chlamydial infection. Penicillin is ineffective. Azithromycin is the preferred choice in pregnancy.[3] Simultaneous antibiotic treatment of both sexual partners is recommended. Abstinence from sexual activity is encouraged to facilitate cure.

Gonorrhea

Gonorrhea is a reportable STI caused by the bacterium *N. gonorrhoeae*. In 2017, 555,608 cases were reported an increase of 67% since 2013. Rates were higher among males, being highest in those 20 to 24 years (705.2 cases per 100,000 males) and 25 to 29 years (645.9 cases per 100,000 males).[18] Like chlamydial infection, gonorrhea is frequently underdiagnosed.

The gonococcus is a pyogenic (*i.e.*, pus-forming), gram-negative diplococcus.[18] Humans are the only natural host for *N. gonorrhoeae*. The organism grows best in warm, mucus-secreting epithelia. The portal of entry can be the genitourinary tract, eyes, oropharynx, anorectum, or skin.

Transmission is usually by sexual intercourse except for perinatal transmission.[2] Autoinoculation of the organism to the conjunctiva is possible. Neonates born to infected mothers can acquire the infection during passage through the birth canal and are in danger of developing gonorrheal conjunctivitis, with resultant blindness unless treated promptly. An amniotic infection syndrome characterized by premature rupture of the membranes, premature delivery, and increased risk of infant morbidity and mortality has been identified as an additional complication of gonococcal infections in pregnancy. Genital gonorrhea in young children should raise the possibility of sexual abuse.

The infection commonly manifests 2 to 7 days after exposure. It typically begins in the anterior urethra, accessory urethral glands, Bartholin or Skene glands, and the cervix. If untreated, gonorrhea spreads from its initial sites upward into the genital tract. In men, it spreads to the prostate and epididymis. In women, it commonly produces endometritis, salpingitis, and PID.[2] Pharyngitis may follow oral–genital contact. The organism can also invade the bloodstream (*i.e.*, disseminated gonococcal infection), causing serious sequelae such as bacteremic involvement of joint spaces, heart valves, meninges, and other body organs and tissues.[2]

Clinical Manifestations

People with gonorrhea may be asymptomatic and may unwittingly spread the disease to their sexual partners. In men, the initial symptoms include urethral pain and a creamy yellow, sometimes bloody, discharge (Fig. 46-8). The disorder may become chronic and affect the prostate, epididymis, and periurethral glands.[2] Rectal infections are common in homosexual men. In women, recognizable symptoms include unusual genital or urinary discharge, dysuria, dyspareunia, pelvic pain or tenderness, unusual vaginal bleeding (including bleeding after intercourse), fever, and proctitis (Fig. 46-9).[2] Symptoms may occur or increase during or immediately after menses because the bacterium is an intracellular diplococcus that thrives in menstrual blood but cannot survive long outside the human body. There may be infections of the uterus and development of acute or chronic infection of the fallopian tubes (*i.e.*, salpingitis), with ultimate scarring and sterility (Fig. 46-10).

Diagnosis

Diagnosis is based on the history of sexual exposure and symptoms. It is confirmed by identification of the organism on Gram stain or culture. A Gram stain is

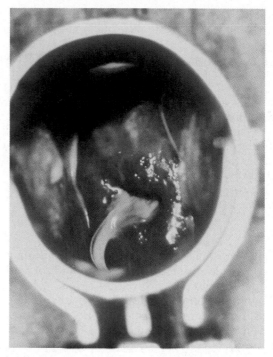

FIGURE 46-9. Gonorrhea—Secretions are yellow and the women report dyspareunia and dysuria. (From Jensen S. (2015). *Nursing health assessment: A best practice approach* (2nd ed., p. 771). Philadelphia, PA: Lippincott Williams & Wilkins.)

usually an effective means of diagnosis in symptomatic men (*i.e.*, those with discharge). In women and asymptomatic men, a culture is usually preferred because the Gram stain is often unreliable. Culture has been the gold standard, particularly when the Gram stain is negative.

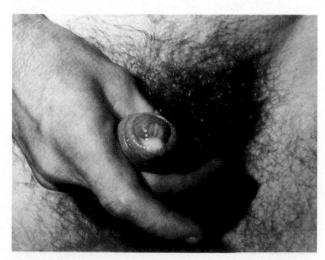

FIGURE 46-8. Purulent penile discharge because of gonorrhea. (From Jensen S. (2015). *Nursing health assessment: A best practice approach* (2nd ed., p. 728). Philadelphia, PA: Lippincott Williams & Wilkins.)

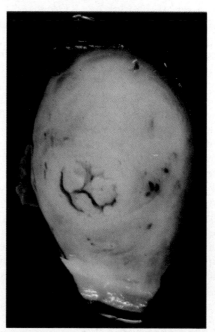

FIGURE 46-10. Gonorrhea of the fallopian tube. Cross-section of a "pus tube" shows thickening of the wall and lumen swollen with pus. (From Rubin R., Strayer D. (Eds.) (2015). *Rubin's pathology: Clinicopathologic foundations of medicine* (7th ed., p. 394). Philadelphia, PA: Lippincott Williams & Wilkins.)

Updated recommendations from the USPSTF suggest that clinicians screen all sexually active women for gonorrhea who are at increased risk for infection (*i.e.,* younger than 25 years of age, new or multiple sexual partners, inconsistent condom use, sex work, or drug use).[20] Testing for other STIs, particularly syphilis and chlamydial infection, is suggested at the time of examination. Pregnant women are routinely screened at the time of their first prenatal visit. High-risk populations should have repeat cultures during the third trimester. Neonates are routinely treated with various antibacterial agents applied to the conjunctiva within 1 hour of birth to protect against undiagnosed gonorrhea and other diseases.

Treatment

Penicillin-resistant strains of *N. gonorrhoeae* are prevalent worldwide and strains with other kinds of antibiotic resistance continue to evolve and spread. The current treatment recommendation to combat tetracycline- and penicillin-resistant strains of *N. gonorrhoeae* has progressively developed resistance to each of the antimicrobials used for treatment of gonorrhea.[18] Most recently, declining susceptibility to cefixime (an oral cephalosporin antibiotic) resulted in a change to the CDC treatment guidelines (2015) so that dual therapy with ceftriaxone (an injectable cephalosporin) and azithromycin is now the only CDC-recommended treatment regimen for gonorrhea.[21]

Syphilis

Syphilis is a reportable systemic STI caused by a spirochete, *Treponema pallidum*. In 2017, there were 30,644 cases of primary and secondary syphilis reported in the United States, a 72.7% increase since 2013. Rates were highest in men aged 25 to 29. However, the rate in women reported a 21.1% increase.

T. pallidum is spread by direct contact with an infectious moist lesion, usually through sexual intercourse. Bacteria-laden secretions may transfer the organism during any type of intimate contact. Skin abrasions provide another possible portal of entry. There is rapid transplacental transmission of the organism from the mother to the fetus after 16 weeks' gestation so that active infection in the mother during pregnancy can produce congenital syphilis in the fetus. Untreated syphilis can cause prematurity, stillbirth, and congenital defects and active infection in the infant. Because the manifestations of maternal syphilis may be subtle, testing for syphilis is mandatory in all pregnancies. Once treated for syphilis, a pregnant woman is usually followed throughout pregnancy by repeat testing of serum titers.

Clinical Manifestations

The clinical disease is divided into three stages: primary, secondary, and tertiary. Primary syphilis is characterized by the appearance of a chancre at the site of exposure, such as on the penis, vulva, anus, or mouth.[2]

Chancres typically appear within an average of 3 weeks of exposure but may incubate up to 3 months.[2] The primary chancre begins as a single, indurated papule up to several centimeters in diameter that erodes to create a clean-based ulcerated lesion on an elevated base. They also are solitary and have discrete raised borders.[2] These lesions are usually painless and located at the site of sexual contact. Primary syphilis is readily apparent in the male, where the lesion is on the scrotum or penis (Fig. 46-11). Although chancres can develop on the external genitalia in females, they are more common on the vagina or cervix, and primary syphilis therefore may go untreated since they are not visible without a speculum examination. Often there is an accompanying inguinal lymphadenopathy.[2] The infection is highly contagious at this stage, but because the symptoms are mild, it frequently goes unnoticed. The chancre usually heals within 3 to 12 weeks, with or without treatment.

The timing of the second stage of syphilis varies even more than that of the first, lasting from 1 week to 6 months. The symptoms of a rash (especially on the palms, mucous membranes, meninges, lymph nodes, stomach, soles, and liver)[2] (Fig. 46-12), fever, sore throat, stomatitis, nausea, loss of appetite, and inflamed eyes may come and go for a year but usually last for 3 to 6 months. Secondary manifestations may include some loss of hair and condylomata lata. These lesions are elevated, red-brown lesions that may ulcerate and produce a foul discharge. They are 2 to 3 cm in diameter, contain many spirochetes, and are highly infectious.

After the second stage, syphilis frequently enters a latent phase that may last the lifetime of the person or progress to tertiary syphilis at some point. Persons can be infective during the first 1 to 2 years of latency.

Tertiary syphilis is a delayed response to the untreated disease. It can occur decades after the initial infection.[2] When syphilis does progress to the symptomatic tertiary stage, it commonly takes one of three forms: development of localized destructive granuloma-like lesions called *gummas*, development of cardiovascular lesions, or development of central nervous system lesions.

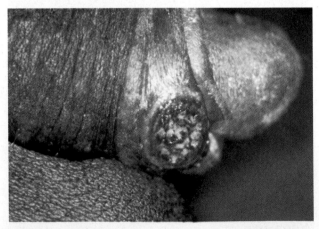

FIGURE 46-11. Syphilitic chancre of the penis shaft. (From Jensen S. (2015). *Nursing health assessment: A best practice approach* (2nd ed., p. 729). Philadelphia, PA: Lippincott Williams & Wilkins.)

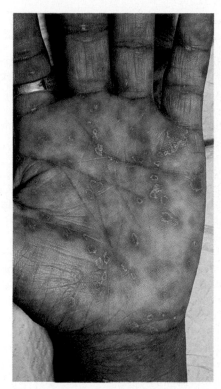

FIGURE 46-12. Secondary syphilis. A maculopapular rash is present on the palm. (From Rubin E., Gorstein F., Rubin R., et al. (Eds.) (2015). *Rubin's pathology: Clinicopathologic foundations of medicine* (7th ed., p. 414). Philadelphia, PA: Lippincott Williams & Wilkins.)

The syphilitic gumma is a peculiar, rubbery, necrotic lesion that is caused by noninflammatory tissue necrosis. Gummas can occur singly or multiply and vary in size from microscopic lesions to large, tumorous masses. They are most commonly found in the liver, testes, and bone. Central nervous system lesions can produce dementia, blindness, or injury to the spinal cord, with ataxia and sensory loss. Cardiovascular manifestations usually result from scarring of the medial layer of the thoracic aorta with aneurysm formation. These aneurysms produce enlargement of the aortic valve ring with aortic valve insufficiency.[2]

Diagnosis

T. pallidum is difficult to culture and requires special dark-field microscopy to adequately detect the organism. As it evokes a humoral immune response leading to production of antibodies, serologic testing can be done. Although PCR tests have now been developed for syphilis, serology remains the mainstay for diagnosis.[22] Because the disease's incubation period may delay test sensitivity, serologic tests are usually repeated after 6 weeks if the initial test results were negative.

The nontreponemal tests identify the presence of regain, which is an autoantibody directed against cardiolipin antigens. These antibodies are detected by flocculation tests such as the Venereal Disease Research Laboratory (VDRL) test or the rapid plasma reagin (RPR) test.[22] Because these tests are nonspecific, positive results can occur with diseases other than syphilis. The tests are easy to perform, rapid, and inexpensive and are frequently used as screening tests for syphilis. Results become positive 4 to 6 weeks after infection or 1 to 3 weeks after the appearance of the primary lesion. Because these tests are quantitative, they can be used to measure the degree of disease activity or treatment effectiveness. The fluorescent treponemal antibody absorption test is used to detect specific antibodies to *T. pallidum*. These qualitative tests are used to determine whether a positive result on a nonspecific test such as the VDRL or RPR is attributable to syphilis.

Treatment

The treatment of choice for syphilis is long-acting penicillin.[3] Because of the spirochetes' long generation time, effective tissue levels of penicillin must be maintained for several weeks. Tetracycline or doxycycline is used for treatment in people who are sensitive to penicillin. Sexual partners should be evaluated and treated prophylactically even though they may show no sign of infection.

 SUMMARY CONCEPTS

The vaginal–urogenital–systemic STIs—chlamydial infections, gonorrhea, and syphilis—can severely involve the genital structures and manifest as systemic infections. Gonorrheal and chlamydial infections can cause a wide variety of genitourinary complications in men and women, and both can cause ocular disease and blindness in neonates born to infected mothers. Syphilis is caused by a spirochete, *T. pallidum*. It can produce widespread systemic effects and is transferred to the fetus of infected mothers through the placenta.

Other Infections

Zika

Zika is a virus that was discovered in 1947 in the Zika Forest of Uganda and was initially spread by the bite of an infected *Aedes* species mosquito (*A. Aegypti* and *A. Albopictus*).[23,24] The first human cases of Zika were detected in 1952. Zika infection can occur in any of the following ways:

- From a bite from this species of mosquito.[23,24]
- From exposure to an infected sexual partner, including sex (oral, vaginal, or anal sex, or the sharing of sex toys) without a condom.[23,24] (Note that having sex with a partner who traveled to or lives in an area with Zika puts a person at risk of infection.)[23,24]

■ This virus can be passed on by a pregnant woman to her fetus, and this infection during pregnancy can cause certain birth defects.[23,24]

Clinical Manifestations

People infected with the Zika virus show few symptoms.[23] Symptoms reported have included fever, rash, joint pain, conjunctivitis, muscle pain, and headache.[23] Zika infection symptoms can last for several days to a week.

Risk

If a woman is infected by Zika during pregnancy, severe birth defects can occur, such as microcephaly, brain defects, hearing and eye defects, and impaired growth.[23] There have also been reports of Guillain–Barré syndrome.[23]

Diagnosis

A blood, cerebrospinal fluid, or urine test can confirm a Zika infection; it is sent to the CDC, where RNA NAT (nucleic acid testing) and antibody testing are performed.

Treatment

Currently there is no vaccine or treatment available for the Zika infection.[23]

Prevention

Use an insect repellent containing one or more of the following ingredients: N,N-Diethyl-m-toluamide, picaridin, IR3535, oil of lemon eucalyptus, para-menthane-diol, or 2-undecanone.[25] These products are safe for pregnant and breastfeeding women but should not be used on babies younger than 2 months old.[25] Prevent exposure to mosquitoes by using screens and bed netting.[25] Prevent sexual transmission by using condoms or abstinence.[25]

SUMMARY CONCEPTS

The Zika virus has been documented for over 70 years but has recently gained attention following an outbreak of the virus and its link to birth defects for the unborn fetus. Transmission is possible through a bite from an infected Aedes species mosquito, through unprotected sex with an infected partner, and from a pregnant woman to her fetus. Although the virus typically causes mild symptoms, pregnant women or those planning to become pregnant should be tested for the Zika antibody. Prevention is key since there is no treatment currently available.

STIs can be passed from a pregnant woman to the baby before and during the birth process; syphilis and HIV can cross the placenta during pregnancy.

Review Exercises

1. A 25-year-old woman has been told that her Pap test indicates infection with HPV type 16.

   A. What are the possible implications of infection with HPV 16?
   B. How might she have acquired this infection?

2. A 35-year-old woman presents with vulvar pruritus, dysuria, dyspareunia, and an odorless, thick, cheesy vaginal discharge. She has diabetes mellitus and has recently recovered from a respiratory tract infection, which required antibiotic treatment.

   A. Given that these manifestations are consistent with a Candida infection, what tests might be used to confirm the diagnosis?
   B. What risk factors does this woman have that predispose to this type of vaginitis?

3. A 21-year-old woman has recently been to Miami, Florida and is complaining of a low-grade fever, rash, and joint pain. Her last menstrual period was 3 months ago. She is sexually active and her pregnancy test is positive.

   A. Given these symptoms are consistent with Zika virus, what test could be done to confirm the diagnosis?
   B. What is the risk for this woman and her baby?
   C. What can be done to prevent this infection in other childbearing women?

REFERENCES

1. Centers for Disease Control and Prevention. (2014). Sexually transmitted disease surveillance. [Online]. Available: https://www.cdc.gov/std/stats14/. Accessed January 31, 2017.
2. World Health Organization (WHO). (2016). Sexually transmitted infections. Fact sheet. [Online]. Available: http://www.who.int/mediacentre/factsheets/fs110/en/. Accessed January 31, 2017.
3. Centers for Disease Control and Prevention. (2015). Sexually transmitted disease guidelines. [Online]. Available: https://www.cdc.gov/std/tg2015/. Accessed January 31, 2017.
4. Center for Disease Control and Prevention. (2013). Self-study STD modules for clinicians: Genital human papillomavirus (HPV) infection. Pathogenesis and microbiology. [Online]. Available: https://www2a.cdc.gov/stdtraining/self-study/hpv/cdc_self_study_hpv_pathogenesis.html. Accessed February 1, 2017.
5. Centers for Disease Control and Prevention. (2016). Questions and answers about HPV. [Online]. Available: https://www.cdc.gov/hpv/parents/questions-answers.html. Accessed February 1, 2017.
6. Morris B. J., Hankins C. A. (2017). Effect of male circumcision on risk of sexually transmitted infections and cervical cancer in women. *The Lancet Global Health* 5(11), e1054–e1055. Available: http://www.thelancet.com/journals/langlo/article/PIIS2214-109X%2817%2930386-8/fulltext.

7. Centers for Disease Control and Prevention. (2015). Molluscum contagiosum. [Online]. Available: https://www.cdc.gov/poxvirus/molluscum-contagiosum/index.html. Accessed February 2, 2017.

8. Centers for Disease Control and Prevention. (2016). Genital herpes: CDC fact sheet. [Online]. Available: https://www.cdc.gov/std/herpes/stdfact-herpes.htm. Accessed February 1, 2017.

9. Centers for Disease Control and Prevention. (2015). Candidiasis. [Online]. Available: https://www.cdc.gov/fungal/diseases/candidiasis/index.html. Accessed February 2, 2017.

10. Center for Disease Control and Prevention. (2015). Trichomoniasis: CDC fact sheet. [Online]. Available: https://www.cdc.gov/std/trichomonas/STDFact-Trichomoniasis.htm. Accessed February 2, 2017.

11. Centers for Disease Control and Prevention. (2015). Lymphogranuloma venereum (LGV). [Online]. Available: https://www.cdc.gov/std/tg2015/lgv.htm. Accessed February 2, 2017.

12. Afsar F., Seremet S., Afsar I., et al. (2017). A case of scrofuloderma complicated with genital elephantiasis and saxophone penis. *Reviews in Medical Microbiology* 28(1), 5–8.

13. Centers for Disease Control and Prevention. (2015). Bacterial vaginosis: CDC fact sheet. [Online]. Available: https://www.cdc.gov/std/bv/stdfact-bacterial-vaginosis.htm. Accessed February 2, 2017.

14. Centers for Disease Control and Prevention. (2015). Chlamydia: CDC fact sheet. [Online]. Available: https://www.cdc.gov/std/chlamydia/STDFact-Chlamydia.htm. Accessed February 2, 2017.

15. Centers for Disease Control and Prevention. (2015). Chlamydial infections. [Online]. Available: https://www.cdc.gov/std/tg2015/chlamydia.htm. Accessed February 2, 2017.

16. U.S. Preventive Services Task Force. (May, 2019). Final recommendation statement: Sexually transmitted infections: Behavioral counseling. Available: https://www.uspreventiveservicestaskforce.org/Page/Document/RecommendationStatementFinal/sexually-transmitted-infections-behavioral-counseling1

17. Centers for Disease Control and Prevention. (2015). Gonorrhea. [Online]. Available: https://www.cdc.gov/std/gonorrhea/default.htm

18. U.S. Preventive Services Task Force. (May, 2019). Final recommendation statement: Chlamydia and gonorrhea: Screening. [Online]. Available: https://www.uspreventiveservicestaskforce.org/Page/Document/RecommendationStatementFinal/chlamydia-and-gonorrhea-screening

19. Centers for Disease Control and Prevention. (2017). Syphilis. [Online]. Available: https://www.cdc.gov/std/stats17/Syphilis.htm Accessed April 29, 2019. Centers for Disease Control and Prevention. (2017). Collecting and submitting fluid specimens for Zika virus testing. [Online]. Available: https://www.cdc.gov/zika/laboratories/test-specimens-bodyfluids.html. Accessed February 24, 2017.

20. Center for Disease Control and Prevention. (2017). HIV among people aged 50 and over. Available: https://www.cdc.gov/hiv/group/age/olderamericans/index.html. Accessed July 8, 2019.

21. Centers for Disease Control and Prevention. (2017). Prevent mosquito bites. [Online]. Available: https://www.cdc.gov/zika/prevention/prevent-mosquito-bites.html. Accessed February 24, 2017.

22. Stewart A., Graham S. (2013). Sexual risk behavior among older adults. *Clinical Advisor* 16(4), 28–38.

23. Centers for Disease Control and Prevention. (2017). About Zika. [Online]. Available: https://www.cdc.gov/zika/about/index.html. Accessed February 24, 2017.

24. Office of Women's Health, U.S. Department of Health and Human Services. (2014). STIs, pregnancy, and breastfeeding. Available: https://www.womenshealth.gov/a-z-topics/stis-pregnancy-and-breastfeeding. Accessed July 8, 2019.

25. Hornor G. (2017). Sexually transmitted infections and children: What the PNP should know. *Journal of Pediatric Health Care* 31(2), 222–229.

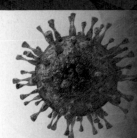
C H A P T E R 47

Structure and Function of the Musculoskeletal System

Learning Objectives

After completing this chapter, the learner will be able to meet the following objectives:

1. Describe the characteristics including one location of elastic cartilage, hyaline cartilage, and fibrocartilage.
2. Characterize the function of the four types of bone cells.
3. State the function of parathyroid hormone, calcitonin, and vitamin D in terms of bone formation and metabolism.
4. Describe the source of blood supply to a synovial joint.
5. Explain why pain is often experienced in all the joints of an extremity when a disease process affects only a single joint.

The bones of the skeletal system are a framework for the attachment of muscles, tendons, and ligaments. The skeletal system protects soft tissues and maintains them in their proper position, provides stability for the body, and maintains the body's shape. Bones act as a storage reservoir for calcium, and the central cavity of some bones contains the hematopoietic connective tissue in which blood cells are formed. Coordinated movement of the skeleton is made possible by the tendons and ligaments that join bones at joints.

The skeletal system includes the bones and cartilage of the skeletal system, as well as the connective tissue structures (*i.e.*, ligaments and tendons) that connect the bones and join muscles to bone.

Bony Structures of the Skeletal System

The skeletal system consists of the axial and appendicular skeleton. The *axial skeleton*, which is composed of the bones of the skull, thorax, and vertebral column, forms the axis of the body. The *appendicular skeleton* consists of the bones of the upper and lower extremities, including the shoulder and hip. The skeletal system contains both bone and cartilage tissue. Bones provide protection for internal organs and rigid support for the extremities. Cartilage provides flexibility for and cushioning of bony structures and for prenatal and postnatal skeletal development.

Bone Structures

There are two types of mature bones: cortical and cancellous bone (Fig. 47-1). Cortical (compact) bone comprises 80% of the skeleton and forms the outer shell of a bone; it has a densely packed, calcified intercellular matrix that makes it more rigid than cancellous bone.[1] Cancellous (spongy) bone is found in the interior of bones and is composed of *trabeculae* and *spicules*, of bone that form a lattice-like pattern.[1] These lattice-like structures are lined with osteogenic cells and filled with red or yellow bone marrow. Cancellous bone is relatively light, but its structure is such that it has considerable tensile strength and weight-bearing properties. Although bones contain both cancellous and cortical elements, their proportions vary in different bones throughout the body and in different parts of the same bone, depending on the relative needs for strength and lightness. Cortical bone is the major component of tubular bones. It is also found along the lines of stress on long bones and forms an outer protective shell on other bones.

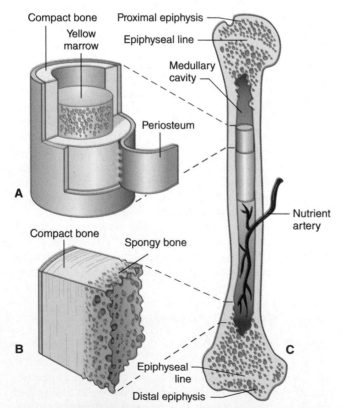

FIGURE 47-1. A long bone shown in longitudinal section. **(A)** Periosteum and bone marrow. **(B)** Compact and cancellous bone. **(C)** Epiphysis and source of blood supply from epiphyseal and nutrient arteries.

KEY POINTS

The Skeletal System

- Two types of connective tissue are found in the skeletal system: (1) cartilage, a semirigid and slightly flexible structure that plays an essential role in prenatal and childhood skeletal development and as a surface for the articulating ends of skeletal joints and (2) bone, which provides for the firm structure of the skeleton and serves as a reservoir for calcium and phosphate storage.

- Bone matrix is maintained by four types of cells: osteoblasts, which synthesize and secrete the constituents of bone; osteoclasts, which resorb surplus bone and are required for bone remodeling; osteocytes, which make up the osteoid tissue of bone; and osteoprogenitor cells, which are the source of all bone cells, except osteoclasts.

Types of Bones

Bones are classified by shape as long, short, flat, or irregular. *Long bones* are found in the upper and lower extremities. *Short bones* are irregularly shaped bones located in the ankle and in the wrist. Except for their surface, which is compact bone, these bones are spongy throughout. *Flat bones* are composed of a layer of cancellous bone between two layers of compact bone.[2] They are found in areas such as the skull and rib cage, where extensive protection of underlying structures is needed, or, as in the scapula, where a broad surface for muscle attachment must be provided. *Irregular bones*, because of their shapes, cannot be classified in any of the previous groups. This group includes bones such as the vertebrae and ethmoid bone.[2]

A typical long bone has a shaft, or *diaphysis*, and two ends, called *epiphyses* (Fig. 47-2). Long bones usually are narrow in the midportion and broad at the ends so weight can be distributed over a wider surface. The shaft of a long bone is formed mainly of compact bone roughly hollowed out to form a marrow-filled medullary canal.[2] The ends of long bones are covered with articular cartilage.[2]

In growing bones, the part of the bone shaft that funnels out as it approaches the epiphysis is called the *metaphysis*.[2] It is composed of bony trabeculae that have cores of cartilage.[2] In the child, the epiphysis is separated from the metaphysis by the cartilaginous growth plate. After puberty, the metaphysis and epiphysis merge, and the growth plate is obliterated.[2]

Periosteum and Endosteum

The *periosteum* covers the bones, except at their articular ends (see Fig. 47-1). The periosteum has an outer fibrous layer and an inner layer that contains the osteoprogenitor cells needed for bone growth and development.[3] The

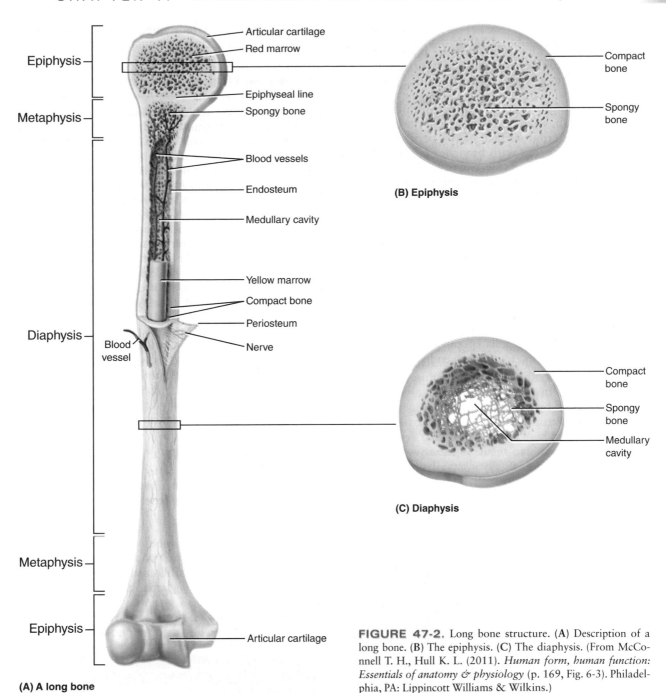

Articular cartilage
Red marrow

Epiphysis

Epiphyseal line
Spongy bone

Metaphysis

Compact bone

Spongy bone

(B) Epiphysis

Blood vessels

Endosteum

Medullary cavity

Yellow marrow

Compact bone

Periosteum

Diaphysis

Blood vessel

Nerve

Compact bone

Spongy bone

Medullary cavity

(C) Diaphysis

Metaphysis

Epiphysis

Articular cartilage

(A) A long bone

FIGURE 47-2. Long bone structure. (**A**) Description of a long bone. (**B**) The epiphysis. (**C**) The diaphysis. (From McConnell T. H., Hull K. L. (2011). *Human form, human function: Essentials of anatomy & physiology* (p. 169, Fig. 6-3). Philadelphia, PA: Lippincott Williams & Wilkins.)

periosteum contains blood vessels and acts as an anchor for vessels as they enter and exit the bone. The endosteum is the membrane that lines the spaces of spongy bone, the marrow cavities, and the Haversian canals of cortical bone. It is composed mainly of osteoprogenitor cells that contribute to the growth and remodeling of bone and are necessary for bone repair.[2]

Bone Marrow

Bone marrow occupies the medullary cavities of the long bones throughout the skeleton and the cavities of cancellous bone in the vertebrae, ribs, sternum, and flat bones of the pelvis. The cellular composition of the bone marrow varies with age and skeletal location. Red bone marrow contains developing red blood cells and is the site of blood cell formation. Yellow bone marrow is composed largely of adipose cells.[3] At birth, nearly all marrow is red and hematopoietically active. As the need for red blood cell production decreases during postnatal life, red marrow is gradually replaced with yellow bone marrow in most of the bones.

 Concept Mastery Alert

In the adult, red marrow persists in the vertebrae, ribs, sternum, and ilia.

symphysis pubis, and insertions of joint capsules. It is also essential for growth before and after birth. In the embryo, most of the axial and appendicular skeleton is formed first as a cartilage model and then replaced by bone. In postnatal life, cartilage continues to play an essential role in the growth of long bones and persists as articular cartilage in the adult.

As a tissue, cartilage both resembles and differs from bone. Both of these connective tissue types consist of living cells, nonliving intercellular fibers, and an amorphous ground substance. The tissue cells are responsible for secreting and maintaining the intercellular substances in which they are housed. However, cartilage consists of more extracellular substance than does bone, and its fibers are embedded in a firm gel rather than a calcified cement-like substance.[2] Hence, cartilage has the flexibility of a firm plastic material rather than the rigid characteristics of bone. In fact, articular cartilage has many advantageous characteristics and is considered resilient. Although resilient, it has poor healing properties and is challenging to repair when injured.[6]

There are three types of cartilage: elastic cartilage, hyaline cartilage, and fibrocartilage.[4] *Elastic cartilage* contains some elastin in its intercellular substance. It is found in areas such as the ear, where some flexibility is important. Pure cartilage is called *hyaline cartilage* (from a Greek word meaning "glass") and is pearly white and opaque. *Fibrocartilage* has characteristics that are between dense connective tissue and hyaline cartilage. It is found in the intervertebral disks, areas where tendons are connected to bone, and the symphysis pubis.[4] In pregnancy, the flexibility of the fibrocartilage allows the symphysis pubis to widen.[7]

Hyaline cartilage is the most abundant type of cartilage. It forms much of the cartilage of the fetal skeleton. In the adult, hyaline cartilage forms the costal cartilages that join the ribs to the sternum and vertebrae, many of the cartilages of the respiratory tract, the articular cartilages, and the epiphyseal plates.

Cartilage cells, which are called **chondrocytes**, are located in lacunae. The lacunae are surrounded by an uncalcified, gellike intercellular matrix of collagen fibers and ground substance. Cartilage is devoid of blood vessels and nerves.[3] The free surfaces of most hyaline cartilage, with the exception of articular cartilage, are covered by a layer of fibrous connective tissue called the *perichondrium*.

It has been estimated that approximately 80% of the wet weight of cartilage is water held in its gel structure. Because cartilage has no blood vessels, this tissue fluid allows the diffusion of gases, nutrients, and wastes between the chondrocytes and blood vessels outside the cartilage.[4] Diffusion cannot take place if the cartilage matrix becomes impregnated with calcium salts, and cartilage dies if it becomes calcified. The other 20% of cartilage consists of two types of macromolecules: type II collagen and proteoglycans.[4]

Hormonal Control of Bone Formation and Metabolism

The process of bone formation and mineral metabolism is complex. It involves the interplay among the actions of

PTH, calcitonin, and vitamin D. Other hormones, such as cortisol, growth hormone, thyroid hormone, and the sex hormones, also influence bone formation directly or indirectly (Table 47-2).

Parathyroid Hormone

PTH is an important regulator of calcium and phosphate levels in the blood.[5] In addition, PTH has been found to be advantageous in fracture healing and prevention of further deterioration of osteoporosis if given as a supplement.[8,9] PTH prevents serum calcium levels from falling below and serum phosphate levels from rising above normal physiologic concentrations.[5] The secretion of PTH is regulated by negative feedback; increased serum levels of ionized calcium inhibit PTH release. PTH maintains serum calcium levels by initiation of calcium release from bone, by conservation of calcium by the kidney, by enhanced intestinal absorption of calcium through activation of vitamin D, and by reduction of serum phosphate levels (Fig. 47-4).[2,4] PTH also increases the movement of calcium and phosphate from bone into the extracellular fluid. Calcium is immediately released from the canaliculi and bone cells. A more prolonged release of calcium and phosphate is mediated by increased osteoclast activity. In the kidney,

TABLE 47-2 Actions of Parathyroid Hormone, Calcitonin, and Vitamin D

Actions	Parathyroid Hormone	Calcitonin	Vitamin D
Intestinal absorption of calcium	Increases indirectly through increased activation of vitamin D	Probably not affected	Increases
Intestinal absorption of phosphate	Increases	Probably not affected	Increases
Renal excretion of calcium	Decreases	Increases	Probably increases, but less effective than PTH
Renal excretion of phosphate	Increases	Increases	Increases
Bone resorption	Increases	Decreases	$1,25\text{-}(OH)_2D_3$ increases
Bone formation	Decreases	Uncertain	$24,25\text{-}(OH)_2D_3$ increases
Serum calcium levels	Produces a prompt increase	Decreases with pharmacologic doses	No effect
Serum phosphate levels	Prevents an increase	Decreases with pharmacologic doses	No effect

PTH, parathyroid hormone.

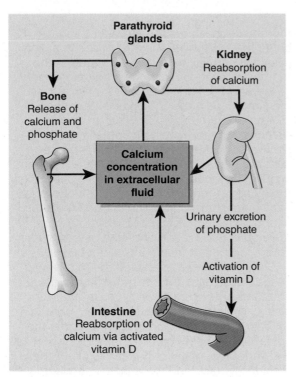

FIGURE 47-4. Regulation and actions of PTH. The PTH drives the serum calcium level by triggering release of calcium from the bone, appropriately conserving calcium by the kidney, and by further increasing calcium in the intestine by activating vitamin D. PTH, parathyroid hormone.

PTH stimulates tubular reabsorption of calcium while reducing the reabsorption of phosphate. The latter effect ensures that increased release of phosphate from bone during mobilization of calcium does not produce an elevation in serum phosphate levels. This is important because an increase in calcium and phosphate levels could lead to crystallization in soft tissues. PTH increases intestinal absorption of calcium because of its ability to stimulate activation of vitamin D by the kidney.

Calcitonin

PTH increases blood calcium levels, whereas the hormone calcitonin lowers blood calcium levels.[5] Calcitonin, sometimes called *thyrocalcitonin*, is secreted by the parafollicular, or C cells of the thyroid gland. Calcitonin inhibits the release of calcium from bone into the extracellular fluid.[5] It is thought to act by causing calcium to sequester in bone cells and inhibiting osteoclast activity. Calcitonin also reduces the renal tubular reabsorption of calcium and phosphate.[2]

The major stimulus for calcitonin synthesis and release is an increase in serum calcium.[5] The role of calcitonin in overall mineral homeostasis is uncertain. There are no clearly definable syndromes of calcitonin deficiency or excess, which suggests that calcitonin does not directly alter calcium metabolism. It has been suggested that the physiologic actions of calcitonin are related to the postprandial handling and processing of dietary calcium. This theory proposes that after meals, calcitonin maintains PTH secretion at a time when it normally would be reduced by calcium entering the blood from the digestive tract. Although states of excess or deficiency associated with alterations in physiologic levels of calcitonin have not been observed, it has been shown that pharmacologic doses of the hormone reduce osteoclastic activity. Because of this action, calcitonin has proved effective in the treatment of Paget disease. The hormone is also used to reduce serum calcium levels during hypercalcemic crises.

Vitamin D

Vitamin D and its metabolites are not true vitamins but steroid hormones. There are two forms of vitamin D: vitamin D_2 (ergocalciferol) and vitamin D_3 (cholecalciferol).[5] The two forms differ by the presence of a double bond, but they have identical biologic activity. The term *vitamin D* is used to indicate both forms.[10]

Vitamin D has little or no activity until it has been converted to be physiologically active and metabolized to compounds that mediate its activity. Figure 47-5 depicts sources of vitamin D and pathways for activation.

The two sources of vitamin D are intestinal absorption and skin production. Intestinal absorption occurs mainly in the jejunum and includes vitamin D_2 and vitamin D_3.

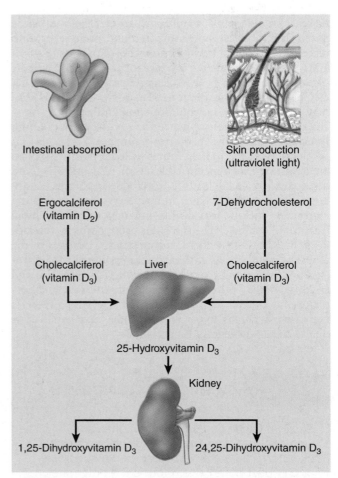

FIGURE 47-5. Sources and pathways for activation of vitamin D. The vitamin D source comes from the skin and the intestine. Vitamin D is then hydroxylated into 25-hydroxyvitamin D_3 in the liver and then goes to the kidneys where it is converted into 24,25-dihydroxyvitamin D_3.

The most important dietary sources of vitamin D are fish, liver, and irradiated milk. Because vitamin D is fat soluble, its absorption is mediated by bile salts and occurs by means of the lymphatic vessels.[5] In the skin, ultraviolet radiation from sunlight spontaneously converts 7-dehydrocholesterol D_3 to vitamin D_3. A circulating vitamin D–binding protein provides a mechanism to remove vitamin D from the skin and make it available to the rest of the body.

With adequate exposure to sunlight, the amount of vitamin D that can be produced by the skin is usually sufficient to meet physiologic requirements. The importance of sunlight exposure is evidenced by population studies that report lower vitamin D levels in countries such as England, which have less sunlight than does the United States. Older adults who are housebound or institutionalized frequently have low vitamin D levels. The deficiency often goes undetected until there are problems such as pseudofractures or electrolyte imbalances. Seasonal variations in vitamin D levels probably reflect changes in sunlight exposure.

The most potent of the vitamin D metabolites is $1,25\text{-}(OH)_2D_3$.[5] This metabolite increases intestinal absorption of calcium and promotes the actions of PTH on resorption of calcium and phosphate from bone.[5] Bone resorption by the osteoclasts is increased, and bone formation by the osteoblasts is decreased. There is also an increase in acid phosphatase and a decrease in alkaline phosphatase. Intestinal absorption and bone resorption increase the amount of calcium and phosphorus available to the mineralizing surface of the bone. The role of $24,25\text{-}(OH)_2D_3$ is less clear. There is evidence that $24,25\text{-}(OH)_2D_3$, in conjunction with $1,25\text{-}(OH)_2D_3$, may be involved in normal bone mineralization.

Several hormones influence the regulation of vitamin D activity. PTH and prolactin stimulate $1,25\text{-}(OH)_2D_3$ production by the kidney. States of hyperparathyroidism are associated with increased levels of $1,25\text{-}(OH)_2D_3$, and hypoparathyroidism leads to lowered levels of this metabolite.[5] Prolactin may have an ancillary role in regulating vitamin D metabolism during pregnancy and lactation. Calcitonin inhibits $1,25\text{-}(OH)_2D_3$ production by the kidneys. In addition to hormonal influences, changes in the concentration of ions such as calcium, phosphate, hydrogen, and potassium exert an effect on $1,25\text{-}(OH)_2D_3$ and $24,25\text{-}(OH)_2D_3$ production. Under conditions of phosphate and calcium deprivation, $1,25\text{-}(OH)_2D_3$ levels are increased, whereas hyperphosphatemia and hypercalcemia decrease the levels of metabolite.

SUMMARY CONCEPTS

Skeletal tissue consists of the bones and cartilage that form the appendicular and axial skeleton. There are two types of bone: cortical or compact bone, which forms the outer shell of a bone, and cancellous or spongy bone that forms the interior. The endosteum is the membrane that lines the spaces of spongy bone, the marrow cavities, and the Haversian canals of cortical bone. The periosteum, the membrane that covers bones, contains blood vessels and acts as an anchor for vessels as they enter and leave the bone. Mature bone is largely made up of cylindrical units called *osteons*, formed from concentric layers or lamellae of bone matrix and surrounding a central *Haversian canal*. The Haversian canals contain the blood vessels and nerve supply for the osteon. There are four types of bone cells: osteocytes, or mature bone cells; osteoblasts, or bone-building cells; osteoclasts, which function in bone resorption; and osteoprogenitor cells, which differentiate into osteoblasts.

Cartilage is a firm, flexible type of skeletal tissue that is essential for growth before and after birth. There are three types of cartilage: elastic, hyaline, and fibrocartilage. Hyaline cartilage, the most abundant type, forms the costal cartilages that join the ribs to the sternum and vertebrae, many of the cartilages of the respiratory tract, and the articular cartilages.

The process of bone formation and mineral metabolism involves the interplay of PTH, calcitonin, and vitamin D. PTH acts to maintain serum levels of ionized calcium; it increases the release of calcium and phosphate from bone; the conservation of calcium and elimination of phosphate by the kidney; and the intestinal reabsorption of calcium through vitamin D. Calcitonin inhibits the release of calcium from bone and increases renal elimination of calcium and phosphate, thereby serving to lower serum calcium levels. Vitamin D functions as a hormone in regulating body calcium. It increases absorption of calcium from the intestine and promotes the actions of PTH on bone.

Articulations and Joints

Articulations, or joints, are areas where two or more bones meet. The term *arthro* is the prefix used to designate a joint; for example, *arthrology* is the study of joints, and *arthroplasty* is the repair of a joint.

Tendons and Ligaments

In the skeletal system, tendons and ligaments are dense connective tissue structures that connect muscles and bones. The dense connective tissue found in tendons and ligaments has a limited blood supply and is composed largely of intercellular bundles of collagen fibers arranged in the same direction and plane (Fig. 47-6). Collagen is a strong, flexible protein.[2] Because of its molecular

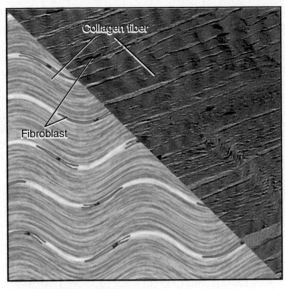

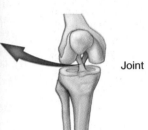

Form
- Cells: a few fibroblasts
- Extracellular matrix: collagenous fibers arranged in bundles (shown here) or irregular networks

Function
- Withstands strong forces
- Attaches structures together
- Forms scar tissue, ligaments, tendons, joint capsules, organ coverings (fascia)

Joint

Dense connective tissue

FIGURE 47-6. Dense connective tissue in tendons and ligaments. This dense connective tissue shows the collagen fibrous tissue and the fibroblasts. Both of these types of cells withstand strong forces and are found in tendons and ligaments. (From McConnell T. H., Hull K. (2011). *Human form, human function: Essentials of anatomy & physiology* (p. 104). Philadelphia, PA: Lippincott Williams & Wilkins.)

configuration, collagen has great tensile strength; the breaking point of collagenous fibers found in human tendons is reached with a force of several hundred kilograms per square centimeter. Fresh collagen is colorless, and tissues that contain large numbers of collagenous fibers generally appear white.

Tendons, which attach skeletal muscles to bone, are relatively inextensible because of their richness in collagen fibers. The collagen bundles of tendons aggregate into bundles that are enveloped by loose connective tissue, blood vessels, and nerves. Tendons that may rub against bone or other friction-generating surfaces are enclosed in double-layered sheaths. An outer connective tissue tube is attached to the structures surrounding the tendon, and an inner sheath encloses the tendon and is attached to it.[3] The space between the inner and outer sheath is filled with a fluid similar to synovial fluid.[3] Overuse can result in *tendonitis* or inflammation of the tendon.

Ligaments are fibrous thickenings of the articular capsule that join one bone to its articulating mate.[3] They vary in size and shape depending on their specific role. Although most ligaments are considered inelastic, they are pliable enough to permit movement at the joints. However, ligaments tear rather than stretch when exposed to excess stress. Torn ligaments are extremely painful and accompanied by local swelling.

Types of Joints

Joints exhibit a variety of movements. Some joints have no movement; others allow only slight movement; and some are freely moveable, such as the shoulder joint. There are two classes of joints depending on their movement and the presence or absence of a joint cavity: solid or synarthroses and synovial joints.[4]

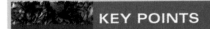

KEY POINTS

Skeletal Joints

- Articulations, or joints, are sites where two or more bones meet to hold the skeleton together and give it mobility.

- There are two types of joints: solid joints, which are immovable, have no cavity, and are bound by connective tissue or cartilage, and synovial joints, which are freely movable and contain a cavity.[11]

Solid or Synarthroses Joints

Solid joints, also called synarthroses, are either fibrous or cartilaginous.[12] The fibrous joints are divided into sutures, gomphoses, and syndesmoses. Sutures are only found in the skull. Gomphoses connect teeth to the jaw. Syndesmoses are where a ligament connects two adjacent bones. These include the ligamentum flavum, which connect vertebral laminae, and the interosseous membrane that connect the radius and ulna in the forearm. Cartilaginous joints can be divided into synchondroses and symphyses. Synchondroses are where a layer of cartilage separates two ossification centers in a developing bone such as the growth plate found in developing long bone. These are designed for bone growth and eventually ossify. Symphyses are joints in which two separate bones are connected by cartilage. These include the pubic symphysis intervertebral disks.[13]

Synovial (Diarthrodial) Joints

Synovial or diarthrodial joints are freely movable.[3] Most joints in the body are of this type. Although they are classified as freely movable, their movement ranges from almost none (*e.g.*, sacroiliac joint), to simple hinge movement (*e.g.*, interphalangeal joint), to movement in many planes (*e.g.*, shoulder or hip joint). The bony surfaces of these joints are covered with thin layers of articular cartilage, and the cartilaginous surfaces of these joints slide past each other during movement. Diarthrodial joints are the joints most frequently affected by rheumatic disorders.

In a diarthrodial joint, the articulating ends of the bones are not connected directly but are indirectly linked by a strong fibrous capsule (*i.e.*, joint capsule) that surrounds the joint and is continuous with the periosteum (Fig. 47-7). This capsule supports the joint and helps hold the bones in place. Additional support may be provided by ligaments that extend between the bones of the joint.

The joint capsule consists of two layers: an outer fibrous layer and an inner membrane, the synovium.[3] The synovium surrounds the tendons that pass through the joints and the free margins of other intra-articular structures such as ligaments and menisci. The synovium forms folds that surround the margins of articulations but do not cover the weight-bearing articular cartilage. These folds permit stretching of the synovium so that movement can occur without tissue damage.

The synovium secretes a slippery fluid called *synovial fluid*.[3] This fluid acts as a lubricant and facilitates the movement of the articulating surfaces of the joint. Normal synovial fluid is clear or pale yellow, does not clot, and contains fewer than 100 cells/mm^3. The cells are predominantly mononuclear cells derived from the synovium. The composition of the synovial fluid is altered in many inflammatory and pathologic joint disorders. Aspiration and examination of the synovial fluid play an important role in the diagnosis of joint diseases.

The articular cartilage is an example of hyaline cartilage and is unique in that its free surface is not covered with perichondrium.[3] It has only a peripheral rim of perichondrium, and calcification of the portion of cartilage abutting the bone may limit or preclude diffusion from blood vessels supplying the **subchondral** bone. Articular cartilage is apparently nourished by the diffusion of substances contained in the synovial fluid bathing the cartilage. Regeneration of most cartilage is slow. It is accomplished primarily by growth that requires the activity of perichondrium cells. In articular cartilage, which has no perichondrium, superficial injuries heal slowly.

Blood Supply and Innervation

All the tissues of synovial joints, except the articulating surfaces of the articulating cartilage, receive nourishment either directly or indirectly from blood vessels.[14] The articulating areas are nourished indirectly by the synovial fluid that is distributed over the surface of the articular cartilage.

The blood supply to a joint arises from blood vessels that enter the subchondral bone at or near the attachment of the joint capsule and form an arterial circle around the joint. The synovial membrane has a rich blood supply, and constituents of plasma diffuse rapidly between these vessels and the joint cavity. Because many of the capillaries are near the surface of the synovium, blood may escape into the synovial fluid after relatively minor injuries. Healing and repair of the synovial membrane are usually rapid and complete. This is important because synovial tissue is often injured during surgical procedures that involve the joint.

The nerve supply to joints is provided by the same nerve trunks that supply the muscles that move the joints. These nerve trunks also supply the skin over the joints. As a rule, all the peripheral nerves that cross the articulation innervate each joint of an extremity. This accounts for the referral of pain from one joint to another. For example, pain from injury to the knee is often experienced as pain in the hip. The synovial membrane is only innervated by autonomic fibers that control blood flow. It is relatively free of pain fibers, as evidenced by the fact that surgical procedures on the joint are often done under local anesthesia. The joint capsule and the ligaments have pain receptors. These receptors are more easily stimulated by stretching and twisting than are other joint structures. Pain arising from the capsule tends to be diffuse and poorly localized.

The tendons and ligaments of the joint capsule are sensitive to position and movement, particularly stretching and twisting.[14] These structures are supplied by the large sensory nerve fibers that form proprioceptor endings. The proprioceptors function reflexively to adjust the tension of the muscles that support the joint and are particularly important in maintaining muscular support for the joint. For example, when a weight is lifted, there is a proprioceptor-mediated reflex contraction and relaxation of appropriate muscle groups to support the joint and protect the joint capsule and other joint structures.

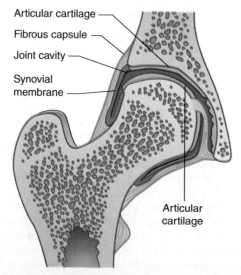

Articular cartilage —
Fibrous capsule —
Joint cavity —
Synovial membrane —

Articular cartilage

FIGURE 47-7. Synovial (diarthrodial) joint, showing the articular cartilage, fibrous joint capsule, joint cavity, and synovial membrane.

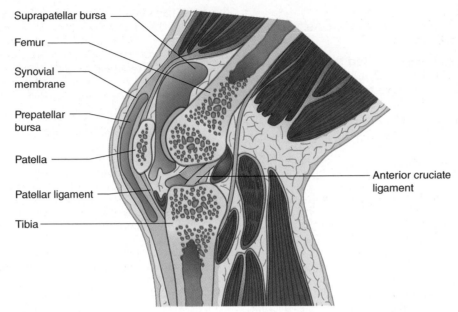

Suprapatellar bursa

Femur

Synovial membrane

Prepatellar bursa

Patella

Patellar ligament

Tibia

Anterior cruciate ligament

FIGURE 47-8. Sagittal section of knee joint, showing prepatellar and suprapatellar bursae.

Loss of proprioception and reflex control of muscular support leads to destructive changes in the joint.

Bursae

In some diarthrotic joints, the synovial membrane forms closed sacs that are not part of the joint. These sacs, called *bursae*, contain synovial fluid.[3] Their purpose is to prevent friction on a tendon. Bursae occur in areas where pressure is exerted because of close approximation of joint structures (Fig. 47-8). Such conditions occur when tendons are deflected over bone or where skin must move freely over bony tissue. Bursae may become injured or inflamed, causing discomfort, swelling, and limitation in movement of the involved area.[3] A bunion is an inflamed bursa of the metatarsophalangeal joint of the great toe.

Intra-Articular Menisci

Intra-articular menisci are fibrocartilage structures that occur in some synovial joints. In the joint capsule, fibrocartilage grows inward to create a pad between articulating bones.[3] Menisci may extend part way through the joint and have a free inner border, as at the lateral and medial articular surfaces of the knee, or they may extend through the joint, separating it into two separate cavities, as in the sternoclavicular joint. The menisci of the knee joint may be torn as the result of an injury.

to bones and ligaments connect the movable bones of joints.

Synarthroses are joints in which bones are joined together by fibrous tissue, cartilage, or bone; they lack a joint cavity and have little or no movement. Synovial or diarthrodial joints are freely movable. The surfaces of the articulating ends of bones in synovial joints are covered with a thin layer of articular cartilage, and they are enclosed in a fibrous joint capsule. The joint capsule consists of two layers: an outer fibrous layer and an inner membrane, the synovium. The synovial fluid, which is secreted by the synovium into the joint capsule, acts as a lubricant and facilitates movement of the joint's articulating surfaces. **Bursae**, which are closed sacs containing synovial fluid, prevent friction in areas where tendons are deflected over bone or where skin must move freely over bony tissue.

Menisci are fibrocartilaginous structures that develop from portions of the articular disk that occupied the space between articular cartilage surfaces during fetal development. The menisci may have a free inner border, or they may extend through the joint, separating it into two cavities.

SUMMARY CONCEPTS

Articulations or joints are areas where two or more bones meet. Tendons and ligaments are dense connective tissue structures that connect muscles and bones. Tendons connect muscles

Review Exercises

1. Often, pain from injury to the knee is experienced as pain in the hip.
   A. Explain why this might occur.

2. Persons with end-stage kidney disease have a deficiency of activated vitamin D.

A. Explain why this occurs and what effect it would have on their bones.

3. Recent studies have revealed that estrogen deficiency as well as normal aging may produce a decrease in osteoblast activity.
   A. Explain how this would contribute to the development of osteoporosis.

REFERENCES

1. Selitz I. A., Teven C. M., Reid R. R. (2018). Repair and grafting of bone. In Gurtner G. C., Neligan P. C. (Eds.), *Plastic surgery, Vol. 1: Principles* (4th ed., pp. 18, 284–314.e.10). London/New York/Philadelphia/St. Louis/Sydney: Elsevier.
2. Ross M. H., Pawlina W. (2016). *Histology: A text and atlas: With correlated cell and molecular biology.* Philadelphia, PA: Lippincott Williams & Wilkins.
3. Saladin K. S. (2015). *Anatomy & physiology: The unity of form and function* (7th ed.). New York, NY: McGraw Hill Education.
4. Rubin R., Strayer D. (Eds.). (2012). *Rubin's pathology: Clinicopathologic foundations of medicine* (6th ed.). Philadelphia, PA: Lippincott Williams & Wilkins.
5. Hall J. E. (2016). *Guyton and Hall textbook of medical physiology* (13th ed.). Philadelphia, PA: Saunders.
6. Vinatier C., Guicheux J. (2016). Cartilage tissue engineering: From biomaterials and stem cells to osteoarthritis treatments. *Annals of Physical and Rehabilitation Medicine* 59(3), 139–144.
7. Eickmeyer S. M. (2017). Anatomy and physiology of the pelvic floor. *Physical Medicine and Rehabilitation Clinics of North America* 28, 455–460.
8. Chan K. Y., Mason A., Cooper C., et al. (2016). Novel advances in the treatment of osteoporosis. *British Medical Bulletin* 119(1), 129–142.
9. Collinge C., Favela J. (2016). Use of teriparatide in osteoporotic fracture patients. *Injury* 47(S1), s36–s38.
10. Deluca H. F., Plum L. (Eds.). (2012). The many faces of vitamin D. *Archives of Biochemistry and Biophysics* 523(1), 1–134.
11. Drake R. L., Vogl A. W., Mitchell A. W. M. (2015). *Gray's anatomy for students* (3rd ed.). Philadelphia, PA: Churchill Livingstone.
12. Kumar V., Abbas A. K., Aster J. C. (2015). *Robbins and Cotran pathologic basis of disease* (9th ed.). Philadelphia, PA: Elsevier Saunders.
13. Drake R. L., Vogl A. W., Mitchell A. W. M. (2015). *Gray's basic anatomy.* Philadelphia, PA: Churchill Livingstone.
14. Moore K. L., Dalley A. F., Agur A. M. R. (2017). *Clinically oriented anatomy* (8th ed.). Baltimore, MD: Lippincott Williams & Wilkins.

CHAPTER 48

Disorders of Musculoskeletal Function: Trauma, Infection, Neoplasms

Learning Objectives

After completing this chapter, the learner will be able to meet the following objectives:

1. Describe the healing process of soft-tissue injuries.
2. Describe the fracture healing process.
3. Differentiate the early complications of fractures from later complications of fracture healing.
4. Explain the implications of bone infection.
5. Differentiate among osteomyelitis due to spread from a contaminated wound, hematogenous osteomyelitis, and osteomyelitis due to vascular insufficiency in terms of etiologies, manifestations, and treatment.
6. Describe the most common sites of tuberculosis of the bone.
7. Describe the four major causes of osteonecrosis.
8. Characterize the blood supply of bone as it relates to the pathologic features of the condition.
9. Differentiate between the properties of benign and malignant bone tumors.
10. Contrast osteogenic sarcoma, Ewing sarcoma, and chondrosarcoma in terms of the most common age groups and anatomic sites that are affected.
11. List the primary sites of tumors that frequently metastasize to the bone.

The musculoskeletal system includes the bones, joints, and muscles as well as associated structures such as ligaments and tendons. A human infant is born with over 300 bones. As humans age, some bones fuse, leaving an adult with approximately 206 bones.[1] The musculoskeletal system is subject to a large number of disorders. These disorders affect people in all age groups and walks of life, causing pain and disability. The discussion in this chapter focuses on the effects of trauma, infection, ischemia, and neoplasms on the musculoskeletal structures of the body.

Injury and Trauma of Musculoskeletal Structures

A broad spectrum of musculoskeletal injuries result from physical forces, including blunt tissue trauma, disruption of tendons and ligaments, and fractures of bony structures. Many of the forces that cause injury to the musculoskeletal system are typical for a particular environmental setting, activity, or age group.

Unintentional falls are the number one cause of nonfatal injuries in children and adolescents between 0 and 14 years of age in the United States.[2] Childhood falls cause approximately 2.8 million emergency department visits each year.[2] Sports- and recreation-related injuries send 2.6 million children between the ages of 0 and 19 to the emergency room each year.[3]

Falls are the most common cause of injury in people 65 years of age and older. Three million older adults are treated in the emergency department for fall injuries each year, and 95% of all hip fractures are caused by falls.[4] Falls among older adults are often due to physiologic changes such as alteration in balance, vision and hearing decline, and unsteady gait. Environmental risks such as inadequate lighting, spills, or even the use of stools or ladders to reach objects in high places can increase the number of falls. Osteoporosis is also a known risk for injury with falls.[5,6] Fall prevention in older adults should focus on strength and balance exercises and vitamin D supplements to improve mobility and bone strength. Polypharmacy, another risk factor for falls, can be mitigated by review of medications. Although most injuries associated with a fall are not serious, mortality following a hip fracture ranges from 18% to 33%.[6]

Athletic Injuries

Athletic injuries are either acute injuries or overuse injuries. Acute injuries are caused by sudden trauma and include injuries to soft tissues (contusion, strains, and sprains) and to bone (fractures). Overuse injuries occur when physical activity applies ongoing and excessive stress to normal musculoskeletal tissue, which fails to adapt.[7] Overuse injuries represent the majority of sports-related injuries among children and adolescents.[7] They commonly occur in the elbow and in tissue where tendons attach to the bone; particularly vulnerable are the apophyses and cartilaginous growth plates in sites such as the heel, elbow, and knee.[8] Because of the vulnerability of growing bones, the consequences of overuse injury are much greater among children and adolescents than among adults.[8] Many factors contribute to the potential for injury among adolescent athletes including height and weight, muscle growth and strength, motor skills and performance, body composition, flexibility, growth plate bone structure, and psychological maturity.[7] The treatment of overuse injuries is focused on rest and modification of activities prevention, and education and early diagnosis are essential.[8]

Soft-Tissue Injuries

Most skeletal injuries are accompanied by soft-tissue (muscle, tendon, or ligament) injuries. These injuries include contusions, hematomas, and lacerations. They are discussed here because of their association with musculoskeletal injuries.

A *contusion* is an injury to soft tissue that results from direct trauma and is usually caused by striking a body part against a hard object. With a contusion, the skin overlying the injury remains intact. Initially, the area becomes ecchymotic because of local hemorrhage; later, the discoloration gradually changes to brown and then to yellow as the blood is reabsorbed. A large area of local hemorrhage is called a *hematoma*. Hematomas cause pain because blood accumulates and exerts pressure on nerve endings. The pain increases with movement or when pressure is applied to the area. The pain and swelling of a hematoma take longer to subside than do those accompanying a contusion. A hematoma may become infected because of bacterial growth. Unlike a contusion, which does not drain, a hematoma may eventually split the skin because of increased pressures and produce drainage. Treatment of a contusion or hematoma consists of elevating the affected part and applying cold compresses every 4 hours for about 20 minutes at a time to reduce the bleeding into the area. A hematoma may need to be aspirated.

A *laceration* is an injury in which the skin is torn or its continuity is disrupted. The seriousness of a laceration depends on the size and depth of the wound and on whether there is contamination from the object that caused the injury. Puncture wounds from nails or rusted material provide the setting for growth of anaerobic bacteria such as those that cause tetanus and gas gangrene.

Lacerations are usually treated by wound closure, which is done after the area is sufficiently cleaned. The closed wound is then covered with a sterile dressing. It is important to minimize contamination of the wound and control bleeding. Contaminated wounds and open fractures are copiously irrigated and debrided, and the skin usually is left open to heal to prevent the development of an anaerobic infection or a sinus tract. Antimicrobial agents are selectively used depending on the suspected nature of the contaminants.

Joint (Musculotendinous) Injuries

Joints, or articulations, are sites where two or more bones meet. Joints (*i.e.*, diarthrodial joints) are supported by tough bundles of collagenous fibers called *ligaments* that attach to the joint capsule and bind the articular ends of bones together, and by *tendons* that join muscles to the periosteum of the articulating bones.[9] Joint injuries involve mechanical overloading or forcible twisting or stretching.

Strains and Sprains

Strains

A *strain* is a stretching injury to a muscle or a musculotendinous unit caused by mechanical overloading. This type of injury may result from an unusual muscle contraction or an excessive forcible stretch. Although there usually is no external evidence of a specific injury, pain, stiffness, and swelling exist. The most common sites for muscle strains are the lower back and the cervical region of the spine. The elbow and the shoulder are also supported by musculotendinous units, which are subject to strains. Foot strain is associated with the weight-bearing stresses of the feet. It may be caused by inadequate muscular and ligamentous support, being overweight, or excessive standing, walking, or running.

In the lumbar and cervical spine regions, muscle strains are more common than are sprains. Mechanical low back pain is becoming increasingly common in the adolescent athlete.[10] Overuse, especially hyperextension of the lumbar spine in such sports as track, wrestling, gymnastics, and diving, can tear the muscles, fascia, and ligaments. Careful diagnosis is necessary because chronic low back pain may indicate spondylolysis (stress fracture of the pars intra-articularis) or spondylolisthesis (vertebral displacement), which are the most commonly occurring causes.[11] Determining the location of the pain during motion helps in diagnosis and treatment.[12] Fractures near the top and bottom surface of the vertebrae can occur when the growing lumbar spine is overstressed, causing the disks to push into the spinal nerve roots. Early detection and treatment are important to prevent complications and disability. Treatment of back strains consists of a short period of rest and mild analgesics followed by a gradual return to activities. Cold packs or ice should be used to reduce pain and swelling of the affected area. Exercises, correct posture, and good body mechanics help reduce the risk of reinjury.

Sprains

A *sprain*, which involves the ligamentous structures (strong bands of connective tissue) surrounding the joint, resembles a strain, but the pain and swelling subside more slowly. It usually is caused by abnormal or excessive movement of the joint. With a sprain, the ligaments may be incompletely torn or, as in a severe sprain, completely torn or ruptured (Fig. 48-1).[13] Occasionally, a chip of bone is evident when the entire ligament, including part of its bony attachment, has been ruptured or torn from the bone. The signs of sprain are

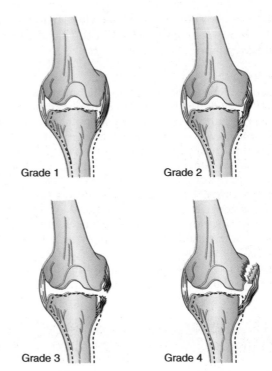

FIGURE 48-1. Degrees of sprain on the medial side of the right knee: grade 1, mild sprain of the medial collateral ligament; grade 2, moderate sprain with hematoma formation; grade 3, severe sprain with total disruption of the ligament; and grade 4, severe sprain with avulsion of the medial femoral condyle at the insertion of the medial collateral ligament.

pain, rapid swelling, heat, disability, discoloration, and limitation of function.

Any joint may be sprained, but the ankle joint is most commonly involved, especially in fast-moving injuries in which the ankle or knee can be suddenly twisted.[13] Most ankle sprains occur in the lateral ankle when the foot is turned inward under a person, forcing the ankle into inversion beyond the structural limits.[13] Other common sites of sprain are the knee (the collateral ligament and anterior cruciate ligament [ACL]) and elbow (the ulnar side). As with a strain, the soft-tissue injury that occurs with a sprain is not evident on the radiograph. Wrist sprains most often occur with a fall on an outstretched hand.

Healing

If properly treated, musculotendinous injuries usually heal with the restoration of the original tensile strength. Repair is accomplished by fibroblasts from the inner tendon sheath or, if the tendon has no sheath, from the loose connective tissue that surrounds the tendon. Capillaries infiltrate the injured area during the initial healing process and supply the fibroblasts with the materials they need to produce large amounts of collagen. Formation of the long collagen bundles occurs within the first 2 weeks, and although tensile strength increases steadily thereafter, it is not sufficient to permit strong tendon pulls for approximately 2 months. During the healing process, there is a danger that muscle contraction will pull the injured ends apart, causing the tendon to heal in the lengthened position. There is also a danger that adhesions will develop in areas where tendons pass through fibrous channels, such as in the distal palm of the hands, rendering the tendon useless.

Treatment

The treatment of muscle strains and ligamentous sprains is similar in several ways. For an injured extremity, elevation of the part followed by local application of cold compresses may be sufficient. Compression, accomplished using adhesive wraps or a removable splint, helps reduce swelling and provides support. A cast is applied for severe sprains, especially those severe enough to warrant surgical repair. Immobilization for a muscle strain is continued until the pain and swelling have subsided. In a sprain, the affected joint is immobilized for several weeks. Immobilization may be followed by graded active exercises. Early diagnosis, treatment, and rehabilitation are essential in preventing chronic ligamentous instability.

KEY POINTS

Joint Injuries

■ Joints are the weakest part of the skeletal system and common sites of injury because of mechanical overloading or forcible twisting or stretching.

■ Injury can include damage to the tendons, which connect muscle to bone; ligaments, which hold bones together; or the cartilage that covers the articular surface.

■ Healing of the dense connective tissue involved in joint injuries requires time to restore the structures so that they are strong enough to withstand the forces imposed on the joint. Ligamentous injuries may require surgical intervention with approximation of many fibrous strands to facilitate healing.

■ Injuries involving the articular cartilage may predispose to later joint disease.

Dislocations

A *dislocation* involves the displacement or separation of the bone ends of a joint with loss of articulation. It usually follows a severe trauma that disrupts the holding ligaments. Dislocations are seen most often in the shoulder and acromioclavicular joints. The shoulder is a complex and unstable joint.[14,15] Most traumatic shoulder dislocations are anterior or are recurrent episodes of a previous injury: either a dislocation or a subluxation.[16] A *subluxation* is a partial dislocation in which the bone ends in the joint are still in partial contact with each other. The first occurrence of an anterior dislocation happens most often in young males and as a result of contact, with recurrence being common.[14,15]

Dislocations can be congenital, traumatic, or pathologic. Congenital dislocations occur in the hip and knee. Traumatic dislocations occur after falls, blows, or rotational injuries. In the shoulder and patella, dislocations may become recurrent, especially in athletes. They recur with the same motion but require less and less force each time to cause the damage.

Pathologic dislocation in the hip is a late complication of infection, rheumatoid arthritis, paralysis, and neuromuscular diseases. Dislocations of the phalangeal joints are not serious and are usually reduced by manipulation. Less common sites of dislocation, seen mainly in young adults, are the wrist and midtarsal region. They usually are the result of direct force, such as a fall on an outstretched hand. Diagnosis of a dislocation is based on history, physical examination, and radiologic findings. The symptoms are pain, deformity, and limited movement.

The treatment depends on the site, mechanism of injury, and associated injuries such as fractures. Dislocations that do not reduce spontaneously usually require manipulation or surgical repair. Various surgical procedures also can be used to prevent redislocation of the patella, shoulder, or acromioclavicular joints. Immobilization is necessary after reduction of a dislocation to allow healing of the joint structures. In dislocations affecting the knee, closed reduction with knee immobilization may be prescribed, although open reduction may be required in the case of vascular or soft-tissue damage.[17]

Loose Bodies

Loose bodies are small pieces of bone or cartilage within a joint space. These can result from trauma to the joint or may occur when cartilage has worn away from the articular surface, causing a necrotic piece of bone to separate and become free floating. The symptoms are painful and often cause catching and locking of the joint. Loose bodies are commonly seen in the knee, elbow, hip, and ankle. The loose body repeatedly gets caught in the crevice of a joint, pinching the underlying healthy cartilage. Unless the loose body is removed, it may cause osteoarthritis and restricted movement. The treatment consists of removal using operative arthroscopy.

Shoulder and Rotator Cuff Injuries

The shoulder is a complex series of joints that produce extraordinary range of motion. The extreme mobility is accomplished at the expense of relative instability. This instability, combined with its relatively exposed position, makes the shoulder extremely vulnerable to injuries such as sprains and dislocations and degenerative processes such as rotator cuff disorders.

The shoulder is composed of three bones: the scapula, the clavicle, and the humerus. The scapula articulates with the humerus by way of the glenoid cavity and with the clavicle at the **acromion** process as well as closely with the chest wall. Clavicle fractures are among the most common fractures of childhood. The typical mechanism of fracture is a fall on the point of the shoulder.

Four articulations form the shoulder joint—the acromioclavicular joint that joins the clavicle to the acromion of the scapula, the sternoclavicular joint that joins the sternum to the clavicle, the glenohumeral joint that connects the head of the humerus to the relatively shallow glenoid cavity in the scapula, and the thoracoscapular joint that joins the posterior thoracic cage and the anterior scapula.[16] The stability of these joints is provided by a series of muscles and tendons. Sprains of the acromioclavicular joint can occur as a result of direct or indirect forces such as contact sports or a fall.[18] The most common site of shoulder dislocation is the glenohumeral joint.[19] Most acute dislocations involve anterior displacement of the humeral head with respect to the glenoid cavity, the result of the shoulder being abducted and forcefully extended and rotated. Other mechanisms include a fall on an outstretched arm or a blow to the posterior shoulder.

Motion of the arm involves the coordinated movement of muscles of the rotator cuff (supraspinatus, teres minor, infraspinatus, subscapularis) and their musculotendinous attachments.[17,20] These muscles are separated from the overlying coracoacromial arch by two bursae, the subdeltoid and subcoracoid. These two bursae, sometimes referred to as the *subacromial bursae*, often communicate and are affected by lesions of the rotator cuff.

The rotator cuff (Fig. 48-2) is like other muscle groups of the body in that its risk of injury increases when it is required to perform a high-stress function in an unconditioned state. Rotator cuff injuries and impingement disorders can result from many causes, including excessive use, a direct blow, or stretch injury, usually involving throwing or swinging, as with baseball pitchers or tennis players.

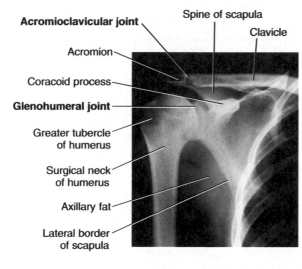

A AP View

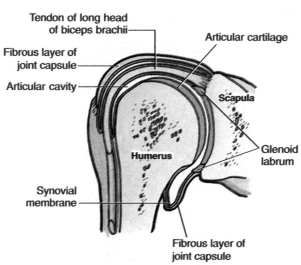

B Coronal section

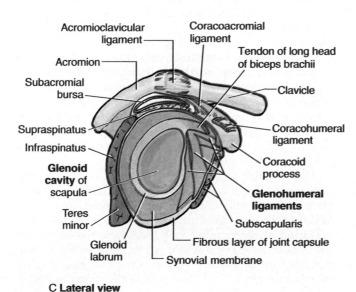

C Lateral view

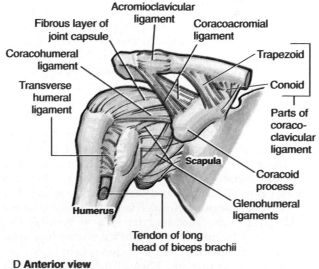

D Anterior view

FIGURE 48-2. The rotator cuff injury. (A) Radiograph. (B) Coronal section of the shoulder's acromioclavicular joint and glenohumeral joint. (C) Lateral view of glenoid cavity. (D) Anterior view of ligaments. (From Moore K. L., Agur A. M., Dalley A. F. (2011). *Essential clinical anatomy* (4th ed., p. 478). Philadelphia, PA: Wolters Kluwer/Lippincott Williams & Wilkins.)

Overuse and degenerative disorders have a slower onset and are seen in older adults with minor or no trauma.[21] The tendons of the rotator cuff fuse together near their insertions into the tuberosities of the humerus to form the musculotendinous cuff. Degeneration of these tendons can result from a number of factors, including repetitive microtrauma, impairment of vascularity as a result of aging, or shoulder instability with secondary overload of the cuff, but incidence does significantly increase with age.[22] Degeneration is most severe near the tendon insertion, with the supraspinous being affected most often. Thickening of the musculotendinous unit decreases the distance between the cuff and the overlying coracoacromial arch. Pain and impingement may be noted when motions of the arm squeeze and pinch these tissues between the humerus and the overlying arch. Overall, rotator cuff injury is caused by a multitude of factors—extrinsic and intrinsic.[17,22]

Several physical examination maneuvers are used to define shoulder pathologic processes.[19,22,23] The history and mechanism of injury are important. In addition to standard radiographs, arthrography, computed tomography (CT), or magnetic resonance imaging (MRI) may be used. Because of the number of rotator cuff injuries, shoulder ultrasound is the most common of the musculoskeletal ultrasound applications.[20] Arthroscopic examination under anesthesia may be used for diagnostic purposes, and operative arthroscopy may be done to repair severe tears. Conservative treatment with anti-inflammatory agents, corticosteroid injections, and physical therapy often is undertaken. A period of rest is followed by a customized exercise and rehabilitation program to improve strength, flexibility, and endurance.[17]

Knee Injuries

The knee is a common site of injury, particularly sports-related injuries in which the knee is subjected to abnormal twisting and compression forces. These forces can result in injury to the menisci, patellar subluxation and dislocation, and chondromalacia. Knee injuries in young adulthood and both knee and hip injuries in middle age are major factors in the development of osteoarthritis.[24]

Meniscus Injuries
The menisci are C-shaped plates of fibrocartilage that are superimposed between the condyles of the femur and tibia. There are two menisci in each knee, a lateral and medial meniscus (Fig. 48-3). The menisci are thicker at their external margins and taper to thin, unattached edges at their interior margin. They are firmly attached at their ends to the intercondylar area of the tibia and are supported by the coronary and transverse ligaments of the knee. The menisci play a major role in load bearing and shock absorption. They also help stabilize the knee by deepening the tibial socket and maintaining the femur and tibia in proper position. In addition, the meniscus assists in joint lubrication and serves as a source of nutrition for articular cartilage in the knee.

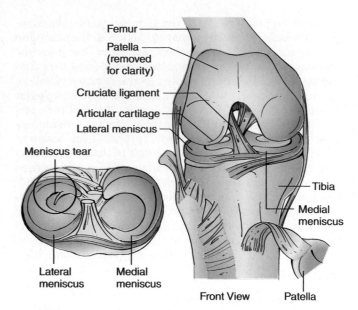

FIGURE 48-3. The knee, showing the lateral and medial meniscus (with the patella removed for clarity). *Inset (lower left)* shows meniscus tear.

Meniscus injury commonly occurs as the result of a rotational injury from a sudden or sharp pivot or a direct blow to the knee, as in hockey, basketball, or football. It is often associated with other injuries, such as a torn ACL. The type and location of the meniscal tear are determined by the magnitude and direction of the force that acts on the knee and the position of the knee at the time of injury. Meniscus tears can be described by their appearance or location.[17] The injured knee is edematous and painful, especially with hyperflexion and hyperextension.

Diagnosis is made by examination and confirmed by MRI. A regular radiograph may be needed to rule out osteoarthritis.[16] Initial treatment of meniscal injuries may be conservative. The knee may be placed in a removable knee immobilizer. Isometric quadriceps exercises may be prescribed. Activity usually is restricted until complete motion is recovered. Arthroscopic meniscectomy may be performed when there are mechanical symptoms, but it is unclear if there is a degenerative or a traumatic tear. For middle-aged adults, it may be difficult to determine whether the tear was the result of osteoarthritis or it will lead to osteoarthritis.[16]

There is evidence that loss of meniscal function is associated with progressive deterioration of knee function.[16] Damaged articular cartilage has a limited capacity to heal because of its avascular nature and inadequate mobilization of regenerative cells. Meniscal reconstruction procedures have been developed to preserve these functions before significant degenerative changes develop, thus preventing a total joint replacement later in life.

Patellar Subluxation and Dislocations
Dislocation of the patella (*i.e.*, knee cap) accounts for approximately 3% of knee injuries, with the first episode often occurring in people under the age of 20.[25]

A recent population-based study found the incidence to be 23.2 per 100,000, with the highest incidence in those between ages 14 and 18, and no major difference between females and males.[26] Dislocation of the patella is often the result of trauma experienced during sports or physical activity.[27] Congenital knee variations are also a predisposing factor.

There is often a sensation of the patella "popping out" when the dislocation occurs.[17] Other complaints include the knee giving out, swelling, crepitus, stiffness, and loss of range of motion. Treatment can be difficult, but nonsurgical methods are used first. They include immobilization with the knee extended, bracing, administration of anti-inflammatory agents, and isometric quadriceps-strengthening exercises. Surgical intervention often is necessary, with numerous options available.[28]

Chondromalacia

Chondromalacia, or degeneration of the articular cartilage, is seen most commonly on the undersurface of the patella.[13] It can be the result of recurrent subluxation of the patella or overuse in strenuous athletic activities. People with this disorder typically complain of pain, particularly when climbing stairs or sitting with the knees bent. Occasionally, the person experiences weakness of the knee.

Treatment consists of rest, isometric exercises, and application of ice after exercise. Part of the patella may be surgically removed in severe cases. In less severe cases, the soft portion is shaved through an arthroscope. Articular cartilage maintenance and repair is a complex process. Polypeptide growth factors that direct cells to divide, differentiate, migrate, and produce matrix appear to have a role in the preservation and degradation of the articular cartilage matrix.

Hip Injuries

The hip is a ball-and-socket joint in which the femoral head articulates deeply in the acetabulum (Fig. 48-4).[9] The proximal part of the femur consists of a head, neck, and greater trochanter. The vascular anatomy of the femoral head is of critical importance in any disorder of the hip. The main sources of blood supply are the intramedullary vessels and the retinacular arteries arising from the circumflex femoral arteries, both of which course from the intertrochanteric region proximally to nourish the femoral head. Disease or injuries that compromise the circulation may damage the viability of the femoral head and lead to avascular necrosis or osteonecrosis. Disorders of the hip include dislocations and fractures of the hip.

Dislocations of the Hip

Dislocations of the hip are the result of severe trauma and can be anterior or posterior, with the posterior being more common.[29] Associated injuries will also impact the outcome of the dislocation.[29]

Hip dislocation is an emergency.[29] In the dislocated position, great tension is placed on the blood supply to the femoral head and avascular necrosis may result.[17,29] Hip osteoarthritis is also a potential long-term

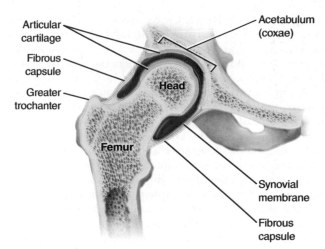

(A) Sectional view

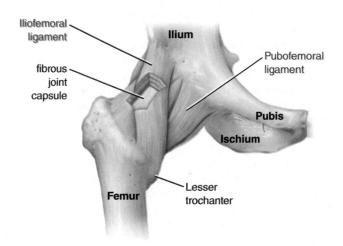

(B) Anterior view

FIGURE 48-4. Right hip joint. **(A)** Sectional view. **(B)** Anterior view. (From McConnell T. H., Hull K. L. (2011). *Human form, human function: Essentials of anatomy & physiology* (p. 218). Philadelphia, PA: Lippincott Williams & Wilkins.)

complication. To prevent these complications, early reduction is indicated.[29] Weight bearing is usually limited after reduction to prevent dislocation from recurring and allow healing to occur.

Fractures of the Hip

Hip fracture is a major public health problem in the Western world, particularly among older adults. It is accompanied by risk of death and impact on function and quality of life.[30] The incidence of hip fractures increases with age. The incidence is also higher in white women as compared to nonwhite women. Risk factors for hip fracture vary with age and sex. For those younger than age 80, greater risk is associated with skeletal issues, whereas for those older than age 80, falls are the greatest risk factor.[31] Osteoporosis and osteopenia are also important contributing factors.

Most hip fractures result from falls. Occasionally, the person may actually fracture the hip before falling, the fracture being caused by twisting or excessive force on a femur that has been weakened by osteoporosis or neoplasms. The characteristics of the fall (the direction, site of impact, and protective response) and environmental factors are important factors influencing the risk of hip fracture from a fall.

A hip fracture is classified according to the anatomic part of the hip where the fracture occurs. Generally, it is a fracture of the proximal femur. Femoral neck fractures are located in the area distal to the femoral head but proximal to the greater and lesser trochanters and are considered intracapsular because they are located within the capsule of the hip joint. Intertrochanteric fractures occur in the metaphyseal region between the greater and lesser trochanter. Subtrochanteric fractures are those that occur just below the greater trochanter. Femoral neck and intertrochanteric fractures account for the majority of hip fractures, occurring in approximately equal proportions.[16,32]

The location of a hip fracture is important in terms of blood flow to the femoral head, which receives its blood supply from vessels that course proximally up the femoral neck (see Fig. 48-4). Subtrochanteric and intertrochanteric fractures that occur distal to these vessels do not usually disturb the blood supply to the femoral head, whereas femoral neck fractures, particularly those involving marked displacement, often disrupt the blood supply to the femoral head and are therefore associated with increased incidence of complications (nonunion and avascular necrosis).[33,34]

Most hip fractures are diagnosed on the basis of clinical findings and standard radiographs. A bone scan or an MRI may be done when the radiograph result is negative, but the clinical findings support the diagnosis of hip fracture. Avascular necrosis often occurs with hip trauma but can also occur without trauma, so it needs to be diagnosed with an MRI.[16]

Impacted fractures have a better prognosis in terms of healing and are often treated nonoperatively or by simple internal fixation to provide stability. Displaced intracapsular fractures in the elderly are usually best treated by surgical hip replacement and early mobilization. Young, healthy people are treated by reduction of the fracture and internal fixation. This method allows for preservation of the femoral head if possible, so a prosthetic is not needed. Intertrochanteric fractures are usually treated with open reduction and internal fixation. Nonunion in this type of fracture is much less common than it is with intracapsular fractures. Weight bearing, however, is usually restricted for 3 months until union of the fracture has occurred.

Fractures

Fracture, or discontinuity of the bone, is the most common type of bone lesion.[33] Normal bone can withstand considerable compression and shearing forces and, to a lesser extent, tension forces. A fracture occurs when more stress is placed on the bone than it can absorb. Grouped according to cause, fractures can be divided into three major categories: fractures caused by sudden injury, fatigue or stress fractures, and pathologic fractures.[33] The most common fractures are those resulting from sudden injury. The force causing the fracture may be direct, such as a fall or blow, or indirect, such as a massive muscle contraction or trauma transmitted along the bone. For example, the head of the radius or clavicle can be fractured by the indirect forces that result from falling on an outstretched hand. A fatigue fracture results from repeated wear on a bone. Pain associated with overuse injuries of the lower extremities, especially posterior medial tibial pain, is one of the most common symptoms that physically active people, such as runners, experience. Stress fractures in the tibia may be confused with "shin splints," a nonspecific term for pain in the lower leg from overuse in walking and running, because they frequently do not appear on x-ray until 2 weeks after the onset of symptoms.

A pathologic fracture occurs in bones that already are weakened by disease or tumors. Fractures of this type may occur spontaneously with little or no stress. The underlying disease state can be local, as with infections, cysts, or tumors, or generalized, as in osteoporosis, Paget disease, or cancer metastasis.[33]

Classification

Fractures usually are classified according to location, type, and direction or pattern of the fracture line (Fig. 48-5). A long bone is divided into three parts: proximal, midshaft, and distal. A fracture of the long bone is described in relation to its position in the bone.

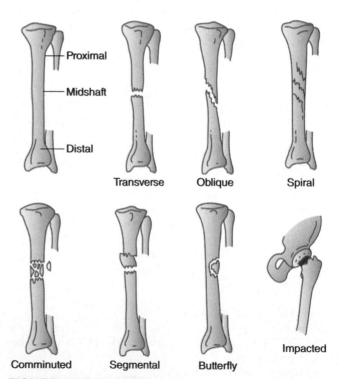

FIGURE 48-5. Classification of fractures. Fractures are classified according to location (proximal, midshaft, or distal), the direction of fracture line (transverse, oblique, spiral), and type (comminuted, segmental, butterfly, or impacted).

Other descriptions are used when the fracture affects the head or neck of a bone, involves a joint, or is near a prominence such as a condyle or malleolus.

The type of fracture is determined by its communication with the external environment, the degree of break in continuity of the bone, and the character of the fracture pieces. When the bone fragments have broken through the skin, the fracture is called an *open* or a *compound fracture*.[35] Open fractures often are complicated by infection, osteomyelitis, delayed union, or nonunion. In a closed fracture, there is no communication with the outside skin.

Concept Mastery Alert

People with compound fractures are more likely to experience complications in bone healing than those with other types of fractures.

The degree of a fracture is described in terms of a partial or complete break in the continuity of bone. A *greenstick fracture*, which is seen in children, is an example of a partial break in bone continuity and resembles that seen when a young sapling is broken. This kind of break occurs because children's bones, especially until approximately 10 years of age, are more resilient than are the bones of adults.

The character of a fracture is determined by its pieces. A *comminuted fracture* has more than two pieces. A *compression fracture*, as occurs in the vertebral body, involves two bones that are crushed or squeezed together. A fracture is called *impacted* when the fracture fragments are wedged together. This type usually occurs in the humerus, is less serious, and is treated without surgery.

The direction of the trauma or mechanism of injury produces a certain configuration or pattern of fracture. The pattern of a fracture indicates the nature of the trauma and provides information about the easiest method for reduction. *Reduction* is the restoration of a fractured bone to its normal anatomic position. *Transverse fractures* are caused by simple angular forces. A *spiral fracture* results from a twisting motion, or torque. A transverse fracture is not likely to become displaced or lose its position after it is reduced. On the other hand, spiral, oblique, and comminuted fractures often are unstable and may change position after reduction.

Clinical Manifestations

The signs and symptoms of a fracture include pain, tenderness at the site of bone disruption, swelling, loss of function, deformity of the affected part, and abnormal mobility. The deformity varies according to the type of force applied, the area of the bone involved, the type of fracture produced, and the strength and balance of the surrounding muscles.

In long bones, three types of deformities—angulation, shortening, and rotation—are seen. Severely angulated

fracture fragments may be felt at the fracture site and often push up against the soft tissue to cause a tenting effect on the skin. Bending forces and unequal muscle pulls cause angulation. Shortening of the extremity occurs as the bone fragments slide and override each other because of the pull of the muscles on the long axis of the extremity (Fig. 48-6).

Rotational deformity occurs when the fracture fragments rotate out of their normal longitudinal axis; this can result from rotational strain produced by the fracture or unequal pull by the muscles that are attached to the fracture fragments. A crepitus or grating may be felt as the bone fragments rub against each other. In the case of an open fracture, there is bleeding from the wound where the bone protrudes. Blood loss from a pelvic fracture or multiple long bone fractures can cause hypovolemic shock in a person who has had a trauma.

Shortly after the fracture has occurred, nerve function at the fracture site may be temporarily lost. The area may become numb, and the surrounding muscles flaccid. This condition has been called *local shock*. During this period, which may last for a few minutes to half an hour, fractured bones may be reduced with little or no pain. After this brief period, the pain returns and, with it, muscle spasms and contractions occur in the surrounding muscles.

The early complications of fractures are associated with loss of skeletal continuity, injury from bone fragments, pressure from swelling and hemorrhage, involvement of nerve fibers, or development of fat emboli. The extent of early complications depends on the severity of the fracture and the area of the body that is involved.

Diagnosis

Diagnosis is the first step in the care of fractures and is based on history and physical manifestations. X-ray examination is used to confirm the diagnosis and direct the treatment. The ease of diagnosis varies with the location and severity of the fracture. In a person who has had a trauma, the presence of other, more serious injuries may make diagnosis more difficult. A thorough history includes the mechanism, time, and place of the injury; first recognition of symptoms; and any treatment initiated. A complete history is important because a delay in seeking treatment or a period of weight bearing on a fracture may cause further injury or displacement of the fracture.

Determination of the severity of injury to soft tissue is an important component of assessment and management of closed fractures. The response of the soft tissue to blunt injury involves microvascular and inflammatory responses that produce localized tissue hypoxia and

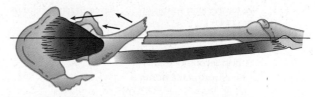

FIGURE 48-6. Displacement and overriding of fracture fragments of a long bone (femur) caused by severe muscle spasm.

acidosis. Incisions placed through such compromised tissue can lead to wound breakdown and infections. Therefore, recognizing the signs of soft-tissue injury is the foundation for successful management of closed fractures. The classification of Oestern and Tscherne can be used to characterize the severity of closed fractures[36,37] (Table 48-1). This system remains the only published classification system for the soft-tissue injury associated with closed fractures. Fractures are assigned one of four grades, from 0 to 3. The presence of deep skin abrasions, muscle contusion, fracture blisters, and massive soft-tissue swelling suggests the need to use external fixation methods to limit further soft-tissue injury and facilitate rapid recovery before surgical intervention.

Treatment

There are three objectives for treatment of fractures: reduction of the fracture, immobilization, and preservation and restoration of the function of the injured part. Also, it is important to prevent complications during the management of the fracture treatment. Preventive care is vital to avoiding fracture complications.

Reduction and Internal Fixation

When bones are realigned to restore their original structure, it is referred to as reduction. This can be accomplished by closed manipulation or surgical (open) reduction.

Immobilization and External Fixation

Immobilization prevents movement of the injured parts and is the single most important element in obtaining union of the fracture fragments. Immobilization can be accomplished using external devices, such as splints, casts, traction, or external fixation devices, or by internal fixation devices inserted during surgical reduction of the fracture.

Splints are made from many different materials including metal, air, or plaster. Splinting should be done if there is any suspicion of a fracture because motion of the fracture site can cause pain, bleeding, more soft-tissue damage, and nerve or blood vessel compression. *Casts*, which are made of plaster or synthetic material such as fiberglass, are commonly used to immobilize fractures of the extremities. They often are applied with a joint in partial flexion to prevent rotation of the fracture fragments. Without this flexion, the extremity, which is essentially a cylinder, tends to rotate within the cylindrical structure of the cast. *Traction* is another method for achieving immobility, maintaining alignment of the bone ends, and maintaining the reduction, particularly if the fracture is unstable or comminuted. Traction is a pulling force applied to an extremity or a part of the body while a counterforce, or countertraction, pulls in the opposite direction. The five goals of traction therapy are to correct and maintain the skeletal alignment of entire bones or joints; reduce pressure on a joint surface; correct, lessen, or prevent deformities such as contractures and dislocations; decrease muscle spasm; and immobilize the fracture site to promote healing (Fig. 48-7).

With *external fixation devices*, pins or screws are inserted directly into the bone above and below the fracture site. They are secured to a metal frame and adjusted to align the fracture. This method of treatment is used primarily for open fractures, infections such as osteomyelitis and septic joints, unstable closed fractures, and limb lengthening.

Limb-Lengthening Systems

Limb-lengthening systems, such as the Ilizarov external fixator (Fig. 48-8), are used to lengthen or widen bones, correct angular or rotational defects, or immobilize fractures.[35] The continuous pulling activates regeneration of bone, soft tissue, nerves, and blood vessels. Newly formed bone fills the posttraumatic defects and eliminates the need for bone grafting. The apparatus is left on until the desired length is achieved and consolidation is complete.

Preservation and Restoration of Function

During the period of immobilization required for fracture healing, muscles tend to atrophy because of lack of use. Joints stiffen as muscles and tendons contract and shorten. The degree of muscle atrophy and joint stiffness depends on several factors. In adults, the degree of atrophy and muscle stiffness is directly related to the length of immobilization, with longer periods of immobility resulting in greater stiffness. Children have a natural tendency to move on their own, and this movement maintains muscle and joint function. They usually have less atrophy and recover sooner after the source of immobilization has been removed. Associated soft-tissue injury, infection, and preexisting joint disease increase the risk of stiffness. Although limbs are immobilized in a functional position, casts are removed as soon as fracture healing has taken place so that joint stiffness does not occur.

TABLE 48-1 Oestern and Tscherne Classification of Closed Fractures		
Grade	**Soft-Tissue Injury**	**Bony Injury**
Grade 0	Minimal soft-tissue damage Indirect injury to limb	Simple fracture pattern
Grade 1	Superficial abrasion/contusion	Mild fracture pattern
Grade 2	Deep abrasion with skin or muscle contusion Direct trauma to limb	Severe fracture pattern
Grade 3	Extensive skin contusion or crush Severe damage to underlying muscle Subcutaneous avulsion Compartmental syndrome may be present	Severe fracture pattern

From Bucholz R. W., Heckman J. D. (2010). *Rockwood & Green's fractures in adults* (7th ed., Table 2-2, p. 45). Philadelphia, PA: Lippincott Williams & Wilkins.

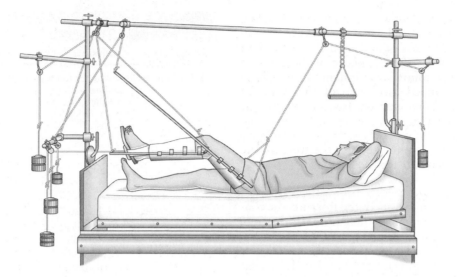

FIGURE 48-7. Balanced suspension skeletal traction with Thomas leg splint. The person can move vertically as long as the resultant line of pull is maintained. Note the use of the overhead trapeze. (From Hinkle J. L., Cheever K. H. (2018). *Brunner & Suddarth's textbook of medical-surgical nursing* (14th ed., Fig. 40-6, p. 1140). Philadelphia, PA: Lippincott Williams & Wilkins.)

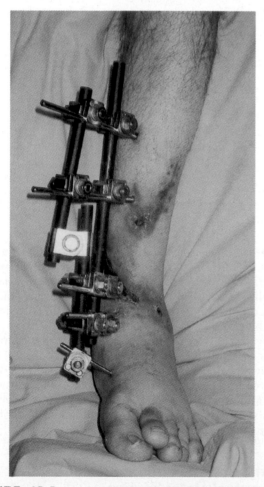

FIGURE 48-8. External fixation device. Pins are inserted into bone. The fracture is reduced and aligned and then stabilized by attaching the pins to a rigid portable frame. The device facilitates treatment of soft tissue damaged in complex fractures. (From Hinkle J. L., Cheever K. H. (2018). *Brunner & Suddarth's textbook of medical-surgical nursing* (14th ed., Fig. 40-3, p. 1138). Philadelphia, PA: Lippincott Williams & Wilkins.)

Exercises designed to preserve function, maintain muscle strength, and reduce joint stiffness in the unaffected and affected extremities should be started early. Active range of motion, in which the person moves the extremity, is done on unaffected extremities, and isometric, or muscle-tensing, exercises are done on the affected extremities. In some instances, an electrical muscle stimulator is applied directly to the skin to stimulate isometric muscle contraction as a means of preventing disuse atrophy.

Bone Healing

Bone healing occurs in a manner similar to soft-tissue healing. It is, however, a more complex process and takes longer. Although the exact mechanisms of bone healing are open to controversy, four stages of the healing process have been identified:

1. Hematoma formation
2. Inflammatory phase
3. Reparative phase
4. Remodeling phase[33]

The degree of response during each of these stages is in direct proportion to the extent of trauma.

The first stage, hematoma formation, occurs during the first 1 to 2 days after the fracture. It develops from torn blood vessels in the periosteum and adjacent muscles and soft tissue. Disruption of blood vessels also leads to death of bone cells at the fracture site. In 2 to 5 days, the hemorrhage forms a large blood clot. The second phase is called inflammation and is characterized by neovascularization, which begins to occur peripheral to the blood clot.[33] By the end of the first week, most of the clot is organized by invasion of blood vessels and early fibrosis. As the result of hematoma formation, clotting factors remain in the injured area to initiate the formation of a fibrin meshwork, which serves as a framework for the ingrowth of fibroblasts and new capillary buds. The woven bone spicules start to appear around the clot and osteoblasts begin to synthesize the bone.[33] There is granulation tissue forming and this is referred to as the beginning of the callus.[33] The reparative phase follows the inflammatory phase and allows the continued formation of the callus of cartilage and woven bone near the fracture site.[33] The final phase is remodeling, which gives the cortex time to be reestablished. The osteoclastic and osteoblastic functions continue at a rapid rate until the fracture site is healed and bone is reconstructed.[33]

Healing Time

Healing time depends on the site of the fracture, the condition of the fracture fragments, hematoma formation, and other local and host factors. In general, fractures of long bones, displaced fractures, and fractures with less surface area heal more slowly. Function usually returns within 6 months of union being completed. However, return to complete function may take longer. Stress fractures usually require less time to heal, usually 2 to 4 weeks, during which time reduction in activity and protection of the area are needed.

Union of a fracture has occurred when the fracture is solid enough to withstand normal stresses and it is clinically and radiologically safe to remove the external fixation. In children, fractures usually heal quicker than they do in adults. The increased rate of healing among children compared with that among adults may be related to the increased cellularity and vascularity of the child's periosteum.

Factors that influence bone healing are specific to the person, the type of injury sustained, and local factors that disrupt healing. Individual factors that may delay bone healing are the person's age; current medications; debilitating diseases, such as diabetes and rheumatoid arthritis; level of immunocompetency, local stress around the fracture site; circulatory problems and coagulation disorders; and poor nutrition.

Impaired Healing

Many factors can contribute to impaired bone healing, including the nature and extent of the injury, the health of the person with the fracture and his or her responses to injury, the adequacy of initial treatment, and pharmacologic factors. For large bone defects caused by trauma or a tumor, bone regeneration may need enhancement.

Malunion is healing with deformity, angulation, or rotation that is visible on x-ray films. Early, aggressive treatment, especially of the hand, can prevent malunion and result in earlier alignment and return of function. Malunion is caused by inadequate reduction or alignment of the fracture. *Delayed union* is the failure of a fracture to unite within the normal period.[35] Intra-articular fractures (*i.e.*, those through a joint) may heal more slowly and may eventually produce arthritis. *Nonunion* is failure to produce union and cessation of the processes of bone repair.[35] It is seen most often in the tibia, especially with open fractures or crushing

TABLE 48-2 Complications of Fracture Healing

Complication	Manifestations	Contributing Factors
Delayed union	Failure of fracture to heal within predicted time as determined by x-ray	Large displaced fracture
		Inadequate immobilization
		Large hematoma
		Infection at fracture site
		Excessive loss of bone
		Inadequate circulation
Malunion	Deformity at fracture site	Inadequate reduction
	Deformity or angulation on x-ray	Malalignment of fracture at time of immobilization
Nonunion	Failure of bone to heal before the process of bone repair stops	Inadequate reduction
	Evidence on x-ray	Mobility at fracture site
	Motion at fracture site	Severe trauma
	Pain on weight bearing	Bone fragment separation
		Soft tissue between bone fragments
		Infection
		Extensive loss of bone
		Inadequate circulation
		Malignancy
		Bone necrosis
		Noncompliance with restrictions

injuries. It is characterized by mobility of the fracture site and pain on weight bearing. Muscle atrophy and loss of range of motion may occur. Nonunion usually is established 6 to 12 months after the time of the fracture. The complications of fracture healing are summarized in Table 48-2.

Treatment methods for impaired bone healing include surgical interventions, such as bone grafts, bracing, external fixation, or electrical stimulation of the bone ends. The treatment for delayed union consists of determining and correcting the cause of the delay. Electrical stimulation is thought to stimulate the osteoblasts to lay down a network of bone.

Complications of Fractures and Other Musculoskeletal Injuries

The complications of fractures and other orthopedic injuries are associated with loss of skeletal continuity, injury from bone fragments, pressure from swelling and hemorrhage (*e.g.*, fracture blisters and compartment syndrome), involvement of nerve fibers (*e.g.*, complex regional pain syndrome [CRPS]) or development of venous thromboembolism and fat embolism syndrome (FES).

Fracture Blisters

Fracture blisters are skin **bullae** and blisters representing areas of epidermal necrosis with separation of the epidermis from the underlying dermis by edema fluid. They occur when the intracompartmental pressure is too high to be relieved through normal means. They are seen with more severe, twisting types of injuries but can also occur after excessive joint manipulation, dependent positioning, and heat application, or from peripheral vascular disease. They can be solitary, multiple, or massive depending on the extent of injury. Most fracture blisters occur in the ankle, elbow, foot, knee, or areas where there is little soft tissue between the bone and the skin. Prevention of fracture blisters is important because they pose an additional risk of infection. They also constitute a warning sign of compartment syndrome.

Compartment Syndrome

Compartment syndrome is a condition of increased pressure within a limited space (*e.g.*, abdominal and limb compartments) that compromises the circulation and function of the tissues in the space. Abdominal compartment syndrome alters cardiovascular hemodynamics, respiratory mechanics, and renal function. The discussion in this chapter is limited to a discussion of limb compartment syndromes.

Etiology and Pathogenesis

The muscles and nerves of an extremity are enclosed in tough, inelastic fascia often termed a *muscle compartment* (Fig. 48-9). If the pressure in the compartment is sufficiently high, tissue circulation is compromised, causing the death of nerve and muscle cells. Permanent loss of function may occur. The amount of pressure required to produce compartment syndrome depends on many factors, including the duration of the pressure elevation, the metabolic rate of the tissues, vascular tone, and local blood pressure. Less tissue pressure is required to stop circulation when hypotension or vasoconstriction is present.

Compartment syndrome can result from a decrease in compartment size, an increase in the volume of its contents, or a combination of the two factors. Among the causes of decreased compartment size are constrictive dressings and casts, closure of fascial defects, and burns. In people with circumferential third-degree burns, the inelastic and constricting eschar decreases the size of the underlying compartments.

An increase in compartment volume can be caused by trauma, swelling, vascular injury and bleeding, and venous obstruction. One of the most important causes of compartment syndrome is bleeding and edema caused by fractures and bone surgery. Contusions and soft-tissue injury also are common causes of compartment syndrome. Increased compartment volume may also follow ischemic events, such as arterial occlusion, that are of sufficient duration to produce capillary damage, causing increased capillary permeability and edema. Infiltration of intravenous fluids or bleeding from an arterial puncture can also cause compartment ischemia and postischemic swelling. During unattended coma caused by drug overdose or carbon monoxide poisoning, high compartment pressures are produced when an extremity is compressed by the weight of the overlying head or torso.

Compartment syndrome can be acute or chronic. Acute compartment syndrome can occur after a fracture or crushing injury, when excessive swelling around the site of injury results in increased pressure in a closed compartment. This increase in pressure occurs because fascia, which covers and separates muscles, is inelastic and unable to stretch and compensate for the extreme swelling. Chronic compartment syndrome may develop from exertion in long-distance runners and others involved in a major change in activity level. Exertional compartment syndrome is an increase in compartment size and intramuscular pressure during exercise that causes ischemia, pain, and, rarely, neurologic symptoms and signs.

Clinical Manifestations and Diagnosis

The hallmark symptom of an acute compartment syndrome is severe pain that is out of proportion to the original injury or physical findings. Nerve compression may cause changes in sensation (*e.g.*, paresthesias such as burning or tingling or loss of sensation), diminished reflexes, and eventually the loss of motor function. These symptoms generally begin quickly after injury but can also occur in a few days.

Because muscle necrosis can occur quickly, anyone at risk for compartment syndrome needs close surveillance.

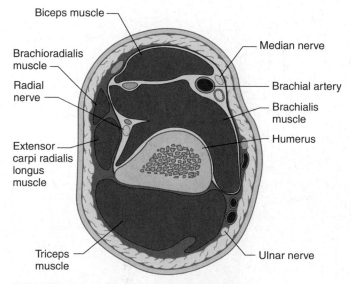

Biceps muscle

Brachioradialis muscle

Radial nerve

Extensor carpi radialis longus muscle

Triceps muscle

Median nerve

Brachial artery

Brachialis muscle

Humerus

Ulnar nerve

FIGURE 48-9. The proximal muscle compartment of the arm, showing the location of fascia, muscles, nerves, and blood vessels.

UNDERSTANDING ➡ Fracture Healing

A fracture, which is any break in a bone, undergoes a healing process to reestablish bone continuity and strength. The repair of simple fractures is commonly divided into four phases: **(1)** hematoma formation, **(2)** inflammation, **(3)** reparative phase, and **(4)** remodeling.

❶

Hematoma Formation When a bone breaks, blood vessels in the bone and surrounding tissues are torn and bleed into and around the fragments of the fractured bone, forming a blood clot, or hematoma. The hematoma facilitates the formation of the fibrin meshwork that seals off the fracture site and serves as a framework for the influx of inflammatory cells, the ingrowth of fibroblasts, and the development of new capillary buds (vessels). It is also the source of signaling molecules that initiate the cellular events that are critical to the healing process.

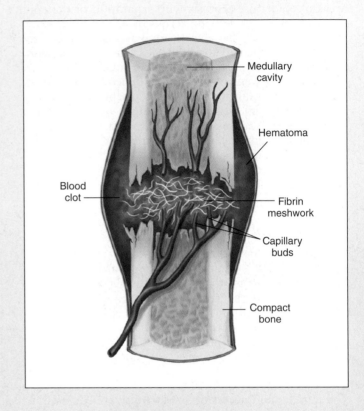

❷

Fibrocartilaginous Callus Formation As new capillaries infiltrate the hematoma at the fracture site, it becomes organized into a form of granulation tissue called *procallus*. Fibroblasts from the periosteum, endosteum, and red bone marrow proliferate and invade the procallus. The fibroblasts produce a fibrocartilaginous soft callus bridge that connects the bone fragments. Although this repair tissue usually reaches its maximum girth at the end of the second or third week, it is not strong enough for weight bearing.

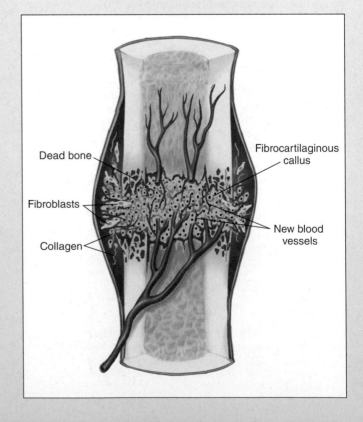

3

Bony Callus Formation

Ossification represents the conversion of the fibrocartilaginous cartilage to bony callus. In areas close to well-vascularized bone tissue, osteogenic cells develop into osteoblasts, or bone-building cells, which produce spongy bone trabeculae. The newly formed osteoblasts first deposit bone on the outer surface of the bone some distance from the fracture site. The formation of bone progresses toward the fracture site until a new bony sheath covers the fibrocartilaginous callus. In time, the fibrocartilage is converted to spongy bone, and the callus is then referred to as bony callus. Gradually, the bony callus calcifies and is replaced by mature bone. Bony callus formation begins 3 to 4 weeks after injury and continues until a firm bony union is formed months later.

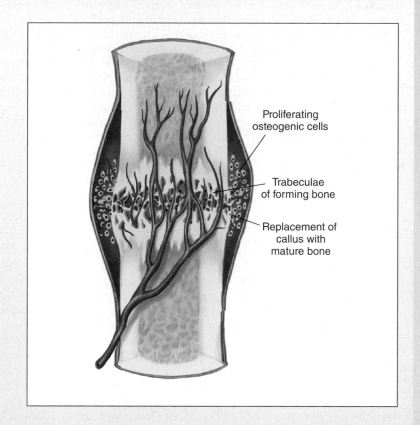

Proliferating osteogenic cells

Trabeculae of forming bone

Replacement of callus with mature bone

4

Remodeling During remodeling of the bony callus, dead portions of the bone are gradually removed by osteoclasts. Compact bone replaces spongy bone around the periphery of the fracture, and there is reorganization of mineralized bone along the lines of mechanical stress. During this period, the excess material on the outside of the bone shaft and within the medullary cavity is removed and compact bone is laid down to reconstruct the shaft. The final structure of the remodeled area resembles that of the original unbroken bone; however, a thickened area on the surface of the bone may remain as evidence of a healed fracture.

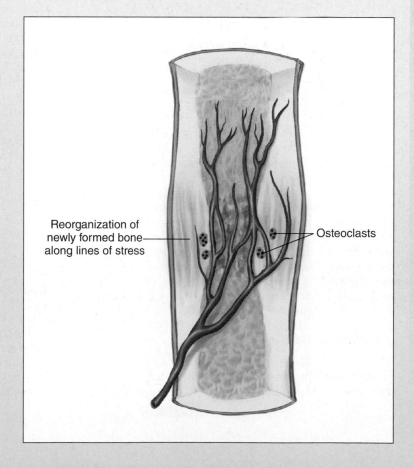

Reorganization of newly formed bone along lines of stress

Osteoclasts

Assessment should include pain assessment, examination of sensory (*i.e.*, light touch and two-point discrimination) and motor function (*i.e.*, movement and muscle strength), as well as tests of passive stretch and palpation of the muscle compartments. Peripheral pulses frequently are normal in the presence of compartment syndrome because the major arteries are located outside the muscle compartments. Although edema may make it difficult to palpate the pulse, the increased compartment pressure seldom is sufficient to occlude flow in a major artery. Doppler methods usually confirm the existence of a pulse. Disagreement exists regarding the pressure at which ischemic damage occurs; it should not be the only factor in diagnosis.[38,39] A recommended measure is pulse pressure (diastolic blood pressure–tissue pressure), where inadequate perfusion occurs at less than 30 mm Hg.[39]

Treatment

Treatment consists of reducing compartmental pressures. This entails cast splitting or removal of restrictive dressings. Elevating the extremity on pillows can help reduce edema. However, excessive elevation should be avoided because the effects of gravity can lower the arterial pressure in the limb, thereby decreasing compartment perfusion. A fasciotomy may be needed to relieve the pressure in an acute situation. During this procedure, the fascia is incised longitudinally and separated so that the compartment volume can expand and blood flow can be reestablished. Because of potential problems with wound infection and closure, this procedure is usually performed as a last resort.

Complex Regional Pain Syndrome

CRPS, previously referred to as *reflex sympathetic dystrophy* and *causalgia*, is a neurologic condition that impacts limbs and results from surgery or injury.[40-42] The classic complaint is pain that seems out of proportion to the injury, increased sweating, and vasomotor instability.

Pain, which is the prominent symptom of the disorder, is described as severe, aching, or burning. It usually increases in intensity with movement and with noxious and nonnoxious stimuli. The pathophysiologic cause of the pain is unclear, but it is thought to have a sympathetic nervous system component. Muscle wasting, thin and shiny skin, and abnormalities of the nails and bone can occur. Decreased muscle strength and disuse can lead to contractures and osteoporosis. Treatment focuses on pain management, prevention of disability, and improving quality of life with physical and occupational therapy considered to be first-line treatment.[40]

Thromboemboli

The person with a lower extremity fracture is at risk for the development of venous thromboembolic disorders, which include pulmonary embolism and deep vein thrombosis. Age and surgery increase these risks.[43,44] Recommended thromboprophylaxis with pharmacologic and mechanical interventions depends on the type of surgery and risk factors.[44]

The majority of symptomatic venous thromboemboli associated with hospital admissions occur at least 2 months after hospital discharge. Venous Doppler ultrasonography is the accepted test for the diagnosis of lower extremity deep vein thrombosis. A lung scan may be used in the diagnosis of a pulmonary embolus, but it may not differentiate between a thrombus and a fat embolus, especially in an individual with a long bone fracture.

Fat Embolism Syndrome

The FES refers to multiple life-threatening manifestations resulting from the presence of fat droplets in the small blood vessels of the lung, kidneys, brain, and other organs after a long bone or pelvic fracture.[35] The fat emboli are thought to be released from the bone marrow or adipose tissue at the fracture site into the venous system through torn veins.

Pathogenesis

The pathophysiologic process of FES is unclear. Fat embolization involves the presence of fat emboli in the circulation, and FES, an identifiable clinical pattern of organ dysfunction associated with fat emboli in the circulation.

Clinical Manifestations

The main clinical features of FES are respiratory failure, cerebral dysfunction, and skin and mucosal petechiae. Cerebral manifestations include encephalopathy, seizures, and focal neurologic deficits unrelated to head injury. Usually, initial symptoms of FES begin to develop within 12 to 72 hours of the injury.[45] The first symptoms include a subtle change in behavior and signs of disorientation resulting from emboli in the cerebral circulation combined with respiratory depression. There may be complaints of substernal chest pain and dyspnea accompanied by tachycardia and a low-grade fever. Diaphoresis, pallor, and cyanosis become evident as respiratory function deteriorates. A petechial rash that does not blanch with pressure often occurs 2 to 3 days after the injury. This rash usually is found on the anterior chest, axillae, neck, and shoulders. It also may appear on the soft palate and conjunctiva. The rash is thought to be related to embolization of the skin capillaries or thrombocytopenia.

Diagnosis and Treatment

An important part of the treatment of FES is early diagnosis. Arterial blood gases should be assayed immediately after recognition of clinical manifestations. Treatment is directed toward correcting hypoxemia, inflammation, and maintaining adequate fluid balance. The only preventive approach to FES is early stabilization of the fracture.

SUMMARY CONCEPTS

Many external physical agents can cause trauma to the musculoskeletal system. Factors such as environment, activity, or age can place a person at greater risk for injury. Some soft-tissue injuries, such as contusions, hematomas, and lacerations, are relatively minor and easily treated. Muscle strains and ligamentous sprains are caused by mechanical overload on the connective tissue. They heal more slowly than do the minor soft-tissue injuries and require some degree of immobilization. Healing of soft tissue begins within 4 to 5 days of the injury and is primarily the function of fibroblasts, which produce collagen. Joint dislocation is caused by trauma to the supporting structures. Repeated trauma to the joint can cause articular softening (*i.e.*, chondromalacia) or the separation of small pieces of bone or cartilage, called *loose bodies*, in the joint.

   Fractures occur when more stress is placed on a bone than the bone can absorb. The nature of the stress determines the type of fracture and the character of the resulting bone fragments. Healing of fractures is a complex process that takes place in four stages: hematoma formation, inflammatory phase, reparative process, and the remodeling stage.[33] For satisfactory healing to take place, the affected bone has to be reduced and immobilized. Immobilization is accomplished with the use of external devices, such as splints, casts, traction, or an external fixation apparatus, or with a surgically implanted internal fixation device. The complications associated with fractures can occur early because of soft-tissue and nerve damage, or later when the healing process of the fracture is interrupted. The early complications of fractures and other orthopedic injuries are associated with swelling and hemorrhage (fracture blisters and compartment syndrome), involvement of nerve fibers (reflex sympathetic dystrophy and causalgia), and development of fat emboli. Impaired healing of a fracture can cause malunion with deformity, angulation, or rotation; delayed union, in which the healing process is prolonged; or nonunion, in which the fracture fails to heal.

Bone Infections

Bone infections, including acute and chronic osteomyelitis, are known for their ability to cause pain, disability, and deformity. Despite the common use of antibiotics,

they remain difficult to treat and eradicate. A resurgence of tubercular bone infections is occurring in industrialized parts of the world, attributed in part to immigration from developing countries and greater numbers of immunocompromised people.

KEY POINTS

Bone Infections

■ Bone infections may be caused by a wide variety of microorganisms introduced during injury or operative procedures, or through the bloodstream.

■ Once localized in bone, the microorganisms proliferate, produce cell death, and spread within the bone shaft, inciting a chronic inflammatory response with further destruction of bone.

■ Bone infections are difficult to treat and eradicate. Measures to prevent infection include careful cleaning and debridement of skeletal injuries and strict operating room protocols.

Osteomyelitis

Osteomyelitis represents an acute or chronic infection of the bone. *Osteo* refers to bone, and *myelo* refers to the marrow cavity, both of which are involved in this disease. The infection can be caused by the following:

■ Direct penetration or contamination of an open fracture or wound (exogenous origin)
■ Seeding through the bloodstream (hematogenous spread)
■ Extension from a contiguous site
■ Skin infections in people with vascular insufficiency

Osteomyelitis can occur as an acute, subacute, or chronic condition. All types of organisms, including viruses, parasites, fungi, and bacteria, can produce osteomyelitis, but infections caused by certain pyogenic bacteria and mycobacteria are the most common.

   The specific agents isolated in pyogenic bacterial osteomyelitis are often associated with the age of the person or the inciting condition (*e.g.*, trauma or surgery). *Staphylococcus aureus* is the most common cause, but organisms such as *Escherichia coli*, *Neisseria gonorrhoeae*, *Haemophilus influenzae*, and *Salmonella* species are also seen.[33,46]

Hematogenous Osteomyelitis

Hematogenous osteomyelitis originates with infectious organisms that reach the bone through the bloodstream. Acute hematogenous osteomyelitis occurs predominantly in children.[47] In adults, it is seen most commonly in people who are debilitated and in those with a history of chronic skin infections, chronic urinary tract infections, and intravenous drug use and in those who are immunologically suppressed. Intravenous drug users are at risk for infections with *Streptococcus* and *Pseudomonas*.[33]

Pathogenesis

The pathogenesis of hematogenous osteomyelitis differs in children and adults. In children, the infection usually affects the long bones of the appendicular skeleton. It starts in the metaphyseal region close to the growth plate, where termination of nutrient blood vessels and sluggish blood flow favor the attachment of blood-borne bacteria (Fig. 48-10). With advancement of the infection, purulent exudate collects in the rigidly enclosed bony tissue. Because of the bone's rigid structure, there is little room for swelling and the purulent exudate finds its way beneath the periosteum, shearing off the perforating arteries that supply the cortex with blood, thereby leading to necrosis of cortical bone. Eventually, the purulent drainage may penetrate the periosteum and skin to form a draining sinus. In children 1 year of age and younger, the adjacent joint is often involved because the periosteum is not firmly attached to the cortex.[33] From 1 year of age to puberty, subperiosteal abscesses are more common.[33] As the process continues, periosteal new bone formation and reactive bone formation in the marrow tend to wall in the infection. *Involucrum* refers to a lesion in which bone formation forms a sheath around the necrotic sequestrum. It is seen most commonly in cases of chronic osteomyelitis.

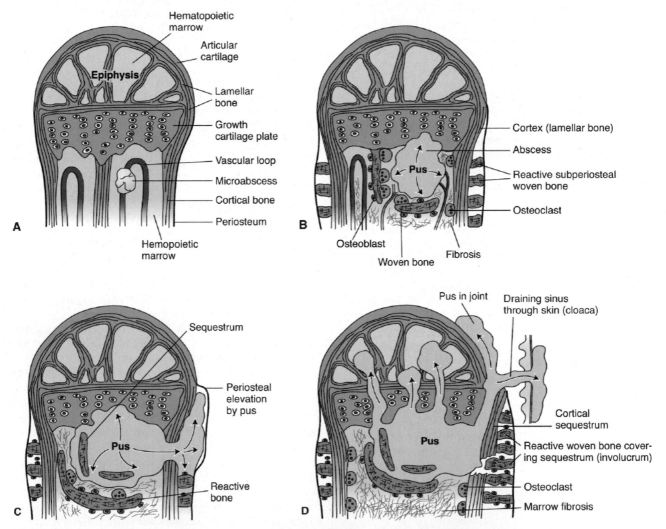

FIGURE 48-10. Pathogenesis of hematogenous osteomyelitis. **(A)** This epiphysis, metaphysis, and growth plate are normal. A small, septic microabscess is developing at the capillary loop. **(B)** Expansion of the septic focus stimulates resorption of adjacent bony trabeculae. Woven bone begins to surround this focus. The abscess expands into the cartilage and stimulates reactive bone formation by the periosteum. **(C)** The abscess, which continues to expand through the cortex into the subperiosteal tissue, shears off the perforating arteries that supply the cortex with blood, thereby leading to necrosis of the cortex. **(D)** The extension of this process into the joint space, the epiphysis, and the skin produces a draining sinus. The necrotic bone is called a sequestrum. The viable bone surrounding a sequestrum is termed the involucrum. (From Strayer D. S., Rubin R. (Eds.). (2015). *Rubin's pathology: Clinicopathologic foundations of medicine* (7th ed., Fig. 30-17, p. 1325). Philadelphia, PA: Lippincott Williams & Wilkins.)

In adults, the long bone microvasculature no longer favors seeding, and hematogenous infection rarely affects the appendicular skeleton. Instead, vertebrae, sternoclavicular and sacroiliac joints, and the symphysis pubis are involved. Infection typically first involves subchondral bone, then spreads to the joint space.[33] With vertebral osteomyelitis, this causes sequential destruction of the endplate, adjoining disk, and contiguous vertebral body. Infection less commonly begins in the joint and spreads to the adjacent bone.

Clinical Manifestations

The signs and symptoms of acute hematogenous osteomyelitis are those of bacteremia accompanied by symptoms referable to the site of the bone lesion. Bacteremia is characterized by chills, fever, and malaise. There often is pain on movement of the affected extremity, loss of movement, and local tenderness followed by redness and swelling. X-ray studies may appear normal initially, but they show evidence of periosteal elevation and increased osteoclast activity after an abscess has formed.

Treatment

The treatment of hematogenous osteomyelitis begins with identification of the causative organism through blood and bone aspiration cultures.[33,47] Antimicrobial agents are given first parenterally and then orally. The length of time the affected limb needs to be rested and pain control measures used are based on symptoms. Debridement and surgical drainage also may be necessary.

Direct Penetration and Contiguous Spread Osteomyelitis

Direct penetration or extension of bacteria from an outside (exogenous) source is now the most common cause of osteomyelitis in the United States.[33] Bacteria may be introduced directly into the bone by a penetrating wound, an open fracture, or a surgery. Inadequate irrigation or debridement, introduction of foreign material into the wound, and extensive tissue injury increase the bone's susceptibility to infection.

Iatrogenic bone infections are those inadvertently brought about by surgery or other treatments. These complications include pin tract infection in skeletal traction, septic (infected) joints in joint replacement surgery, and wound infections after surgery. Staphylococci and streptococci are still commonly implicated, but in 25% of postoperative infections, gram-negative organisms are detected.[33] Measures to prevent these infections include preparation of the skin to reduce bacterial growth before surgery or insertion of traction devices or wires, strict operating room protocols, prophylactic use of antibiotics immediately before and for 24 hours after surgery and as a topical wound irrigation, and maintenance of sterile technique after surgery when working with drainage tubes and dressing changes.

Pathogenesis

The pathogenesis of osteomyelitis resulting from direct penetration or contiguous spread differs from hematogenous infection in that virtually any traumatized bone may be involved. Although healthy bone is highly resistant to infection, injury from local inflammation and trauma may devitalize bone and surrounding tissue, providing an inert matrix on which microorganisms introduced during trauma thrive.

Clinical Manifestations

Osteomyelitis after trauma or bone surgery usually is associated with persistent or recurrent fever, increased pain at the operative or trauma site, and poor incisional healing, which often is accompanied by continued wound drainage and wound separation. Prosthetic joint infections often present with joint pain, fever, and cutaneous drainage.

Diagnosis and Treatment

Diagnosis requires both confirming the infection and identifying the offending microorganism with culture and sensitivity studies. The diagnosis of skeletal infection entails use of various imaging strategies, including conventional radiology, nuclear imaging studies, CT scans, and MRI.[47] Bone biopsy may be used to identify the causative microorganisms.

Treatment includes antibiotics and selective use of surgical interventions. Antimicrobial agents are usually used prophylactically in people undergoing bone surgery. For people with osteomyelitis, early antimicrobial treatment, before there is extensive destruction of bone, produces the best results. The choice of agents and method of administration depend on the microorganisms causing the infection. In acute osteomyelitis that does not respond to antibiotic therapy, surgical decompression is used to release intramedullary pressure and remove drainage from the periosteal area. Prosthesis removal may be necessary in cases of an infected prosthetic joint.

Chronic Osteomyelitis

Chronic osteomyelitis usually occurs in adults. Generally, these infections occur secondary to an open wound, most often to the bone or surrounding tissue. Chronic osteomyelitis has long been recognized as a disease. However, the incidence has decreased in the past century because of improvements in surgical techniques and the advent of broad-spectrum antibiotic therapy. Chronic osteomyelitis includes all inflammatory processes of bone, excluding those in rheumatic diseases that are caused by microorganisms. It may be the result of delayed or inadequate treatment of acute hematogenous osteomyelitis or osteomyelitis caused by direct contamination of bone by exogenous organisms. Chronic osteomyelitis can persist for years; it may appear spontaneously, after a minor trauma, or when resistance is lowered.

The hallmark feature of chronic osteomyelitis is the presence of infected dead bone, a *sequestrum*, that has separated from the living bone.[33] A sheath of new bone, called the *involucrum*, forms around the dead bone. Radiologic techniques such as x-ray films, bone scans, and sinograms are used to identify the infected site. Chronic osteomyelitis or infection around a total joint prosthesis can be difficult to diagnose because the classic signs of infection are not apparent and the blood leukocyte count may not be elevated. A subclinical infection may exist for years. Bone scans are used with bone biopsy for a definitive diagnosis.

The treatment of chronic bone infections begins with wound cultures to identify the microorganism and its sensitivity to antibiotic therapy. The goal in selecting antimicrobial treatment for osteomyelitis is to use the drug with the highest bactericidal activity and least toxicity, and at the lowest cost. Initial antibiotic therapy is followed by surgery to remove foreign bodies (*e.g.,* metal plates and screws) or sequestra and by long-term antibiotic therapy. Immobilization of the affected part usually is necessary, with restriction of weight bearing on a lower extremity. External fixation devices are sometimes used. Chronic refractory osteomyelitis may be diagnosed in those who do not respond after 4 to 6 weeks of appropriate therapy.[48]

Osteomyelitis with Vascular Insufficiency

In people with vascular insufficiency, osteomyelitis may develop from a skin lesion. It is most commonly associated with chronic or ischemic foot ulcers in people with long-standing diabetes. Neuropathy causes a loss of protective reflexes, and impaired arterial circulation and repetitive trauma are the major contributors to skin fissure and ulcer formation.

People with vascular insufficiency osteomyelitis often present with seemingly unrelated problems such as ingrown toenails, cellulitis, or a perforating foot ulcer, making diagnosis difficult. Furthermore, pain is often muted by peripheral neuropathy. Osteomyelitis is confirmed when bone is exposed in the ulcer bed or after debridement. Radiologic evidence is a late sign.

Treatment depends on the oxygen tension of the involved tissues. Debridement and antibiotic therapy may benefit people who have good oxygen tension in the infected site. Hyperbaric oxygen therapy may be used as an adjunctive treatment.

Tuberculosis of the Bone or Joint

For those at risk, the spread of tuberculosis to the bone occurs through a variety of means but generally through the bloodstream. Although it may occur during primary infection, it is more likely to occur through reactivated latent bacilli.[49]

Tuberculosis can spread from one part of the body, such as the lungs or the lymph nodes, to the musculoskeletal system. Tubercular osteomyelitis tends to be more destructive and difficult to control than pyogenic osteomyelitis. The infection spreads through large areas of the medullary cavity and causes extensive necrosis. In tuberculosis of the spine, also known as *Pott disease or tuberculous spondylitis,* the infection spreads through the intervertebral disks to involve multiple vertebrae and extends into the soft tissue, forming abscesses.

Local symptoms include pain, immobility, and muscle atrophy; joint swelling, mild fever, and leukocytosis

also may occur. The most feared complication of spinal tuberculosis is neurologic compromise because of spinal deformity and epidural abscess formation. Because there are no specific radiographic findings in tubercular osteomyelitis, the diagnosis is usually made by tissue biopsy or culture findings. In spinal tuberculosis, a CT-guided biopsy is often used. The mainstay of treatment for tubercular osteomyelitis is similar to the guidelines for respiratory tuberculosis.

SUMMARY CONCEPTS

Bone infections occur because of the direct or indirect invasion of the musculoskeletal system by microorganisms, most commonly *S. aureus.* Osteomyelitis, or infection of the bone and marrow, can be an acute or chronic disease. Acute osteomyelitis is seen most often as a result of the direct contamination of bone by a foreign object. Chronic osteomyelitis represents an infection that continues beyond 6 to 8 weeks and may persist for years. The incidence of all types of bone infection has been dramatically reduced since the advent of antibiotic therapy. Iatrogenic infections are those inadvertently brought about by surgery or other treatments. Tuberculosis of the bone, which is characterized by bone destruction and abscess formation, is caused by spread of the infection from the lungs or lymph nodes.

Osteonecrosis

Osteonecrosis, or death of a segment of bone, is a condition caused by the interruption of blood supply to the marrow, medullary bone, or cortex in the absence of infection[33] (Fig. 48-11). It is a relatively common disorder and can occur in the medullary cavity of the metaphysis and the subchondral region of the epiphysis, especially in the proximal femur, distal femur, and proximal humerus. It is a common complicating disorder of Legg–Calvé–Perthes disease, slipped capital femoral epiphysis, sickle cell disease, steroid therapy, alcohol abuse, and hip trauma, fracture, or surgery. People treated with corticosteroids and/or bisphosphonates are more vulnerable to developing osteonecrosis.[50,51]

Etiology and Pathogenesis

Although bone necrosis results from ischemia, the mechanisms producing the ischemia are varied and include mechanical vascular interruption such as occurs with trauma or a fracture; thrombosis and embolism

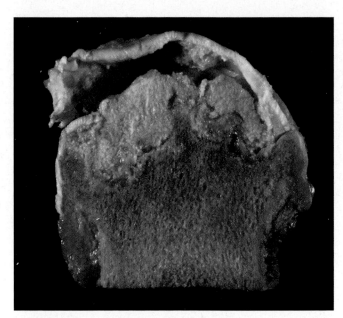

FIGURE 48-11. Osteonecrosis of the head of the femur. A coronal section shows a circumscribed area of subchondral infarction with partial detachment of the overlying articular cartilage and subarticular bone. (From Strayer D. S., Rubin R. (Eds.). (2015). *Rubin's pathology: Clinicopathologic foundations of medicine* (7th ed., Fig. 30-14A, p. 1321). Philadelphia, PA: Lippincott Williams & Wilkins.)

(*e.g.*, sickle cell disease, nitrogen bubbles caused by inadequate decompression during deep sea diving); and vessel injury (*e.g.*, vasculitis, radiation therapy). In many cases, the cause of the necrosis is uncertain. Other than fracture, the most common causes of bone necrosis are idiopathic (*i.e.*, those of unknown cause) and prior steroid therapy. Chart 48-1 lists disorders associated with osteonecrosis.

Bone has a rich blood supply that varies from site to site.[33] The flow in the medullary portion of bone originates in nutrient vessels from an interconnecting plexus that supplies the marrow, trabecular bone, and endosteal half of the cortex. The outer cortex receives its blood supply from periosteal, muscular, metaphyseal, and epiphyseal vessels that surround the bone. Some bony sites, such as the head of the femur, have only limited collateral circulation, so that interruption of the flow, such as with a hip fracture, can cause necrosis of a substantial portion of medullary and cortical bone and irreversible damage.

One of the most frequent causes of osteonecrosis is that associated with administration of corticosteroids.[33] The mechanism of steroid-induced osteonecrosis remains unclear. The condition may develop after the administration of very high, short-term doses; during long-term treatment; or even from intra-articular injection. Although the risk increases with the dose and duration of treatment, it is difficult to predict who will be affected. The interval between corticosteroid administration and onset of symptoms rarely is less than 6 months and may be more than 3 years. There is no satisfactory method for preventing progression of the disease. Osteonecrosis of the jaw has been reported after long-term use of bisphosphonates.[50]

The pathologic features of bone necrosis are the same, regardless of cause. The site of the lesion is related to the vessels involved. There is necrosis of cancellous bone and marrow. The cortex usually is not involved because of collateral blood flow. In subchondral infarcts (*i.e.*, ischemia below the cartilage), a triangular or wedge-shaped segment of tissue that has the subchondral bone plate as its base and the center of the epiphysis as its apex undergoes necrosis. When medullary infarcts occur in fatty bone marrow, the death of bone cells causes calcium release and necrosis of fat cells, with the formation of free fatty acids. Released calcium forms an insoluble "soap" with free fatty acids. Because bone lacks mechanisms for resolving the infarct, the lesions remain for life.

Clinical Manifestations, Diagnosis, and Treatment

The symptoms associated with osteonecrosis are varied and depend on the extent of infarction. Typically, subchondral infarcts cause chronic pain that is initially associated with activity but that gradually becomes more progressive until it is experienced at rest. Subchondral infarcts often collapse and predispose the person to severe secondary osteoarthritis.

Diagnosis of osteonecrosis is based on history, physical findings, radiographic findings, and results of special imaging studies, including CT scans and technetium-99m bone scans. Treatment of osteonecrosis depends on the underlying pathologic process. In some cases, only short-term immobilization, nonsteroidal anti-inflammatory drugs, exercises, and limitation in weight bearing are used. Osteonecrosis of the hip is particularly difficult to treat. In people with early disease, limitation of weight bearing using crutches may allow the condition to stabilize. Although several surgical approaches have been used, the most definitive treatment of advanced osteonecrosis of the knee or hip is total joint replacement.

SUMMARY CONCEPTS

Osteonecrosis is a common condition that has long been recognized but is not fully understood. Death of bone is caused by disruption of the blood supply from intravascular or extravascular processes. Sites with poor collateral circulation, such as the femoral head, are most seriously affected. Causative factors include corticosteroid therapy. Symptoms include pain that varies in severity, depending on the extent of infarction. Total joint replacement is the most frequently used treatment for advanced osteonecrosis.

Neoplasms

Neoplasms in the skeletal system are referred to as *bone tumors*. Primary malignant tumors of the bone are uncommon, constituting less than 0.2% of all cancers.[52] The National Cancer Institute projectes 3500 new cases of bone cancer and approximately 1660 deaths in 2019.[53] Metastatic disease of the bone, however, is relatively common. Primary bone tumors may arise from any of the skeletal components, including osseous bone tissue, cartilage, and bone marrow. The discussion in this section focuses on primary benign and malignant bone tumors of osseous or cartilaginous origin and metastatic bone disease.

Like other types of neoplasms, bone tumors may be benign or malignant. Benign tumors far outnumber malignant tumors. The benign types, such as osteochondromas, tend to grow rather slowly and usually do not destroy the supporting or surrounding tissue or spread to other parts of the body. Malignant tumors, such as osteosarcoma, grow rapidly and can spread to other parts of the body through the bloodstream or lymphatics. The two major forms of bone cancer in children and young adults are osteosarcoma and Ewing sarcoma.[52] Chondrosarcomas tend to occur during adulthood, with 51 being the average age of diagnosis.[52] The classification of benign and malignant bone tumors is described in Table 48-3.

Characteristics of Bone Tumors

There are three major manifestations of bone tumors: pain, presence of a mass, and impairment of function. Pain is a feature common to almost all malignant tumors

TABLE 48-3 Classification of Primary Bone Neoplasms

Tissue Type	Benign Neoplasm	Malignant Neoplasm
Bone	Osteoid osteoma Benign osteoblastoma	Osteosarcoma Parosteal osteogenic sarcoma
Cartilage	Osteochondroma Chondroma Chondroblastoma Chondromyxoid fibroma	Chondrosarcoma
Lipid	Lipoma	Liposarcoma
Fibrous and fibro-osseous tissue	Fibrous dysplasia	Fibrosarcoma Malignant fibrous histiocytoma
Miscellaneous	Giant cell tumor	Malignant giant cell Ewing sarcoma
Bone marrow		Multiple myeloma Reticulum cell sarcoma

but may or may not occur with benign tumors. For example, a benign bone cyst usually is asymptomatic until a fracture occurs. Pain that persists at night and is not relieved by rest suggests malignancy. A mass or hard lump may be the first sign of a bone tumor. A malignant tumor is suspected when a painful mass that is enlarging or eroding the cortex of the bone exists. The ease of discovery of a mass depends on the location of the tumor; a small lump arising on the surface of the tibia is easy to detect, whereas a tumor that is deep in the medial portion of the thigh may grow to a considerable size before it is noticed. Benign and malignant tumors may cause the bone to erode to the point at which it cannot withstand the strain of ordinary use. In such cases, even a small amount of bone stress or trauma precipitates a pathologic fracture. A tumor may produce pressure on a peripheral nerve, causing decreased sensation, numbness, a limp, or limitation of movement.

KEY POINTS

Bone Neoplasms

- Neoplasms of the skeletal system can affect bone tissue, cartilage, or bone marrow.

- Benign tumors tend to grow slowly, do not spread to other parts of the body, and exert their effects through the space-occupying nature of the tumor and their ability to weaken bone structures.

- Malignant bone tumors are rare before 10 years of age, have their peak incidence in the teenage years, tend to grow rapidly, and have a high mortality rate.

Benign Neoplasms

Benign bone tumors usually are limited to the confines of the bone, have well-demarcated edges, and are surrounded by a thin rim of sclerotic bone. An *osteoma* is a small bony tumor found on the surface of a long bone, flat bone, or the skull. It usually is composed of hard, compact (ivory osteoma), or spongy (cancellous) bone. It may be excised or left alone.

A *chondroma* is a tumor composed of hyaline cartilage. It may arise on the surface of the bone (*i.e.,* ecchondroma) or in the medullary cavity (*i.e.,* endochondroma). These tumors may become large and are especially common in the hands and feet. A chondroma may persist for many years and then take on the attributes of a malignant chondrosarcoma. A chondroma usually is not treated unless it becomes unsightly or uncomfortable.

An *osteochondroma* is the most common form of a benign tumor in the skeletal system, representing 50% of all benign bone tumors and approximately 15% of all primary skeletal lesions. It grows only during periods of skeletal growth, originating in the epiphyseal cartilage plate and growing out of the bone like a mushroom. An osteochondroma is composed of cartilage and bone and usually occurs singly but may affect several bones in a condition called *multiple exostoses*. Malignant changes are rare, and excision of the tumor is done only when necessary.

A *giant cell tumor*, or *osteoclastoma*, is an aggressive tumor of multinucleated cells that often behaves like a malignant tumor, metastasizing through the bloodstream and recurring locally after excision. It arises most often in people in their 20s to 40s and is found most commonly in the knee, wrist, or shoulder. The tumor begins in the metaphyseal region, grows into the epiphysis, and may extend into the joint surface. Pathologic fractures are common because the tumor destroys the bone substance. Clinically, pain may occur at the tumor site, with gradually increasing swelling. X-ray films show destruction of the bone with expansion of the cortex.

The treatment of giant cell tumors depends on their location. If the affected bone can be eliminated without loss of function, such as the clavicle or fibula, the entire bone or part of it may be removed. When the tumor is near a major joint, such as the knee or shoulder, a local excision is done. Irradiation may be used to prevent recurrence of the tumor.

Malignant Bone Tumors

In contrast to benign tumors, primary malignant tumors tend to be ill defined, lack sharp borders, and extend beyond the confines of the bone. Primary bone tumors occur in all age groups and may arise in any part of the body. However, certain types of tumors tend to target certain age groups and anatomic sites (Fig. 48-12). For example, most osteogenic sarcomas occur in adolescents and are particularly common around the knee joint. Also, people with certain conditions such as Paget disease are at increased risk for development of bone cancer.

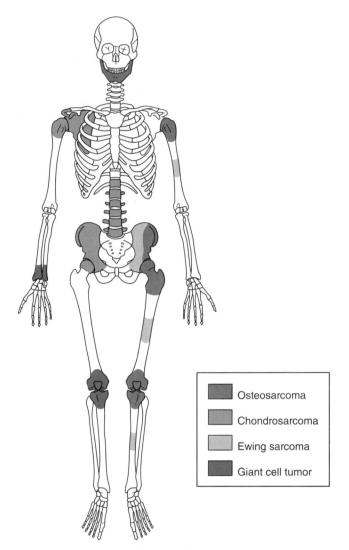

Osteosarcoma

Chondrosarcoma

Ewing sarcoma

Giant cell tumor

FIGURE 48-12. Common sites of primary malignant bone tumors (chondrosarcoma, osteosarcoma, and Ewing sarcoma) and giant cell tumor, a locally aggressive benign tumor.

The diagnosis of bone tumors includes radiologic staging and biopsy.[54] Radiographs give the most general diagnostic information, such as malignant versus benign and primary versus metastatic status. The radiograph demonstrates the region of bone involvement, extent of destruction, and amount of reactive bone formed. Radioisotope scans are used to estimate the local intramedullary extent of the tumor and screen for other skeletal areas of involvement. CT scans further aid diagnosis and anatomic localization and can identify small pulmonary metastases not seen by conventional radiographs. MRI is the most accurate method of evaluating the intramedullary extent of bone tumor and can demarcate the soft structures in relation to neurovascular structures without the use of contrast media. It is best used in conjunction with a CT scan. Radionuclide bone scans are used to assess for metastasis. A biopsy also is done because the definitive treatment of most bone tumors is based on pathologic interpretation of the biopsy specimen.

the diagnosis or treatment. A closed-needle biopsy with CT localization is particularly useful with spine lesions. Serum levels of alkaline phosphatase and calcium often are elevated in people with metastatic bone disease.

Treatment

The primary goals in treatment of metastatic bone disease are to prevent pathologic fractures and promote survival with maximum functioning and pain control. Standard treatment methods include chemotherapy, irradiation, and surgical stabilization.

SUMMARY CONCEPTS

Bone tumors, like any other type of neoplasm, may be benign or malignant. Benign bone tumors grow slowly and usually do not destroy the surrounding tissues. Malignant tumors can be primary or metastatic. Primary bone tumors are rare, grow rapidly, metastasize to the lungs and other parts of the body through the bloodstream, and have a high mortality rate. Metastatic bone tumors usually are multiple, originating primarily from cancers of the breast, lung, and prostate. The incidence of metastatic bone disease probably is increasing because improved treatment methods enable people with cancer to live longer. Advances in chemotherapy, radiation therapy, and surgical procedures have substantially increased the survival and cure rates for many types of bone cancers. A primary goal in metastatic bone disease is the prevention of pathologic fractures.

Review Exercises

1. A 39-year-old man is in intensive care after a motorcycle crash in which he skidded across the pavement on his right side. He has fractures of his right femur, pelvis, and several ribs on the right side. His leg was crushed beneath the motorcycle. He is beginning to lose movement in his leg.

   A. What are the priorities in treating his orthopedic injuries? What are the options for stabilizing his leg?

   B. What risk factors for complications of fractures are present?

   C. What are the symptoms of compartment syndrome?

2. A 73-year-old woman sustained a comminuted fracture in the middiaphysis of her left humerus when her husband lifted her up in bed. She has multiple lucent lesions scattered throughout her proximal humerus, radius, and ulna. She was recently hospitalized for confusion and was found to have diffuse bone metastases. Her bone marrow biopsy showed adenocarcinoma. She has a history of breast cancer 30 years ago, but her most recent mammogram returned a negative result.

   A. What would you consider to be the most likely cause of her fracture?

   B. What are the most common sites for bone metastasis?

3. A 14-year-old boy has complained of recent pain and swelling of his knee, with some restriction in movement. Although he thinks he may have injured his knee playing football, his mother insists that he be seen by an orthopedic specialist, who raises the possibility that the boy may have an osteosarcoma.

   A. Use the theory that osteosarcoma has its origin in sites of maximal growth velocity to explain the site of this boy's possible tumor.

   B. What diagnostic tests could be used to establish a diagnosis of osteosarcoma?

REFERENCES

1. Horvai A. (2015). Bones, joints, and soft tissue tumors. In Kumar V., Abbas A., Aster J. (Eds.), *Robbins & Cotran pathologic basis of disease* (9th ed., pp. 1179–1226). Philadelphia, PA: Elsevier/Saunders; Chapter 26.
2. Centers for Disease Control and Prevention Protect the Ones You Love: Child Injuries are Preventable CDC Childhood Injury Report. [Online]. Available: https://www.cdc.gov/safechild/child_injury_data.html. Accessed October 28, 2017.
3. Centers for Disease Control and Prevention Protect the Ones You Love: Child Injuries are Preventable. [Online]. Available: https://www.cdc.gov/safechild/sports_injuries/index.html. Accessed October 28, 2017.
4. Centers for Disease Control and Prevention, National Center for Injury Prevention and Control. Web–based Injury Statistics Query and Reporting System (WISQARS) [online]. Available: https://www.cdc.gov/injury/wisqars/index.html. Accessed August 5, 2016.
5. Vieira L. S., Gomes A. P., Bierhals I. O., et al. (2018). Falls among older adults in the South of Brazil: Prevalence and determinants. *Revista de Saúde Pública* 52, 22. http://doi.org.ezproxy.uthsc.edu/10.11606/S1518-8787.2018052000103.
6. Rubenstein L. Z. (2016). Falls in the elderly. [Online]. Available: https://www.merckmanuals.com/professional/geriatrics/falls-in-the-elderly/falls-in-the-elderly. Accessed May 5, 2018.
7. Patel D., Yamaski A., Brown K. (2017). Epidemiology of sports-related musculoskeletal injuries in young athletes in United States. *Translational Pediatrics* 6(3), 160–166.
8. Hoang Q., Mortazavi M. (2012). Pediatric overuse injuries in sports. *Advances in Pediatrics* 59(1), 359–393.
9. Saladin K. S. (2015). *Anatomy & physiology: The unity of form and function* (7th ed.). New York, NY: McGraw Hill Education.

10. Patel D., Kinsella E. (2017). Evaluation and management of lower back pain in young athletes. *Translational Pediatrics* 6(3), 225–235.

11. Mataliotakis G., Tsirikos A. (2017). Spondylolysis and spondylolisthesis in children and adolescents: Current concepts and treatment. *Spine* 31(6), 395–401.

12. Sairyo K., Nagamachi A. (2016). State-of-the-art management of low back pain in athletes: Instructional lecture. *Journal of Orthopaedic Science* 21(3), 263–272.

13. Gorroll A. H., Mulley A. G. (2014). *Primary care medicine: Office evaluation and management of the adult patient* (7th ed.). Philadelphia, PA: Lippincott Williams & Wilkins.

14. Rosa J., Checchia C., Miyazaki A. (2017). Traumatic instability of the shoulder. *Revista Brasileira de Ortopedia* 52(5), 513–520.

15. Carpinteiro E., Barros A. (2017). Natural history of anterior shoulder instability. *The Open Orthapaedics Journal* 11(Suppl-6, M9), 909–918.

16. Dunphy L. M., Windland-Brown J. E., Porter B. O., et al. (2015). *Primary care: The art and science of advanced practice nursing* (4th ed.). Philadelphia, PA: FA Davis.

17. National Association of Orthopedic Nurses (NAON). (2013). *Core curriculum for orthopaedic nursing* (7th ed.). Boston, MA: Pearson.

18. Hibberd E. E., Kerr Z. Y., Roos K. G., et al. (2016). Epidemiology of acromioclavicular joint sprains in 25 national collegiate association sports: 2009–2020 to 2014–2015 academic years. *The American Journal of Sports Medicine* 44(10), 2667–2674.

19. Monica J., Vredenburgh Z., Korsh J., et al. (2016). Acute shoulder injuries in adults. *American Family Physician* 94(2), 119–127.

20. Gupta H., Robinson P. (2015). Normal shoulder ultrasound: Anatomy and technique. *Seminars in Musculoskeletal Radiology* 19(3), 203–211.

21. Lazarides A., Alentorn E., Choi J., et al. (2015). Rotator cuff tears in young patients: A different disease than rotator cuff tears in elderly patients. *Journal of Shoulder and Elbow Surgery* 24, 1834–1843.

22. Oliva F., Piccirilli E., Bossa M., et al. (2015). I.S.Mu.L.T. Rotator cuff tears guidelines. *Muscles, Ligaments and Tendons Journal* 5(4), 227–263.

23. Jensen S. (2015). *Nursing health assessment: A best practice approach* (2nd ed.). Philadelphia, PA: Wolters Kluwer Health.

24. Antonelli M., Starz T. (2012). Assessing for risk and progression of osteoarthritis: The nurse's role. *American Journal of Nursing* 112(3), S26–S31.

25. Vetrano M., Oliva F., Bisschia S., et al. (2017). I.S.Mu.L.T. first-time patellar dislocation guidelines. *Muscles, Ligaments and Tendons Journal* 7(1), 1–10.

26. Sanders T., Pareek A., Hewett T., et al. (2018). Incidence of first-time lateral patellar dislocation: A 21-year population-based study. *Sports Health* 10(2), 146–151. doi:10.1177/1941738117725055.

27. Duthon V. (2015). Acute traumatic patellar dislocation. *Orthopaedics & Traumatology: Surgery & Research* 101, S59–S67.

28. Laidlaw M., Diduch D. (2017). Current concepts in the management of patellar instability. *Indian Journal of Orthopaedics* (serial online) (cited March 7 2017) 51, 493–504. Available: http://www.ijoonline.com/text.asp?2017/51/5/493/214211. Accessed May 31, 2019.

29. Dortaj H., Emamifar A. (2015). Case report: Traumatic hip dislocation with associated femoral head fracture. *Case Reports in Orthopedics* 2015(865786), 1–3.

30. Dyer S., Crotty M., Fairhill N., et al. (2016). A critical review of the long-term disability outcomes following hip fracture. *BMC Geriatrics* 16(158), 1–18.

31. Anpalahan M., Morrison S. G., Gibson S. J. (2014). Hip fracture risk factors and the discriminability of hip fracture risk vary by age: A case-control study. *Geriatrics & Gerontology International* 14, 413–419. doi:10.1111/ggi.12117.

32. Mangram A., Moeser P., Corneille M. G., et al. (2014). Geriatric hip trauma hip fractures: Is there a difference in outcomes based on fracture patterns? *World Journal of Emergency Surgery* 9(59), 1–8.

33. Rubin R., Strayer D. (Eds.). (2012). *Rubin's pathology: Clinicopathologic foundations of medicine* (6th ed.). Philadelphia, PA: Lippincott Williams & Wilkins.

34. Drake R. L., Vogl A. W., Mitchell A. W. M. (2015). *Gray's anatomy for students* (3rd ed.). Philadelphia, PA: Churchill Livingstone.

35. Hinkle J. L., Cheever K. H. (2018). *Brunner & Suddarth's textbook of medical-surgical nursing* (14th ed.). Philadelphia, PA: Lippincott Williams & Wilkins.

36. Browner B., Jupiter J., Krettek K., et al. (2015). *Skeletal trauma: Basic science, management and reconstruction* (5th ed.). Philadelphia, PA: Elsevier Saunders.

37. Valderama-Molina C. O., Estrada-Castrillón M., Hincapie J. A., et al. (2014). Intra- and interobserver agreement on the Oestern and Tscherne classification of soft tissue injury in periarticular lower-limb closed fractures. *Colombia Médica* 45(4), 173–178.

38. Lollo L., Grabinsky A. (2016). Clinical and functional outcomes of acute lower extremity compartment syndrome at a major trauma hospital. *International Journal of Critical Illness and Injury Science* 6(3), 133–142.

39. Garner M. R., Taylor S. A., Gausden E., et al. (2014). Compartment syndrome: Diagnosis, management, and unique concerns in the twenty-first century. *The Musculoskeletal Journal of Hospital for Special Surgery* 10, 143–152.

40. Goh E. L., Chidambaram S., Daqing M. (2017). Complex regional pain syndrome: A recent update. *Burns & Trauma* 5(2), 1–11. doi:10.1186/s41038-016-0066-4.

41. Tajerian M., Clark J. D. (2016). New concepts in complex regional pain syndrome. *Hand Clinics* 32(1), 41–49.

42. Pons T., Shipton E. A., Williman J., et al. (2015). Potential risk factors for the onset of complex regional pain syndrome type 1: A systematic literature review. *Anesthesiology Research and Practice* 2015(956539), 1–15.

43. Whiting P. S., Jahangir A. A. (2016). Thromboembolic disease after orthopedic trauma. *Orthopedic Clinics of North America* 47, 335–344.

44. Falck-Ytter Y., Francis C. W., Johanson N. A., et al. (2012). Prevention of VTE in orthopedic surgery patients: Antithrombotic therapy and prevention of thrombosis, 9th ed.: American College of Chest Physicians Evidence-based Clinical Practice Guidelines. *Chest* 141(2 suppl), e278S–e325S.

45. Kosova E., Bergmark B., Piazza G. (2015). Fat embolism syndrome. *Circulation* 131, 317–320.

46. Tyagi R. (2016). Spinal infections in children: A review. *Journal of Orthopaedics* 13, 254–258.

47. Schmitt S. K. (2017). Osteomyelitis. *Infectious Disease Clinics of North America* 31, 325–338.

48. Hanley M. E., Cooper J. S. (2017). Hyperbaric, chronic refractory osteomyelitis. [Online]. Available https://www.ncbi.nlm.nih.gov/books/NBK430703/. Accessed April 22, 2018.

49. Hogan J. I., Hurtado R. M., Nelson S. B. (2017). Mycobacterial musculoskeletal infections. *Infectious Disease Clinics of North America* 31, 369–382.

50. Brown J. P., Morin S., Leslie W., et al. (2014). Bisphosphonates for the treatment of osteoporosis: Expected benefits, potential harms, and drug holidays. *Canadian Family Physician* 60, 324–333.

51. Liu L. H., Zhang Q. Y., Sun W., et al. (2017). Corticosteroid-induced osteonecrosis of the femoral head: Detection, diagnosis, and treatment in earlier stages. *Chinese Medical Journal* 130, 2601–2607.

52. American Cancer Society. (2018). Bone cancer. [Online]. Available: http://www.cancer.org/cancer/bonecancer/detailed-guide/bone-cancer-key-statistics. Accessed March 4, 2018.

53. National Cancer Institute. (2019). Cancer stat facts: Bone and joint cancer. Available: https://seer.cancer.gov/statfacts/html/bones.html. Accessed July 8, 2019.

54. American Cancer Society. (2018). Bone cancer. [Online]. Available: https://www.cancer.org/cancer/bone-cancer/detection-diagnosis-staging/how-diagnosed.html. Accessed March 4, 2018.

55. American Cancer Society. (2018). Bone cancer. [Online]. Available: https://www.cancer.org/cancer/osteosarcoma/about/what-is-osteosarcoma.html. Accessed March 4, 2018.

56. Cronin K., Bui M., Caracciolo J. T. (2015). Osteoblastic osteosarcoma. *Applied Radiology* 44(7), 38–41.

57. Haddox C. L., Han G., Anijar L., et al. (2014). Osteosarcoma in pediatric patients and young adults: A single institution retrospective review of presentation, therapy, and outcome. *Sarcoma* 2014, 402509.

58. Brown H. K., Schiavone K., Gouin F., et al. (2018). Biology of bone sarcomas and new therapeutic developments. *Calcified Tissue International* 102, 174–195.

59. Freeman A. K., Sumathis V., Jeys L. (2014). Primary malignant tumors of the bone. *Orthopaedics 1: General Principles Surgery* 33(1), 26–33.

60. The ESMO/European Sarcoma Network Working Group. (2014). Bone sarcomas: ESMO clinical practice guidelines for diagnosis, treatment and follow-up. *Annals of Oncology* 25(Suppl 3), iii13–iii123.

61. Bharma J. S., Malik A. A., Aresti N. A., et al. (2012). The perioperative management of skeletal metastases. *Journal of Perioperative Practice* 22(1), 24–29.

62. American Cancer Society. (2018). Understanding advanced cancer, metastatic cancer, and bone metastasis. [Online]. Available: https://www.cancer.org/treatment/understanding-your-diagnosis/advanced-cancer/what-is.html. Accessed March 4, 2018.

63. Hernandez R. K., Wade S. W., Reich A., et al. (2018). Incidence of bone metastases in patients with solid tumors: Analysis of oncology electronic medical records in the United States. *BMC Cancer* 18(44), 1–11.

64. Li S., Peng Y., Weinhandl E. D., et al. (2012). Estimated number of prevalent cases of metastatic bone disease on the US adult population. *Clinical Epidemiology* 4, 87–93.

65. American Cancer Society. (2018). Finding bone metastases. [Online]. Available: https://www.cancer.org/treatment/understanding-your-diagnosis/advanced-cancer/finding-bone-metastases.html. Accessed March 4, 2018.

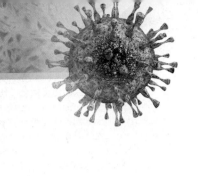

Disorders of Musculoskeletal Function: Developmental and Metabolic Disorders, Activity Intolerance, and Fatigue

Learning Objectives

After completing this chapter, the learner will be able to meet the following objectives:

1. Describe the function of the epiphyseal growth plate in skeletal growth.
2. Characterize the abnormalities associated with developmental dysplasia of the hip and methods of diagnosis and treatment.
3. Differentiate between congenital, idiopathic, and neuromuscular scoliosis.
4. Describe risk factors that contribute to the development of osteopenia, osteoporosis, osteomalacia, rickets, and Paget disease, and relate them to the prevention of the disorder.
5. Define fatigue and describe its manifestations.
6. Differentiate acute from chronic fatigue.
7. Define myalgic encephalomyelitis/chronic fatigue syndrome and describe assessment findings, presenting symptoms, and laboratory values associated with the disorder.

The development of skeletal structures begins in utero and continues to change throughout life. During childhood, skeletal structures grow in length and diameter and sustain a large increase in bone mass. The term *modeling* refers to the formation of the macroscopic skeleton, which ceases at maturity, usually between 18 and 20 years of age. Once skeletal growth has attained its adult size, the process of bone remodeling is responsible for skeletal maintenance. It involves bone resorption and formation and is responsible for skeletal maintenance at sites that require replacement or repair. With aging, bone resorption and formation are no longer perfectly coupled, and there is loss of bone.

Skeletal disorders may develop because of abnormal growth and developmental processes because of hereditary or congenital influences. Other skeletal disorders can occur later in life because of nutritional deficiencies, metabolic disorders, hormonal influences, or the aging process. This chapter is divided into two parts including altered skeletal growth and development and metabolic bone diseases.

Alterations in Skeletal Growth and Development

Bone Growth and Remodeling

Embryonic and Fetal Development

The skeletal system is generated from the mesodermal and neural crest cells of the developing embryo.[1] Development of the vertebrae of the axial skeleton begins at approximately the fourth week in utero. During the ninth week, ossification begins with the appearance of ossification centers in the lower thoracic and upper lumbar vertebrae. The paddle-shaped limb buds of the lower extremities make their appearance late in the fourth week of development; the hand pads are developed by days 33 to 36; and the finger rays are evident on days 41 to 43.[1]

Abnormalities originating from the embryonic stage of development are relatively uncommon. When they do occur, they are usually limited to defined embryonic structures (*e.g.*, congenital absence of a **phalanx**; formation of extra bones [supernumerary digits], or fusion of adjacent digits [syndactylism]). In utero positioning during fetal development causes the more common problems. In the newborn, the imprint of in utero positioning may be evident and confused with an abnormality. The effects of in utero positioning are usually physiologic in origin, rather than anatomic.

Bone Growth in Childhood

During the first two decades of life, the skeleton undergoes general overall growth. The long bones of the skeleton, which grow at a relatively rapid rate, are provided with a specialized structure called the *epiphyseal growth plate*[2] (Fig. 49-1). The chondrocytes are involved in synthesizing the cartilage of the epiphyseal plate.[2] As long bones grow in length, the deeper layers of cartilage cells in the growth plate multiply and enlarge and ultimately calcify. The embedded cartilage cells then die, attracting the osteoblasts to migrate into the area. Osteoid is secreted from the osteoblasts, which assists the mature bone in forming. Therefore, in the epiphyseal plates, there is continuous cartilage synthesis, calcification, erosion, and osteoblast invasion so that there is always active bone formation[2] (Fig. 49-2). This process allows bone growth to proceed without changing the shape of the bone or causing disruption of the articular cartilage.

The cells in the growth plate stop dividing at puberty, at which time the epiphysis and metaphysis fuse.

Several factors can influence the growth of cells in the epiphyseal growth plate. Epiphyseal separation can occur in children because of trauma. The separation usually occurs in the zone of the mature enlarged cartilage cells, which is the weakest part of the growth plate. The blood vessels that nourish the epiphysis pass through the growth plate. These vessels are ruptured when the growth plate separates. This can cause cessation of growth and a shortened extremity. The growth plate also is sensitive to nutritional and metabolic changes. Scurvy (*i.e.*, vitamin C deficiency) impairs the formation of the organic matrix of bone, causing slowing of growth at the epiphyseal plate and decreased diaphyseal growth. In rickets (*i.e.*, vitamin D deficiency), calcification of the newly developed bone on the metaphyseal side of the growth plate is impaired. Thyroid hormone, insulin-like growth factor, and insulin are required for normal growth. Alterations in these and other hormones can also affect growth. A few years after reaching puberty, the epiphyseal plates in the long bones become less responsive to the hormones and then become totally unresponsive.[2] Generally, people reach the end of bone growth by the age of 20 as the epiphyseal plate closes. However, some bones remain responsive to hormones and continue to grow. Examples include the skull, fingers, feet, and jaw.[2]

Growth in the diameter of bones occurs as new bone is added to the outer surface of existing bone along with an accompanying resorption of bone on the endosteal or inner surface. Such oppositional growth allows for widening of the marrow cavity while preventing the cortex from becoming too thick and heavy. In this way, the shape of the bone is maintained. As a bone grows in diameter, concentric rings are added to the bone surface, much as rings are added to a tree trunk. These rings form the lamellar structure of mature bone. Osteocytes, which develop from osteoblasts, become buried in the rings. Haversian canals form as periosteal vessels running along the long axis become surrounded by bone.[3]

Alterations during Normal Growth Periods

Infants and children undergo changes in muscle tone and joint motion during growth and development. Toeing-in, toeing-out, bowlegs, and knock-knees occur frequently in infancy and childhood.[4] They usually cause a few problems and are corrected during normal growth processes. There may be physiologic flexion contractures of the hips, which tend to be externally rotated and the patellae point outward, whereas the feet appear to point forward because of the internal pulling force of the tibiae. During the first year of life, the lower extremities begin to straighten out in preparation for walking. Internal and external rotations become equal, and the hips extend.

Musculoskeletal assessment of the newborn is important to identify abnormalities that require early intervention, facilitate treatment, establish baselines for future reference, and educate and counsel parents.[5,6] There are many clinical deviations that are easily correctable in a newborn and others that correct spontaneously as the child grows.

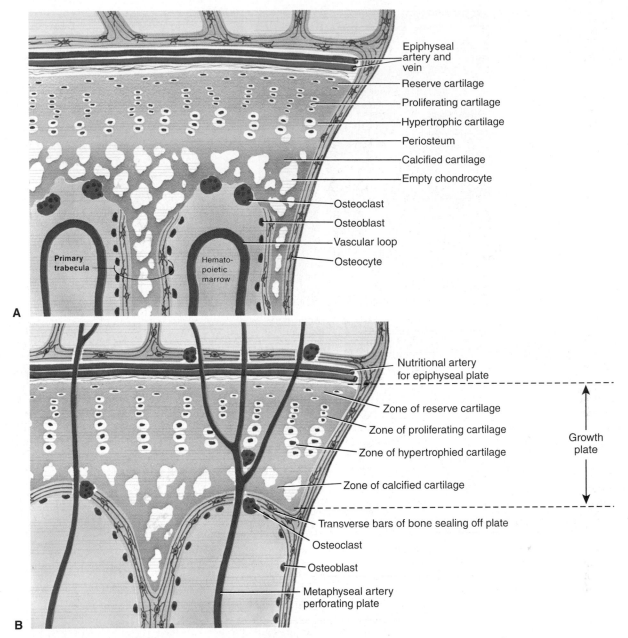

FIGURE 49-1. Anatomy of the epiphyseal growth plate. (**A**) Normal growing epiphyseal plate. The epiphysis is separated from the plate by transverse plates of bone that seal the plate so that it grows only toward the metaphysis. There are multiple zones of cartilage. (**B**) Normal closure. The epiphyseal cartilage has stopped growing. There are metaphyseal vessels penetrating the cartilage plate. Transverse bars of bone separate the plate from the metaphysis. (From Rubin R., Strayer D. S. (Eds.). (2015). *Rubin's pathology: Clinicopathologic foundations of medicine* (7th ed., p. 1314). Philadelphia, PA: Lippincott Williams & Wilkins.)

KEY POINTS

Developmental Skeletal Disorders

■ Many disorders of early infancy are caused by intrauterine positions and resolve as the child grows.

■ Nutritional and metabolic disorders can impair the formation of the organic matrix of bone, causing slowing of growth at the epiphyseal plate.

Torsional Deformities

All infants and toddlers have lax ligaments that become tighter with age and assumption of the weight-bearing posture. The hypermobility that accompanies joint laxity, coupled with the torsional (*i.e.*, rotational) forces exerted on the limbs during growth, is responsible for many variants seen in young children. Torsional forces caused by intrauterine positions or sleeping and sitting patterns twist the growing bones and can produce the deformities as a child grows and develops.

In infants, the femur normally is rotated to an anteverted position, with the femoral head and neck rotated anteriorly with respect to the femoral condyles. Femoral

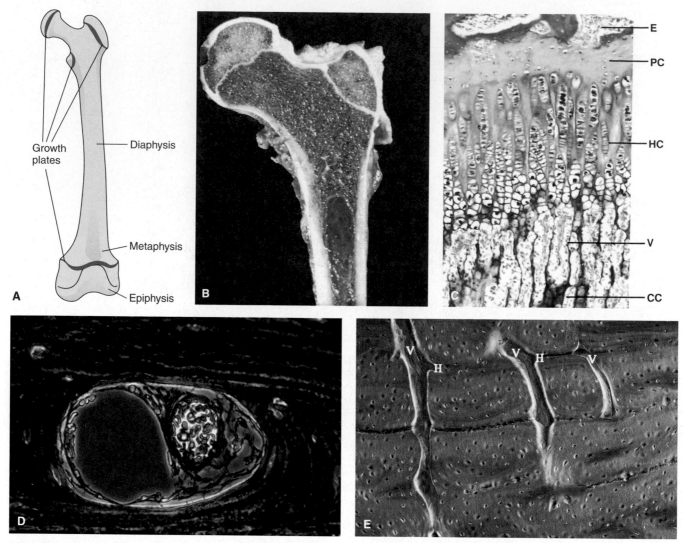

FIGURE 49-2. Anatomy of the long bone. **(A)** Diagram of femur illustrating the various compartments. **(B)** Coronal section of the proximal femur illustrates the various anatomic parts of a long bone. The epiphysis of the femoral head and the apophysis of the greater trochanter are separated from the metaphysis by their respective growth plates. The cortex and medullary cavity are well visualized. The medullary cavity contains cancellous bone until the metaphysis narrows into the diaphysis (shaft) of the bone, at which point the medullary cavity is completely devoid of bone and filled with marrow. **(C)** A section of the epiphysis with a zone of proliferating cartilage cells. Beneath this zone, the hypertrophic cartilage cells are arranged in columns. At the bottom, the calcifying matrix is invaded by blood vessels. **(D)** Haversian canal has a venule (thin-walled wider vessel on left) and an arteriole (thicker walled narrow vessel on the right). **(E)** Volkmann canals. There are three Volkmann canals visible running parallel to each other and perpendicular to the cortex. The openings of two of the haversian canals are also visible. CC, calcified cartilage; E, epiphysis; HC, hypertrophic cartilage; PC, proliferative cartilage; V, vascular invasion. (From Rubin R., Strayer D. S. (Eds.). (2015). *Rubin's pathology: Clinicopathologic foundations of medicine* (7th ed., p. 1308). Philadelphia, PA: Lippincott Williams & Wilkins.)

anteversion (*i.e.*, medial rotation) decreases from approximately 40 degrees at birth to approximately 15 degrees at maturity (Fig. 49-3). The normal tibia is externally rotated approximately 5 degrees at birth and approximately 15 degrees at maturity. Torsional abnormalities frequently demonstrate a familial tendency.[5]

The foot progression angle describes the angle between the axis of the foot and the line of progression.[4,5] It is determined by watching the child walking and running, although it is usually less noticeable when the child is running or barefoot. Figure 49-4 illustrates the position of the foot in toeing-in and toeing-out, and the line of progression, when a child is walking.

Toeing-In

Toeing-in (*i.e.*, metatarsus adductus) is the most common congenital foot deformity, with an incidence of approximately 1 per every 1000 to 2000 live births.[5] It is sometimes called pigeon toe. The forefoot commonly is adducted and gives the foot a kidney-shaped appearance, whereas the hindfoot is normal[6] (Fig. 49-5). It can be caused by torsion in the foot, lower leg, or in the entire leg. Toeing-in because of adduction of the forefoot (*i.e.*, congenital metatarsus adductus) usually is the result of the fetal position maintained in utero. It may occur in one foot or in both feet. Diagnostic methods include examination of the plantar aspect of

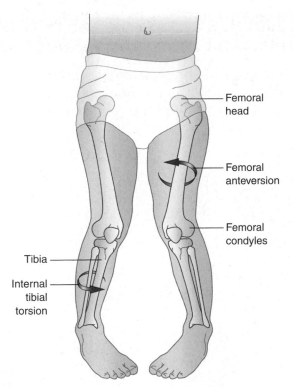

FIGURE 49-3. Femoral anteversion and internal tibial rotation. Femoral anteversion normally decreases from about 40 degrees at birth to 15 degrees at maturity, and internal tibial rotation from 5 degrees at birth to 15 degrees at maturity.

the foot, noting the overall shape of the foot and the presence or absence of an arch.[6] The presence of a skin crease indicates a congenital deformity (see Fig. 49-5). Metatarsus adductus is graded on the basis of the foot's flexibility while applying pressure to the medial

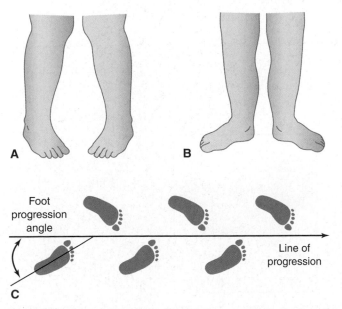

FIGURE 49-4. (A) Toeing-in. (B) Toeing-out. (C) Toeing-in and toeing-out can be determined by watching a child walk and comparing the long axis of the foot with the direction in which the child is walking. If the foot is directed inward, the angle is negative and indicative of toeing-in; if it is positive, it is indicative of toeing-out.

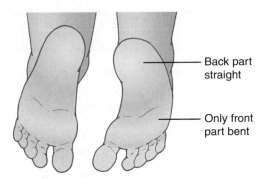

FIGURE 49-5. Shape of foot. The left foot is normal, whereas the right foot has metatarsus adductus.

forefoot. The defect is defined as grade I, II, or III. Grade I is a supple deformity that can be passively manipulated into a straight position and requires no treatment. A grade II deformity corrects only to a straight lateral border, and a grade III deformity is more rigid and may require further treatment.[6] Treatment consisting of serial long leg casting or a brace that pushes the metatarsals (not the hindfoot) into abduction usually is required in a fixed (rigid) deformity (*i.e.*, one in which the forefoot cannot be passively manipulated into a straight position).[6]

Toeing-Out

Toeing-out (slew foot) is a common problem in children and is caused by external femoral torsion. It is less common than toeing-in and occurs sometimes with calcaneovalgus and pes planovalgus.[5] This occurs when the femur can be externally rotated to approximately 90 degrees but internally rotated only to a neutral position or slightly beyond. Because the femoral torsion persists when a child habitually sleeps in the prone position, an external tibial torsion also may develop. If external tibial torsion is present, the feet point lateral to the midline of the medial plane. External tibial torsion rarely causes toeing-out; it only intensifies the condition. Toeing-out usually corrects itself as the child becomes proficient in walking. Occasionally, a night splint is used.

Tibial Torsion

Tibial torsion is determined by measuring the thigh–foot angle, which is done with the ankle and knee positioned at 90 degrees. In this position, the foot normally rotates outward. *Internal tibial torsion* (*i.e.*, bowing of the tibia) is a rotation of the tibia that makes the feet appear to turn inward (see Fig. 49-3). It is the most common cause of toeing-in in children younger than 2 years of age. It is present at birth and may fail to correct itself if children sleep on their knees with the feet turned in or sit on in-turned feet.[5] It is thought to be caused by genetic factors and intrauterine compression, such as an unstretched uterus during a first pregnancy or intrauterine crowding with twins or multiple fetuses. Tibial torsion generally improves naturally with growth, but this may take years.

External tibial torsion, a much less common disorder, is associated with calcaneovalgus foot and is caused by a

UNDERSTANDING ➡ Bone Remodeling

Bone remodeling constitutes a process of skeletal maintenance once skeletal growth is complete. Significant progress has been made in understanding the phenomenon of bone remodeling because it relates to the coupling of bone resorption with bone formation.

1

Bone Remodeling Cycle Mature bone is made up of units called *osteons* in which concentric lamellae (bone layers) surround a central, *haversian* canal. Bone remodeling consists of a sequence of bone resorption within an osteon by osteoclasts, followed by new bone formation by osteoblasts. In the adult, the length of one sequence (*i.e.*, bone resorption and formation) is approximately 4 months. Ideally, the replaced bone should equal the resorbed bone. If it does not, there is net loss of bone. In the elderly, for example, bone resorption and formation no longer are perfectly coupled, and bone mass is lost.

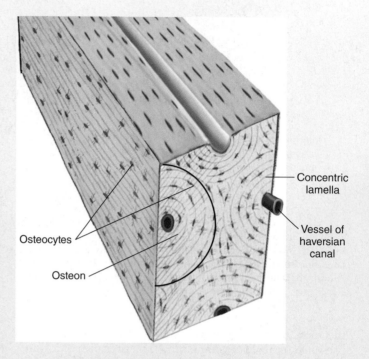

Concentric lamella

Vessel of haversian canal

Osteocytes

Osteon

2

Bone Resorption The osteoclasts, which are bone-resorbing cells derived from monocyte/macrophage precursors, are the cells involved in the initiation of bone remodeling. The sequence of bone resorption and bone formation is activated by many stimuli, including the action of parathyroid hormone and calcitonin. It begins with osteoclastic resorption of existing bone, during which the organic (protein matrix) and inorganic (mineral) components are removed, creating a tunnel-like space in the osteon. Soluble factors released during resorption aid in the recruitment of osteoblasts to the site, thereby linking bone resorption to bone formation.

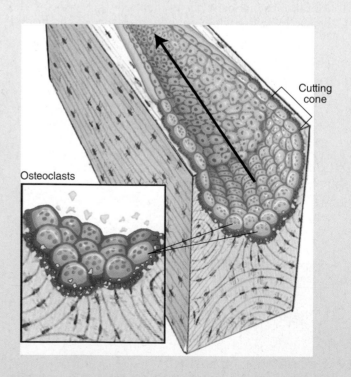

Cutting cone

Osteoclasts

3

Bone Formation After osteoclastic activity has ceased, osteoblasts begin to deposit the organic matrix (osteoid) on the wall of the osteon canal. As successive lamellae of bone are deposited, the canal ultimately attains the relative proportions of the original osteon. In the formation and maintenance of bone, osteoblasts provide much of the local control because not only do they produce new bone matrix but they also play an essential role in mediating osteoclast activity. Many of the primary stimulators of bone resorption, such as parathyroid hormone, have minimal or no direct effects on osteoclasts. Once the osteoblast, which has receptors for these substances, receives the appropriate signal, it releases a soluble mediator called *RANKL* (receptor activator of nuclear factor kappa-B ligand) that induces osteoclast activity.

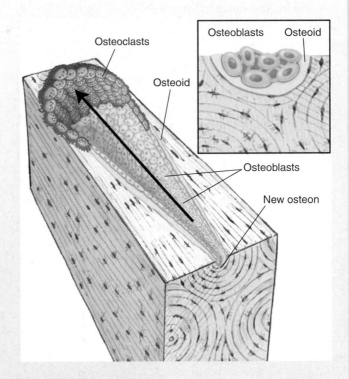

4

Control of Bone Metabolism and Remodeling The pivotal pathway linking osteoclast-mediated bone resorption with osteoblast-mediated bone formation consists of a paracrine system that includes the RANKL, its receptor RANK, and a soluble protein called *osteoprotegerin* (OPG). RANKL, which is produced by osteoblasts and their precursors, binds to RANK, promoting osteoclast differentiation and proliferation. The soluble OPG molecule, which is produced by many tissues, acts as a decoy receptor to block the action of RANKL. This system ensures the tight coupling of bone formation and resorption and provides a means whereby a wide variety of biologic mediators (*e.g.*, hormones, cytokines, and growth factors) influence the homeostasis of bone.

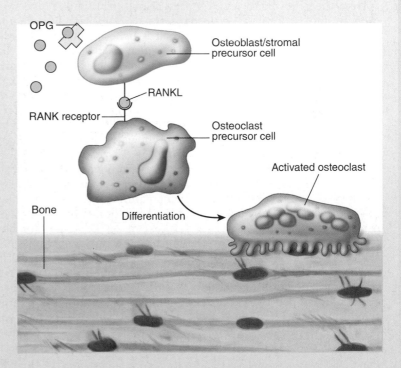

normal variation of intrauterine positioning or a neuro-muscular disorder. It is characterized by an abnormally positive thigh–foot angle of 30 to 50 degrees.[5] The condition corrects itself naturally, and treatment is observational. Significant improvement begins during the first year with the onset of ambulation and usually is complete by 2 to 3 years of age.[5] The normal adult exhibits about 20 degrees of tibial torsion.

Femoral Torsion

Femoral torsion refers to abnormal variations in hip rotation. Hip rotation is measured at the pelvic level with the child in the prone position and the knees flexed at a 90-degree angle. In this position, the hip is in a neutral position. Rotating the lower leg outward produces internal or medial femoral rotation; rotating it inward produces external or lateral rotation. During measurement of hip rotation, the legs are allowed to fall to full internal rotation by gravity alone; lateral rotation is measured by allowing the legs to fall inward and cross. Hip rotation in flexion and extension also can be measured with computed tomography (CT). By 1 year of age, there is normally approximately 45 degrees of internal rotation and 45 degrees of external rotation.

Internal femoral torsion, also called *femoral anteversion* (see Fig. 49-3), is a normal variant commonly seen during the first 6 years of life, especially in 3- and 4-year-old girls.[6] Characteristically, there is 80 to 90 degrees of internal rotation of the hip in the prone position. The condition is thought to be related to increased laxity of the anterior capsule of the hip such that it does not provide the stable pressure needed to correct the anteversion that is present at birth. Children are most comfortable sitting in the "W" position, with their hips between their knees. It is believed that this position allows the lower leg to act as a lever, producing torsional changes in the femur. When the child stands, the knees turn in and the feet appear to point straight ahead. When the child walks, the knees and toes point in. Children with this problem are encouraged to sit cross-legged or in the so-called *tailor position*. If left untreated, the tibiae compensate by becoming externally rotated so that by 8 to 12 years of age, the knees may turn in but the feet no longer do so. This can result in patellofemoral malalignment with patellar subluxation or dislocation and pain.[6] A derotational osteotomy may be done in severe cases or if there is functional disability.

External femoral torsion is an uncommon disorder characterized by excessive external rotation of the hip. Bilateral external torsion is usually a benign condition, and treatment is observational. When the disorder is unilateral, slipped capital femoral epiphysis should be ruled out.

Genu Varum and Genu Valgum

Genu varum, or *bowlegs*, is an outward bowing of the knees greater than 1 inch when the medial malleoli of the ankles are touching (Fig. 49-6). As children grow, lower limb alignment usually follows a predictable pattern (Fig. 49-7). Most infants and toddlers have some bowing

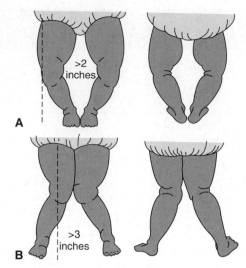

FIGURE 49-6. (A) Genu varum. (B) Genu valgum. (From Silbert-Flagg J., Pillitteri A. (2018). *Maternal and child health nursing: Care of the childbearing and child rearing family* (8th ed., Fig. 51.9, p. 1444). Philadelphia, PA: Lippincott Williams & Wilkins.)

of their legs up to 18 months of age. If there is a large separation between the knees (>15 degrees) after 2 years of age, the child may require bracing. The child also should be evaluated for diseases such as rickets or tibia vara[6] (Fig. 49-8).

Genu valgum, or *knock-knees*, is a deformity in which there is decreased space between the knees (Fig. 49-6). The medial malleoli in the ankles cannot be brought in contact with each other when the knees are touching. Valgus gradually develops after age 24 months and is most apparent between 3 and 4 years of age. The condition usually is the result of lax medial collateral ligaments of the knee. Obesity is also associated with the development of genu valgum and is becoming almost epidemic in the United States.[7] By 7 years of age, the lower limb is in slight valgus and changes very little thereafter. Genu valgum can be ignored up to 7 years of age, unless it is a larger angle, one sided, or associated with short stature. It usually resolves spontaneously and rarely requires treatment. If genu varum or genu valgum persists and is not corrected, osteoarthritis may develop in adulthood as a result of abnormal intra-articular stress. There is a new surgical treatment for both knock-knees and bowlegs, which includes the use of extraphyseal tension band plates that manipulate the angle of the growth plate.[8] Genu varum can cause gait awkwardness and increased risk for sprains and fractures. Uncorrected genu valgum may cause subluxation and recurrent dislocation of the patella, with a predisposition to chondromalacia and joint pain and fatigue. Therefore, new challenges such as obesity need to become a priority management outcome in pediatric orthopedics.[7,9]

Flatfoot

Flatfoot (*i.e.*, pes planus) is a deformity characterized by the absence of the longitudinal arch of the foot. Infants

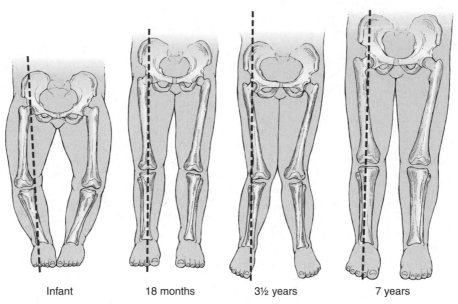

Infant   18 months   3½ years   7 years

FIGURE 49-7. Lower limb alignment follows a predictable pattern. Infants typically have a gentle varus bow throughout the femur and tibia. By 18 to 24 months, the lower leg is nearly straight, with a neutral mechanical axis. Valgus gradually develops and is most apparent between 3 and 4 years of age. By 7 years of age, the lower limb is in slight valgus and changes very little thereafter. Varus should not recur, nor should valgus increase. (From Morissy R. T., Weinstein S. L. (Eds.). (2006). *Lovell & Winter's pediatric orthopaedics* (6th ed.). Philadelphia, PA: Lippincott Williams & Wilkins.)

normally have a wider and fatter foot than do adults. The fat pads that normally are accentuated by pliable muscles with young children create the appearance of fullness often mistaken for flatfoot.[10,11] Until the longitudinal arch develops around 2 years of age, most children appear to have flat feet. The true criterion for flatfoot is that with weight-bearing, the talus points medially and downward, so that the heel is everted and the forefoot is inverted.

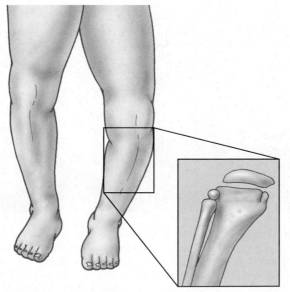

FIGURE 49-8. Rotational deformity of the proximal tibia, especially when unilateral, suggests tibia vara (Blount disease).

Obesity, ligament laxity (which is genetically linked), and the wearing of nonsupportive shoes over time are other possible etiologies of pes planus.[10,11] Overweight children have lower plantar arch height because of the excessive body weight putting increased pressure on the child's feet.[10,11]

There are two types of flatfoot—flexible and rigid. Most children with flexible flatfoot have loose ligaments, allowing the feet to sag when they gain weight. With this type of flatfoot, the arch disappears only with weight-bearing. No special treatment is needed for flexible flatfoot. People with flexible flatfoot are less prone to pain and injury than those with normal or high arches. The rigid flatfoot is fixed, with no apparent arch in any position. It is seen in conjunction with neuromuscular diseases such as cerebral palsy.

In the adult, treatment of flatfoot is conservative and aimed at relieving fatigue and discomfort. Supportive, well-fitting shoes with arch supports may be helpful and prevent ligaments from becoming overstretched. Surgery may be done in cases of severe and persistent symptoms.

Hereditary and Congenital Deformities

Congenital deformities are abnormalities that are present at birth. They range in severity from mild limb deformities, which are relatively common, to major limb malformations, which are relatively rare. The most common anomaly of the toes or fingers is *polydactyly* or the presence of an extra digit on the hand or foot.

Macrodactyly occurs when one or more toes or fingers are hypertrophied and are significantly larger than the surrounding toes or fingers.

There may also be a simple webbing of the fingers or toes (syndactyly) or the absence of a bone such as the phalanx, rib, or clavicle. Joint contractures and dislocations produce more severe deformity, as does the absence of entire bones, joints, or limbs. Surgery is done to relieve functional symptoms, such as pain or difficulty in fitting shoes. The cosmetic goal is to alter the grotesque appearance of the hand or foot and to achieve a size similar to that of the opposite extremity.

Congenital deformities are caused by many factors, some unknown. These factors include hereditary influences, external agents that injure the fetus (*e.g.*, radiation, alcohol, drugs, such as thalidomide taken by pregnant women with morning sickness in the 1960s, and viruses), and intrauterine environmental factors. Many of the organic bone matrix components have been identified only recently, and their interactions were found to be more complex than were originally thought. Hand and foot disorders associated with abnormalities in bone matrix include those with deficient collagen synthesis and decreased bone mass.[12]

Osteogenesis Imperfecta

Osteogenesis imperfecta (OI) is a hereditary disease characterized by defective synthesis of type I collagen[13,14] (Fig. 49-9). It is one of the most common hereditary bone diseases, with an estimated 20,000 to 50,000 people with OI in the United States.[13] OI is usually transmitted as an autosomal dominant trait. However, the type III form of OI, which is the most progressively deforming type with multiple life-threatening defects, is sometimes, although rarely, inherited as an autosomal recessive trait.[14]

Mutations in the genes connected with type I collagen, which impacts the development of bones, joints, ears, ligaments, teeth, sclerae, and skin, cause the problems.[14] The genes are *COL1A1* and *COL1A2*, which encode the alpha$_1$ and alpha$_2$ chains of type I procollagen.[14] These genes are found in chromosome 17 and 7 and cause different structural and clinical changes in the types of OI.

Clinical Manifestations

The clinical manifestations of OI include a spectrum of disorders marked by extreme skeletal fragility. Four major subtypes of the disorder have been identified, each with their specific manifestations[14] (Table 49-1).

The disorder is characterized by thin and poorly developed bones that are prone to multiple fractures. These children have short limbs and a soft, thin cranium with bifrontal prominences that give a triangular appearance to the face. Other problems associated with defective connective tissue synthesis include wormian bone in the skull, thin skin, blue or gray sclera, abnormal tooth development, hypotonic muscles, loose-jointedness, and scoliosis.[15] Hearing loss because of otosclerosis of the tiny bones in the middle ear is common in affected adults. The most serious defects occur with type II. Severely affected fetuses have multiple intrauterine fractures and bowing and shortening of the extremities. Many of these infants are stillborn or die during infancy.

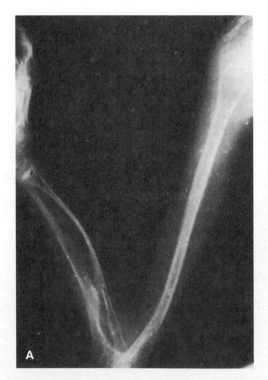

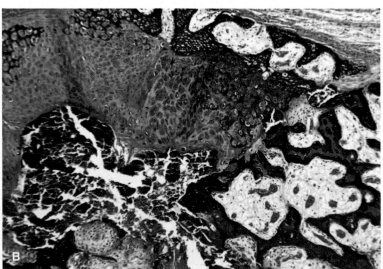

FIGURE 49-9. Osteogenesis imperfecta. (**A**) A radiograph illustrates the thin humerus and bones of the forearm. There is a fracture callus in the proximal ulna. (**B**) A photomicrograph of the fracture callus with prominent cartilage in the upper left. The cortex is thin and composed of hypercellular woven bone. (From Rubin R., Strayer D. S. (Eds.). (2015). *Rubin's pathology: Clinicopathologic foundations of medicine* (7th ed., p. 1318). Philadelphia, PA: Lippincott Williams & Wilkins.)

TABLE 49-1 Types of OI			
Type	**Subtype**	**Inheritance**	**Manifestations**
I	Postbirth—manifestations are mildest of the OI types	Autosomal dominant	Multiple fractures, blue sclera, hearing problems, and possible dental problems
II	Perinatal—lethal disorder ending in early death	Autosomal dominant	Infant dies within a few days or is stillborn
III	Perinatal and postbirth—sclerae are blue at birth and turn white soon after, most progressive and severely deforming type	Usually autosomal dominant, but can be recessive	Multiple bone fractures, growth retardation, severe skeletal deformities
IV	Postbirth—manifestations are similar to type I except that sclerae are white	Autosomal dominant	Multiple fractures, possible dental and hearing disorders; sclerae are normal
Other type IV (V, VI, VII, and VIII)	Distinct clinical, genetic, and bone histologic features	Both autosomal dominant and recessive	Heterogeneous type IV

OI, Osteogenesis Imperfecta.
From Rubin R., Strayer D. S. (Eds.). (2015). Rubin's pathology: Clinicopathologic foundations of medicine (7th ed., pp. 1318–1319). Philadelphia, PA: Lippincott Williams & Wilkins.

Treatment

There is no definitive treatment for correction of the defective collagen synthesis that is characteristic of OI. However, the bisphosphonates have been shown to produce an increase in cortical bone width and cancellous bone volume, as well as increased bone strength and mineral content.[15] Prevention and treatment of fractures are important. Precise alignment is necessary to prevent deformities. Nonunion is common, especially with repeated fractures. Surgical intervention is often needed to stabilize fractures and correct deformities.

Developmental Dysplasia of the Hip

Developmental dysplasia of the hip (DDH), formerly known as *congenital dislocation of the hip*, is an abnormality in hip development that leads to a wide spectrum of hip problems in infants and children, including hips that are unstable, malformed, subluxated, or completely dislocated.[16] In less severe cases, the hip joint may be unstable, with excessive laxity of the joint capsule, or subluxated, so that the joint surfaces are separated and there is a partial dislocation (Fig. 49-10). With dislocated hips, the head of the femur is located outside of the acetabulum.

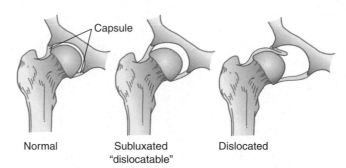

FIGURE 49-10. Normal (*left*) and abnormal relationships of hip joint structure in subluxation (*middle*) and dislocation (*right*).

The results of newborn screening programs have shown that 1 in 100 infants have some evidence of hip instability, whereas dislocation of the hip is seen in 1 in every 1000 live births.[10] The left hip is involved more frequently than is the right hip because of the left occipital intrauterine positioning of most infants.[10] The disorder occurs most frequently in first-born children and is six times more common in female than in male infants.[16]

Etiology

The cause of DDH is multifactorial, with heredity, environmental, and mechanical factors playing a role. A positive family history and generalized laxity of the ligaments are related. The increased frequency in girls is thought to result from their susceptibility to maternal estrogens and other hormones associated with pelvic relaxation. Dislocation also may result from environmental factors such as fetal position, a tight uterus that prevents fetal movement, and breech delivery. The presence of other congenital abnormalities is associated with an increased incidence of DDH. Thus, the hips of children presenting with congenital abnormalities should be examined carefully.

Diagnosis

Early diagnosis of DDH is important because treatment is easiest and most effective if begun during the first 6 months of life.[16] Also, repeated dislocations cause damage to the femoral head and the acetabulum. There is no uniformly accepted method for diagnosis of DDH during the newborn period. However, there is evidence that ultrasound is most effective during the first month of life for screening hip joint problems.[17] However, the U.S. Preventive Services Task Force (USPSTF) states that 90% of the hip abnormalities identified by ultrasound resolve on their own.[17] Clinical examination of the hips is recommended at birth and every several months during the first year of life.[17] Research states that 60% to 80% of hip deformities identified in children from clinical examination resolve on their own.[16] Follow-up clinical examinations should be done in the presence of an abnormality. In infants, signs of DDH include asymmetry of the hip or gluteal folds, shortening of the thigh so that one knee (on the affected side) is higher than the other hip, and limited abduction of the affected hip (Fig. 49-11). The asymmetry of gluteal folds is not definitive but indicates the need for further evaluation. The USPSTF states that

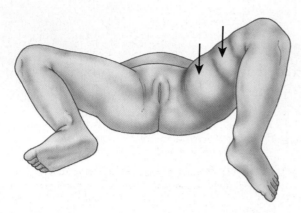

FIGURE 49-11. Congenital dysplasia of the left hip with shortening of the femur, as indicated by legs in abduction and asymmetric gluteal and thigh folds (*arrows*).

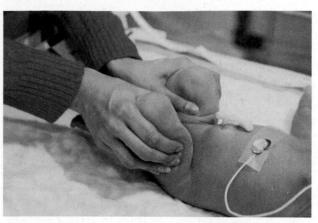

FIGURE 49-13. Barlow maneuver. (From Jensen S. (2015). *Nursing health assessment: A best practice approach* (2nd ed., Fig. 26.9, p. 836). Philadelphia, PA: Lippincott Williams & Wilkins.)

evidence is insufficient to recommend routine screening of asymptomatic infants as a means of preventing adverse outcomes.[16]

Several examination techniques can be used to screen for a dislocatable hip.[5,16,18] Two specific maneuvers for assessing hip stability in the newborn are the Ortolani maneuver (for reducible dislocation) (Fig. 49-12) and the Barlow maneuver (for the dislocatable hip) (Fig. 49-13).[5,16,18] The Barlow maneuver involves a manual attempt to dislocate and reduce the abnormal hip while the infant is in the supine position with both knees flexed. With gentle downward pressure being applied to the knees, the knee and thigh are manually abducted as an upward and medial pressure is applied to the proximal thigh. In infants with the disorder, the initial downward pressure on the knee produces a dislocation of the hip, a positive Barlow sign. This is followed by a palpable or audible click (*i.e.,* Ortolani sign) as the hip is reduced and moves back into the acetabulum. The sensitivity of these tests is improved significantly with the use

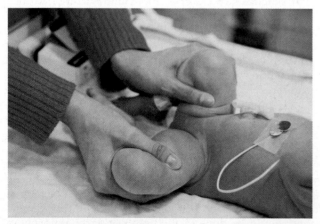

FIGURE 49-12. Examination for developmental dysplasia of the hip. In the newborn, both hips can be equally flexed, abducted, and externally rotated without producing a "click." A diagnosis of congenital dislocation of the hip may be confirmed by the Ortolani "click" test. The involved hip cannot be abducted as far as the opposite one, and there is a "click" as the hip reduces. (From Jensen S. (2015). *Nursing health assessment: A best practice approach* (2nd ed., Fig. 26.9A, p. 836). Philadelphia, PA: Lippincott Williams & Wilkins.)

of trained and experienced examiners. The Galeazzi test is a measurement of the length of the femurs that is done by comparing the height at the knees while they are flexed at 90 degrees. An inequality in the height of the knees is a positive Galeazzi sign and is usually caused by hip dislocation or congenital femoral shortening. This test is not useful in detecting bilateral DDH because both leg lengths will be equal. In an older child, instability of the hip may produce a delay in standing or walking and eventually cause a characteristic waddling gait. When the thumbs are placed over the anterior iliac crest and the hands are placed over the lateral pelvis in examination, the levels of the thumbs are not even; the child is unable to elevate the opposite side of the pelvis (positive Trendelenburg test).

Diagnosis of DDH is confirmed by ultrasonography or radiography. Ultrasonography is used in infants with high-risk factors (*e.g.,* female infants born in the breech position) or an abnormal result on examination.[18,19] Radiographs of newborns with suspected DDH are of limited value because the femoral heads do not ossify until 4 to 6 months of age. After 6 months of age, the increasing ossification of the femur renders ultrasonography less reliable, and radiographs are preferred.

Treatment

Treatment of DDH should be individualized and depends on whether the hip is subluxated or dislocated. Subluxation of the hip at birth often resolves without treatment and should be observed for 2 weeks. When subluxation persists beyond this time, treatment may be indicated and referral is recommended. The best results are obtained if the treatment is begun before changes in the hip structure (*e.g.,* 2 to 3 months) prevent it from being reduced by gentle manipulation or abduction devices. Treatment at any age includes reduction of the dislocation and immobilization of the legs in an abducted position.

Congenital Clubfoot

Clubfoot, or talipes, is one of the most common pediatric orthopedic conditions. It has an incidence of approximately 1 to 2 cases per 1000 live births, is bilateral in about 50% of cases, and affects boys more often than it does girls.[20] Like congenital dislocation of the hip, its occurrence follows a multifactorial inheritance pattern. Clubfoot may be associated with chromosomal abnormalities or congenital syndromes that are transmitted by Mendelian inheritance patterns (Fig. 49-14). However, it is most commonly idiopathic and found in normal infants in whom no genetic or chromosomal abnormality or other extrinsic cause can be found.

In forefoot adduction, which accounts for approximately 95% of idiopathic cases, the foot is plantar flexed and inverted. This is the so-called *equinovarus type* in which the foot resembles a horse's hoof. The other 5% of cases are of the calcaneovalgus type, or reverse clubfoot, in which the foot is dorsiflexed and everted. The reverse clubfoot can occur as an isolated condition or in association with multiple congenital defects. At birth, the feet of many infants assume one of these two positions, but they can be passively overcorrected or brought back into the opposite position. If the foot cannot be overcorrected, some type of correction may be necessary.

Treatment of clubfoot is begun as soon as the diagnosis is made. One screening tool for equinovarus type clubfoot is the clubfoot assessment protocol, which is also helpful in developing a management plan.[20] When treatment is initiated during the first few weeks of life, a nonoperative procedure may be effective. Serial manipulations and casting are used gently to correct each component of the deformity. Surgery may be required for severe deformities or when nonoperative treatment methods are unsuccessful.

Juvenile Osteochondroses

The term *juvenile osteochondroses* is used to describe a group of children's diseases in which one or more

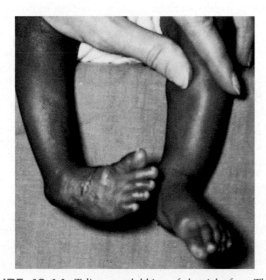

FIGURE 49-14. Talipes or clubbing of the right foot. The foot is turned to the side, and the involved foot, calf, and leg are smaller and shorter than the normal side. One or both feet may be affected. This condition is not painful; however, if left untreated, significant discomfort and disability will develop. Treatment ranges from braces or casts to surgery. (From Jensen S. (2015). *Nursing health assessment: A best practice approach* (2nd ed., Fig. 21.3, p. 648). Philadelphia, PA: Lippincott Williams & Wilkins.)

growth ossification centers undergo a period of degeneration, necrosis, or inactivity that is followed by regeneration and usually deformity. The osteochondroses are separated into two groups according to their causes. The first group consists of the true osteonecrotic osteochondroses, so called because the diseases are caused by localized osteonecrosis of an apophyseal or epiphyseal center (*e.g.*, Legg–Calvé–Perthes disease, Freiberg infraction, Panner disease, and Kienböck disease). The second group of juvenile osteochondroses is caused by abnormalities in ossification of cartilaginous tissue resulting from a genetically determined normal variation or from trauma (*e.g.*, Osgood–Schlatter disease, Blount disease, Sever disease, and Scheuermann disease). The discussion in this section focuses on Legg–Calvé–Perthes disease from the first group and Osgood–Schlatter disease from the second group. Slipped capital femoral epiphysis is a disorder of the growth plate.

Legg–Calvé–Perthes Disease

Legg–Calvé–Perthes disease is an idiopathic osteonecrotic disease of the proximal (capital) femoral epiphysis.[21] It occurs in 1 of 1200 children, affecting primarily those, mostly boys, between ages 3 and 12 years, with a median age of 7 years.[22] It occurs primarily in boys and is much more common in whites than in African Americans. Although no definite genetic pattern has been established, it occasionally affects more than one family member.

Etiology and Pathogenesis
The cause of Legg–Calvé–Perthes disease is unknown. The disorder is usually insidious at onset and occurs in otherwise healthy children. It may, however, be associated with acute trauma. Evidence suggests a correlation between acquiring Legg–Calvé–Perthes disease and some procoagulation parameters with boys.[22] Affected children usually have a short stature. Undernutrition has been suggested as a causative factor. When girls are affected, they usually have a poorer prognosis than do boys because they are skeletally more mature and have a shorter period for growth and remodeling than do boys of the same age.[22]

The primary pathologic feature of Legg–Calvé–Perthes disease is an avascular necrosis of the bone and marrow involving the epiphyseal growth center in the femoral head.[21] The disorder may be confined to part of the epiphysis, or it may involve the entire epiphysis. In severe cases, there is a disturbance in the growth pattern that leads to a broad, short femoral neck. The necrosis is followed by slow absorption of the dead bone over 2 to 3 years. Although the necrotic trabeculae eventually are replaced by healthy new bone, the epiphysis rarely regains its normal shape. The process occurs in four predictable stages.[21,22] The *first stage*, which lasts for 6 to 12 months, is the avascular stage when the ossification center is becoming necrotic. Damage to the femoral head is determined by the amount of necrosis occurring during this stage. The *second stage*, lasting about 1 to 3 years, is the revascularization stage, during which resorption of the necrotic bone takes place. The *third stage* is the reossification stage, during which radiolucent areas become dense, whereas the shape of the femoral head improves. The *fourth stage*, which is the healed stage, involves the forming of immature bone cells by normal bone cells and the resulting femoral head.[21,22]

Clinical Manifestations

The main symptoms of Legg–Calvé–Perthes disease are pain in the thigh or knee and difficulty in walking. The child may have a painless limp with limited abduction and internal rotation and a flexion contracture of the affected hip. The age of onset is important because young children have a greater capability for remodeling of the femoral head and acetabulum, and thus, less flattening of the femoral head occurs.

Diagnosis and Treatment

Early diagnosis is important and is based on correlating physical symptoms with radiographic findings (*e.g.*, magnetic resonance imaging [MRI], CT scan, ultrasound, arthrography, bone scintigraphy, and radiography), which are related to the stage of the disease.[21]

The goal of treatment is to reduce deformity and preserve the integrity of the femoral head while the necrotic bone is resorbed.[21]

Conservative and surgical interventions are used in the treatment of Legg–Calvé–Perthes disease. Children younger than 4 years of age with little or no involvement of the femoral head may require only periodic observation. In all other children, some intervention is needed to relieve the force of weight-bearing, muscular tension, and subluxation of the femoral head. It is important to maintain the femur in a well-seated position in the concave acetabulum to prevent deformity. This is done by keeping the hip in abduction and mild internal rotation. Treatment involves periods of rest, use of assistive devices for walking, nonweight-bearing, and abduction braces to keep the legs separated in abduction with mild internal rotation.

Surgery may be done to contain the femoral head in the acetabulum. This treatment usually is reserved for children older than 6 years of age who at the time of diagnosis have more serious involvement of the femoral head. Some children with Legg–Calvé–Perthes disease may require total hip replacement surgery at some point in time depending on the degree of avascular necrosis.[22]

Osgood–Schlatter Disease

Osgood–Schlatter disease involves microfractures in the area where the patellar tendon inserts into the tibial tubercle, which is an extension of the proximal tibial epiphysis.[23] This area is particularly vulnerable to injury caused by sudden or continued strain from the patellar tendon during periods of growth, particularly in athletic adolescents.

The patellar tendon is inflamed and thickened from the continuous inflammation and causes pain in front of the knee. There is swelling, tenderness, and increased prominence of the tibial tubercle. The symptoms usually are self-limiting. They may recur during growth periods but usually resolve after closure of the tibial growth plate. In some cases, limitations on activity, tibial bands, or braces to immobilize the knee; anti-inflammatory agents; and application of cold are necessary to relieve the pain.[23] The objective of treatment is to release tension on the quadriceps to permit revascularization and reossification of the tibial tubercle. Complete resolution of symptoms through healing (physical closure) of the tibial tubercle can extend to a year or even 2 years.[23]

 Concept Mastery Alert

Osgood–Schlatter disease is characterized by thickening of the patellar tendon. Pain occurs during activity and is focused in the front of the knee.

Slipped Capital Femoral Epiphysis

Slipped capital femoral epiphysis, or coxa vara, is a disorder of the growth plate that occurs near the age of skeletal maturity. It involves a three-dimensional displacement of the epiphysis (posteriorly, medially, inferiorly), meaning that the femur is rotated externally from under the epiphysis. The condition is rare, with an estimated frequency of 10 in 10,000.[24]

The cause of slipped capital femoral epiphysis is obscure, but it may be related to the child's susceptibility to stress on the femoral neck as a result of genetics or structural abnormalities.[24] Boys are affected twice as often as are girls, and in approximately half the cases the condition is bilateral. Affected children often are overweight with poorly developed secondary sex characteristics or, in some instances, are extremely tall and thin. In many cases, there is a history of rapid skeletal growth preceding displacement of the epiphysis. The condition also may be affected by nutritional deficiencies or endocrine disorders such as hypothyroidism, hypopituitarism, and hypogonadism.[24]

Children with the condition often complain of referred knee pain accompanied by difficulty in walking, fatigue, and stiffness.[24] The diagnosis is confirmed by radiographic studies in which the degree of slipping is determined and graded according to severity (mild, <33%; moderate, 33% to 50%; and severe, >50%).[9] Early treatment is imperative to prevent lifelong crippling. In situ fixation is recommended.[24] Avoidance of weight-bearing on the femur and bed rest are essential parts of the treatment. Traction or gentle manipulation under anesthesia is used to reduce the slip. Surgical insertion of pins to keep the femoral neck and head of the femur aligned is a common method of treatment for children with moderate or severe slips. Crutches are used for several months after surgical correction to prevent full weight-bearing until the growth plate closes.

Children with the disorder must be followed up closely until the epiphyseal plate closes. Long-term prognosis depends on the amount of displacement that occurs. Complications include avascular necrosis, leg shortening, malunion, and problems with the internal fixation.[24] Degenerative arthritis may develop, requiring joint replacement later in life.

Scoliosis

Scoliosis is a lateral deviation of the spinal column commonly in the coronal or frontal plane that may or may not include rotation or deformity of the vertebrae.[25] Scoliosis, a three-dimensional deformity of the spine, often affects the entire skeletal torso.[25] It can be classified with regard to age of onset and etiology. Generally, girls are affected.[14] The majority of scoliotic deformities are idiopathic.[25] Others can be congenital, associated with neuromuscular disorders (cerebral palsy or muscular dystrophy), a result of intraspinal deformities, or caused by uneven lower limb length.[25]

Idiopathic Scoliosis

Idiopathic scoliosis is classified into three types:

1. Infantile: When the deformity curve is manifested before 3 years of age. This type is rare.
2. Juvenile: When the curve(s) present between 4 and 9 years of age. This type is uncommon.
3. Adolescent: When the deformity manifests after 10 years of age until the end of growth. This type represents approximately 80% of scoliosis cases.[26]

Idiopathic scoliosis is a structural spinal curvature for which no cause has been established. It occurs in healthy, neurologically normal children. The cause is most likely complex and multifactorial. It seems likely that heredity is involved because mother–daughter pairings are common, but identical twins are not uniformly affected. The magnitude of the curvature in an affected child is not related to magnitude of curvature in relatives. A recent study of the melatonin receptor 1B (*MTNR1B*) gene in people with adolescent idiopathic scoliosis suggests that *MTNR1B* may serve as a susceptibility gene for adolescent idiopathic scoliosis.[27] Also, evidence suggests that many people with neurofibromatosis type 1 have some type of scoliosis.[28] One new screening tool available for diagnosis and determination of treatment especially with adolescent idiopathic scoliosis is the ScoliScore assessment (a collection of genetic markers correlated with scoliosis), which is a genetic testing that studies the person's DNA sample and predicts the curve progression risk for people with scoliosis.[25]

Although a scoliotic curve may be present in any area of the spine, the most common curve is a right thoracic curve, which produces a rib prominence on the convex side and hypokyphosis from rotation of the vertebral column around its long axis as the spine begins to curve.

Congenital Scoliosis

Congenital scoliosis is caused by disturbances in vertebral development during the sixth to eighth weeks of embryologic development.[28] Congenital scoliosis may be divided into failures of formation and failures of segmentation. Failures of formation indicate the absence of a portion of the vertebra, such as hemivertebra (absence of a whole side of the vertebra) and wedge vertebra (missing only a portion of the vertebra). Failure of segmentation is the absence of the normal separation between the vertebrae.[25] The child may have other anomalies and neurologic complications if the spine is involved. Early diagnosis and treatment of progressive curves are essential for children with congenital scoliosis. Surgical intervention is the treatment of choice for progressive congenital scoliosis.[6,25]

Neuromuscular Scoliosis

Neuromuscular scoliosis develops from neuropathic or myopathic diseases. It is seen with cerebral palsy, muscular dystrophy, myelodysplasia, and poliomyelitis. There is often a long, C-shaped curve from the cervical to the sacral region. In children with cerebral palsy, severe deformity may make treatment difficult. Myopathic neuromuscular scoliosis develops with Duchenne muscular dystrophy and usually is not severe.

Clinical Manifestations

Scoliosis is usually first noticed because of the deformity it causes. A high shoulder, prominent hip, or projecting scapula may be noticed by a parent or in a school-based screening program. In girls, difficulty in hemming or fitting a dress may call attention to the deformity. Idiopathic scoliosis usually is a painless process, although pain may be present in severe cases, usually in the lumbar region. The pain may be caused by pressure on the ribs or on the crest of the ilium. There may be shortness of breath because of diminished chest expansion and gastrointestinal disturbances from crowding of the abdominal organs. Adults with less severe deformity may experience mild backache. If scoliosis is left untreated, the curve may progress to an extent that compromises cardiopulmonary function and creates a risk for neurologic complications.

Diagnosis

Early diagnosis of scoliosis can be important in the prevention of severe spinal deformity. The cardinal signs of scoliosis are uneven shoulders or iliac crest, prominent scapula on the convex side of the curve, malalignment of spinous processes, asymmetry of the flanks, asymmetry of the thoracic cage, and rib hump or paraspinal muscle prominence when bending forward. A complete physical examination is necessary for children with scoliosis because the defect may be indicative of other, underlying pathologic processes.

Diagnosis of scoliosis is made by physical examination and confirmed by radiography. A scoliometer should be used at the apex of the curvature to quantify a prominence; a scoliometer reading of greater than 5 degrees requires referral to a physician.[25] The curve is measured by determining the amount of lateral deviation present on radiographs and is labeled "right" or "left" for the convex portion of the curve. Other radiographic procedures may be done, including CT scanning, MRI, and myelography.

Although school screening continues to be mandated in a number of states, the *USPSTF* recommends against the routine screening of asymptomatic adolescents for idiopathic scoliosis, indicating that the potential harms from screening include unnecessary follow-up visits and evaluations because of false-positive results, and adverse psychological effects, especially related to brace wear.[25,26] Although routine screening is not recommended, health care professionals should be prepared to evaluate idiopathic scoliosis when it is discovered incidentally or when the adolescent or parent expresses concern about scoliosis.[25]

Treatment

The treatment of scoliosis depends on the severity of the deformity and the likelihood of progression. Larger curves are more likely to progress. Age of presentation also is important. Curves that are detected before menarche are more likely to progress than those detected after menarche. For people with lesser degrees of curvature (10 to 20 degrees), the trend has been away from aggressive treatment and toward a "wait and see" approach, taking advantage of the more sophisticated diagnostic methods that now are available.[25] Treatment is considered for physically immature children with curves between 20 and 30 degrees. Curves between 30 and 40 degrees usually are considered for bracing, and those greater than 40 to 45 degrees are considered for surgery.[25]

SUMMARY CONCEPTS

Skeletal disorders can result from congenital or hereditary influences or from factors that occur during normal periods of skeletal growth and development. Newborn infants undergo normal changes in muscle tone and joint motion, causing torsional conditions of the femur or tibia. Many of these conditions are corrected as skeletal growth and development take place. OI is a rare autosomal hereditary disorder characterized by defective synthesis of connective tissue, including bone matrix. It results in poorly developed bones that fracture easily. DDH includes a range of structural abnormalities. Dislocated hips are always treated to prevent changes in the anatomic structure. Other childhood skeletal disorders, such as the osteochondroses, slipped capital femoral epiphysis, and scoliosis, are not corrected by the growth process. These disorders are progressive, can cause permanent disability, and require treatment. Disorders such as DDH and congenital clubfoot are present at birth. Both disorders are best treated during infancy. Regular examinations during the first year of life are recommended as a means of achieving early diagnosis of such disorders.

Metabolic Bone Disease

Metabolic bone disease refers to a group of diseases that cause bone demineralization or dysmineralization, usually because of a defect in bone absorption that interferes with the parathyroid hormone, calcium, and vitamin D leading to bone fragility, rickets, or osteoarthritis. As discussed earlier in this chapter, metabolic bone diseases have their origin in the bone remodeling process, which involves an orderly sequence of osteoclastic bone reabsorption, the formation of new bone by the osteoblasts, and mineralization of the newly formed osteoid tissue.

Osteopenia

Osteopenia is a condition that is common to all metabolic bone diseases. It is characterized by a reduction in bone mass greater than expected for age, race, or sex that occurs because of a decrease in bone formation, inadequate bone mineralization, or excessive bone deossification.

Osteopenia is not a diagnosis but a term used to describe an apparent lack of bone seen on x-ray studies. The major causes of osteopenia are osteoporosis, osteomalacia, malignancies such as multiple myeloma, and endocrine disorders such as hyperparathyroidism and hyperthyroidism. Approximately 44 million people in the United States have osteopenia or osteoporosis.[29]

Osteoporosis

Osteoporosis is a metabolic bone disease characterized by a loss of mineralized bone mass causing increased porosity of the skeleton and susceptibility to fractures.[30] According to the World Health Organization (WHO), bone density is reported using a T score. This score compares the bone density of a healthy 30-year-old adult to the patient's bone density.[30] The World Health Organization Osteoporosis Guidelines recommends that postmenopausal women and men over 50 years of age be treated according to the following guidelines:

- Those who have a hip or vertebral fracture
- Those who have T scores less than −2.5 at the neck of the femur or spine after appropriate evaluation to exclude secondary causes
- Those who have a 10-year probability of a hip fracture greater than 3% and a T score between −1.0 and −2.5 at the spine or neck of the femur
- Those who have a 10-year probability of a major osteoporosis-related fracture greater than 20%[30]

Although osteoporosis can occur as the result of several disorders, it most often is associated with the aging process. Because bone loss is positively associated with age, the prevalence of osteoporosis and low bone mass is expected to increase.

Pathogenesis

The pathogenesis of osteoporosis is unclear, but most data suggest an imbalance between bone resorption and formation such that bone resorption exceeds bone formation. Although both of these factors play a role in most cases of osteoporosis, their relative contribution to bone loss may vary depending on age, gender, genetic predisposition, activity level, and nutritional status. Exercise may prevent or delay the onset of osteoporosis by increasing peak bone mineral density (BMD) during periods of growth. Poor nutrition or an age-related decrease in intestinal absorption of calcium because of deficient activation of vitamin D may contribute to the development of osteoporosis, particularly in older adults.

Under normal conditions, bone mass increases steadily during childhood, reaching a peak in the young adult years. The peak bone mass, or BMD, is an important determinant of the subsequent risk for osteoporosis. It is determined in part by genetic factors, estrogen levels, exercise, calcium intake and absorption, and environmental factors. Genetic factors are linked, in large part, to the maximal amount of bone in each person, referred to as *peak bone mass*. Race is a key determinant of BMD and the risk of fractures. Incidence rates obtained from studies among racial and ethnic groups demonstrate that although women have higher fracture rates compared with men overall, these differences vary by race and age. White and Asian women had higher rates for all age groups older than 50 years.[30] The highest BMD values and lowest fracture rates have been reported for black women.[30] Body size is another factor affecting the risk of osteoporosis and risk of fractures. Women with smaller body builds are at increased risk of hip fracture because of lower hip BMD.

Hormonal factors play a significant role in the development of osteoporosis, which leads to an imbalance in osteoclast and osteoblast activity, particularly in postmenopausal women.[31,32] Postmenopausal osteoporosis, which is caused by an estrogen deficiency, is manifested by a loss of cancellous bone and a predisposition to fractures of the vertebrae and distal radius. The loss of bone mass is greatest during early menopause, when estrogen levels are withdrawing. Several factors appear to influence the increased loss of bone mass associated with an estrogen deficiency. Decreased estrogen levels are associated with an increase in cytokines (*e.g.*, interleukin-1, interleukin-6, and tumor necrosis factor [TNF]) that stimulate the production of osteoclast precursors. Estrogen deficiency also influences osteoclast differentiation through the RANK receptor pathways.[32] Estrogen stimulates the production of OPG and thus inhibits the formation of osteoclasts; it also blunts the responsiveness of osteoclast precursors to RANKL.[32] With menopause and its accompanying estrogen deficiency, this inhibition of osteoclast production is lost.[32] Compensatory osteoblastic activity and new bone formation occurs, but it does not keep pace with the bone that is lost.

Sex hormone deficiency may contribute to bone loss in men with senile osteoporosis, although the effect is not of the same magnitude as that caused by estrogen deficiency. Unlike women, men do not have a midlife loss of sex hormone production.[33] Another factor that provides relative protection for men is the fact that they achieve 8% to 10% more peak bone mass than do women. Although androgens have long been assumed to be critical for growth and maintenance of the male skeleton, estrogens obtained from peripheral conversion of testicular and adrenal hormone precursors may be even more important than androgens in the maintenance of bone mass in men.

Age-related changes in bone density occur in all people and contribute to the development of osteoporosis in both genders.[33] Age-related changes in bone cells and matrix have a strong impact on bone metabolism. Osteoblasts from older adults have reduced replicative and biosynthetic potential compared with those of younger people. Growth factors that stimulate osteoblastic activity also lose their potential over time. The result is a skeleton that has decreased ability to make bone. Reduced physical activity increases the rate of bone loss because mechanical forces are important stimuli for normal bone remodeling. Thus, the decreased physical activity that often accompanies aging may also contribute to the loss of bone mass in older adults.

Secondary osteoporosis is associated with many conditions, including endocrine disorders, malabsorption disorders, malignancies, alcoholism, and certain medications.[34] People with endocrine disorders such as hyperthyroidism, hyperparathyroidism, Cushing syndrome, or diabetes mellitus are at high risk for development of osteoporosis. Hyperthyroidism causes an acceleration of bone turnover. Some malignancies (*e.g.*, multiple myeloma) secrete the osteoclast-activating factor, causing significant bone loss. Alcohol is a direct inhibitor of osteoblasts and may also inhibit calcium absorption. Corticosteroid use is the most common cause of drug-related osteoporosis, and long-term corticosteroid use in the treatment of disorders such as rheumatoid arthritis and chronic obstructive lung disease is associated with a high rate of fractures. With the increased use of prednisone and other drugs that act like cortisol for the treatment of many inflammatory and autoimmune diseases, this form of bone loss has become a major clinical concern. The prolonged use of medications that increase calcium excretion, such as aluminum-containing antacids, corticosteroids, and anticonvulsants, also is associated with bone loss.

Several groups of children and adolescents are at increased risk for decreased bone mass, including premature infants and those with low birth weight who have lower than expected bone mass in the early weeks of life, children who require treatment with corticosteroid drugs (*e.g.*, those with asthma, inflammatory diseases, and transplant recipients), children with cystic fibrosis, and those with hypogonadal states (*e.g.*, anorexia nervosa and the female athlete triad).[35] Children with cystic fibrosis often have impaired gastrointestinal function that reduces the absorption of calcium and other nutrients, and many also require the frequent use of corticosteroid drugs.

Premature osteoporosis is increasingly being seen in female athletes owing to an increased prevalence of eating disorders and amenorrhea.[35] It most frequently affects women engaged in endurance sports, such as running and swimming; in activities where appearance is important, such as figure skating, diving, and gymnastics; or in sports with weight categories, such as horse racing, martial arts, and rowing. The *female athlete triad* refers to a pattern of disordered eating that leads to amenorrhea and eventually to osteoporosis. Poor nutrition, combined with intense training, can decrease the critical body fat-to-muscle ratio needed for normal menses and estrogen production by the ovary. The decreased levels of estrogen combined with the lack of calcium and vitamin D from dietary deficiencies result in a loss of bone density and increased risk for fractures. There is a concern that athletes with low BMD will be at increased risk for fractures during their competitive years. It is unclear whether osteoporosis induced by amenorrhea is reversible. Data that confirm that having only one or two elements of the triad greatly increases the risk of long-term morbidity in these women are emerging.[35]

Clinical Manifestations

Osteoporotic changes occur in the diaphysis and metaphysis of bone. In severe osteoporosis, the bones begin to resemble the fragile structure of a fine porcelain vase. There is loss of trabeculae from cancellous bone and thinning of the cortex to such an extent that minimal stress causes fractures. The changes that occur with osteoporosis have been explained by two distinct disease processes: postmenopausal and senile osteoporosis. In postmenopausal women, the increase in osteoclastic activity affects mainly bones or portions of bone that have increased surface area, such as the cancellous compartment of the vertebral bodies. The osteoporotic trabeculae become thinned and lose their interconnections, leading to microfractures and eventual vertebral collapse. In senile osteoporosis, the osteoporotic cortex is thinned by subperiosteal and endosteal resorption and the haversian systems are widened. In severe cases, the haversian systems are so enlarged that the cortex resembles cancellous bone (Fig. 49-15). Hip fractures, which are seen later in life, are more commonly associated with senile osteoporosis.

Osteoporosis is usually a silent disorder. Often, the first manifestations of the disorder are those that accompany a skeletal fracture—a vertebral compression fracture or fractures of the hip, pelvis, humerus, or any other bone (Fig. 49-16). Typically, the fractures occur with less force than usual, such as when a postmenopausal woman is in a crowded area such as a subway and is pushed slightly by the crowd. If the pushing occurs several times such as by someone brushing up alongside the woman as the crowd moves from the door and to the door of the subway, enough pressure could cause the woman to sustain a fracture. Women who present with fractures are much more likely to sustain another fracture than are women of the same age without osteoporosis. Wedging and collapse of vertebrae cause a loss of height in the vertebral column and kyphosis, a condition commonly referred to as *dowager hump*. Usually, there is no generalized bone tenderness. When pain occurs, it is related to fractures. Systemic symptoms such as weakness and weight loss suggest that the osteoporosis may be caused by underlying disease.

Diagnosis

The National Osteoporosis Foundation (NOF) and the WHO adapted the WHO Working Group on Osteoporosis

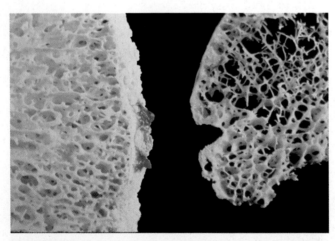

FIGURE 49-15. Osteoporosis. Femoral head of an 82-year-old woman with osteoporosis and femoral neck fracture (*right*), compared with a normal control bone cut to the same thickness (*left*). (From Rubin R., Strayer D. S. (Eds.). (2015). *Rubin's pathology: Clinicopathologic foundations of medicine* (7th ed., Fig. 30.24A, p. 1331). Philadelphia, PA: Lippincott Williams & Wilkins.)

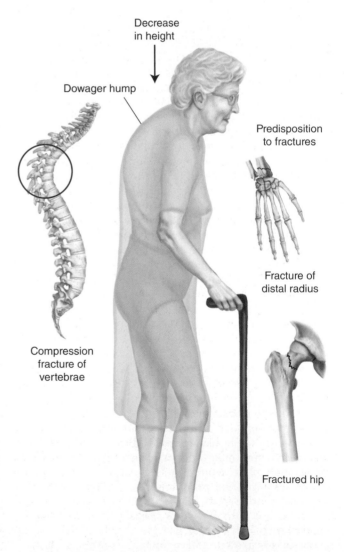

Decrease in height

Dowager hump

Predisposition to fractures

Fracture of distal radius

Compression fracture of vertebrae

Fractured hip

FIGURE 49-16. Clinical manifestations of osteoporosis.

Screening Tool, Fracture Risk Assessment Algorithm, to identify future hip fracture possibility depending on a person's risk possibility.[30] BMD assessment is most commonly undertaken with dual-energy x-ray absorptiometry (DXA) of the spine and hip. Current practice is to perform DXA on the total hip, the femoral neck, and the anterior lumbar spine (L1 to L4). The site with the lowest score should be used to make a diagnosis. Measurement of BMD has become increasingly common for early detection and fracture prevention. Measurement of serial heights in older adults is another simple way to screen for osteoporosis. A further advance in the diagnosis of osteoporosis is the refinement of risk factors. Testing for BMD should be performed on the basis of individual person's risk. The NOF has recommended that all women should have a measurement of BMD at 65 years of age unless they have risk factors, which means earlier screening should be performed.[30] Risk factors that may indicate a need for testing women at a younger age include the following:

- A delayed menarche (*i.e.*, age 15 years or later)
- Low body weight (*i.e.*, <21 kg/m^2, or 127 lb at menopause)
- Current smoker
- History of fractures after menopause (other than skull, facial bone, ankle, finger, or toe)
- History of a hip fracture in a parent[30]

Treatment

Prevention and early detection of osteoporosis are essential to the prevention of associated deformities and fractures. It is important to identify people in high-risk groups so that treatment can begin early (Chart 49-1). Regular exercise and adequate calcium intake are important factors in preventing osteoporosis. Weight-bearing exercises such as walking, jogging, rowing, and weight lifting are important in the maintenance of bone mass.

Studies have indicated that premenopausal women need more than 1000 mg/day of calcium, and postmenopausal women should take 1500 mg of calcium daily. Because most older American women do not consume a sufficient quantity of dairy products to meet their calcium needs, calcium supplementation is recommended. Calcium tablets vary in content of elemental calcium. Vitamin D deficiency may be an important factor in the impaired intestinal absorption of calcium in the older adult. On the basis of this evidence, 1,25-dihydroxyvitamin D$_3$ is being studied as a treatment for osteoporosis.[36] A daily intake of 400 to 800 International Unit of vitamin D is recommended because vitamin D optimizes calcium absorption and inhibits parathyroid secretion.[36]

Pharmacologic treatment of osteoporosis includes antiresorptive drugs and anabolic agents. There are three main types of antiresorptive agent: estrogens and selective estrogen receptor modulators (SERMs), bisphosphonates, and calcitonin. Although estrogen is one of the most effective interventions for reducing the incidence and progression of osteoporosis in postmenopausal women, the use of hormone therapy (estrogen plus progestin) has come under scrutiny since the Women's Health Initiative.[37] Raloxifene, a SERM that acts only on specific estrogen

CHART 49-1

RISK FACTORS ASSOCIATED WITH OSTEOPOROSIS

Personal Characteristics

Advanced age

Female

White (fair, thin skin)

Small bone structure

Postmenopausal

Family history

Lifestyle

Sedentary

Calcium deficiency (long term)

High-protein diet

Excessive alcohol intake

Excessive caffeine intake

Smoking

Drug and Disease Related

Aluminum-containing antacids

Anticonvulsants

Heparin

Corticosteroids or Cushing disease

Gastrectomy

Diabetes mellitus

Chronic obstructive lung disease

Malignancy

Hyperthyroidism

Hyperparathyroidism

Rheumatoid arthritis

receptors, is effective in the prevention and treatment of osteoporosis in postmenopausal women.

In men, testosterone appears to play an important role in bone homeostasis by stimulating osteoblasts and inhibiting osteoclasts. The use of testosterone is contraindicated in men with prostate cancer. Men with osteoporosis may also benefit from bisphosphonate, calcitonin, or parathyroid hormone therapy. Like women, they have the same need for calcium and vitamin D supplementation.

People with osteoporosis have many special needs. Walking and swimming are encouraged. Surgical intervention is done for stable fracture fixation that allows early restoration of mobility and function; for fractures of the lower extremities, this means early weight-bearing. Vertebral fractures are treated symptomatically. Vertebroplasty and kyphoplasty are minimally invasive spinal procedures that use bone cement to restore vertebral height and relieve pain.

Osteomalacia and Rickets

In contrast to osteoporosis, which causes a loss of total bone mass and results in brittle bones, osteomalacia and rickets produce a softening of the bones but do not involve a loss of bone matrix.[38,39] Approximately 60% of bone is mineral content, approximately 30% is organic matrix, and the remainder is living bone cells. The organic matrix and the inorganic mineral salts are needed for normal bone consistency. The term *rickets* refers to the disorder in children in which changes in bone growth produce characteristic skeletal abnormalities, and *osteomalacia* is used in adults because the bone that forms during the remodeling process is undermineralized.[14]

Osteomalacia

Osteomalacia is a generalized bone condition in which there is inadequate mineralization of bone. There are two main causes of osteomalacia:

1. Insufficient calcium absorption from the intestine because of a lack of dietary calcium or a deficiency of or resistance to the action of vitamin D
2. Phosphate deficiency caused by increased renal losses or decreased intestinal absorption

Vitamin D deficiency is caused most commonly by reduced vitamin D absorption as a result of biliary tract or intestinal diseases that impair fat and fat-soluble vitamin absorption. Lack of vitamin D in the diet is rare in the United States because many foods are fortified with the vitamin. Anticonvulsant medications, such as phenobarbital and phenytoin, induce hepatic hydroxylases that accelerate breakdown of the active forms of vitamin D.

The incidence of osteomalacia is high among older adults because of diets deficient in calcium and vitamin D, a problem often compounded by the intestinal malabsorption that accompanies aging. Osteomalacia often is seen in cultures in which the diet is deficient in vitamin D, such as in northern China, Japan, and in northern India. Women in these areas have a higher incidence of the disorder than do men because of the combined effects of pregnancy, lactation, and more indoor confinement. Osteomalacia occasionally is seen in strict vegetarians, people who have had a gastrectomy, and those on long-term anticonvulsants, tranquilizers, sedatives, muscle relaxants, or diuretic drugs. There also is a greater incidence of osteomalacia in the colder regions of the world, particularly during the winter months, probably because of lessened exposure to sunlight.

A form of osteomalacia called *renal rickets* occurs in people with chronic renal failure.[38] It is caused by the inability of the kidney to activate vitamin D and excrete phosphate and is accompanied by hyperparathyroidism, increased bone turnover, and increased bone resorption. Long-standing primary hyperparathyroidism causes increased calcium resorption from bone and hypophosphatemia, which can lead to rickets in children and osteomalacia in adults.

Clinical Manifestations

The clinical manifestations of osteomalacia are bone pain, tenderness, and fractures as the disease progresses.

In severe cases, muscle weakness often is an early sign. The cause of muscle weakness is unclear. Osteomalacia predisposes a person to pathologic fractures in the weakened areas, especially in the distal radius and proximal femur. In contrast to osteoporosis, it is not a significant cause of hip fractures. There may be delayed healing and poor retention of internal fixation devices. Osteomalacia usually is accompanied by a compensatory or secondary hyperparathyroidism stimulated by low serum calcium levels. Parathyroid hormone reduces renal absorption of phosphate and removes calcium from the bone. Serum calcium levels are only slightly reduced in osteomalacia.

Diagnosis and Treatment

Diagnostic measures are directed toward identifying osteomalacia and establishing its cause. Diagnostic methods include x-ray studies, laboratory tests, bone scan, and bone biopsy. X-ray findings typical of osteomalacia are the development of transverse lines or pseudofractures. These apparently are caused by stress fractures that are inadequately healed. A bone biopsy may be done to confirm the diagnosis of osteomalacia in a person with nonspecific osteopenia who shows no improvement after treatment with exercise, vitamin D, and calcium.

The treatment of osteomalacia is directed at the underlying cause.[38,39] If the problem is nutritional, restoring adequate amounts of calcium and vitamin D to the diet may be sufficient. The elderly with intestinal malabsorption also may benefit from vitamin D. The least expensive and most effective long-term treatment is a diet rich in vitamin D (*i.e.*, fish, dairy products, and margarine) along with careful exposure to the midday sun.

Rickets

Rickets is a metabolic bone disease characterized by a failure or delay in calcification of the cartilaginous growth plate in children whose epiphyses have not yet fused.[39] It is also manifested by widening and deformation of the metaphyseal regions of long bones and a delay in the mineralization of trabecular, endosteal, and periosteal bone surfaces. There are several forms of rickets, including nutritional rickets, vitamin D–dependent rickets, and vitamin D–resistant rickets.

Etiology

As with osteomalacia in the adult, rickets can result from kidney failure; malabsorptive syndromes such as celiac disease and cystic fibrosis; and medications such as anticonvulsants, which cause target organ resistance to vitamin D, and aluminum-containing antacids, which bind phosphorus and prevent its absorption.

Nutritional rickets results from inadequate sunlight exposure or inadequate intake of vitamin D, calcium, or phosphate. Nutritional rickets occurs primarily in underdeveloped areas of the world and among immigrants to developed countries. The causes are inadequate exposure to sunlight (*e.g.*, children are often kept clothed and indoors) and prolonged breast-feeding without vitamin D supplementation. Although the vitamin D content of human milk is low, the combination of breast milk and sunlight exposure usually provides sufficient vitamin D. Another cause of rickets is the use of commercial alternative milks (*e.g.*, soy or rice beverages) that are not fortified with vitamin D. Vitamin D–dependent rickets can result from abnormalities in the gene coding for the enzyme that converts inactive vitamin D to the active vitamin D–resistant rickets and involves hypophosphatemia or a decrease in serum phosphate levels, the most common form being caused by mutations of the phosphate-regulating gene on the X chromosome.[39] Gene mutation causes renal wasting of phosphate at the proximal tubular level of the kidney.

Clinical Manifestations

Rickets is characterized by changes in the growing bones of children with overgrowth of the epiphyseal cartilage because of inadequate provisional calcification and failure of the cartilage cells to disintegrate. Bones become deformed; ossification at the epiphyseal plates is delayed and disordered, resulting in widening of the epiphyseal cartilage plate. Any new bone that does grow is unmineralized. During the nonmobile stage of infancy, the head and chest undergo the greatest stresses. The skull is enlarged and soft, and closure of the fontanels is delayed. Teeth are slow to develop, and the child may have difficulty standing. When an ambulating child develops rickets, deformities are likely to affect the spine, pelvis, and long bones (*i.e.*, tibia), causing, most notably, lumbar **lordosis** and bowing of the legs. The ends of long bones and ribs are enlarged. The thorax may be abnormally shaped, with prominent rib cartilage (*i.e.*, rachitic rosary). The child usually has stunted growth, with a height sometimes far below the normal range. Weight often is not affected so that the children, many of whom present with a protruding abdomen (*i.e.*, rachitic potbelly), have been described as presenting a Buddha-like appearance when sitting.

Treatment

Nutritional rickets is treated with a balanced diet sufficient in calcium, phosphorus, and vitamin D. Exposure to sunlight also is important, especially for premature infants and those on artificial milk feedings. Supplemental vitamin D exceeding normal daily requirements is given for several months. Maintenance of good posture, positioning, and bracing in older children are used to prevent deformities. After the disease is controlled, deformities may have to be surgically corrected as the child grows.

Children with vitamin D–dependent and vitamin D–independent rickets require special treatment measures. Children with vitamin D–dependent rickets caused by lack of the enzyme needed to convert vitamin D to its active form are treated with calcitriol, the active form of vitamin D.[39] Vitamin D–resistant forms of rickets are treated with oral phosphorus or oral phosphorus and calcitriol.

Paget Disease

Paget disease (*i.e.*, osteitis deformans) is the second most common bone disease after osteoporosis.[14,39,40] The disease tends to occur in people in their fourth decade and is characterized by local areas of excessive bone turnover and disorganized osteoid formation. The disease is more common in people of Northern European heritage.

Paget disease is a focal process with considerable variation in its stage of development in separate sites. At the onset, the disease is marked by regions of rapidly occurring osteoclastic bone resorption, followed by a period of hectic bone formation with increased numbers of osteoblasts rapidly depositing bone in a chaotic manner such that the newly formed bone is of poor quality and is disorganized rather than lamellar. The poor quality of bone accounts for the bowing and fractures that occur in bones affected by the disease. The bone marrow adjacent to the bone-forming surface is replaced by loose connective tissue that contains osteoprogenitor cells and numerous blood vessels, which transport blood to and from these metabolically active sites.[39] The lesions of Paget disease may be solitary or may occur in multiple sites. They tend to localize to the bones of the axial skeleton, including to the spine, skull, hips, and the pelvis. The proximal femur and tibia may be involved in more widespread forms of the disease. Histologically, Paget lesions show increased vascularity and bone marrow fibrosis with intense cellular activity. The bone has a somewhat mosaic-like pattern caused by areas of density outlined by heavy blue lines, called *cement lines* (Fig. 49-17).

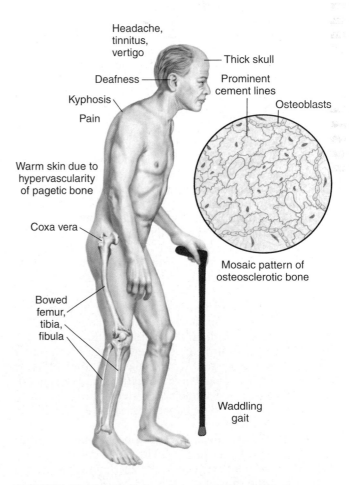

FIGURE 49-17. Clinical manifestations of Paget disease.

Etiology

Although the cause of Paget disease remains unclear, there is evidence of both genetic and environmental influences. It has been reported that 15% to 40% of people with the disease have a first-degree relative with Paget disease, and numerous studies have described extended family members with the disease.[39,40] In addition, evidence supports that people with Paget disease have been found to have a mutation of the *SQSM1/p62* gene in their diseased bone and tumor samples.[39,40] It is possible that factors other than genetics are also involved in the pathogenesis of the disease such as a paramyxovirus.[39] This has been supported by the observation of viral particles resembling the paramyxovirus nucleocapsid in the cytoplasm of osteoclasts in people with Paget disease.

In children, hyperostosis corticalis deformans juvenilis (a rare autosomal recessive disorder), hyperphosphatemia, and diseases that cause diaphyseal stenosis may mimic Paget disease and sometimes are referred to as *juvenile Paget disease*.[40] The disorder presents in infancy or early childhood with pain from debilitating fractures and deformities because of a markedly accelerated rate of bone remodeling throughout the skeleton.

Clinical Manifestations

The disease varies in severity from a simple lesion to involvement of many bones. It may be present long before it is detected clinically. In fact, many people have no symptoms and their disease is found when managing another health problem. The clinical manifestations of Paget disease depend on the specific area involved (see Fig. 49-17). Involvement of the skull can cause headaches, intermittent tinnitus, vertigo, and eventual hearing loss. In the spine, collapse of the anterior vertebrae causes kyphosis of the thoracic spine. The femur and tibia become bowed. Softening of the femoral neck can cause coxa vara (*i.e.*, reduced angle of the femoral neck). Coxa vara, in combination with softening of the sacral and iliac bones, causes a waddling gait. When the lesion affects only one bone, it may cause only mild pain and stiffness. Progressive deossification weakens and distorts the bone structure. The deossification process begins along the inner cortical surfaces and continues until the substance of the bone disappears. Pathologic fractures may occur, especially in the bones subjected to the greatest stress (*e.g.*, upper femur, lower spine, pelvic bones). These fractures often heal poorly, with excessive and poorly distributed callus.

Other manifestations of Paget disease include nerve palsy syndromes from lesions in the upper extremities, mental deterioration, and cardiovascular disease because of high-output heart failure (HF). Cardiovascular disease is the most serious complication and the most common cause of death in those with advanced generalized Paget disease. Calcific aortic stenosis may occur in severe cases. Ventilatory capacity may be limited by rib and spine involvement.

Osteogenic sarcomas have also been found to occur in people with Paget disease. The bones most often affected, in order of frequency, are the femur, pelvis, humerus, and the tibia.

Diagnosis and Treatment

Diagnosis of Paget disease is based on characteristic bone deformities and x-ray changes. Elevated levels of serum alkaline phosphatase and urinary hydroxyproline support the diagnosis and continued surveillance of these levels may be used to monitor the effectiveness of treatment. Bone scans are used to detect the rapid bone turnover indicative of active disease and to monitor the response to treatment. The scan cannot identify bone activity resulting from malignant lesions. Bone biopsy may be done to differentiate the lesion from osteomyelitis or a primary or metastatic bone tumor.

The treatment of Paget disease is based on the degree of pain and the extent of the disease. Pain can be reduced with nonsteroidal or other anti-inflammatory agents. Suppressive agents such as the bisphosphonates and calcitonin are used to manage pain and prevent further spread of the disease and neurologic defects. Early diagnosis and bisphosphonate therapy are the most effective ways to manage Paget disease because of the ability to decrease bone resorption.[39,40]

SUMMARY CONCEPTS

In addition to its structural function, the skeleton is a homeostatic organ. Metabolic bone diseases such as osteoporosis, osteomalacia, rickets, and Paget disease are the result of a disruption in the equilibrium of bone formation and resorption. Osteoporosis, which is the most common of the metabolic bone diseases, occurs when the rate of bone resorption is greater than that of bone formation. It is seen frequently in postmenopausal women and is the major cause of fractures in people older than 45 years of age. Osteomalacia and rickets are caused by inadequate mineralization of bone matrix, primarily because of a deficiency of vitamin D. Paget disease results from excessive osteoclastic activity and is characterized by the formation of poor-quality bone. The success rate of the various drugs and hormones that are used to treat metabolic bone diseases varies.

Activity Intolerance and Fatigue

Activity tolerance is the amount of physical activity a person can perform without injury or excessive exertion. Activity tolerance can be measured by having the person describe his or her normal activities, perceived activity tolerance, or level of fatigue. One method of assessing activity tolerance involves the administration of a screening tool in which participants describe their normal activities, their perceived level of activity tolerance, or their level of fatigue. An example of such a tool is the Human Activity

Profile (HAP).[41] The HAP originally was developed to assess the quality of life for the people participating in a rehabilitation program for chronic obstructive pulmonary disease. After investigating numerous physiologic and psychological measures, it was noted that the most important aspect of quality of life was the amount of daily activity the person was able to perform. Activity intolerance can be viewed as not having sufficient physical or psychological energy reserves to endure or complete required or desired daily activities. Fatigue is the sensation that comes with having exhausted those energy reserves. It is a state experienced by everyone at some time in life. Fatigue can be a normal physical response, such as that following extreme exercise in healthy people, or it can be a symptom experienced by people with limited energy reserve, such as people with cardiac or respiratory disease, anemia, or malnutrition, or those on certain types of drug therapy. Fatigue also may be related to lack of sleep or mental stress.

Like dyspnea and pain, fatigue is a subjective symptom. It often is described as a feeling of just not feeling right and having a lack of energy and motivation to do anything. Fatigue is different from the normal tiredness that people experience at the end of the day. Tiredness is relieved by a good night's sleep, whereas fatigue persists despite sufficient or adequate sleep. Although fatigue is one of the most common symptoms reported to health care professionals, it is one of the least understood of all health problems. Fatigue cannot be explained using a measurement such as amount of activity or exercise.[42]

The physiologic basis of fatigue includes factors such as diaphragmatic, motor, and neurologic mechanisms. Diaphragmatic fatigue occurs in both acute and chronic respiratory conditions where the force and duration of muscle work exceeds muscle energy stores. Neuromuscular fatigue involves the loss of maximal capacity to generate force during exercise.

KEY POINTS

- Acute fatigue is fatigue with a rapid onset resulting from short-term sleep loss or heavy exercise. Adequate sleep and nutrition allow for recovery from acute fatigue.

- Myalgic encephalomyelitis (ME)/chronic fatigue syndrome (CFS) is characterized by disabling fatigue and many nonspecific symptoms, including cognitive impairments, sleep disturbances, and musculoskeletal pain. The etiology of CFS is unknown, but it is associated with several chronic diseases such as fibromyalgia, depression, and irritable bowel syndrome.

Mechanisms of Fatigue

The origin or cause of fatigue can be physiologic, psychological, pathologic, or unknown (*e.g.*, CFS or ME).

It can be caused by environmental factors (*e.g.*, excessive noise, temperature extremes, changes in weather), drug-related incidents (*e.g.*, use of tranquilizers, alcohol, toxic chemical exposure), treatment-related causes (*e.g.*, chemotherapy, radiation therapy, surgery, anesthesia, diagnostic testing), physical exertion (*e.g.*, exercise), and psychological factors (*e.g.*, stress, monotony).

Clinically, fatigue can be described by how it begins, what seems to trigger it, and how it is managed. This information can sometimes assist in determining the etiology of the pain. It is thought that both acute and chronic fatigue can exist in the same person, similar to acute and chronic pain.

Acute Physical Fatigue

Acute fatigue has a rapid onset and is often defined as muscle fatigue associated with increased activity, or exercise, that is carried out to the point of exhaustion. It also is frequently associated with a viral or bacterial infection and may present with other systemic symptoms such as fever or malaise.[42] If it is associated with muscle fatigue, it is relieved shortly after the activity ceases and serves as a protective mechanism. Physical conditioning can influence the onset of acute fatigue. People who engage in regular exercise compared with sedentary people can perform an activity for longer periods before acute fatigue develops. They can do so in part because their muscles use oxygen and nutrients more efficiently, and their circulatory and respiratory systems are better able to deliver oxygen and nutrients to the exercising muscles.

Acute physical fatigue occurs more rapidly in deconditioned muscle. For example, acute fatigue often is seen in people who have been on bed rest because of a surgical procedure or in people who have had their activity curtailed because of chronic illness, such as heart or respiratory disease (see Fig. 49-18). In such cases, the acute fatigue often is out of proportion to the activity that is being performed (*e.g.*, dangling at the bedside, sitting in a chair for the first time). When resuming activity after a prolonged period of bed rest or inactivity, the person may experience tachycardia and hypotension. Unless these parameters are changed by medications such as β-adrenergic blocking drugs, heart rate and blood pressure become particularly sensitive indicators of activity tolerance or intolerance.

Another example of acute fatigue is that which occurs in people who require the use of assistive devices such as wheelchairs, walkers, or crutches. The upper arm muscles are less well adapted to prolonged exercise than are the leg muscles. This is because arm muscles are primarily composed of type II muscle fibers. Type II muscle fibers, which are used when the body requires short bursts of energy, fatigue quickly. As a result, people who use wheelchairs or crutches may quickly experience fatigue until their arms become conditioned to the increased activity.

Chronic Fatigue

Chronic fatigue differs from acute fatigue in terms of onset, intensity, perception, duration, and relief. Chronic

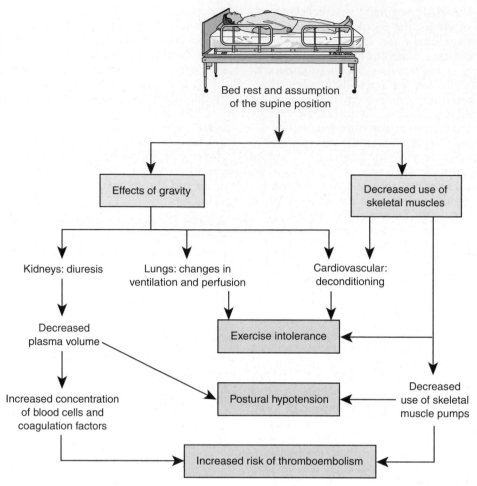

FIGURE 49-18. The effects of gravity and decreased use of the skeletal muscles during bed rest and assumption of the supine position on cardiovascular, respiratory, and renal function and their impact on exercise tolerance and the risk of complications such as thromboembolism and postural hypotension.

fatigue is much more complex and difficult to diagnose. There are several possible causes such as hypothyroidism, anemia, heart disease, Lyme disease, fibromyalgia, lung disease, electrolyte dysfunction, tuberculosis, hepatitis, and cancer.[42] It is a common problem experienced by people with chronic health problems (Table 49-2). In the primary care setting, many people complain of chronic fatigue. Chronic fatigue with HF or emphysema is accepted given the pathophysiology of these conditions. Others may have a transient fatigue that can be managed with vitamin or other medication supplementation.

Although acute fatigue often serves a protective function, chronic fatigue does not. It limits the amount of activity that a person can perform and may interfere with employment, performance of activities of daily living, and quality of life. Although fatigue often is viewed as a symptom of anxiety and depression, it is important to recognize that the anxiety and depression may instead be symptoms of the fatigue. For example, people with persistent fatigue because of a chronic illness may have to curtail their work schedules, decrease social activities, and limit their usual family responsibilities. These lifestyle changes may be the reasons for the depression rather than the depression being a cause of the fatigue.

Chronic fatigue occurs across a broad spectrum of disease states. It is a common complaint of people with cancer, cardiac disease, end-stage renal disease, chronic lung disease, hepatitis C, arthritis, human immunodeficiency virus (HIV) infection and acquired immunodeficiency syndrome (AIDS), and neurologic disorders such as multiple sclerosis, postpolio syndrome, and Parkinson disease.

Chronic fatigue is an almost universal phenomenon in people with cancer. Of people undergoing treatment for cancer, 14% to 96% percent experience fatigue.[43] In addition, post treatment, 19% to 82% of people experience fatigue.[43] Cancer-related fatigue may be caused by the disease itself or by the treatment. Cancer-related fatigue involves a number of physiologic, sensory, affective, and cognitive dimensions. There is often a sensation of feeling unusually tired, with generalized weakness and a greater need for rest. There may also be a disturbing lack of motivation, anxiety, and sadness, as well as an inability to concentrate or difficulty in thinking.

There are several types of cancer-related factors that may cause fatigue, the most prominent of which are factors related to energy imbalance from the following disorders: anemia, cachexia, stress, pain, infection, medications, and metabolic disorders. The cytokine theory of cancer-related fatigue is based in part on the observation that people

TABLE 49-2 Chronic Illnesses and Causes of Chronic Fatigue

Chronic Illness	Cause of Fatigue
Acquired immunodeficiency syndrome	Impaired immune function, anorexia, muscle weakness, and psychosocial factors associated with the disease
Anemia	Decreased oxygen-carrying capacity of blood
Arthritis	Pain and joint dysfunction lead to impaired mobility, loss of sleep, and emotional factors
Cancer	Presence of chemical products and catabolic processes associated with tumor growth; anorexia and difficulty eating; effects of chemotherapy and radiation therapy; and psychosocial factors such as depression, grieving, hopelessness, and fear
Cardiac Disease	
Myocardial infarction	Death of myocardial tissue results in decreased cardiac output, poor tissue perfusion, and impaired delivery of oxygen and nutrients to vital organs
Congestive HF	Impaired pumping ability of the heart results in poor perfusion of muscle tissue and vital organs
Neurologic Disorders	
Multiple sclerosis	Demyelinating disease of CNS characterized by slowing of nerve conduction, resulting in lower extremity weakness and fatigue
Myasthenia gravis	Disorder of postsynaptic acetylcholine receptors of the myoneural junction, resulting in muscle weakness and fatigue
Chronic lung disease	Increased work of breathing and impaired gas exchange
Chronic renal failure	Accumulation of metabolic wastes; fluid, electrolyte, and acid–base disorders; decreased red blood cell count and oxygen-carrying capacity because of impaired erythropoietin production
Metabolic Disorders	
Hypothyroidism	Decrease in basal metabolic rate manifested by fatigue
Diabetes mellitus	Impaired cellular use of glucose by muscle cells
Obesity	Imbalance in nutritional intake and energy expenditure; increased workload because of excess weight
Steroid myopathy	Glucocorticosteroids interfere with protein and glycogen synthesis, which leads to muscle wasting

CNS, *central nervous system; HF, heart failure.*

receiving agents such as interferon-α as part of their treatment plan experienced devastating fatigue that appears dose limited. Interferon-α and other agents used to treat cancer also influence the release of other cytokines that are related to fatigue. Cancer cells and the immune system appear to produce or express a number of cytokines with the potential for manufacturing many of the factors that contribute to fatigue, particularly interleukin-1 beta and TNF-α.[44] One of these cytokines, TNF-α, is thought to be associated with morning fatigue and sleep disturbances.[44,45] Another study demonstrates that the performance of specific skeletal exercises by people with cancer results in the release of interleukin-6, which can decrease the levels of TNF-α and interleukin 1 beta.[44,45]

Management of Chronic Fatigue

Many of the pathologic factors associated with fatigue, including insomnia, anemia, psychological stress, and weakness, respond to appropriate treatment measures. Anemia, which is common among people with HIV/AIDS, people with end-stage renal disease, and people with cancer receiving chemotherapy, causes fatigue by interfering with the oxygen-carrying capacity of the blood. It is sometimes treated with recombinant forms of erythropoietin (epoetin alfa), an endogenous hormone normally produced by the kidney. Insomnia—which occurs for several reasons including anxiety and depression, hot flashes, nocturia, and pain—is treatable with nonpharmacologic and pharmacologic methods. Psychological disturbances, such as anxiety and depression, which are frequently associated with fatigue, can be treated with selected pharmacologic agents. Another cause of fatigue is loss of muscle mass, muscle strength, and endurance. It may be that the person needs to have a thorough physical examination with laboratory studies to determine whether there are any musculoskeletal or neurologic problems that may be impacting the person's stamina, such as myositis, Guillain–Barré, or polymyalgia, or whether the person needs to build endurance with a consistent exercise program.

Myalgic Encephalomyelitis/Chronic Fatigue Syndrome

ME/CFS is a condition of disabling fatigue of at least 6 months' duration that is typically accompanied by an array of self-reported, nonspecific symptoms such as cognitive impairments, sleep disturbances, and musculoskeletal pain. This disorder continues to be a relatively common problem.

Definition

Because the etiology of CFS is unknown, there are no biologic markers for the diagnosis of CFS and there are no definitive treatments. Furthermore, the overlap of symptoms of CFS with other functional disorders such as fibromyalgia, multiple chemical sensitivities, depression, and irritable bowel syndrome, which also are characterized by fatigue, complicates the ability to define the syndrome with any degree of certainty. In fact, CFS may describe a group of similar symptoms that develop with different pathophysiologic disturbances.

Because of the need for diagnostic criteria, the case definition for CFS was established in 1988 by the Centers for Disease Control and Prevention (CDC) and revised through its International Chronic Fatigue Syndrome Study Group in 1994.[46] To be classified as CFS, the fatigue must be clinically evaluated, cause severe mental and physical exhaustion, and result in a significant reduction in the individual's premorbid activity level. Table 49-3 illustrates examples of conditions that may mimic CFS. Chart 49-2 outlines the CDC's symptoms of CFS and the criteria for diagnosis of CFS.[46,47]

Pathophysiology

Theories of the pathogenesis of CFS include genetic expression, infections, stress and prior psychological disorders, a dysfunction in the hypothalamic–pituitary–adrenal axis, nutritional deficiencies, or increased oxidative and nitrosative stress.[47] Despite much research and the development of several theories, the underlying pathophysiology of CFS remains elusive. Many people with CFS attribute the onset of their disease to an influenza-like infection. Thus, the link between infectious agents such as Epstein–Barr virus, human herpesvirus 6, *Candida* yeast, *Borrelia* bacteria, and others has been extensively studied. To date, however, none of these agents has been conclusively linked in a cause-and-effect relationship with the development of CFS.[47] It is hypothesized that the immune system may overreact to an environmental agent (most likely an infectious agent) or internal stimuli and be unable to self-regulate after the infectious insult is over.

Psychological disorders often are associated with CFS, especially anxiety and depression, but this is difficult to evaluate. People with CFS are more likely than are the general population to have experienced a psychological disorder such as major depression or panic disorder before the development of CFS. However, it also is true that a significant proportion of those people with CFS have not had such episodes, either before or after the development of CFS.[47]

Abnormalities of the hypothalamic–pituitary–adrenal axis, such as attenuated activity of corticotropin-releasing hormone and changes in the circadian rhythm of cortisol secretion, have been documented. Although low thyroid hormones, dehydroepiandrosterone, and cortisol levels have been found in people with CFS, these parameters are not decreased in all people with CFS.[47]

TABLE 49-3 Examples of Conditions That May Present as Chronic Fatigue

Psychological	Depression
	Anxiety
	Somatization disorder
Pharmacologic	Hypnotics
	Antihypertensives
	Tranquilizers
	Drug abuse and drug withdrawal
Endocrine—Metabolic	Hypothyroidism
	Diabetes mellitus
	Apathetic hyperthyroidism of the elderly
	Pituitary insufficiency
	Hyperparathyroidism of hypercalcemia of any origin
	Addison disease
	Chronic renal failure
	Hepatocellular failure
Neoplastic—Hematologic	Occult malignancy (*e.g.*, pancreatic cancer)
	Severe anemia
Infectious	Endocarditis
	Tuberculosis
	Mononucleosis
	Hepatitis
	Parasitic disease
	HIV infection
	Cytomegalovirus infection
Cardiopulmonary	Chronic congestive heart failure
	Chronic obstructive pulmonary disease
Connective tissue disease—immune	Rheumatoid disease
Hyperreactivity	Myalgic encephalomyelitis/chronic fatigue syndrome
Disturbed sleep	Sleep apnea
	Esophageal reflux
	Allergic rhinitis
	Psychological etiologies (see earlier entries)

HIV, human immunodeficiency virus.

Genetic links with CFS include a gene associated with Huntington disease neurodegenerative protein, abnormalities in the way genes affect mitochondrial cell energy production, and connections to depression and anxiety.[46] In addition, connections with people with CFS and a persistent inflammatory state have been determined.[48]

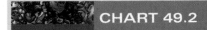

CHART 49.2

CENTERS FOR DISEASE CONTROL AND PREVENTION SYMPTOMS OF MYALGIC ENCEPHALOMYELITIS/CHRONIC FATIGUE SYNDROME

ME/CFS has three primary symptoms required for diagnosis, with additional common symptoms, which may or may not be experienced with all people with ME/CFS. The primary symptoms include the following:

1. Decreased ability to participate in activities that were common before the disease, accompanied by fatigue lasting 6 months or longer. The fatigue associated with ME/CFS is severe, does not improve with sleep/rest, was not present before the disease, and is not related to performing difficult activities.

2. Increased symptoms following physical or mental activity that were not present before the disease; this "postexertional malaise" may last days, weeks, or longer.

3. Alterations in sleep, such as being tired after a full night of sleep.

   In addition to these primary symptoms, *one* of the following must be present for a diagnosis of ME/CFS:

- Difficulty thinking/remembering
- Orthostatic intolerance, in which symptoms become worse when standing or sitting upright.

   Other common symptoms include the following:

- Aches and pain in muscles
- Pain in the joints without swelling or erythema
- New or more severe headaches
- Recurring sore throat
- Night sweats/chills
- New sensitivities/allergies to substances such as food or noise
- Tenderness in neck/armpit lymph nodes

Adapted from CDC. (2017). Myalgic encephalomyelitis/chronic fatigue syndrome. [Online]. Available: https://www.cdc.gov/me-cfs/symptoms-diagnosis/symptoms.html. Accessed February 20, 2018.

Clinical Manifestations

One of the most important findings in people with CFS is the complaint of fatigue. Often, the symptom of fatigue is preceded by a cold or flulike illness. Frequently, the person describes the illness as recurring, with periods of exacerbations and remissions. With each subsequent episode of the illness, the fatigue increases.

Physical findings include low-grade fever. The fever is intermittent and occurs only when the illness recurs. Other findings include nonexudative pharyngitis, palpable and tender cervical lymph nodes, a mildly enlarged thyroid gland, wheezing, splenomegaly, myalgia, arthralgia, and heme-positive stool with subsequent negative sigmoidoscopy.

Psychological problems include impaired cognition, which the person describes as an inability to concentrate and perform previously mundane tasks. There are reports of mood and sleep disturbances, balance problems, visual disturbances, and various degrees of anxiety and depression.

Diagnosis and Treatment

The diagnosis of CFS is based on integration of the entire clinical picture of the person's symptoms, physical assessment findings, and the results of diagnostic tests. Laboratory investigations are used to detect other disorders. Usually, the final diagnosis is based on the definition of CFS provided by the CDC[47] (see Chart 49-2). There is some discussion that people with less associated symptoms of CFS may be able to be accurately diagnosed with CFS at an earlier state.[47]

Because there is no known cause of CFS, current treatment tends to remain symptomatic, with a focus on management rather than on cure. It centers on education, emotional support, treatment of symptoms, and overall management of general health. Symptom management includes development of an exercise program that helps the person regain strength. Along with a structured activity program, people should be encouraged to be as active as possible as they resume their activities of daily living.

SUMMARY CONCEPTS

Fatigue is a nonspecific, self-recognized state of physical and psychological exhaustion. It results in the persons not being able to perform routine activities and is not relieved with sleep or rest. Acute fatigue results from excessive use of the body or specific muscle groups and often is related to depletion of energy sources. Chronic fatigue often is associated with a specific disease or chronic illness and may be relieved when the effects of the disease are corrected. CFS is a complex illness that has physiologic and psychological manifestations. It is characterized by debilitating fatigue. Diagnosis often is made by a process of elimination, and treatment requires a holistic approach.

Review Exercises

1. A newborn girl was found to have DDH during a routine screening examination.
   A. Describe the anatomic abnormalities that are present in the disorder.
   B. Explain the need for early treatment of DDH.

2. A 12-year-old girl was noted to have asymmetry of the shoulders, scapular height, and pelvic height during routine physical examination. On x-ray examination, she is found to have a 30-degree curvature of the spine.

   A. Describe the physical problems associated with progressive scoliosis.

3. A 60-year-old postmenopausal woman presents with a compression fracture of the vertebrae. She has also noticed increased backache and loss of height over the past few years.

   A. Explain how the lack of estrogen and aging contribute to the development of osteoporosis.

   B. What other factors should be considered when assessing the risk for development of osteoporosis?

   C. What is one way to measure bone density?

   D. Name the two most important factors in preventing osteoporosis.

4. A 40-year-old woman who is being treated with chemotherapy for breast cancer complains of excessive fatigue and activity intolerance. She claims she has so little energy she can hardly get up in the morning and has difficulty concentrating and doing such simple activities as shopping.

   A. What are some explanations for this woman's excessive fatigue?

   B. What independent interventions might be used to decrease her fatigue?

REFERENCES

1. Sadler T. (2015). *Langman's medical embryology* (3rd ed.). Philadelphia, PA: Wolters Kluwer.
2. Rhoades R. A., Bell D. R. (2012). *Medical physiology: Principles for clinical medicine* (4th ed.). Philadelphia, PA: Lippincott Williams & Wilkins.
3. Ross M. H., Pawlina W. (2015). *Histology: A text and atlas* (7th ed.). Philadelphia, PA: Lippincott Williams & Wilkins.
4. Hockenberry M., Wilson D., Rodgers C. (2016). *Wong's essentials of pediatric nursing* (10th ed.). St. Louis, MO: Mosby.
5. Staheli L. (2015). *Fundamentals of pediatric orthopedics* (5th ed.). Philadelphia, PA: Lippincott Williams & Wilkins.
6. Cramer K., Scherl S., Tornetta P., et al. (Eds.). (2003). *Pediatrics (orthopedic surgery essential series)*. Philadelphia, PA: Lippincott Williams & Wilkins.
7. Gilbert S. (2013). Obesity in pediatric orthopedics. *Current Orthopaedic Practice* 24(6), 576–580. Available: http://www.medscape.com/viewarticle/813428. Accessed August 1, 2017.
8. Whitaker A., Vuillermin C. (2016). Lower extremity growth and deformity. *Current Reviews in Musculoskeletal Medicine* 9(4), 454–461.
9. Carr J., Yang S., Lather L. (2016). Pediatric pes planus: A state-of-the-art review. *Pediatrics* 137(3), 1–10. Available: http://pediatrics.aappublications.org/content/137/3/e20151230. Accessed August 1, 2017.
10. Stoltzman S., Irby M., Callahan A., et al. (2015). Pes planus and paediatric obesity: A systematic review of the literature. *Clinical Obesity* 5(2), 52–59.
11. Malik S. (2013). Polydactyly: Phenotypes, genetics and classification. *Clinical Genetics* 85(3), 203–212.
12. National Institutes of Health. (2014). What is osteogenesis imperfecta? [Online]. Available: http://www.niams.nih.gov/Health_Info/bone/Osteogenesis_Imperfecta/osteogenesis_imperfecta_ff.asp. Accessed August 1, 2017.
13. Rubin R., Strayer D. S. (Eds.). (2014). *Rubin's pathology: Clinicopathologic foundations of medicine* (7th ed.). Philadelphia, PA: Lippincott Williams & Wilkins.
14. Van Dijk F., Sillence D. (2014). Osteogenesis imperfecta: Clinical diagnosis, nomenclature and severity assessment. *American Journal of Medical Genetics* 164(6), 1470–1481.
15. Wright J., James K. (2016). Developmental dysplasia of the hip. In Aresti N., Ramachandran M., Paterson M., Barry M. (Eds.), *Paediatric orthopaedics in clinical practice*. London, UK: Springer.
16. U.S. Preventive Services Task Force. (2015). Developmental hip dysplasia: Screening. [Online]. Available: https://www.uspreventiveservicestaskforce.org/Page/Document/UpdateSummaryFinal/developmental-hip-dysplasia-screening. Accessed February 11, 2018.
17. Jensen S. (2014). *Nursing health assessment: A best practice approach* (2nd ed.). Philadelphia, PA: Lippincott Williams & Wilkins.
18. Delaney L. R., Karmazyn B. (2011). Developmental dysplasia of the hip: Background and the utility of ultrasound. *Seminars in Ultrasound, CT, and MR* 32(2), 151–156.
19. Hossain M., Davis N. (2017). Evidence-based treatment for clubfoot. In Alshryda S., Huntley J., Banaszkiewicz P. (Eds.), *Paediatric orthopaedics*. Cham, Switzerland: Springer.
20. Hernandez J. (2015). Legg-Calve-Perthes disease in emergency medicine treatment and management. Available: http://emedicine.medscape.com/article/826935-overview. Accessed August 1, 2017.
21. Chaudhry S., Phillips D., Feldman D. (2014). Legg-Calvé-Perthes disease: An overview with recent literature. *Bulletin of the Hospital for Joint Diseases* 72(1), 18–27. Available: http://presentationgrafix.com/_dev/cake/files/archive/pdfs/2.pdf. Accessed August 1, 2017.
22. Gregory J. (2017). Osgood-Schlatter disease. Available: http://emedicine.medscape.com/article/1993268-overview. Accessed August 1, 2017.
23. Makhni M. C., Makhni E. C., Swart E. F., et al. (2017). Slipped capital femoral epiphysis. In Makhni M., Makhni E., Swart E., Day C. (Eds.), *Orthopedic emergencies*. Cham, Switzerland: Springer International Publishing.
24. El-Hawary R., Chukwunyerenwa C. (2014). Update on evaluation and treatment of scoliosis. *Pediatric Clinics of North America* 61(6), 1223–1241.
25. Mehlman C. T. (2016). Idiopathic scoliosis. Available: http://emedicine.medscape.com/article/1265794-overview. Accessed August 1, 2017.
26. Morningstar M. W., Strauchman M. N., Stitzel C. J., et al. (2016). Methylenetetrahydrofolate reductase (MTHFR) gene mutations in patients with idiopathic scoliosis: A clinical chart review. Available: http://file.scirp.org/pdf/OJGen_2017033015113499.pdf. Accessed September 1, 2017.
27. Weinstein S. (2005). The thoracolumbar spine. In Weinstein S. L., Buckwalter J. A. (Eds.), *Turek's orthopaedics: Principles and their application* (6th ed., pp. 477–518). Philadelphia, PA: Lippincott Williams & Wilkins.
28. Looker A., Frenk S. (2015). Percentage of adults aged 65 and over with osteoporosis or low bone mass at the femur

neck or lumbar spine: United States, 2005–2010. Available: https://www.cdc.gov/nchs/data/hestat/osteoporsis/osteoporosis2005_2010.pdf. Accessed August 26, 2019.

29. Sigl V., Penninger J. (2014). RANKL/RANK—From bone physiology to breast cancer. *Cytokine & Growth Factor Reviews* 25(2), 205–214.

30. Cosman F., de Beur S., LeBoff M., et al. (2014). Clinician's guide to prevention and treatment of osteoporosis. *Osteoporosis International* 25(10), 2359–2381.

31. Naylor K. (2016). Response of bone turnover markers to raloxifene treatment in postmenopausal women with osteopenia. *Osteoporosis International* 27(8), 2585–2592.

32. Martin T. J., Sims N. A. (2016). RANKL/OPG: Critical role in bone physiology. *Reviews in Endocrine & Metabolic Disorders* 16(2), 131–139.

33. Willson T., Nelson S., Newbold J., et al. (2015). The clinical epidemiology of male osteoporosis: A review of the recent literature. *Clinical Epidemiology* 7, 65–76.

34. Bethel M., Carbone L., Lohr K., et al. (2017). Osteoporosis. Available: http://emedicine.medscape.com/article/330598-overview. Accessed August 2, 2017.

35. Thralls K., Nichols J., Barrack M., et al. (2016). Body mass-related predictors of the female athlete triad among adolescent athletes. *International Journal of Sport Nutrition and Exercise Metabolism* 26(1), 17–25.

36. Aspray T. J., Bowring C., Fraser W., et al. (2014). National Osteoporosis Society Vitamin D guideline summary. *Age and Ageing* 43(5), 592–595.

37. Seton M. (2017). Review: Breaking from bisphosphonates. *Arthritis and Rheumatology* 69(3), 494–498.

38. Plotkin H., Finberg L. (2017). Disorders of bone mineralization. Available: http://emedicine.medscape.com/article/985766-overview. Accessed August 2, 2017.

39. Alikhan M., Driver K., Lohr K. (2016). Paget disease. Available: http://emedicine.medscape.com/article/334607-overview Accessed August 2, 2017.

40. Grasemann C., Unger N., Hövel M., et al. (2017). Loss of functional osteoprotegerin: More than a skeletal problem. *Journal of Clinical Endocrinology and Metabolism* 102(1), 210–219.

41. Davidson M., Morton N. (2007). A systematic review of the Human Activity Profile. *Clinical Rehabilitation* 21(2), 151–162.

42. Dunphy L. M., Winland-Brown J. E., Porter B. O., et al. (2015). *Primary care: The art and science of advanced practice nursing* (4th ed.). Philadelphia, PA: Lippincott Williams & Wilkins.

43. National Cancer Institute. (2015). Fatigue. [Online]. Available: http://www.cancer.gov/cancertopics/pdq/supportivecare/fatigue/HealthProfessional/page1. Accessed September 29, 2017.

44. Kwak S., Choi Y., Yoon H., et al. (2012). The relationship between interleukin-6, tumor necrosis factor-α, and fatigue in terminally ill cancer patients. *Palliative Medicine* 26(3), 275–282.

45. Doong S., Dhruva A., Dunn L. B., et al. (2014). Associations between cytokine genes and a symptom cluster of pain, fatigue, sleep disturbance, and depression in patients prior to breast cancer surgery. *Biological Research for Nursing* 17(3), 237–247.

46. Centers for Disease Control and Prevention. (2015). Chronic fatigue syndrome. [Online]. Available: http://www.cdc.gov/cfs/general/index.html. Accessed September 19, 2017.

47. Yancey J. R., Thomas S. A. (2012). Chronic fatigue syndrome: Diagnosis and treatment. *American Family Physician* 86(8), 741–746. Available: http://www.aafp.org/afp/2012/1015/p741.pdf. Accessed September 19, 2017.

48. Centers for Disease Control and Prevention. (2017). Evidence of inflammatory immune signaling in chronic fatigue syndrome: A pilot study of gene expression in peripheral blood. [Online]. Available: https://www.cdc.gov/me-cfs/about/possible-causes.html. Accessed September 19, 2017.

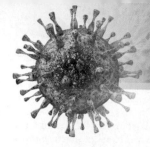

Disorders of Musculoskeletal Function: Rheumatic Disorders

Learning Objectives

After completing this chapter, the learner will be able to meet the following objectives:

1. Characterize the common characteristics of the different systemic autoimmune rheumatic disorders.
2. Describe the pathologic changes that may be found in the joint of a person with rheumatoid arthritis (RA).
3. Describe the immunologic process that occurs in systemic lupus erythematosus.
4. Cite a definition of the seronegative spondyloarthropathies.
5. Describe the primary features of ankylosing spondylitis (AS).
6. Compare AS, reactive arthritis, and psoriatic arthritis in terms of cause, pathogenesis, and clinical manifestations.
7. Compare RA and osteoarthritis (OA) in terms of joint involvement, level of inflammation, and local and systemic manifestations.
8. Describe the pathologic joint changes associated with OA.
9. Relate the metabolism and elimination of uric acid to the pathogenesis of crystal-induced arthropathy.

10. Describe the clinical manifestations, diagnostic measures, and methods used in the treatment of gouty arthritis.
11. Differentiate among the major characteristics of the different types of juvenile arthritis.

Arthritis is a descriptive term applied to more than 100 rheumatic diseases, ranging from localized, self-limiting conditions to those that are systemic autoimmune processes. More than 30 million Americans have osteoarthritis (OA).[1] This type of arthritis impacts people in all age groups and is the leading cause of disability in the United States. Approximately 1.5 million Americans have rheumatoid arthritis (RA) and about 300,000 children younger than 18 years of age have juvenile arthritis or some type of rheumatic condition.[1]

The common use of the term *arthritis* can oversimplify the nature of the varied disease processes, the difficulty in differentiating one form of arthritis or rheumatic disease from another, and the complexity of treatment of these usually chronic conditions. These conditions share inflammation of the joint as a prominent or an accompanying symptom. In the systemic rheumatic diseases—those affecting body systems in addition to the musculoskeletal system—the inflammation is primary, resulting from an immune response. In rheumatic conditions limited to a single or a few diarthrodial joints, the inflammation is secondary, resulting from a degenerative process and the resulting joint irregularities that occur as the bone attempts to remodel itself. Although arthritis cannot be cured, much can be done to control its progress.

This chapter focuses on systemic autoimmune rheumatic diseases, arthritis associated with spondylitis, OA syndrome, metabolic diseases associated with arthritis, and rheumatic disease in children and older adults.

Systemic Autoimmune Rheumatic Diseases

Systemic autoimmune rheumatic diseases are a group of chronic disorders characterized by diffuse inflammatory lesions and degenerative changes in connective tissue.[2] These disorders share similar clinical features and may affect many of the same organs. RA, systemic lupus erythematosus (SLE), polymyalgia rheumatica, temporal arteritis, and juvenile arthritis and dermatomyositis, which share an autoimmune systemic pathogenesis, are discussed in this section.

Rheumatoid Arthritis

RA is a systemic inflammatory disease that affects 1% to 2% of the population.[2] Females are affected approximately three times more frequently than are males.[1,2] Although the disease occurs in all age groups, its prevalence increases with age.[1] RA occurring after age 65 is known as elderly onset rheumatoid.[3]

Etiology and Pathogenesis

Although the cause of RA remains uncertain, evidence points to a genetic predisposition and the development of joint inflammation that is immunologically mediated. It has been suggested that the disease is initiated in a genetically predisposed person by the activation of a T-cell–mediated response to an immunologic trigger, such as a microbial agent (Fig. 50-1). The importance of genetic factors in the pathogenesis of RA is supported by the increased frequency of the disease among first-degree relatives.[2] In addition, it is generally agreed that certain major histocompatibility complex (MHC) genes are expressed in a nonrandom manner in people with RA. An important genetic locus that predisposes to RA is present on the human leukocyte antigen (HLA) loci on the MHC class II molecules, with a specific focus on the DRB1 locus.[4] This *HLA-DRB1* gene, which forms a rheumatoid pocket on the HLA molecule, may influence the types of peptides that can be bound by the RA-associated HLA-DR molecules, thereby affecting the immune response.[2]

The pathogenesis of RA can be viewed as an aberrant immune response that leads to synovial inflammation and destruction of the joint architecture. It has been suggested that the disease is initiated by the activation of helper T cells, release of cytokines (*e.g.*, tumor necrosis factor [TNF], interleukin [IL]-1), and antibody formation. Approximately 70% to 80% of people with the disease have a substance called the *rheumatoid factor* (RF), which is an autologous (self-produced) antibody (immunoglobulin [Ig] RF) that reacts with a fragment of IgG to form immune complexes.[2] Immune complexes (Ig RF + IgG) and complement components are found in the synovium, synovial fluid, and extra-articular lesions of people with RA. Although people with RA may be seronegative (not have Ig RF in their serum), the presence of a high RF titer is frequently associated with severe and unremitting disease, mainly systemic complications. Across people with RA, the presence of autoantibodies is inconsistent; thus, a multimarker panel may be more useful for diagnosis and prediction of treatment response.[5]

The role of the autoimmune process in the joint destruction of RA remains obscure. At the cellular level, neutrophils, macrophages, and lymphocytes are attracted to the area. The neutrophils and macrophages phagocytize the immune complexes and, in the process, release lysosomal enzymes capable of causing destructive changes in the joint cartilage (see Fig. 50-1). The inflammatory response that follows attracts additional inflammatory cells, setting in motion a chain of events that perpetuates the condition. As the inflammatory process progresses, the synovial cells and subsynovial tissues undergo reactive hyperplasia. Vasodilation and increased blood flow cause warmth and redness. The joint swelling that occurs is the result of the increased capillary permeability that accompanies the inflammatory process.

Characteristic of RA is the development of an extensive network of new blood vessels in the synovial membrane that contributes to the advancement of the rheumatoid synovitis. This destructive vascular granulation tissue, which is called *pannus*, extends from the synovium to involve a

Clinical Manifestations

RA often is associated with extra-articular as well as articular manifestations (see Fig. 50-2). It usually has an insidious onset marked by systemic manifestations such as fatigue, anorexia, weight loss, and generalized aching and stiffness. The disease, which is characterized by exacerbations and remissions, may involve only a few joints for brief durations, or it may become relentlessly progressive and debilitating.

Joint Manifestations

Joint involvement usually is symmetric and polyarticular. Any diarthrodial joint can be involved. The person may complain of joint pain and stiffness that lasts for 30 minutes and frequently for several hours. The limitation of joint motion that occurs early in the disease usually is because of pain; later, it is because of fibrosis. The most frequently affected joints initially are the fingers, hands, wrists, knees, and feet. Later, other diarthrodial joints may become involved, but recent research has shown a decline in RA-related joint replacements because of more effective RA drug treatment.[4,7] Spinal involvement usually is limited to the cervical region. In the hands, there usually is bilateral and symmetric involvement of the proximal interphalangeal (PIP) and metacarpophalangeal (MCP) joints in the early stages of RA; later disease affects the distal interphalangeal (DIP) joints.[4] Progressive joint destruction may lead to subluxation (i.e., dislocation of the joint resulting in misalignment of the bone ends) and instability of the joint and limitation of movement. Swelling and thickening of the synovium can result in stretching of the joint capsule and ligaments. When this occurs, muscle and tendon imbalances develop, and mechanical forces applied to the joints through daily activities produce joint deformities (Fig. 50-3). In the MCP joints, the extensor tendons can slip to the ulnar side of the metacarpal head, causing ulnar deviation of the fingers (see Fig. 50-2A). Subluxation of the MCP joints may develop when this deformity is present. Hyperextension of the PIP joint and partial flexion of the DIP joint is called a *swan neck deformity*.[8,9] After this

condition becomes fixed, severe loss of function occurs because the person can no longer make a fist. Flexion of the PIP joint with hyperextension of the DIP joint is called a *boutonnière deformity*.[8,9]

The knee is one of the commonly affected joints associated with the disease.[4] Active synovitis may be apparent as visible swelling that obliterates the normal contour over the medial and lateral aspects of the patella. The *bulge sign*, which involves milking fluid from the lateral to the medial side of the patella, may be used to determine the presence of excess fluid when it is not visible. Joint contractures, instability, and genu valgus (knock-knee) deformity are other possible manifestations. Severe quadriceps atrophy can contribute to the disability. A *Baker cyst* may develop in the popliteal area behind the knee. This is caused by enlargement of the bursa but does not usually cause symptoms unless the cyst ruptures, in which case symptoms mimicking thrombophlebitis appear.

Ankle involvement can limit flexion and extension, which can create difficulty in walking. Involvement of the metatarsophalangeal joints can cause subluxation, hallux valgus, and hammer toe deformities. Neck discomfort is common. In rare cases, long-standing disease can lead to neurologic complications such as occipital headaches, muscle weakness, and numbness and tingling in the upper extremities.

Extra-Articular Manifestations

Although characteristically a joint disease, RA can affect many other tissues. Extra-articular manifestations probably occur with a fair degree of frequency but usually are mild enough to cause only a few problems. They are most likely to occur in people who have RF.

Because RA is a systemic disease, it may be accompanied by complaints of fatigue, weakness, anorexia, weight loss, and low-grade fever when the disease is active. The erythrocyte sedimentation rate (ESR), which commonly is elevated during inflammatory processes, has been found to correlate with the amount of disease

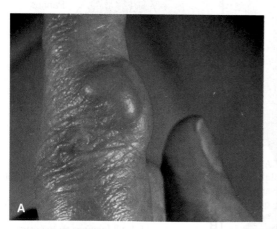
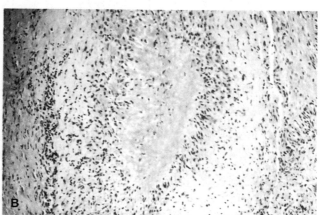

FIGURE 50-3. Rheumatoid nodule. **(A)** A person with rheumatoid arthritis has a subcutaneous mass on a digit. **(B)** Microscopic view of a rheumatoid nodule shows a central area of necrosis surrounded by palisaded macrophages and a chronic inflammatory infiltrate. (From Strayer D., Rubin R. (Eds.) (2015). *Rubin's pathology: Clinicopathologic foundations of medicine* (7th ed., Fig. 30-58, p. 1365). Philadelphia, PA: Lippincott Williams & Wilkins.)

activity.[4] Hematologic effects include thrombocytosis or anemia of chronic disease.[4] This anemia usually is resistant to iron therapy. Felty syndrome, although rare, is characterized by RA, splenomegaly, and neutropenia.[4,10] Rheumatoid nodules are granulomatous lesions that develop around small blood vessels. The nodules may be tender or nontender, movable or immovable, and small or large. Typically, they are found over pressure points such as the extensor surfaces of the ulna. The nodules may remain unless surgically removed, or they may resolve spontaneously.

Vasculitis, or inflammation of small and medium-sized arteries, is an uncommon manifestation of RA in people with a long history of active arthritis and high titers of RF. Manifestations include ischemic areas in the nail fold and digital pulp that appears as brown spots. Ulcerations may occur in the lower extremities, particularly around the malleolar areas. In some cases, neuropathy may be the only symptom of vasculitis. The visceral organs, such as the heart, lungs, and gastrointestinal tract, also may be affected.

Manifestations affecting the eyes include keratoconjunctivitis sicca, episcleritis, uveitis, and nodular scleritis, which can cause visual impairment.[4,11] A small number of people have splenomegaly and lymph node enlargement.

KEY POINTS

Rheumatoid Arthritis

- RA is a chronic systemic inflammatory disease with bilateral involvement of synovial or diarthrodial joints.

- The initial joint changes involve the synovial cells lining the joint. Inflammatory cells accumulate, and angiogenesis and formation of pannus, which proceed to cover the articular cartilage and isolate it from its nutritional synovial fluid, take place.

Diagnosis

The diagnosis of RA is based on findings of the history, physical examination, and laboratory tests. Information should be elicited regarding the duration of symptoms, systemic manifestations, stiffness, and family history. The criteria for RA, updated in 2010 by the American College of Rheumatology (ACR) and the European League Against Rheumatism, are useful in establishing the diagnosis of RA earlier than what has been done in the past.[12,13] At least 6 out of 10 possible points must be present to make a diagnosis of RA. These criteria consisting of four categories (joint involvement, serology, acute phase reactants, and duration of symptoms) were developed for use in facilitating earlier recognition of RA so people could begin treatment earlier to prevent recurrences or decrease disease severity.[12,13]

In the early stages, the disease often is difficult to diagnose. On physical examination, the affected joints show signs of inflammation, swelling, tenderness, and possibly warmth and reduced motion. The joints have a soft, spongy feeling because of synovial thickening and inflammation. Body movements may be guarded to prevent pain. Changes in joint structure usually are not visible early in the disease.

The RF test results are not diagnostic for RA, but they can be of value in differentiating RA from other forms of arthritis. A small percentage of healthy people have a positive RF. Also, a person can have RA without the presence of RF. Evidence suggests a stronger linkage of RA and anticitrullinated protein/peptide antibodies, which are measured as anticyclic citrullinated peptide (anti-CCP) autoantibodies.[4] This test has a higher specificity than does RF, and identification is possible very early in the RA process but may not be as predictive of disease severity or prognosis.[4] The term *citrullination* defines the posttranslational change of arginine into citrulline.[14]

RA is linked with the HLA-DRB1 locus,[15] which is thought to be the result of local antigens that trigger an inflammatory response in the joint space leading to joint destruction.[4] T-cell response is activated and these cells make up almost half of the immune cells present in an inflamed joint.[4] The challenge has been to understand the antigen specificity of first set of T cells that initiate the immune response.[4]

Radiologic findings also are not diagnostic in RA because joint erosions often are not seen on radiographic images in the early stages of the disorder. Synovial fluid analysis can be helpful in the diagnostic process. The synovial fluid has a cloudy appearance, the white blood cell count is elevated because of inflammation, and the complement components are decreased because of the inflammatory process.

Treatment

The treatment goals for a person with RA are to prevent and/or reduce the pain, decrease stiffness and swelling, maximize mobility, and possibly halt the pathologic process.[4] The treatment plan includes education about the disease and its treatment, rest, therapeutic exercises, and medications. Because of the chronicity of the disease and the need for continuous, long-term adherence to the prescribed treatment modalities, it is important that the treatment be integrated with the person's lifestyle.

The goals of pharmacologic therapy for RA are to reduce pain, decrease inflammation, maintain or restore joint function, and prevent bone and cartilage destruction. Ideally, disease-modifying antirheumatic drug (DMARD) therapy should be used when the diagnosis of RA is established and before erosive changes appear on radiography but must be balanced with the potential risks of anti-inflammatory and immunosuppressive interventions.[4,16] Early treatment is based on the theory that T-cell–dependent pathways, which manifest early in the inflammatory process are more responsive to treatment than those that manifest later in the process, when disease progression is controlled by activated fibroblasts and macrophages, and the disease may be more resistant to treatment.

Nonsteroidal anti-inflammatory drugs (NSAIDs) usually are used early in the treatment of RA and provide analgesic and anti-inflammatory effects.

Corticosteroid drugs may be used to reduce discomfort. These agents interrupt the inflammatory and immune cascade at several levels, such as interfering with inflammatory cell adhesion and migration, impairing prostaglandin synthesis, and inhibiting neutrophil superoxide production.

Other first-line antirheumatic drugs include biologics such as anti-TNFs. TNF-α is a cytokine, present in inflammation but overly present in the bloodstream and joints of those with RA.[17]

Surgery also may be a part of the treatment of RA. Synovectomy may be indicated to reduce pain and joint damage when synovitis does not respond to medical treatment.

Systemic Lupus Erythematosus

SLE is a chronic inflammatory disease that can affect virtually any organ system, including the musculoskeletal system. It is a major rheumatic disease, with approximately 1.5 million Americans and over 5 million people worldwide diagnosed with lupus.[18] Prevalence is related to gender, race, age, and genetics.[4] SLE is more common in females (85% of cases) than in males; is more common in African Americans, Hispanics, and Asians than in Caucasians; most cases occur between the ages of 15 and 44[4,19,18]; and it appears to have a genetic component.[4] There are four types of lupus erythematosus: SLE, cutaneous lupus erythematosus, drug-induced lupus erythematous, and neonatal lupus. The most common one is SLE.[16] Cutaneous lupus erythematosus only affects the skin, but 5% to 10% of those who have cutaneous lupus will develop SLE.[19,20] Drug-induced lupus is caused by particular prescription drugs including hydralazine, procainamide and isoniazid, and about 6 months after the drugs are stopped the person's lupus completely resolves.[19,20] Neonatal lupus is the result of mothers (not all of whom have lupus) with particular antibodies, and usually affects the neonate's skin, which clears up during the first few months and rarely lasts until childhood. In a small number of cases (1% to 2%), the infant is born with heart block and requires a pacemaker. Congenital heart block is usually permanent because of altered transfer of conduction of nerve impulses to heart muscles.[19,20]

Etiology and Pathogenesis

The cause of SLE is unknown. It is characterized by the formation of autoantibodies and immune complexes. People with SLE appear to have B-cell hyperreactivity and increased production of antibodies against self (*i.e.*, autoantibodies) and nonself antigens. These B cells are polyclonal, each producing a different type of antibody. The autoantibodies can directly damage tissues or combine with corresponding antigens to form tissue-damaging immune complexes. Autoantibodies have been identified against an array of nuclear and cytoplasmic cell components. Some autoantibodies that have been identified in SLE are antinuclear antibodies (ANA), including anti-deoxyribonucleic acid (anti-DNA) antibodies, antiphospholipid antibodies, and anti-Smith (Sm) antibodies. In addition to ANAs, people with lupus have a host of other self-autoantibodies including those directed against elements of the blood (red cells, platelets, lymphocytes) and plasma proteins (clotting and complement factors).

The development of autoantibodies can result from a combination of factors, including genetic, hormonal, immunologic, and environmental factors.[4] Genetic predisposition is evidenced by the occurrence of familial cases of SLE, especially among identical twins. The increased incidence among African Americans compared with Caucasians also suggests genetic factors. As many as four genes may be involved in the expression of SLE in humans. Genes linked to the HLA-DR and HLA-DQ loci in the MHC class II molecules show strong support for a genetic link in the development of SLE.[4] The disease is so prevalent among females.[4] It has been suggested that an imbalance in sex hormone levels may lead to heightened helper T-cell and weakened suppressor T-cell immune responses that could in turn lead to the development of autoantibodies.[4]

Possible environmental triggers include ultraviolet (UV) light, chemicals (*e.g.*, drugs, hair dyes), some foods, and infectious agents (Fig. 50-4).[19] UV light, specifically UVB associated with exposure to the sun or unshielded fluorescent bulbs, may trigger exacerbations. Photosensitivity occurs in approximately one third of people with SLE. Certain drugs may also provoke a lupus-like disorder in susceptible people, particularly in older adults. The most common of these drugs are hydralazine, minocycline, and procainamide.[4] The disease usually recedes when the drug is discontinued.[19,20]

Clinical Manifestations

SLE can manifest in a variety of ways. The disease has been called the *great imitator* because it has the capacity to affect many different body systems, including the musculoskeletal system, skin, cardiovascular system, lungs, kidneys, central nervous system (CNS), and red blood cells and platelets (Fig. 50-5). The onset may be acute or insidious, and the course of the disease is characterized by exacerbations and remissions.

Arthralgias and arthritis are among the most commonly occurring early symptoms of SLE. Approximately 90% of all people with the disease complain of joint pain, and this is often the symptom that they present with.[4] The polyarthritis of SLE initially can be confused with other forms of arthritis, especially RA, because of the symmetric arthropathy. However, on radiologic examination, articular destruction rarely is found. Ligaments, tendons, and the joint capsule may be involved, causing varied deformities of people with the disease. Flexion contractures, hyperextension of the interphalangeal

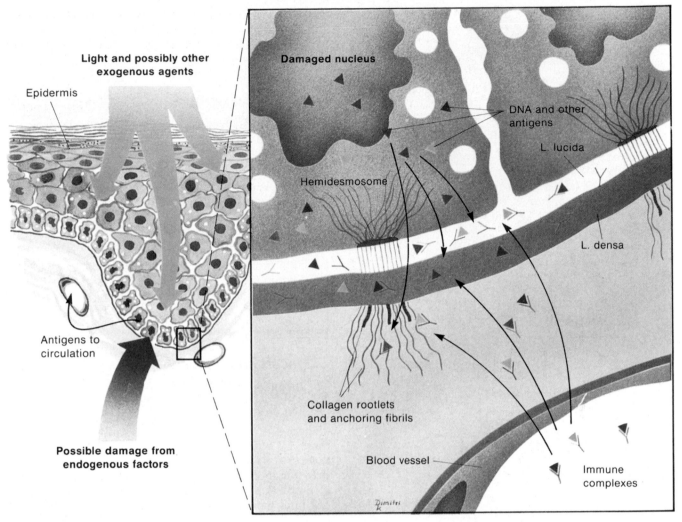

FIGURE 50-4. Lupus erythematosus. A cell-mediated immune reaction leads to epidermal cellular damage when initiated by light or other exogenous agents as well as endogenous ones. Such injury releases a large number of antigens, some of which may return to the skin in the form of immune complexes. Immune complexes are also formed in the skin by a reaction of local DNA with antibody that may also be deposited beneath the epidermal basement membrane zone. L, lamina. (From Strayer D., Rubin R. (Eds.) (2015). *Rubin's pathology: Clinicopathologic foundations of medicine* (7th ed., Figure 28-27, p. 1241). Philadelphia, PA: Lippincott Williams & Wilkins.)

joints, and subluxation of the carpometacarpal joints contribute to the deformity and subsequent loss of function in the hands. Other musculoskeletal manifestations of SLE include tenosynovitis, rupture of the intrapatellar and Achilles tendons, and avascular necrosis, frequently of the femoral head.

Skin manifestations can vary greatly and may be classified as acute, subacute, or chronic. The acute skin lesions include the classic malar or "butterfly" rash on the nose and cheeks (see Fig. 50-5). This rash is seen in SLE, but may be associated with other skin lesions, such as hives or livedo reticularis (*i.e.*, reticular cyanotic discoloration of the skin, often precipitated by cold) and fingertip lesions, such as periungual erythema, nail fold infarcts, and splinter hemorrhages. Hair loss is common. Mucous membrane lesions tend to occur during periods of exacerbation. Sun sensitivity may occur in SLE even after mild sun exposure.

Renal involvement occurs in close to 50% of people with SLE.[4] Several forms of glomerulonephritis may

occur, including mesangial, focal proliferative, diffuse proliferative, and membranous.[4] Of these, diffuse proliferative has the worst prognosis and presents with hypertension and, in up to 50% of cases, can lead to end-stage renal disease or death.[4] Interstitial nephritis also may occur. Nephrotic syndrome causes proteinuria with resultant edema in the legs and abdomen, and around the eyes. Kidney biopsy is the best determinant of renal damage and the extent of treatment needed.

Pulmonary involvement in SLE is manifested primarily by pleural effusions or pleuritis. Less frequently occurring pulmonary problems include acute pneumonitis, pulmonary hemorrhage, chronic interstitial lung disease, and pulmonary embolism.

Pericarditis is the most common of the cardiac manifestations, and is often accompanied by pleural effusions. Myocarditis affects as much as 25% of those with SLE. Secondary heart disease also is a problem in those with SLE. Hypertension may be associated with

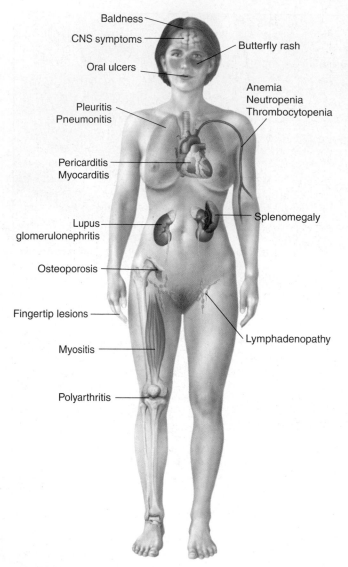

Baldness
CNS symptoms
Oral ulcers
Butterfly rash
Anemia
Neutropenia
Thrombocytopenia
Pleuritis
Pneumonitis
Pericarditis
Myocarditis
Splenomegaly
Lupus glomerulonephritis
Osteoporosis
Fingertip lesions
Myositis
Lymphadenopathy
Polyarthritis

FIGURE 50-5. Clinical manifestations of systemic lupus erythematosus. CNS, central nervous system.

These lesions first appear as red, swollen patches of skin, and later there can be scarring, depigmentation, and plugging of hair follicles. Most people with discoid lupus have disease that involves only the skin.

KEY POINTS

Clinical Manifestations of Systemic Lupus Erythematosus

- SLE is a chronic autoimmune disorder characterized by production of a wide array of autoantibodies against nuclear and cytoplasmic cell components.

- SLE is often described as the great imitator because it can affect almost any organ system, including the joints of the musculoskeletal system, the skin, kidneys, lungs, nervous system, and the heart.

Diagnosis and Treatment

The diagnosis of SLE can be complicated and difficult. The 1982 ACR (updated in 1997 and currently in review) has defined 11 criteria to be considered in the diagnosis of the disease.[21] If a person has at least 4 of these 11 criteria, the individual has SLE.[21] However, these criteria are intended for use in clinical trials rather than for individual diagnosis.[22] Diagnosis is based on a complete history, physical examination, and analysis of blood work. No single test can diagnose SLE in all people.

The most common laboratory test performed is the immunofluorescence test for ANA. Ninety-five percent of people with untreated SLE have high ANA levels. The ANA test is not specific for SLE, and positive ANA results may be found in healthy people or may be associated with other disorders. The anti-DNA antibody test is more specific for the diagnosis of SLE.[4] Other serum tests may reveal moderate to severe anemia, thrombocytopenia, and leukocytosis or leukopenia. Additional immunologic tests may be done to give support to the diagnosis or to differentiate SLE from other connective tissue diseases.[4]

Treatment of SLE focuses on managing the acute and chronic symptoms of the disease. The goals of treatment include preventing progressive loss of organ function, reducing the possibility of exacerbations, minimizing disability from the disease process, and preventing complications from medication therapy. Treatment with medications may be as simple as a drug to reduce inflammation, such as an NSAID to control fever, arthritis, and mild pleuritis. An antimalarial drug is generally the next medication considered to treat cutaneous and musculoskeletal manifestations of SLE. Corticosteroids are used to treat more significant symptoms of SLE, such as renal and CNS disorders.[4] Immunosuppressive drugs are used in cases of severe disease.

lupus nephritis and long-term corticosteroid use. Ischemic heart disease can occur in older adults with longer duration SLE.

The pathologic basis for the CNS symptoms is not entirely clear. It has been related to an acute vasculitis that impedes blood flow, causing strokes or hemorrhage; an immune response involving antineuronal antibodies that attack nerve cells; or production of antiphospholipid antibodies that damage blood vessels and cause blood clots in the brain. Seizures can occur and are more frequent when renal failure is present. Psychotic symptoms, including depression and unnatural euphoria, as well as decreased cognitive functioning, confusion, and altered levels of consciousness, may develop.

Hematologic disorders may manifest as hemolytic anemia, leukopenia, lymphopenia, or thrombocytopenia. Lymphadenopathy also may occur in many people with SLE and is evidence of systemic disease.[4] Discoid SLE involves plaquelike lesions on the head, scalp, and neck.

Systemic Sclerosis/Scleroderma

Systemic sclerosis, sometimes called *scleroderma*, is an autoimmune disease of connective tissue characterized by excessive collagen deposition in the skin and internal organs such as the lungs, gastrointestinal tract, heart, and kidneys. In this disorder, the skin is thickened through fibrosis, with an accompanying fixation of subdermal structures, including the sheaths or fascia covering tendons and muscles.[2] Systemic sclerosis affects females four times as frequently as it does males, with a peak incidence in the 25- to 50-year-old age group.[2] The cause of this rare disorder is poorly understood. There is correlation between the development of autoantibodies of scleroderma and HLA-DQBI.[2] There is evidence of both humoral and cellular immune system abnormalities.

Clinical Manifestations

Scleroderma presents as two distinct clinical entities: the diffuse or generalized form of the disease and the limited or CREST variant. CREST syndrome is an acronym for several different symptoms that tend to occur with scleroderma:

- C stands for calcinosis.
- R equals Raynaud phenomenon.
- E is esophageal dysmobility.
- S equals sclerodactyly.
- T stands for telangiectasias.

In 2004, another four letters were added to the CREST acronym so that it is known now as ABCDCREST:

- A stands for antibodies to centromeric protein A (CENP), anti-topo1, or fibrillarin.
- B stands for bibasilar pulmonary fibrosis.
- C stands for contractures of digital joints.
- D stands for dermal thickening proximal to wrists.[23]

Generally, a person would have to have four of these symptoms to be diagnosed with CREST type of scleroderma.

Diffuse scleroderma is characterized by severe and progressive disease of the skin and the early onset of organ involvement. The typical person has "stone facies" because of tightening of the facial skin with restricted motion of the mouth. Involvement of the esophagus leads to hypomotility and difficulty in swallowing. Malabsorption may develop if the submucosal and muscular atrophy affect the intestine. Pulmonary involvement leads to dyspnea and eventually respiratory failure. Vascular involvement of the kidneys is responsible for malignant hypertension and progressive renal insufficiency. Cardiac problems include pericarditis, heart block, and myocardial fibrosis.

Diagnosis and Treatment

Diagnostics for systemic scleroderma is more difficult than it is for the CREST variant. The measurement of the autoantibody, Scl-70, is most diagnostic, although only about 60% of people with systemic scleroderma have this.

Treatment of systemic sclerosis is largely symptomatic and supportive. Advances in treatment, primarily the use of angiotensin-converting enzyme inhibitors in renal involvement, have led to a substantial decrease in the mortality from hypertensive renal disease.

Polymyositis and Dermatomyositis

Polymyositis and dermatomyositis are chronic inflammatory myopathies. The pathogenesis is multifactorial and includes cellular and humoral immune mechanisms. Systemic manifestations can occur with an impact on morbidity and mortality.[23] These conditions are characterized by symmetric proximal muscle weakness and occasional muscle pain and tenderness. The Bohan and Peter criteria are used for the classification of polymyositis and dermatomyositis.[24,25] Careful diagnosis is important because there are many potential differential diagnoses.[23] Treatment for the inflammatory myopathies should seek to control inflammation and prevent long-term damage to muscles, joints, and internal organs. Corticosteroids are the mainstay of treatment for these conditions.

SUMMARY CONCEPTS

RA is a systemic inflammatory disorder that affects 1% to 2% of the population. Females are affected more frequently than are males. This form of arthritis, the cause of which is unknown, has a chronic course and usually is characterized by remissions and exacerbations. Joint involvement is symmetric and begins with inflammatory changes in the synovial membrane. As joint inflammation progresses, structural changes can occur, leading to joint instability and eventual deformity. Systemic manifestations include weakness, anorexia, weight loss, and low-grade fever. Some extra-articular features include rheumatoid nodules and vasculitis. The treatment goals are to prevent and/or reduce pain, decrease stiffness and swelling, maximize mobility, and possibly halt the pathologic process.

SLE is a chronic autoimmune disorder that affects multiple body systems. There is no known cause of SLE, but the disease may result from an immunoregulatory disturbance brought about by a combination of genetic, hormonal, and environmental factors. Some drugs have been shown to induce SLE, especially in older adults. There is an exaggerated production of autoantibodies, which interact with antigens to produce an immune complex. These immune complexes produce an inflammatory response in affected tissues. Treatment focuses on preventing loss of organ function, controlling inflammation, and minimizing complications of medication therapy.

Systemic sclerosis, often prefixed by the term *progressive*, is sometimes called *scleroderma*. In this disorder, the skin is thickened through fibrosis with an accompanying fixation to the subdermal structures, including the sheaths or fascia covering tendons and muscles. Polymyositis and dermatomyositis are chronic inflammatory myopathies. Its pathogenesis is multifactorial and includes cellular and humoral immune mechanisms.

Seronegative Spondyloarthropathies

The *spondyloarthropathies* (SpA) are an interrelated group of multisystem inflammatory disorders that primarily affect the axial skeleton, particularly the spine. Typically, the inflammation begins at sites where tendon and ligament insert into bone rather than in the synovium. Sacroiliitis is a pathologic hallmark of the disorders.[2] People with SpA may also have inflammation and involvement of the peripheral joints, in which case the signs and symptoms overlap with other inflammatory types of arthritis. Because there is an absence of RF, these disorders often are referred to as *seronegative SpA* and are recognized as specific disease entities.[2]

The seronegative SpA include ankylosing spondylitis (AS), reactive arthritis, arthritis related to inflammatory bowel disease, and psoriatic arthritis.[2] Although they differ in terms of factors such as age and type of onset and extent of joint involvement, there is clinical evidence of overlap between the various seronegative SpA. In none of these disorders is the cause or pathogenesis well understood. There is a striking association with the HLA-B27 antigen, but the presence of the HLA-B27 antigen by itself is neither necessary nor sufficient for the development of any of the diseases.[2]

Ankylosing Spondylitis

AS is a chronic, systemic inflammatory disease of the joints of the vertebral column and sacroiliac joints manifested by pain and progressive stiffening of the spine.[26] Clinical manifestations usually begin in late adolescence or in early adulthood and are slightly more common in males than in females. The disease usually evolves more slowly and is less severe in females. AS can occur later in life and, when it does, initial symptoms commonly include more involvement of the cervical spine and arthritis of the upper and lower limbs. The late-onset group also demonstrates a higher amount of missed presentations (axial and peripheral joints) as the disease progresses.[27]

AS produces an inflammatory erosion of the sites where tendons and ligaments attach to bone.[26] Typically, the disease process begins with bilateral involvement of the sacroiliac joints and then moves to the smaller joints of the posterior elements of the spine. The result is ultimate destruction of these joints with ankylosis or posterior fusion of the spine. The vertebrae take on a squared appearance and bone bridges fuse one vertebral body to the next across the intervertebral disks. Progressive spinal changes usually follow an ascending pattern beginning with the sacroiliac area and then moving up the spine to involve the costovertebral joints and cervical spine. Occasionally, large synovial joints (*i.e.*, hips, knees, and shoulders) may be involved. The small peripheral joints usually are not affected. The disease spectrum ranges from an asymptomatic **sacroiliitis** to a progressive disease that can affect many body systems.

Etiology and Pathogenesis

Although the pathogenesis of AS has not been established, the presence of mononuclear cells in the acutely involved tissue suggests an immune response. Epidemiologic findings indicate that genetic and environmental factors play a role in the pathogenesis of the disease. Approximately 90% of those with AS possess the HLA-B27 antigen and nearly 100% of those who also have uveitis or aortitis have the marker; the HLA-B27 antigen also is present in approximately 8% of the normal population.[2] An autoimmune reaction to an antigenic determinant site in the host's tissues may occur as a consequence of an immunologic response to an identical or closely related antigen of a foreign agent, usually an infectious agent.[28]

Clinical Manifestations

The person with AS typically complains of lower back pain, which may be persistent or intermittent. The pain, which becomes worse when resting, particularly when lying in bed, initially may be attributed to muscle strain or spasm from physical activity. Lumbosacral pain also may be present, with discomfort in the buttocks and hip areas. Sometimes, pain can radiate to the thigh in a manner like that of sciatic pain. Prolonged stiffness is present in the morning and after periods of rest. Walking or exercise may be needed to provide the comfort needed to return to sleep. Loss of motion in the spinal column is characteristic of the disease (Fig. 50-6). The severity and duration of disease activity influence the degree of mobility. Loss of lumbar lordosis occurs as the disease progresses, and this is followed by kyphosis of the thoracic spine and extension of the neck. A spine fused in the flexed position is the end result in severe AS. A kyphotic spine makes it difficult for the person to look ahead and to maintain balance while walking. The image is of a person bent over looking at the floor and unable to straighten up. X-ray films show a rigid, bamboo-like spine. The heart and lungs are constricted in the chest cavity. Abnormal weight-bearing can lead to degeneration and destruction of the hips, necessitating joint replacement procedures. Peripheral arthritis is more common in the hips and shoulders.

The most common extraskeletal involvement is acute anterior uveitis and may be the first indication of the

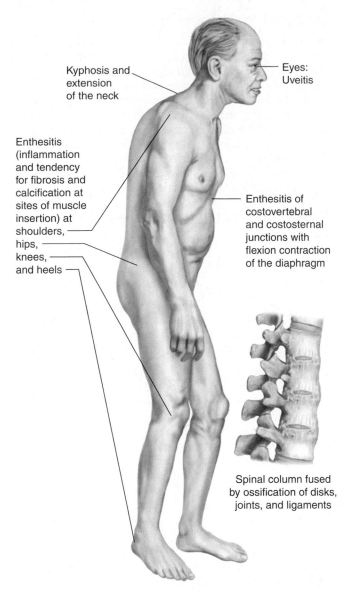

Kyphosis and extension of the neck

Eyes: Uveitis

Enthesitis (inflammation and tendency for fibrosis and calcification at sites of muscle insertion) at shoulders, hips, knees, and heels

Enthesitis of costovertebral and costosternal junctions with flexion contraction of the diaphragm

Spinal column fused by ossification of disks, joints, and ligaments

FIGURE 50-6. Clinical manifestations of ankylosing spondylitis.

disease.[27] Systemic features of weight loss, fever, and fatigue may be apparent. Sometimes, the fatigue is a greater problem than is pain or stiffness. Osteoporosis can occur, especially in the spine, which contributes to the risk of spinal fracture. Fusion of the costovertebral joints can lead to reduced lung volume.

The disease process varies considerably among people. Exacerbations and remissions are common. The unpredictability of the disease can create uncertainty in planning daily activities and in setting goals. Fortunately, most of those affected can lead productive lives. The prognosis for AS in general is good. The first decade of disease predicts the remainder. Severe disease usually occurs early and is marked by peripheral arthritis, especially of the hip.

Diagnosis

The diagnosis of AS is based on history and physical and x-ray examinations. The early and precise diagnosis of

AS is closely related to a favorable prognosis. Early recognition allows for implementation of a conservative and usually effective treatment program on a lifelong basis.

Several methods are available to assess spinal mobility, detect sacroiliitis, and diagnose AS. These methods include assessment of sacroiliitis through imaging, spinal flexion including chest expansion, modified Schöber test, lateral lumber flexion, cervical rotation and the Bath Ankylosing Spondylitis Metrology Scale, and laboratory values such as C-reactive protein and ESR.[26,28,29] Although these measures alone do not provide a diagnosis of AS or other SpA, they can provide useful measurements for monitoring the disease status. Measurement of chest expansion may be used as an indirect indicator of thoracic involvement, which usually occurs late in the disease course.

Laboratory findings frequently include an elevated ESR. Radiologic evaluations help differentiate AS from sacroiliitis because of other diseases. However, x-ray images may show a negative result in early disease. Vertebrae normally are concave on the anterior border. In AS, the vertebrae take on a squared appearance (see Fig. 50-6).

Treatment

Treatment of AS is directed at controlling pain and maintaining mobility by suppressing inflammation. Proper posture and positioning are important. Therapeutic exercises are important to assist in maintaining motion in peripheral joints and in the spine. Muscle-strengthening exercises for extensor muscle groups also are prescribed. Maintaining ideal weight reduces the stress on weight-bearing joints. Smoking should be discouraged because it can exaccrbate respiratory problems. Occupational counseling or job evaluation may be warranted because of postural abnormalities.

Pharmacologic treatment includes the use of NSAIDs to reduce inflammation, relieve pain, and reduce muscle spasm. In high disease activity not responsive to conventional therapy, DMARDs may be considered.

Current practice is to use anti–TNF-α therapies, including etanercept, infliximab, and adalimumab, which have demonstrated positive effects on disease activity.[26,30]

Reactive Arthropathies

The reactive arthropathies may be defined as sterile inflammatory joint disorders that are distant in time and place from the initial inciting infective process. The infecting agents cannot be cultured and are not viable once they reach the joints. The list of triggering agents is continuously increasing and may be divided into urogenic, enterogenic, and respiratory tract associated, and the idiopathic arthritides.

Reactive arthritis also has been observed in people with acquired immunodeficiency syndrome. SpA such as Reiter syndrome and psoriatic arthritis are more severe and frequent in people infected with human immunodeficiency virus than in the general population. Reactive arthritis may also result from the presence of a foreign substance in the joint tissue, as in silicone implants in the small joints of the hands or feet or after exposure to industrial gases and oils. However, there is no evidence of antigenicity of the causative substance.

Similarities exist between reactive arthritis and bacterial arthritis. Several bacteria cause both diseases. When cultured bacteria are isolated from the synovial fluid, the diagnosis is bacterial arthritis. When they cannot be isolated, even though there has been a preceding infection, the diagnosis of reactive arthritis is made.

Reactive arthritis may follow a self-limited course. It may involve recurrent episodes of arthritis or, in a small number of cases, may follow a continuous and unremitting course. The treatment is largely symptomatic. NSAIDs are used in treating the arthritic symptoms. Vigorous treatment of possible triggering infections is thought to prevent relapses of reactive arthritis, but in many cases the triggering infection passes unnoticed or is mild, and the person contacts a physician only with the onset of definite arthritis. Short antibiotic courses at this time are not effective.

Reiter Syndrome

Reiter syndrome is considered to be a clinical manifestation of reactive arthritis that may be accompanied by extra-articular symptoms such as uveitis, bowel inflammation, and nonspecific urethritis.[2] The disease often develops in a genetically susceptible host after a bacterial infection (*e.g.*, a sexually transmitted infection).[2]

KEY POINTS

Seronegative Spondyloarthropathies

- The seronegative SpA represent a group of related multisystem disorders that lack the RF.

- The inflammatory process associated with the disorders commonly affects the axial skeleton, involving areas where ligaments and tendons attach to bone.

- Although the cause of the disorders is unknown, there is a striking association between the HLA-B27 antigen and the development of SpA.

Psoriatic Arthritis

Psoriatic arthritis is a seronegative inflammatory arthropathy that occurs in 7% of people with psoriasis.[2] It is a heterogeneous disease with features of the SpA in some people, RA in others, and features of both coexisting in yet others.

Etiology and Pathogenesis

The etiology of psoriasis and psoriatic arthritis is unknown. Genetic, environmental, and immunologic factors appear to affect susceptibility and play a role in expression of the psoriatic skin disease and the arthritis. Environmental factors that may play a role in the pathogenesis of the disorder include infectious agents and physical trauma. T-cell–mediated immune responses seem to play an important role in the skin and joint manifestations of the disease, as indicated by the observation that there is improvement in disease status after treatment with immunosuppressant agents such as cyclosporine.

Clinical Manifestations and Treatment

Although the arthritis can antedate a detectable skin rash, the definitive diagnosis of psoriatic arthritis cannot be made without evidence of skin or nail changes typical of psoriasis. Psoriatic arthritis falls into five subgroups:

1. Asymmetric—about 35% of cases, often mild
2. Spondylitis—pain and stiffness in the spine and neck
3. Symmetric—about 50% of cases
4. DIP—inflammation and stiffness near the ends of the fingers
5. Mutilans—most severe—only about 5% of cases[31]

This heterogeneous clinical presentation suggests that more than one disease is associated with psoriasis or various clinical responses to a common cause. Some with psoriatic arthritis have an elevated serum level of uric acid. The abnormally elevated serum uric acid level is caused by the rapid skin turnover of psoriasis and the subsequent breakdown of nucleic acid followed by its metabolism to uric acid. This finding may lead to a misdiagnosis of gout. Psoriatic arthritis tends to be slowly progressive, but it has a more favorable prognosis than does RA.

Basic management is similar to the treatment of RA. Suppression of the skin disease may be important in controlling the arthritis. Often, affected joints are surprisingly functional and only minimally symptomatic. If there are musculoskeletal symptoms, NSAIDs may be used.[32] DMARDs such as methotrexate, sulfasalazine, and leflunomide should be considered early in those with active disease.[32] Methotrexate is indicated in psoriatic arthritis and significant psoriasis.[32] TNF inhibitors are indicated when there is an inadequate response to indicated DMARDs, NSAIDs, or steroid injections.[32]

Enteropathic Arthritis

Arthritis that is associated with an inflammatory bowel disease usually is considered an **enteropathic** arthritis because the intestinal disease is directly involved in the pathogenesis. Most cases of enteropathic arthritis are classified among the SpA. These include cases in which the arthritis is associated with inflammatory bowel disease (*i.e.*, ulcerative colitis and Crohn disease), which is generally 20%, spondylitis (10%), and a few with the reactive arthritides triggered by bacterial infections of the gut, and Whipple disease.[2]

SUMMARY CONCEPTS

The seronegative arthropathies are a group of rheumatic disorders that lack RF. The *seronegative SpA* affect the axial skeleton, particularly the spine. Inflammation develops at sites where tendons and ligaments insert into bone. They include AS, reactive arthritis, psoriatic arthritis, and enteropathic arthritis. AS is considered a prototype of this classification category. Bilateral sacroiliitis is the primary feature of AS. The disease spectrum ranges from asymptomatic sacroiliitis to a progressive disorder affecting many body systems. The cause remains unknown. However, a strong association between the HLA-B27 antigen and AS has been identified. Loss of motion in the spinal column is characteristic of the disease. Peripheral arthritis may occur in some people. Another form of spondyloarthritis is reactive arthritis. Although there are overlapping features for each of the SpA, identifying etiologic differences and clinical manifestations is important for determining treatment.

Osteoarthritis Syndrome

OA, formerly called *degenerative joint disease*, is the most prevalent form of arthritis and is a leading cause of disability and pain in older adults. OA is more of a disease process than a specific entity and is considered to have an inflammatory component along with the degenerative aspect. OA is a slowly progressive destruction of articular cartilage of weight-bearing joints and fingers of older adults and the joints of younger people who have experienced trauma.[2] It can occur as a primary disorder or as a secondary disorder, although this distinction is not always clear. Primary variants of OA occur due to intrinsic defects in the articular cartilage that cause joint narrowing, subchondral bone thickening, and, ultimately, a painful joint.[2] Secondary OA has a known underlying cause such as congenital or acquired defects of joint structures, trauma, infection, endocrinopathies, crystal deposits, osteonecrosis, metabolic disorders, or inflammatory diseases (Chart 50-1).

The joint changes associated with OA, which include a progressive loss of articular cartilage and synovitis, result from the inflammation caused when cartilage attempts to repair itself, creating **osteophytes** or spurs. These changes are accompanied by joint pain, stiffness, and limitation of motion, and in some cases by joint instability and deformity.

Epidemiology and Risk Factors

Age, gender, and race interact to influence the time of onset and the pattern of joint involvement in OA.

CHART 50-1

CAUSES OF OSTEOARTHRITIS

Postinflammatory disorders
    Rheumatoid arthritis
    Septic joint
Posttraumatic disorders
    Acute fracture
    Ligament or meniscal injury
    Cumulative occupational or recreational trauma
Anatomic or bony disorders
    Hip dysplasia
    Avascular necrosis
    Paget disease
    Slipped capital femoral epiphysis
    Legg–Calvé–Perthes disease
Metabolic disorders
    Calcium crystal deposition
    Hemochromatosis
    Acromegaly
    Endocrinopathies
    Wilson disease
    Ochronosis
Neuropathic arthritis
    Charcot joint
Hereditary disorders of collagen
Idiopathic or primary variants

Primary OA affects 4% of people between 18 and 24 years of age; 85% of people with OA are in their 70s.[2] Males are affected more commonly at a younger age, such as 45 years. However, by 55 years of age, females are more frequently affected by OA.[2] Heredity influences the occurrence of hand OA in the DIP joint. Hand OA is more likely to affect Caucasian females, whereas knee OA is more common in African American females. The incidence of hip OA is lower among the Chinese than among the Europeans, perhaps representing the influence of other factors such as occupation, obesity, or heredity. Bone mass may also influence the risk of developing OA. In theory, thinner subchondral bone mass may provide a greater shock-absorbing function than does denser bone, allowing less direct trauma to the cartilage.

Obesity is a risk factor for OA of the knee in females and a contributory biomechanical factor in the pathogenesis of the disease. Excess fat may have a direct metabolic effect on cartilage beyond the effects of excess joint stress.

Pathogenesis

The pathogenesis of OA resides in the homeostatic mechanisms that maintain the articular cartilage. Articular cartilage plays two essential mechanical roles in joint physiology. First, the articular cartilage serves as a remarkably smooth weight-bearing surface. In combination with synovial fluid, the articular cartilage provides extremely low friction during movement of the joint. Second, the cartilage transmits the load down to the bone, dissipating the mechanical stress.[2] Thus, the subchondral bone protects the overlying articular cartilage, providing it with a pliable bed and absorbing the energy of the force (Fig. 50-7).

Cartilage is a specialized type of connective tissue. As with other types of tissue, it consists of cells (*i.e.*, chondrocytes) nested in an extracellular matrix. In articular cartilage, the extracellular matrix is composed of water, proteoglycans, collagen, and ground substance. The proteoglycans, which are large macromolecules made up of disaccharides and amino acids, afford elasticity and stiffness, permitting articular cartilage to resist compression. The ground substance constitutes a highly hydrated, semisolid gel. Collagen molecules consist of polypeptide chains that form long, fibrous strands. They provide form and tensile strength. The primary function of the collagen fibers is to provide a rigid scaffold to support the chondrocytes and ground substance of cartilage. The hydrated proteoglycan molecules, because of their size and charge, are trapped in the collagen meshwork of the extracellular matrix and prevented from expanding to their maximum size. Because of this process, there is high interstitial osmotic pressure and enough fluid available for joint lubrication. As in the case of adult bone, articular cartilage is not static. It undergoes turnover and its "worn out" matrix components are continually degraded and replaced. This turnover is maintained by the chondrocytes, which not only synthesize the matrix but also secrete matrix-degrading enzymes. Thus, the health of the chondrocytes determines joint integrity. In OA, this integrity can be disturbed by many influences.

Popularly known as *wear-and-tear* arthritis, OA is characterized by significant changes in both the composition and mechanical properties of cartilage. Early during the disease, the cartilage contains increased water and decreased concentrations of proteoglycans compared with healthy cartilage. In addition, there appears to be a weakening of the collagen network, presumably caused by a decrease in the local synthesis of new collagen and an increase in the breakdown of existing collagen. It is thought that the injured articular cartilage is due to cytokine release, which triggers destruction of the joint[2] (Fig. 50-8). The resulting damage predisposes the chondrocytes to more injury and impairs their ability to repair the damage by producing new collagen and proteoglycans. The combined effects of inadequate repair mechanisms and imbalances between the proteases and their inhibitors contribute further to disease progression.

The earliest structural changes in OA include enlargement and reorganization of the chondrocytes in the superficial part of the articular cartilage. This is accompanied by edematous changes in the cartilaginous matrix, principally the intermediate layer. The cartilage loses its smooth aspect and surface cracks or microfractures occur, allowing synovial fluid to enter and widen the crack (Fig. 50-9). As the crack deepens and clefts form, it eventually extends through the articular surface and into the subchondral aspect of the bone.[2] Portions of the articular cartilage eventually become completely eroded and the exposed surface of the subchondral bone becomes thickened and polished to an ivory-like consistency. Fragments of cartilage and bone often become dislodged, creating free-floating osteocartilaginous bodies ("joint mice") that enter the joint cavity. As the disease progresses, the underlying trabecular bone becomes sclerotic in response to increased pressure on the surface of the joint, rendering it less effective as a shock absorber. Sclerosis, or formation of new bone and cysts, usually occurs at the joint margins, forming abnormal bony outgrowths called *osteophytes*, or *spurs* (Fig. 50-7). As the joint begins to lose its integrity, there is trauma to the synovial membrane, which results in nonspecific inflammation. Compared with RA, however, the changes in the synovium that occur in OA are not as pronounced, nor do they occur as early.

In secondary forms of OA, repetitive impact loading contributes to joint failure, accounting for the high prevalence of OA specific to vocational or avocational sites, such as the shoulders and elbows of baseball pitchers, ankles of ballet dancers, and knees of basketball players. Immobilization also can produce degenerative changes in articular cartilage. Cartilage degeneration because of immobility may result from loss of the pumping action of lubrication that occurs with joint movement. These changes are more marked and appear earlier in areas of contact but occur also in areas not subject to mechanical compression. Although cartilage atrophy is rapidly reversible with activity after a period of immobilization, impact exercise during the period of remobilization can prevent reversal of the atrophy. Therefore, slow and gradual remobilization may be important in preventing cartilage injury. Clinically, this has implications for instructions concerning the recommended level of physical activity after removal of a cast.

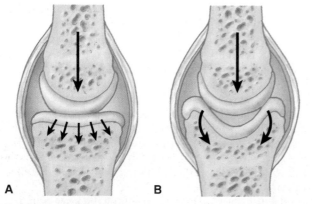

FIGURE 50-7. (A) A joint normally undergoes deformation of the articular cartilage and the subchondral bone when carrying a load. This maximizes the contact area and spreads the force of the load. (B) If the joint does not deform with a load, the stresses are concentrated and the joint breaks down.

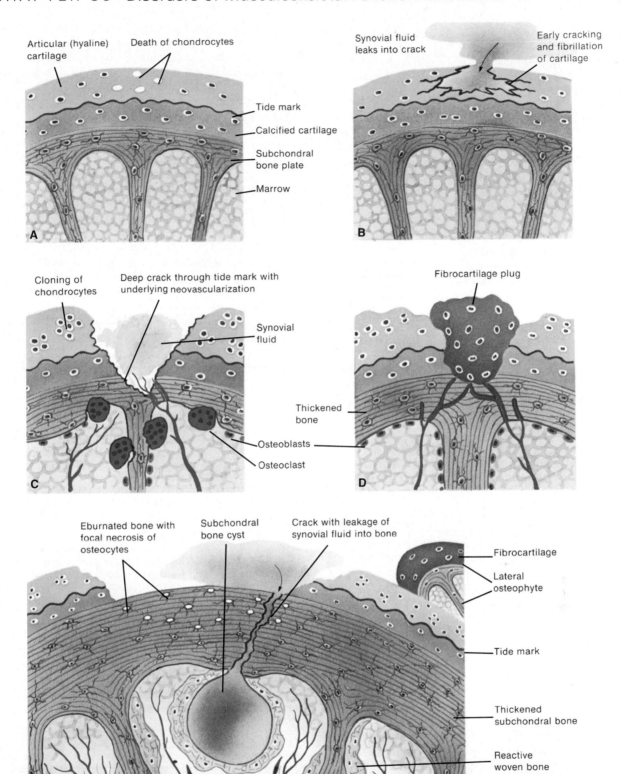

FIGURE 50-8. Histogenesis of osteoarthritis. (**A and B**) The death of chondrocytes leads to a crack in the articular cartilage that is followed by an influx of synovial fluid and further loss of cartilage. (**C**) As a result of this process, cartilage is gradually worn away. Below the tidemark, new vessels grow in from the epiphysis, and fibrocartilage (**D**) is deposited. (**E**) The fibrocartilage plug is not mechanically sufficient and may be worn away, thus exposing the subchondral bone plate, which becomes thickened and eburnated. If there is a crack in this region, synovial fluid leaks into the marrow space and produces a subchondral bone cyst. Focal regrowth of the articular surface leads to the formation of osteophytes. (From Strayer D., Rubin R. (Eds.) (2015). *Rubin's pathology: Clinicopathologic foundations of medicine* (7th ed., Fig. 30-53, p. 1361). Philadelphia, PA: Lippincott Williams & Wilkins.)

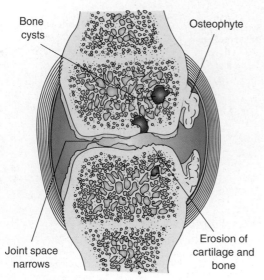

FIGURE 50-9. Joint changes in osteoarthritis. The left side denotes early changes and joint space narrowing with cartilage breakdown. The right side shows more severe disease progression with lost cartilage and osteophyte formation.

KEY POINTS

Osteoarthritis

- OA can present as a primary disease of unknown etiology or as a secondary disorder related to congenital or acquired defects that affect the distribution of joint stress.

- The pathogenesis of OA includes the progressive disruption of the smooth surface of the articular cartilage with development of surface cracks that deepen to involve the subchondral bone, followed by complete erosion of the articular cartilage with exposure of ivory-like polished subchondral bone, dislodgment of fragments of free-floating osteocartilaginous bodies, development of bone cysts, and formation of abnormal bony spurs at the joint margins.

Clinical Manifestations

The manifestations of OA may arise suddenly or insidiously. Initially, the pain may be described as aching and may be somewhat difficult to localize. It usually worsens with use or activity and is relieved by rest. In later stages of disease activity, night pain may be experienced during rest. Pain can occur at rest, several hours after the use of the involved joints. Crepitus and grinding may be evident when the joint is moved. As the disease advances, even minimal activity may cause pain because of the limited range of motion resulting from intra-articular and periarticular structural damage.

The most frequently affected joints are the hips, knees, lumbar and cervical vertebrae, proximal and distal joints of the hands, the first carpometacarpal joint, and the first metatarsophalangeal joints of the feet.[2] Table 50-1 identifies the joints that commonly are affected by OA and the common clinical features correlated with the disease activity of each particular joint. A single joint or several joints may be affected. Although a single weight-bearing joint may be involved initially, other joints often become affected because of the additional stress placed on them while trying to protect the initial joint. It is not unusual for a person having a knee replacement to discover soon after the surgery is done that the second knee also needs to be replaced. Other clinical features are limitations of joint motion and joint instability. Joint enlargement usually results from new bone formation; the joint feels hard, in contrast to the soft, spongy feeling characteristic of the joint in RA. Sometimes, mild synovitis or increased synovial fluid can cause joint enlargement.

TABLE 50-1 Clinical Features of Osteoarthritis

Joint	Clinical Features
Cervical spine	Localized stiffness; radicular or nonradicular pain; posterior osteophyte formation may cause vascular compression
Lumbar spine	Low back pain and stiffness; muscle spasm; decreased back motion; nerve root compression causing radicular pain; spinal stenosis
Hip	Most common in older males; characterized by insidious onset of pain, localized to groin region or inner aspect of the thigh; may be referred to buttocks, sciatic region, or knee; reduced hip motion; leg may be held in external rotation with hip flexed and adducted; limp or shuffling gait; difficulty getting in and out of chairs
Knee	Localized discomfort with pain on motion; limitation of motion; crepitus; quadriceps atrophy because of lack of use; joint instability; genu varus or valgus; joint effusion
First carpometacarpal joint	Tenderness at base of the thumb; squared appearance to joint
PIP joint—Bouchard nodes	Same as for DIP joint disease
DIP joint—Heberden nodes	Occurs more frequently in females; usually involves multiple DIPs, lateral flexor deviation of joint, spur formation at joint margins, pain and discomfort after joint use
First metatarsophalangeal joint	Insidious onset; irregular joint contour; pain and swelling aggravated by tight shoes

DIP, distal interphalangeal; PIP, proximal interphalangeal.

Diagnosis and Treatment

The diagnosis of OA usually is determined by history and physical examination, x-ray studies, and laboratory findings that exclude other diseases. Although OA often is contrasted with RA for diagnostic purposes, the differences are not always readily apparent. Other rheumatic diseases may be superimposed on OA.

Characteristic radiologic changes initially include medial joint space narrowing, followed by subchondral bony sclerosis, formation of spikes on the tibial eminence, and osteophytes.[2,32] The results of laboratory studies usually are normal because the disorder is not a systemic disease but can be helpful for differential diagnosis.[4] The ESR may be slightly elevated in older adults.[4] If inflammation is present, there may be a slight increase in the white blood cell count. The synovial fluid usually is normal. The ACR (2018) website has guidelines for classification of Hand, Knee, and Hip Criteria for OA.[33]

Because there is no cure, the focus of treatment of OA is symptomatic and includes physical rehabilitative, pharmacologic, and surgical measures. Physical measures are aimed at improving the supporting structures of the joint and strengthening opposing muscle groups involved in cushioning weight-bearing forces. This includes a balance of rest and exercise, use of splints to protect and rest the joint, use of heat and cold to relieve pain and muscle spasm, and adjusting the activities of daily living. Weight reduction is helpful when the knee is involved. The involved joint should not be further abused, and steps should be taken to protect and rest it. These include weight reduction (when weight-bearing surfaces are involved) and the use of a cane or walker if the hips and knees are involved.

Oral medications are aimed at reducing inflammation or providing analgesia. Popular medications used in the treatment of OA are the NSAIDs. The pain of OA may arise from factors other than an inflamed synovium. These factors include stretching of the joint capsule, ligaments, or nerve endings in the periosteum over osteophytes; nontrabecular microfractures; intraosseous hypertension; bursitis or tendinitis; and muscle spasm.

Intra-articular corticosteroid injections may be used when other treatment measures have been unsuccessful in adequately relieving symptoms. They are especially helpful in people who have an effusion of the joint.

Viscosupplementation is another treatment and is based on the hypothesis that joint lubrication is abnormal in OA.[4]

Surgery is considered when the person has severe pain and joint function is severely reduced. Procedures include joint replacement, arthroscopic lavage and debridement, bunion resections, osteotomies to change alignment of the knee and hip joints, and decompression of the spinal roots in osteoarthritic vertebral stenosis. Arthrodesis (surgical stiffening of a joint) is used in advanced disease to reduce pain. However, this results in loss of motion.

SUMMARY CONCEPTS

OA, the most common form of arthritis, is a localized condition affecting primarily the weight-bearing joints. Risk factors for OA progression include older age, OA in multiple joints, neuropathy, and, for knees, obesity. The disorder is characterized by degeneration of the articular cartilage and subchondral bone. It has been suggested that the cellular events responsible for the development of OA begin with some type of abnormal mechanical insult or stimulus, including hormones and growth factors, drugs, mechanical stresses, and the extracellular environment. Studies also implicate immunologic factors in the perpetuation and acceleration of the osteoarthritic change. As cartilage ages, biochemical events such as collagen fatigue and fracture occur with less stress. Attempts at repair by increased matrix synthesis and cellular proliferation maintain the integrity of the cartilage until failure of reparative processes allows the degenerative changes to progress. Joint enlargement usually results from new bone formation, which causes the joint to feel hard. Pain and stiffness are primary features of the disease. Inflammatory mediators (*e.g.,* prostaglandins) may increase the inflammatory and degenerative response.

Treatment is directed toward the relief of pain and maintenance of mobility while preserving the articular cartilage. Although there is no known cure for OA, appropriate treatment can reduce pain, maintain or improve joint mobility, and limit functional disability.

Crystal-Induced Arthropathies

Metabolic bone and joint disorders result from biochemical and metabolic disorders that affect the joints. Metabolic and endocrine diseases associated with joint symptoms include amyloidosis, osteogenesis imperfecta, diabetes mellitus, hyperparathyroidism, thyroid disease, AIDS, and hypermobility syndromes. The discussion in this chapter is limited to the crystal-induced arthropathy caused by monosodium urate deposition, or gout.

Crystal deposition in joints produces arthritis. In gout, monosodium urate or uric acid crystals are found in the joint cavity. Another condition in which calcium pyrophosphate dihydrate crystals are found in the joints sometimes is referred to as *pseudogout* or *chondrocalcinosis*. A brief discussion of pseudogout is found in the section on rheumatic diseases in older adults.

Gout

Gout is a group of disorders characterized by increased serum uric acid and urate crystal deposits in the kidneys and joints.[2] Gout is more prevalent in males (70% of cases), particularly in males of African American descent, and the peak age of occurrence is between ages 40 and 50.[4] High uric acid levels or hyperuricemia (>7 mg/dL in males and 6 mg/dL in females) are present in 5% to 10% of the population of the United States.[4] Asymptomatic hyperuricemia is a laboratory finding and not a disease. About one in five people with hyperuricemia will develop gout.[4] Most people with hyperuricemia do not develop gout. Only one third of people with hyperuricemia have primary gout and the other two thirds have secondary gout.[2]

Gout disorders include acute gouty arthritis with recurrent attacks of severe articular and periarticular inflammation; tophi or the accumulation of crystalline deposits in articular surfaces, bones, soft tissue, and cartilage; gouty nephropathy or renal impairment; and uric acid kidney stones.

The term *primary gout* is used to designate cases in which the cause of the disorder is unknown or it is caused by an inborn error in metabolism and characterized primarily by hyperuricemia and gout. Primary gout is predominantly a disease of males, with a peak incidence in the fourth to sixth decade.[2] In secondary gout, the cause of the hyperuricemia is known but the gout is not the main disorder.

Pathogenesis

The pathogenesis of gout resides in an elevation of serum uric acid levels. Uric acid is the end product of purine metabolism.[34] Two pathways are involved in purine synthesis:

1. A de novo pathway in which purines are synthesized from nonpurine precursors
2. The salvage pathway in which purine bases are recaptured from the breakdown of nucleic acids derived from exogenous (dietary) or endogenous sources

The elevation of uric acid and the subsequent development of gout can result from overproduction of purines, decreased salvage of free purine bases, augmented breakdown of nucleic acids because of increased cell turnover, or decreased urinary excretion of uric acid (Fig. 50-10). Primary gout, which constitutes 90% of cases, may be a consequence of enzyme defects that result in an overproduction of uric acid or inadequate elimination of uric acid by the kidney.[34] In most cases, the reason is unknown. In secondary gout, the hyperuricemia may be caused by the increased breakdown of nucleic acids, as occurs with rapid tumor cell lysis during treatment for lymphoma or leukemia. Other cases of secondary gout result from chronic renal disease. Some of the diuretics, including the thiazides, can interfere with the excretion of uric acid.

An attack of gout occurs when monosodium urate crystals precipitate in the joint and initiate an inflammatory response. Synovial fluid is a poorer solvent for uric acid than is plasma, and uric acid crystals are even less soluble at temperatures below 37°C. Crystal deposition usually occurs in peripheral areas of the body, such as

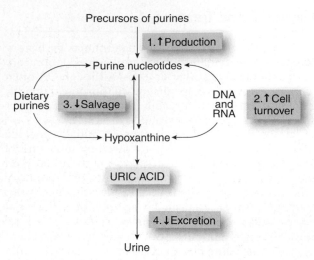

FIGURE 50-10. Pathogenesis of hyperuricemia and gout. Purine nucleotides are synthesized de novo from nonpurine precursors or derived from preformed purines in the diet. Purine nucleotides are catabolized to hypoxanthine or incorporated into nucleic acids. The degradation of nucleic acids and dietary purines also produces hypoxanthine. Hypoxanthine is converted into uric acid, which in turn is excreted into the urine. Hyperuricemia and gout from (*1*) increased de novo purine synthesis, (*2*) increased cell turnover, (*3*) decreased salvage of dietary purines and hypoxanthine, and (*4*) decreased uric acid excretion by the kidneys. (From Strayer D., Rubin R. (Eds.) (2015). *Rubin's pathology: Clinicopathologic foundations of medicine* (7th ed., Fig. 30-60, p. 1367). Philadelphia, PA: Lippincott Williams & Wilkins.)

the great toe, where the temperatures are cooler than in other parts of the body. With prolonged hyperuricemia, crystals and microtophi (*i.e.*, small, hard nodules with irregular surfaces that contain crystalline deposits of monosodium urate) accumulate in the synovial lining cells and in the joint cartilage.[4] The released crystals are chemotactic to leukocytes and also activate complements. Phagocytosis of urate crystals by polymorphonuclear leukocytes occurs and leads to polymorphonuclear cell death with the release of lysosomal enzymes. As this process continues, the inflammation causes destruction of the cartilage and subchondral bone.

Repeated or untreated attacks of acute arthritis eventually lead to chronic arthritis and the formation of the large, hard nodules called *tophi*[4,34] (Fig. 50-11). They are found most commonly in the synovium, olecranon bursa, Achilles tendon, subchondral bone, and extensor surface of the forearm and may be mistaken for rheumatoid nodules. Tophi usually do not appear until 10 years or more after the first gout attack. This stage of gout, called *chronic tophaceous gout*, is characterized by more frequent and prolonged attacks, which often are polyarticular.

Clinical Manifestations

Gout is categorized into four phases:

1. The asymptomatic hyperuricemia
2. Acute gout arthritis
3. Intercritical gout
4. Chronic tophaceous gout[2]

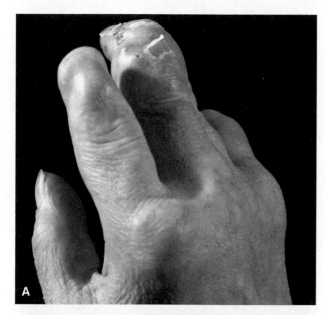

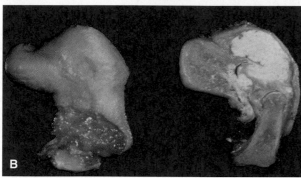

FIGURE 50-11. Gout. **(A)** Gouty tophi of the hands appear as multiple rubbery nodules, one of which is ulcerated. **(B)** A cross section of a digit demonstrates a tophaceous collection of toothpaste-like urate crystals. (From Strayer D., Rubin R. (Eds.) (2015). *Rubin's pathology: Clinicopathologic foundations of medicine* (7th ed., Fig. 30-61A and B, p. 1368). Philadelphia, PA: Lippincott Williams & Wilkins.)

The first phase may not even be identified or may be detected during an annual physical examination because the person has no symptoms. The typical acute attack of gout is monoarticular and usually affects the first metatarsophalangeal joint. The tarsal joints, insteps, ankles, heels, knees, wrists, fingers, and elbows also may be initial sites of involvement. Acute gout often begins at night and may be precipitated by excessive exercise, certain medications or foods, alcohol, or dieting. The onset of pain typically is abrupt, and redness and swelling are observed. The attack may last for days or weeks. Pain may be severe enough to be aggravated even by the weight of a bedsheet covering the affected area.

In the early stages of gout after the initial attack has subsided, the person is asymptomatic, and joint abnormalities are not evident. This is the third phase or *intercritical gout*. After the first attack, it may be months or years before another attack. Because attacks recur with increased frequency, joint changes occur and become permanent. This fourth phase is called chronic tophaceous gout.

Gout has been linked with cardiovascular disease, obesity, metabolic syndrome, hyperlipidemia, excessive alcohol use, and renal insufficiency. Therefore, these potential comorbidities need to be ruled out and, if they are ruled out, should be prevented.[35]

Diagnosis and Treatment

Although hyperuricemia is the biochemical hallmark of gout, the presence of hyperuricemia cannot be equated with gout because many people with this condition never develop gout. A definitive diagnosis of gout can be made only when monosodium urate crystals are in the synovial fluid or in the tissue sections of tophaceous deposits. Synovial fluid analysis is useful in excluding other conditions, such as septic arthritis, pseudogout, and RA. Measurement of serum uric acid levels and collection of a 24-hour urine sample for determination of urate excretion in the urine is diagnostic.[34,36] The objectives for treatment of gout include the termination and prevention of the acute attacks of gouty arthritis and the correction of hyperuricemia, with consequent inhibition of further precipitation of sodium urate and absorption of urate crystal deposits already in the tissues.

Pharmacologic management of acute gout is directed toward reducing joint inflammation. Hyperuricemia and related problems of tophi, joint destruction, and renal problems are treated after the acute inflammatory process has subsided. NSAIDs, particularly indomethacin and ibuprofen, are used for treating acute gouty arthritis. Alternative therapies include colchicine and intra-articular deposition of corticosteroids.

Treatment of hyperuricemia is aimed at maintaining normal uric acid levels and is lifelong.

Education about the disease and its management are fundamental to the treatment and management of gout. Some changes in lifestyle may be needed, such as maintenance of ideal weight, moderation in alcohol consumption, smoking cessation, and avoidance of purine-rich foods, particularly by people with excessive tophaceous deposits.[34,36]

 SUMMARY CONCEPTS

Crystal-induced arthropathy is characterized by crystal deposition in the joint. Gout is the prototype of this group. Acute attacks of arthritis occur with gout and are characterized by the presence of monosodium urate crystals in the joint. The disorder is accompanied by hyperuricemia, which results from overproduction of uric acid or from the reduced ability of the kidney to rid the body of excess uric acid. Management of acute gout is directed first toward the reduction of joint inflammation, after which the hyperuricemia is treated. Hyperuricemia is treated with uricosuric agents, which prevent the tubular reabsorption of urate, or with medication that inhibits the production of uric acid. Although gout is chronic, most people can control it with appropriate lifestyle changes.

Rheumatic Diseases in Children and Older Adults

Rheumatic Diseases in Children

Children can be affected with almost all the rheumatic diseases. In addition to disease-specific differences, these conditions affect not only the child but also the family. Growth and development require special attention. Adherence to the treatment program requires intervention with the child and parents.

Juvenile Idiopathic Arthritis

Juvenile idiopathic arthritis (JIA), also known as juvenile RA, is characterized by joint inflammation as well as possible impacts on other areas of the body and occurs most frequently among arthritis of childhood.[35,37] In the United States, close to 300,000 children have a type of arthritis.[37] JIA is characterized by synovitis and can influence epiphyseal growth by stimulating growth of the affected side. Generalized stunted growth also may occur. JIA can be regarded not as a single disease, but as a category of diseases with subtypes:

- Systemic JIA
- Oligoarticular JIA
- Polyarticular JIA
- Enthesitis-related JIA
- Juvenile psoriatic arthritis
- Undifferentiated arthritis[4]

The symptoms of systemic JIA include a daily intermittent high fever, which usually is accompanied by a rash, generalized lymphadenopathy, hepatosplenomegaly, leukocytosis, and anemia. Most of these children also have joint involvement, which develops concurrently with fever and rash. Systemic symptoms usually subside in 6 to 12 months. This form of JIA also can make an initial appearance in adulthood. Infections, heart disease, and adrenal insufficiency may cause death. Systemic JIA accounts for about 10% of JIA cases.[37]

Oligoarticular arthritis affects no more than four joints. Uveitis is more common in this subgroup and is seen more often in those with positive ANA results.[37] The third subgroup, accounting for approximately 25% of the total cases of JIA, is polyarticular disease. This third classification affects five or more joints. In this form of arthritis, RF may or may not be present but when it is, the disease process may be more severe and likely to resemble adult RA.[37]

Enthesitis-related JIA is characterized by enthesitis or pain between bones and tendons, ligaments or other connective tissue as well as inflammation in other parts of the body. It may also be called spondyloarthritis and occurs more frequently in boys, beginning between 8 and 15 years of age. Often, the children will present with a positive *HLA-B27* gene test result.[37] Juvenile psoriatic arthritis often occurs with psoriasis that may begin long before joint symptoms occur. Undifferentiated arthritis refers to a juvenile arthritis that either spans two or more subtypes or does not fit into any of the listed subtypes.[37]

The prognosis for most children with JIA is variable and dependent on clinical factors. These factors vary depending on the subtype and whether the disease is systemic.[35] Treatment also varies depending on the subtype and clinical factors.[35] NSAIDs generally are the first-line drugs used in treating JIA.[35] Second-line agents are methotrexate, glucocorticoid joint injection, and TNF-α inhibitors.[35] Other aspects of treatment of children with JIA require careful attention to growth and development as well as to nutritional issues.

Systemic Lupus Erythematosus

The features of SLE in children are similar to those in adults. The incidence in children is 0.5 to 0.6 cases per 100,000 in children younger than 15 years.[38] African Americans, especially girls, are the most frequently affected by SLE. Most children who are diagnosed with SLE are 8 years or older, although SLE has been seen from infancy throughout the age cycle.[38] The clinical manifestations of SLE in children reflect the extent and severity of systemic involvement. The best prognostic indicator in children is the extent of renal involvement, which is more common and more severe in children than in adults with SLE.

Children with SLE may present with symptoms including fever, malaise, anorexia, and weight loss. Symptoms of the integumentary, musculoskeletal, central nervous, cardiac, pulmonary, and hematopoietic systems are like those in adults. Endocrine abnormalities include Cushing syndrome from long-term corticosteroid use and autoimmune thyroiditis.

Treatment of SLE in children is like that in adults. The use of NSAIDs, corticosteroids, antimalarial drugs, and immunosuppressive agents depends on the symptoms. Corticosteroids may cause stunting of growth and necrosis of femoral heads and other joints. Immunization schedules should be maintained using attenuated rather than live vaccines. The diversity of the clinical manifestations of SLE in the young requires the establishment of a comprehensive treatment or management program.

Juvenile Dermatomyositis

Juvenile dermatomyositis (JDMS) is a rare inflammatory myopathy primarily involving skin and muscle and associated with a characteristic rash. JDMS is the most frequently occurring disorder among the group of heterogeneous immune-mediated disorders called juvenile idiopathic inflammatory myopathies.[39] JDMS can affect children of all ages, with a mean age at onset of 7.5 years.[39] There is an increased incidence among girls. The cause is not known. Symmetric proximal muscle weakness, elevated muscle enzymes, evidence of vasculitis, and electromyographic changes confirming an inflammatory myopathy are diagnostic for JDMS. Generalized vasculitis is not seen in the adult form of the disease. In children, weak proximal muscles, a heliotrope rash around the eyes, Gottron papules, and vasculopathy are characteristic symptoms.[39] The rash may precede or follow the onset of proximal muscle weakness. Periorbital edema, erythema, and eyelid telangiectasia are common. The criteria of Bohan and Pila are used to diagnose this disorder. A child must have three out of the five criteria (progressive proximal symmetrical weakness, increased muscle enzyme levels, abnormal muscle biopsy results, abnormal electromyogram results, and compatible cutaneous disease) to be diagnosed with JDMS.[25]

Calcifications can occur in 30% to 50% of children with JDMS and are by far the most debilitating symptom. The calcifications appear at pressure points or sites of previous trauma. JDMS is treated primarily with corticosteroids to reduce inflammation.

Juvenile Spondyloarthropathies

AS, reactive arthritis, psoriatic arthritis, and SpA associated with ulcerative colitis and regional enteritis can affect children as well as adults. In children, spondyloarthropathy manifests in peripheral joints first, mimicking oligoarticular JIA. There is no evidence of sacroiliac or spine involvement until later in the disease, such as months to years after onset. The SpA are more common in boys and commonly occur in children who have a positive family history. HLA-B27 typing is helpful in diagnosing children because of the unusual presentation of the disease.

Management of the disease involves physical therapy, education, and attention to school and growth and development issues. Medication includes the use of salicylates, NSAIDs, and biologic modifiers.

Rheumatic Diseases in Older Adults

Arthritis is the most common complaint of older adults. The pain, stiffness, and muscle weakness affect daily life, often threatening independence and quality of life. Symptoms of the rheumatic diseases can also have an indirect effect on and even threaten the duration of life for older adults. The weakness and gait disturbance that often accompany rheumatic diseases can contribute to the likelihood of falls and fracture, causing suffering, increased health care costs, further loss of independence, and the potential for a decreased life span.

Older adults cope less well with mild to moderately severe disease, which, in younger people, is less likely to lead to serious disability for the same degree of impairment. Unfortunately, older adults, and often their health care providers, think the problems associated with arthritis are an inevitable consequence of aging and fail to take advantage of measures that can improve the quality of life.

Older adults often have multiple problems complicating diagnosis and management. The diagnosis of an older adult with a musculoskeletal problem must consider a wide variety of disorders that usually are regarded as outside the range of typical rheumatic disease. Among these are metastatic malignancy, multiple myeloma, musculoskeletal disorders accompanying endocrine or metabolic disorders, orthopedic conditions, and neurologic disease. The diagnosis may be missed if the assumption is that musculoskeletal problems in the older adult are caused by OA.

There is an increased incidence of false-positive test results for RF and ANA in the older adult population with or without rheumatic disease because older adults are better producers of autoantibodies than are younger people. There are differences in the manifestations, diagnosis, and treatment of some of the rheumatic diseases in older adults. The usual presentation of these conditions was discussed earlier in this chapter. One form of rheumatic disease that has a predilection for older adults is polymyalgia rheumatica, which generally affects people older than 60 years of age.

Rheumatoid Arthritis

The prevalence of RA increases with age.[4] Seropositive people are more likely to have had an acute onset with systemic features and higher disease activity. People with seronegative, elderly onset RA have a disease that usually follows a mild course. It may be that RA in older adults is a broad disorder that includes many distinct subsets with characteristic manifestations, courses, and outcomes.

Systemic Lupus Erythematosus

SLE is another condition with different manifestations in older adults. The disease is accompanied less frequently by renal involvement. However, pleurisy, pericarditis, arthritis, and symptoms closely resembling polymyalgia rheumatica are more common than in younger people. The characteristics of SLE in older adults closely resemble those of drug-induced SLE.

Osteoarthritis

OA is by far the most common form of arthritis among older adults. It is the greatest cause of disability and limitation of activity in older populations worldwide. Disease prevention and early intervention is the current focus but has proved difficult because of the multifactorial epidemiology of the disorder including biologic, biomechanical, and genetic factors.[32]

Crystal-Induced Arthropathies

Gout

The incidence of clinical gout increases with advancing age, in part because of the increased involvement of joints after years of continued hyperuricemia. High serum urate levels rarely occur in females, especially before menopause, because of estrogen's uricosuric effects.[34] Gouty attacks in older adults are sometimes precipitated by the use of diuretics. The treatment of gout is often more difficult in older adults.

Pseudogout

As part of the tissue-aging process, OA develops with associated cartilage degeneration and the shedding of calcium pyrophosphate crystals into the joint cavity. These crystals may produce a low-grade chronic inflammation—the chronic pseudogout syndrome. The accumulation of calcium pyrophosphate and related crystalline deposits in articular cartilage is common in the elderly. There are no medications that can remove the crystals from the joints. Although it may be asymptomatic, the presence of the crystals may contribute to more rapid cartilage deterioration. This condition may coexist with severe OA.

Polymyalgia Rheumatica

Polymyalgia rheumatica is an inflammatory condition of unknown origin characterized by aching and morning stiffness in the shoulder and pelvic areas.[40,41] Of the forms of arthritis affecting older adults, it is one of the more difficult to diagnose and one of the most important to identify. Older females are especially at risk. Polymyalgia rheumatica is a common syndrome of older adults, rarely occurring before 50 years with a peak between 70 and 79 years of age.[40] The onset can be abrupt, with the person going to bed feeling well and awakening with pain and stiffness in the neck, shoulders, and hips.

Diagnosis is based on the pain and stiffness persisting for at least 1 month and an elevated ESR. The diagnosis is confirmed when the symptoms respond dramatically to a small dose of prednisone, a corticosteroid. Biopsies have shown that the muscles are normal, despite the name, but that a nonspecific inflammation affecting the synovial tissue is present. It is possible that a number of people are erroneously diagnosed as having RA or OA. For symptomatic people with an elevated ESR, the diagnosis usually is made. Generally, the person is given oral steroids. People with polymyalgia rheumatica typically exhibit striking clinical improvement approximately on the second day after beginning the oral steroid, and this response adds to confirmation of the diagnosis.[41] People with RA also show improvement, although usually not as quickly.

Treatment with NSAIDs provides relief for some people, but most require continuing therapy with prednisone, with gradual reduction of the dose over the course of 2 to 6 years, using the person's symptoms as the primary guide. People need close monitoring during the maintenance phase with prednisone therapy.

A certain percentage of people with polymyalgia rheumatica also develop giant cell arteritis (*i.e.*, temporal arteritis) with involvement of the ophthalmic arteries. The two conditions are considered as representing different manifestations of the same disease. Giant cell arteritis, a form of systemic vasculitis, is a systemic inflammatory disease of large and medium-sized arteries.[41] The inflammatory response seems to be a T-cell response to an antigen.

Clinical manifestations of giant cell arteritis usually begin insidiously and may exist for some time before being recognized.[40,41] It is potentially dangerous if missed or mistreated, especially if the temporal artery or other vessels supplying the eye are involved, in which case blindness can ensue quickly without treatment. Initial treatment consists of large doses of prednisone. This dosage is continued for 4 to 6 weeks and then decreased gradually.

Management of Rheumatic Diseases in Older Adults

In addition to diagnosis-specific treatment, older adults require special considerations. Management techniques that rely on modalities other than drugs are particularly important. These include assistive devices, muscle-building exercise, and local heat. Muscle-strengthening and stretching exercises are particularly effective in the older adult with age-related losses in muscle function and should be instituted early.

Joint arthroplasty can also be used for pain relief and increased function. Chronologic age is not a contraindication to surgical treatment of arthritis. In appropriately selected older candidates, survival and functional outcome after surgery are equivalent to those in younger age groups. The more sedentary activity level of the older adult makes them even better candidates for joint replacement because they put less stress and demand on the new joint.

SUMMARY CONCEPTS

Rheumatic diseases that affect children can be like the adult diseases, but there are also manifestations unique to the younger population. Children with chronic diseases also must be approached with priorities different from those used in adults. Managing rheumatic diseases in children requires a team approach to address issues of the family, school, growth and development, and coping strategies and requires a comprehensive disease management program.

Arthritis is the most common complaint of the older adult population. The pain, stiffness, and muscle weakness affect daily life, often threatening independence and quality of life. There is a difference in the manifestations, diagnosis, and treatment of some of the rheumatic diseases in older adults compared with those in the younger population. OA is the most common form of arthritis among older adults. The prevalence of RA and gout increases with advancing age. One form of rheumatic disease that has a predilection for older adults is polymyalgia rheumatica. A certain percentage of people with polymyalgia rheumatica also have giant cell arteritis, frequently with involvement of the ophthalmic arteries. If this condition is untreated, it carries a serious threat of blindness.

Review Exercises

1. A 30-year-old woman, recently diagnosed with RA, complains of general fatigue and weight loss along with symmetric joint swelling, stiffness, and pain. The stiffness is more prominent in the morning and subsides during the day. Laboratory measures reveal an RF of 120 IU/mL (nonreactive, 0–39 IU/mL; weakly reactive, 40–79 IU/mL; reactive, >80 IU/mL) and a positive anti-CCP antibody.

A. Describe the immunopathogenesis of the joint changes that occur with RA.

B. How do these changes relate to this woman's symptoms?

C. What is the significance of her RF test results?

D. What is the significance of her positive anti-CCP antibody test?

E. How do her complaints of general fatigue and weight loss relate to the RA disease process?

2. A 65-year-old obese woman with a diagnosis of OA has been having increasing pain in her right knee that worsens with movement and weight-bearing and is relieved by rest. Physical examination reveals an enlarged joint with a varus deformity; coarse crepitus is felt over the joint on passive movement.

A. Compare the pathogenesis and articular structures involved in OA with those of RA.

B. What is the origin of the enlargement of the affected joint, the varus deformity, and the crepitus that is felt on movement of the affected knee?

C. Explain the predilection for involvement of the knee in people such as this woman.

3. A 75-year-old woman is seen by her health care provider because of complaints of fever, malaise, and weight loss. She is having trouble combing her hair, putting on a coat, and getting out of chairs because of the stiffness and pain in her shoulders, hip, and lower back. Because of her symptoms, the health care provider suspects the woman has polymyalgia rheumatica.

A. What laboratory test can be used to substantiate the diagnosis?

B. What other diagnostic strategies are used to confirm the diagnosis?

REFERENCES

1. Arthritis Foundation. (2018). Exercise benefits for hip osteoarthritis. [Online]. Available: https://www.arthritis.org/about-arthritis/types/osteoarthritis/articles/hip-oa-exercises.php. Accessed March 14, 2018.

2. Strayer D., Rubin R. (Eds.) (2015). *Rubin's pathology: Clinicopathologic foundations of medicine* (7th ed.). Philadelphia, PA: Lippincott Williams & Wilkins.

3. Arnold M. B., Bykerk V. P., Boire G., et al. (2014). Are there differences between young- and older-onset early inflammatory arthritis and do these impact outcomes? An analysis from the CATCH cohort. *Rheumatology* 53, 1075–1086.

4. Dunphy L. M., Windland-Brown J. E., Porter B. O., et al. (2015). *Primary care: The art and science of advanced practice nursing* (4th ed.). Philadelphia, PA: FA Davis.

5. Schulte-Pelkum J. S., Schulz-Knappe P. S. (2015). A multimarker approach to diagnosing autoimmune diseases. *MLO: Medical Laboratory Observer* 47(10), 44–46.

6. Liu Q., Zhao J., Zhou H., et al. (2015). Parthenolide inhibits pro-inflammatory cytokine production and exhibits protective effects on progression of collagen-induced arthritis in a rat model. *Scandinavian Journal of Rheumatology* 44(3), 182–191.

7. Jämsen E., Virta L. J., Hakala M., et al. (2013). The decline in joint replacement surgery in RA is associated with a concomitant increase in the intensity of anti-rheumatic therapy: A nationwide register-based study from 1995–2010. *Acta Orthopaedica* 84(4), 331–337.

8. Jensen S. (2014). *Nursing health assessment: A best practice approach* (2nd ed.). Philadelphia, PA: Lippincott Williams & Wilkins.

9. American Academy of Orthopaedic Surgeons; Armstrong A. D., Hubbard M. C. (Eds.) (2016). *Essentials of musculoskeletal care* (5th ed.). Rosemont, IL: American Academy of Orthopaedic Surgeons.

10. Woolston W., Connelly L. M. (2017). Felty's syndrome: A qualitative case study. *Medsurg Nursing* 26(2), 105–118.

11. Schuler S., Brunner M., Bernauer W. (2016). Rituximab and acute retinal necrosis in a patient with scleromalacia and rheumatoid arthritis. *Ocular Immunology and Inflammation* 24(1), 96–98.

12. American College of Rheumatology and European League against Rheumatism Association. (2010). 2010 ACR–EULAR classification criteria of rheumatoid arthritis. [Online]. Available: https://www.rheumatology.org/Portals/0/Files/2010%20Rheumatoid%20Arthritis%20Classification_EXCERPT%202010.pdf. Accessed March 16, 2018.

13. Aletaha D., Neogi T., Silman A. J., et al. (2010). 2010 Rheumatoid arthritis classification criteria: An American college of rheumatology/European league against rheumatism collaborative initiative. *Arthritis and Rheumatism* 62(9), 2569–2581.

14. Mastrangelo A., Colasanti T., Barbati C., et al. (2015). The role of posttranslational protein modifications in rheumatological diseases: Focus on rheumatoid arthritis. *Journal of Immunology Research* 2015, 1–10.

15. Scally S.W., Petersen J., Law S. C., et al. (2013). A molecular basis for the association of the HLA-DRB1 locus, citrullination, and rheumatoid arthritis. *Journal of Experimental Medicine* 210(12), 2569–2582.

16. Arthritis Foundation. (2018). Rheumatoid arthritis treatment. [Online]. Available: https://www.arthritis.org/about-arthritis/types/rheumatoid-arthritis/treatment.php. Accessed March 17, 2018.

17. National Rheumatoid Arthritis Society. (2018). Anti-TNFα treatment in rheumatoid arthritis. [Online]. Available: https://www.nras.org.uk/anti-tnfa-treatment-in-rheumatoid-arthritis. Accessed March 17, 2018.

18. American College of Rheumatology. Lupus. [Online]. Available: https://www.rheumatology.org/I-Am-A/Patient-Caregiver/Diseases-Conditions/Lupus. Accessed March 17, 2018

19. Lupus Foundation of America. What is lupus? [Online]. Available: https://resources.lupus.org/entry/what-is-lupus?utm_source=lupusorg&utm_medium=answersFAQ. Accessed March 17, 2018.

20. The Johns Hopkins Lupus Center. Lupus primer: Types of lupus. [Online]. Available: https://www.hopkinslupus.org/lupus-info/types-lupus/. Accessed March 17, 2018.

21. American College of Rheumatology. (2011). Systemic lupus erythematosus. [Online]. Available: https://www.rheumatology.org/Portals/0/Files/1997%20Update%20of%201982%20Revised.pdf. Accessed March 17, 2018.

22. Singh J. A., Solomon D. H., Dougados M., et al.; Classification and Response Criteria Subcommittee of the American College of Rheumatology Committee on Quality Measures. (2006). Development of classification and response criteria for rheumatic diseases. *Arthritis and Rheumatism (Arthritis Care and Research)* 55(2), 348–352.

23. Oldroyd A., Lilleker J., Chinoy H. (2017). Idiopathic inflammatory myopathies: A guide to subtypes, diagnostic approach and treatment. *Clinical Medicine* 17(4), 322–328.

24. Bohan A., Peter J. B. (1975). Polymyositis and dermatomyositis (first of two parts). *New England Journal of Medicine* 292, 344–347.

25. Bohan A., Peter J. B. (1975). Polymyositis and dermatomyositis (second of two parts). *New England Journal of Medicine* 292, 403–407.

26. Bond D. (2013). Ankylosing spondylitis: Diagnosis and treatment. *Nursing Standard* 28(16–18), 52–59.

27. Montilla C., Del Pino-Montes J., Collantes-Estevez E., et al. (2012). Clinical features of late-onset ankylosing spondylitis: Comparison with early-onset disease. *Journal of Rheumatology* 39(5), 1008–1012.

28. Calvo-Gutiérrez J., Garrido-Castro J. L., González-Navas C., et al. (2016). Inter-rater reliability of clinical mobility measures in ankylosing spondylitis. *BMC Musculoskeletal Disorders* 17, 1–6.

29. Rudwaleit M., van der Heijde D., Landewé R., et al. (2009). The development of Assessment of Spondylo Arthritis International Society classification criteria for axial spondyloarthritis (part II): Validation and final selection. *Annals of the Rheumatic Diseases* 68(6), 777–783.

30. Van der Heijde D., Ramiro S., Landew R., et al. 2016 Update of the ASAS-EULAR managements recommendations for axial spondyloarthritis. *Annals of the Rheumatic Diseases* 76, 978–991.

31. Arthritis Foundation. (2018). What is psoriatic arthritis? [Online]. Available: https://www.arthritis.org/about-arthritis/types/psoriatic-arthritis/what-is-psoriatic-arthritis.php. Accessed March 18, 2018.

32. Glyn-Jones S., Palmer A. J. R., Agricola R., et al. (2015). Osteoarthritis. *Lancet* 386, 376–387.

33. American College of Rheumatology. (2018). Osteoarthritis. [Online]. Available: https://www.rheumatology.org/Practice-Quality/Clinical-Support/Clinical-Practice-Guidelines/Osteoarthritis. Accessed March 18, 2018.

34. Abhishek A., Roddy E., Doherty M. (2017). Gout: A guide for the general and acute physicians. *Clinical Medicine* 17(1), 54–59.

35. American College of Rheumatology. (2011). 2011 American College of Rheumatology recommendations for the treatment of juvenile idiopathic arthritis: Initiation and safety monitoring of therapeutic agents for the treatment of arthritis and systemic features. *Arthritis Care and Research* 63(4), 465–482.

36. Khanna D., Fitzgerald J. D., Khanna P. P., et al. (2012). 2012 American College of Rheumatology guidelines for management of gout. Part 1: Systemic nonpharmacologic and pharmacologic therapeutic approaches to hyperuricemia. *Arthritis Care and Research* 64(10), 1431–1446.

37. Arthritis Foundation. (2018). What is juvenile idiopathic arthritis? [Online]. Available: https://www.arthritis.org/about-arthritis/types/juvenile-idiopathic-arthritis-jia/what-is-juvenile-idiopathic-arthritis.php. Accessed March 18, 2018

38. Klein-Gitelman M. S. (2015). Pediatric systemic lupus erythematosus. [Online]. *Medscape*. Available: http://emedicine.medscape.com/article/1008066-overview#showall. Accessed March 18, 2018.

39. Rider, L. G., Katz, J. D., Jones, O. Y. (2013). Developments in the classification and treatment of juvenile idiopathic inflammatory myopathies. *Rheumatic Diseases Clinics of North America* 39(4), 877–904.

40. Kennedy S. (2012). Polymyalgia rheumatica and giant cell arteritis: An in-depth look at diagnosis and treatment. *Journal of the American Academy of Nurse Practitioners* 24(5), 277–285.

41. Werner R. (2017) Polymyalgia rheumatica and giant cell arteritis: Common, dangerous, treatable. *Massage & Bodywork* 32(6), 36–39.

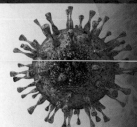

C H A P T E R 51

Structure and Function of the Skin

Learning Objectives

After completing this chapter, the learner will be able to meet the following objectives:

1. Characterize the changes in a keratinocyte from its inception in the basal lamina to its arrival on the outer surface of the skin.
2. Describe the following skin appendages and their functions: sebaceous gland, eccrine gland, apocrine gland, nails, and hair.
3. Characterize the skin in terms of sensory and immune functions.

The skin, also called the *integumentum*, is one of most versatile organs of the body, accounting for roughly 16% of the body's weight. It forms the major interface between the internal organs and the external environment. The thickness of the skin can range from less than 1 to greater than 5 mm.[1] As the body's first line of defense, the skin is continuously subjected to potentially harmful environmental agents, including solid matter, liquids, gases, sunlight, and microorganisms. Although it may become bruised, lacerated, burned, or infected, it has remarkable properties that allow for a continuous cycle of shedding, healing, and cell regeneration.

As the outer covering of the body, the skin may demonstrate outwardly what occurs inside the body. A number of systemic diseases are manifested by skin disorders (*e.g.*, malar rash associated with systemic lupus erythematosus, bronze skin with Addison disease, and jaundice with liver disease). Thus, it is important to recognize that although skin eruptions are frequently caused by primary disorders of the skin, they may also represent manifestations of systemic disease.

Structure and Function of the Skin

Skin Structures

There are great variations in skin structure on different parts of the body. Therefore, "normal skin" on any one surface of the body is difficult to describe. Variations are found in the properties of the skin, such as the thickness of skin layers, the distribution of sweat glands, and the number and size of hair follicles. For example, the epidermis is thicker on the palms of the hands and soles of the feet than it is elsewhere on the body. The dermis, on the other hand, is thickest on the back, whereas the subcutaneous fat layer is thickest on the abdomen and buttocks. Hair follicles are densely distributed on the scalp, axillae, and genitalia, but they are sparse on the inner arms and abdomen. The apocrine sweat glands are confined to the axillae and the anogenital area. Nevertheless, certain structural properties are common to the skin on all areas of the body.

The skin is composed of the following three layers:

1. Epidermis (outer layer)
2. Dermis (inner layer)
3. Subcutaneous fat layer

The basement membrane divides the first two layers. The subcutaneous tissue, a layer of loose connective and adipose connective tissues, binds the dermis to the underlying tissues of the body (Fig. 51-1).

> **KEY POINTS**
>
> ### Organization of Skin Structures
>
> - The epidermis, which is avascular, is composed of four to five layers of stratified squamous keratinized epithelial cells that are formed in the deepest layer of the epidermis and migrate to the skin surface to replace cells that are lost during normal skin shedding.

> - The basement membrane is a thin adhesive layer that cements the epidermis to the dermis.
>
> - The dermis is a connective tissue layer that separates the epidermis from the underlying subcutaneous fat layer. It contains the blood vessels and nerve fibers that supply the epidermis.

Epidermis

The functions of the skin depend on the properties of its outermost layer, the epidermis. The epidermis covers the body. It is specialized to form the various skin appendages, which include the hair, nails, and glandular structures.[2] The keratinocytes of the epidermis produce a fibrous protein called *keratin*, which is essential for the protective function of the skin. The epidermis also has three other types of cells that arise from its basal layer—melanocytes, Merkel cells, and Langerhans cells. Melanocytes produce a pigment called *melanin*, which is responsible for skin color, tanning, and protection against ultraviolet radiation. Merkel cells provide sensory information and Langerhans cells link the

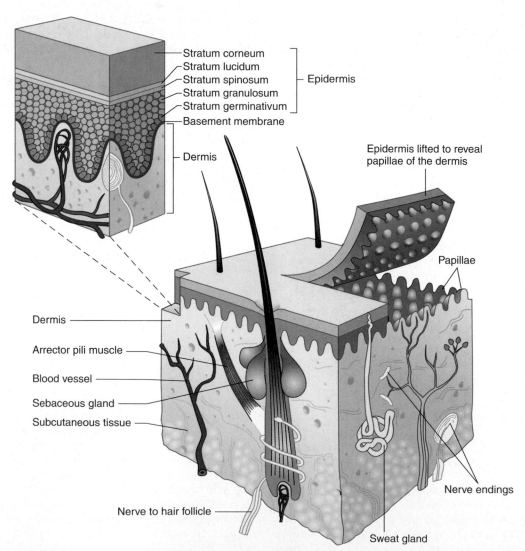

FIGURE 51-1. Three-dimensional view of the skin.

epidermis to the immune system. The epidermis contains openings for two types of glands—sweat glands, which produce watery secretions, and sebaceous glands, which produce an oily secretion called *sebum*.

Keratinocytes

The *keratinocyte* is the major cell of the epidermis, comprising approximately 85% of the cells of this layer. The epidermis is composed of stratified squamous keratinized epithelium, which, when viewed under the microscope, is seen to consist of five distinct layers, or strata, that represent a progressive differentiation or maturation of the keratinocytes:

1. Stratum germinativum or stratum basale
2. Stratum spinosum
3. Stratum granulosum
4. Stratum lucidum
5. Stratum corneum

The deepest layer, the *stratum germinativum* or *stratum basale*, consists of a single layer of basal cells that are attached to the basal lamina. The basal cells, which are columnar, undergo mitosis to produce new keratinocytes that move toward the skin surface to replace cells lost during normal skin shedding.

The next layer, the *stratum spinosum*, is formed as a result of the cell division in the stratum basale. The stratum spinosum is two to four layers thick, and its cells become differentiated as they migrate toward the surface of the epidermis. Because they develop a spiny appearance where their cell borders interconnect, the cells of this layer are commonly referred to as *prickle cells*.[1]

The *stratum granulosum* is only a few cells thick (thickness varies between one and three cells).[1] It consists of granular cells that are the most differentiated cells of the living skin. The cells in this layer are unique in that two opposing functions occur simultaneously. Although some cells lose cytoplasm and nuclear structures, others continue to synthesize keratin. Keratinocytes in this layer secrete lamellar bodies into the next layer of the epidermis, the stratum lucidum, providing the skin with its important water-impermeable properties.

The *stratum lucidum*, which lies just superficial to the stratum granulosum, is a thin, transparent layer found primarily on the thick skin such as over the palms of the hands and soles of the feet.[1] It consists of transitional cells that retain some of the functions of living skin cells from the layers below and provide a barrier to water.

The most superficial layer, the *stratum corneum*, consists of dead, keratinized cells, which shed intermittently. This layer contains the most cell layers and the largest cells of the epidermis. This layer blocks microbes from entering the skin and prevents dehydration of tissues.

The keratinocytes that originate in the basal layer change morphologically as they are pushed toward the outer layer of the epidermis. In the basal layer, keratinocytes are cuboidal to low columnar. As it is pushed into the stratum spinosum, the keratinocyte becomes multisided. It becomes flatter in the granular layer and is flattened and elongated in the stratum corneum (Fig. 51-2). Keratinocytes also change cytoplasmic structure and composition as they are pushed toward the surface of the epidermis. This transformation from viable cells to the dead cells of

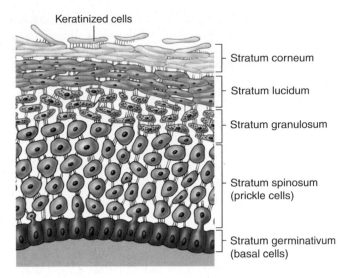

FIGURE 51-2. Epidermal cells. The basal cells undergo mitosis, producing keratinocytes that change their size and shape as they move upward, replacing cells that are lost during normal cell shedding.

the stratum corneum is called *keratinization*. The migration time of a keratinocyte from the basal layer to the stratum corneum is 20 to 30 days. The rate of production of new keratinocytes needs to be consistent with the rate of shedding old keratinocytes. When these rates are not in balance, skin anomalies occur.

Keratinocytes are connected by minute points of attachment called **desmosomes.** They are terminal end points on the cell walls of keratinocytes, made up of fibrous material that is bound into bundles, called *tonofilaments*. Desmosomes keep the cells from detaching and provide some structure to the skin while it is in perpetual motion. The basal layer provides the underlying structure and stability for the epidermis.

Besides desmosomes, there are three other types of cellular junctions that bind keratinocytes—adherens junctions, gap junctions, and tight junctions. *Adherens junctions* are specialized structures that provide strong mechanical connections between cells. They are responsible for adhesion between cells, communicate about the presence of neighboring cells, and anchor the skin cells. *Gap junctions* are cylindrical channels that permit ions and small molecules to pass between cells. They are composed of proteins called *connexins*. *Tight junctions* are made of transmembrane proteins that function to prevent substances passing between cells.

Keratinocytes are active secretory cells that play an important role in the immunobiology of the skin by communicating and regulating cells of the immune response and secreting cytokines and inflammatory mediators.

Melanocytes

Melanocytes are pigment-synthesizing cells that are scattered in the basal layer and are responsible for skin color.[1,3] They function to produce pigment granules called *melanin*, the substance that gives the skin its color. There are two major forms of melanin—*eumelanin* and *pheomelanin*. The two forms of eumelanin are brown and black; pheomelanin is yellow to red. The type of melanin produced depends on the stimulation of specific hormones or proteins and the binding of these substances to receptors on the melanocyte. Eumelanin is the most abundant in humans. Exposure to the sun's ultraviolet rays increases the production of eumelanin, causing tanning to occur. The primary function of such melanin is to protect the skin by absorbing and scattering harmful ultraviolet rays, which are associated with skin cancers. Localized concentrations of eumelanin are also responsible for the formation of freckles and moles.

Pheomelanin, the yellow to red pigment, is found in all humans. It is particularly concentrated in the lips, nipples, glans penis, and vagina. Besides the skin, it is found in the hair, particularly red hair. The ability to synthesize melanin depends on the ability of the melanocytes to produce an enzyme called *tyrosinase*, which converts the amino acid tyrosine to a precursor of melanin. A genetic lack of this enzyme results in a clinical condition called *albinism*, or lack of pigmentation in the skin, hair, and the iris of the eye. Tyrosinase is synthesized in the rough endoplasmic reticulum of the melanocytes and then routed to membranous vesicles in the Golgi complex called *melanosomes*. Melanin is subsequently synthesized in the melanosomes. Melanocytes have long, cytoplasm-filled dendritic processes that contain accumulated melanosomes and extend between the keratinocytes. Although the melanocytes remain in the basal layer, the melanosomes are transferred to the keratinocytes through their dendritic processes. The dendrite tip containing the melanosome is engulfed by a nearby keratinocyte, and the melanin is transferred (Fig. 51-3).

The amount of melanin in the keratinocytes determines a person's skin color.[3] Dark-skinned and light-skinned people have approximately the same number of melanocytes, but the production and packaging of pigment are different. In dark-skinned people, *larger* melanin-containing melanosomes are produced and transferred individually to the keratinocyte. In light-skinned people, *smaller* melanosomes are produced and then packaged together in a membrane before being transferred to the keratinocyte. All people, regardless of skin color, have relatively few or no melanocytes in the epidermis of the palms of the hands or the soles of the feet. In light-skinned people, the number of melanocytes decreases with age, and the skin becomes lighter and is more susceptible to skin cancer when exposed to ultraviolet light. However, people with vitiligo, a skin problem where the melanocytes are destroyed, have a significantly reduced risk of developing nonmelanoma skin cancers, whereas people with albinism have a significantly increased risk.[4]

Merkel Cells

Merkel cells are clear cells found in the stratum basale of the epidermis. They are connected to other skin cells by desmosomes. Each Merkel cell is connected to an afferent nerve terminal, forming a structure known as a *Merkel disk*. They are the sparsest cells of the epidermis and are found over the entire body, but are most plentiful in the basal layer of the fingers, toes, lips, and oral cavity, and in the outermost sheath of hair follicles (*i.e.*, the touch areas). All functions of Merkel cells are unclear, but they serve as sensory touch receptors and are believed to be neuroendocrine cells (*i.e.*, they release hormones into the blood in response to neural stimuli).[1]

Langerhans Cells

Langerhans cells are scattered in the suprabasal layers of the epidermis among the keratinocytes. They are less numerous (3% to 5% of epidermal cells) than are the keratinocytes. They are derived from precursor cells originating in the bone marrow and continuously repopulate the epidermis. Like melanocytes, they have a dendritic shape and clear cytoplasm. *Birbeck granules* that often resemble tennis racquets are their most distinguishing characteristic microscopically.[1]

Langerhans cells are the immunologic cells responsible for recognizing foreign antigens harmful to the body (Fig. 51-4). As such, Langerhans cells play an important role in defending the body against foreign antigens. Langerhans cells bind antigen to their surface and process it, and, bearing the processed antigen, migrate from the epidermis into lymphatic vessels and then into regional lymph nodes, where they are known as *dendritic cells*. During their migration in the lymph system, the Langerhans cells become potent antigen-presenting cells.[1] Langerhans cells are innervated by sympathetic nerve fibers, which may explain why the skin's immune system is altered under stress. An example of this is the exacerbations of acne seen in people under stress. Langerhans cells and the keratinocytes produce a number of cytokines that stimulate maturation of skin-localizing T lymphocytes.

Basement Membrane

The terms *basement membrane* and *basal lamina* are often used interchangeably. Technically, however, the basal lamina is a component of the basement membrane. The basement membrane is a layer of intercellular and extracellular matrices that serves as an interface between the dermis and the epidermis (Fig. 51-5). It separates the epithelium from the underlying connective

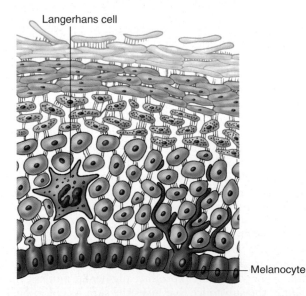

FIGURE 51-3. The melanocytes, which are located in the basal layer of the skin, produce melanin pigment granules that give the skin its color. The melanocytes have threadlike, cytoplasm-filled extensions that are used in passing the pigment granules to the keratinocytes.

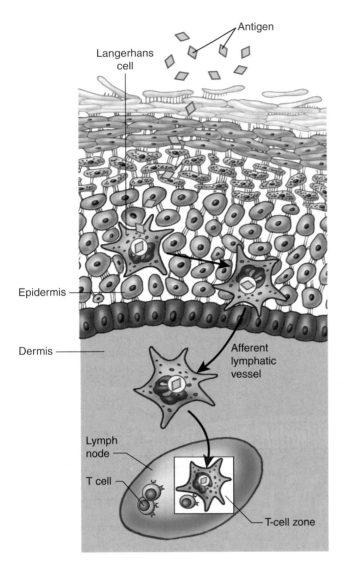

FIGURE 51-4. Langerhans cells.

that insert into the lamina densa and the superficial dermis, where they are known as *anchoring fibrils*. Type VII collagen, another adherent substance, has been found in the anchoring fibrils and plaques. Another component of the lamina fibroreticularis are elastic fiber bundles that extend to the dermis.[2]

Hemidesmosomes are like half desmosomes in both structure and function. They lie immediately at the basal plasma membrane and form the site or source of tonofilaments, which attach the dermis and epidermis (see Fig. 51-5).[2] Because they form a continuous link between the intracellular keratin filament network and the extracellular basement membrane, they are also involved in relaying signals between the skin layers.

Dermis

The dermis is the connective tissue layer that separates the epidermis from the subcutaneous fat layer (see Fig. 51-1). It supports the epidermis and serves as its primary source of nutrition. The two layers of the dermis, the papillary dermis and the reticular dermis, are composed of cells, fibers, ground substances, nerves, and blood vessels. The main component of the dermis is collagen, a group of fibrous proteins. The collagen is enmeshed in a ground substance called *hyaluronic acid*.[2] Collagen fibers are loosely arranged in the papillary dermis, but are tightly bundled in the reticular dermis.

The pilar (hair) and glandular structures are embedded in this layer and continue through the epidermis. In general, a dark dermis is more compact than is a white dermis, and consequently darker skinned people show less wrinkling.

Papillary Dermis

The *papillary dermis* (pars papillaris) is a thin, superficial layer that lies adjacent to the epidermis. It consists of collagen fibers and ground substance. This layer is densely covered with conical projections called *dermal papillae* (see Fig. 51-1). The basal cells of the epidermis project into the papillary dermis, forming *rete ridges*. Microscopically, the junction between the epidermis and the dermis appears like undulating ridges and valleys. It is believed that the dense structure of the dermal papillae serves to minimize the separation of the dermis and the epidermis. Dermal papillae contain capillaries, end arterioles, and venules that nourish the epidermal layers of the skin. This layer of the dermis is richly vascularized. Lymph vessels and nerve tissue also are found in this layer.

Reticular Dermis

The *reticular dermis* (pars reticularis) is the thicker area of the dermis and forms the bulk of the dermal layer. The reticular dermis is characterized by a complex meshwork of three-dimensional collagen bundles interconnected with large elastic fibers and ground substance, a viscid gel that is rich in mucopolysaccharides. The collagen fibers are oriented parallel to the body's surface in any given area. Collagen bundles may be organized lengthwise, as on the abdomen, or in round clusters, as on the heel. The direction of surgical incisions is often determined by this organizational pattern.

tissue, it anchors the epithelium to the loose connective tissue underneath, and it serves as a selective filter for molecules moving between the two layers. It is also a major site of immunoglobulin and complement deposition in skin disease. The basement membrane is involved in skin disorders that cause bullae or blister formation.[1]

The basement membrane consists of three distinct zones or layers—lamina lucida, lamina densa, and lamina fibroreticularis—all of which contribute to the adhesion of the two skin layers. The *lamina lucida* is an electron-lucent layer where adherence proteins are located. It consists of fine anchoring filaments and a cell adhesion glycoprotein, called *laminin*, which plays a role in the organization of the macromolecules in the basement membrane zone and promotes attachment of cells to the extracellular matrix. The *lamina densa* contains an adhesive called *type IV collagen* as well as laminin. It is important in dermal–epidermal attachment. Combined, the lamina lucida and the lamina densa comprise what is known as the *basal lamina*. The *lamina fibroreticularis* then completes the basement membrane. This layer contains many anchoring microfibrils. These are short, curved structures

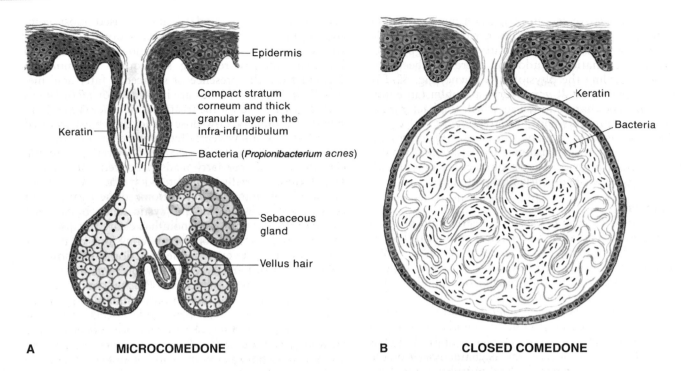

A   **MICROCOMEDONE**   B   **CLOSED COMEDONE**

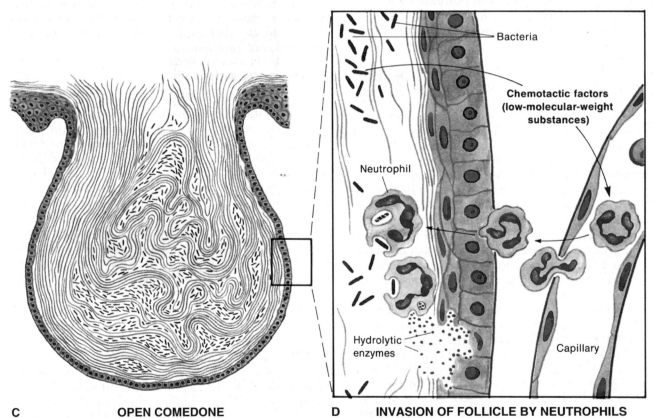

C   **OPEN COMEDONE**   D   **INVASION OF FOLLICLE BY NEUTROPHILS**

FIGURE 52-12. Acne vulgaris. The pathogenesis of follicular distension, rupture, and inflammation is illustrated. Microcomedones (**A**) and closed (**B**) and open (**C**) comedones form. Excessive sebum can be secreted, and the *Propionibacterium acnes* proliferates. Neutrophilic enzymes are released, and the comedone ruptures causing a cycle of intense inflammation (**D and E**). (From Strayer D., Rubin R. (2015). *Rubin's pathology: Clinicopathologic foundations of medicine* (7th ed., p. 1250). Philadelphia, PA: Wolters Kluwer.)

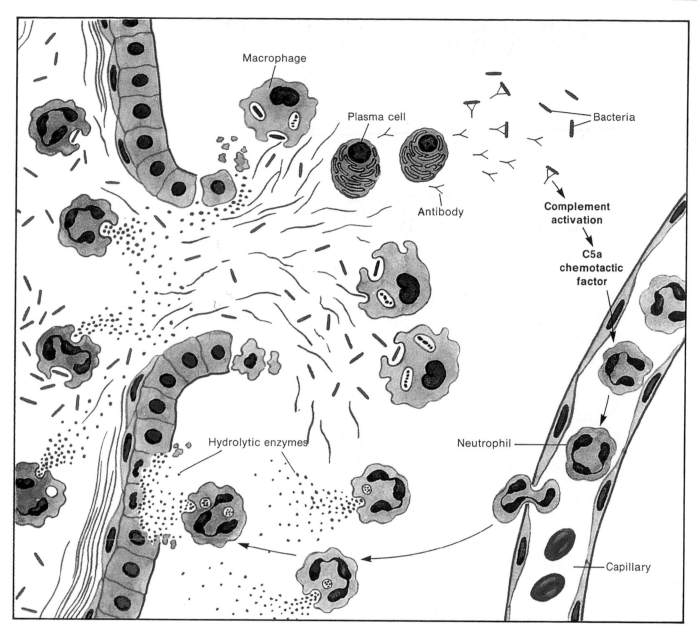

E   **INFLAMMATION AND RUPTURE OF SEBACEOUS FOLLICLE**

FIGURE 52-12. (*Continued*)

by gastrointestinal symptoms. *Helicobacter pylori* infection has been implicated as a possible cause, with studies showing an improvement in rosacea after eradication of *H. pylori*.[26] Other causes suggested have been genetic, environmental, and vascular.

Types and Clinical Manifestations

Rosacea is classified into four types:

1. Erythematotelangiectatic (flushing and persistent central facial erythema)
2. Papulopustular (inflammatory)
3. Phymatous (thickening of the skin with irregular surface nodularities and enlargement)
4. Ocular (involving the eyes)[26]

In the early stage of rosacea development, there are repeated episodes of blushing. The blush eventually becomes a permanent dark red erythema on the nose and cheeks that sometimes extends to the forehead and chin. This stage often occurs before 20 years of age. Ocular problems occur in at least 50% of people with rosacea, which may lead to visual losses.[26-29] Prominent symptoms include eyes that are itchy, burning, or dry; a gritty

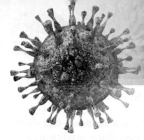

Appendix

Lab Values

TABLE A-1 Prefixes Denoting Decimal Factors

Prefix	Symbol	Factor	Prefix	Symbol	Factor
deka	da	10^{1}	deci	d	10^{-1}
hecto	h	10^{2}	centi	c	10^{-2}
kilo	k	10^{3}	milli	m	10^{-3}
mega	M	10^{6}	micro	μ	10^{-6}
giga	G	10^{9}	nano	n	10^{-9}
tera	T	10^{12}	pico	p	10^{-12}
peta	P	10^{15}	femto	f	10^{-15}
exa	E	10^{18}	atto	a	10^{-18}
zetta	Z	10^{21}	zepto	z	10^{-21}
yotta	Y	10^{24}	yocto	y	10^{-24}

TABLE A-2 Hematology

Test	Conventional Units	SI Units
Erythrocyte count (RBC count)	Male: $4.2–5.4 \times 10^{6}/mm^{3}$	Male: $4.2–5.4 \times 10^{12}/L$
	Female: $3.6–5.0 \times 10^{6}/mm^{3}$	Female: $3.6–5.0 \times 10^{12}/L$
Hematocrit (Hct)	Male: 42%–52%	Male: 0.42–0.52
	Female: 36%–48%	Female: 0.36–0.48
Hemoglobin (Hb)	Male: 14.0–17.4 g/dL	Male: 140–174 g/L
	Female: 12.0–16.0 g/dL	Female: 120–160 g/L
Mean corpuscular hemoglobin (MCH)	26–34 pg/cell	0.40–0.53 fmol/cell
Mean corpuscular hemoglobin concentration (MCHC)	32–36 g/dL or 4.9–5.5 mmol/L	
Mean corpuscular volume (MCV)	82–98 mm^{3} or 82–98 fL/cell	
Reticulocyte count	0.5%–1.5% total RBC (women may be slightly higher)	
Platelet count	$140–400 \times 10^{3}/\mu L$	$140–400 \times 10^{9}/L$
Leukocyte count (WBC count)	$4.5–10.5 \times 10^{3}$ cells/mm^{3} or $4.5–10.5 \times 10^{9}/L$	4500–10,500 cells/mm^{3}
	Black adults: $3.2–10.0 \times 10^{3}$ or $\times 10^{9}$	3200–10,000 cells/mm^{3}
Basophils	15–50/mm^{3}	$0.02–0.05 \times 10^{9}/L$
	Differential: 0%–1.0% of total WBC	
Eosinophils	Differential: 0%–3% of total WBC	$0.07 \times 10^{9}/L$
Lymphocytes	24%–40% of total leukocytes count or 1500–4000 cells/mm^{3}	$1.5–4.0 \times 10^{9}/L$
Monocytes	100–500 mm^{3}	0.03–0.07 of total WBC count
	Differential: 3%–7% of total WBC	
Neutrophils (segmented [Segs])	3000–7000/mm^{3}	$3–7 \times 10^{9}/L$
Polymorphonuclear neutrophils (PMN)	Differential: 50% of total of WBC	Black adults: $1.2–6.6 \times 10^{9}/L^{*}$
Neutrophils (bands)	0%–3% of total PMN	

Ethnic difference occurs for neutrophils only.

TABLE A-3 Blood Chemistry*

Test	Conventional Units	SI Units
Alanine aminotransferase (ALT)	Males: 10–40 U/L	Males: 0.17–0.68 µkat/L
	Females: 7–35 U/L	Females: 0.12–0.60 µkat/L
Albumin	3.9–5.0 g/dL	39–50 g/L
Alkaline phosphatase	52–142 U/L[†,‡]	
Ammonia	15–60 µg/dL	11–35 µmol/L
Amylase	25–125 units/L[†]	0.4–2.1 µkat/L[†]
Arterial blood gas	pH 7.35–7.45	
	$PaCO_2$ 35–45 mm Hg	
	PaO_2 > 80 mm Hg	
	Base excess > 2 mEq/L	
	Base deficit < –2 mEq/L	
	HCO_3 22–26 mEq/L	
Aspartase aminotransferase (AST)	Males: 14–20 U/L	Males: 0.23–0.33 µkat/L[†]
	Females: 10–36 U/L[†]	Females: 0.17–0.60 µkat/L[†]
Bilirubin (total)	0.3–1.0 mg/dL	5–17 µmol/L
Bilirubin (direct or conjugated)	0.0–0.2 mg/dL	0.0–3.4 µmol/L
Blood urea nitrogen (BUN)	6–20 mg/dL	2.1–7.1 mmol/L
Calcium (Ca^{2+}) (total)	8.8–10.4 mg/dL	2.20–2.60 mmol/L
Chloride	96–106 mEq/L	96–106 mmol/L
Creatine kinase (CK, CPK)	Males: 38–174 units/L[†]	Males: 0.63–2.90 µkat/L[†]
	Females: 26–140 U/L	Females: 0.46–2.38
Creatine kinase isoenzymes:		
MB (CK_2)	0%–6%	0.00–0.06
MM (CK_3)	96% or 100%	0.96–1.0
BB (CK_1)	0%	0.00
Creatinine (serum)	Males: 0.6–1.2	Males: 71–106 µmol/L
	Females: 0.4–1.0 mg/dL[‡]	Females: 39–90 µmol/L[‡]
Gamma-glutamyl-transpeptidase (GGT)	Males: 7–47 U/L	Males: 0.12–1.80 µkat/L[†]
	Females: 5–25 U/L	Females: 0.08–0.42 µkat/L
Glucose (plasma, fasting)	<100 mg/dL	<5.6 mmol/L
Glycosylated hemoglobin (HbA_{1c})	5.0%–7.0%	5.5–9.3 mmol/L
Lactate dehydrogenase (LDH)	140–280 U/L	2.34–4.68 µkat/L[†]
Lipids		
Cholesterol (fasting)	140–199 mg/dL (desirable)	3.63–5.15 mmol/L (optimal)
	200–239 mg/dL (borderline high)	5.18–6.19 mmol/L (borderline)
	≥240 mg/dL (high)	>6.20 mmol/L (high)
LDL cholesterol	<100 mg/dL (optimal)	<2.6 mmol/L
	100–129 mg/dL (near optimal)	2.6–3.3 mmol/L
	130–159 mg/dL (borderline high)	3.4–4.1 mmol/L
	160–189 mg/dL (high)	4.2–4.9 mmol/L
	>190 mg/dL	>5.0 mmol/L
HDL cholesterol	Male: 35–65 mg/dL	Male: 0. 91–1.68 mmol/L
	Female: 35–80 mg/dL	Female: 0.91–2.07 mmol/L
Triglycerides	<150 mg/dL (desirable)	<1.70 mmol/L (desirable)
	150–199 mg/dL (borderline high)	1.70–2.25 mmol/L
	200–499 mg/dL	2.26–5.64 mmol/L
	≥500 mg/d:	≥5.65 mmol/L
Lipase	10–140 U/L[†]	0.17–2.3 µkat/L[†]
Magnesium	1.8–2.6 mg/dL	0.74–1.07 mmol/L
Osmolality (24-hour urine specimen)	300–900 mOsm/kg H_2O	
Osmolality (serum)	280–303 mOsm/kg H_2O	
Phosphorus (inorganic)	2.7–4.5 mg/dL	0.87–1.45 mmol/L
Potassium	3.5–5.2 mEq/L	3.5–5.2 mmol/L
Prostate-specific antigen (PSA)	<2.5 ng/mL	<2.5 µg/L
Protein total	6.0–8.0 g/dL	60–80 g/L
Immunoglobulin		
IgG	700–1500 mg/dL	7.0–15.0 g/L
IgA	60–400 mg/dL	600–4000 mg/dL
IgM	60–300 mg/d:	600–3000 mg/dL
IgE	3–423 IU/mL	3–423 kIU/L

(*continued*)

TABLE A-3 Blood Chemistry* (*continued*)

Test	Conventional Units	SI Units
Thyroid tests		
Thyroxine (T_4) total	5.4–11.5 µg/dL	57–148 nmol/L
Thyroxine, free (FT_4)	0.7–2.0 ng/dL	10–26 pmol/L[†]
Triiodothyronine (T_3) total	80–200 ng/dL	1.2–3.1 nmol/L
Thyroid stimulating hormone (TSH)	0.45–4.5 µU/mL	0.45–4.5 mU/L
Thyroglobin	2–55 ng/mL	2–55 µg/L
Sodium	136–145 mEq/L	136–145 mmol/L
Uric acid	Male: 3.4–7.0 mg/dL	Male: 202–416 µmol/L
	Female: 2.4–6.0 mg/dL	Female: 143–357 µmol/L

*Values provided are for adults unless otherwise specified. Values may vary with laboratory. The values supplied by the laboratory performing the test should always be used since the ranges may be method specific.

[†]Laboratory and/or method specific.

[‡]Varies with pregnancy, puberty, age, and muscle mass.

Values obtained from Fischbach F. T., Fischbach, M. A. (2018). *Fischbach's manual of laboratory and diagnostic tests* (10th ed.). Philadelphia, PA: Lippincott Williams & Wilkins.

Glossary

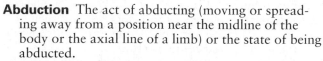

Abduction The act of abducting (moving or spreading away from a position near the midline of the body or the axial line of a limb) or the state of being abducted.

Abrasion The wearing or scraping away of a substance or structure, such as the skin, through an unusual or abnormal mechanical process.

Abscess A collection of pus that is restricted to a specific area in tissues, organs, or confined spaces.

Accommodation The adjustment of the lens (eye) to variations in distance.

Acromion The lateral extension of the spine of the scapula, forming the highest point of the shoulder. (Adjective: acromial)

Active transport The movement of molecules from an area of lower concentration to higher concentration (opposite of diffusion).

Acuity The clearness or sharpness of perception, especially of vision.

Adaptation The adjustment of an organism to its environment, physical or psychological, through changes and responses to stress of any kind.

Adduction The act of adducting (moving or drawing toward a position near the midline of the body or the axial line of a limb) or the state of being adducted.

Adenylyl cyclase An enzyme that converts AMP from ATP.

Adhesin The molecular components of the bacterial cell wall that are involved in adhesion processes.

Adrenarche Beginning of augmented adrenal androgen production.

Adrenergic Activated by or characteristic of the sympathetic nervous system or its neurotransmitters (*i.e.*, epinephrine and norepinephrine).

Aerobic Growing, living, or occurring only in the presence of air or oxygen.

Afferent Bearing or conducting inward or toward a center, as an afferent neuron.

Agenesis Failure of an organ to develop at all.

Agglutination The clumping together of particles, microorganisms, or blood cells in response to an antigen–antibody reaction.

Agonist A muscle whose action is opposed by another muscle (antagonist) with which it is paired, or a drug or other chemical substance that has affinity for or stimulates a predictable physiologic function.

Akinesia An abnormal state in which there is an absence or poverty of movement.

Allele One of two or more different forms of a gene that can occupy a particular locus on a chromosome.

Alveolus A small saclike structure, as in the alveolus of the lung.

Amblyopia A condition of vision impairment without a detectable organic lesion of the eye.

Amine An organic compound containing nitrogen.

Amorphous Without a definite form; shapeless.

Amphoteric Capable of reacting chemically as an acid or a base.

Ampulla A saclike dilatation of a duct, canal, or any other tubular structure.

Anabolism A constructive metabolic process characterized by the conversion of simple substances into larger, complex molecules.

Anaerobic Growing, living, or occurring only in the absence of air or oxygen.

Analog A part, organ, or chemical having the same function or appearance but differing in respect to a certain component, such as origin or development.

Anaplasia A change in the structure of cells and in their orientation to each other that is characterized by a loss of cell differentiation, as in cancerous cell growth.

Anastomose The joining of normally separate parts, which occurs during embryonic development.

Anastomosis The connection or joining between two vessels; or an opening created by surgical, traumatic, or pathologic means.

Androgen Any substance, such as a male sex hormone, that increases male characteristics.

Anergy A state of absent or diminished reaction to an antigen or group of antigens.

Aneuploidy A variation in the number of chromosomes within a cell involving one or more missing chromosomes rather than entire sets.

Aneurysm An outpouching or dilation in the wall of a blood vessel or the heart.

Angiogenesis The growth of new blood vessels; in cancer new blood vessels are needed to allow tumors to grow.

Ankylosis Stiffness or fixation of separate bones of a joint, resulting from disease, injury, or surgical procedure. (Verb: ankylose)

Anoikis Programed cell death that occurs when anchorage-dependent cells detach from cell or extracellular matrix.

Anorexia Lack or loss of appetite for food. (Adjective: anorexic)

Anoxia An abnormal condition characterized by the total lack of oxygen.

Antagonist A muscle whose action directly opposes that of another muscle (agonist) with which it is paired, or a drug or other chemical substance that can diminish or nullify the action of a neuromediator or body function.

Anterior Pertaining to a surface or part that is situated near or toward the front.

Antigen A substance that generates an immune response by causing the formation of an antibody or reacting with antibodies or T-cell receptors.

Antiport Movement of two different molecules across a membrane by a common carrier.

Apex The uppermost point, the narrowed or pointed end, or the highest point of a structure, such as an organ.

Aphagia A condition characterized by the refusal or the loss of ability to swallow.

Aplasia The absence of an organ or tissue due to a developmental failure.

Apnea The absence of spontaneous respiration.

Apoptosis A mechanism of programmed cell death, marked by shrinkage of the cell, condensation of chromatin, formation of cytoplasmic blebs, and fragmentation of the cell into membrane-bound bodies eliminated by phagocytosis.

Apraxia Loss of the ability to carry out familiar, purposeful acts or to manipulate objects in the absence of paralysis or other motor or sensory impairment.

Aquaporins A water channel that forms pores in membranes of cells allowing water to pass.

Articulation The place of connection or junction between two or more bones of a skeletal joint.

Ascites An abnormal accumulation of serous fluid in the peritoneal cavity.

Asepsis The condition of being free or freed from pathogenic microorganisms.

Astereognosis A neurologic disorder characterized by an inability to identify objects by touch.

Asterixis A motor disturbance characterized by a hand-flapping tremor, which results when the prolonged contraction of groups of muscles lapses intermittently.

Ataxia An abnormal condition characterized by an inability to coordinate voluntary muscular movement.

Athetosis A neuromuscular condition characterized by the continuous occurrence of slow, sinuous, writhing movements that are performed involuntarily. (Adjective: athetoid)

Atopy Genetic predisposition toward the development of a hypersensitivity or an allergic reaction to common environmental allergens.

Atresia The absence or closure of a normal body orifice or tubular organ, such as the esophagus.

Atrophy A wasting or diminution of size, often accompanied by a decrease in function, of a cell, tissue, or organ.

Autocrine A mode of hormone action in which a chemical messenger acts on the same cell that secretes it.

Autophagy Segregation of part of the cell's own damaged cytoplasmic material within a vacuole and its disposal.

Autosome Any chromosome other than a sex chromosome.

Avascular The lack of blood vessels.

Axillary Of or pertaining to the axilla, or armpit.

Bacteremia The presence of bacteria in the blood.

Bactericide An agent that destroys bacteria. (Adjective: bactericidal)

Bacteriostat An agent that inhibits bacterial growth. (Adjective: bacteriostatic)

Ballismus An abnormal condition characterized by violent flailing motions of the arms and, occasionally, the head, resulting from injury to or destruction of the subthalamic nucleus or its fiber connections.

Baroreceptor A type of sensory nerve ending such as those found in the aorta and the carotid sinus that is stimulated by changes in pressure.

Basal Pertaining to, situated at, or forming the base, or the fundamental or the basic.

Basal lamina The basement membrane.

Basement membrane Keeps the epithelium in place and separates the epithelial cells from the underlying tissue.

Benign Not malignant or of the character that does not threaten health or life.

Bipolar neuron A nerve cell that has a process at each end—an afferent process and an efferent process.

Bolus A rounded mass of food ready to swallow or such a mass passing through the gastrointestinal tract, or a concentrated mass of medicinal material or other pharmaceutical preparation injected all at once intravenously for diagnostic purposes.

Borborygmus The rumbling, gurgling, or tinkling noise produced by the propulsion of gas through the intestine.

Bronchiectasis Damage to the bronchial tubes due to inflammation.

Bruit A sound or murmur heard while auscultating an organ or blood vessel, especially an abnormal one.

Buccal Pertaining to or directed toward the inside of the cheek.

Buffer A substance or group of substances that prevents change in the concentration of another chemical substance.

Bulla A thin-walled blister of the skin or mucous membranes greater than 5 mm in diameter containing serous or seropurulent fluid.

Bursa A fluid-filled sac or saclike cavity situated in places in the tissues at which friction would otherwise develop, such as between certain tendons and the bones beneath them.

Cachexia A condition of general ill health and malnutrition, marked by weakness and emaciation.

Calculus A stony mass formed within body tissues, usually composed of mineral salts.

Capsid The protein shell that envelops and protects the nucleic acid of a virus.

Carcinogen Any substance or agent that causes the development or increases the incidence of cancer.

Carpal Of or pertaining to the carpus, or wrist.

Caseation A form of tissue necrosis in which the tissue is changed into a dry, amorphous mass resembling crumbly cheese.

Caspase pathway Involved in apoptosis or programmed cell death.

Catabolism A metabolic process through which living organisms break down complex substances to simple compounds, liberating energy for use in work, energy storage, or heat production.

Catalyst A substance that increases the velocity of a chemical reaction without being consumed by the process.

Catecholamines Any one of a group of biogenic amines having a sympathomimetic action and composed of a catechol molecule and the aliphatic portion of an amine.

Caudal Signifying an inferior position, toward the distal end of the spine.

Cell The smallest basic unit of any living organism surrounded by a membrane, which contains a nucleus and cytoplasm.

Cell cycle The stages that cells undergo to divide and produce new cells.

Cell differentiation The process by which cells become specialized.

Cellular respiration Metabolic reactions that take place in cells to generate energy by converting biochemical energy into adenosine triphosphate (ATP).

Cellulitis An acute, diffuse, spreading, edematous inflammation of the deep subcutaneous tissues and sometimes muscle, characterized most commonly by an area of heat, redness, pain, and swelling, and occasionally by fever, malaise, chills, and headache.

Cephalic Of or pertaining to the head, or to the head end of the body.

Cerumen The waxlike secretion produced by vestigial apocrine sweat glands in the external ear canal.

Channelopathies Diseases due to a malfunction of an ion channel.

Cheilosis A noninflammatory disorder of the lips and mouth characterized by chapping and fissuring.

Chelate A chemical compound composed of a central metal ion and an organic molecule with multiple bonds, arranged in ring formation, used especially in treatment of metal poisoning.

Chemoreceptor A sensory nerve cell activated by chemical stimuli, as a chemoreceptor in the carotid artery that is sensitive to changes in the oxygen content in the blood and reflexly increases or decreases respiration and blood pressure.

Chemotaxis A response involving cell orientation or cell movement that is either toward (positive chemotaxis) or away from (negative chemotaxis) a chemical stimulus.

Chimeric Relating to, derived from, or being an individual possessing one's own immunologic characteristics and that of another individual; a phenomenon that can occur as the result of procedures such as a bone marrow graft.

Chondrocyte Any one of the mature polymorphic cells that form the cartilage of the body.

Chromatid One of the paired threadlike chromosome filaments, joined at the centromere, that makes up a metaphase chromosome.

Chromosome Any one of the structures in the nucleus of a cell containing a linear thread of DNA, which functions in the transmission of genetic information.

Chyme The creamy, viscous, semifluid material produced during digestion of a meal that is expelled by the stomach into the duodenum.

Cilia A minute, hairlike process projecting from a cell, composed of nine microtubules arrayed around a single pair. Cilia beat rhythmically to move the cell around in its environment, or they move mucus or fluids over the surface.

Circadian Being, having, pertaining to, or occurring in a period or cycle of approximately 24 hours.

Circumduction The active or passive circular movement of a limb or of the eye.

Cisterna An enclosed space, such as a cavity, that serves as a reservoir for lymph or other body fluids.

Clone One or a group of genetically identical cells or organisms derived from a single parent.

Coagulation The process of transforming a liquid into a semisolid mass, especially of blood clot formation.

Coarctation A condition of stricture or contraction of the walls of a vessel.

Cofactor A substance that must unite with another substance in order to function.

Colic Sharp, intermittent abdominal pain localized in a hollow or tubular organ, resulting from torsion, obstruction, or smooth muscle spasm. (Adjective: colicky)

Collagen The protein substance of the white, glistening, inelastic fibers of the skin, tendons, bone, cartilage, and all other connective tissue.

Collateral Secondary or accessory rather than direct or immediate, or a small branch, as of a blood vessel or nerve.

Columnar cells Tall thin epithelial cells.

Complement Any one of the complex, enzymatic serum proteins that are involved in physiologic reactions, including antigen–antibody reaction and anaphylaxis.

Confluent Flowing or coming together, not discrete.

Congenital Present at, and usually before, birth.

Conjugate To pair and fuse in conjugation, or a form of sexual reproduction seen in unicellular organisms in which genetic material is exchanged during the temporary fusion of two cells.

Contiguous In contact or nearly so in an unbroken sequence along a boundary or at a point.

Contralateral Affecting, pertaining to, or originating in the opposite side of a point or reference.

Cotransport The process by which two substances are transported across a membrane at the same time.

Contusion An injury of a part without a break in the skin, characterized by swelling, discoloration, and pain.

Convolution An elevation or tortuous winding, such as one of the irregular ridges on the surface of the brain, formed by a structure being infolded upon itself.

Corpuscle Any small mass, cell, or body, such as a red or white blood cell.

Costal Pertaining to a rib or ribs.

Countertransport The process by which a substance moves across a membrane in opposite directions.

Crepitus A sound or sensation that resembles a crackling or grating noise.

Cristae The infolding of the inner membrane of the mitochondria.

Cuboidal cells The closely packed cells of the epidermis.

Cutaneous Pertaining to the skin.

Cyanosis A bluish discoloration, especially of the skin and mucous membranes, caused by an excess of deoxygenated hemoglobin in the blood.

Cystic fibrosis An inherited disease causing thick mucus to develop in the lung and other organs.

Cytochromes Hemoproteins which transports electrons.

Cytokine Any of a class of polypeptide immunoregulatory substances that are secreted by cells, usually of the immune system, that affect other cells.

Cytology The study of cells, including their origin, structure, function, and pathology.

Cytoplasm The fluid contained within the cell membrane.

Cytosol Cytoplasm exclusive of membranous components (*e.g.*, mitochondria, endoplasmic reticulum) and nonmembranous insoluble components.

Decibel A unit for expressing the relative power intensity of electric or acoustic signal power that is equal to one tenth of a bel.

Defecation The evacuation of feces from the digestive tract through the rectum.

Deformation The process of adapting in form or shape; also the product of such alteration.

Degeneration The deterioration of a normal cell, tissue, or organ to a less functionally active form. (Adjective: degenerative)

Deglutition The act or process of swallowing.

Degradation The reduction of a chemical compound to a compound less complex, usually by splitting off one or more groups.

Dehydration The condition that results from excessive loss of water from the body tissues.

Delirium An acute, reversible organic mental syndrome characterized by confusion, disorientation, restlessness, incoherence, fear, and often illusions.

Dendrite One of the branching processes that extends and transmits impulses toward a cell body of a neuron. (Adjective: dendritic)

Depolarization The reduction of a cell membrane potential to a less negative value than that of the potential outside the cell.

Dermatome The area of the skin supplied with afferent nerve fibers of a single dorsal root of a spinal nerve.

Desmosome A small, circular, dense area within the intercellular bridge that forms the site of adhesion between intermediate filaments and cell membranes.

Desquamation A normal process in which the cornified layer of the epidermis is shed in fine scales or sheets.

Dialysis The process of separating colloids and crystalline substances in solution, which involves the two distinct physical processes of diffusion and ultrafiltration, or a medical procedure for the removal of urea and other elements from the blood or lymph.

Diapedesis The outward passage of red or white blood corpuscles through the intact walls of the vessels.

Diaphoresis Perspiration, especially the profuse perspiration associated with an elevated body temperature, physical exertion, exposure to heat, and mental or emotional stress.

Diarthrosis A specialized articulation that permits, to some extent, free joint movement. (Adjective: diarthrodial)

Diastole The dilatation of the heart, or the period of dilatation, which is the interval between the second and the first heart sound and is the time during which blood enters the relaxed chambers of the heart from the systemic circulation and the lungs.

Differentiation The act or process in development in which unspecialized cells or tissues acquire more specialized characteristics, including those of physical form, physiologic function, and chemical properties.

Diffusion The process of becoming widely spread, as in the spontaneous movement of molecules or other particles in solution from an area of higher concentration to an area of lower concentration, resulting in an even distribution of the particles in the fluid.

Dimer A compound or unit formed by the combination of two identical molecules or radicals of a simpler compound. (Adjective: dimeric)

Diopter A unit of measurement of the refractive power of lenses equal to the reciprocal of the focal length in meters.

Diploid Pertaining to an individual, organism, strain, or cell that has two full sets of homologous chromosomes.

Disseminate To scatter or distribute over a considerable area.

Distal Away from or being the farthest from a point of reference.

Diurnal Of, relating to, or occurring in the daytime.

Diverticulum A pouch or sac of variable size occurring naturally or through herniation of the muscular wall of a tubular organ.

Dorsum The back or posterior. (Adjective: dorsal)

Down-regulation Depressing the response to a stimuli due to a fewer numbers of receptors.

Dysgenesis Defective or abnormal development of an organ or part, typically occurring during embryonic development. (Also called dysgenesia.)

Dyslexia A disturbance in the ability to read, spell, and write words.

Dyspepsia The impairment of the power or function of digestion, especially epigastric discomfort following eating.

Dysphagia A difficulty in swallowing.

Dysphonia Any impairment of the voice that is experienced as a difficulty in speaking.

Dysplasia The alteration in size, shape, and organization of adult cell types.

Eburnation The conversion of bone or cartilage, through thinning or loss, into a hard and dense mass with a worn, polished, ivory-like surface.

Ecchymosis A small hemorrhagic spot, larger than a petechia, in the skin or mucous membrane caused by the extravasation of blood into the subcutaneous tissues.

Ectoderm The outermost of the three primary germ layers of the embryo, and from which the epidermis and epidermal tissues, such as nails, hair, and glands of the skin, develop.

Ectopic Relating to or characterized by an object or organ being situated in an unusual place, away from its normal location.

Edema The presence of an abnormal accumulation of fluid in interstitial spaces of tissues. (Adjective: edematous)

Efferent Conveyed or directed away from a center.

Effusion The escape of fluid from blood vessels into a part or tissue, as an exudation or a transudation.

Elastin A protein that has the ability to coil and uncoil giving many structures such as the skin elasticity.

Embolus A mass of clotted blood or other formed elements, such as bubbles of air, calcium fragments, or a bit of tissue or tumor, that circulates in the bloodstream until it becomes lodged in a vessel, obstructing the circulation. (Plural: emboli)

Empyema An accumulation of pus in a cavity of the body, especially the pleural space.

Emulsify To disperse one liquid throughout the body of another liquid, making a colloidal suspension, or emulsion.

Endocrine glands Release substances into the blood or tissues of the body.

Endocytosis The uptake or incorporation of substances into a cell by invagination of its plasma membrane, as in the processes of phagocytosis and pinocytosis.

Endoderm The innermost of the three primary germ layers of the embryo, and from which epithelium arises.

Endogenous Growing within the body, or developing or originating from within the body or produced from internal causes.

Endoscopy The visualization of any cavity of the body with an endoscope.

Endothelium The inner most layer of cells in blood and lymphatic vessels.

Enteropathic Relating to any disease of the intestinal tract.

Enzyme A protein molecule produced by living cells that catalyzes chemical reactions of other organic substances without itself being destroyed or altered.

Epiphysis The expanded articular end of a long bone (head) that is separated from the shaft of the bone by the epiphyseal plate until the bone stops growing, the plate is obliterated, and the shaft and the head become united.

Epithelium The covering of the internal and the external surfaces of the body, including the lining of vessels and other small cavities.

Epitope The simplest form of an antigenic determinant that combines with an antibody or a T-cell receptor to cause a specific reaction by an immunoglobulin.

Erectile Capable of being erected or raised to an erect position.

Erythema The redness or inflammation of the skin or mucous membranes produced by the congestion of superficial capillaries. (Adjective: erythematous)

Etiology The study or theory of all factors that may be involved in the development of a disease, including susceptibility of an individual, the nature of the disease agent, and the way in which an individual's body is invaded by the agent, or the cause of a disease.

Eukaryotic Pertaining to an organism with cells having a true nucleus; that is, a highly complex, organized nucleus surrounded by a nuclear membrane containing organelles and exhibiting mitosis.

Euploid Pertaining to an individual, organism, strain, or cell with a balanced set or sets of chromosomes, in any number, that is an exact multiple of the normal, basic haploid number characteristic of the species; or such an individual, organism, strain, or cell.

Evisceration The removal of the viscera from the abdominal cavity or disembowelment, or the extrusion of an internal organ through a wound or surgical incision.

Exacerbation An increase in the severity of a disease as marked by greater intensity in any of its signs and symptoms.

Exfoliation Peeling and sloughing off tissue cells in scales or layers. (Adjective: exfoliative)

Exocrine glands Release substances such as digestive enzymes to the outside of the body or another surface in the body.

Exocytosis The discharge of cell particles, which are packaged in membrane-bound vesicles, by fusion of the vesicular membrane with the plasma membrane and subsequent release of the particles to the exterior of the cell.

Exogenous Developed or originating outside the body, as a disease caused by a bacterial or viral agent foreign to the body.

Exophthalmos A marked or abnormal protrusion of the eyeball.

Extension A movement that allows the two elements of any jointed part to be drawn apart, increasing the angle between them, as extending the leg increases the angle between the femur and the tibia.

Extrapyramidal Pertaining to motor systems supplied by fibers outside the corticospinal or pyramidal tracts.

Extravasation A discharge or escape, usually of blood, serum, or lymph, from a vessel into the tissues.

Extubation The process of withdrawing a previously inserted tube from an orifice or cavity of the body.

Exudate Fluids, cells, or other substances that have been slowly exuded or have escaped from blood vessels and have been deposited in tissues or on tissue surfaces.

Fascia A sheet or band of fibrous connective tissue that may be separated from other specifically organized structures, as the tendons, the aponeuroses, and the ligaments.

Febrile Pertaining to or characterized by an elevated body temperature, or fever.

Fibrillation A small, local, involuntary contraction of muscle, resulting from spontaneous activation of a single muscle fiber or of an isolated bundle of nerve fibers.

Fibrin A stringy, insoluble protein formed by the action of thrombin on fibrinogen during the clotting process.

Fibrosis The formation of fibrous connective tissue, as in the repair or replacement of parenchymatous elements.

Filtration The process of passing a liquid through or as if through a filter, which is accomplished by gravity, pressure, or vacuum.

Fimbria Any structure that forms a fringe, border, or edge or the processes that resemble such a structure.

Fissure A cleft or a groove, normal or otherwise, on the surface of an organ or a bony structure.

First messengers Extracellular factors that can cause a response within a cell.

Fistula An abnormal passage or communication from an internal organ to the body surface or between two internal organs.

Flaccid Weak, soft, and lax; lacking normal muscle tone.

Flagella and cilia Thin threadlike structures that allow cells to move.

Flatus Air or gas in the intestinal tract that is expelled through the anus. (Adjective: flatulent)

Flexion A movement that allows the two elements of any jointed part to be brought together, decreasing the angle between them, as bending the elbow.

Flora The microorganisms, such as bacteria and fungi, both normally occurring and pathologic, found in or on an organ.

Focal Relating to, having, or occupying a focus.

Follicle A sac or pouchlike depression or cavity.

Fontanelle A membrane-covered opening in bones or between bones, such as the soft spot covered by tough membranes between the bones of an infant's incompletely ossified skull.

Foramen A natural opening or aperture in a membranous structure or bone.

Fossa A hollow or depressed area, especially on the surface of the end of a bone.

Fovea A small pit or depression in the surface of a structure or an organ.

Fundus The base or bottom of an organ or the portion farthest from the mouth of an organ.

G-proteins Bind guanine nucleotides and interact with cell surface receptors to transmit stimuli to inside the cell.

Ganglion One of the nerve cell bodies, chiefly collected in groups outside the central nervous system. (Plural: ganglia)

Gene penetrance Penetrance is expressed in mathematical terms: a 50% penetrance indicates that a person who inherits the defective gene has a 50% chance of expressing the disorder.

Genotype The entire genetic constitution of an individual, as determined by the particular combination and location of the genes on the chromosomes, or the alleles present at one or more sites on homologous chromosomes.

Glia The neuroglia, or supporting structure of nervous tissue.

Globulin One of a broad group of proteins classified by solubility, electrophoretic mobility, and size.

Gluconeogenesis The formation of glucose from any of the substances of glycolysis other than carbohydrates.

Glycolysis A series of enzymatically catalyzed reactions, occurring within cells, by which glucose is converted to adenosine triphosphate (ATP) and pyruvic acid during aerobic metabolism.

Glycosaminoglycans Polysaccharides that contain amino acids and attract water serving as a lubricant.

Goblet cells They have the primary role of mucus secretion.

Gonad A gamete-producing gland, as an ovary or a testis.

Gradient The rate of increase or decrease of a measurable phenomenon expressed as a function of a second, or the visual representation of such a change.

Granuloma A small mass of nodular granulation tissue resulting from chronic inflammation, injury, or infection. (Adjective: granulomatous)

GTPase cycle Occurs when hydrolase enzymes break down guanosine triphosphate.

Hapten A small, nonproteinaceous substance that is not antigenic by itself but that can act as an antigen when combined with a larger molecule.

Haustrum A structure resembling a recess or sacculation. (Plural: haustra)

Hematoma A localized collection of extravasated blood trapped in an organ, space, or tissue, resulting from a break in the wall of a blood vessel.

Hematopoiesis The normal formation and development of blood cells.

Hemianopia Defective vision or blindness in half of the visual field of one or both eyes.

Heterogeneous Consisting of or composed of dissimilar elements or parts, or not having a uniform quality throughout. (Noun: heterogeneity)

Heterophagy The taking into the cell of an exogenous substance by phagocytosis or pinocytosis and the subsequent digestion of the newly formed vacuole by a lysosome.

Heterozygous Having two different alleles at corresponding loci on homologous chromosomes.

Histology The branch of anatomy that deals with the minute (microscopic) structure, composition, and function of cells and tissue. (Adjective: histologic)

Homolog Any organ or part corresponding in function, position, origin, and structure to another organ or part, as the flippers of a seal that correspond to human hands. (Adjective: homologous)

Homozygous Having two identical alleles at corresponding loci on homologous chromosomes.

Humoral Relating to elements dissolved in the blood or body fluids.

Hybridoma A tumor of hybrid cells produced by fusion of normal lymphocytes and tumor cells.

Hydrolysis The chemical alteration or decomposition of a compound into fragments by the addition of water.

Hydrophilic A substance that has a strong affinity for water; a molecule that absorbs, mixes, and dissolves in water.

Hydrophobic A substance that repels water and does not readily dissolve in water.

Hypercapnia Excess amount of carbon dioxide in the blood.

Hyperemia An excess or engorgement of blood in a part of the body.

Hyperesthesia An unusual or pathologic increase in sensitivity of a part, especially the skin, or of a particular sense.

Hyperglycemia High blood sugar or excess of glucose in the blood.

Hyperplasia An abnormal multiplication or increase in the number of normal cells of a body part.

Hypertonic A solution having a greater concentration of solute than another solution with which it is compared, hence exerting more osmotic pressure than that solution.

Hypertrophy The enlargement or overgrowth of an organ that is due to an increase in the size of its cells rather than the number of its cells.

Hypesthesia An abnormal decrease of sensation in response to stimulation of the sensory nerves. (Also called hypoesthesia.)

Hypocapnia A deficiency of carbon dioxide in the blood.

Hypotonic A solution having a lesser concentration of solute than another solution with which it is compared, hence exerting less osmotic pressure than that solution.

Hypoxia An inadequate supply of oxygen to tissue that is below physiologic levels despite adequate perfusion of the tissue by blood.

Iatrogenic Induced inadvertently through the activity of a physician or by medical treatment or diagnostic procedures.

Idiopathic Arising spontaneously or from an unknown cause.

Idiosyncrasy A physical or behavioral characteristic or manner that is unique to an individual or to a group. (Adjective: idiosyncratic)

Immotile cilia syndrome Also known as Kartagener syndrome is a rare autosomal recessive genetic disorder that results in the inability of the cilia of the respiratory track to move.

Incidence The rate at which a certain event occurs (*e.g.*, the number of new cases of a specific disease during a particular period of time in a population at risk).

Inclusion The act of enclosing or the condition of being enclosed, or anything that is enclosed.

Indigenous Native, or natural, to the particular country or region where found.

Infarction Necrosis or death of tissues due to local ischemia resulting from obstruction of blood flow.

Inotropic Influencing the force or energy of muscular contractions.

In situ In the natural or normal place, or something, such as cancer, that is confined to its place of origin and has not invaded neighboring tissues.

Interferon Any one of a group of small glycoproteins (cytokines) produced in response to viral infection and which inhibit viral replication.

Integral proteins Proteins that are permanently attached to the cell membrane.

Intercostal retraction Pulling in of the intercostal spaces due to decreased air pressure within the chest, as the person takes in a breath the intercostal muscles are sucked inward.

Interleukin Any of several multifunctional cytokines produced by a variety of lymphoid and nonlymphoid cells, including immune cells, that stimulate or otherwise affect the function of lymphopoietic and other cells and systems in the body.

Interstitial Relating to or situated between parts or in the interspaces of a tissue.

Intermembrane space The space between the inner and outer membrane of a mitochondrion.

Intramural Situated or occurring within the wall of an organ.

Intrinsic Pertaining exclusively to a part or situated entirely within an organ or tissue.

In vitro A biologic reaction occurring in an artificial environment, such as a test tube.

In vivo A biologic reaction occurring within the living body.

Involuntary muscle An automatic response to a stimulus.

Involution The act or instance of enfolding, entangling, or turning inward.

Ionize To separate or change into ions.

Ipsilateral Situated on, pertaining to, or affecting the same side of the body.

Ischemia Decreased blood supply to a body organ or part, usually due to functional constriction or actual obstruction of a blood vessel.

Juxta-articular Situated near a joint or in the region of a joint.

Juxtaglomerular Near to or adjoining a glomerulus of the kidney.

Karyoplasm (nucleoplasm) Also known as nucleoplasm is enveloped by the nuclear membrane and includes chromosomes and the nucleus.

Karyotype The total chromosomal characteristics of a cell, or the micrograph of chromosomes arranged in pairs in descending order of size.

Keratin A fibrous, sulfur-containing protein that is the primary component of the epidermis, hair, and horny tissues. (Adjective: keratinous)

Keratinocytes The most common cell in the epidermis and produces keratin.

Keratosis Any skin condition in which there is overgrowth and thickening of the cornified epithelium.

Ketosis A condition characterized by the abnormal accumulation of ketones (organic compounds with a carboxyl group attached to two carbon atoms) in the body tissues and fluid.

Kinesthesia The sense of movement, weight, tension, and position of body parts mediated by input from joint and muscle receptors and hair cells. (Adjective: kinesthetic)

Krebs cycle The process by which living cells release energy through aerobic respiration.

Kwashiorkor A form of malnutrition resulting from severe protein deficiencies that leads to severe edema or swelling.

Kyphosis An abnormal condition of the vertebral column, characterized by increased convexity in the curvature of the thoracic spine as viewed from the side.

Lacuna A small pit or cavity within a structure, especially bony tissue, or a defect or gap, as in the field of vision.

Lateral A position farther from the median plane or midline of the body or a structure, or situated on, coming from, or directed toward the side.

Lesion Any wound, injury, or pathologic change in body tissue.

Lethargy The lowered level of consciousness characterized by listlessness, drowsiness, and apathy, or a state of indifference.

Ligament One of many predominantly white, shiny, flexible bands of fibrous tissue that binds joints together and connects bones or cartilages.

Ligand A group, ion, or molecule that binds to the central atom or molecule in a chemical complex.

Lipid Any of the group of fats and fatlike substances characterized by being insoluble in water and soluble in nonpolar organic solvents, such as chloroform and ether.

Lipoprotein Any one of the conjugated proteins that is a complex of protein and lipid.

Lobule A small lobe.

Lordosis The anterior concavity in the curvature of the lumbar and cervical spine as observed from the side.

Lumen A cavity or the channel within a tube or tubular organ of the body.

Luteal Of or pertaining to or having the properties of the corpus luteum.

Lysis Destruction or dissolution of a cell or molecule through the action of a specific agent.

Lysosomal storage disorders Inherited metabolic diseases due to lysomal dysfunction allowing sugars, fats, and toxic materials to accumulate.

Maceration Softening of tissue by soaking, especially in acidic solutions.

Macroscopic Large enough to be visible with the unaided eye or without the microscope.

Macula A small, flat blemish, thickening, or discoloration that is flush with the skin surface. (Adjective: macular)

Malaise A vague feeling of bodily fatigue and discomfort.

Manometry The measurement of tension or pressure of a liquid or gas using a device called a manometer.

Marasmus A condition of extreme protein-calorie malnutrition that is characterized by growth retardation and progressive wasting of subcutaneous tissue and muscle and occurs chiefly during the first year of life.

Matrix The intracellular substance of a tissue or the basic substance from which a specific organ or kind of tissue develops.

Matrix space The material in which specialized structures are implanted.

Meatus An opening or passage through any body part.

Medial Pertaining to the middle, or situated or oriented toward the midline of the body.

Mediastinum The mass of tissues and organs in the middle of the thorax, separating the pleural sacs containing the two lungs.

Meiosis The division of a sex cell as it matures, so that each daughter nucleus receives one half of the number of chromosomes characteristic of the somatic cells of the species.

Membrane potentials The voltage generated by the differences of ions on opposite side of the cell membrane.

Menarche First menstrual cycle.

Mesoderm The middle layer of the three primary germ layers of the developing embryo, lying between the ectoderm and the endoderm.

Mesothelium Flat cells derived from the mesoderm and line body cavities such as the thoracic and abdominal cavity.

Metabolism The sum of all the physical and chemical processes by which living organisms are produced and maintained, and also the transformation by which energy is provided for vital processes and activities.

Metaplasia Change in type of adult cells in a tissue to a form that is not normal for that tissue.

Metastasis The transfer of disease (*e.g.*, cancer) from one organ or part to another not directly connected with it. (Adjective: metastatic)

Miosis Contraction of the pupil of the eye.

Mitosis A type of indirect cell division that occurs in somatic cells and results in the formation of two daughter nuclei containing the identical complements of the number of chromosomes characteristic of the somatic cells of the species.

Molecule The smallest mass of matter that exhibits the properties of an element or compound.

Morbidity A diseased condition or state; the relative incidence of a disease or of all diseases in a population.

Morphology The study of the physical form and structure of an organism, or the form and structure of a particular organism. (Adjective: morphologic)

Mosaicism In genetics, the presence in an individual or in an organism of cell cultures having two or more cell lines that differ in genetic constitution but are derived from a single zygote.

Multiunit smooth muscle Muscle fibers not closely jointed and contract as separate units.

Mutagen Any chemical or physical agent that induces a genetic mutation (an unusual change in form, quality, or some other characteristic) or increases the mutation rate by causing changes in DNA.

Mydriasis Physiologic dilatation of the pupil of the eye.

Myoclonus A spasm of a portion of a muscle, an entire muscle, or a group of muscles.

Myofibrils Fine threads in striated muscle cells and can contract.

Myoglobin The oxygen-transporting pigment of muscle consisting of one heme molecule containing one iron molecule attached to a single globin chain.

Myopathy Any disease or abnormal condition of skeletal muscle, usually characterized by muscle weakness, wasting, and histologic changes within muscle tissue.

Myotome The muscle plate or portion of an embryonic somite that develops into a voluntary muscle, or a group of muscles innervated by a single spinal segment.

Necrosis Localized tissue death that occurs in groups of cells or part of a structure or an organ in response to disease or injury.

Neurofibrillary tangles Formed of tau protein and are an indicator of Alzheimer disease and tauopathies.

Neutropenia An abnormal decrease in the number of neutrophilic leukocytes in the blood.

Nidus The point where a morbid process originates, develops, or is located.

Nociception The reception of painful stimuli from the physical or mechanical injury to body tissues by nociceptors (receptors usually found in either the skin or the walls of the viscera).

Nonenveloped Nonenveloped viruses have an outer cover made of proteins. These viruses are more virulent and resistant producing antibodies in the host.

Nosocomial Pertaining to or originating in a hospital, such as a nosocomial infection: an infection acquired during hospitalization.

Nuclear envelope A double-layered membrane that surrounds the nucleus and controls passage of substances into and out of the nucleus.

Nucleotide The building blocks of nucleic acids (5-carbon sugar, phosphate group, and nitrogenous base).

Nystagmus Involuntary, rapid, rhythmic movements of the eyeball.

Oncogene A gene that is capable of causing the initial and continuing conversion of normal cells into cancer cells.

Oncotic Relating to, caused by, or marked by edema or any swelling.

Oocyte A primordial or incompletely developed ovum.

Oogenesis The process of the growth and maturation of the female gametes or ova.

Opsonization The process of making cells, such as bacteria, more susceptible to the action of phagocytes.

Organelle Any one of the various membrane-bound particles of distinctive morphology and function present within most cells, as the mitochondria, the Golgi complex, and the lysosomes.

Orthopnea An abnormal condition in which a person must be in an upright position in order to breathe deeply or comfortably.

Orthosis An external orthopedic appliance or apparatus, as a brace or splint, used to support, align, prevent or correct deformities, or to improve the function of movable parts of the body.

Osmolality The concentration of osmotically active particles in solution expressed in osmols or milliosmols per kilogram of solvent.

Osmolarity The concentration of osmotically active particles in solution expressed in osmols or milliosmols per liter of solution.

Osmosis The movement or passage of a pure solvent, such as water, through a semipermeable membrane from a solution that has a lower solute concentration to one that has a higher solute concentration.

Osmotic pressure The pressure required to prevent osmosis into a solution.

Osteophyte A bony project or outgrowth.

Oxidative phosphorylation The biochemical process by which ATP is formed in the mitochondria from phosphate and ADP.

Palpable Perceptible by touch.

Papilla A small nipple-shaped projection, elevation, or structure, as the conoid papillae of the tongue.

Papule A small, circumscribed, solid elevation of the skin less than 1 cm in diameter. (Adjective: papular)

Paracrine A mode of hormone action in which a chemical messenger that is synthesized and released from a cell acts on nearby cells of a different type and affects their function.

Paralysis An abnormal condition characterized by the impairment or loss of motor function due to a lesion of the neural or muscular mechanism.

Paraneoplastic Relating to alterations produced in tissue remote from a tumor or its metastases.

Parenchyma The basic tissue or elements of an organ as distinguished from supporting or connective tissue or elements. (Adjective: parenchymal)

Paresis Slight or partial paralysis.

Paresthesia Any abnormal touch sensation, which can be experienced as numbness, tingling, or a "pins and needles" feeling, often in the absence of external stimuli.

Parietal Pertaining to the outer wall of a cavity or organ, or pertaining to the parietal bone of the skull or the parietal lobe of the brain.

Parous Having borne one or more viable offspring.

Passive transport The movement of substances across a cell membrane with the need for energy.

Pathogen Any microorganism capable of producing disease.

Pedigree A systematic presentation, such as in a table, chart, or list, of an individual's ancestors that is used in human genetics in the analysis of inheritance.

Pedunculated Tumor or growth on a stalk.

Peptide Any of a class of molecular chain compounds composed of two or more amino acids joined by peptide bonds.

Perfusion The process or act of pouring over or through, especially the passage of a fluid through a specific organ or an area of the body.

Peripheral Pertaining to the outside, surface, or surrounding area of an organ or other structure, or located away from a center or central structure.

Peripheral proteins Proteins found on the membrane, which can easily disconnect.

Permeable A condition of being pervious or permitting passage, so that fluids and certain other substances can pass through, as a permeable membrane.

Peroxisomes Found in cytoplasm are responsible for carrying out oxidative reactions.

Pervasive Pertaining to something that becomes diffused throughout every part.

Petechia A tiny, perfectly round, purplish red spot that appears on the skin as a result of minute intradermal or submucous hemorrhage. (Plural: petechiae)

Phagocytosis The process by which certain cells engulf and consume foreign material and cell debris.

Phagocytosis The ingestion of other cells.

Phagosome A vacuole that contains engulfed or ingested particles.

Phalanx Any one of the bones composing the fingers of each hand and the toes of each foot.

Phenotype The complete physical, biochemical, and physiologic makeup of an individual, as determined by the interaction of both genetic makeup and environmental factors.

Pheresis A procedure in which blood is withdrawn from a donor, a portion (plasma, leukocytes, etc.) is separated and retained, and the remainder is reperfused into the donor. It includes plasmapheresis and leukapheresis.

Pili Hair, or in microbiology, the minute filamentous appendages of certain bacteria. (Singular: pilus)

Pinocytosis The process by which cells ingest liquid.

Plasma membrane or cell membrane A thin membrane made of fats and proteins that separate the cell's cytoplasm from the external environment.

Plethoric Relating to an excess of any of the body fluids, especially blood; the term used to describe the beefy red coloration of a newborn.

Plexus A network of intersecting nerves, blood vessels, or lymphatic vessels.

Pluripotent stem cells Are considered to be "master" or "true" stems due to their potential to differentiate into almost any cell in the body.

Polycystic kidney disease An inherited disease in which many cysts grow in the kidneys causing hypertrophy and leads to kidney failure.

Polygene Any of a group of nonallelic genes that interact to influence the same character in the same way so that the effect is cumulative, usually of a quantitative nature, as size, weight, or skin pigmentation. (Adjective: polygenic)

Polymorph One of several, or many, forms of an organism or cell. (Adjective: polymorphic)

Polyp A small, tumor-like growth that protrudes from a mucous membrane surface.

Polypeptide A molecular chain of more than two amino acids joined by peptide bonds.

Presbyopia A visual condition (farsightedness) that commonly develops with advancing years or old age in which the lens loses elasticity causing defective accommodation and inability to focus sharply for near vision.

Prevalence The number of new and old cases of a disease that is present in a population at a given time, or occurrences of an event during a particular period of time.

Primary active transport The energy needed to move molecules are derived from the breakdown of ATP.

Primary lysosomes Produced by the Golgi complex and fuse with phagosomes or pinosomes and become **secondary lysosomes** where lysis occurs due to hydrolytic enzymes.

Prodrome An early symptom indicating the onset of a condition or disease. (Adjective: prodromal)

Progenitors An ancestor.

Prokaryotic Pertaining to an organism, such as bacterium, with cells lacking a true nucleus and nuclear membrane that reproduces through simple fission.

Prolapse The falling down, sinking, or sliding of an organ from its normal position or location in the body.

Proliferation The reproduction or multiplication of similar forms, especially cells.

Pronation Assumption of a position in which the ventral, or front, surface of the body or part of the body faces downward. (Adjective: prone)

Propagation The act or action of reproduction.

Proprioception The reception of stimuli originating from within the body regarding body position and muscular activity by proprioceptors (sensory nerve endings found in muscles, tendons, joints).

Prosthesis An artificial replacement for a missing body part, or a device designed and applied to improve function, such as a hearing aid.

Proteasome Breaks down protein especially when not needed.

Protein kinases Modify proteins by adding phosphate groups causing a function change.

Proteoglycans Any one of a group of polysaccharide–protein conjugates occurring primarily in the matrix of connective tissue and cartilage.

Proteolysis The breakdown of proteins such as during digestion.

Proto-oncogene A normal cellular gene that with alteration, such as by mutation, becomes an active oncogene.

Protoplasm The liquid substances of the interior of living cells, which contains both organic and inorganic substances.

Proximal Closer to a point of reference, usually the trunk of the body, than other parts of the body.

Pruritus The symptom of itching, an uncomfortable sensation leading to the urge to rub or scratch the skin to obtain relief. (Adjective: pruritic)

Pseudostratified A layer of epithelial cells in direct contact with the basement membrane.

Pseudostratified epithelium A single layer of epithelial cells that give the appearance of being stratified.

Purpura A small hemorrhage, up to about 1 cm in diameter, in the skin, mucous membrane, or serosal surface, or any of several bleeding disorders characterized by the presence of purpuric lesions.

Purulent Producing or containing pus.

Quiescent Quiet, causing no disturbance, activity, or symptoms.

Receptor-mediated endocytosis The process by which the cells absorbs, get nutrients and other materials into the cell through invagination.

Reflux An abnormal backward or return flow of a fluid, such as stomach contents, blood, or urine.

Regurgitation A flow of material that is in the opposite direction from normal, as in the return of swallowed food into the mouth or the backward flow of blood through a defective heart valve.

Remission The partial or complete disappearance of the symptoms of a chronic or malignant disease, or the period of time during which the abatement of symptoms occurs.

Residual bodies Cytoplasmic vacuoles contain undigestable substances.

Resorption The loss of substance or bone by physiologic or pathologic means, for example, the loss of dentin and cementum of a tooth.

Retrograde Moving backward or against the usual direction of flow, reverting to an earlier state or worse condition (degenerating), catabolic.

Retroversion A condition in which an entire organ is tipped backward or in a posterior direction, usually without flexion or other distortion.

Rhabdomyolysis Destruction or degeneration of muscle, associated with myoglobinuria (excretion of myoglobin in the urine).

Rigor mortis The stiffening of the muscles and joints postmortem due to chemic changes primarily in the muscles.

Rostral Situated near a beak (oral or nasal region).

Rough endoplasmic reticulum A tubular membrane studded with ribosomes giving the uneven appearance and plays a role in synthesizing and storing proteins.

Sacroiliitis Inflammation in the sacroiliac joint.

Sarcolemma The cell membrane that covers striated muscle fiber cells.

Sarcomeres The foundational unit of striated muscle tissue.

Sarcoplasm The cytoplasm of a muscle fiber.

Sarcoplasmic reticulum The storage unit in muscle cells for calcium.

Sclerosis A condition characterized by induration or hardening of tissue resulting from any of several causes, including inflammation, diseases of the interstitial substance, and increased formation of connective tissues.

Scotopic vision Describes vision, especially night vision, when the eye is dark adapted.

Second messengers Intracellular substances released by the cell in response to a first messenger.

Secondary active transport The energy needed to move molecules is derived from stored energy rather than the breakdown of ATP.

Secretory granules A vesicle in which neuropeptides and hormones are stored for secretion.

Semipermeable Partially but not wholly permeable, especially a membrane that permits the passage of some (usually small) molecules but not of other (usually larger) particles.

Senescence The process or condition of aging or growing old.

Sepsis The presence in the blood or other tissues of pathogenic microorganisms or their toxins, or the condition resulting from the spread of microorganisms or their products. (Adjective: septic)

Serous Relating to or resembling serum, or containing or producing serum, such as a serous gland.

Shunt To divert or bypass bodily fluid from one channel, path, or part to another; a passage or anastomosis between two natural channels, especially between blood vessels, established by surgery or occurring as an abnormality.

Signal transduction A chemical reaction that occurs when a signal such as a hormone interacts with a receptor.

Simple cell Converts chemical energy into electrical energy.

Simple columnar epithelium Cells that are taller than wide and are one layer. They line most organs of the digestive track and some other organs such as the respiratory bronchioles and their primary function is secretion and absorption.

Simple cuboidal epithelium A single layer of cuboidal epithelium cells and specializes in secretion.

Single-unit smooth muscle A large number of cells that contract as a unit.

Skeletal muscle Striated muscle connected to the skeleton and under voluntary control.

Smooth endoplasmic reticulum Serves as a storage unit and plays a role in the creating and storage of lipids and steroids.

Smooth muscle Muscle tissue that contracts involuntarily.

Soma The body of an organism as distinguished from the mind; all of an organism, excluding germ cells; the body of a cell.

Spasticity The condition characterized by spasms or other uncontrolled contractions of the skeletal muscles. (Adjective: spastic)

Spatial Relating to, having the character of, or occupying space.

Sphincter A ringlike band of muscle fibers that constricts a passage or closes a natural orifice of the body.

Squamous cells They are flat and make up most of the cells of the epidermis, respiratory, and digestive tract.

Stem cells Undifferentiated cells that are able to become specialized cells.

Stenosis An abnormal condition characterized by the narrowing or stricture of a duct or canal.

Stochastic Involving a random process.

Stratified epithelium Flat cells arranged in layers with only one being in contract with the basement membrane.

Stratified squamous keratinized Dead squamous cells.

Stria A streak or a linear scarlike lesion that often results from rapidly developing tension in the skin, or a narrow bandlike structure, especially the longitudinal collections of nerve fibers in the brain.

Stricture An abnormal temporary or permanent narrowing of the lumen of a duct, canal, or other passage, as the esophagus, because of inflammation, external pressure, or scarring.

Stroma The supporting tissue or the matrix of an organ as distinguished from its functional element or parenchyma.

Stupor A lowered level of consciousness characterized by lethargy and unresponsiveness in which a person seems unaware of his or her surroundings.

Subchondral Beneath a cartilage.

Subcutaneous Beneath the skin.

Subluxation An incomplete or partial dislocation in which the relationship between joint surfaces is altered, but contact remains.

Sulcus A shallow groove, depression, or furrow on the surface of an organ, as a sulcus on the surface of the brain, separating the gyri.

Supination Assuming the position of lying horizontally on the back or with the face upward. (Adjective: supine)

Suppuration The formation of pus or purulent matter.

Symbiosis Mode of living characterized by close association between organisms of different species, usually in a mutually beneficial relationship.

Sympathomimetic An agent or substance that produces stimulating effects on organs and structures similar to those produced by the sympathetic nervous system.

Symport The process by which two molecules move through a membrane by a common carrier or cotransporter.

Synapses Gaps between two nerve cells allowing an electrical or chemic impulse to pass.

Syncope A brief lapse of consciousness due to generalized cerebral ischemia.

Syncytium A multinucleate mass of protoplasm produced by the merging of a group of cells.

Syndrome A complex of signs and symptoms that occur together to present a clinical picture of a disease or inherited abnormality.

Synergist An organ, agent, or substance that aids or cooperates with another organ, agent, or substance.

Synthesis An integration or combination of various parts or elements to create a unified whole.

Systemic Pertaining to the whole body rather than to a localized area or regional portion of the body.

Systole The contraction, or period of contraction, of the heart that drives the blood onward into the aorta and pulmonary arteries.

T tubules The small tubules that run across striated muscle fiber and conduct electrical impulses.

Tachyarrhythmias An abnormal heart rate of greater than 100 bpm.

Tamponade Stoppage of the flow of blood to an organ or a part of the body by pathologic compression, such as the compression of the heart by an accumulation of pericardial fluid.

Tenesmus The feeling of not being able to completely evacuate the bowel.

Teratogen Any agent or factor that induces or increases the incidence of developmental abnormalities in the fetus.

Thelarche Breast development in girls marking development of puberty prior to age 8.

Thrombus A stationary mass of clotted blood or other formed elements that remains attached to its place of origin along the wall of a blood vessel, frequently obstructing the circulation. (Plural: thrombi)

Tinnitus A tinkling, buzzing, or ringing noise heard in one or both ears.

Tissue Composed of similar cells performing a specific function.

Tophus A chalky deposit containing sodium urate that most often develops in periarticular fibrous tissue, typically in individuals with gout. (Plural: tophi)

Torsion The act or process of twisting in either a positive (clockwise) or negative (counterclockwise) direction.

Trabecula A supporting or anchoring stand of connective tissue, such as the delicate fibrous threads connecting the inner surface of the arachnoid to the pia mater.

Transitional epithelium Epithelial cells that can contract and expand.

Transmembrane proteins A type of integral membrane proteins and cover the cell membrane.

Transmural Situated or occurring through the wall of an organ.

Transudate A fluid substance passed through a membrane or extruded from the blood.

Transverse A right angle to the long axis of the body or lying across.

Tremor Involuntary quivering or trembling movements caused by the alternating contraction and relaxation of opposing groups of skeletal muscles.

Tricarboxylic acid Known as the citric acid cycle are chemical reactions allowing cells to break down energy in the presence of oxygen.

Trigone A triangular-shaped area.

Tropomyosin A muscle protein that controls muscle contraction and prevents muscle contraction when not needed.

Troponin A protein in skeletal and cardiac muscle causing contraction. When elevated, heart muscle damage has most likely occurred.

Tubulin A protein found in cell cytoplasm that serves as the building block for microtubules.

Ubiquitous The condition or state of existing or being everywhere at the same time.

Ulcer A circumscribed excavation of the surface of an organ or tissue, which results from necrosis that accompanies some inflammatory, infectious, or malignant processes. (Adjective: ulcerative)

Up-regulation An increase response to a stimuli due to an increased number of receptors.

Urticaria A pruritic skin eruption of the upper dermis, usually transient, characterized by wheals (hives) of various shapes and sizes.

Uveitis An inflammation of all or part of the uveal tract of the eye.

Vector An invertebrate animal (*e.g.*, tick, mite, mosquito) that serves as a carrier, transferring an infective agent from one vertebrate host to another.

Ventral Pertaining to a position toward the belly of the body, or situated or oriented toward the front or anterior of the body.

Vertigo An illusory sensation that the environment or one's own body is revolving.

Vesicle A small bladder or sac, as a small, thin-walled, raised skin lesion, containing liquid.

Visceral Pertaining to the viscera or internal organs of the body.

Viscosity Pertaining to the physical property of fluids, caused by the adhesion of adjacent molecules, that determines the internal resistance to shear forces.

Zoonosis A disease of animals that may be transmitted to humans from its primary animal host under natural conditions.

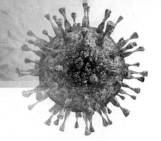

Index

Note: Page numbers followed by the letter "*f*" refer to figures; those followed by the letter "*t*" refer to tables; those followed by the letter *b* refer to boxes; and those followed by the letter "*c*" refer to charts.